Pediatric Images

Pediatric Images
Casebook of
Differential Diagnosis

Eugene Blank, M.D.

Professor Emeritus, Departments of Pediatrics and Radiology,
Oregon Health Sciences University School of Medicine, Portland, Oregon

with Photography by

Paul D. Miller

Department of Photography,
Oregon Health Sciences University School of Medicine, Portland, Oregon

Steven Frick

Department of Photography,
Oregon Health Sciences University School of Medicine, Portland, Oregon

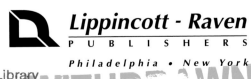

Lippincott - Raven
P U B L I S H E R S

Philadelphia • New York

Editorial Production and Composition: Silverchair Science + Communications, Inc.
Cover Designer: Marsha Cohen
Printer: Quebecor Kingsport

Printed in the United States of America

9 8 7 6 5 4 3 2 1

Library of Congress Cataloging-in-Publication Data

Blank, Eugene.
    Pediatric images : casebook of differential diagnosis / Eugene
Blank ; with photography by Steven Frick, Paul D. Miller.
        p.   cm.
    Includes bibliographical references and index.
    ISBN 0-316-09991-0
    1. Pediatrics--Case studies.   2. Diagnosis, Differential.
3. Pediatric diagnostic imaging--Case studies.   I. Title.
    [DNLM: 1. Pediatrics--case studies.   2. Diagnosis, Differential.
3. Diagnostic Imaging--in infancy & childhood.   WS 200 B642p 1997]
RJ58.B53   1997
618.92'00754--dc21
DNLM/DLC
for Library of Congress   97-4093
                                                                          CIP

Care has been taken to confirm the accuracy of the information presented and to describe generally accepted practices. However, the authors, editors, and publisher are not responsible for errors or omissions or for any consequences from application of the information in this book and make no warranty, express or implied, with respect to the concerns of the publication.

The authors, editors, and publisher have exerted every effort to ensure that drug selection and dosage set forth in this text are in accordance with current recommendations and practice at the time of publication. However, in view of ongoing research, changes in government regulations, and the constant flow of information relating to drug therapy and drug reactions, the reader is urged to check the package insert for each drug for any change in indications and dosage and for added warnings and precautions. This is particularly important when the recommended agent is a new or infrequently employed drug.

Some drugs and medical devices presented in this publication have Food and Drug Administration (FDA) clearance for limited use in restricted research settings. It is the responsibility of the health care provider to ascertain the FDA status of each drug or device planned for use in their clinical practice.

Faultes escaped in the Printing, correcte with your pennes; omitted by my neglygence, overslippe with patience; committed by ignorance, remit with favour.

John Lyly, *Euphues and His England*, 1580

epigraph to *The Plant-Lore & Garden-Craft of Shakespeare*, Henry N. Ellacombe, 1884

Contents

Commonly Used Abbreviations

ALL	acute lymphoblastic leukemia
AT III	antithrombin III
AU	arbitrary units
ASO	antistreptolysin O
BCG	Bacille Calmette-Guérin
C1–7	cervical vertebrae
CALLA	common acute lymphocytic leukemia antigen
CF	complement fixation
CK	creatine kinase
CNS	central nervous system
CSF	cerebrospinal fluid
CT	computed tomography
ECG	electrocardiogram
EEG	electroencephalogram
ESR	erythrocyte sedimentation rate
FEV	forced expiratory volume
FiO_2	fraction of inspired oxygen
FSH	follicle-stimulating hormone
GGT	γ-glutamyl transferase
GI	gastrointestinal
HBcAg	hepatitis B core antigen
HBsAb	hepatitis B surface antibody
HBsAg	hepatitis B surface antigen
HCG	human chorionic gonadotropin
βHCG	beta subunit of human chorionic gonadotropin
HDL	high-density lipoprotein
HIV	human immunodeficiency virus
HPF	high-power field
IFA	indirect fluorescent antibody
IM	intramuscular
IV	intravenous
L1–5	lumbar vertebrae
LDH	lactate dehydrogenase
LDL	low-density lipoprotein
LH	luteinizing hormone
LPF	low-power field
MCH	mean corpuscular hemoglobin
MCHC	mean corpuscular hemoglobin concentration
MCV	mean corpuscular volume
MRI	magnetic resonance imaging
PAS	periodic acid–Schiff
PET	positron emission tomography
PPD	purified protein derivative (tuberculin)
PT	prothrombin time
PTT	partial thromboplastin time
S1–5	sacral vertebrae
SD	standard deviation
SGOT	serum glutamic-oxalate transaminase
SGPT (ALT)	serum glutamic pyruvic transaminase (alanine aminotransferase)
T1–12	thoracic vertebrae
T_3	triiodothyronine
T_4	thyroxine
TdT	terminal deoxynucleotidyl transferase
TSH	thyrotropin (previously thyroid-stimulating hormone)

Preface

This book belongs to the children. They tell us their story, and they teach us. The library for the book has been the medical records room at the Oregon Health Sciences University. The book consists of brief biographies of children in clinico-pathologic form. It presents the symptoms, signs, evolution of disease, normal findings, and resolution of apparent abnormalities in children and a few adults examined in a busy x-ray department over several decades. The cases are presented as they might be in the emergency room at midnight. They are arranged in the order taught in medical school: chief complaint, history, and physical examination from head to foot. They contain laboratory data in SI units and, in a few cases, include laboratory errors. The data are accompanied by the images requested by clinicians and, sometimes, complementary images that were added in the x-ray department. The cases include, whenever available, the findings at operation, biopsy, and necropsy.

Russell J. Blattner, who wrote monthly "Comments on Current Literature" in the *Journal of Pediatrics* four decades ago, once used the phrase, "the scientific world of changing uncertainty." We were taught then that humans had 48 chromosomes, that the spleen had no particular function, and that Halsted's radical mastectomy was the only way to treat breast cancer. Patient biographies are as close to the truth as we can come and do not change.

The material in this book is as free of opinion and pronouncement as possible so that readers may decide for themselves. If their diagnoses differ, then the case presentation is even more successful. This book does not contain charts, tables, algorithms, or diagrams, and the physician in the emergency room at midnight is not likely to have them either.

A quotation from an editorial by Faith T. Fitzgerald expresses the purpose of *Pediatric Images:*

> Teaching should return to the bedside . . . the demonstration by the attending physician of the ineffable skills of the diagnostician and therapist—the careful illumination of the history with the directed physical examination, the comparison of these findings with the laboratory results at hand, and the richness of interpretation of all these "clues" to the central reality of the patient—can be done nowhere else as well as in the presence of the patient and with his or her participation.*

There is the thrill of medicine. *Pediatric Images* is my attempt to pass it on.

E.B.

---

*FT Fitzgerald. The case for internal medicine. N Engl J Med 328:654, 1993.

Acknowledgments

The words of the Chorus at the start of Shakespeare's *Henry V*, "Into a thousand parts divide one man," apply here, where a few names must stand for many. First are the teachers, the children who come in trust and in need of help. Then are the teachers in the classroom and at bedside. A few names for the many are James Templeman, who taught Latin in a high school in Baltimore many years ago and showed us the joy of learning; Melchijah Spragins, pediatrician and academician in practical, happy combination, who made 22 housecalls one Sunday and maybe more on other Sundays; John Caffey, the wisest, wittiest, and most humane physician I have known, who, on his seventy-ninth birthday, was skimming flat stones across Oregon's Eagle Creek, and who almost two decades after his death remains a shining example; and Bertram Girdany, whose enthusiasm one February day long ago was immediately contagious and who taught me the value of a teaching file, which is really, as Steven Ross told me, a learning file.

The librarians in the medical records room at Oregon Health Sciences University helped me with charts, smiles, and kindness almost every day for years. Let two names stand for many: Tiebo Muratha and Sandy Jones. Roentgenograms were photographed and often bad ones were made into better photographs by Paul D. Miller and Steven Frick. The debt is deep to countless individuals: students, nurses, and physicians, who listened, observed, and recorded; laboratory and x-ray technicians, who performed with devotion and skill and often too little appreciation; and the administration at Oregon Health Sciences University, who encouraged. I am grateful to the x-ray department for its support.

This book would not be if it were not for the encouragement, help, and guidance, sometimes seeming harsh, sometimes hard to take, but always improving the work, that came from Thomas Manning, former Publisher at Little, Brown and Company, who could hear the stories in distant words; Deeth Ellis, former Development Editor at Little, Brown, who saw that the garden needed a lot of weeding; Marie Salter, former Senior Production Editor at Little, Brown, who guided the book along its arcane journey and was always there with encouragement when needed; and Jenn Nagaj, Production Editor at Silverchair Science + Communications, who, like Theseus in *A Midsummer Night's Dream*, found words that were "like a tangled chain, nothing impaired, but all disordered" and untangled and ordered them.

Inexpressible debt is to my mother, Fannie Jacob, who gave me childhood and young adulthood that lacked nothing of real value; Freda and Harry Honikberg, who gave me Esther; our daughters and their families—Lisa and Isaac Bankman and Judy and Danny, Anne and Peter Mathers and Emma, and Linda and Kurt Hofgard—who give me the future; and Esther—without her, nothing.

E.B.

Skull and Brain

Case 1

A 4½-month-old boy has a bruised forehead several hours after hitting his head when he fell off a bed. The rest of the physical findings are normal.

Figures 1-1 and 1-2 show a midline longitudinal cleft in the frontal bone. An interparietal bone (inca bone) is in the posterior fontanel at lambda (Figures 1-1A and 1-2). In Figure 1-2, a separate ossification center is in the supraoccipital part of the occipital bone behind the foramen magnum, a synchondrosis is between the exoccipital part in front and supraoccipital part in back on each side of the separate ossification center, and a cleft is in each side of squamous part of occipital bone at lambdoid suture.

Diagnosis: Metopic suture in frontal bone, Kerckring's ossification center (Kerckring's ossicle) in occipital bone, mendosal suture in occipital bone, normal skull.

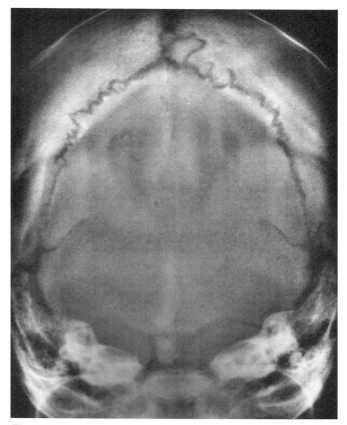

Fig. 1-2

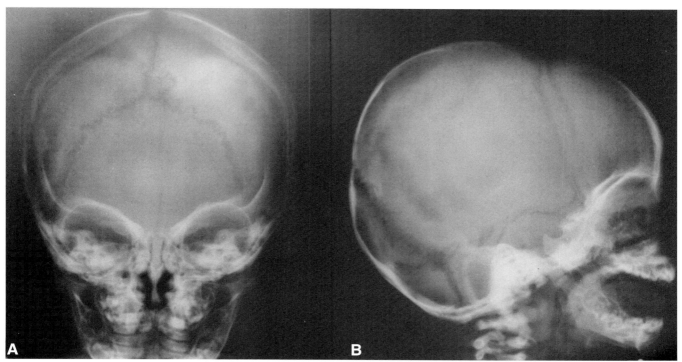

Fig. 1-1

Case 2

A 1-day-old boy is unresponsive.

Pregnancy of mother (18 years old) was normal; labor lasted 12 hours, during which she was given 200 mg meperidine and 25 mg chlorpromazine. Birth weight was 3.8 kg and cry immediate. He was slightly hypotonic. Cry became squeaky. He would not nurse at 17 hours. He was stiff for several minutes at 19½ hours and then unresponsive.

Weight at 1 day is 3.6 kg, temperature 33.9°C, heart rate 110, respiratory rate 60, and blood glucose 2.2 mmol/liter. Deep tendon reflexes in legs are diminished. The rest of the physical findings are normal. He soon responds.

Hematocrit is 0.58. White cell count is 8.1 × 10⁹/liter. Serum sodium is 129 mmol/liter, potassium 6.2, carbon dioxide 23, and calcium 1.90. On the fourth day, peak total bilirubin is 308 μmol/liter, and direct bilirubin 46. Urine specific gravity is 1.005, pH 5. Urine is normal.

Head circumference is 47 cm at 27½ months. He has occasional generalized seizures. He uses sentences, feeds and helps dress himself, and goes up and down stairs. At 33 months, his weight is 13 kg, height 86 cm, temperature 37.8°C, heart rate 100, and blood pressure 82/50 mm Hg. He is small. The rest of the physical findings are normal.

Width of lambdoid suture near lambda is approximately 7 mm at 1 day (Figure 2-1A). Small bones are in lambdoid and sagittal sutures at 33 months (Figure 2-1B).

Diagnosis: Epilepsy of questionable cause; small skull, normal wormian (intrasutural) bones.

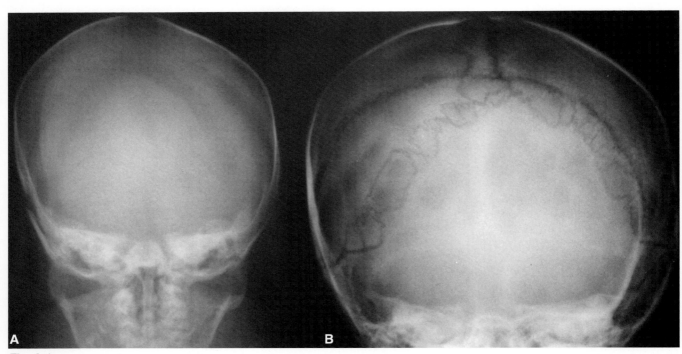

Fig. 2-1

Case 3

A 2-month-old boy has a bulge at occiput and another bulge below it. The rest of the physical findings are normal.

Figures 3-1 and 3-2 show paired bones in the supraoccipital part of occipital bone behind the foramen magnum. External occipital protuberance is prominent in Figure 3-1.

Diagnosis: Bathrocephaly, Schulz's ossicles, normal skull.

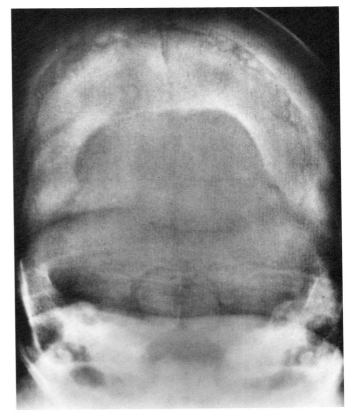

Fig. 3-2

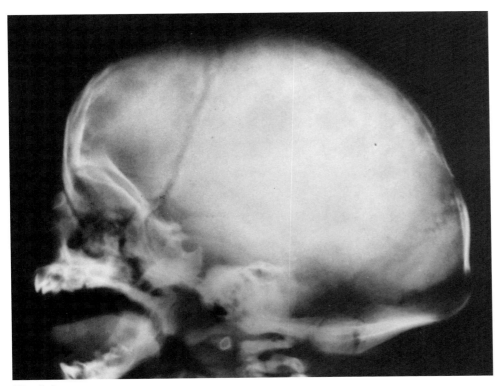

Fig. 3-1

Case 4

A 7-month-old girl vomits and is not gaining weight.

Birth weight was 3.2 kg. She began to vomit at 2 months. At 7 months, she is breast-fed and can sit up.

Weight is 5.4 kg, length 62 cm. Neither anterior nor posterior fontanel is palpable. Muscles seem weak. The rest of the physical findings are normal.

Figure 4-1 shows a bone in anterior fontanel and another in lambda. A suture bisects the frontal bone.

She does not vomit during the next 6 days, gains 240 g, and, a month later, pulls herself to stand.

Diagnosis: Anterior fontanel bone, interparietal bone (inca bone), metopic suture, normal skull.

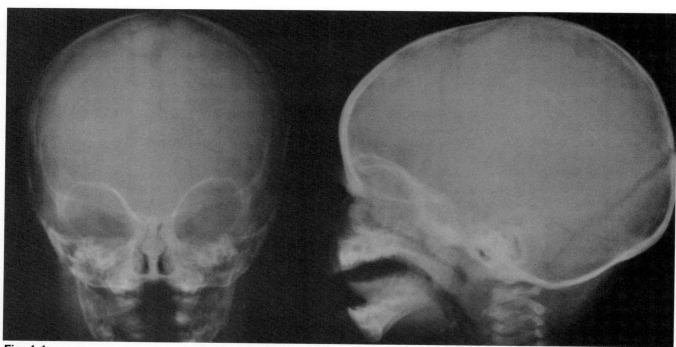

Fig. 4-1

Case 5

A 4½-month-old boy is vomiting.

Birth weight was 3.6 kg, Apgar score 8/9 at 1 and 10 minutes. Skin was loose and wrinkled on the neck and backs of hands and feet. He was a "very quiet baby who hardly ever fussed." He lifted his head at 1 month. His head "wobbled around" when he tried to lift it at 3 months. He was "soggy and flaccid" at 3 months. Eyes did not "function together." Eyes and mouth twitched for 3 days at 3½ months. Inguinal hernias were present at 4 months. Vomiting began a week ago. He has vomited several times today.

Parents, sister (7 years old), and brother (4 years old) are well. Maternal grandmother had stillborn baby with a ruptured aorta and a mentally retarded daughter with brittle bones. Maternal great-grandmother had a stillborn boy.

Temperature is 37.4°C, heart rate 140, respiratory rate 56, systolic blood pressure 80 mm Hg, and weight 5 kg. He is floppy. Skin is dry and scaly, turgor poor, subcutaneous tissue thin. Hair is dry, coarse, and brittle. Eyebrows are white. Eyes are sunken. Sternum is depressed. Liver edge is 2 cm below costal margin. A mass is in left flank. Joints are loose, reflexes weak. Thumbs are fisted. First and second toes are widely separated. The rest of the physical findings are normal.

Hematocrit is 0.34. White cell count is 8.4×10^9/liter. Urine specific gravity is 1.007, pH 6.5. Urine has trace glucose, 1+ hemoglobin/myoglobin, 4–6 white cells and >100 red cells/HPF. Serum sodium is 114 mmol/liter, potassium 4.5, chloride 88, carbon dioxide 7, urea nitrogen 13.6, calcium 2.32, phosphorus 1.58, cholesterol 3.31, and glucose 6.7. Creatinine is 70 μmol/liter, uric acid 460, total bilirubin 2, direct bilirubin 2, zinc 14.4 (normal: 11.5–18.5). Total protein is 59 g/liter, albumin 40. Alkaline phosphatase is 248 U/liter, LDH 286, and SGOT 43.

Figure 5-1 shows wormian bones in lambdoid suture, mosaic rarefactions in parietal, occipital, and temporal bones. Parietal scalp is wrinkled.

Cystogram shows displacement of collecting system of left kidney. Left kidney is in normal place in excretory urogram at 6½ months. Part of bladder is in left inguinal canal.

Microscopic examination shows twisted hairs of varying diameter.

Serum copper is 3.1, 4.4, and 22.5 μmol/liter (normal: 11–22), ceruloplasmin <200 and 1,500 mg/liter (normal: 200–350), urine copper 2.4 μmol/day (normal: <0.6).

Diagnosis: Menkes' kinky hair syndrome.

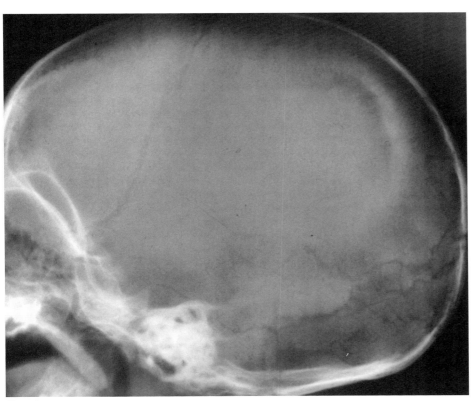

Fig. 5-1

Case 6

A 3-year-old boy has a large soft spot in his head.

Pregnancy was normal, birth weight 3.1 kg. Head was soft. He walked at 9 months.

Mother (28 years old), father, and five half siblings are well.

Weight at 3 years is 13.6 kg, height 93 cm, head circumference 52 cm, temperature 37.2°C, heart rate 90, respiratory rate 20, and blood pressure 100/60 mm Hg. Anterior fontanel is 5 cm wide and 10–15 cm long. He can almost bring his shoulders together in front. Lower ribs flare. Adduction and internal rotation at hips are limited. The rest of the physical findings are normal.

Hematocrit is 0.38. White cell count is 7.6 × 10⁹/liter with 0.24 polymorphonuclear cells, 0.07 bands, 0.47 lymphocytes, 0.07 monocytes, 0.11 eosinophils, and 0.04 basophils.

Urine specific gravity is 1.008, pH 5. Urine has 0–1 white cell/HPF. Serum sodium is 135 mmol/liter, potassium 3.8, and chloride 102.

In Figure 6-1, sutures, especially sagittal suture, are wide, fontanels large, and parasutural serrations prominent. Anterior arch of C1 is not ossified, posterior arch only partly ossified in Figure 6-1. Only medial fragments of clavicles are ossified in Figure 6-2. In Figure 6-3A, carpal bones are not ossified, pseudoepiphyses are in metacarpal bones, and phalanges are dysplastic. In Figure 6-3B, pubic bones are not ossified, femoral epiphyses are dysplastic, and neck-shaft angle of femurs is less than normal.

Diagnosis: Cleidocranial dysostosis.

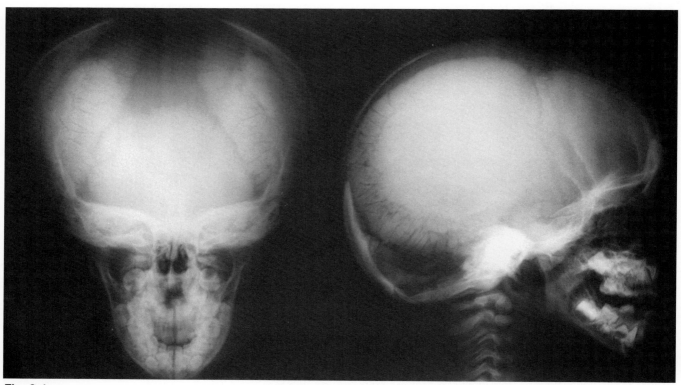

Fig. 6-1

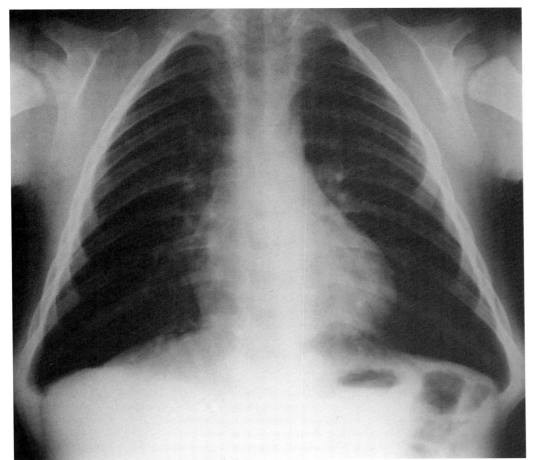

Fig. 6-2

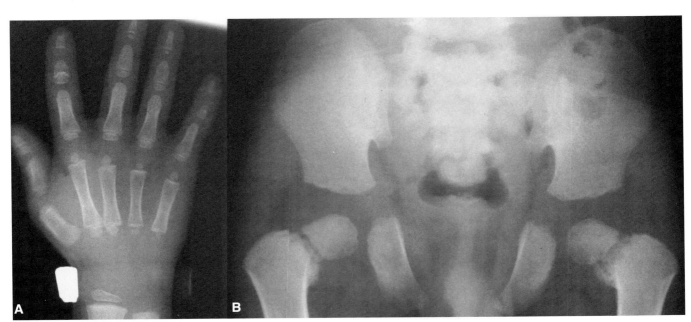

Fig. 6-3

Case 7

A 19-year-old woman has abnormal teeth.

She had no teeth and a large soft spot in her skull at 2 years, caries, malocclusion, and only deciduous teeth at 9 years. Carious deciduous teeth were pulled at 14 years. Upper incisors and canines were exposed by removing overlying bone.

Pregnancy of mother was normal, birth weight 3.7 kg. She began to walk at 9 months, to talk at 1 year. Osteotomies for femoral abnormality were performed at 5 years. Tonsils and adenoids were removed at 8 years. She had a grand mal seizure at 9 years and several more seizures until 16 years. Menarche was at 15 years.

Mother, father, and brother (16 years old) are well. Maternal grandfather had cancer of the pancreas.

Weight was 36 kg at 14 years, height 144 cm. Head was wide, face flat and square, sternum depressed. Scapulas were displaced forward. She could bring shoulders together in front. A hard lump was palpable at symphysis pubis. Scars were on thighs. The rest of the physical findings were normal. Weight is 57 kg at 19 years, height 152 cm.

Cranial sutures are prominent at 19 years (Figure 7-1). In Figure 7-1B, a parasagittal suture is in each parietal bone and parasutural serrations or wormian bones are in lambdoid suture. Panoramic view of jaws shows unerupted teeth at odd angles (Figure 7-2A). Lateral half of left clavicle is not ossified; lateral half of the right clavicle is fragmented (Figure 7-2B).

Diagnosis: Cleidocranial dysostosis.

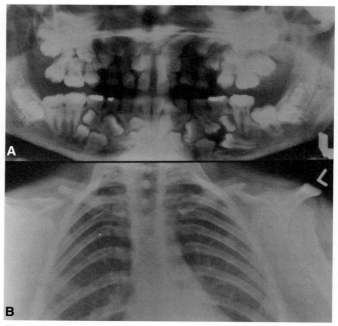

Fig. 7-2

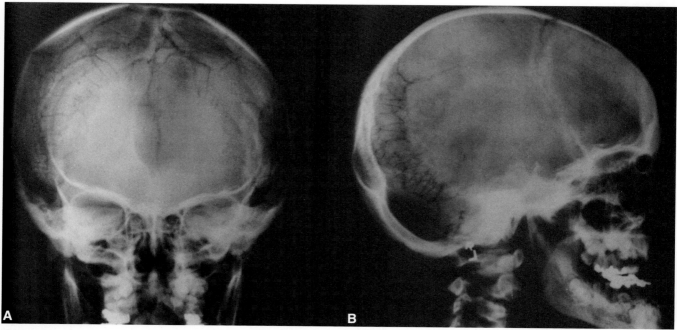

Fig. 7-1

Case 8

A newborn girl has a sacral meningomyelocele.

Pregnancy of mother (28 years old) was normal, presentation vertex. Birth weight is 4 kg, head circumference 36 cm, and Apgar score 8/9 at 1 and 5 minutes. Anus does not contract during perianal stimulation. The rest of the physical findings are normal.

Figure 8-1 shows a depression in the left parietal bone.

She develops normally but lacks bowel and bladder control.

Diagnosis: Congenital depression, left parietal bone.

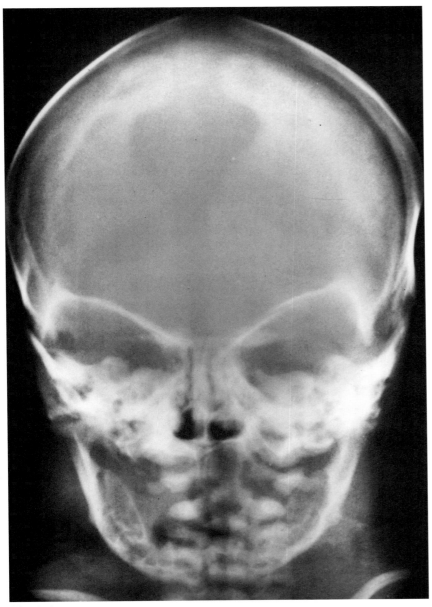

Fig. 8-1

Case 9

A 2½-year-old girl who fell and hit the back of her head 2 hours ago is sleepy and will not eat. She was not unconscious. She is easy to rouse.

Temperature is 36.7°C, heart rate 87, and blood pressure 110/72 mm Hg. She resists examination. Physical findings are normal.

A radiolucent cleft and a small, round defect are in occipital bone (Figure 9-1).

Diagnosis: Normal median fissure and normal inioendinial canal in occipital bone.

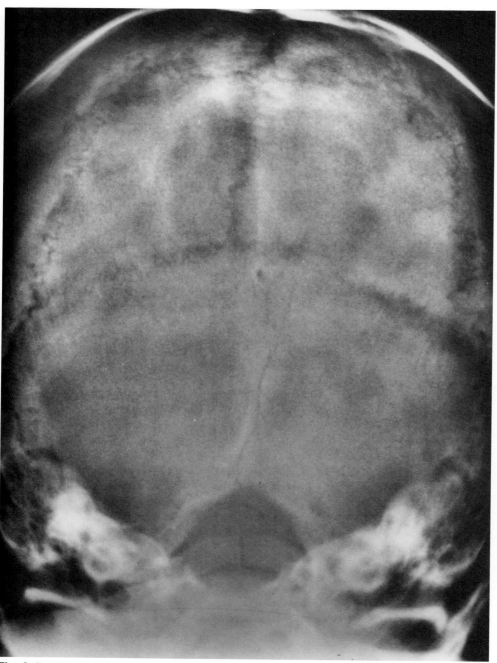

Fig. 9-1

Case 10

A 24-year-old man is vomiting and dizzy after being hit on back of the head. He thinks he was unconscious for a little while. He has a headache.

Temperature is 37.3°C, heart rate 84, respiratory rate 16, blood pressure 122/70 mm Hg, weight 61 kg, and height 178 cm. Back of head is slightly swollen. A bruised cut is over left eye. The rest of the physical findings are normal.

In Figure 10-1, a radiolucent strip bisects occipital bone to foramen magnum, where dorsum sellae is apparent because of brow-down projection in Towne's view.

Diagnosis: Normal median fissure, occipital bone.

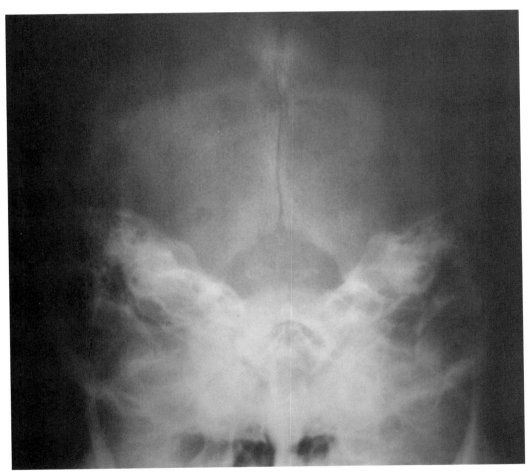

Fig. 10-1

Case 11

A 7½-year-old girl is too small.

Birth weight was 4.1 kg, length 52 cm.

Weight is 21 kg, height 115 cm, head circumference 51 cm, heart rate 80, respiratory rate 16, and blood pressure 84/40 mm Hg. Neck is broad, sternum slightly depressed. The rest of the physical findings are normal.

Chromosomes are 46,XX.

Convolutional markings are prominent in Figure 11-1.

Diagnosis: Normal skull, probable Noonan's syndrome.

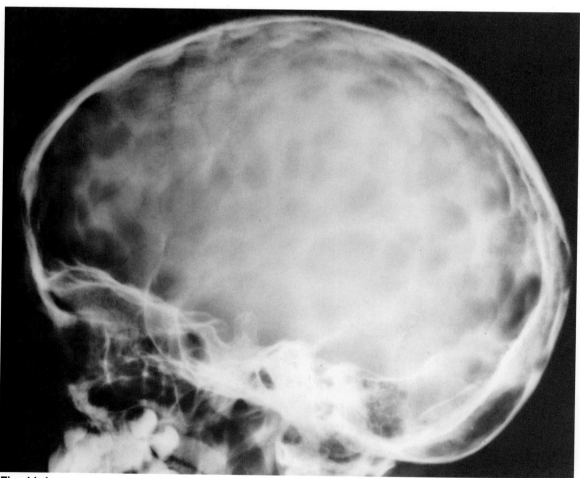

Fig. 11-1

Case 12

A 3½-year-old girl has a bump on top of her head that was first noticed when she was 2 years old and has not gotten larger.

The rest of the physical findings are normal.

Figure 12-1A shows thinned diploë and skull bulging on both sides of sagittal suture. Pneumoencephalogram (Figure 12-1B) and angiogram (Figure 12-1C) show normal findings. Superior sagittal sinus follows bulge in Figure 12-1C.

Diagnosis: Pacchionian depressions, normal skull.

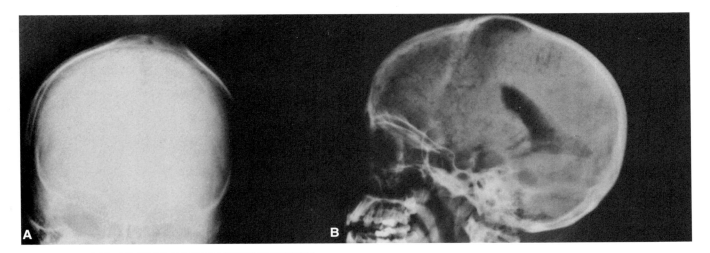

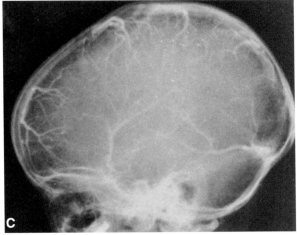

Fig. 12-1

Case 13

A 3-year-old girl, her 2-year-old brother, and 7-month-old sister have big heads.

Mother (34 years old) and father (40 years old) are well and of normal intelligence. Mother's hearing is bad. A maternal uncle is deaf in one ear. Mother's head circumference is 60 cm, father's is 61 cm.

The 3-year-old girl sat at 9 months, stood at 12 months, used about a dozen words at 17 months, climbed out of a crib, and turned the knob to open a door at 2 years. Weight was 15 kg at 26 months, height 88 cm, and head circumference 52 cm. The rest of the physical findings were normal.

Her brother is clumsy at 25 months. His weight is 14.7 kg, height 89 cm, and head circumference 54 cm. The rest of the physical findings are normal.

The younger sister's weight at 7 months is 8.7 kg, length 67 cm, and head circumference 46 cm. A flame nevus is on bridge of nose, a hemangioma on lower lip, and a tan macule on buttock. The rest of the physical findings are normal.

Roentgenograms of 3-year-old girl in Figure 13-1 show normal skull with overhanging brow (as do those of younger siblings).

Diagnosis: Benign familial macrocephaly.

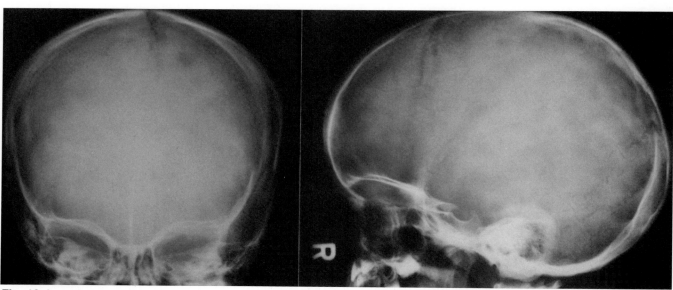

Fig. 13-1

Case 14

A 16-year-old girl has headaches that were occasional when they began 3 years ago and have been frequent for the last 6 months. Headaches are accompanied by a whirling sensation until she closes her eyes or sits down. She also has blurred vision and ringing in her ears.

Tonsils and adenoids were removed at 8 years, tubes put in ears at 11 years. Her back was injured in a car crash at 12 years. Menarche was at 12 years, and periods are regular.

Parents and six siblings are well.

Weight at 16 years is 59 kg, height 160 cm, head circumference 60 cm, temperature 37.2°C, heart rate 70, respiratory rate 20, and blood pressure 130/70 mm Hg. Eyes are widely separated and have an antimongoloid slant. One eye or the other turns out occasionally. The rest of the physical findings are normal.

Hematocrit is 0.41. White cell count is 8.1×10^9/liter with 0.56 polymorphonuclear cells, 0.42 lymphocytes, and 0.02 monocytes. Urine specific gravity is 1.005, pH 6. Urine is normal. Serum sodium is 144 mmol/liter, potassium 3.7, chloride 106, carbon dioxide 24, urea nitrogen 6.4, calcium 2.50, phosphorus 1.13, cholesterol 4.16, and glucose 4.9. Creatinine is 100 µmol/liter, uric acid 310, total bilirubin 3, and direct bilirubin 2. Total protein is 68 g/liter, albumin 42. Alkaline phosphatase is 90 U/liter, LDH 212, SGOT 37, and CK 164.

Figure 14-1 shows large skull. Orbits are widely separated. Inner table of frontal bone is irregularly thickened.

Diagnosis: Macrocephaly and orbital hypertelorism; hyperostosis frontalis interna (Morgagni-Stewart-Morell syndrome).

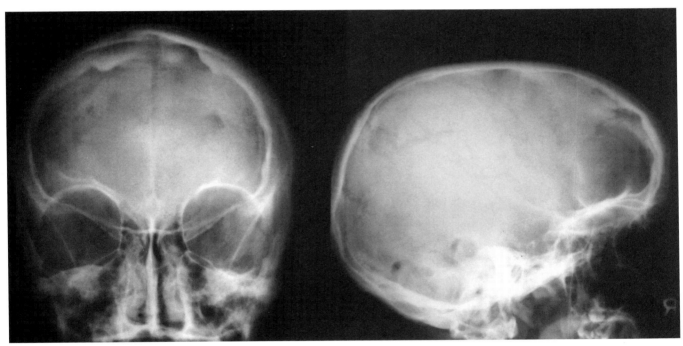

Fig. 14-1

Case 15

A newborn girl is convulsing.

Pregnancy of mother (18 years old) was normal, onset of labor spontaneous, progress slow and associated with meconium-stained amniotic fluid, fetal bradycardia, and loss of variability in fetal heart rate, and delivery by cesarean section. Birth weight is 3.1 kg, length 54 cm, Apgar score 1/5 at 1 and 5 minutes, temperature 37.2°C, heart rate 150, respiratory rate 80, and systolic blood pressure 52 mm Hg. She does not respond to stimuli. Limbs are flexed. Scalp is bruised. Bones overlap at sutures. Skin and nails are meconium stained. Reflexes are poor. Thick meconium is aspirated from stomach. The rest of the physical findings are normal.

Capillary blood pH is 7.15. At 8 hours, hematocrit is 0.68, serum sodium 130 mmol/liter, potassium 3.8, chloride 91, urea nitrogen 8.6, calcium 2.07, and glucose 2.8. Total bilirubin is 36 µmol/liter.

In Figure 15-1A, suture width, including width of metopic suture from anterior fontanel to nasion at frontonasal suture, is normal. In Figure 15-1B, parietal bones overlap at sagittal suture, scalp wrinkles are in parietal areas, and prognathism suggests brain undergrowth.

At 12 hours, arms twitch, legs bicycle, fists clench, back arches, and seizures persist. EEG shows low-voltage background activity and paroxysmal high-voltage discharges. She dies at 26 hours.

At necropsy, subcutaneous blood is down to pericranium at left pterion. The rest of the findings are normal.

Diagnosis: Intrauterine asphyxia, normal molding of newborn skull, and scalp wrinkles.

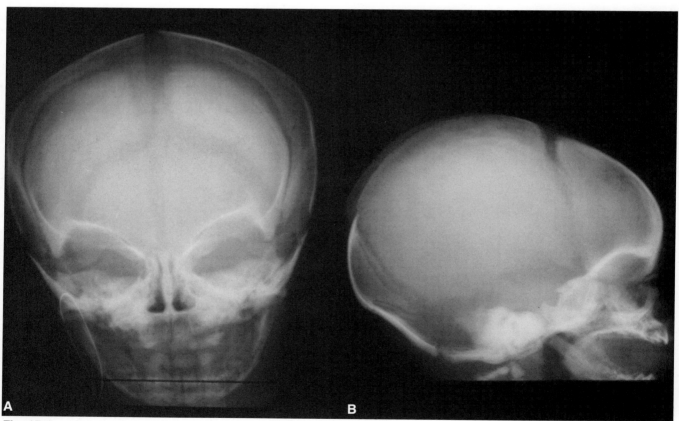

Fig. 15-1

Case 16

A girl is born after pregnancy of mother (31 years old) is marred by premature rupture of membranes.

Birth weight is 1.7 kg, length 43 cm, Apgar score 5/7 at 1 and 5 minutes, temperature 36°C, heart rate 156, respiratory rate 48, and blood pressure 43/26 mm Hg. Caput succedaneum is over right occiput. The rest of the physical findings are normal.

Hematocrit is 0.51, blood glucose 4.2 mmol/liter, arterial blood pH 7.21, P_{CO_2} 48 mm Hg, P_{O_2} 225 mm Hg, and total carbon dioxide 20 mmol/liter. Bilirubin peak is 195 μmol/liter at 5 days.

An ultrasound examination of head in Figure 16-1 at 8 days shows normal lateral ventricles, choroid plexus in lateral ventricles, and continuous cava front to back (reader's left to right) of septum pellucidum, Verga, and velum interpositum.

Diagnosis: Prematurity, normal brain.

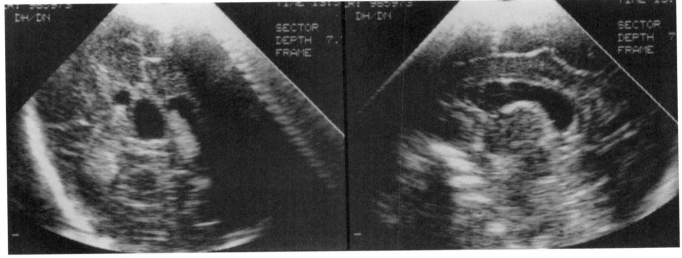

Fig. 16-1

Case 17

A 4-month-old boy has a flat occiput.

Pregnancy of mother was normal. Left foot was clubbed at birth.

Mother is American, father Japanese. He says it is a Japanese custom to put babies to sleep on their backs.

Head circumference is 41 cm. Left side of occiput is flat. A cast is on the left foot. The rest of the physical findings are normal.

CT in Figure 17-1 shows broad head and confirms occipital flattening along left side.

At 6 months, head circumference is 44 cm and occiput is not as flat.

Diagnosis: Postural flattening.

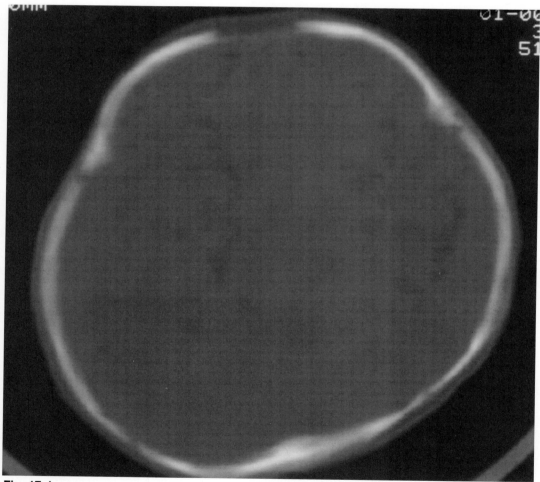

Fig. 17-1

Case 18

A 14-year-old boy who fell this afternoon has a laceration on back of head.

Blood is caked around a 5-cm laceration of scalp over occiput. Neurologic findings are normal.

Figure 18-1 shows paired deposits of calcium density in the posterior cranial fossa.

Diagnosis: Normal calcification in choroid plexuses of lateral ventricles.

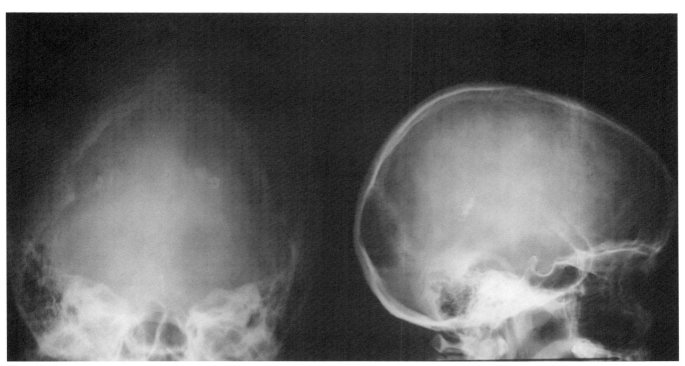

Fig. 18-1

Case 19

A 4⅓-year-old boy, who was put in a foster home last night, eats until he vomits and continues to ask for food.

Weight is 11.8 kg, height 84 cm, and head circumference 50 cm. Scars, scratches, and bruises are on body. Limbs are thin. Abdomen is distended and tense, liver edge 5 cm below costal margin. Bowel sounds are increased. The rest of the physical findings are normal.

Hematocrit is 0.37. White cell count is 6.7×10^9/liter with 0.21 polymorphonuclear cells, 0.05 bands, 0.68 lymphocytes, 0.04 monocytes, and 0.02 eosinophils. Platelet estimate is normal. Urine specific gravity is 1.015, pH 7. Urine has 0–1 white cell/HPF and 0.2 urobilinogen. Serum sodium is 136 mmol/liter, potassium 5.1, chloride 100, carbon dioxide 21, urea nitrogen 6.8, calcium 2.37, phosphorus 1.19, cholesterol 5.64, and glucose 4.3. Creatinine is 40 μmol/liter, uric acid 120, total bilirubin 5, and direct bilirubin 2. Total protein is 79 g/liter, albumin 55. Alkaline phosphatase is 148 U/liter, LDH 348, and SGOT 57. TSH is 2 mU/liter, free T_4 is 33 pmol/liter (normal: 10–36).

He hides food, takes food from other children, drinks from toilet, and has headaches during the next 9 days. Figure 19-1 shows that sutures have widened.

Weight is 12.9 kg on the tenth day, height is 86 cm, head circumference 51 cm, and temperature 38.3°C. He does not have headaches.

Diagnosis: Abuse, starvation, fatty liver.

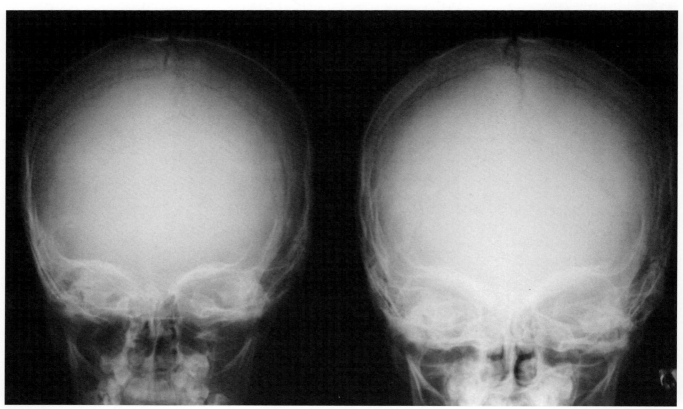

Fig. 19-1

Case 20

A 3½-year-old girl has a skull deformity that was present at birth and is subsiding.

Forehead is flattened on both sides of a midline ridge. The rest of the physical findings are normal.

Long axis of orbits is normal and no longer converges superiorly in Figure 20-1A. CT scan in Figure 20-1B shows a ridge in middle of frontal bone.

Diagnosis: Subsiding trigonocephaly.

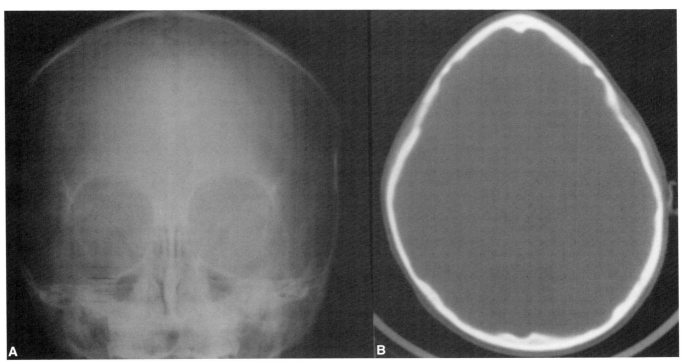

Fig. 20-1

Case 21

A newborn boy has flattened right side of forehead.

Presentation was vertex, delivery vaginal. Birth weight is 4 kg, head circumference 36 cm. Right coronal suture is ridged and forward. Caput succedaneum is over the right side of the occiput. Nose is flattened and pushed left. The rest of the physical findings are normal.

Maternal grandmother and great-grandmother say that members of five generations of their family have been born with abnormal bulge of one side and flattening of other side of forehead.

Roentgenograms show asymmetry of orbits and upward angulation of right orbital surface of frontal bone in infant's skull (Figure 21-1); similar, less obvious deformity in mother's skull (Figure 21-2A); and similar, least obvious deformity in maternal grandmother's skull (Figure 21-2B).

Diagnosis: Plagiocephaly, familial unilateral coronal synostosis.

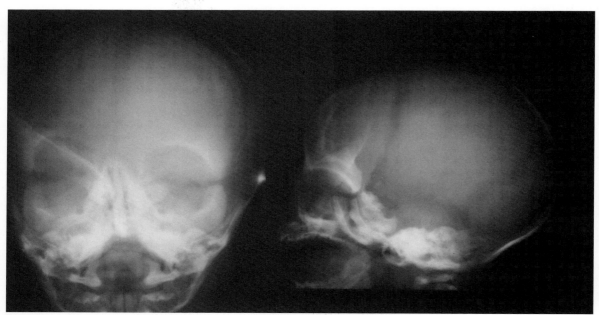

Fig. 21-1

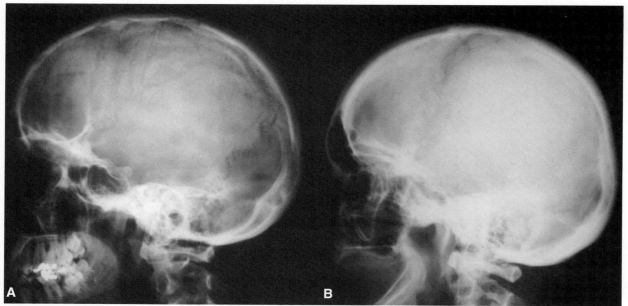

Fig. 21-2

Case 22

A 9-month-old girl has broad, flat forehead, recessed nasal bridge, and fused fingers and toes.

Pregnancy of mother was normal, birth weight 3.1 kg. She sits alone and reaches for toys.

Mother's parents are fourth cousins. Sister and two cousins of mother have fused fingers; a niece has two fused toes. A cousin of father has fused digits.

Weight at 9 months is 6.9 kg, length 71 cm, and head circumference 45 cm. Anterior fontanel is 6 × 4 cm. Eyeballs protrude. Fingers and toes are fused; thumbs are fused to palms. First toes stick out medially. The rest of the physical findings are normal.

Shape of skull and orbits in Figure 22-1 is that of coronal synostosis. In Figure 22-2, bones are abnormal in hands and feet, digits are fused.

Diagnosis: Apert's syndrome (acrocephalosyndactyly).

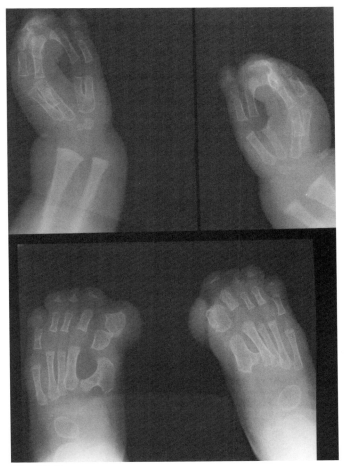

Fig. 22-2

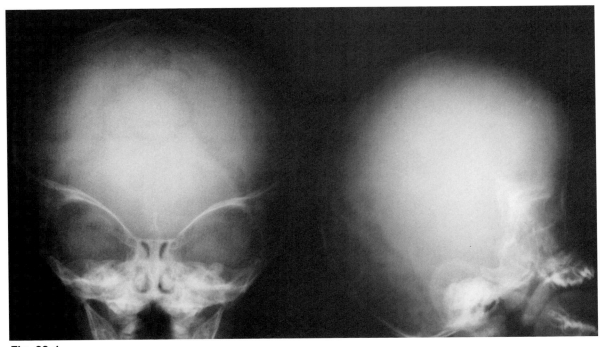

Fig. 22-1

Case 23

A newborn infant has a bulging forehead and arms fixed in half flexion.

Father and sister (4 years old) are well. Sister has had seizures.

Mother (23 years old) was thought to have fatty liver during pregnancy because of increased amounts of alkaline phosphatase and LDH in serum. Her gallbladder was removed a month before birth. Labor began spontaneously, but slow progress led to cesarean section. Birth weight is 2.0 kg, length 49 cm, head circumference 30 cm, and Apgar score 5/6 at 1 and 5 minutes. Infant improves with brief exposure to oxygen. Temperature is 39°C at 2 hours, heart rate 130, respiratory rate 40, blood pressure 63/39 mm Hg, hematocrit 0.42, and blood glucose 3.4 mmol/liter. Lids close over prominent eyeballs. Ophthalmologic findings are normal. Auricles are small. Bridge of nose is depressed. A no. 6 French catheter barely passes through each side of nose. Mouth is small. Arms are flexed. Length of phallus is 1.5 cm. Testes are not in small scrotum. Fingers and toes are long. The rest of the physical findings are normal. Brain stem auditory-evoked responses are normal at 5 days.

Serum 11-deoxycortisol is 26 nmol/liter (normal: 0–60), 17-alpha-hydroxyprogesterone 9 (normal: 0.5–4.5). Urine 17-ketosteroids are 0.7 μmol/liter (normal: ≤3.5 for infant 1–14 days) at 1 week. Chromosomes are 46,XX.

Figure 23-1 shows closed coronal sutures. Humeri and radii are fused at elbows in Figure 23-2. Cystogram in Figure 23-3 shows vagina, uterus, and normal bladder and urethra.

Diagnosis: Coronal synostosis, Antley-Bixler syndrome.

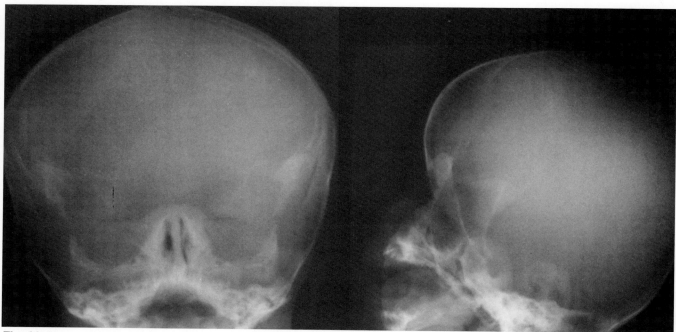

Fig. 23-1

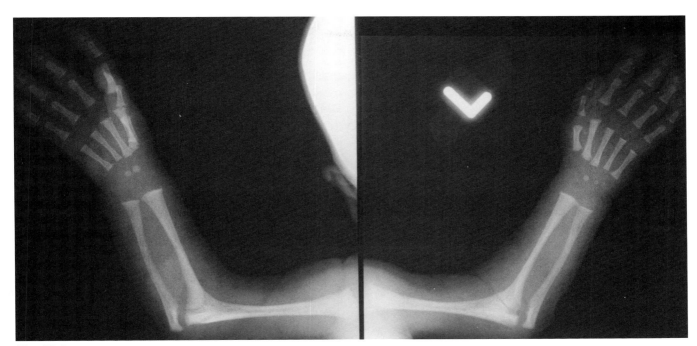

Fig. 23-2

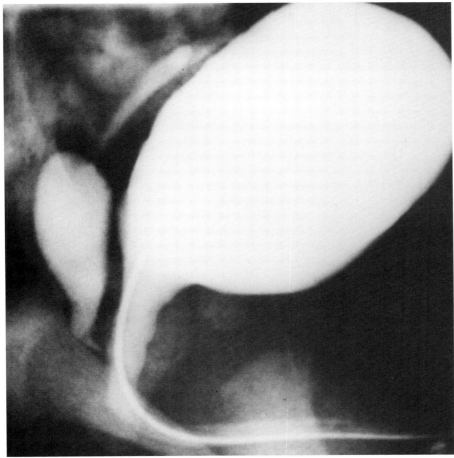

Fig. 23-3

Case 24

A newborn boy is thought to have a chromosomal abnormality.

Pregnancy of mother (19 years old) was normal. Birth weight is 3 kg, length 50 cm, head circumference 32 cm, Apgar score 8/9 at 1 and 5 minutes, temperature 36°C, heart rate 142, and respiratory rate 48. Hands and feet are blue. Fifth fingers curve in. Third and fourth toes of each foot are partly fused by soft tissues. A small umbilical hernia is present. The rest of the findings are normal.

Orbits are close together in Figure 24-1A. In Figure 24-1B, sphenoid bone is more oblique than normal so that sella turcica opens towards occiput and not vertex, and prognathism suggests brain undergrowth.

Diagnosis: Down syndrome. (Chromosomes are 47,XY,+21.)

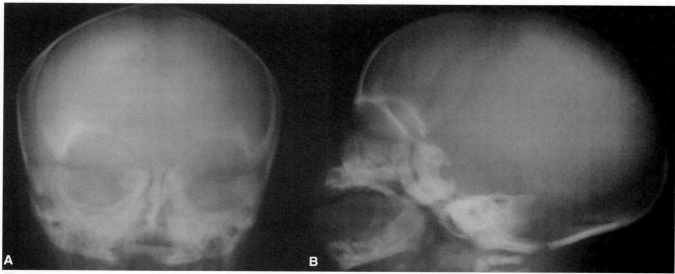

Fig. 24-1

Case 25

A newborn girl has bulging eyeballs, stiff arms, and broad thumbs and first toes.

Mother (32 years old), father (37 years old), and four siblings are well.

Pregnancy of mother was normal. Birth weight is 3.6 kg, length 50 cm, head circumference 36 cm, Apgar score 4/8 at 1 and 5 minutes, temperature 36.5°C, heart rate 152, respiratory rate 44, and blood pressure 61/37 mm Hg. Lids are swollen and red. Eyeballs bulge, right eyeball so much—especially when she cries—that lids cannot close (lagophthalmos). Upper lids are notched in medial third. Optic discs are pale. Bridge of nose is depressed. A no. 8 French catheter passes through left side of the nose but not right. Auricles are normal. External acoustic meatuses are absent. A systolic murmur is present. Anus ends at posterior labial commissure of vagina. Arms are fixed in extension at elbows. Thumbs are bent laterally. The rest of the physical findings are normal.

Hematocrit is 0.42. White cell count is 18.8×10^9/liter with 0.54 polymorphonuclear cells, 0.04 bands, 0.32 lymphocytes,

0.09 monocytes, and 0.01 eosinophils. Platelet count is 340×10^9/liter. At 2 days, serum sodium is 137 mmol/liter, potassium 4.3, chloride 104, carbon dioxide 20, urea nitrogen 3.6, calcium 2.35, phosphorus 2.13, cholesterol 1.60, and glucose 4.7. Creatinine is 90 µmol/liter, uric acid 530, total bilirubin 41, and direct bilirubin 3. Total protein is 54 g/liter, albumin 33. Alkaline phosphatase is 167 U/liter, LDH 724, and SGOT 124. Chromosomes are 46,XX.

In Figure 25-1, coronal sutures seem prematurely closed and farther back in skull, sphenoid bone is tipped back, and enchondral bone at base of skull is thick. Little muscle is in arms, and bones of arms seem to have formed in a rod of cartilage with synostosis at elbow (Figure 25-2). Thumbs are bent, first toes broad (Figures 25-3 and 25-4).

Diagnosis: Radioulnohumeral synostosis and questionable coronal synostosis, Pfeiffer's syndrome.

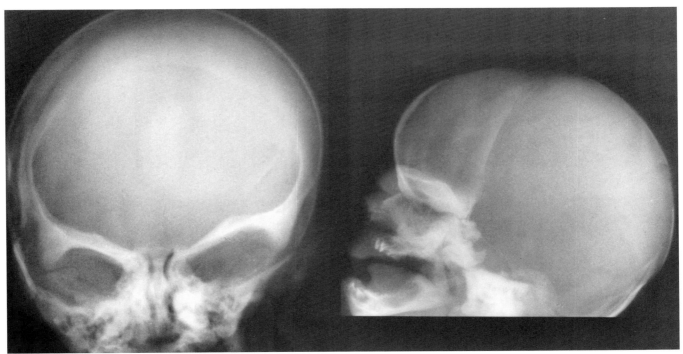

Fig. 25-1

(Continued)

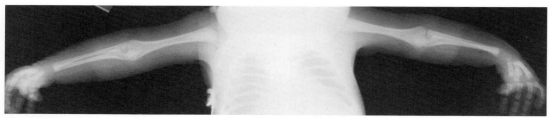

Fig. 25-2

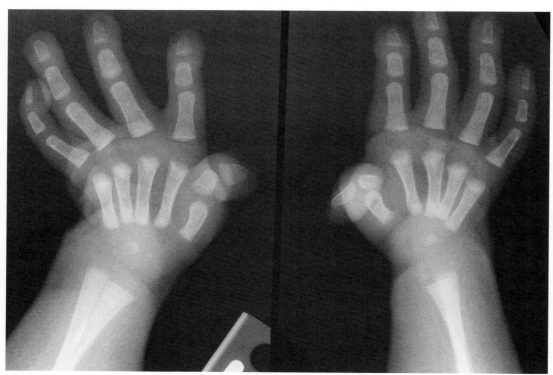

Fig. 25-3

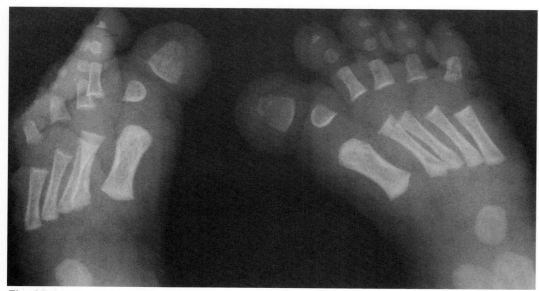

Fig. 25-4

Case 26

A newborn girl has omphalocele, brachycephaly, and polydactyly.

Mother (22 years old) and father (39 years old) are well. She is their only child.

Pregnancy of mother was normal. Birth weight is 4.1 kg, length 50 cm, head circumference 35 cm, Apgar score 8/9 at 1 and 5 minutes, temperature 36.6°C, heart rate 137, respiratory rate 40, and blood pressure 80/35 mm Hg. Forehead is narrow. Lids with epicanthi close easily over slightly proptotic eyes. Inner canthal distance is 2.5 cm. Nose is flat. Diameter of omphalocele is 5 cm. Fingers are short. Feet have six toes. The rest of the physical findings are normal. Ophthalmologic findings are normal.

Hematocrit is 0.57, white cell count 23.3×10^9/liter, and platelet count 261×10^9/liter.

In Figure 26-1, orbital surface of frontal bone is oblique, coronal suture is open and forward, and shape of orbits suggests trigonocephaly. Middle phalanges of fingers are hypoplastic or absent (Figure 26-2). Forefeet are adducted, have an extra first toe and five metatarsals, the first metatarsal dysplastic (Figure 26-3). CT scan in Figure 26-4 shows midline ridge of forehead and normal brain with cavum septi pellucidi.

Omphalocele is repaired. Operations on head and feet are performed later.

She is alert at 5 years. Weight is 25 kg, height 115 cm, and head circumference 54 cm. Physical findings are normal except for surgical scars.

Diagnosis: Carpenter's syndrome.

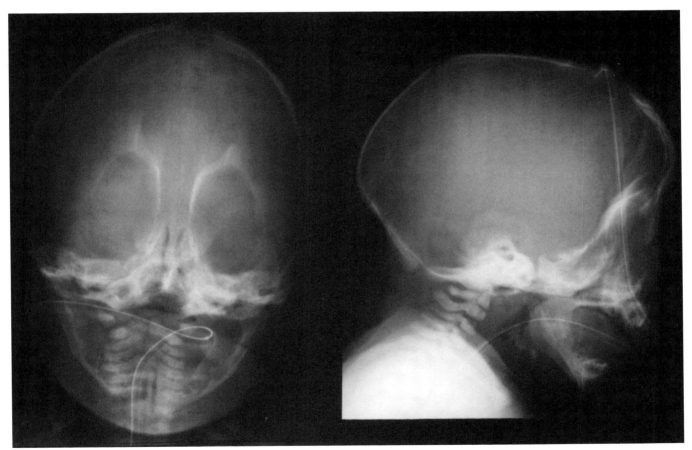

Fig. 26-1

(Continued)

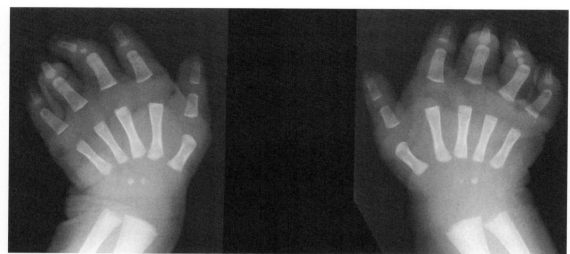

Fig. 26-2

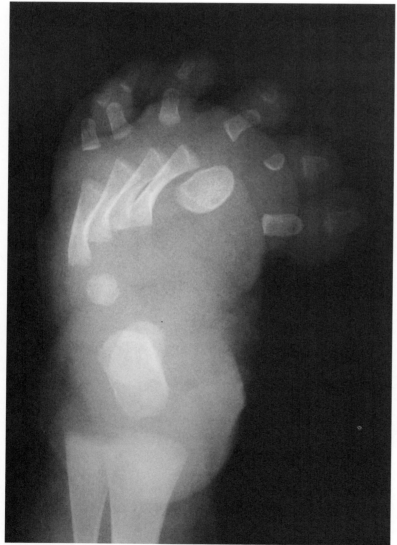

Fig. 26-3

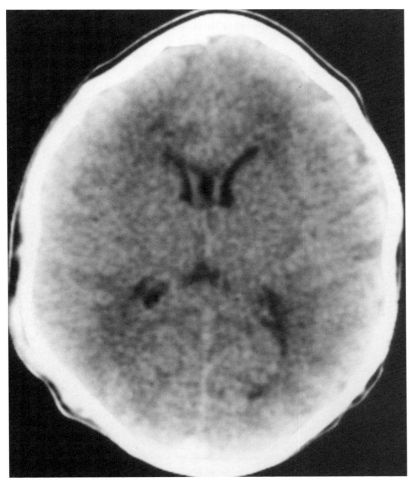

Fig. 26-4

Case 27

A 3-month-old boy has a ridge "like a spine" along the middle of his head front to back that was noticed by his mother right after he was born. Pregnancy was normal.

Weight is 6.9 kg, head circumference 42 cm. The rest of the physical findings are normal.

Towne's view of skull, in Figure 27-1A, shows sagittal ridge. Lateral view, in Figure 27-1B, shows scaphocephaly. CT scan shows long skull and normal brain.

Diagnosis: Sagittal synostosis.

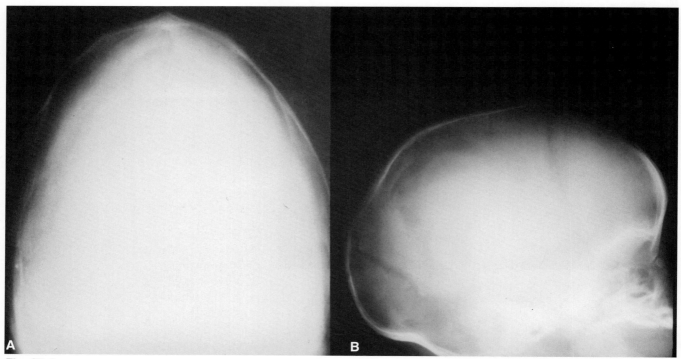

Fig. 27-1

Case 28

A 2-week-old boy has an abnormally shaped head.

Mother (24 years old), a carrier of hepatitis B, smoked half a pack of cigarettes per day during pregnancy, took an antidepressant during first month of pregnancy, and occasionally used amphetamines, cocaine, wine, and aspirin during rest of the pregnancy.

Weight 3.4 kg, length 50 cm, and head circumference 36 cm. Left side of occiput is flat. A ridge is along sagittal and left side of lambdoid suture. The rest of the physical findings are normal.

Figure 28-1 shows that sagittal suture is thin, left side of lambdoid suture discontinuous, and lambda displaced to the right. CT scan in Figure 28-2 shows left occipital flattening and overlap of bones at left side of lambdoid suture.

Diagnosis: Sagittal and left lambdoid synostosis.

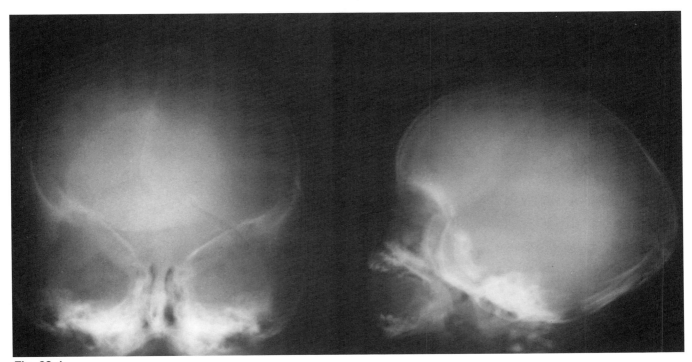

Fig. 28-1

(Continued)

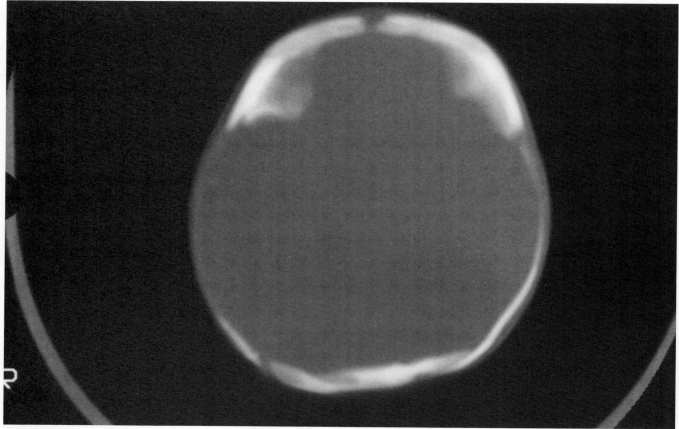

Fig. 28-2

Case 29

A newborn boy has a skull deformity that was discovered in prenatal ultrasound examination.

Mother (19 years old), father, and sibling (1½ years old) are well.

Pregnancy was normal. Birth weight is 4 kg, Apgar score 8/9 at 1 and 5 minutes, temperature 36.7°C, heart rate 135, respiratory rate 30, and blood pressure 65/50 mm Hg. Head bulges at top and sides. Eyelids are behind protruding eyeballs. Conjunctival vessels are swollen, corneas rough, pupils small, anterior chambers shallow, discs cupped, and maculae and retinal vessels normal. Ears are low, slanted toward shoulders, and without external acoustic meatuses. A no. 5 French catheter does not pass through either side of nose. A midline groove is in palate. Extension at elbows and movement at other joints are restricted. Slight hypospadias is present. Little fingers curve in. First toes are large. The rest of the physical findings are normal.

Chromosomes are 46,XY.

Figure 29-1 shows thin, ridged calvarial bulges. CT scan in Figure 29-2 shows dilated ventricles and lateral bulges. Radiohumeral joints appear fused in Figure 29-3.

Diagnosis: Cloverleaf skull (Kleeblattschädel), Antley-Bixler syndrome.

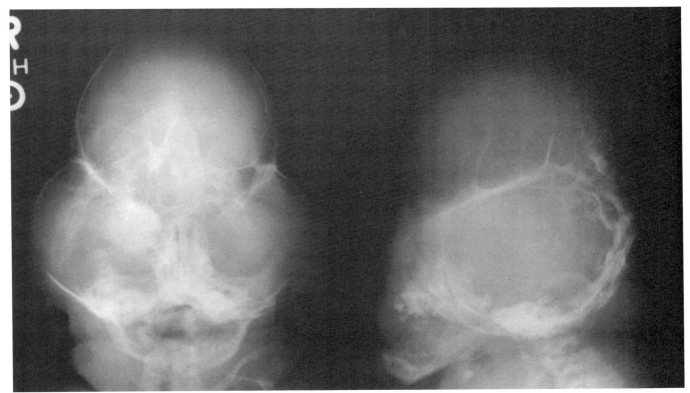

Fig. 29-1

(Continued)

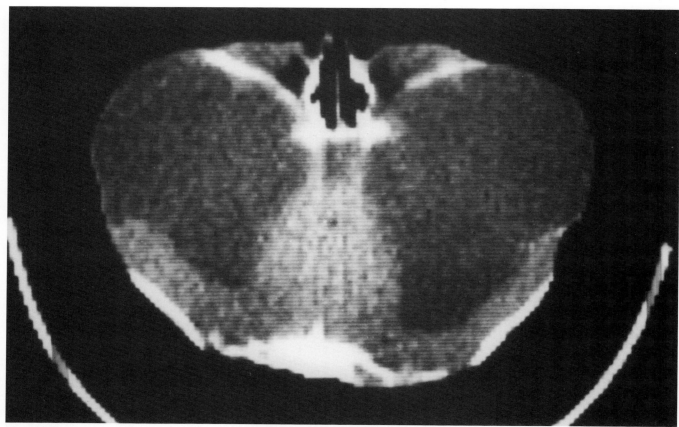

Fig. 29-2

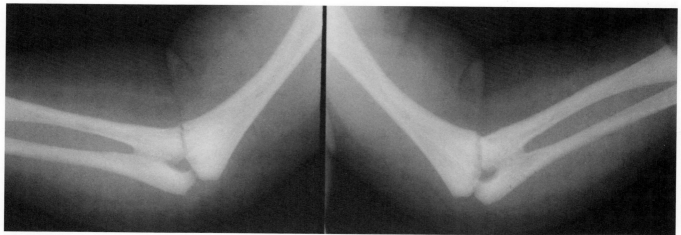

Fig. 29-3

Case 30

An 8-day-old girl is to have placement of a ventriculoperitoneal shunt. She had a low meningomyelocele repaired the day of birth.

Mother (28 years old) took levothyroxine daily during pregnancy and an antibiotic briefly for urinary tract symptoms.

Weight at 8 days is 3.1 kg, length 49 cm, head circumference 34 cm, temperature 36.6°C, heart rate 140, respiratory rate 48, and systolic blood pressure 82 mm Hg. She does not respond to pain below L5–S1. The rest of the physical findings are normal.

Hematocrit is 0.46. White cell count is 31.4×10^9/liter with 0.53 polymorphonuclear cells, 0.03 bands, 0.25 lymphocytes, and 0.19 monocytes. Platelet count is 528×10^9/liter. Urine specific gravity is 1.007, pH 6. Urine has few squamous epithelial cells/HPF. Serum sodium is 143 mmol/liter, potassium 4.1, chloride 107, and calcium 2.42.

Lacunar rarefactions in calvaria at 8 days (Figure 30-1A) are shown in CT scan (Figure 30-2) to be caused by ridges and hollows along inner table. Examination in Figure 30-1B at 3 months for a lump behind right ear shows smooth calvaria and a tangle of nonfunctioning shunt tube, which includes distal end at operation. Examination in Figure 30-3 after revision of shunt shows peritoneal tube and abnormal pedicles in sacrum and L5.

Diagnosis: Meningomyelocele, hydrocephalus, and lacunar rarefactions (Lückenschädel) that disappear in early months regardless of intracranial pressure.

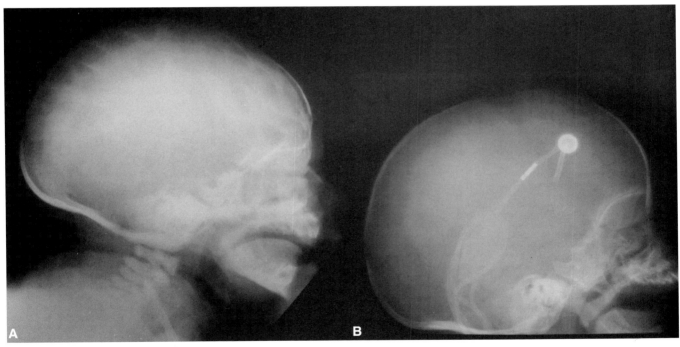

Fig. 30-1

(Continued)

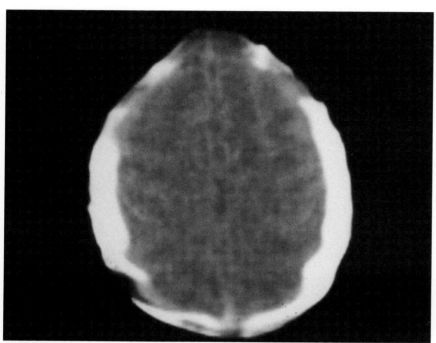

Fig. 30-2

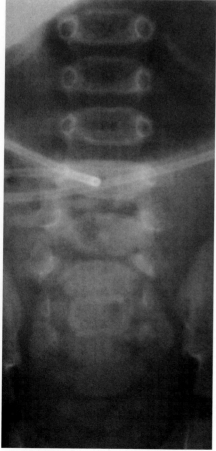

Fig. 30-3

Case 31

A girl is delivered from 26-year-old mother by cesarean section for prolapsed umbilical cord and slowing of fetal heart rate to 80.

Birth weight is 3.2 kg, length 51 cm, Apgar score 4/6 at 1 and 10 minutes, temperature 36.8°C, heart rate 215, respiratory rate 50, and blood pressure 49/27 mm Hg. She is intubated and given oxygen. She is jittery. The rest of the physical findings are normal.

Hematocrit is 0.53. Umbilical venous blood pH is 7.07. P_{CO_2} is 53 mm Hg, P_{O_2} 78. Bicarbonate is 15 mmol/liter. Serum calcium is 2.35 mmol/liter, glucose 6.7.

CT scan at 8 days (Figure 31-1A) shows normal findings; CT scan at 2 months (Figure 31-1B) shows widened interhemispheric fissure.

She does not sit at 1 year. She walks stiffly on toes at 22 months. Right eye turns out at 6 years. Leg muscles are tight. Abduction at hips is limited. Feet have equinus deformity and Babinski's sign.

Neck-shaft angle of femurs in Figure 31-2 is greater than normal at 6 years.

Diagnosis: Cerebral palsy with spastic diplegia (Little's disease).

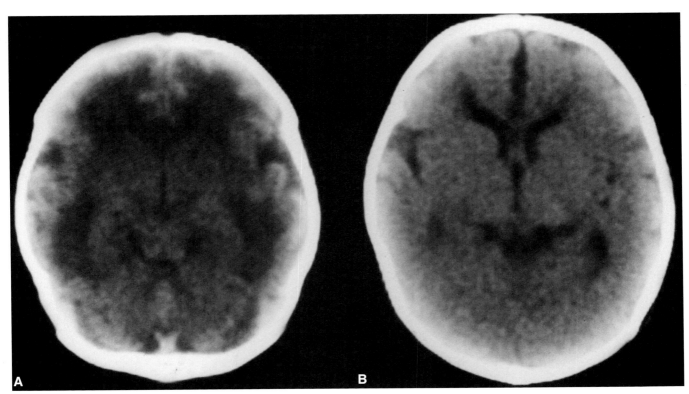

Fig. 31-1

(Continued)

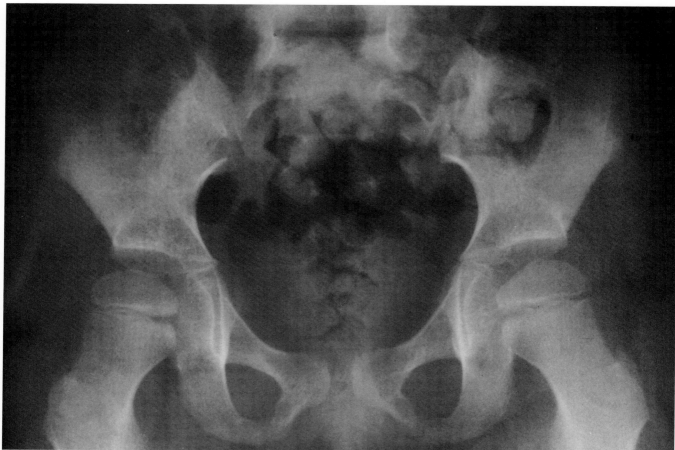

Fig. 31-2

Case 32

Twin girls are delivered by cesarean section for intrauterine growth retardation found in prenatal ultrasound examination. Gestational age is 36 weeks by dates.

Mother (27 years old), father (25 years old), and sister (3 years old) are well. Mother did not smoke or use drugs or alcohol during pregnancy. Parents are not consanguineous.

Birth weight of first girl is 1.6 kg, length 42 cm, head circumference 26 cm, Apgar score 7/9 at 1 and 5 minutes, temperature 36.6°C, heart rate 128, respiratory rate 48, and blood pressure 60/34 mm Hg. Head is small, nose big, chin small, and body stiff. The rest of the physical findings are normal.

Hematocrit of first girl is 0.43. White cell count is 9.3 × 10⁹/liter with 0.42 polymorphonuclear cells, 0.07 bands, 0.40 lymphocytes, 0.07 monocytes, 0.01 eosinophils, and 0.03 metamyelocytes. Platelet count is 186 × 10⁹/liter.

Birth weight of second girl is 1.7 kg, length 42 cm, head circumference 30 cm, Apgar score 5/9 at 1 and 5 minutes, temperature 35.5°C, heart rate 140, and respiratory rate 42. Nose is big, chin small. She is floppy at delivery. She arches her back and clamps jaws tightly at 30 minutes and again at 1 hour. Heart rate slows to 110. The rest of the physical findings are normal.

Hematocrit of second girl is 0.49. White cell count is 11.2 × 10⁹/liter with 0.28 polymorphonuclear cells, 0.06 bands, 0.43 lymphocytes, 0.11 monocytes, 0.11 eosinophils, and 0.01 metamyelocytes. Platelet count is 214 × 10⁹/liter.

Both girls suck from a nipple but swallow poorly. They are stiff. Thumbs are adducted tightly across palms. First girl has hypoplastic optic nerves. Three EEGs in second girl show normal findings. Chromosomes of both girls are 46,XX, with identical quinacrine banding.

First girl has microcephaly. She has small mandible (Figure 32-1), as does second girl. CT scan of the head on day of delivery shows symmetric absence of the back part of both cerebral hemispheres in microcephalic first girl (Figure 32-2A) and normal findings in the second girl (Figure 32-2B).

Diagnosis: Seckel's syndrome, probable identical twins.

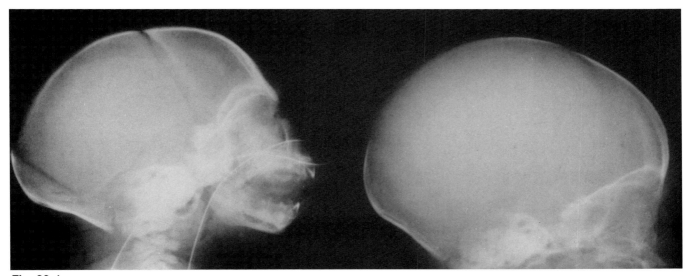

Fig. 32-1

(Continued)

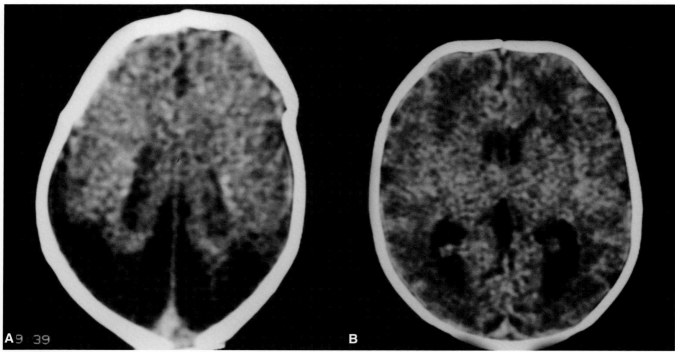

Fig. 32-2

Case 33

A 20-month-old girl is "like a newborn." She sleeps most of the time. She cries when hurt but not when hungry or wet. She drinks from a bottle and eats and turns away when full. She does not hold toys.

Mother (31 years old), a dentist's assistant, was exposed to nitrous oxide during pregnancy. Birth weight was 2.6 kg, Apgar score 6/7 at 1 and 5 minutes. She did not react to cuddling at 6 weeks. She lay limp on back, arms at sides, but stiffened when disturbed. She arched back when touched, especially on face, at 4 months. She had convulsions for 1–2 minutes at 18 months. Eyes rolled side to side, jaws clenched, and arms stiffened and twitched.

Parents and sister (5 years old) are well.

Weight at 20 months is 8.2 kg, length 75 cm, and head circumference 45 cm. She is limp but resists movement of head. She tracks poorly. She drools. Muscles of limbs are thin. Fists are clenched. Deep tendon reflexes are hyperactive. Bilateral ankle clonus and Babinski's sign are present. The rest of the physical findings are normal.

EEG shows high-voltage, rhythmic activity over both cerebral hemispheres.

Symmetrically malformed brain (Figure 33-1) is without gyri, sulci, and gray-white distinction. Lateral and third ventricles and cistern of great cerebral brain are dilated (see Figure 33-1).

Diagnosis: Lissencephaly.

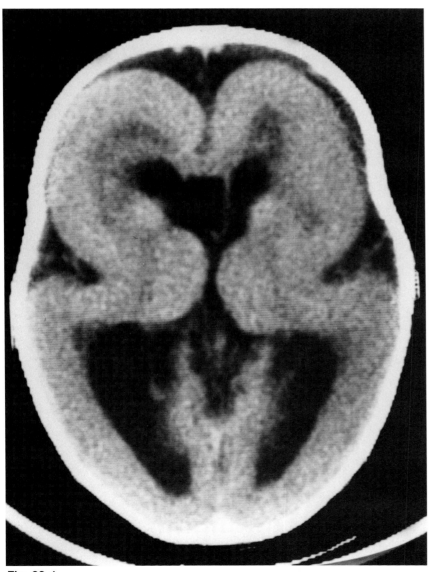

Fig. 33-1

Case 34

A newborn boy, who is dusky, pale, tachypneic, and limp, becomes twitchy and irritable when stimulated.

Mother (23 years old) is HBsAg positive and anti-HBc positive and took cephalosporin during third trimester for cyst of Bartholin's gland. Father (25 years old) is well. The boy is their only child.

Birth weight is 3.5 kg, head circumference 32 cm, Apgar score 3/7 at 1 and 5 minutes, temperature 38.2°C, heart rate 135, respiratory rate 93, and blood pressure 53/46 mm Hg. Pupils are dilated and nonreactive. Ophthalmologic examination shows bulge at back of right lens; pale, cupped optic discs; and faint double ring around left disc. Legs are mottled. Deep tendon reflexes are hyperactive and accompanied by twitches and grimaces. The rest of the physical findings are normal.

Hematocrit is 0.37. White cell count is 13.9×10^9/liter with 0.35 polymorphonuclear cells, 0.05 bands, 0.49 lymphocytes, 0.08 monocytes, 0.02 eosinophils, and 0.01 basophils. Blood glucose is 3.3 mmol/liter. Urine specific gravity is 1.005, pH 5. Urine has trace protein, bacteria, 0–2 white cells and few squamous epithelial cells/HPF, and 0–2 hyaline casts/LPF. Chromosomes are 46,XY.

EEG shows high-voltage spikes over both cerebral hemispheres.

CT scan in Figure 34-1 shows deep clefts in cerebral hemispheres, no lateral and third ventricles, and subarachnoid blood along falx cerebri.

Diagnosis: Schizencephaly, subarachnoid blood, right posterior keratoconus, and coloboma of optic nerves.

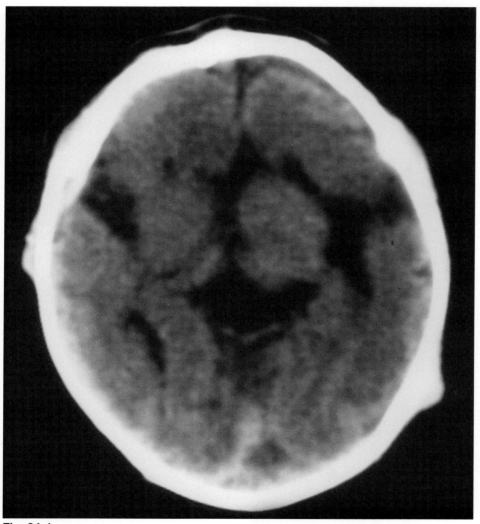

Fig. 34-1

Case 35

A 3½-month-old girl has a brain abnormality that was discovered in prenatal ultrasound examination at 5 months' gestation.

Mother (22 years old), father (21 years old), and brother (1 year old) are well.

Pregnancy was normal, marred only by findings in ultrasound examination to confirm dates. Birth weight was 2.6 kg, head circumference 35 cm, and Apgar score 8/9 at 1 and 5 minutes. Head transilluminated. Infant was tremulous. She receives only nursing care. She takes 2 oz formula every 3 hours.

Head circumference at 3½ months is 45 cm, weight 4.2 kg, temperature 37.5°C, heart rate 110, respiratory rate 32, and blood pressure 101/67 mm Hg. She lies stiffly and cries when disturbed. Fontanels are large and tense. Head transilluminates. Sclerae show above iris. Breathing is snorty. Knee jerks are brisk. The rest of the physical findings are normal.

Hematocrit is 0.30. White cell count is 22.0×10^9/liter with 0.31 polymorphonuclear cells, 0.06 bands, 0.56 lymphocytes, 0.05 monocytes, and 0.02 eosinophils. Platelet count is 391×10^9/liter. Urine specific gravity is 1.011, pH 6. Urine is normal. Serum sodium is 156 mmol/liter, potassium 4.2, chloride 124, carbon dioxide 15, urea nitrogen 3.2, calcium 2.40, phosphorus 2.16, cholesterol 3.65, and glucose 6.4. Creatine is 50 μmol/liter, uric acid 420, total bilirubin 24, and direct bilirubin 10. Total protein is 61 g/liter, albumin 38. Alkaline phosphatase is 1,014 U/liter, LDH 512, and SGOT 81. Cortisol is 330 nmol/liter (normal: 193–690). FSH is <2 IU/liter, LH 5. Serum osmolality is 308 mOsm/kg.

CT scan in Figure 35-1 shows no cerebral mantel. Thalami, cerebellum, midbrain, brain stem, falx cerebri, and tentorium cerebelli are normal.

Much CSF drains at incision of dura to place ventriculoperitoneal shunt. CSF has 111×10^6/liter red cells, $<1 \times 10^6$/liter white cells, 0.41 lymphocytes, 0.12 histiocytes, 0.12 ependymal cells, 0.35 atypical lymphocytes, 3.5 mmol/liter glucose, and 1.47 g/liter protein, and is sterile.

Diagnosis: Hydranencephaly.

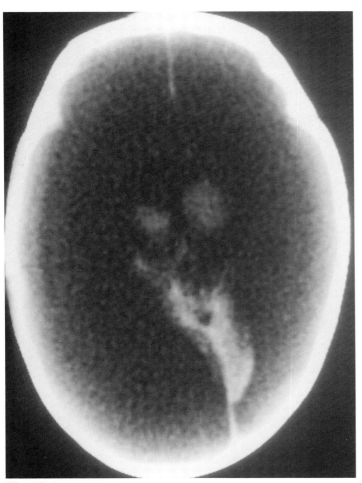

Fig. 35-1

Case 36

A newborn girl has closely set, bulging eyeballs; flat nose; and cleft lip.

Mother (24 years old) has been taking thyroid pills since age 17. A sibling is normal.

Pregnancy was normal. Birth weight is 2.4 kg, length 48 cm, head circumference 30 cm, Apgar score 5/6 at 1 and 5 minutes, temperature 36.3°C, heart rate 136, and respiratory rate 36. She is dusky, depressed, meconium stained, and twitching. She has no nasal bridge and no septum. A wide cleft is in palate. Skin is loose, especially on back of neck. Breath sounds are noisy. Liver edge is 2 cm below costal margin. Muscle tone and reflexes are depressed. The rest of the physical findings are normal.

Urine specific gravity is 1.011 at 3 days, pH 6. Urine has 1+ protein, many squamous epithelial cells, 1–2 nonsquamous epithelial cells, rare red cells, and 1–2 white cells/HPF, uric acid crystals, and bacteria. At 3 days, serum sodium is 137 mmol/liter, potassium 5.8, chloride 84, and glucose 2.0. Chromosomes are 46,XX.

In Figure 36-1, orbits are close together, nasal bone is absent, a midline gap is in maxilla and hard palate, and a metopic suture bisects frontal bone.

At 8 days, she has convulsions as often as every 10 minutes. She cries out. Eyes roll, head turns right, tongue protrudes, fists clench, body stiffens. Temperature varies between 33.5 and 38.1°C during the first few weeks, heart rate between 80 and 160, and respiratory rate between 20 and 76.

Diagnosis: Cebocephaly.

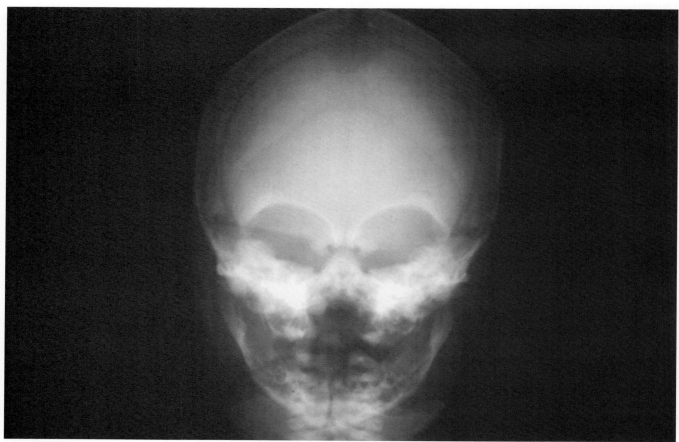

Fig. 36-1

Case 37

A 7-year-old boy gags and chokes when he swallows and then vomits.

Mother used cocaine during pregnancy. Membranes ruptured a week before birth. Birth weight was 1.3 kg. He did not suck or swallow until he was a month old. He was stiff at 5 months. Legs scissored and feet extended when he was picked up at 10 months. He followed with his eyes and turned to sound at 1 year. He had Moro's reflex at 1 year and assumed fencer's position when head was turned left. Babinski's sign was in feet. He has had ear infections, pneumonia, tonsillectomy and adenoidectomy, tracheostomy, gastrostomy, and adductor transfers at the hips. He is not toilet trained. He does not stand. He sits in a wheelchair. He grinds his teeth. He bites his hands when upset. He sweats and becomes pale several times a day. He has begun to use a few words in the past year.

Temperature at 7 years is 36.5°C, heart rate 104, respiratory rate 20, blood pressure 70/54 mm Hg, weight 14 kg, and head circumference 44 cm. He smiles and follows with his eyes. Auricles are simple and turned out. Mouth is open and full of spit. He does not move tongue or limbs in a deliberate manner. Scar is on neck, gastrostomy button on abdomen, livedo reticularis on limbs. Scars are at hips. Elbows, wrists, knees, and ankles are flexed. Ankle clonus is present. The rest of the physical findings are normal.

Hematocrit is 0.41. White cell count is 10.2×10^9/liter with 0.58 polymorphonuclear cells, 0.34 lymphocytes, 0.07 monocytes, 0.01 eosinophils, and 0.01 basophils. Platelet count is 179×10^9/liter. Urine specific gravity is 1.015, pH 9. Urine has 3–5 white cells and occasional squamous epithelial cells/HPF, and 0.2 AU urobilinogen. Serum sodium is 186 mmol/liter, potassium 3.9, chloride 147, carbon dioxide 34, urea nitrogen 16.1, calcium 2.45, phosphorus 1.00, cholesterol 2.02, and glucose 7.2. Creatinine is 80 μmol/liter, uric acid 654, total bilirubin 3, and direct bilirubin 0. Total protein is 57 g/liter, albumin 35. Alkaline phosphatase is 197 U/liter, LDH 204, and SGOT 58.

Figure 37-1 shows a single midline ventricle in brain. Falx cerebri and corpus callosum are absent.

Diagnosis: Holoprosencephaly.

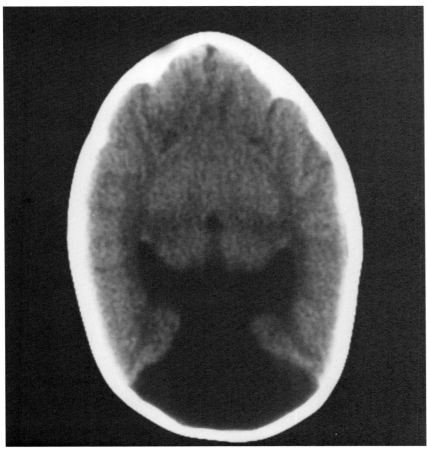

Fig. 37-1

Case 38

An 11-year-old girl has fever, diarrhea, and abdominal pain.

Mother was 21 years old, father 25 years old when girl was born. Both were well.

Pregnancy of mother was normal. Birth weight was 3.4 kg. She was born with imperforate anus, cloaca, atrial septal defect, bicornuate uterus, dysplastic kidneys, and skin tags on face. Colostomy, later sacroperineal pull-through operation, and closure of atrial septal defect were performed. She had gram-negative meningitis at 3 weeks. Hemodialysis was begun at 8 years. Renal transplantation at 9 years was followed by acute rejection and peritoneal dialysis. She had a convulsion at 9 years. She did well in school at 10 years. She had peritonitis caused by *Candida parapsilosis* 1 month ago.

Temperature at 11 years is 37.9°C, heart rate 160, respiratory rate 18, and blood pressure 100/68 mm Hg. Skin is mottled. Chest is scarred. Abdomen is distended, tender, and scarred. Papules are on legs. The rest of the physical findings are normal.

Hematocrit is 0.26, white cell count 0.5×10^9/liter, and platelet count 74×10^9/liter. Bacteroides grows in culture of peritoneal aspirate. She dies 2 weeks later.

In Figure 38-1, a radiolucent mass with plaque of calcium density in left front part is in midline above third ventricle at age 11 years.

At necropsy a soft tan mass ($2 \times 2 \times 1$ cm) replaces splenium of corpus callosum and extends beyond frontal poles of lateral ventricles. Locus ceruleus and substantia nigra are hypopigmented. Microscopic examination shows fat in mass, calcium in cingulate gyrus, and deficit of pigmented neurons in locus ceruleus and substantia nigra.

Diagnosis: Partial agenesis and lipoma of corpus callosum.

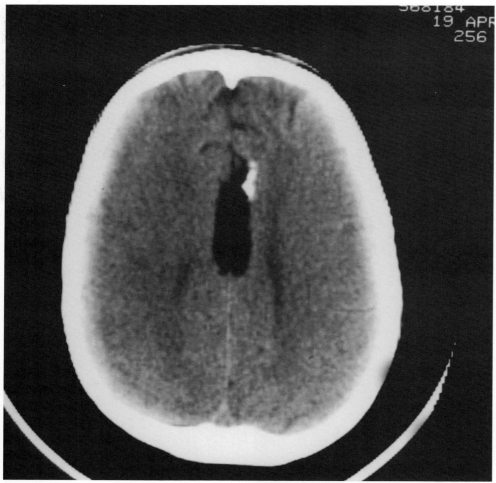

Fig. 38-1

Case 39

A 7-month-old boy has seizures that began at 4 months with limbs jerking and eyes turning right. At 7 months, he trembles for a few minutes once or twice a day. At other times he is unresponsive with staring eyes for 30 seconds. Eyes move rapidly in all directions several times a day. He has been fussy and vomiting for 2 weeks.

Pregnancy was marred by polyhydramnios; birth weight was 2.3 kg, length 47 cm, head circumference 31 cm, and Apgar score 4/8 at 1 and 5 minutes. Mandible was small. Simian creases were on palms. Feet were everted. He fed poorly. Chromosomes were 46,XY,del(1)(q43). He lifted and turned head at 1½ months and sometimes smiled but does so no longer. Head circumference was 36 cm at 3 months.

Mother (19 years old) and father (23 years old) are well. Her chromosomes are 46,XX; his are 46,XY. The boy is their only child.

Temperature at 7 months is 37°C, heart rate 145, respiratory rate 36, systolic blood pressure 100 mm Hg, and weight 5.2 kg. He holds head turned to right. Occiput is prominent and has a tuft of thick hair above a small swelling. Nose is small, mouth large. Legs are turned out at knees, feet rocker-bottom with fusion of second and third toes. The rest of the physical findings are normal.

Hematocrit is 0.37, white cell count 14.7 × 10⁹/liter, and platelet count 566 × 10⁹/liter. Urine specific gravity is 1.015, pH 6. Urine has ketones and occasional squamous epithelial cells and 0–1 white cell/HPF. Serum sodium is 141 mmol/liter, potassium 4.8, chloride 107, carbon dioxide 19, urea nitrogen 2.1, calcium 2.62, phosphorus 1.49, cholesterol 4.30, and glucose 5.2. Creatinine is 40 µmol/liter, uric acid 330, total bilirubin 3, and direct bilirubin 0. Total protein is 58 g/liter, albumin 43. Alkaline phosphatase is 279 U/liter, LDH 321, and SGOT 51.

Ultrasound examination at 1 day shows dilated third ventricle high between dilated, separated lateral ventricles in coronal view (Figure 39-1A) and fanning of sulci instead of cingulate sulcus in lateral view (Figure 39-1B). Normal echoes are in posterior fossa. Findings in CT scan at 1 day are similar. CT scan at 7 months (Figure 39-2) shows cyst in posterior fossa, dilated lateral ventricles with large occipital horns, and dilated, high third ventricle. Plain film after placement of shunt between cyst in posterior fossa and peritoneum shows orbital hypotelorism (Figure 39-3).

Clear liquid obtained from cyst has <1 × 10⁶/liter white cells, 7 × 10⁶/liter red cells, 0.34 g/liter protein, and 2.8 mmol/liter glucose.

He has frequent respiratory infections, seizures, and vomiting. At 4 years, he smiles, sometimes follows with eyes, lifts head from prone, sucks thumb, and is fed by gastrostomy.

Diagnosis: Agenesis of corpus callosum, arachnoid cyst, small terminal deletion on long arm of chromosome 1.

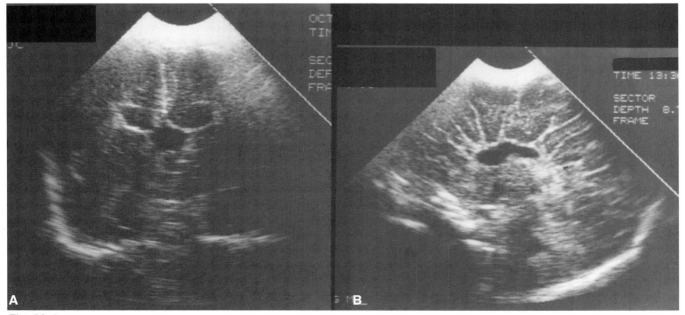

Fig. 39-1

(Continued)

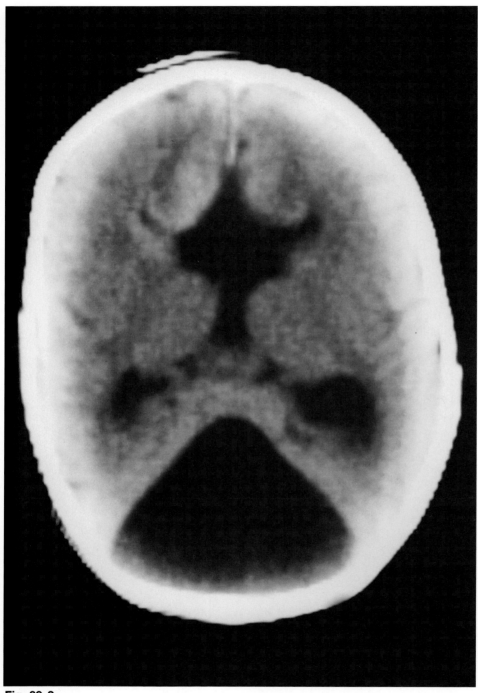

Fig. 39-2

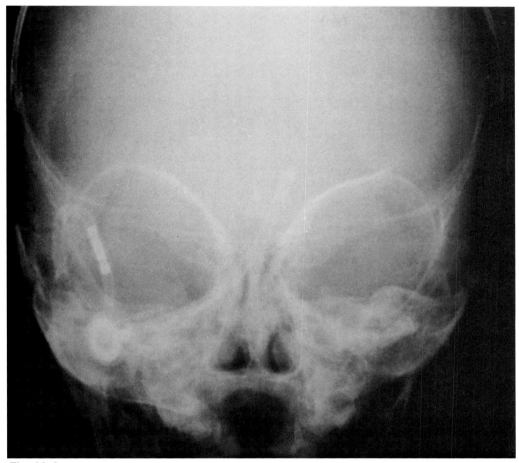

Fig. 39-3

Case 40

A 4-year-old boy who cannot be roused this morning has blood glucose 1.5 mmol/liter and revives with IV glucose. He has had a cold for a week.

Birth weight was 4.7 kg. He had an operation for squint at 8 months. He was hard to rouse when he got out of bed one morning at age 2½. He was hard to rouse one morning a month ago after he had been raiding the sugar bowl for 3 days.

Mother and brother (2 years old) are well. Father has kidney trouble.

Weight at 4 years is 16 kg, height 98 cm, temperature 38.0°C, heart rate 114, respiratory rate 20, and systolic blood pressure 94 mm Hg. Right pupil reacts sluggishly. Right disc is pale and one-third the size of left disc. Margin of right disc is blurred. The rest of the physical findings are normal. At 7 years, visual acuity in right eye is 20/400, 20/30 in left eye.

Hematocrit is 0.36. White cell count is 6.8×10^9/liter with 0.35 polymorphonuclear cells, 0.02 bands, 0.50 lymphocytes, 0.05 monocytes, 0.05 eosinophils, and 0.03 basophils. Urine specific gravity is 1.022, pH 5. Urine has 1+ ketones and few white cells/HPF. Fasting blood glucose is 4.6 mmol/liter at start of glucose tolerance test; its nadir is 2.9 mmol/liter at 3 hours.

CT scan of brain in Figure 40-1 shows absence of septum pellucidum.

Diagnosis: Septo-optic dysplasia (De Morsier's syndrome), hypoglycemia.

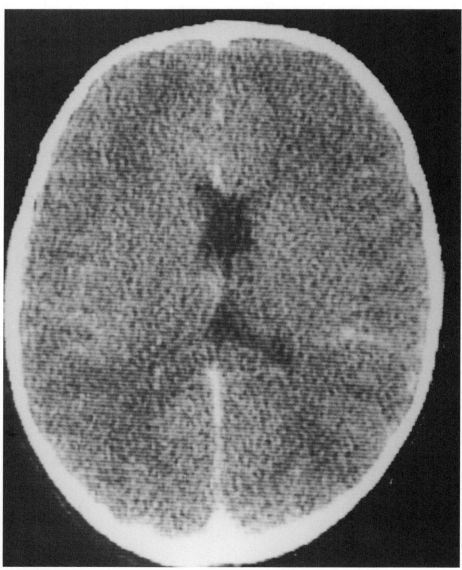

Fig. 40-1

Case 41

A 9-year-old girl is no taller than her 6-year-old sister and barely taller than her 4-year-old brother.

Mother had toxemia during pregnancy. Birth weight was 3.7 kg, length 52 cm. Blood glucose was low the first few days. Growth was slow at 1½ years. First baby tooth fell out at 7 years. She has had several ear infections and has occasional afternoon headaches. She does well in school.

Mother's height is 163 cm, father's 183 cm, sister's 117 cm, and brother's 116 cm.

Height at 9 years is 117 cm, weight 33 kg, temperature 37.3°C, heart rate 104, respiratory rate 20, and blood pressure 88/60 mm Hg. Maxillary central incisors are partly erupted. Elbow extension is limited. Fingernails are hyperconvex. The rest of the physical findings are normal.

Hematocrit is 0.37. White cell count is 6.3×10^9/liter with 0.52 polymorphonuclear cells, 0.38 bands, 0.07 monocytes, and 0.03 eosinophils. Platelet count is 276×10^9/liter. Urine specific gravity is 1.020, pH 5. Urine has 0–1 red cell, 25–50 white cells, 1–5 squamous epithelial cells/HPF, and mucus. Serum sodium is 143 mmol/liter, potassium 4.1, chloride 105, carbon dioxide 24, urea nitrogen 4.6, calcium 2.32, phosphorus 1.58, cholesterol 4.89, triglycerides 2.30, and glucose 5.1.

Creatinine is 50 µmol/liter, uric acid 300, total bilirubin 2, and direct bilirubin 0. Total protein is 74 g/liter, albumin 42. Alkaline phosphatase is 192 U/liter, LDH 224, and SGOT 27. Chromosomes are 46,XX.

MRI in Figure 41-1 shows (1) bright signal above pituitary fossa behind optic chiasm, (2) threadlike pituitary stalk, and (3) lack of normal bright signal of neurohypophysis in pituitary fossa. Bone age in the left hand is 7 years.

Serum-free T_4 is 19 pmol/liter (normal: 10–36). TSH is 1 mU/liter. Blood glucose nadir is 2.3 mmol/liter 15 minutes after IV insulin. Serum cortisol is 320 nmol/liter before insulin, 160 sixty minutes after insulin (normal: 193–690). Serum growth hormone is <1.5 mg/liter at all times after insulin and arginine (except 15 minutes after insulin, when level is 2.3). Serum growth hormone is 2.0 mg/liter at 60 minutes and 1.8 at 90 minutes after oral levodopa (normal: >10).

She is treated with growth hormone and levothyroxine until age 13 when height is 161 cm and weight 85 kg.

Diagnosis: Growth hormone deficiency, pituitary dwarfism.

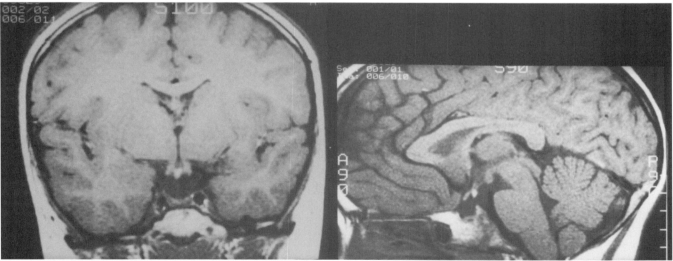

Fig. 41-1

Case 42

A 1-month-old girl has a big head.

Mother (22 years old) took occasional antihistamines during normal pregnancy. Birth weight was 3.8 kg, head circumference 38 cm. Right clavicle was fractured. She takes 4–5 oz formula every 4 hours. She cries when hungry or wet and stops crying when attended to. She does not lift her head from prone.

Head circumference is 44 cm, temperature 37.4°C, heart rate 120, respiratory rate 32, and systolic blood pressure 88 mm Hg. Anterior fontanel is large and tense. Eyes are widely separated. A yellow crust is in inner canthus of right eye. The rest of the physical findings are normal.

Hematocrit is 0.37. White cell count is 8.4×10^9/liter with 0.23 polymorphonuclear cells, 0.57 lymphocytes, 0.13 eosinophils, 0.04 monocytes, 0.01 basophils, and 0.02 atypical lymphocytes. Platelet count is 496×10^9/liter.

CT scan in Figure 42-1 shows dilated lateral ventricles separated by cavum septi pellucidi and cavum vergae, dilated third ventricle, and dilated fourth ventricle that communicates with a large cyst.

CSF is under moderate pressure during placement of a ventriculoperitoneal shunt. The fluid is clear and colorless; it has 2×10^6/liter white cells, 121×10^6/liter red cells, 2.7 mmol/liter glucose, 0.31 g/liter protein, and is sterile.

Diagnosis: Hydrocephalus, Dandy-Walker syndrome.

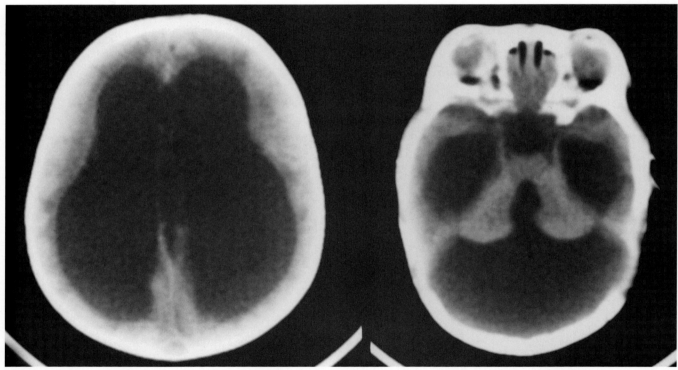

Fig. 42-1

Case 43

A newborn boy breathes hard and irregularly.

Mother (27 years old) smoked a pack of cigarettes a day during pregnancy. Delivery was by cesarean section. Birth weight is 3.2 kg, length 47 cm, head circumference 37 cm, Apgar score 6/7 at 1 and 5 minutes, temperature 37.1°C, heart rate 100, and, at 5 hours, blood pressure 67/35 mm Hg. Head is large, face flat. Colobomas are in retinas; coloboma involves left optic nerve. Depressed tip of nose covers philtrum. A midline cleft is in upper lip and hard palate. Tongue is small, grooved, and lobulated. A systolic murmur is present. Penis is small. Testes are not in scrotum. Polydactyly is present in hands and feet. The rest of the physical findings are normal.

Blood glucose is 5.5 mmol/liter at 50 minutes. At 9 hours, serum sodium is 146 mmol/liter, potassium 3.8, chloride 107, and calcium 2.62. At 11 hours, hematocrit is 0.71. White cell count is 18.7×10^9/liter with 0.68 polymorphonuclear cells, 0.16 bands, 0.14 lymphocytes, 0.01 monocytes, and 0.01 eosinophils. Platelet count is 79×10^9/liter.

Echocardiogram shows left superior vena cava, large coronary sinus, right ventricular hypertrophy, bicuspid aortic valve, and hypoplasia of aortic arch, which is confirmed by aortography.

Polydactyly is associated with extra metacarpal and metatarsal bones (Figures 43-1 and 43-2). CT scan of brain in Figure 43-3 shows right parietal cyst, dilation of ventricles, hypoplasia of vermis cerebelli, and isodense mass in hypothalamus. Roentgenogram of chest shows crooked left seventh and eighth ribs.

A Gore-Tex (Artex, Scarborough, Ontario) conduit is placed between ascending and descending aorta at one week. The boy dies at 3 months.

Necropsy shows additional abnormalities: (1) Meckel's diverticulum, (2) congestion and focal intra-alveolar blood in lungs, (3) no olfactory bulbs or tracts, (4) no olfactory groove in straight gyrus of frontal lobes, (5) hypoplasia of vermis and splenium of corpus callosum, (6) cyst in place of pineal gland, (7) right parietal cyst, (8) hypoxic changes in hippocampi, (9) congestion of cortical capillaries, (10) Purkinje's cells in cerebellar white matter, and (11) hypothalamic hamartoma of poorly organized brain tissue with increase in number of glial cells, scattered clusters of ganglion cells, and irregular growth of capillaries.

Diagnosis: Joubert's syndrome.

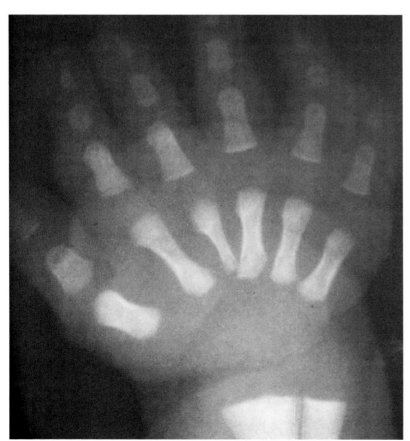

Fig. 43-1

(Continued)

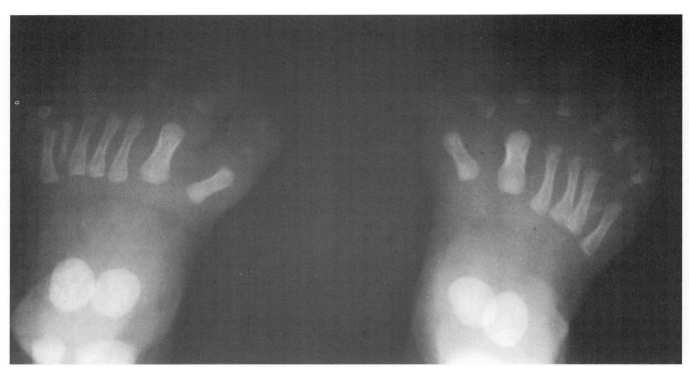

Fig. 43-2

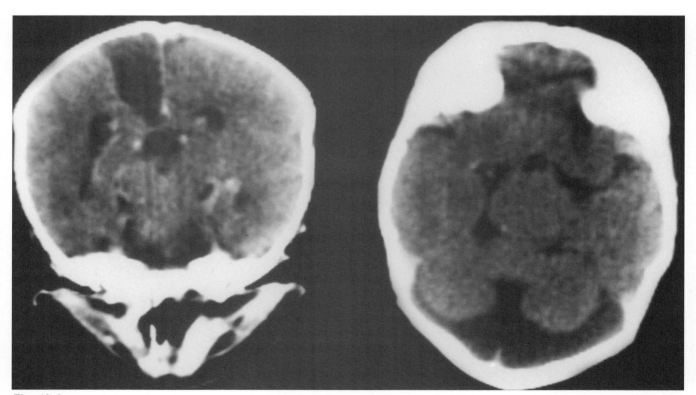

Fig. 43-3

Case 44

A newborn girl cries at birth and then does not breathe.

Pregnancy of the mother (32 years old) was normal, onset of labor spontaneous, and delivery by second cesarean section. Heart rate is less than 60, Apgar score 1/6 at 1 and 5 minutes, weight 1.7 kg, length 42 cm, and head circumference 30 cm. After intubation—when meconium is seen in airway—and administration of oxygen at FIO_2 0.71, temperature is 37°C, heart rate 120, respiratory rate 30, and blood pressure 88/48 mm Hg. Eyes are close together. Occiput is prominent and has much dark hair. Heart sounds and systolic murmur are in right side of chest. Two vessels are in umbilical cord. Left thumb and first toes are short. Fingers are ulnar deviated. The rest of the physical findings are normal.

Hematocrit is 0.52. White cell count is 10.4×10^9/liter with 0.53 polymorphonuclear cells, 0.02 bands, 0.44 lymphocytes, and 0.01 monocytes. Platelet count is 200×10^9/liter.

Capillary blood glucose is 5.0 mmol/liter. Chromosomes are 47,XX,+18.

Prenatal ultrasound examination in Figure 44-1 shows cyst in posterior cranial fossa of fetus. Roentgenogram of chest and abdomen at 2½ hours (Figure 44-2) shows heart in right side of chest, elevation of left side of diaphragm, umbilical vascular catheter in midline, endotracheal tube, and gas and liquid in gut. CT scan of head in Figure 44-3 shows fusion of occipital horns of lateral ventricles, large cisterna magna, and hypoplasia of cerebellum.

Echocardiogram shows double-outlet right ventricle, ventricular septal defect with overriding aorta, and atrial septal defect.

Diagnosis: Trisomy 18 with cerebellar hypoplasia and other defects.

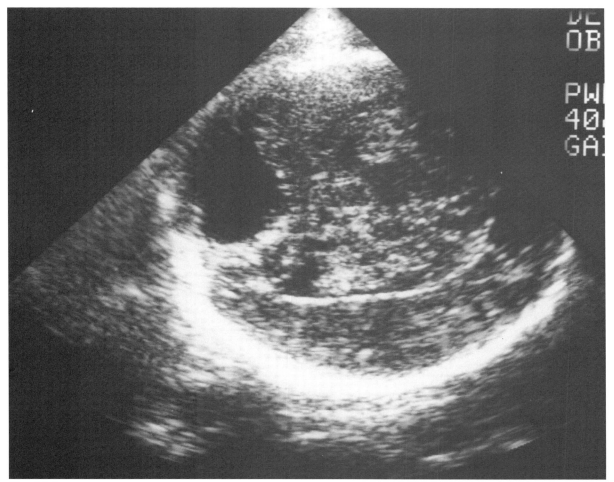

Fig. 44-1

(Continued)

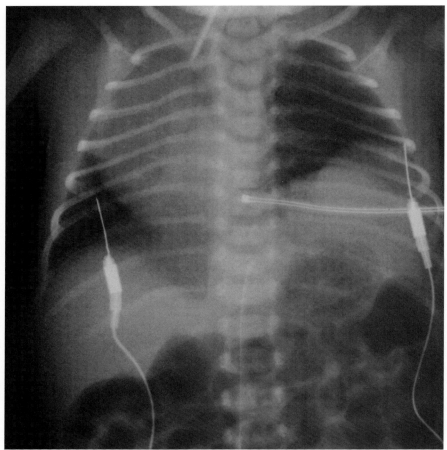

Fig. 44-2

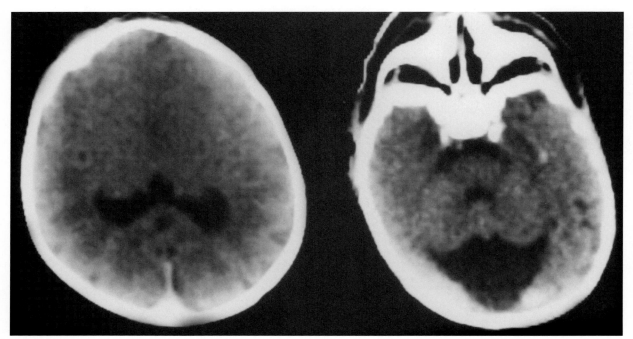

Fig. 44-3

Case 45

A 1-year-old boy is fussy, vomiting, and crying unless held. He had meningitis caused by *Escherichia coli* at 4 months.

Weight at 1 year is 8.4 kg, head circumference 47 cm, temperature 37.2°C, heart rate 114, respiratory rate 22, and blood pressure 120/75 mm Hg. Anterior fontanel bulges. A swelling with central dimple is on back of head. Babinski's sign is present. The rest of the physical findings are normal.

Hematocrit is 0.36. White cell count is 11.9×10^9/liter with 0.45 polymorphonuclear cells, 0.05 bands, 0.37 lymphocytes, 0.07 monocytes, and 0.06 atypical lymphocytes. Platelet count is 579×10^9/liter, ESR 76 mm/hour. CSF has 1×10^6/liter white cells, 112×10^6/liter red cells, 3.8 mmol/liter glucose, and 0.18 g/liter protein. Gram's stain of CSF is negative, culture sterile.

Occipital bone is thin and bulges at external occipital protuberance (Figure 45-1). MRI in Figure 45-2 shows mass in cerebellum and mass above and behind cerebellum.

At operation through an incision to right of midline dimple on back of head, a cyst that contains hair and pus is below and medial to right transverse sinus and continues through tentorial notch into a cerebellar abscess. Roof of fourth ventricle is part of wall of abscess.

Wall of cyst is tan to red-brown. Cyst contains hair and keratinous debris. Culture of cyst grows *E. coli*; culture of abscess grows *E. coli*, *Citrobacter freundii*, and *Enterobacter agglomerans*.

Diagnosis: Occipital dermoid cyst and cerebellar abscess.

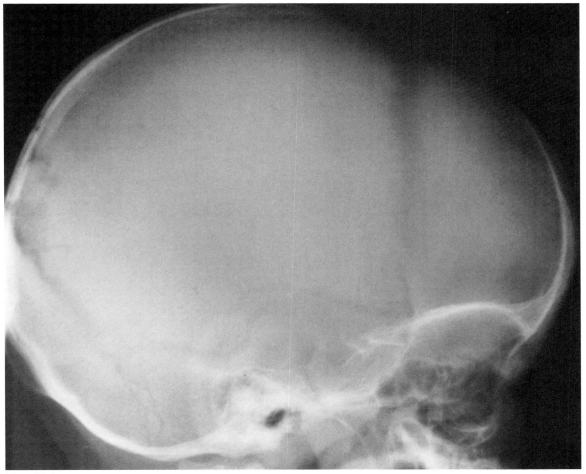

Fig. 45-1

(Continued)

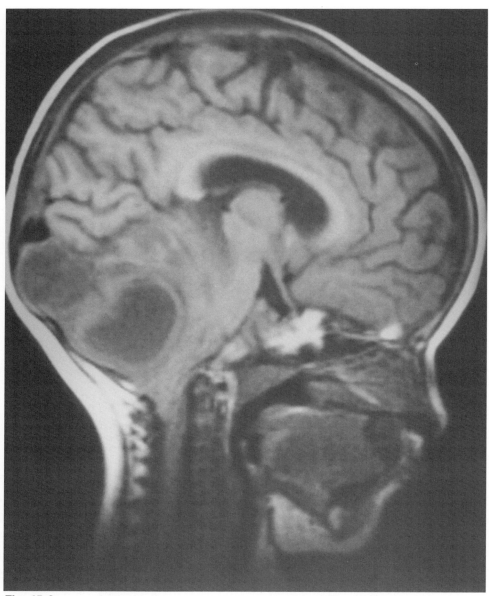

Fig. 45-2

Case 46

A 4-year-old girl has a lump on right side of head that was noticed at 3 years. It gets larger when she cries and smaller when she stands.

Slight thickening of scalp over right parietal bone when she stands becomes a soft mass (3 × 1 cm) when she lies down. No bruit can be heard. The rest of the physical findings are normal.

In Figure 46-1, a parasagittal defect is in right parietal bone. CT scan after IV injection of contrast medium in Figure 46-2 shows superior sagittal sinus and an enhancing focus on right side of sinus. CT scan also shows thinning of right parietal bone (not shown).

Diagnosis: Sinus pericranii.

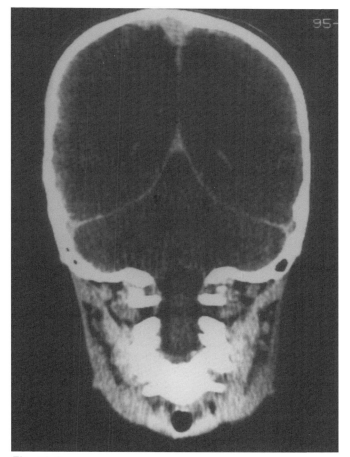

Fig. 46-2

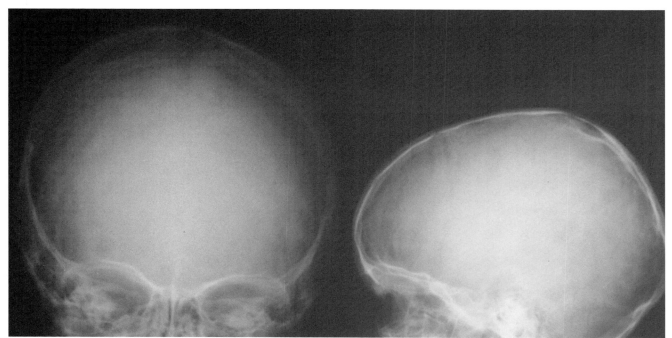

Fig. 46-1

Case 47

A newborn girl has a cyst on back of head and neck.

Pregnancy of mother (22 years old) was normal. Birth weight is 2.5 kg, Apgar score 8/10 at 1 and 5 minutes, length 50 cm, head circumference 31 cm, temperature 37.6°C, and systolic blood pressure 60 mm Hg. A cyst (8 × 5 cm) that is covered by skin and transilluminates is on back of head and neck. A systolic murmur is present. Moro's reflex is weak. The rest of the physical findings are normal.

Hematocrit is 0.52, white cell count 28×10^9/liter. Urine specific gravity is 1.006, pH 5. Urine has squamous epithelial cells. Chromosomes are 46,XX.

Figure 47-1 shows lacunar rarefactions in skull. A defect is in occipital bone and cervical and upper thoracic neural arches. A mass of water density is behind head and neck. Neck is short and retroflexed.

At operation, dura, arachnoid, and vascular connective tissue are under skin, and nerve tissue is at bony defect.

Cardiac catheterization at 4 months shows ventricular septal defect, ductus arteriosus, left superior vena cava to coronary sinus, and pulmonary hypertension.

Diagnosis: Iniencephaly.

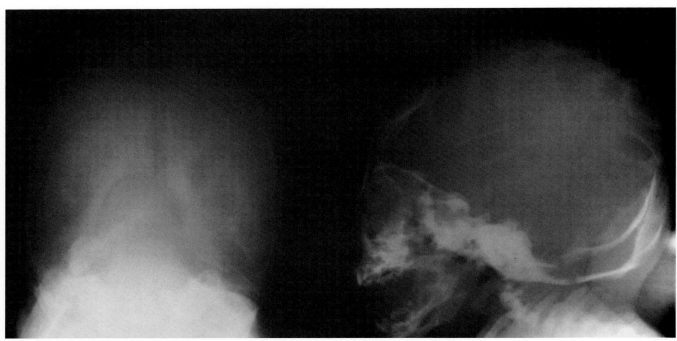

Fig. 47-1

Case 48

An 8-year-old girl has swollen, bruised arms and legs after being hit by her father, a gambler. The mortgage on the family home is about to be foreclosed, the car repossessed.

Weight is 38.7 kg, height 141 cm, temperature 37.6°C, heart rate 96, respiratory rate 26, and blood pressure 120/80 mm Hg. The rest of the physical findings are normal.

Hematocrit is 0.38. White cell count is 7.2×10^9/liter with 0.46 polymorphonuclear cells, 0.01 bands, 0.50 lymphocytes, 0.01 monocytes, 0.01 eosinophils, and 0.01 basophils. Platelet count is 317×10^9/liter. Urine specific gravity is 1.005, pH 7. Urine has occasional epithelial cells and 0–1 white cell/HPF. Serum sodium is 141 mmol/liter, potassium 4.2, chloride 107,

carbon dioxide 20, urea nitrogen 5.0, calcium 2.52, phosphorus 1.58, cholesterol 4.01, and glucose 4.9. Creatinine is 60 µmol/liter, uric acid 280, total bilirubin 19, and direct bilirubin 2. Total protein is 71 g/liter, albumin 42. Alkaline phosphatase is 360 U/liter, LDH 355, and SGOT 29.

Radio-opaque strips are almost parallel on parietal bone in Figure 48-1A. In Figure 48-1B, examination with bright light, or here, LogEtronic (LogEtronic, Inc., Springfield, VA) negative, shows that they are caused by hair braids. Roentgenographic findings in the rest of the skeleton are normal.

Diagnosis: Hair braids.

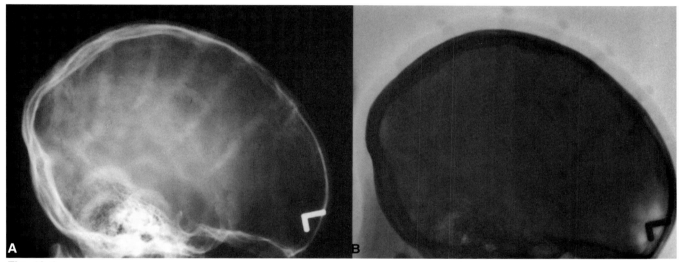

Fig. 48-1

Case 49

A newborn girl has a swollen scalp.

Pregnancy of mother (31 years old) was normal, presentation vertex with vacuum extraction. Birth weight is 3.7 kg, length 53 cm, head circumference 35 cm, and Apgar score 8/9 at 1 and 5 minutes. Scalp is bruised and swollen. Skull clicks with palpation. Feet are clubbed but flexible. The rest of the physical findings are normal.

Scalp is swollen. Swelling crosses sutures and perhaps a fracture (Figure 49-1).

Diagnosis: Caput succedaneum.

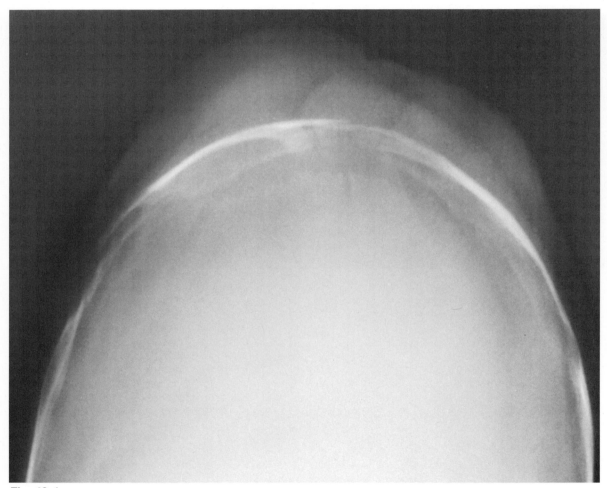

Fig. 49-1

Case 50

A 22-day-old boy has a soft swelling (8 × 5 cm) on back of head.

Mother thinks fetal movements were few and weak during the last 2 months of pregnancy. Onset of labor was spontaneous, presentation breech, delivery by cesarean section, birth weight 2.7 kg, head circumference 37 cm, and Apgar score 1/1 at 1 and 5 minutes. Right humerus and left femur were fractured. Muscle tone was poor.

Weight at 22 days is 3.1 kg. He moves hands and withdraws from pain. Abdomen is flaccid. Testes are not palpable. The rest of the physical findings are normal.

Chromosomes are 46,XY.

Occipital mass bounded by lambdoid and mendosal sutures (fissures between supraoccipital and interparietal parts of squamous part of occipital bone) has a thin shell of bone in lower edge at 22 days (Figure 50-1A). Mass is smaller and has gradually more bone in rim and inside at (2 months, 4 months, and) 9 months (Figure 50-1B).

Diagnosis: Ossifying cephalohematoma.

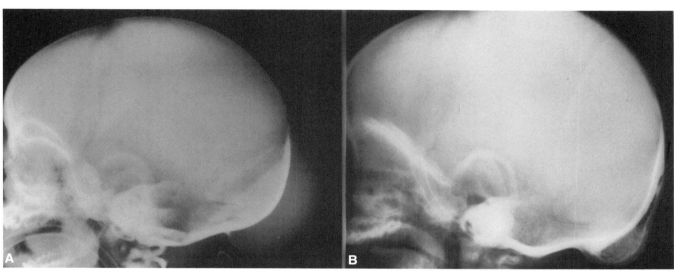

Fig. 50-1

Case 51

A 9-month-old boy has swelling on right side of head that appeared last night right after he fell and hit his head while pulling himself up. The swelling has not gotten larger. He is eating and playing normally.

A fluctuant, nontender swelling (10-cm diameter) with a hard rim is on right side of head. The rest of the physical findings are normal.

In Figure 51-1, deep swelling over right parietal bone stops at sagittal, coronal, and lambdoid sutures. Figure 51-2 shows a linear fracture in right parietal bone, one end of it about halfway down lambdoid suture.

Swelling is about the same 1 week later and a small hard lump with palpable cleft is seen 2 weeks later.

Diagnosis: Right parietal fracture, subpericranial hematoma.

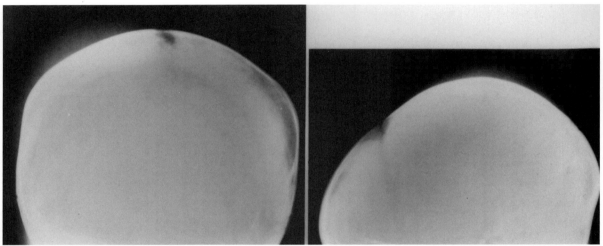

Fig. 51-1

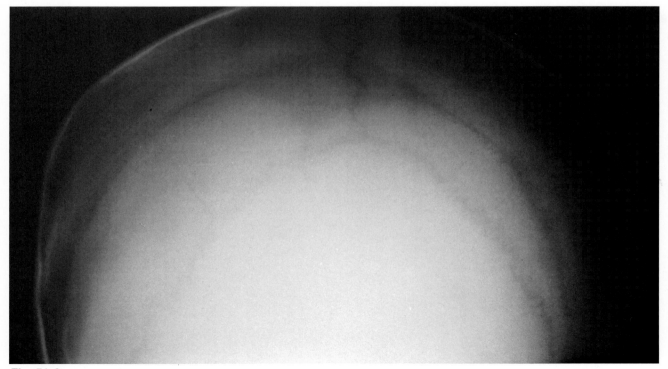

Fig. 51-2

Case 52

An 8-year-old boy, who was hit in the head by an ice ball 6 days ago and saw "stars and black circles" for a while, has a depressed scab on right side of forehead and black right upper eyelid.

Temperature is 37.6°C, heart rate 68, respiratory rate 20, blood pressure 90/56 mm Hg, height 126 cm, and weight 24.5 kg. The depression is tender. A systolic murmur is present. The rest of the physical findings are normal.

Hematocrit is 0.36. White cell count is 7.7×10^9/liter with 0.51 polymorphonuclear cells, 0.02 bands, 0.40 lymphocytes, 0.05 monocytes, 0.01 eosinophils, and 0.01 basophils. Platelet count is 386×10^9/liter. Urine specific gravity is 1.015, pH 7. Urine is normal.

Figure 52-1 shows a stellate fracture with a fragment on end in right side of frontal bone in frontal view and a bone in anterior fontanel in lateral view.

At operation, depressed fragments of a comminuted fracture are elevated. Dura and bridging veins are intact.

Diagnosis: Comminuted, depressed skull fracture; anterior fontanel bone.

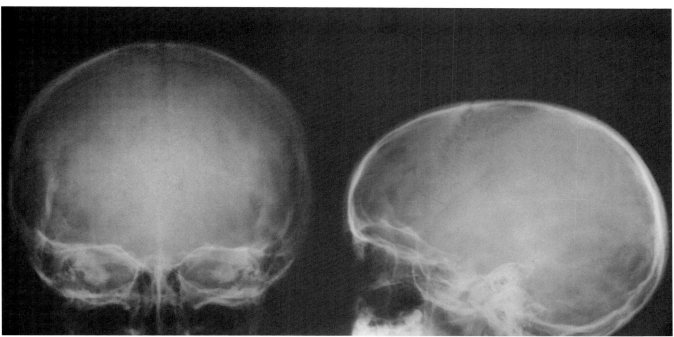

Fig. 52-1

Case 53

A 12-year-old-boy, who was operated on at 8 years for coarctation of the aorta, has thick bones in follow-up examination of the chest.

Pregnancy of mother was normal, birth weight 2.4 kg. He was jaundiced and hypoglycemic for a short time. He sat at 7 months, walked at 17 months, and spoke in sentences at 2½ years. Head was large at 9 months. Ventriculoperitoneal shunt was put in at 11 months. Head circumference was 50 cm at 14 months. Neurologic findings were normal. He had inguinal herniorrhaphies at 18 months, otitis media several times, and systolic murmur at 3 years. Cardiac catheterization at 8 years showed bicuspid aortic valve and coarctation of the aorta. Serum calcium was 2.54 mmol/liter, 2.24, and 2.54; phosphorus 1.84, 1.74, and 1.61. Alkaline phosphatase was 407 U/liter, 227, and 250.

Parents, three brothers, and one sister are well. Father can tell which members of the family have thick bones by their broad foreheads.

Bones of boy's skull are thick at 4 years (Figure 53-1). A shunt catheter goes out through right occipital bur hole. Ribs and clavicles are thick at 12 years; right margin of heart bulges (Figure 53-2). Bones of skull and the mandible of brother (9 years old) are thick (Figure 53-3), and bones of pelvis and shanks sclerotic (Figure 53-4). Mandible and bones of skull of father (36 years old) are thick (Figure 53-5).

Diagnosis: Familial osteosclerosis (hyperostosis corticalis generalisata, benign).

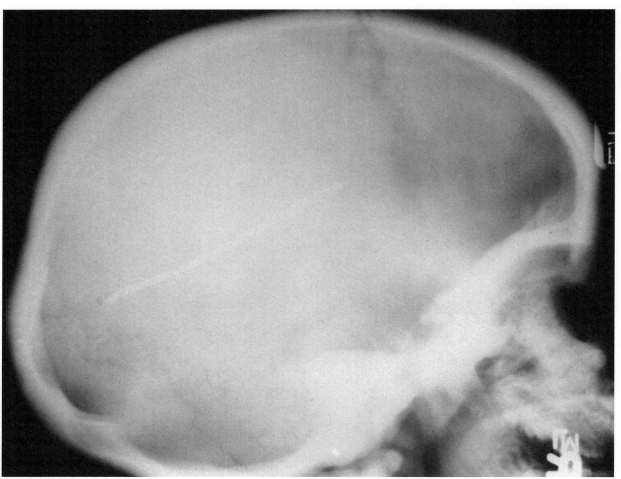

Fig. 53-1

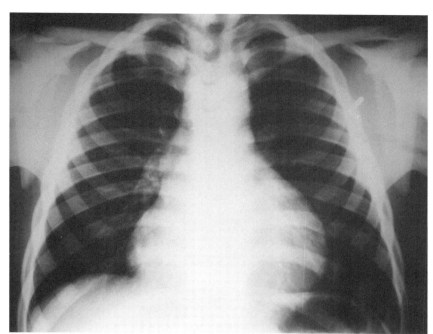

Fig. 53-2

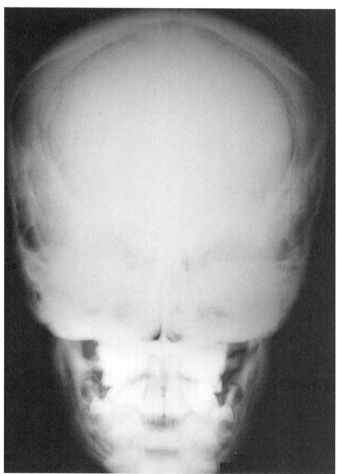

Fig. 53-3

(Continued)

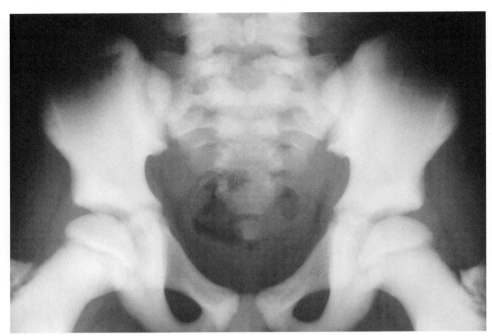

Fig. 53-4

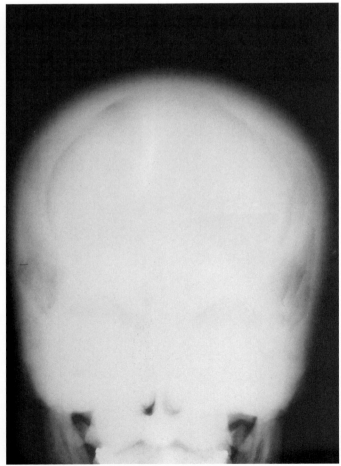

Fig. 53-5

Case 54

A 6-month-old girl has weepy eyes, stuffy nose, and a large head.

She was delivered by cesarean section for placenta previa. Birth weight was 2.7 kg, length 50 cm, head circumference 33 cm, and Apgar score 3/9 at 1 and 5 minutes. She had right facial palsy. Nose was stuffy. Nostrils flared during inspiration. She turned blue when she cried. She slept with right eye open. Eardrums were red at 3 months, red and bulging at 4 months.

Mother (21 years old) and father (34 years old) are well.

Head circumference at 6 months is 44 cm. Nasal bridge is flat and broad. Eyes are widely separated. She follows and reaches for objects. Eardrums are red. The rest of the physical findings are normal.

Hematocrit is 0.39. White cell count is 17.1×10^9/liter with 0.29 polymorphonuclear cells, 0.66 lymphocytes, 0.01 mono-cytes, 0.01 eosinophils, 0.01 basophils, and 0.02 atypical lymphocytes.

Obstruction of nasolacrimal ducts by large inferior nasal conchae is relieved by operation at 7 months. She is deaf at 5 years and has large chin at 10 years.

Figure 54-1 shows thick, sclerotic bones at base of skull, maxilla, and mandible at 6 months. Orbits are widely separated. Diaphyses of long bones are sclerotic, metaphyses undertubulated; some of tubular bones of hands and feet are sclerotic (Figures 54-2 through 54-4). Ribs and clavicles are thick at examination done 1 day after plastic operation on forehead at 10 years (Figure 54-5).

Diagnosis: Craniometaphyseal dysplasia.

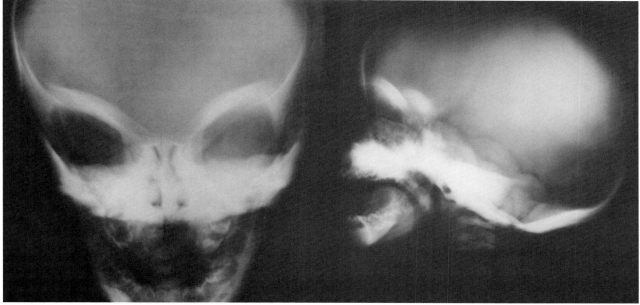

Fig. 54-1

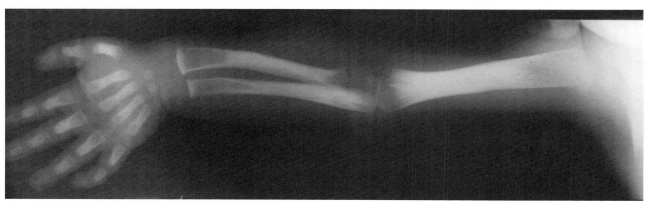

Fig. 54-2

(Continued)

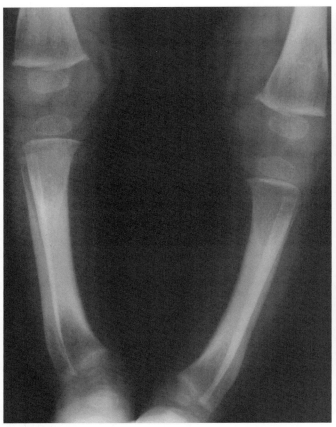

Fig. 54-3

Fig. 54-4

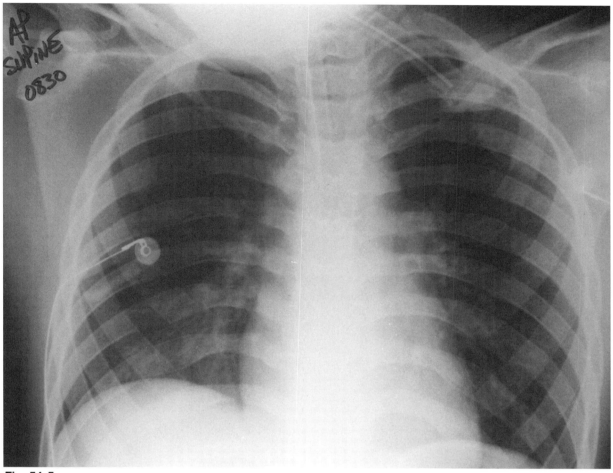

Fig. 54-5

Case 55

A 5½-year-old boy has swelling on left side of head.

He punctured his scalp 6 weeks ago when he hit his head on a nail on a chicken coop. He was given an antibiotic when fever appeared a week later. He was soon well. Swelling appeared 5 days ago.

He had measles at 7 months.

Mother, brother (4 years old), and 2 older half brothers are well. Some members of mother's family have cancer and diabetes mellitus.

Temperature is 36.6°C, heart rate 86, respiratory rate 20, blood pressure 120/72 mm Hg, weight 17 kg, and height 108 cm. Scalp over left side of head is swollen and tender. A systolic murmur is present. The rest of the physical findings are normal.

Hematocrit is 0.36. White cell count is 8.2×10^9/liter with 0.41 polymorphonuclear cells, 0.05 bands, 0.50 lymphocytes, 0.03 monocytes, and 0.01 basophils. Platelet count is 490×10^9/liter. Urine specific gravity is 1.019, pH 5. Urine has occasional red and white cells/HPF. Serum sodium is 139 mmol/liter, potassium 4.6, chloride 104, carbon dioxide 23, urea nitrogen 4.6, calcium 2.50, phosphorus 1.52, and glucose 7.0. Creatinine is 50 µmol/liter, uric acid 240, total bilirubin 5, and direct bilirubin 0. Total protein is 76 g/liter, and albumin 43.

Scalp over left parietal bone is swollen. In Figure 55-1, left parietal bone is mottled from suture to suture.

At operation, pericranium of left parietal bone is lifted and thick, outer table is vascular and motheaten. Pus is in wound. Bone discoloration extends to inner table. Granulation tissue is between inner table and dura. Culture of pus grows group A β-hemolytic streptococci.

Microscopic examination of pink to light tan bits of resected tissue show skin, adherent blood clot, granulation tissue, and acute and chronic inflammation.

Diagnosis: Osteomyelitis, left parietal bone. (He is found to have acute lymphoblastic leukemia at 7 years and dies at 8 years with chickenpox and group A β-hemolytic streptococcemia.)

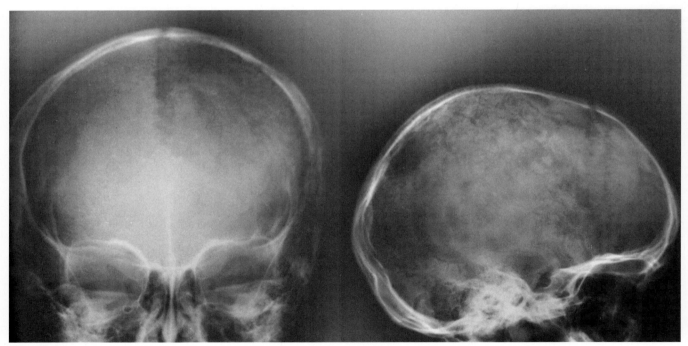

Fig. 55-1

Case 56

An 8-year-old has a lump on his head, discovered 3 years ago; it has gotten larger since he bumped his head a month ago.

Birth weight was 3.9 kg. Mother says that he has always been big and now is overweight, too, because he eats a lot of sugared breakfast cereal and drinks a lot of soda pop.

Weight at 8 years is 51 kg, height 145 cm, and blood pressure 104/60 mm Hg. Right side of forehead bulges. Right upper eyelid is thickened. Visual acuity is 20/20 in both eyes. Pubis is without hair. Volume of each testis is 2 cm³. The rest of the physical findings are normal.

Serum testosterone is <1.04 nmol/liter (normal: <0.10–0.35).

In Figure 56-1, right side of frontal bone and of sphenoid bone is thickened. Bone age in left hand is between 10 and 11 years, about 3 SDs above the mean.

Diagnosis: Fibrous dysplasia. (First signs of puberty, thinning of scrotum and increase in testicular volume to 3 cm³ appear at 9¾ years, early maturation ascribed to his size, not McCune-Albright syndrome.)

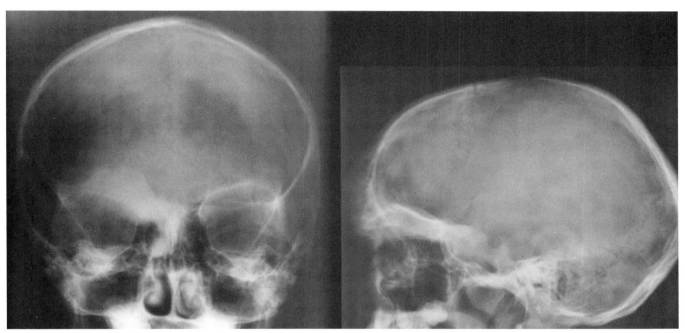

Fig. 56-1

Case 57

A 21-month-old boy has a large spleen.

He was anemic without enlarged spleen when examined at 18 months for anorexia and irritability.

Mother (40 years old) had goiter; father (68 years old) had gallstones. They are Greek. Sister (3 years old) is well.

Temperature at 21 months is 38°C, heart rate 100, respiratory rate 20, blood pressure 100/60 mm Hg, weight 13.6 kg, and height 86 cm. He is sallow and pale. A few small lymph nodes are in neck. Spleen edge is at iliac crest, liver edge 3 cm below costal margin. The rest of the physical findings are normal.

Hematocrit is 0.21. Hemoglobin is 62 g/liter. Red blood cell count is 3.2×10^{12}/liter, reticulocyte count 246×10^9/liter. White cell count is 31.0×10^9/liter with 0.20 polymorphonuclear cells, 0.09 bands, 0.26 lymphocytes, 0.07 monocytes, 0.02 eosinophils, 0.01 basophils, 0.04 metamyelocytes, 0.01 myelocytes, and 0.30 disintegrated cells. Blood smear shows anisocytosis, poikilocytosis, target cells, nucleated red cells, polychromatophilia, and few platelets. Marrow is hyperplastic.

Spleen, removed at 5 years because its bulk makes the boy uncomfortable, weighs 700 g and is $18 \times 12 \times 8$ cm. Lymph follicles are small and few. Cellularity is increased by hematopoiesis. Fibrous bands contain hemosiderin.

Diploë is thick at 9 years (Figure 57-1A), thicker at 17 years (Figure 57-1B). Mandible is swollen at 17 years; vascular grooves are prominent in inner table of parietal bone. Maxillary sinuses are opaque in both examinations (Figure 57-1). In Figure 57-2, a calcified stone is in gall bladder at 13 years, and cortex of ribs, most obvious in top corner, is thickened. Figure 57-3 shows proximal metaphysis of right and left humeri. Right humerus (Figure 57-3A) is hatchet shaped and partly fused at 17 years; left (Figure 57-3B) is normal. In Figure 57-4, bone age in the left hand is between 14 and 15 years at 17 years, and metacarpals and phalanges are expanded and have coarse trabecular pattern and cystic defects.

Diagnosis: β-thalassemia major.

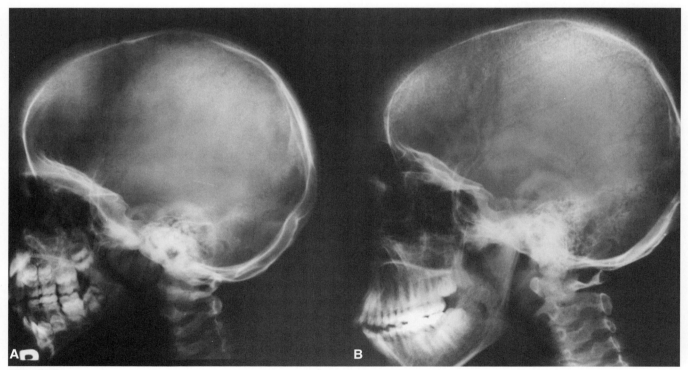

Fig. 57-1

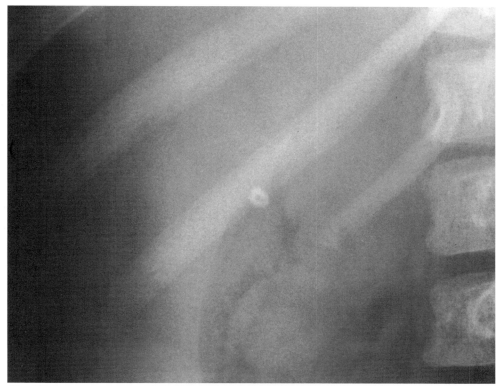

Fig. 57-2

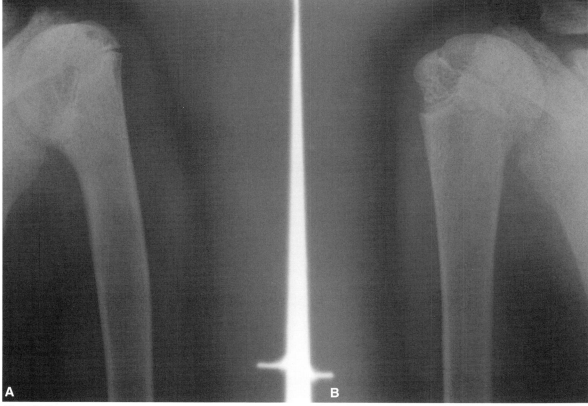

Fig. 57-3

(Continued)

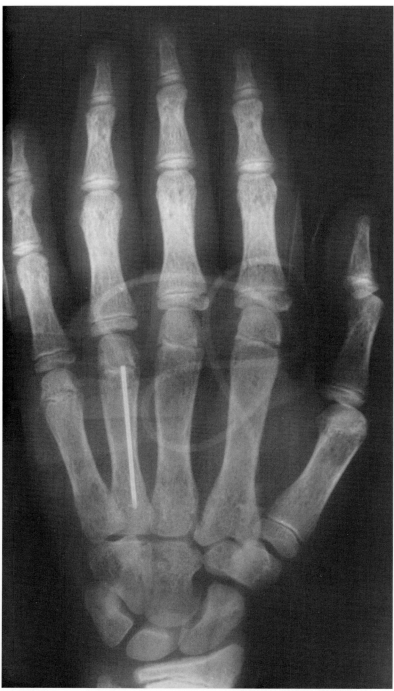

Fig. 57-4

Case 58

A 38-year-old man has convulsions several times a day for up to 30 seconds during which head turns left and body assumes fencer's position. He sometimes falls and is hurt, once breaking a leg. He has convulsions during sleep when legs extend and stiffen. He is sometimes incontinent during the convulsion and sleepy after it. He lives with parents, watches TV, and does small household chores.

Mother had diabetes mellitus during the pregnancy. Delivery was slowed by shoulder dystocia. Birth weight was 4.9 kg. He sat at 9 months, walked at 18 months. IQ was 60 at 8 years. He leaned to left when he stood and dragged the left foot when he walked. Left arm was limp, left forearm with partly clenched fist turned backward. Left arm and left leg were smaller and cooler than right. Clonus was at left ankle; Babinski's sign was in left foot. He began to have convulsions at 9 years.

Weight at 38 years is 94 kg, temperature 36°C, heart rate 80, respiratory rate 16, and blood pressure 100/74 mm Hg. He is alert and pleasant. He knows he is in a hospital but does not know day or year. He can count to 5 but makes mistakes beyond, and he cannot give his medical history. Lateral and up nystagmus, left limb atrophy, and left Babinski's sign are present. The rest of the physical findings are normal.

Hematocrit is 0.37. White cell count is 6.8×10^9/liter with 0.65 polymorphonuclear cells, 0.31 lymphocytes, 0.03 monocytes, and 0.01 eosinophils. Platelet count is 321×10^9/liter. Urine specific gravity is 1.007, pH 5. Urine is normal. Serum sodium is 140 mmol/liter, potassium 4.2, chloride 101, carbon dioxide 25, urea nitrogen 3.2, calcium 2.20, phosphorus 0.97, triglycerides 1.85, cholesterol 4.86, and glucose 5.1. Creatinine is 50 μmol/liter, total bilirubin 5, and direct bilirubin 2. Total protein is 72 g/liter, albumin 39. Alkaline phosphatase is 160 U/liter, LDH 40, SGOT 11, and SGPT 16.

EEG shows generalized frequent spikes and waves for 2–20 seconds intermixed with slow background activity.

Roentgenogram in Figure 58-1 at 15 years shows enlargement of right side of frontal sinus, elevation of petrous part of right temporal bone, thickened right parietal bone, and, in pneumoencephalogram, right displacement of dilated right lateral ventricle and air lateral to right ventricle. Lateral roentgenogram at 15 years shows small head. CT scan in Figure 58-2 at 32 years shows right displacement and dilation of right lateral ventricle and porencephalic cyst lateral to it.

Diagnosis: Dyke-Davidoff syndrome.

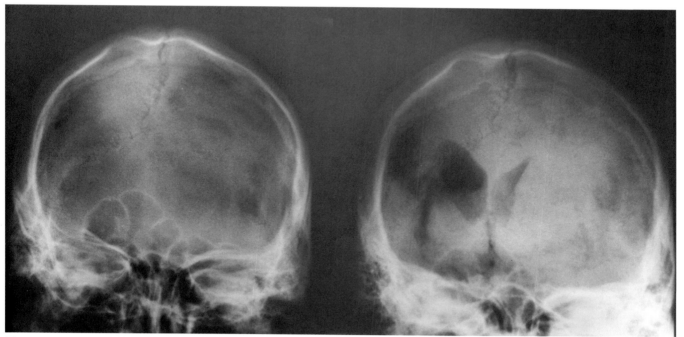

Fig. 58-1

(Continued)

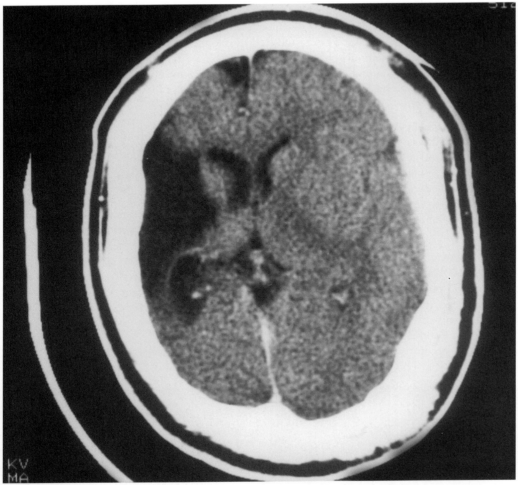

Fig. 58-2

Case 59

A 6-year-old boy has a swelling of the right side of the head that appeared after he fell from a bicycle 3 years ago and has gotten larger. He is usually "up and playing all day."

Temperature is 36°C, heart rate 92, respiratory rate 24, and blood pressure 90/50 mm Hg. A bony, nontender swelling is in right temporoparietal region. The rest of the physical findings are normal.

Right side of calvaria bulges, and its bone is thinned in Figure 59-1. CT scan in Figure 59-2 shows cyst between brain and right inner table, and lateral ventricles displaced to left.

Diagnosis: Arachnoid cyst, traumatic.

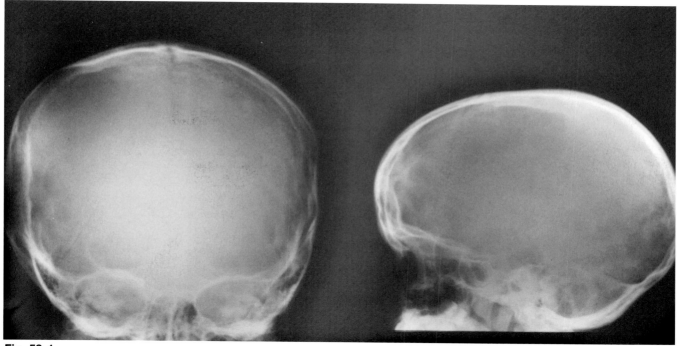

Fig. 59-1

(Continued)

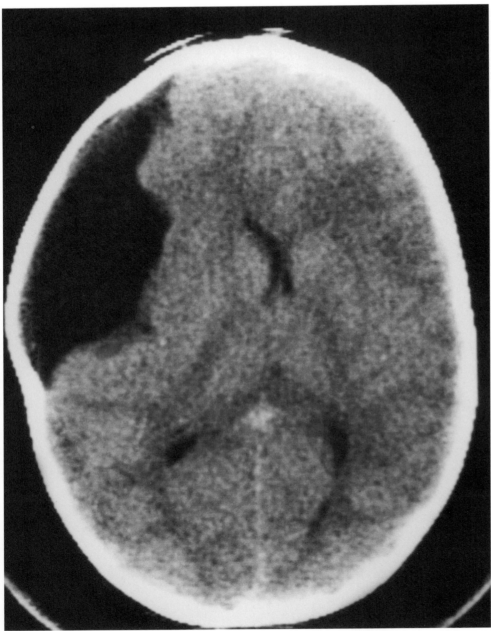

Fig. 59-2

Case 60

A 2-year-old girl has a lump above the right eye.

She has had scalp and body rash for 6 months, swelling and redness of right upper lid for 6 weeks, and a lump that is getting larger. She has been cranky for 2 weeks. She vomits occasionally.

Temperature is 37.8°C, heart rate 120, respiratory rate 28, blood pressure 96/40 mm Hg, weight 18.6 kg, and height 92 cm. A soft, nonfluctuant mass (5 × 5 cm) is above right eye. Right upper lid is swollen, right eyeball displaced downward and inward. A scaly rash is on scalp. A dry, red rash and scratches are on face, trunk, and extensor surfaces of arms and legs. The rest of the physical findings are normal.

Hematocrit is 0.38. White cell count is 18.2×10^9/liter with 0.54 polymorphonuclear cells, 0.01 bands, 0.43 lymphocytes,

0.01 monocytes, and 0.01 eosinophils. Platelet count is 570×10^9/liter. ESR is 47 mm/hr. Urine specific gravity is 1.029.

Roentgenogram in Figure 60-1 shows defect in squamous and orbital surfaces of right side of frontal bone and small defect in left side of skull. CT scan in Figure 60-2 shows soft tissue in bony defect above right orbit and extension into right orbit through frontal bone and its orbital surface.

Biopsy of granular yellow tissue in the lump shows (1) eosinophils, neutrophils, and small lymphocytes; (2) large cells with eosinophilic cytoplasm, large vesicular nuclei, and prominent nucleoli; (3) multinucleated giant cells; and (4) necrosis.

Diagnosis: Eosinophilic granuloma, probable atopic dermatitis.

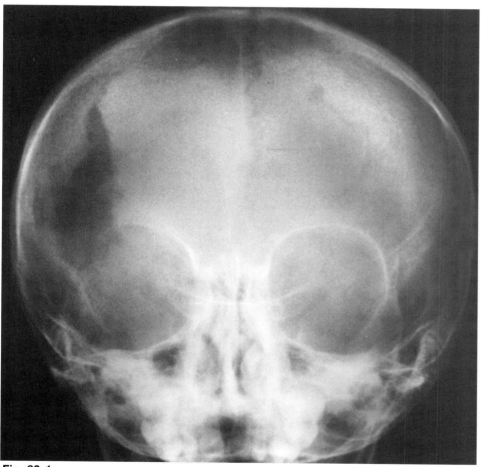

Fig. 60-1

(Continued)

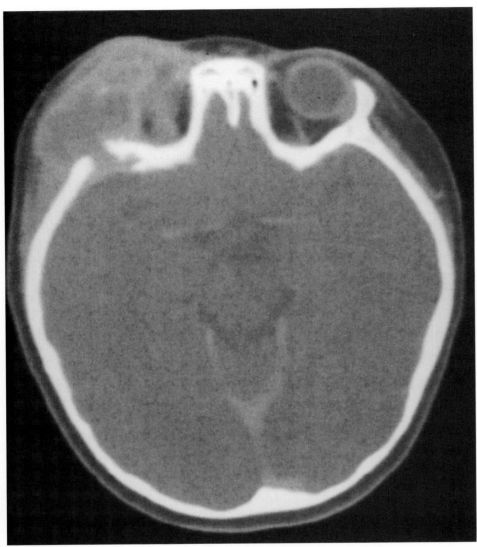

Fig. 60-2

Case 61

A 22-month-old boy drinks and urinates too much.

Pregnancy was normal, birth weight 3.9 kg. He was breast-fed for 13 months. He began to walk at 13 months. He had otitis media at 9 months and has had several colds. He has been drinking excessively and needing diaper changes almost every half hour for 3 months. He has lost 1 kg in the last 2 months.

At 21 months, hemoglobin was 120 g/liter. White cell count was 8.7×10^9/liter. Serum sodium was 143 mmol/liter, potassium 4.3, urea nitrogen 4.0, and glucose 5.0. Creatinine was 40 µmol/liter. Urine specific gravity was 1.003.

Temperature at 22 months is 36.5°C, heart rate 116, respiratory rate 24, and weight 9.8 kg. He is thin, small, and playful. A skin tag is on left cheek. The rest of the physical findings are normal.

Serum osmolality is 275 mmol/kg. He gets agitated during 4-hour water deprivation. Weight changes from 9.8 to 9.2 kg. He voids 600 ml urine, specific gravity 1.001. He does not urinate during 2¼ hours after he is given 10 U aqueous vasopressin (Pitressin) IM.

A defect in right parietal bone (Figure 61-1) is associated with increased signal in T2-weighted MRI (Figure 61-2A). MRI in sagittal section (Figure 61-2B) shows high signal of normal posterior pituitary gland in pituitary fossa.

Diagnosis: Langerhans' cell histiocytosis, diabetes insipidus.

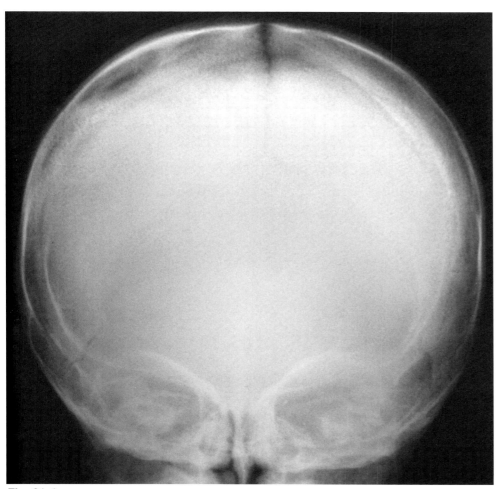

Fig. 61-1

(Continued)

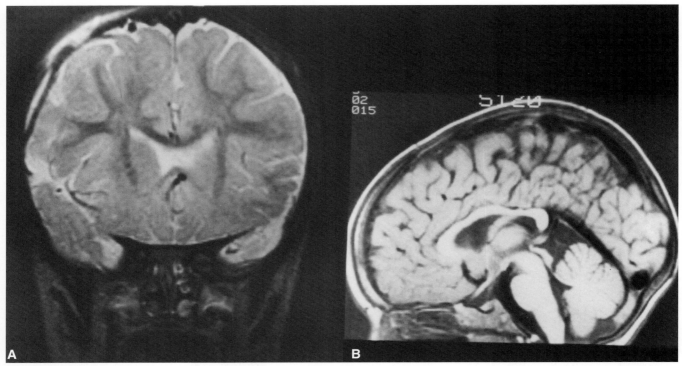

Fig. 61-2

Case 62

A 20-month-old girl has a swollen left cheek.

She had an ear infection several months ago. Blood came from left ear a month ago.

Mother (28 years old), father (29 years old), brother (8 years old), and sister (4 years old) are well.

Temperature at 20 months is 36.6°C, heart rate 114, respiratory rate 24, and systolic blood pressure 51 mm Hg. Left eye stays open. Smile is crooked. Left external acoustic meatus is blocked. The rest of the physical findings are normal.

Hematocrit is 0.32. White cell count is 6.8×10^9/liter with 0.15 polymorphonuclear cells, 0.80 lymphocytes, 0.03 monocytes, and 0.02 eosinophils.

Axial CT scan after IV injection of contrast medium (Figure 62-1A) shows a septate mass with curved margin in left tem-

poral region and an interface between two liquids, the lower, settled liquid more radio-opaque, in medial locule. Coronal MRI (Figure 62-1B) shows mixed signal in the mass.

At operation, soft temporal bone covers a mass of soft tissue that contains pieces of bone and protrudes into left external acoustic meatus.

Microscopic examination of red-brown and tan mass shows dilated and collapsed cysts, extravasated blood, spindle cells, osteoclast-like giant cells, fibroblastic stroma, metaplastic osteoid, loose fibromyxoid reparative tissue, plates of bone, and bits of woven and lamellar bone.

Diagnosis: Aneurysmal bone cyst.

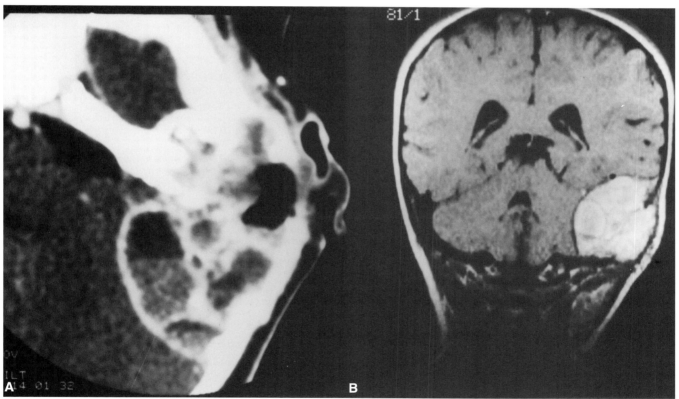

Fig. 62-1

Case 63

A 9-year-old-boy has left earache.

He fell off his bicycle 3 weeks ago because the ear started to hurt so much. Swelling around the left ear appeared 2 weeks ago and is larger. Hearing in left ear is impaired. He has had a cough and a runny nose for a few days.

Temperature is 37.4°C, heart rate 104, respiratory rate 20, and blood pressure 110/70 mm Hg. Soft, nontender swelling under normal skin displaces left auricle outward and downward. Left external acoustic meatus is narrow, red, and edematous, and contains gray-yellow liquid. Left eardrum cannot be seen. Tonsils are large. Warts are on hands. The rest of the physical findings are normal.

Hematocrit is 0.41. White cell count is 4.1×10^9/liter with 0.33 polymorphonuclear cells, 0.02 bands, 0.39 lymphocytes, 0.12 monocytes, 0.06 eosinophils, and 0.08 atypical lymphocytes. Platelet count is 316×10^9/liter. ESR is 5 mm/hr.

CT scan after IV injection of contrast medium (Figure 63-1A) shows an enhancing mass on both sides of left temporal bone and defect in bone. Coronal MRI (Figure 63-1B) shows a mass of varying signal intensity that displaces subcutaneous tissues out and temporal lobe in. Lateral and third ventricles are normal. Cavum septi pellucidi and cavum vergae are between the lateral ventricles.

Biopsy of the red-to-tan lobulated tissue from the tumor shows sheets and clusters of malignant cells with eosinophilic cytoplasm, large pleomorphic nuclei, prominent nucleoli, abnormal mitotic figures, and fibrovascular stroma.

Diagnosis: Rhabdomyosarcoma.

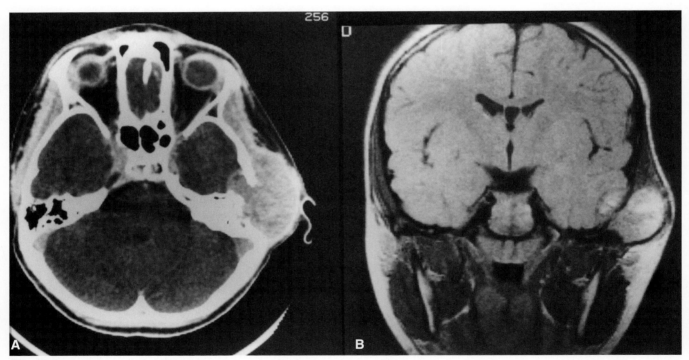

Fig. 63-1

Case 64

A 19-month-old boy will not walk.

He has been cranky and has had fever up to 38°C for several weeks. Upper eyelids have been bruised for 3 weeks. He sleeps with eyes open and sleeps more now.

He began to walk at 11 months. He says a few words.

Weight is 11.6 kg, height 79 cm, head circumference 49 cm, temperature 37°C, heart rate 142, respiratory rate 32, and systolic blood pressure 94 mm Hg. He is pale. Forehead bulges above outer edge of right eye. The rest of the physical findings are normal.

Hematocrit is 0.20. White cell count is 6.8×10^9/liter. Platelet count is 189×10^9/liter.

Sutures of skull are widened in Figure 64-1. CT scan in Figure 64-2 shows spicules of new bone along orbital part of right side of frontal bone and a mass of soft tissue in upper outer part of right orbit. Brain is normal. A mass with calcium in it is above left kidney in Figure 64-3A. A mass is in the spinal canal at a lower level in Figure 64-3B.

Urine homovanillic acid is 115 µmol/day (normal: <45).

Diagnosis: Neuroblastoma.

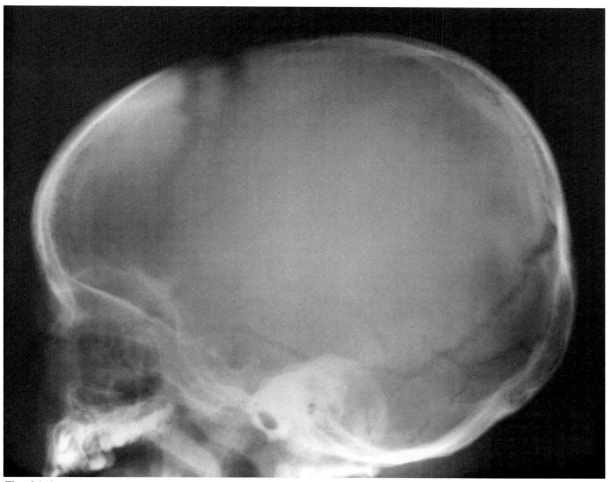

Fig. 64-1

(Continued)

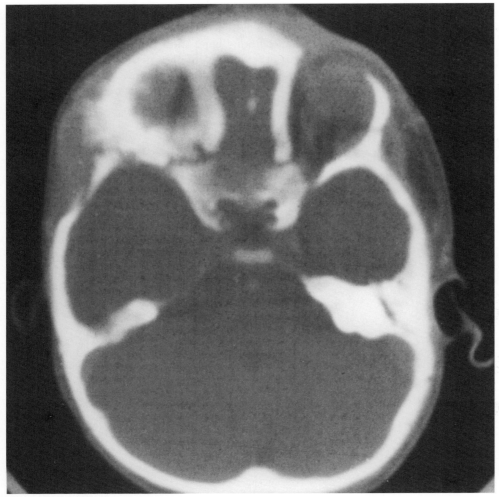

Fig. 64-2

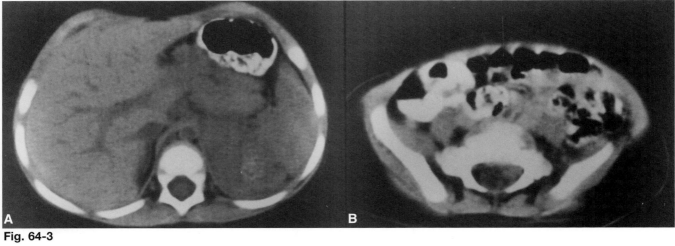

Fig. 64-3

Case 65

A 9-year-old girl has a "squishy" lump on head and shoulder pain.

Right shoulder hurt for a few weeks after she went waterskiing 4 months ago. It began to hurt again a month ago while she was playing soccer. Sometimes left shoulder hurts. Lump on head came up 2 weeks ago. She broke an arm when she fell off a horse at 5 years.

Temperature at 9 years is 37.9°C, heart rate 86, respiratory rate 22, blood pressure 100/68 mm Hg, weight 28.6 kg, and height 139 cm. A soft mass (3×3 cm) is on scalp just behind hairline. Spleen edge is 4 cm below costal margin. The rest of the physical findings are normal.

Hemoglobin is 135 g/liter. Hematocrit is 0.40. White cell count is 14.0×10^9/liter with 0.31 polymorphonuclear cells, 0.10 bands, 0.45 lymphocytes, 0.02 monocytes, 0.03 eosinophils, and 0.09 blasts. Platelet count is 169×10^9/liter. Serum LDH is 711 U/liter, alkaline phosphatase 190. Calcium is 2.84 mmol/liter, phosphorus 1.61.

Figure 65-1 shows irregular mineralization of right humerus and thickened cortex; relation of head to shaft suggests fracture. Defects are in calvaria in Figure 65-2.

Bone marrow has medium-sized blasts with sparse, basophilic, occasionally granular or vacuolated cytoplasm, and finely dispersed chromatin in large, deeply basophilic nuclei. The cells stain with antibody to TdT, CALLA, and B4.

Diagnosis: B-cell lymphoblastic leukemia.

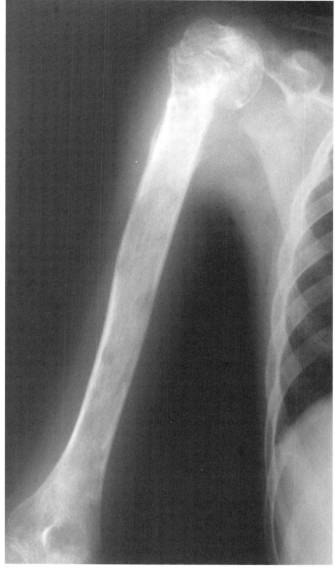

Fig. 65-1

(Continued)

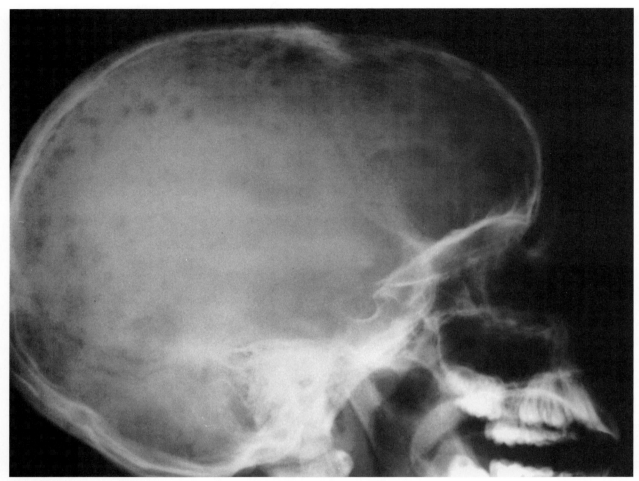

Fig. 65-2

Case 66

A 13-month-old girl has a large soft spot on back of head. She walks and uses about 20 words.

Head circumference is 45 cm. A soft spot (5 cm wide) behind vertex is flat, nontender, pulsating, and covered by normal scalp. The rest of the physical findings are normal.

Figure 66-1 shows a defect in parietal bones. Interparietal (inca) bones and intralambdoid sutural (wormian) bones are present. Smaller defects in similar location are in parietal bones of mother (Figure 66-2) and maternal grandmother (Figure 66-3).

Diagnosis: Parietal foramens (Catlin mark).

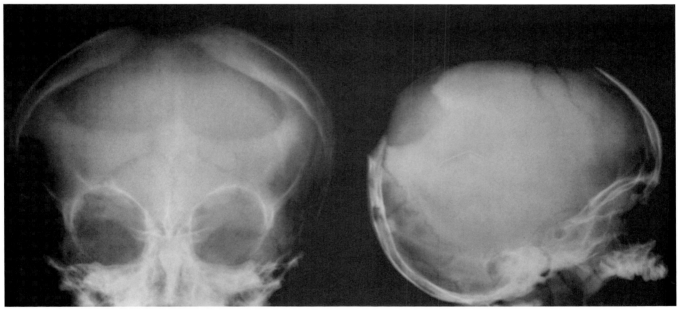

Fig. 66-1

(Continued)

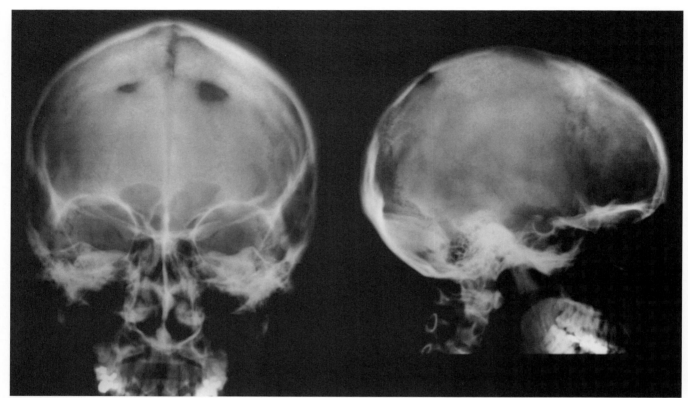

Fig. 66-2

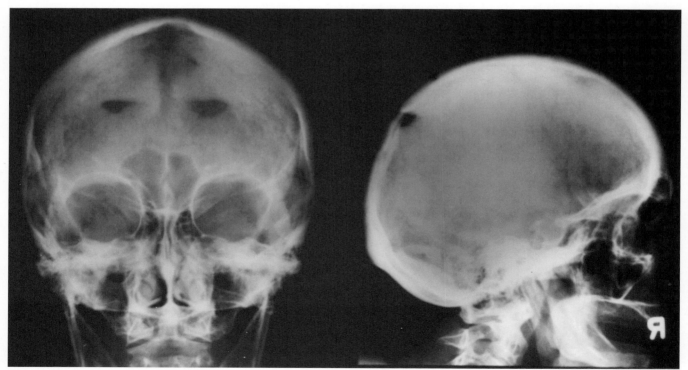

Fig. 66-3

Case 67

An 8-year-old girl is bruised by her father's beating. A scab is in front of the left ear. The rest of the physical findings are normal.

A sclerotic focus is in each parietal bone near sagittal suture in frontal view (Figure 67-1A) and several centimeters behind vertex in lateral view (Figure 67-1B).

Diagnosis: Normal skull, sclerosis at site of parietal foramens.

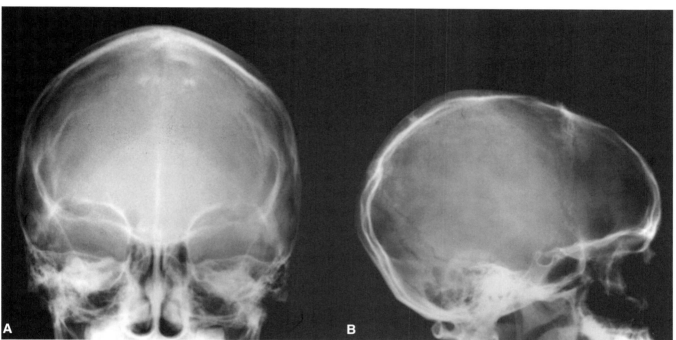

Fig. 67-1

Case 68

A newborn boy has a scab on the top of his head.

Mother (27 years old), father (24 years old), and sister (5 years old) are well.

Pregnancy of mother was normal. Birth weight is 4.1 kg, length 54 cm, head circumference 35 cm, temperature 36.8°C, heart rate 130, and respiratory rate 38. He is meconium stained, depressed at first, active at 10 minutes. A band of granulation tissue, 5 cm wide, is over sagittal suture and lambda. Sagittal suture is 1.5 cm wide. Fingers and toes are short with loose skin at the ends and small nails. Systolic murmur and third heart sound are present. The rest of the physical findings are normal.

Hematocrit is 0.58. White cell count is 34.3×10^9/liter with 0.63 polymorphonuclear cells, 0.21 bands, 0.12 lymphocytes, 0.03 monocytes, and 0.01 metamyelocytes. Platelet count is 225×10^9/liter. Serum sodium is 139 mmol/liter, potassium 7.3, chloride 106, and calcium 2.19. Total bilirubin is 60 μmol/liter, direct bilirubin 34.

Figure 68-1 shows irregular defects (larger near vertex) in parietal bones along sagittal suture. CT scan in Figure 68-2 shows width of skull defect. In Figure 68-3, distal phalanges of fingers are small or unossified, proximal phalanx of first toes is small, and middle and distal phalanges of all toes have small or no ossification centers.

Diagnosis: Adams-Oliver syndrome.

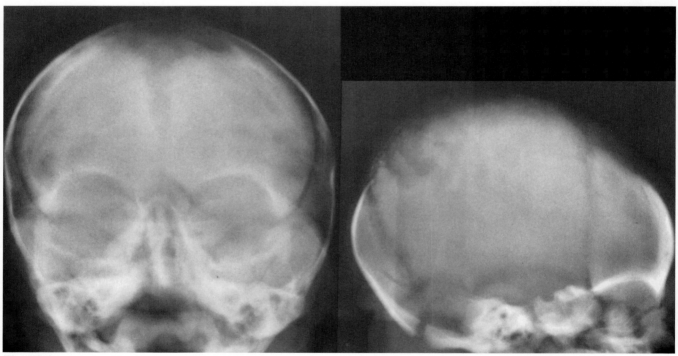

Fig. 68-1

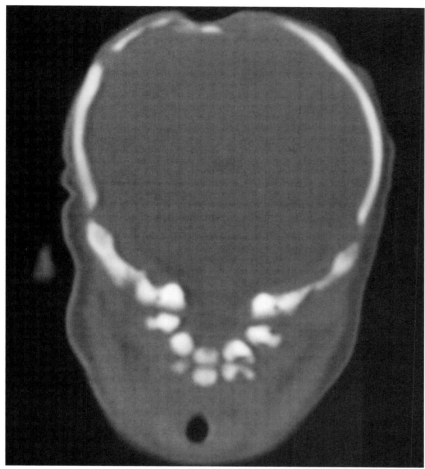

Fig. 68-2

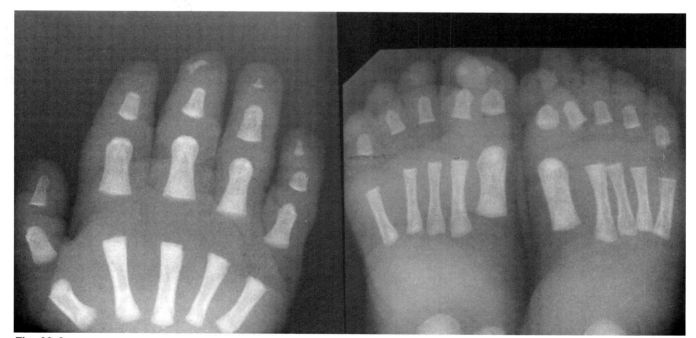

Fig. 68-3

Case 69

A 14-month-old boy is drowsy. He cried and seemed all right after being hit by a slow vehicle 3 hours ago.

Heart rate is 112, respiratory rate 20, and systolic blood pressure 104 mm Hg. He can be roused. Abrasions are on left side of head and face. Left eyelids are swollen and blue. Left pupil is larger than right and less reactive to light. Limbs withdraw from pinprick. The rest of the physical findings are normal. 45 minutes later, he opens his eyes, looks around, and cries.

Hematocrit is 0.34. White cell count is 27.4 × 10⁹/liter with 0.69 polymorphonuclear cells, 0.02 bands, 0.14 lymphocytes, 0.05 monocytes, and 0.10 basophils. Platelet count is 558 × 10^9/liter. Serum sodium is 137 mmol/liter, potassium 5.4, chloride 106, and glucose 11.0. Urine specific gravity is 1.029, pH 6. Urine has 0.05 g/liter ketones and 1–2 white cells/HPF.

CT scan shows a depressed fracture in left side of occipital bone and in left greater wing of sphenoid bone (Figure 69-1A). A wedge of high attenuation is in posterior fossa (Figure 69-1B).

Diagnosis: Skull fractures, subdural blood under tentorium cerebelli.

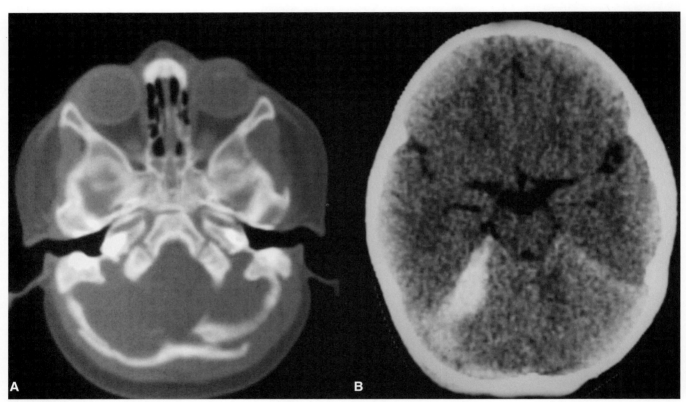

Fig. 69-1

Case 70

An 11-month-old girl, who has been walking for 3 weeks and who just fell 12 feet from a balcony, is comatose and breathing slowly.

Heart rate is 156, systolic blood pressure 100 mm Hg, then 130 mm Hg, then 85 mm Hg. Eyes are turned left. Anterior fontanel is tense. Left side of head is swollen. The rest of the physical findings are normal.

Hematocrit is 0.28. White cell count is 32.8×10^9/liter with 0.24 polymorphonuclear cells, 0.14 bands, 0.56 lymphocytes, 0.04 monocytes, 0.01 eosinophils, and 0.01 basophils. Urine specific gravity is 1.035, pH 6. Urine has trace protein and trace ketones.

She does not move limbs spontaneously the next day but does withdraw from pinprick. She moves limbs spontaneously the second day. She is fussy a week later.

Scalp is swollen, left parietal bone fractured (Figure 70-1); skull defect is larger 6½ months later (Figure 70-2). CT scan 1 month after the fall (Figure 70-3A) shows low attenuation in left frontal lobe, left frontal subdural liquid, and left scalp swelling. CT scan 6½ months after the fall (Figure 70-3B) shows larger defect in brain and skull.

At operation, necrotic dura and bits of bone are found at defect.

Diagnosis: Diastatic skull fracture, leptomeningeal cyst.

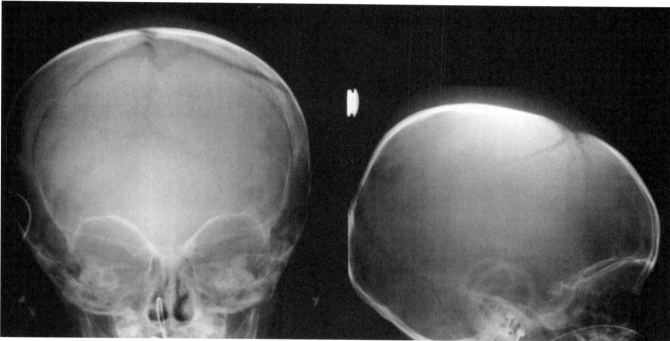

Fig. 70-1

(Continued)

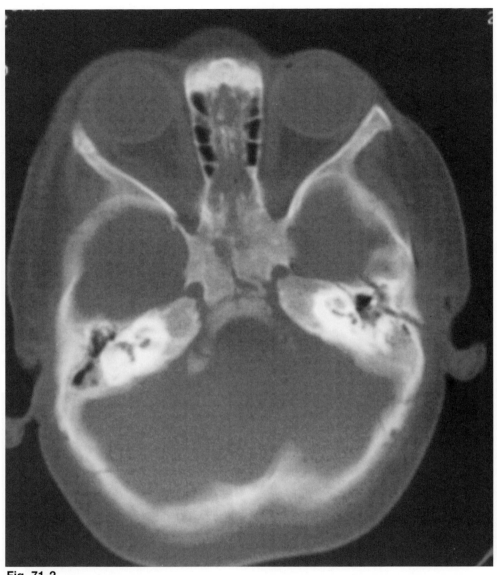

Fig. 71-2

Case 72

An 11-month-old boy has a big head.

He was knocked out when he fell and hit left side of his head a month ago but soon revived.

Weight at 11 months is 16 kg, length 85 cm, head circumference 57 cm, chest circumference 58 cm, temperature 36.6°C, heart rate 116, respiratory rate 24, and blood pressure 105/56 mm Hg. Babinski's sign is in left foot. The rest of the physical findings are normal.

Hematocrit is 0.31. White cell count is 9.6 × 10⁹/liter with 0.33 polymorphonuclear cells, 0.02 bands, 0.60 lymphocytes, 0.04 monocytes, and 0.01 eosinophils. Platelet count is 345 × 10⁹/liter. ESR is 10 mm/hr. Serum sodium is 142 mmol/liter, potassium 4.5, chloride 100, carbon dioxide 23, urea nitrogen 2.1, calcium 2.40, phosphorus 1.97, cholesterol 3.36, and glucose 5.6. Creatinine is 40 μmol/liter, uric acid 260, total bilirubin 3, and direct bilirubin 0. Total protein is 60 g/liter, albumin 41. Alkaline phosphatase is 3,773 U/liter, LDH 256, and SGOT 22.

CT scan in Figure 72-1 shows matter of different radiodensities between cerebral hemispheres and skull and a membrane that enhances after IV injection of contrast medium.

At operation, 200 ml xanthochromic liquid in layers with membranes between them is released through bur holes and cruciate dural incisions.

Head circumference at 5 years is 63 cm, weight 35 kg. Neurologic findings and social interactions are normal.

Diagnosis: Subdural hematomas of different ages.

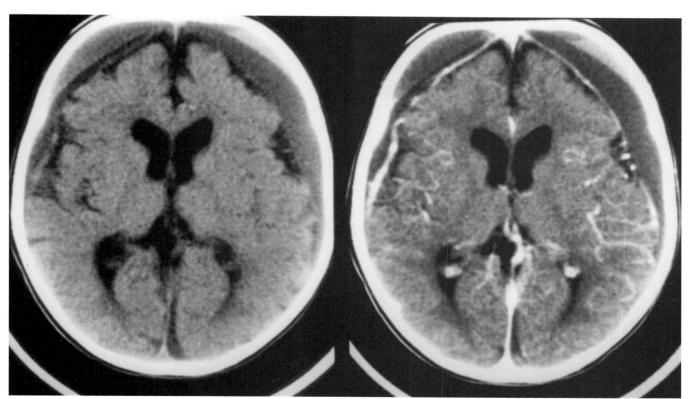

Fig. 72-1

Case 73

A 3-day-old boy has a convulsion. Fists clench and unclench for a few seconds, right arm twitches an hour later, and then hands and right foot twitch.

He was first of twins. Presentation was vertex, delivery assisted by vacuum extraction. Birth weight was 2.6 kg, Apgar score 1/6 at 1 and 10 minutes, temperature 37.2°C, heart rate 140, and respiratory rate 82. He was pale, limp, grunting, and retracting. A cephalohematoma was present. Hemoglobin was 143 g/liter, arterial blood pH 7.14, Pco_2 24 mm Hg, and Po_2 211 mm Hg. At 1 day, he had apneic spells until stimu-

lated. Heart rate was 90–146. He lay with head extended, back arched, and legs flexed the next 2 days.

Cephalohematoma and Babinski's signs are present at 3 days. The rest of the physical findings are normal.

Figure 73-1 shows strips of increased attenuation along occipital sulci and gyri.

Diagnosis: Subarachnoid hemorrhage.

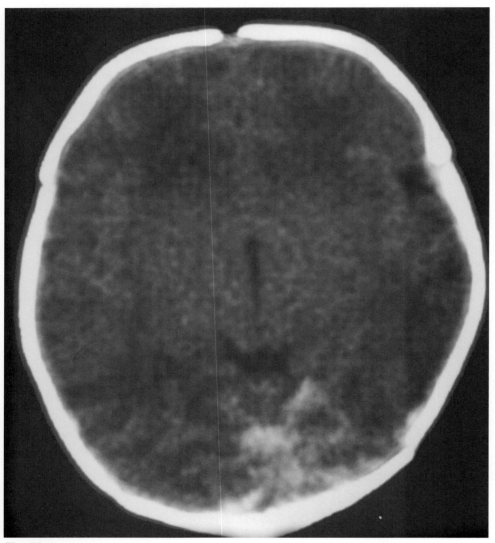

Fig. 73-1

Case 74

An 8-year-old boy is unconscious after being hit by a car and thrown 25 ft.

Heart rate is 80, systolic blood pressure 98 mm Hg. Diameter of right pupil is 8 mm, left pupil 6 mm. Blood is in left side of nose and in left external acoustic meatus. Vomit is on face. An abrasion is on right side of abdomen. Crepitus is in left leg. Right arm and right leg are extended. The rest of the physical findings are normal.

Hematocrit is 0.27. White cell count is 15.0×10^9/liter with 0.55 polymorphonuclear cells, 0.37 bands, 0.06 lymphocytes, 0.01 monocytes, and 0.01 eosinophils. Platelet count is 260×10^9/liter. Urine specific gravity is 1.025, pH 6. Urine has trace blood and 0–1 white cell/HPF. Serum sodium is 139 mmol/liter, potassium 3.4, urea nitrogen 4.3, and glucose 9.2. Creatine is 60 µmol/liter.

Foci of high attenuation are in left thalamus and occipital horn of left lateral ventricle (Figure 74-1A). Air is in basal cisterns in Figure 74-1B. Gas is in front of liver; left ilium, left femur, and left tibia are fractured in other roentgenograms.

At laparotomy, two lacerations, 1 cm long and 5 cm apart, are in ecchymotic jejunum, a small tear and hematoma in mesentery. Blood is in pelvis.

Diagnosis: Intrathalamic and intraventricular blood, pneumocephalus, perforations of jejunum, abdominal blood, fracture of left ilium, left femur, and left tibia.

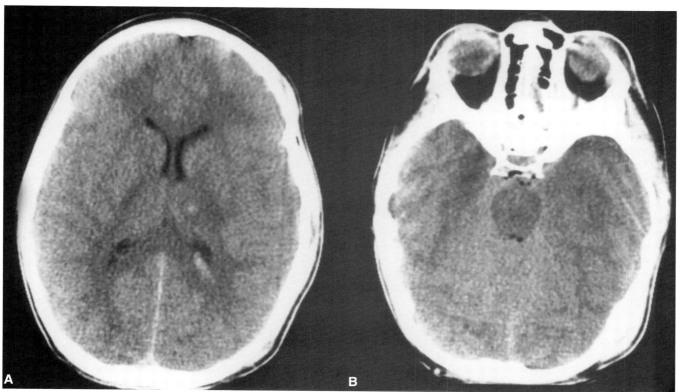

Fig. 74-1

Case 75

A prematurely born boy, who presented as double-footling breech, does not breathe on his own.

Weight is 900 g, Apgar score 1/5 at 1 and 5 minutes, temperature 36.5°C, heart rate 167, and blood pressure 64/40 mm Hg. He is intubated. Anterior fontanel is full, right leg bruised. Heart rate is 60–80 at 20 minutes. He is limp and pale. Head jerks. The rest of the physical findings are normal.

Hematocrit is 0.34, blood glucose 6.7 mmol/liter, arterial blood pH 7.39 at 20 minutes.

CT scan of brain at 2 days (Figure 75-1) shows high attenuation in lateral ventricles and along falx cerebri.

He dies the second day.

Diagnosis: Prematurity, intraventricular and subarachnoid hemorrhage.

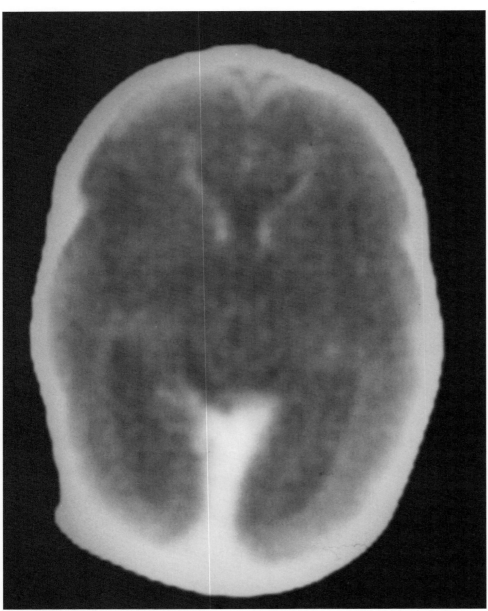

Fig. 75-1

Case 76

A 2½-month-old boy is grunting and unresponsive. Blood is around nose. Limbs are jerking, left more than right. He did not nurse well yesterday.

Pregnancy of mother was normal. Birth weight was 4.5 kg, Apgar score 8/9 at 1 and 5 minutes.

Mother (30 years old), father (31 years old), and brother (4 years old) are well. Sister (22 months old) has hypoplastic optic nerve. Maternal grandmother had goiter and Addison's disease; maternal grandfather had diabetes mellitus.

Temperature at 2½ months is 37.9°C, heart rate 132, respiratory rate 40, systolic blood pressure 120 mm Hg, weight 7.4 kg, and head circumference 42 cm. He is pale. Neck is slightly stiff. Eyes move to midline but not above. Nystagmus to left is briefly present. Eyes do not follow. The rest of the physical findings are normal.

Hematocrit is 0.36. White cell count is 24.3×10^9/liter with 0.66 polymorphonuclear cells, 0.15 bands, 0.17 lymphocytes, 0.01 monocytes, and 0.01 metamyelocytes. Platelet estimate is increased. ESR is 29 mm/hr. Urine specific gravity is 1.029, pH 5. Urine has 4+ glucose, trace ketones, amorphous crystals, and bacteria. Serum sodium is 132 mmol/liter, potassium 5.9, chloride 107, carbon dioxide 16, urea nitrogen 4.3, and glucose 16.3. Creatinine is 40 μmol/liter. Twelve hours later, uric acid is 320 μmol/liter, total bilirubin 7, and direct bilirubin 2. Total protein is 59 g/liter, albumin 39. Alkaline phosphatase is 272 U/liter, LDH 346, and SGOT 31. CSF is bloody; it has 5.2×10^{12}/liter red cells, 400×10^6/liter white cells, 0.88 mononuclear cells, 0+12 polymorphonuclear cells, 6.1 mmol/liter glucose, and 16.30 g/liter protein. PT is 10.9 seconds, activated PTT 15.6.

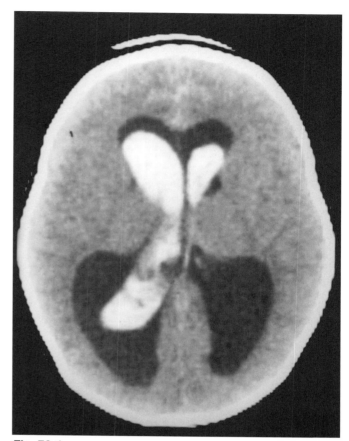

Fig. 76-1

CT scan 12 hours later (Figure 76-1) shows blood clot in dilated lateral ventricles. T1-weighted MRI (Figure 76-2A) 3 days later shows bright rim of free methemoglobin in right lateral ventricle. T2-weighted image (Figure 76-2B) shows absent signal of intracellular deoxyhemoglobin and methemoglobin and high signal of serum. T1-weighted image at lower level (Figure 76-3) shows (1) no signal in left anterior cerebral artery because of blood flow (*flow void*), (2) higher signal in right anterior cerebral artery because of slow or no blood flow, and (3) high signal around right anterior cerebral artery. Cerebral angiograms confirm absence of flow in right anterior cerebral artery.

He walks at 14 months and talks appropriately at 6 years when neurologic findings are normal.

Diagnosis: Cerebral hemorrhage.

(Continued)

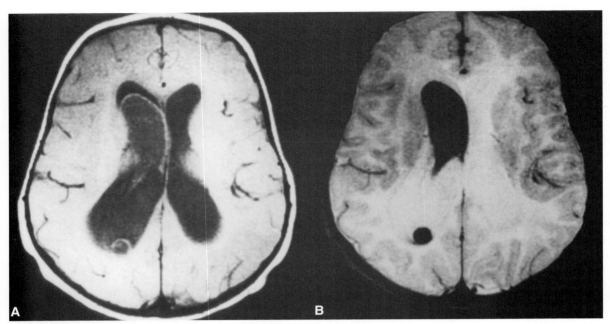

Fig. 76-2

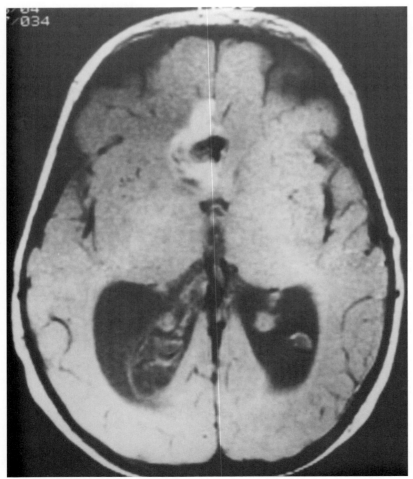

Fig. 76-3

Case 77

An 8-year-old girl felt like she was "spinning around" this morning.

She vomited 16 days ago and had jaw pain for 2 days. She vomited 11 days ago and had headache and jaw pain for 1 day. She felt dizzy while playing today, had headache, went to sleep, and vomited twice while asleep.

She had chickenpox at 2 months. When she began to walk, she walked on her toes "like a ballet dancer." She had otitis media at 6 years.

Mother and brother are well. Father has multiple sclerosis.

Temperature at 8 years is 36.9°C, heart rate 100, respiratory rate 24, blood pressure 100/60 mm Hg, weight 28 kg, and height 130 cm. She is pale. She stares vacantly and moves slowly. Neck hurts when flexed past neutral. Ankles dorsiflex to 90 degrees. The rest of the physical findings are normal.

Hematocrit is 0.37. White cell count is 13.4×10^9/liter with 0.88 polymorphonuclear cells, 0.02 bands, 0.09 lymphocytes, and 0.01 monocytes. Platelet count is 219×10^9/liter. Urine specific gravity is 1.025, pH 7. Urine has 0–1 white cell/HPF, amorphous phosphates, 0.30 g/liter protein, and 0.40 g/liter ketones. Serum sodium is 139 mmol/liter, potassium 4.3, carbon dioxide 21, urea nitrogen 5.0, calcium 2.47, and glucose 7.2. Creatinine is 80 μmol/liter.

CT scan shows calcium in head of right caudate nucleus and blood in occipital horn of right lateral ventricle (Figure 77-1) and in fourth ventricle. MRI in Figure 77-2A shows mass with loculated low signals in right lateral ventricle and contiguous basal ganglia. A lower image shows Swiss cheese–like signals of flow void in part of brain supplied by lenticulostriate arteries (Figure 77-2B). A small amount of blood is in third (see Figure 77-2B) and fourth ventricles. Cerebral angiogram (Figure 77-3) confirms right lenticulostriate hypervascularity.

She feels better and can touch chin to chest the next morning.

Diagnosis: Intracranial bleeding from vascular malformation.

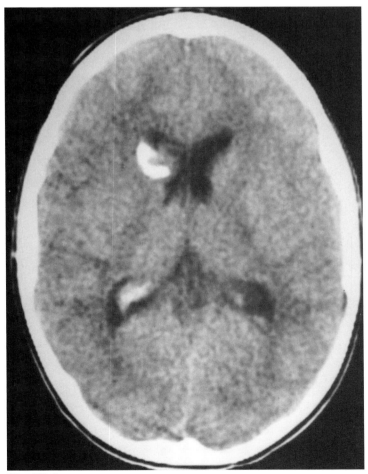

Fig. 77-1

(Continued)

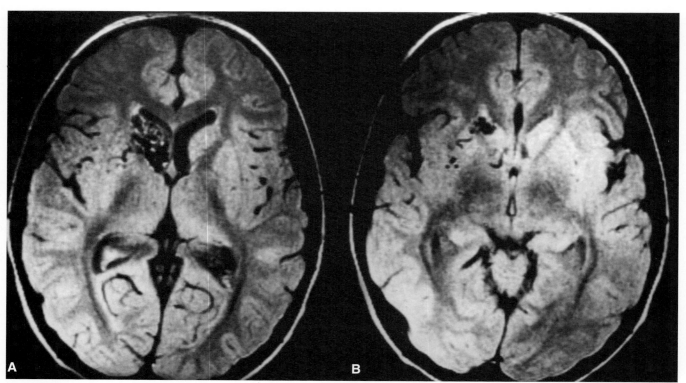

Fig. 77-2

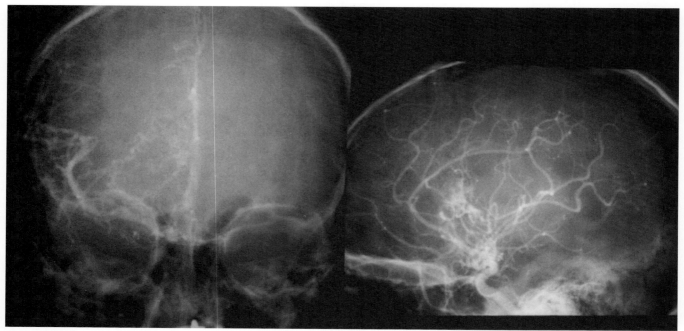

Fig. 77-3

Case 78

A newborn boy is slow to start breathing.

Pregnancy of the mother (21 years old) was normal. Birth weight is 3.4 kg, length 51 cm, head circumference 37 cm, Apgar score 2/5 at 1 and 5 minutes, respiratory rate 80–150 when he starts to breathe on his own, temperature 37°C, heart rate 143, and blood pressure 54/35 mm Hg. Hands and feet are blue. The rest of the physical findings are normal.

Dependent side of face is puffy the second day. He is pale. Systolic murmur and gallop rhythm are present. Liver edge is 3 cm below costal margin. Platelet count is 63×10^9/liter. A small amount of urine is obtained by bladder catheter. At 3 days, a cranial bruit is heard. Hematocrit is 0.54. White cell count is 10.1×10^9/liter. Serum sodium is 143 mmol/liter, potassium 4.6, chloride 109, calcium 2.20, and urea nitrogen 6.1. Creatinine is 110 μmol/liter.

At cardiac catheterization, oxygen saturation in superior vena cava is 0.92, in inferior vena cava 0.78. Angiocardiography shows large right ventricle and quick flow of blood from aorta to superior vena cava.

Heart is large the third day (Figure 78-1). Ultrasound examination of head (Figure 78-2A) shows hypoechoic mass between lateral ventricles. CT scan after IV injection of contrast medium (Figure 78-2B) shows aneurysm, straight sinus, and confluence of sinuses. Findings are similar in examination after injection of contrast medium into aneurysm (Figure 78-3).

Diagnosis: Intracranial arteriovenous malformation (vein of Galen aneurysm).

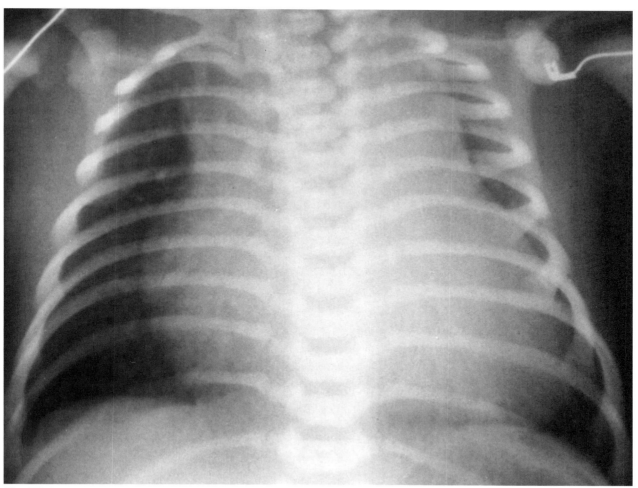

Fig. 78-1

(Continued)

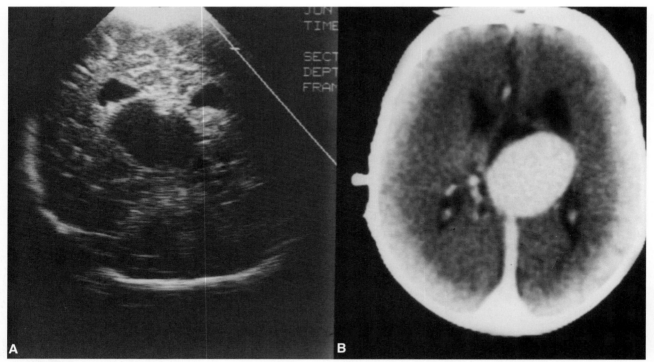

Fig. 78-2

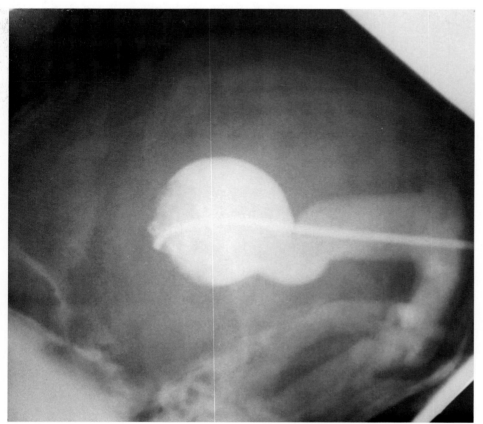

Fig. 78-3

Case 79

A 9-year-old boy, whose right arm has been limp for a week, drags right leg when he walks.

He began to have frontal headache and occasional vomiting 6 weeks ago. Parents had trouble getting him out of bed for school. He began to drag right leg yesterday.

He has had ear infections and placement of tubes.

Temperature is 37°C, heart rate 81, respiratory rate 16, blood pressure 130/96 mm Hg, weight 33 kg, and head circumference 52 cm. Head is tilted to left. Right arm and right leg are weak. Deep tendon reflexes are more active on right side. Metacarpophalangeal joints of right hand are extended, fingers flexed. Finger tapping and toe movement are slow on right side. Babinski's sign is in right foot. The rest of the physical findings are normal.

Serum sodium is 137 mmol/liter, potassium 3.6, chloride 102, and urea nitrogen 4.6. Creatinine is 40 µmol/liter.

MRI after IV injection of gadolinium (Figure 79-1) shows a round mass of mixed signal intensity between medulla and basilar part of occipital bone. Vertebral angiogram (Figure 79-2) shows up and back displacement of intracranial part of dilated left vertebral artery, dilation of nearby segment of right vertebral artery, and right displacement of basilar artery.

At left suboccipital craniotomy, an aneurysm with a clot is present at junction of vertebral and basilar arteries.

Diagnosis: Aneurysm in posterior fossa.

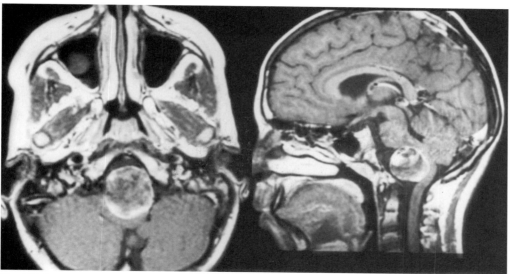

Fig. 79-1

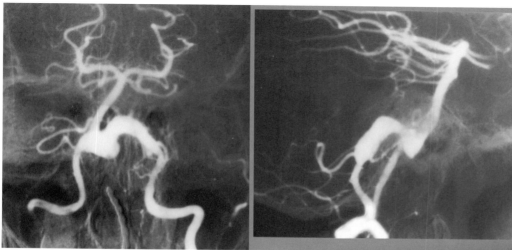

Fig. 79-2

Case 80

A 3-year-old girl who has left hemiparesis is alert and happy.

Pregnancy of mother was normal, birth weight 3.1 kg, and Apgar score 8/9 at 1 and 5 minutes. She has had otitis media twice, the second time 3 months ago, when she was given amoxicillin. She was "whiney" a week and a half later, kept saying, "It hurts," and then slept. Her mother heard her cry approximately 2 hours after she fell asleep and found her lying on the floor beside the bed. The girl kept falling when the mother tried to stand her up. "The left side was not working right."

Mother, father, and two brothers are well. Maternal great-grandparents had heart attacks. Maternal grandfather has headaches. Paternal grandmother died with melanoma of CNS, and a paternal uncle and cousin had tumors of CNS.

At hospital admission 3 months ago, the girl's temperature was 36.9°C, blood pressure 98/53 mm Hg, and weight 13.3 kg. She listed to left and dragged and circled left foot laterally when she walked. Most of movement of left arm was at the shoulder. Left grip was weak. She did not move left hand and left foot spontaneously. Left eye did not close tightly. Left side of mouth drooped and drooled. Sensation was depressed on left side. Babinski's sign was in left foot. Left toes extended when skin over left lateral malleolus was scratched (Chaddock's sign). Left eardrum was slightly retracted. The rest of the physical findings were normal.

Hematocrit was 0.35. White cell count was 10.8×10^9/liter with 0.84 polymorphonuclear cells, 0.15 lymphocytes, and 0.01 monocytes. Urine specific gravity was 1.056, pH 8.

Urine was normal. Serum sodium was 142 mmol/liter, potassium 4.1, chloride 103, carbon dioxide 24, urea nitrogen 4.6, cholesterol 4.14, triglycerides 0.34, HDL 1.11 (mean for girls: 1.42), LDL 2.07 (mean for girls: 2.52), and glucose 8.0. Creatinine was 40 µmol/liter, uric acid 140, total bilirubin 5, and direct bilirubin 0. Total protein was 73 g/liter, albumin 45. Alkaline phosphatase was 191 U/liter, LDH 245, and SGOT 30. CSF had 1×10^9/liter red cells, 0 white cells, 3.4 mmol/liter glucose, 0.21 g/liter protein, and was sterile. Activated PTT was 23.4 seconds (normal: 25–38); PT was normal. Blood levels of AT III and protein C were normal.

EEG showed slowing over right hemisphere. Echocardiogram showed patent foramen ovale. Findings in CT scan of brain with and without IV contrast medium were normal. Angiogram showed occlusion of the right middle cerebral artery at its origin and moderate stenosis of the right anterior cerebral artery near its origin (A1 segment).

CT scan (Figure 80-1) shows atrophy of right cerebral hemisphere 3 months after appearance of left hemiparesis; left cerebral hemisphere is normal.

Total free protein S antigen in the girl's blood at 3 years is 0.27 U/ml, 0.32, and 0.41 (normal: 0.55–1.47). Total protein S is 0.97. Her blood does not contain antiphospholipid antibodies. Free protein S antigen in parents' and 2 brothers' blood, and in girl's blood 1 year later, is normal.

Diagnosis: Cerebral infarction, acquired free protein S deficiency.

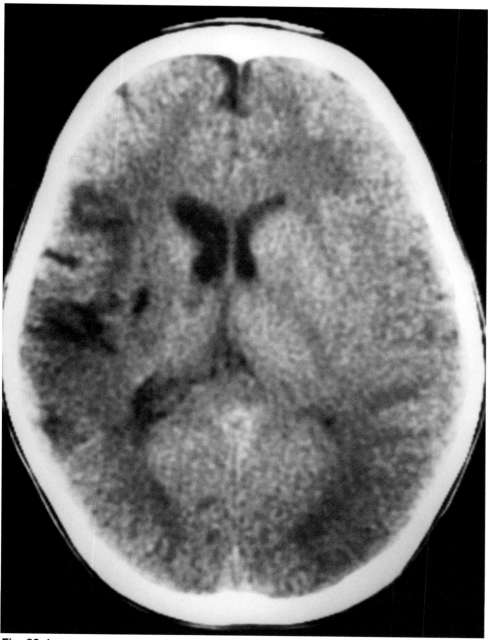

Fig. 80-1

Case 81

An 11-month-old boy is unconscious. He was put into bed for a nap 6 hours ago, was sleeping face down with knees flexed and buttocks up 4 hours ago, and was found face down on a pillow with head caught between bed and wall 3 hours ago. He was limp. Body was pale. Face and neck were blue. No heartbeat was felt. He was intubated and given oxygen by paramedics.

Birth weight was 3 kg, length 49 cm, head circumference 31 cm, and Apgar score 9/9 at 1 and 5 minutes. Weight was 8.5 kg, head circumference 44 cm at 8 months when inguinal hernias were repaired. He has been stuffy and not eating well for 2 days.

Temperature at 11 months is 33.3°C, heart rate 150, and blood pressure 97/34 mm Hg. Pupils are fixed and dilated, fundi normal. The rest of the physical findings are normal.

Venous blood pH is 6.56, P_{CO_2} 139 mm Hg, P_{O_2} 29 mm Hg, and bicarbonate 13 mmol/liter. Hematocrit is 0.36. White cell count is 14.9×10^9/liter with 0.20 polymorphonuclear cells, 0.06 bands, 0.67 lymphocytes, 0.01 eosinophils, 0.05 atypical lymphocytes, and 0.01 metamyelocytes. Platelet count is 374×10^9/liter. Urine specific gravity 1.020, pH 6.5. Urine has 0.1 g/liter protein, 5–10 white cells, and 5–10 red cells/HPF, 1 hyaline cast/LPF, and bacteria. Serum sodium is 151 mmol/liter, potassium 3.1, chloride 119, carbon dioxide 3, urea nitrogen 2.0, and glucose 15.9. Creatinine is 60 μmol/liter.

CT scan in Figure 81-1 shows collapsed lateral ventricles, obliteration of the cistern of the great cerebral vein, and absence of gray-white differentiation.

Diagnosis: Suffocation, cerebral edema.

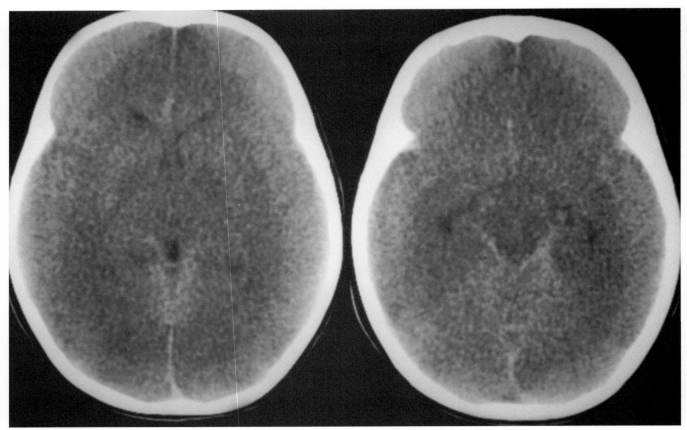

Fig. 81-1

Case 82

A 2-year-old boy is semicomatose.

He was blue and apneic 2½ hours ago. Temperature was 28.9°C, heart rate 60, and systolic blood pressure 70 mm Hg. He was intubated and given oxygen and IV sodium bicarbonate and normal saline. Arterial blood pH was 6.75, P_{CO_2} 37 mm Hg, P_{O_2} 472 mm Hg, and bicarbonate 5 mmol/liter. Hematocrit was 0.27. White cell count was 5.9 × 10^9/liter. Serum sodium was 134 mmol/liter, potassium 4.2, carbon dioxide 4, urea nitrogen 4.6, and glucose 10.7. Creatinine was 80 μmol/liter.

Temperature is now 36.2°C, heart rate 130. He withdraws from pinprick. Back is arched. Legs are stiff. Some scalp hair is gone. Eyes are black, cheeks bruised, pupils dilated and then pinpoint. Subconjunctival hemorrhages are present. Abdomen is tense and quiet. Bruises are on arms and legs, burns on scrotum and buttocks. Body and limbs shake intermittently. The rest of the physical findings are normal.

The second day, serum sodium is 134 mmol/liter, potassium 4.1, chloride 103, carbon dioxide 23, urea nitrogen 2.9, calcium 1.67, phosphorus 0.68, cholesterol 1.40, and glucose 4.1. Creatinine is 40 μmol/liter, uric acid 320, total bilirubin 10, and direct bilirubin 3. Total protein is 34 g/liter, albumin 20. Alkaline phosphatase is 119 U/liter, LDH 2,145, and SGOT 2,805.

CT scan on the third day (Figure 82-1) shows poor differentiation between gray and white matter; low attenuation in head of caudate nucleus, internal capsule, lentiform nucleus, and tail of caudate nucleus; and blood along falx cerebri.

He dies on the fourth day.

Diagnosis: Infarction of basal ganglia. Microscopic examination of brain shows edema, gliosis, and loss of neurons.

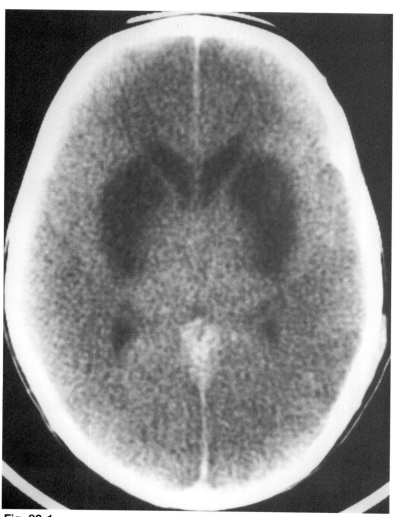

Fig. 82-1

Case 83

A 1-month-old boy is convulsing. Stools have been runny for 2 days. He cried a lot during the night and refused a feeding. He has taken 0.05 oz formula today. Sister (2 years old) has a cold.

Pregnancy of mother (24 years old) was normal, birth weight 3 kg. He had gastroenteritis 2 weeks ago.

Temperature at 1 month is 37.4°C, heart rate 124, respiratory rate 26, blood pressure 70/36 mm Hg, weight 2.8 kg, length 53 cm, and head circumference 36 cm. Right side of face twitches. Eyes turn right or left. Lips smack. Right hand shakes. Legs extend. He cries between seizures. Anterior fontanel is soft. Thrush is in mouth. A systolic murmur is present. The rest of the physical findings are normal.

Hematocrit is 0.31. White cell count is 19.2×10^9/liter with 0.44 polymorphonuclear cells, 0.03 bands, 0.38 lymphocytes, 0.13 monocytes, and 0.02 eosinophils. Platelet count is 146 ×

10^9/liter. Urine specific gravity is 1.025, pH 6. Urine has 0.2 AU urobilinogen and occasional squamous epithelial cells/HPF. CSF has 70×10^6/liter red blood cells, 40×10^6/liter white cells, 1.00 lymphocytes, 1.76 g/liter protein, and 3.6 mmol/liter glucose . Serum sodium is 135 mmol/liter, potassium 6.3, chloride 94, carbon dioxide 28, urea nitrogen 2.1, calcium 2.22, phosphorus 1.58, cholesterol 2.53, and glucose 7.3. Creatinine is 60 μmol/liter, uric acid 170, total bilirubin 10, and direct bilirubin 3. Total protein is 57 g/liter, albumin 29. GGT is 58 U/liter. Four days later, alkaline phosphatase is 128 U/liter, LDH 330, and SGOT 51.

CT scan before IV injection of contrast medium shows high attenuation in straight sinus (Figure 83-1A) and after injection a less dense core in sagittal sinus (*delta sign*) (Figure 83-1B).

Diagnosis: Sagittal sinus thrombosis.

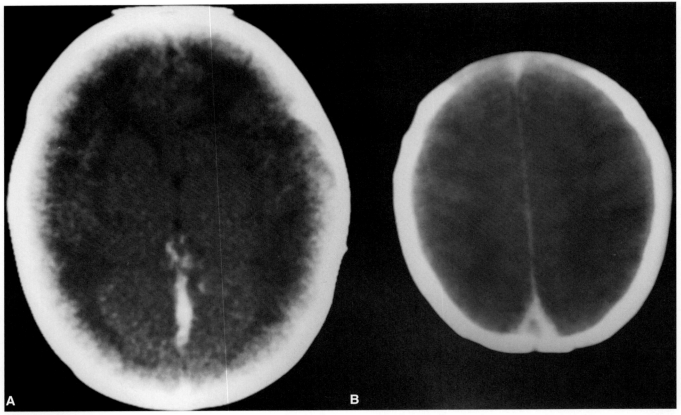

Fig. 83-1

Case 84

A 13-year-old girl is too sleepy.

She was treated for seizures with phenobarbital from age 9 months to 7½ years. Phenobarbital was resumed after a seizure 6 months ago in which she had a staring spell and fell down a flight of stairs. The last "blanking out" was 3 months ago. Five days ago, the dose of phenobarbital was increased from 80 to 300 mg/day. Speech became slurred, movements clumsy. She began to sleep a lot the next day. She had to be awakened to eat. She missed her mouth with the spoon. She fell out of a chair in school yesterday.

Pregnancy of mother was normal. A flat hemangioma was on left cheek and left eyelids at birth. She had a seizure at 9 months in which right limbs jerked and right eyelids and right side of mouth twitched.

Mother and two sisters (11 and 12 years old) are well.

Temperature at 13 years is 37.3°C, heart rate 88, and respiratory rate 18. A hemangioma is on left side of face. A strip of deeper pigment (8 × 2 cm) is on right side of chest. She has right esotropia and mild right amblyopia. Optic fundi are normal. Right quadriceps is slightly weaker than left. Deep ten-don reflexes are brisker in right arm than left. She hops easily on either foot. Right leg is 71 cm long, left 73 cm. Right hand is smaller than left. The rest of the physical findings are normal.

Serum sodium is 140 mmol/liter, potassium 4.1, chloride 104, carbon dioxide 21, urea nitrogen 4.3, calcium 2.30, phosphorus 1.70, cholesterol 4.86, and glucose 4.7. Creatinine is 50 µmol/liter, uric acid 330, total bilirubin 2, and direct bilirubin 0. Total protein is 68 g/liter, albumin 41. Alkaline phosphatase is 472 U/liter, LDH 229, and SGOT 20.

Deposits of calcium are in the left cerebral hemisphere (Figure 84-1).

She is shot with a BB gun at 16 years.

A BB is in left side of the face; calvaria is thicker, frontal sinus larger on left side (Figure 84-2).

Diagnosis: Sturge-Weber syndrome, phenobarbital overdose, Dyke-Davidoff syndrome.

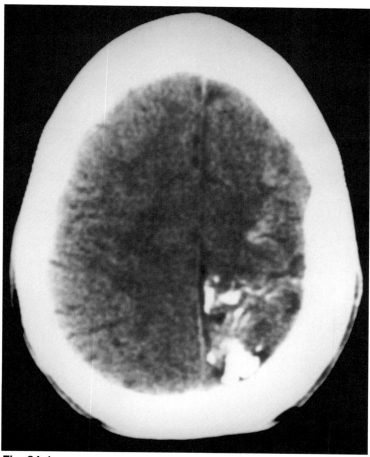

Fig. 84-1

(Continued)

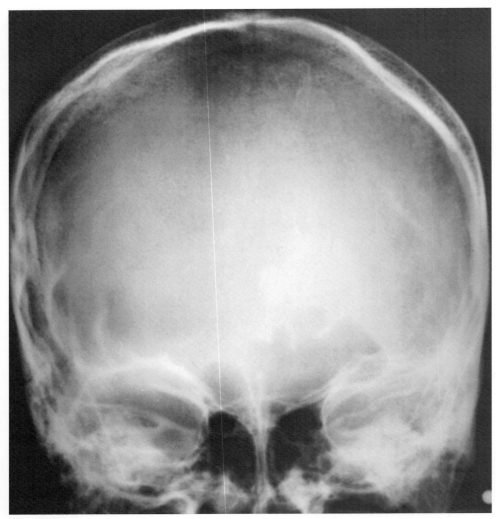

Fig. 84-2

Case 85

A 7-year-old boy drools, staggers, falls, and bumps into walls.

Slurred speech, numbness of right hand, and then brief headache 16 months ago were followed by his being "spacey for a little while." He has had eight similar spells since then, during which right hand, right arm, and right side of face tingle, sometimes followed by headache. Speech is slurred and inappropriate.

Birth weight was 3.9 kg, Apgar score 9/10 at 1 and 5 minutes. He walked at 9 months and began to read at 4 years. Myringotomy tubes were put in at 7 months and at 3 years, when adenoids were removed.

Mother (34 years old) has allergies and had a parotid mucoepidermoid cyst. Father (35 years old) and two brothers (1 and 4 years old) are well. Sister (8 years old) has Down syndrome. Maternal great grandfather had stroke at 32 years. Both grandfathers and paternal grandmother had heart disease.

Temperature at 7 years is 37.4°C, heart rate 108, respiratory rate 24, blood pressure 114/78 mm Hg, weight 23.6 kg, and height 127 cm. Right eardrum is opaque. Right arm, right hand, and right leg are weak. Sensation is impaired on right side. Questionable Babinski's sign is in right foot. The rest of the physical findings are normal.

Hematocrit is 0.38. White cell count is 11.0×10^9/liter with 0.56 polymorphonuclear cells, 0.04 bands, 0.29 lymphocytes, 0.06 monocytes, 0.04 eosinophils, and 0.01 basophils. ESR is 6 mm/hr. Urine specific gravity is 1.024, pH 6. Urine is normal.

Xenon 133 isotope scan shows decreased blood flow in temporal lobes. PET shows foci of hypoperfusion in right frontal lobe, left frontoparietal lobes, and basal ganglia.

MRI (Figure 85-1) shows Swiss cheese–like pattern of flow voids. Carotid angiogram shows no anterior cerebral arteries and a mesh of small vessels (Figure 85-2).

Diagnosis: Moyamoya disease.

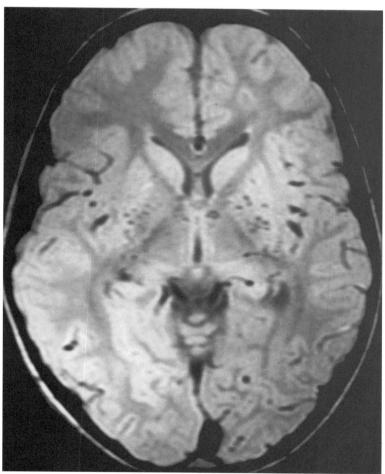

Fig. 85-1

(Continued)

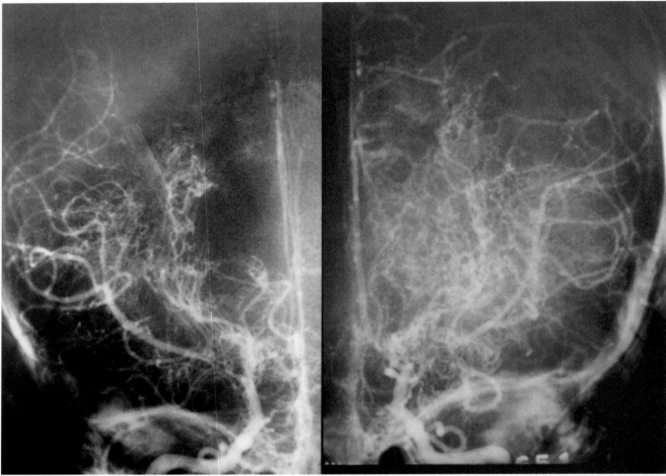

Fig. 85-2

Case 86

A 15-month-old boy has seizures during which neck and trunk flex and arms extend. They began 3 weeks ago, occur once or twice a day, and last seconds.

He had febrile seizure at 9 months. He has had otitis media.

Pregnancy of mother was normal, birth weight 3.5 kg. A dimple on nose at birth is now larger and discharges liquid from a small opening. The boy sat alone at 9 months, crawled at 11 months, and now walks with support.

Parents and older sister are well. Paternal grandfather had a brain tumor and epilepsy; a paternal cousin had paraplegia.

Weight at 15 months is 11.7 kg, height 84 cm, and head circumference 49 cm. At 16 months, heart rate is 180 when he has fever, respiratory rate 42, and blood pressure 140/80 mm Hg. At times he gazes at his left hand and has no interest in his surroundings. Skin of nose is red over a soft mass that extends from frontonasal suture to alar cartilage. A small pit is present at bottom of mass. Abdomen is large. An egg-sized mass is below right costal margin. Left kidney is palpable. Pale spots (1.0–2.5 cm) that appear in Wood's light are on right thigh, right shank, and left forearm. The rest of the physical findings are normal.

Hematocrit is 0.39. White cell count is 15.4 × 10⁹/liter with 0.38 polymorphonuclear cells, 0.54 lymphocytes, 0.04 mono-cytes, 0.03 eosinophils, and 0.01 basophils. Urine specific gravity is 1.010, pH 6. Urine has 0.2 urobilinogen, 0–1 hyaline cast/LPF, occasional squamous epithelial cells/HPF, and 0–1 white cell/HPF. Serum sodium is 141 mmol/liter, potassium 5.0, chloride 114, carbon dioxide 14, urea nitrogen 3.5, calcium 2.54, phosphorus 2.07, cholesterol 3.67, and glucose 5.8. Creatinine is 40 µmol/liter, uric acid 110, total bilirubin 2, and direct bilirubin 0. Total protein is 59 g/liter, albumin 47. Alkaline phosphatase is 445 U/liter, LDH 309, and SGOT 105.

Echocardiogram shows slight left ventricular hypertrophy.

EEG shows high-amplitude polyspike and slow-wave complexes that are diffuse, frequent, and brief on background of 2–4 cycles per second of high-amplitude activity.

T2-weighted MRI (Figure 86-1) shows high signal in right frontal lobe. CT scan shows soft tissue in left side of nose (Figure 86-2A) and defect in frontal bone (Figure 86-2B). CT scan of abdomen shows renal (Figure 86-3A) and perirenal cysts (Figure 86-3B).

Diagnosis: Tuberous sclerosis, hypsarrhythmia, renal and perirenal cysts (angiomyolipomas, lymphangiomatous cysts, lymphangioleiomyomatosis), nasal dermoid.

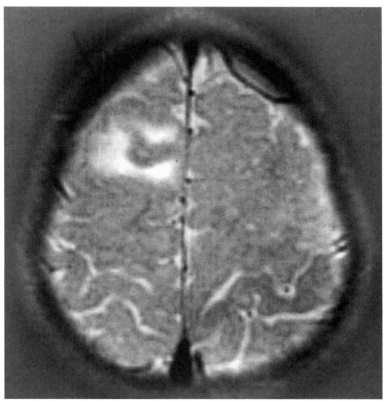

Fig. 86-1

(Continued)

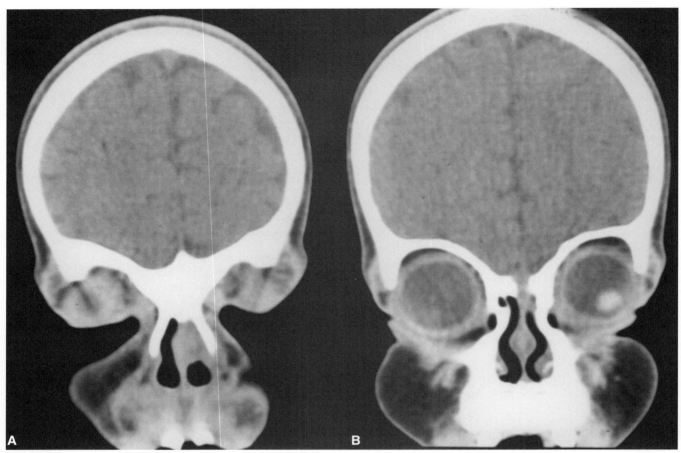

Fig. 86-2

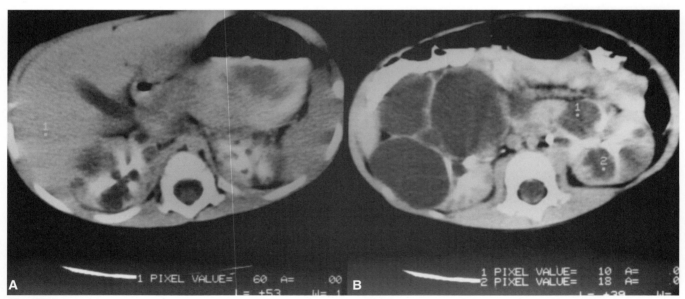

Fig. 86-3

Brain

Case 1

A 3½-year-old boy and his 9-year-old sister are mentally retarded and have convulsions.

At 3½ years, as seldom as once a week and as often as several times a day, the boy becomes glassy eyed, looks left, slumps to floor, flexes limbs, gnashes teeth for a few seconds, and then sleeps 5–10 minutes. He had convulsions from ages 4 months to 2 years, despite anticonvulsants. Convulsions began again 2 months ago. At 9 years, his sister has convulsions despite large doses of anticonvulsants. Her first convulsion was observed at 5 hours. At 5 years, she had major motor seizures with rolling eyes and jerking limbs for long and short periods as well as absence attacks with fluttering eyes and arched back.

The boy's birth weight was 3.5 kg. He sat at 8 months, walked at 18 months, and does not talk at 3½ years. His sister's birth weight was 2.2 kg, Apgar score 9/10 at 1 and 5 minutes. She cannot sit or walk at 9 years and barely perceives pain.

Maternal grandmother had brain tumors, facial angiofibromas, and kidney and lung disease. A maternal aunt, who had convulsions, brain tumors, and scoliosis, died at 36 years with lung disease. Mother had bilateral pneumothorax at 21 years and died at 26 years with lung disease.

The boy's weight at 3½ years is 16.3 kg, height 99 cm, head circumference 54 cm, temperature 38°C, heart rate 120, respiratory rate 28, and blood pressure 140/100 mm Hg. He is crying. A hemangioma is on forehead. Angiofibromas are in nasolabial folds, papules are on back, and hypopigmented spots are on back and legs. A grayish-white raised mass, a benign astrocytoma (one-third size of optic disc) is in right optic fundus. The rest of the physical findings are normal.

His sister's weight is 21 kg at 9 years, length 107 cm, head circumference 49 cm, temperature 36.7°C, heart rate 88, respiratory rate 16, and blood pressure 100/60 mm Hg. Eyes drift to right. Left eardrum is thick and retracted. Angiofibromas are on face. Gums are thick, teeth decayed. Wood's light shows hypopigmented spots. Legs scissor. The rest of the physical findings are normal.

The boy's hematocrit is 0.38. White cell count is 11.3×10^9/liter with 0.33 polymorphonuclear cells, 0.07 bands, 0.54 lymphocytes, 0.04 monocytes, 0.01 eosinophils, and 0.01 basophils. Urine specific gravity is 1.027, pH 6. Urine is normal. Serum sodium is 147 mmol/liter, potassium 5.0, chloride 108, carbon dioxide 23, urea nitrogen 3.6, calcium 2.62, and glucose 5.0. Creatinine is 50 μmol/liter. CSF has 1×10^6/liter white cells (all lymphocytes), 3.4 mmol/liter glucose, and 0.08 g/liter protein.

In Figure 1-1A, at 9 years, the sister's lateral ventricles are dilated, right ventricle more than left; a focus of calcium density is in right frontal lobe; smaller foci of calcium density are in wall of lateral ventricles. Development of left frontal sinus is at approximately 12-year level (Figure 1-1B). Mother has bilateral tension pneumothorax at 21 years and nodules and reticulating strands of water density in the lungs 6 months later. In Figure 1-2, diaphragm is low.

Biopsy of mother's lung at time of pneumothorax showed smooth muscle proliferating around cysts that are continuous with bronchioles, lined in part by small foci of atypical epithelium, which also lines and is present in some alveoli. Biopsy also showed pleural cysts and small parenchymal hemorrhages caused by proliferation of smooth muscle around lymphatics and in venules.

Diagnosis: Tuberous sclerosis. (Microscopic diagnosis of mother's lung at biopsy is pulmonary lymphangioleiomyomatosis.)

(Continued)

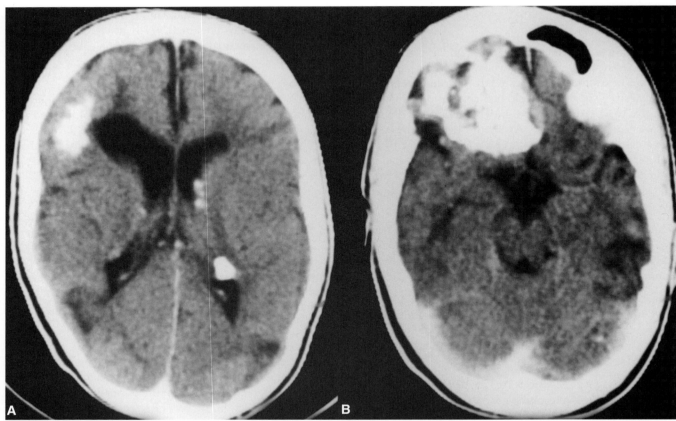

Fig. 1-1

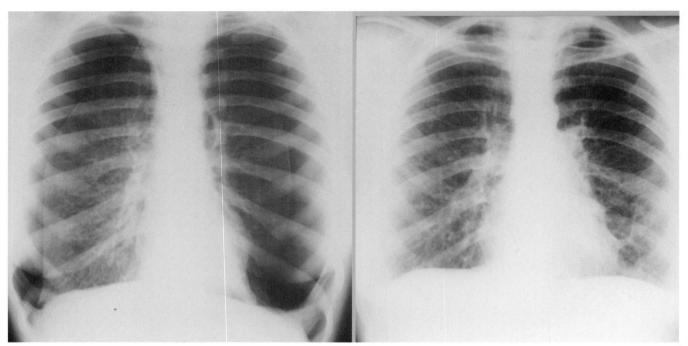

Fig. 1-2

Case 2

A 16-year-old boy shakes too much to work.

He was anemic at 10 years. He was weak 9 months ago and then felt well until 3 months ago, when he became unsteady. Voice became soft. He stopped working in a fast food restaurant 3 weeks ago. Body and limbs trembled. Back of head and neck ached. He has been taking sleeping pills for 1 week.

Parents and eight siblings are well.

Weight at 16 years is 55 kg, temperature 37.3°C, heart rate 68, respiratory rate 16, and blood pressure 104/62 mm Hg. Speech is slurred. He walks slowly and unsteadily; right foot slaps the floor. Alternating movements—palm up, palm down, and finger to nose—are slow. He leaves his arm where movement ends, arm flexed and hand in air. A ring of brown-yellow pigment is in corneas, 2 mm from limbus. Spleen edge is 5 cm below costal margin. Muscle tone is increased. Babinski's sign is in feet. The rest of the physical findings are normal.

Hematocrit is 0.39. White cell count is 1.9×10^9/liter. Platelet count is 27×10^9/liter. Urine specific gravity is 1.010, pH 8. Urine has 0.2 AU urobilinogen and amorphous phosphates. Serum sodium is 140 mmol/liter, potassium 3.8, chloride 122, carbon dioxide 24, urea nitrogen 3.9, calcium 2.40, phosphorus 1.36, cholesterol 3.49, and glucose 4.6. Creatinine is 100 μmol/liter, uric acid 100, total bilirubin 17, direct bilirubin 3, iron 10 (normal: 14–32), and iron-binding capacity 55 (normal: 45–82). Total protein is 65 g/liter, albumin 45. Alkaline phosphatase is 144 U/liter, LDH 146, and SGOT 34. PT is 14.1 seconds (normal: 11–13), activated PTT 33.8 (normal: 24–35).

Bone marrow is slightly hypocellular.

MRI shows low signal in putamen, thin rim of higher signal in T1-weighted image (Figure 2-1), mixed high and low signal in T2-weighted image (Figure 2-2). Apparent crescentic defect in left frontal lobe results from slight tilt of image at junction of brain and frontal bone.

Serum ceruloplasmin is 20 mg/liter (normal: 200–350), copper 4.9 μmol/liter (normal: 11–22). Urine copper excretion, five determinations, ranges from 4.5 to 27.8 μmol/day (normal: <0.6). Urine copper concentration, five determinations, ranges from 3.4 to 28.1 μmol/liter (normal: <0.5).

Diagnosis: Wilson's disease (hepatolenticular degeneration).

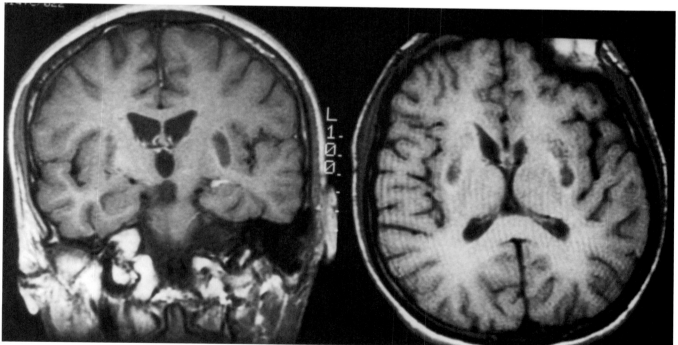

Fig. 2-1

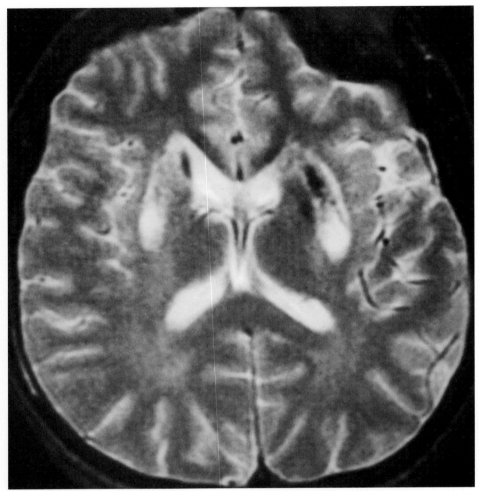

Fig. 2-2

Case 3

A 9-month-old boy does not cry, sit, lift head, or hold bottle. He gags on his spit. Left eye "wanders out."

Birth weight was 3.5 kg.

Mother (28 years old), father (27 years old), and brother (5 years old) are well.

Temperature is 37.2°C, heart rate 140, respiratory rate 40, weight 11.9 kg, length 81 cm, and head circumference 48 cm. He tracks with his eyes. Eye movement is jerky. Left eye turns out. Maculae look like red fried eggs. Muscle tone is poor. Deep tendon reflexes are normal. Babinski's sign is in feet. The rest of the physical findings are normal.

Skull is normal at 9 months. In Figure 3-1, sutures are widened and head circumference is 53 cm at 19 months. Spheno-occipital synchondrosis is also widened (Figure 3-1B).

Serum hexosaminidase A activity is 0. Necropsy soon after second roentgenogram shows ganglioside GM_2 accumulation in brain and a 6% decrease in hexosaminidase activity upon heating of brain tissue at 50°C for 4 hours compared with a 52% decrease for an age-matched control, which has normal amount of heat-labile hexosaminidase A and heat-stable hexosaminidase B.

Diagnosis: Tay-Sachs disease (GM_2 gangliosidosis, hexosaminidase A deficiency).

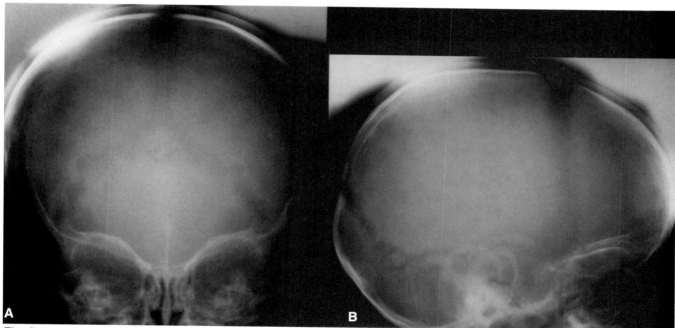

Fig. 3-1

Case 4

A 6-year-old boy stumbles and falls, chokes on his food, says only the first syllable of few words, and "can't do a series of anything."

Mother, 20 years old at his birth and Rh negative, took 200 mg/day phenytoin during pregnancy. Delivery was by cesarean section, birth weight 3 kg, length 53 cm, and Apgar score 7/9 at 1 and 5 minutes. He was floppy. He crawled at 9 months, walked at 17 months, started to feed himself at 18 months, and was toilet trained at 4 years. He can get his clothes off but not on. He cannot run or pedal a bicycle. Intelligence is at level of 2½–3 year old. Tonsils and adenoids have been removed. He had operation at 2 years for ptosis of upper lids. He has had rubeola and rubella.

Mother had first seizure at 12 years, last seizure at 21 years. She was treated by conization for cancer of cervix at 18 years. Father (30 years old) is well. He may have had a seizure in high school. A sister (7 years old) is well. Maternal grandmother had nephrosis and is epileptic. Paternal great-grandmother was epileptic. Maternal grandfather has headaches and arthritis.

Weight at 6 years is 18 kg, height 105 cm, temperature 38.8°C, heart rate 96, respiratory rate 16–36, and blood pressure 98/68 mm Hg. He is cooperative and "unusually happy." Speech is nasal and incomprehensible. Face is without expression. Orbicularis oculi and superior rectus muscles are weak. Upper lip is stretched. He cannot purse his lips. Mouth is open. Limbs are thin and weak. He gets up from the floor by pulling hand over hand on furniture. Gait is stiff and unsteady with arms fixed and flexed at elbows and wrists. Reflexes are brisk. Muscles are rigid and variably hypertonic. Ankles cannot dorsiflex past 90 degrees. A few light and dark spots are on his back. The rest of the physical findings are normal.

Hematocrit is 0.39. White cell is count 7.7×10^9/liter with 0.57 polymorphonuclear cells, 0.04 bands, 0.29 lymphocytes, 0.04 monocytes, and 0.06 eosinophils. Platelet count is 236×10^9/liter. Urine specific gravity is 1.029, pH 5. Urine has 0.30 g/liter protein, 0.15 g/liter ketones, 2+ hemoglobin/myoglobin, mucus, occasional squamous epithelial cells/HPF, 13–15 red cells/HPF, and 4–5 white cells/HPF. Serum sodium is 141 mmol/liter, potassium 4.1, chloride 102, carbon dioxide 15, urea nitrogen 5.0, calcium 2.72, phosphorus 1.19, cholesterol 5.07, and glucose 4.1. Creatinine is 50 μmol/liter, uric acid 370, total bilirubin 7, and direct bilirubin 2. Total protein is 74 g/liter, albumin 51. Alkaline phosphatase is 188 U/liter, LDH 179, and SGOT 22. Serum lactate is 2.3 and 3.6 mmol/liter (normal: 0.9–1.6), pyruvate 0.09 and 0.16 (normal: 0.3–0.7). Ratio of lactate to pyruvate is 26 and 23 (normal: 10 and 33). CSF contains 1×10^6/liter white cells (most lymphocytes), 22×10^6/liter red cells, 3.2 mmol/liter glucose, and 0.23 g/liter protein. Serum alanine is 452 and 627 μmol/liter (normal: 148–475), glutamine 269 (normal: 475–746). Chromosomes are 46,XY.

Putamens and heads of caudate nuclei are radiolucent in CT scan at 4 years (Figure 4-1A). Increased signal is present in the same place and in right thalamus in T1-weighted MRI at 6 years (Figure 4-1B).

Needle muscle biopsy at 7 years shows two to three muscle fibers that have excess granular red material beneath sarcolemma in trichrome preparation, excess intracellular lipid in oil red O preparation, and prominent granularity in succinic dehydrogenase preparation.

His condition deteriorates over next 3 years.

Diagnosis: Leigh's necrotizing encephalopathy.

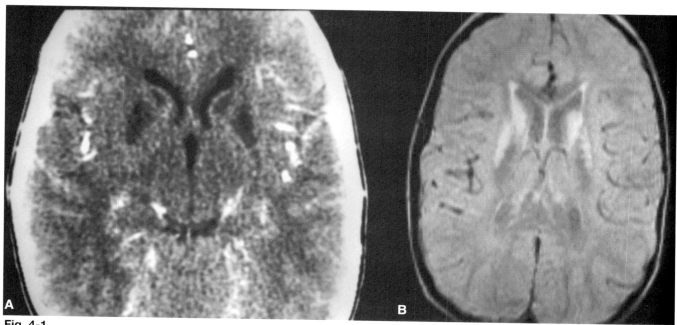

Fig. 4-1

Case 5

A 7-year-old boy, with a cough and temperature of 38.9°C, begins convulsing, first twitching of left arm and left side of face, then generalized, on his way to the hospital.

Pregnancy of mother was normal, birth weight 3.1 kg, Apgar score 8/10 at 1 and 5 minutes. He was cheerful and agreeable when examined at 2 years. He spoke well and was bright at 3 years but was very active and kicked others in the family. He could write the alphabet at 3¼ years but had already been expelled from two nursery schools. A baby-sitter refused to stay at 3¾ years. He had pain in groins and legs at 4½ years. Right eye turned out at 5 years. He was very active at 6 years but could not run as fast as other children. Visual acuity was 20/30 OS, 20/150 OD but not correctable with a +3.00 D lens, a result that perplexed the ophthalmologist. He began to bump into things. He stopped singing, reading, and dressing himself.

Mother (28 years old), father, and brother (2 years old) are well. Three maternal uncles died before they were 10 years old.

He does not blink or react to noise. Deep tendon reflexes are brisk, left more than right. Clonus is present at right ankle; Babinski's sign is in feet. The rest of the physical findings are normal. Several days later, he recognizes his parents by touch or smell, not by sight. When food is brought to him 11 days after the convulsion, he says "You want me to eat? I'll eat if you let me go home."

Roentgenogram of pelvis at 5¾ years shows increased neck-shaft angle of femurs. CT scan of brain at 7 years (Figure 5-1A) shows hypodense white matter, especially in occipital lobes around occipital horns of lateral ventricles and in putamens and posterior limbs of internal capsule. CT scan at 12 years (Figure 5-1B) shows dilated ventricles and deep sulci.

Serum cortisol is 500 nmol/liter before IV injection of corticotropin at 7⅔ years and increases to only 540 nmol/liter during next 2 hours (normal increase: >193). Ratio of plasma C24/C22 fatty acids is 1.58 (normal: 0.84 ± 0.08), C26/C22 0.60 (normal: 0.01 ± 0.01).

His brother has Addison's disease at 5 years.

Diagnosis: Adrenoleukodystrophy.

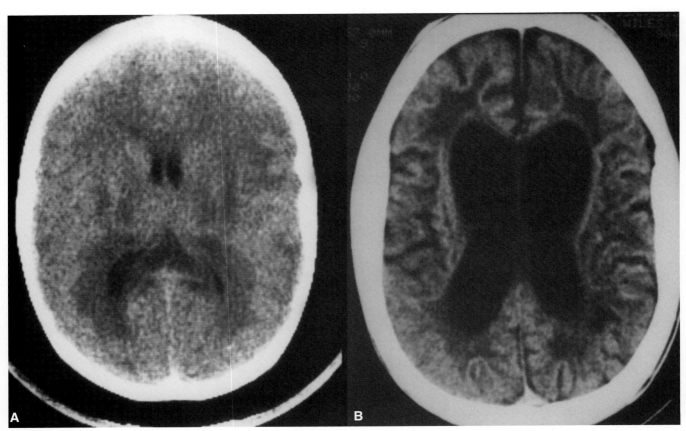

Fig. 5-1

Case 6

A 14-year-old girl has dry heaves and keeps her eyes closed.

She felt that the school room was spinning 3 days ago and has been dizzy and nauseated since then. Vision was blurred for 6 weeks at 12 years. Six months ago, left side of face and left hand were weak, and left hand and left leg tingled for 3 weeks.

Weight at 14 years is 57 kg, height 163 cm, temperature 38°C, heart rate 88, and blood pressure 120/80 mm Hg. She is alert, will not stand up, and has blurred vision and horizontal and vertical nystagmus. Right eyeball does not elevate fully. Thumbs flex when fingernails are flicked (Hoffmann's reflex). The rest of the physical findings are normal.

CT scan with IV contrast medium 6 months ago (Figure 6-1) shows a radiolucent defect in right cerebral hemisphere. T1-weighted MRI at 14 years shows a large focus of increased signal in right cerebral hemisphere (Figure 6-2A) and a small focus of increased signal in left claustrum or retrolenticular part of internal capsule (Figure 6-2B).

She is better but a little uneasy when she walks on the ninth day.

Diagnosis: Multiple sclerosis.

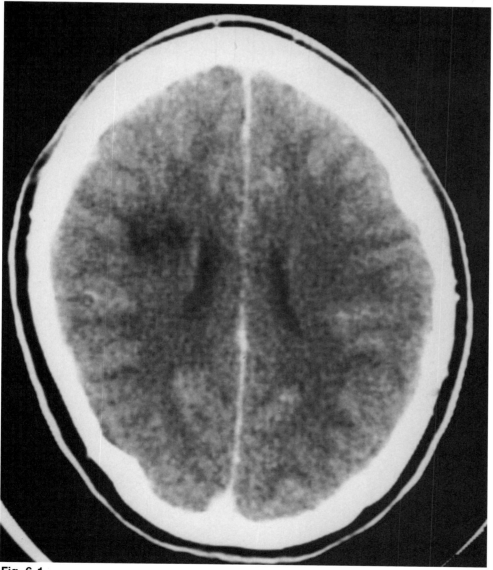

Fig. 6-1

(Continued)

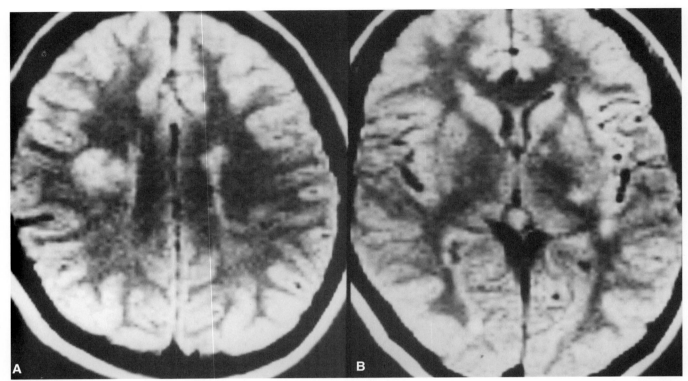

Fig. 6-2

Case 7

A 10-year-old boy who has had diabetes mellitus for 7 years is lethargic. Speech is slurred. He vomited yesterday and has had a backache since last night. He says that he is short of breath and it hurts to breathe.

Heart rate is 148, respiratory rate 30, and blood pressure 100/50 mm Hg. Eyes are sunken with dark circles. Cheeks are pink. Mouth is dry. The rest of the physical findings are normal.

Venus blood pH is 6.9, glucose 38.8 mmol/liter. Serum sodium is 126 mmol/liter, carbon dioxide 6, bicarbonate 5, and urea nitrogen 11.8. Creatinine is 200 μmol/liter.

He feels hot 2 hours after IV infusion of saline and insulin is begun. He is breathing more easily. He is restless at 3 hours, complains of headache, and falls into deep sleep. Blood glucose is 21.6 mmol/liter. At 4 hours, he vomits clear yellow liquid. At 7 hours, he does not respond when blood is taken. Blood glucose is 13.2 mmol/liter. At 9 hours, left pupil is sluggish and larger than right. At 11 hours, he is unresponsive.

Face is flushed. Breathing is slow and deep. Blood glucose is 10.9 mmol/liter, serum sodium 123, and potassium 4.4. He stops breathing 20 minutes later and is intubated. Pupils are 6 mm and fixed. Babinski's sign is in feet. At 15 hours, temperature is 37.2°C, heart rate 170, respiratory rate 15, and blood pressure 125/60 mm Hg. He moves his limbs and withdraws from pinprick. Left pupil is 3 mm and sluggish, right pupil 1.5 mm and reactive. He gags and tries to spit out endotracheal tube. Right leg is immobile, right arm nearly immobile a few hours later. Heart has premature ventricular contractions and bigeminal rhythm for a while the second day. He is lethargic and apathetic.

CT scan on the second day (Figure 7-1) shows small lateral ventricles and hypodense focus in right thalamus. T2-weighted MRI on the eighth day shows high signal in right thalamus in coronal (Figure 7-2A) and axial (Figure 7-2B) planes.

Diagnosis: Diabetic ketoacidosis; infarct, right thalamus.

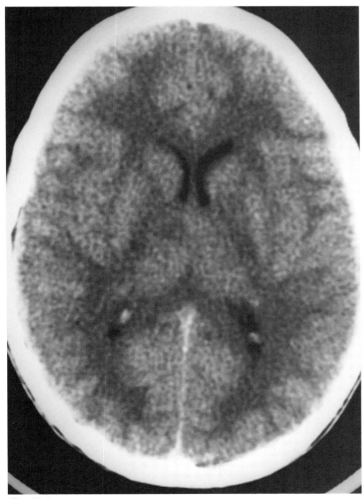

Fig. 7-1

(Continued)

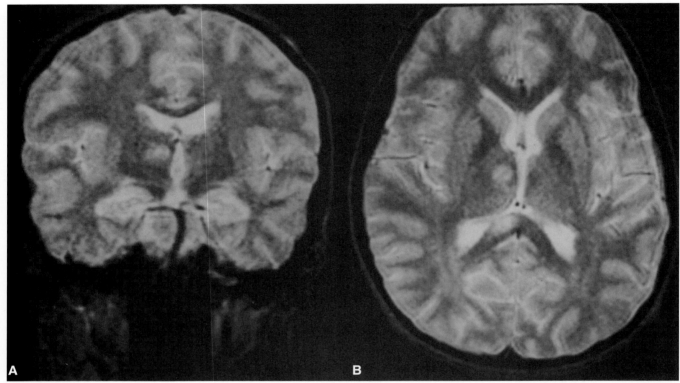

Fig. 7-2

Case 8

A newborn boy's heart rate has slowed from 130 to 40. He is limp, unresponsive, and breathing slowly. Blood glucose is 0. He is intubated and given oxygen and glucose.

Mother (29 years old) and father (36 years old) are well. He is their only child.

Apgar score is 4/8 at 1 and 5 minutes, weight 2 kg, length 42 cm, and head circumference 29 cm. Skin is yellow with purpuric spots (0.1–0.5 cm), like a blueberry muffin. He has circumoral cyanosis and acrocyanosis. Head is small and edematous. Back is arched. Liver edge is 4 cm below costal margin, spleen edge 2 cm. Blood comes from nose and endotracheal tube. The rest of the physical findings are normal.

Hematocrit at 1½ hours is 0.42. White cell count is 37.7 × 10^9/liter with 0.03 polymorphonuclear cells, 0.12 bands, 0.73 lymphocytes, 0.02 monocytes, 0.03 eosinophils, 0.05 metamyelocytes, 0.02 myelocytes, and 70 nucleated red cells/100 white cells. Platelet count is 478 × 10^9/liter (32 × 10^9/liter at 7 hours). At 1½ hours, serum sodium is 142 mmol/liter, potassium 2.7, chloride 97, carbon dioxide 22, urea nitrogen 4.3, calcium 3.04, phosphorus 0.48, cholesterol 1.80, and glucose 4.6. Creatinine is 90 μmol/liter, uric acid 420, total bilirubin 182, and direct bilirubin 88. Total protein is 47 g/liter, albumin 29. Alkaline phosphatase is 102 U/liter, SGOT 860.

Skull is small with intracranial calcification in Figure 8-1. CT scan in Figure 8-2 shows periventricular calcification.

Culture of urine and throat is positive for cytomegalovirus.

At necropsy, weight of liver is two times normal, spleen five times normal, and brain one-third times normal. Blood is clotted in stomach, mucosa hemorrhagic. Brain is soft. Sulci and gyri are immature. Lungs are dense, pleura and parenchyma purpuric. Microscopic examination shows immature lungs with thick, cellular alveolar walls and scattered hyaline membranes. Large epithelial cells with large nuclei and finely stippled basophilic inclusions surrounded by clear halos are found in bile ducts, pancreatic ducts, hepatocytes, and kidney tubules. Kidneys, lungs, and gastric mucosa are hemorrhagic.

Diagnosis: Congenital cytomegalovirus infection.

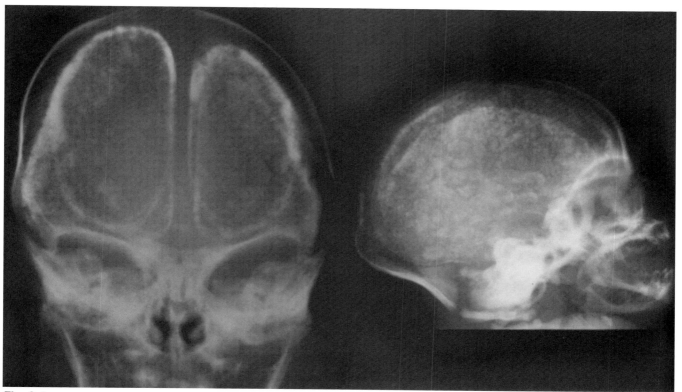

Fig. 8-1

(Continued)

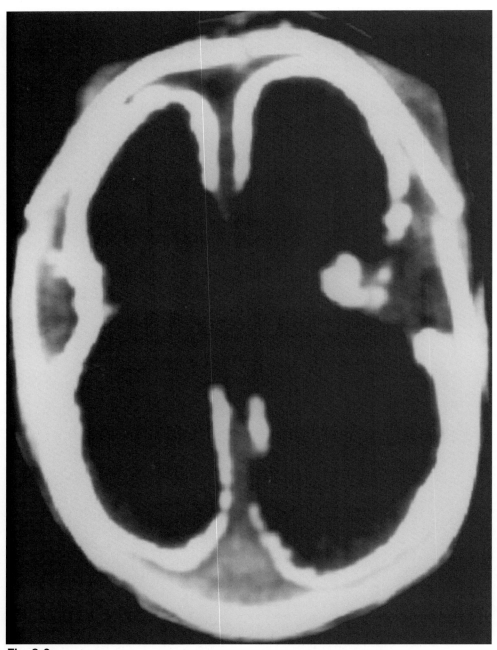

Fig. 8-2

Case 9

A 2½-year-old girl is convulsing. She cried out, hands twitched, and now twitching is generalized.

Mother (23 years old) and father (26 years old) are well. Mother had a miscarriage before the birth of their only child. Father has slight clumping of the infratemporal retinal pigment in the left eye.

Mother smoked a pack of cigarettes per day during pregnancy and bled from vagina during third trimester. Fetal heart rate was 60–90 during labor. Birth weight was 3.3 kg, length 49 cm, head circumference 34 cm, and Apgar score 9/9 at 1 and 5 minutes. Right eye turned out at 6 months. At 9 months, she had a respiratory infection; at 10 months she had otitis media. At 15 months, she had jerk nystagmus. She walked at 17 months. One side of her body twitched at 22 months. Eye examination at 27 months showed scar in the temporal part of each retina, abnormal exit of vessels from the discs, and right cataract and microcornea.

Temperature at 2½ years is 38.8°C, heart rate 150, respiratory rate 28, blood pressure 110/60 mm Hg, weight 11.4 kg, length 93 cm, and head circumference 45 cm. Hypopigmented spots are on back of arms and legs. The rest of the physical findings are normal.

Hematocrit is 0.38. White cell count is 7.0 × 10⁹/liter with 0.60 polymorphonuclear cells, 0.03 bands, 0.34 lymphocytes, 0.01 monocytes, and 0.02 eosinophils. Serum sodium is 132 mmol/liter, potassium 4.2, chloride 98, urea nitrogen 4.6, calcium 2.42, phosphorus 1.97, triglycerides 1.66, cholesterol 4.58, and glucose 9.9. Creatinine is 40 μmol/liter, uric acid 330, total bilirubin 3, direct bilirubin 0, and iron 6 (normal: 9.0–21.5). Total protein is 81 g/liter, albumin 48. Alkaline phosphatase is 186 U/liter, LDH 190, and SGOT 32. CSF is clear and colorless with 2 × 10⁶/liter white cells, no red cells, 0.16 g/liter protein, and 4.1 mmol/liter glucose.

Figure 9-1 shows deposits of calcium density in the brain.

Two weeks before the girl was born, mother's serologic titers for toxoplasmosis were IgM <1:10, IgG 2,040. Neonatal screening test for toxoplasmosis was negative. The girl's indirect hemagglutination titer for toxoplasmosis is 1:4,096 at presentation, IFA-IgM 0, and test for cytomegalovirus antibodies nonreactive.

The girl's IQ on Stanford-Binet test is 58 at 3 years, motor quotient 97.

Diagnosis: Toxoplasmosis.

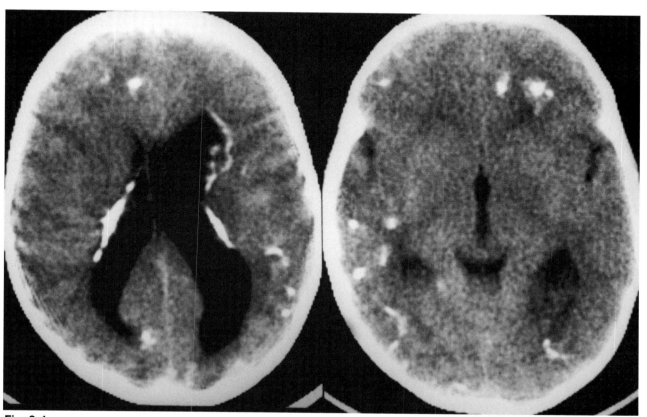

Fig. 9-1

Case 10

A 2½-year-old girl is unconscious.

She vomited blood 1 day ago and had loose stools. She acted as if she could not see this morning, screamed, and became unconscious. She vomited for several days last week. Her sister (4 years old), who is now well, vomited and had loose stools 3 days ago.

Temperature is 36.5°C and soon 40.5°C, heart rate 134, respiratory rate 32, blood pressure 72/40 mm Hg, and weight 10 kg. Right pupil is larger than left. Bowel sounds are absent. The rest of the physical findings are normal. Optic discs are blurred the next day.

Hematocrit is 0.38. White cell count is 12.7×10^9/liter with 0.59 polymorphonuclear cells, 0.03 bands, 0.37 lymphocytes, and 0.01 monocytes. Urine specific gravity is 1.025, pH 5. Urine has ketones and 2–5 white cells/HPF and >100 red cells/HPF. Serum sodium is 143 mmol/liter, potassium 4.7, chloride 106, carbon dioxide 6, calcium 2.40, phosphorus 2.30, and glucose 3.4. Alkaline phosphatase is 183 U/liter, SGOT 66. Serum complement fixation titers are herpes simplex virus 1:32, influenza A <1:8, influenza B <1:8, and varicella-zoster <1:8.

CT scan after IV injection of contrast medium shows small ventricles (Figure 10-1).

Brain herniates when dura is incised at craniotomy.

CSF has 2×10^6/liter white cells, 0.70 lymphocytes and 0.30 monocytes, $<1 \times 10^6$/liter red cells, 11.1 mmol/liter glucose, and 0.19 g/liter protein.

Brain biopsy shows normal microscopic findings and positive direct fluorescent antibody stains for herpes simplex antigen. Culture of throat and brain grows herpes simplex virus 1.

Diagnosis: Herpes simplex 1 encephalitis.

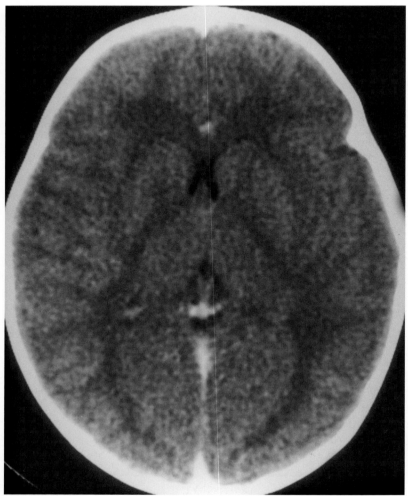

Fig. 10-1

Case 11

An 18-day-old boy has a bulging anterior fontanel.

He cried and refused breast-feeding 9 hours ago, was irritable, and then cried shrilly and jerked as if "someone had stabbed him." He has had loose stools.

Pregnancy of mother was normal, birth weight 3.7 kg. At 13 days, weight was 3.8 kg.

Temperature at 18 days is 40.1°C, heart rate 180 with occasional slowing, respiratory rate 48 and irregular, and systolic blood pressure 80 mm Hg. He is alternately irritable and moaning or lethargic. Eyes are open, pupils small. Neck is not stiff. Legs are flexed at hips. Reflexes are hyperactive. The rest of the physical findings are normal.

Hematocrit is 0.54. White cell count is 4.7×10^9/liter. Blood glucose is 8.0 mmol/liter. CSF is cloudy yellow with 358×10^6/liter white cells (almost all polymorphonuclear), 5.68 g/liter protein, and no glucose. Gram's stain of CSF shows gram-positive cocci in pairs and chains. Fluorescent antibody test is positive for group B streptococci.

In Figure 11-1, anterior fontanel is bulging, coronal sutures are wide.

Diagnosis: Group B β-hemolytic streptococcal meningitis (*Streptococcus agalactiae*).

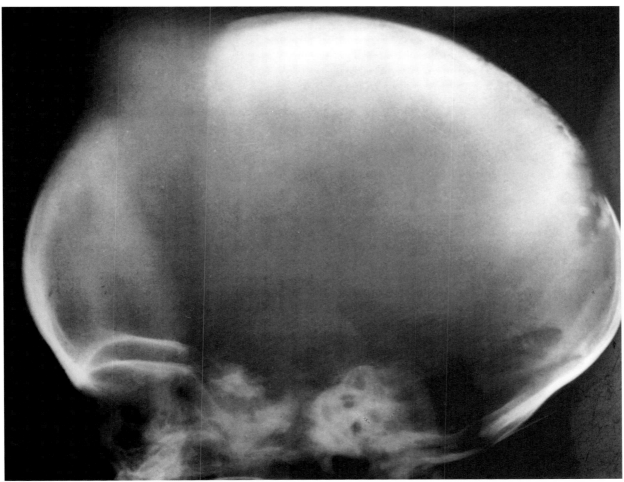

Fig. 11-1

Case 12

An 8-month-old girl is lethargic and febrile.

She has had a cough and runny nose for 6 days and has been treated with amoxicillin for 2 days.

Mother (19 years old) is well.

Temperature is 38.9°C, heart rate 160, respiratory rate 30, systolic blood pressure 74 mm Hg, weight 8.2 kg, and length 66 cm. She lies still with neck extended, follows with her eyes, and cries when moved. She has a moist cough. Limbs are pale. Kernig's and Brudzinski's signs are present. Eardrums are dull red. The rest of the physical findings are normal.

Hematocrit is 0.30. White cell count is 6.7×10^9/liter with 0.53 polymorphonuclear cells, 0.08 bands, 0.30 lymphocytes, and 0.09 monocytes. Platelet count is 100×10^9/liter. Serum sodium is 144 mmol/liter, potassium 4.2, chloride 99, carbon dioxide 29, urea nitrogen 4.3, and glucose 5.3. CSF has no red cells, 8.6×10^9/liter white cells, all polymorphonuclear, 0.2 mmol/liter glucose, 3.75 g/liter protein, and pleomorphic gram-negative rods. Urine specific gravity is 1.010 the next day, pH 5. Urine has trace ketones, 0.03 g/liter protein, urobilinogen, 3–6 white cells/HPF, occasional red cells/HPF, 0–3 squamous epithelial cells/HPF, mucus, and amorphous matter. Culture of CSF and blood grows *Haemophilus influenzae* B, β-lactamase positive.

Fever to 38.9–39.4°C and stiff neck persist. She has a seizure on the fourth day.

On the seventh day, CSF has 3×10^6/liter white cells, 0.98 lymphocytes, 1.2 mmol/liter glucose, 2.2 g/liter protein, and is sterile.

On the tenth day, CT scan shows subdural fluid in Figure 12-1A and enhancing rim in Figure 12-1B.

She is afebrile and well on the twelfth day.

Diagnosis: Meningitis, *H. influenzae* type B infection, and subdural effusion.

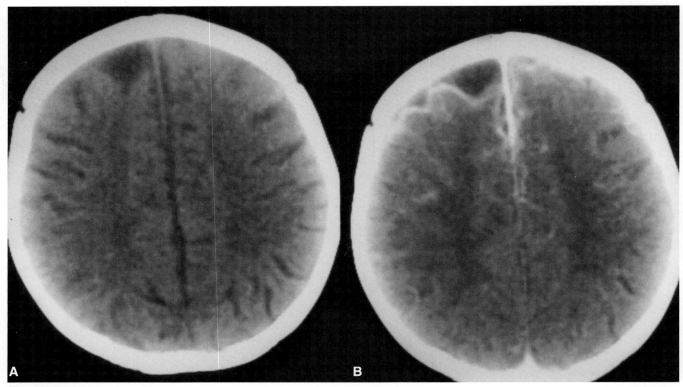

Fig. 12-1

Case 13

A 6-month-old girl has been vomiting and sleeping a lot for 3 days. She was fussy last night.

Birth weight was 3.5 kg, length 51 cm, and head circumference 35 cm. She smiled at 1 month. She is breast-fed. Weight at 5 months was 5.3 kg, length 62 cm.

Mother (24 years old) is well. The girl is her only child.

Weight at 6 months is 5.0 kg, length 64 cm, head circumference 42 cm, temperature 37.6°C, heart rate 140, and respiratory rate 44. She is thin and pale. Lips are dry. The rest of the physical findings are normal.

Hematocrit is 0.34. White cell count is 20.8×10^9/liter with 0.74 polymorphonuclear cells, 0.10 bands, 0.12 lymphocytes, and 0.04 monocytes. Urine specific gravity is 1.018, pH 6. Urine has 1+ ketones, trace reducing substances, few squamous epithelial cells/HPF, and many amorphous urates. Serum sodium is 143 mmol/liter, potassium 4.6, chloride 102, carbon dioxide 21, urea nitrogen 3.2, calcium 2.69, phosphorus 1.19, cholesterol 5.40, and glucose 8.0. Creatinine is 50 μmol/liter, uric acid 360, total bilirubin 3, and direct bilirubin 2. Total protein is 79 g/liter, albumin 46. Alkaline phosphatase is 156 U/liter, LDH 300, and SGOT 19.

She has seizures that last less than 30 seconds on the second day. She stiffens, left arm trembles, eyes turn left. Systolic blood pressure is 108 mm Hg. Liver edge is 2 cm below costal margin. CSF has 32×10^6/liter white cells, 0.07 polymorphonuclear cells, 0.57 lymphocytes, 0.36 pia-arachnoid cells, 1.0 mmol/liter glucose, and 1.00 g/liter protein. Serum sodium is 123 mmol/liter, glucose 9.8. Serum osmolality is 247 mmol/kg, urine 283.

Supracardiac shadow is widened in Figure 13-1.

On the third day, left eye turns downward and inward; she moves left limbs less than right. On the sixth day, anterior fontanel is bulging; left Babinski's sign is present.

On the sixth day, CT scan in Figure 13-2 shows dilation of lateral and third ventricles.

Serum sodium ranges from 128 to 133 mmol/liter from the fourth to twelfth days. Although parents are tuberculin-negative the tenth day, her treatment with antituberculous drugs is begun. CSF culture grows *Mycobacterium tuberculosis* the thirtieth day.

Her father's friend, who visited the family often 2 months ago, is hospitalized for tuberculosis the twelfth day. Father (32 years old) has not felt well for a month and coughs up sputum. He is tuberculin-negative, mother tuberculin-positive the thirty-second day. He has lost weight. His physical findings are normal. His sputum has acid-fast bacilli the thirty-second day.

Chest roentgenogram of father the twenty-seventh day (Figure 13-3) shows nodules of water density in right lung and a shadow of calcium density in mid–left lung at level of pulmonary artery.

Diagnosis: Tuberculous basal meningitis in daughter, pulmonary tuberculosis in father and family friend, questionable recent skin test conversion in mother.

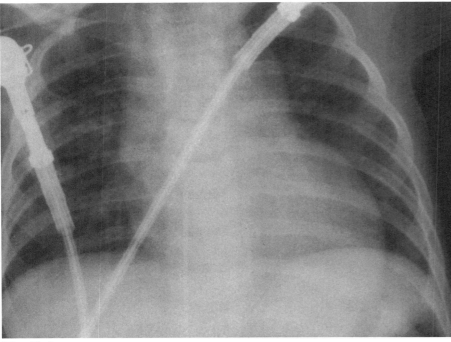

Fig. 13-1

(Continued)

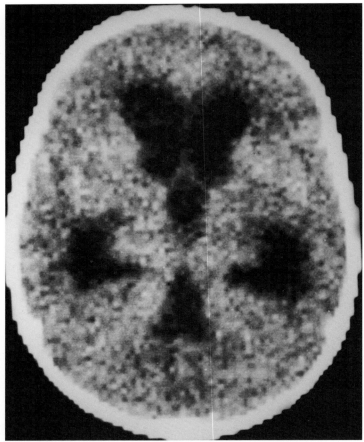

Fig. 13-2

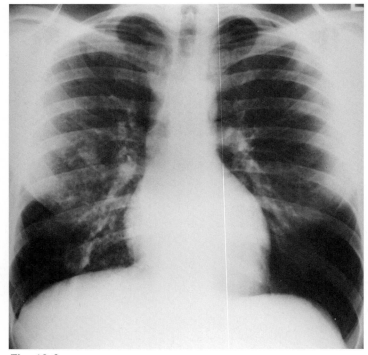

Fig. 13-3

Case 14

A 3-year-old boy is febrile, vomiting, and has had diarrhea for 10 days.

Mother and two siblings (9 months and 6 years old) are well. Father, who used drugs, was murdered 3 months ago.

Weight at 3 years is 11.1 kg, temperature 39.5°C, heart rate 112, and respiratory rate 24. Eyes are sunken. The rest of the physical findings are normal.

Hematocrit is 0.34; white cell count is 11.5×10^9/liter with a "normal differential," according to admitting hospital. Urine is "normal." Admission SMAC is "normal." Roentgenogram of chest shows "normal" findings.

He looks very ill on second day. Right pupil is dilated for 15 minutes.

CT scan in Figure 14-1 shows focus of high attenuation in right occipital lobe and foci of low attenuation elsewhere and enhancement after IV injection of contrast medium.

At operation, dura is tight over right occipital lobe until more IV mannitol is given. A firm mass ($2.2 \times 2 \times 0.9$ cm) is removed from right occipital lobe.

Microscopic examination of the grayish-white to pale-yellow mass shows lymphocytes, plasma cells, multinucleated giant cells, necrosis, and adjacent reactive gliosis. Stains show acid-fast bacilli.

Diagnosis: Tuberculous granulomatous inflammation in occipital lobe with caseation.

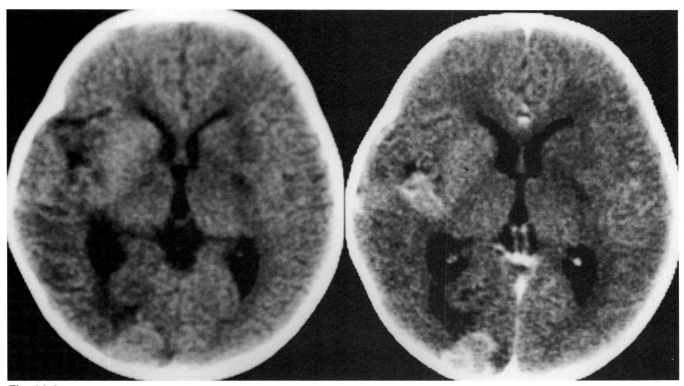

Fig. 14-1

Case 15

A 6-day-old girl is febrile. She cried a lot last night and had watery stools. Her twin is well.

Birth weight was 2.8 kg. Total bilirubin at 5 days was 203 μmol/liter. Temperature at 6 days is 38.3°C, heart rate 180, respiratory rate 48, blood pressure 75/53 mm Hg, and weight 2.7 kg. Left arm twitches briefly. The rest of the physical findings are normal.

Hematocrit at 6 days is 0.56. White cell count is 27.3 × 10^9/liter with 0.62 polymorphonuclear cells, 0.02 bands, 0.26 lymphocytes, and 0.10 monocytes. Urine specific gravity is 1.015, pH 7.5. Urine is normal. CSF is cloudy yellow with 3.6 × 10^9/liter white cells, 0.74 polymorphonuclear cells, 0.10 lymphocytes, 0.16 monocytes, 450 × 10^6/liter red cells, no glucose, and 3.20 g/liter protein. Gram's and India ink stains are negative. Serum sodium is 136 mmol/liter, potassium 5.3, chloride 100, carbon dioxide 35, calcium 2.32, urea nitrogen 3.6, and glucose 4.7. Creatinine is 40 μmol/liter, total bilirubin 210, and direct bilirubin 19.

She is given antibiotics. She is alert and afebrile at 7 days. Culture of umbilicus and CSF at 8 days shows *Citrobacter diversus*. Blood culture is sterile.

At 28 days, she is afebrile and alert. A hemangioma is on right arm. Small purple spots are present on left upper lid, back of head, and groin. The rest of the physical findings are normal.

CSF is clear at 28 days and has 15 × 10^6/liter white cells, 0.41 lymphocytes, 0.57 monocytes, 0.02 polymorphonuclear cells, 2 × 10^6/liter red cells, 1.6 mmol/liter glucose, and 0.79 g/liter protein. ESR is 12 mm/hr.

CT scan at 28 days shows a round, well-defined hypodense focus in left frontal lobe and hypodense rim behind the focus (Figure 15-1). Ultrasound examination at 30 days (Figure 15-2) shows the left frontal mass and a smaller cyst and debris behind it.

Thick yellow pus is aspirated from the mass at 31 days. Cultures for bacteria, including *Mycobacterium tuberculosis*, and fungi are sterile.

Diagnosis: Meningitis, *C. diversus*; brain abscess.

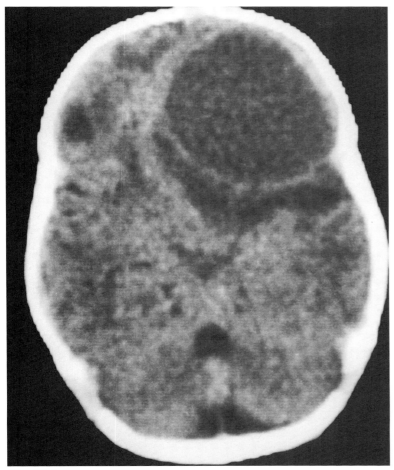

Fig. 15-1

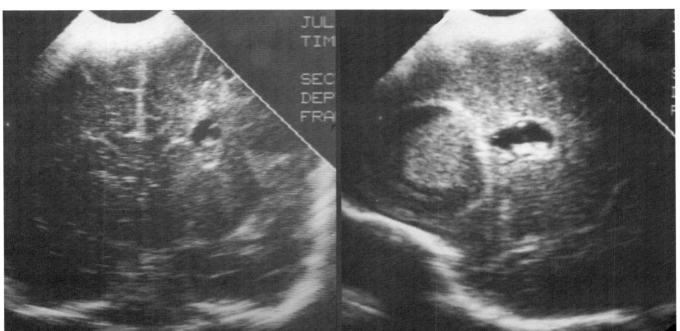

Fig. 15-2

Case 16

A 10-year-old boy has a headache and is vomiting, confused, and feverish.

Headaches began 9 months ago, after he fell and hit his head. They used to occur every 3 weeks and sometimes lasted all day. He has had this one for 2 weeks.

Temperature at 10 years is 38.9°C, blood pressure 122/70 mm Hg, and breathing slow and shallow. Neck is stiff. The rest of the physical findings are normal. Skin test for tuberculosis is negative.

CSF has 5.0×10^9/liter white cells, 0.88 polymorphonuclear, 1.6 mmol/liter glucose, and 0.76 g/liter protein. Cultures, stains, and counterimmune electrophoresis are negative.

CT scan shows hypodensity in left parieto-occipital region (Figure 16-1A) and ring enhancement after IV injection of contrast medium (Figure 16-1B).

He was right-handed before the illness and is left-handed after it, at 11 years. Weight at 11 years is 38 kg, height 139 cm, temperature 37°C, heart rate 104, respiratory rate 18, and blood pressure 100/66 mm Hg. Right arm and leg are weak. Position sense in right foot is diminished. The rest of the physical findings are normal.

Hematocrit at 11 years is 0.46. White cell count is 8.9×10^9/liter with 0.45 polymorphonuclear cells, 0.04 bands, 0.46 lymphocytes, 0.02 monocytes, and 0.03 eosinophils. Platelet count is 398×10^9/liter. Arterial blood pH is 7.39 when F_{IO_2} = 0.20. P_{CO_2} is 35 mm Hg, P_{O_2} 69.

Cardiac catheterization and angiocardiogram show anomalous pulmonary venous drainage, left superior vena cava, and atrial septal defect. At operation, four veins from left upper lobe drain into left superior vena cava and a defect (2 × 2 cm) is found in atrial septum at entrance of right superior vena cava.

Diagnosis: Brain abscess, right-to-left shunt through atrial septal defect.

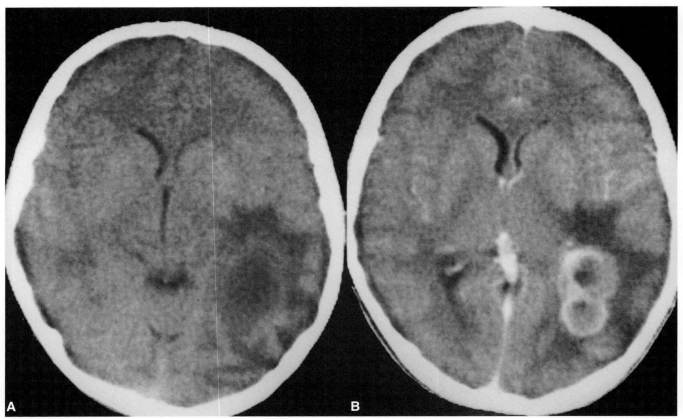

Fig. 16-1

Case 17

A 2-month-old boy has a big head and "strange eye movements." He vomited twice yesterday.

Mother (17 years old) took an antibiotic for bronchitis during fourth month of pregnancy. She bled from the vagina during seventh month. Delivery was by cesarean section for hypertension.

Birth weight was 2.9 kg, length 50 cm, head circumference 34 cm, and Apgar score 8/9 at 1 and 5 minutes.

Temperature at 2 months is 36°C, heart rate 148, respiratory rate 36, blood pressure 120/73 mm Hg, weight 5.3 kg, length 58 cm, and head circumference 45 cm. He cries or whimpers. Cry is high pitched. Eyes deviate downward. Anterior fontanel bulges. Sagittal suture is 1 cm wide. The rest of the physical findings are normal.

Hematocrit is 0.31. White cell count is 10.7×10^9/liter with 0.39 polymorphonuclear cells, 0.03 bands, 0.49 lymphocytes, 0.05 monocytes, 0.02 eosinophils, 0.01 atypical lymphocytes, and 0.01 metamyelocytes. Platelet count is 684×10^9/liter. Serum sodium is 139 mmol/liter, potassium 5.4, chloride 101,

carbon dioxide 20, urea nitrogen 3.2, calcium 2.59, phosphorus 1.94, cholesterol 3.93, and glucose 8.3. Creatinine is 40 µmol/liter, uric acid 190, total bilirubin 8, and direct bilirubin 3. Total protein is 62 g/liter, albumin 44. Alkaline phosphatase is 329 U/liter, LDH 359, and SGOT 73. CSF is clear and sterile with 15×10^6/liter red cells, 2×10^6/liter white cells, 0.01 polymorphonuclear cells, 0.09 lymphocytes, 0.83 monocytes, 0.06 macrophages, 0.01 atypical lymphocytes, 2.1 mmol/liter glucose, and 0.26 g/liter protein.

Ventricles and cisterns are dilated in Figure 17-1A. A lobed mass that enhances after IV injection of contrast medium is in left lateral ventricle (Figure 17-1B).

At operation, dura bulges until 80 ml CSF is removed. A lobed, friable mass with granular surface is in left lateral ventricle.

Microscopic examination shows papillae with thin fibrovascular cores lined by cells with pink cytoplasm and oval nuclei. Loose connective tissue thickens the core in places.

Diagnosis: Papilloma of choroid plexus.

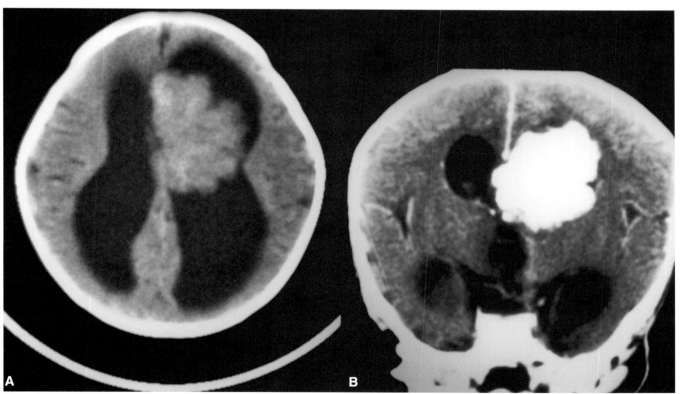

Fig. 17-1

Case 18

A 2-year-old girl, who has asthma and is wheezing, convulses in the emergency room. She looks over left shoulder, drops a toy from limp left hand, and loses consciousness. Treatment with theophylline was started 2 days ago. She vomited this morning.

Birth weight was 3.4 kg, Apgar score 8/9 at 1 and 5 minutes. She had a seizure at 2 weeks, another at 1 year when she had fever. She has had ear infections. Asthma was diagnosed a year ago.

Mother (29 years old) takes thyroid pills. An older sibling is well.

Temperature at 2 years is 36.6°C, heart rate 160–175, respiratory rate 46, blood pressure 104/50 mm Hg, and weight 11 kg. Right pupil is larger than left. Both pupils react slowly to light. Eardrums are dull. She moves right arm and leg from pinprick but not left. The rest of the physical findings are normal. She has another seizure. Head and eyes turn left, teeth chew, limbs jerk. Pupils are pinpoint.

Hematocrit is 0.40. White cell count is 9.5×10^9/liter with 0.68 polymorphonuclear cells, 0.12 bands, 0.16 lymphocytes, and 0.04 monocytes. Platelet count is 237×10^9/liter. Serum sodium is 134 mmol/liter, potassium 3.8, chloride 101, carbon dioxide 19, urea nitrogen 1.4, calcium 2.25, phosphorus 1.23, and glucose 5.4. Creatinine is 40 μmol/liter, theophylline 72 (normal therapeutic range: 55–110).

CT scan in Figure 18-1 shows a calcified, enhancing mass in right cerebral hemisphere.

At operation, a firm, encapsulated tumor (4 × 3 cm) is in right lateral ventricle.

Surface is gray-tan to gray-brown on outside, white in cut-section, and gritty. Microscopic examination shows uniform interlacing fascicles of fibrocytes, thick bands of collagen, psammoma bodies, hyalinized acellular foci, and islands of gliotic brain tissue.

Diagnosis: Meningioma.

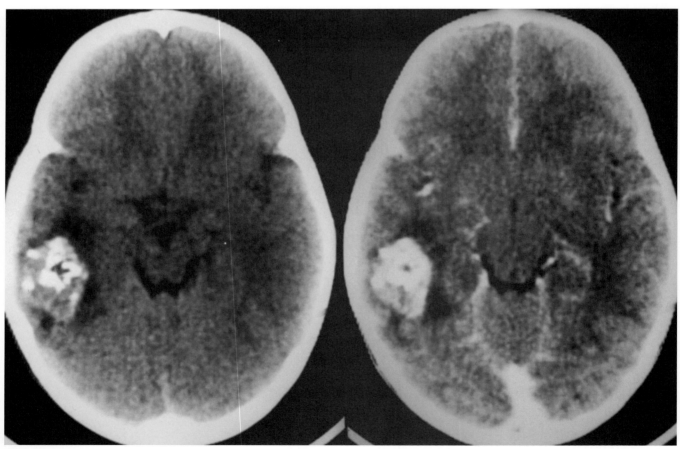

Fig. 18-1

Case 19

A 9-year-old boy is clumsy and dull.

Mother bled from vagina in midpregnancy and was given diazepam, doxylamine-pyridoxine, aspirin, meperidine, and menadione sodium diphosphate. Birth weight was 2.6 kg. He was blue. Large red-purple marks were present on shanks and feet. Feeding was hard, sleeping unpredictable. He cried a lot, had temper tantrums, and showed little response to parents. He sat at 9 months and walked and used single words at 2 years. He had a convulsion at 6 years. Limbs jerked, left side of face twitched, eyes turned downward to the right, and teeth clenched for several minutes. He overeats, wets his pants, forgets things, fears new places and new people, and cannot find or pronounce words.

Mother (32 years old), father (33 years old), sister (12 years old), and brother (2 years old) are well. Maternal grandmother had cancer of uterus; paternal grandfather had a heart attack and paternal grandmother had high blood pressure.

Temperature at 9 years is 36°C, heart rate 68, respiratory rate 16, blood pressure 90/58 mm Hg, weight 34 kg, and height 126 cm. He has bitemporal hemianopsia, hyperactive deep tendon reflexes, and hemangiomas on shanks and feet. The rest of the physical findings are normal.

Hematocrit is 0.37. White cell count is 4.9×10^9/liter with 0.48 polymorphonuclear cells, 0.01 bands, 0.42 lymphocytes, 0.07 monocytes, and 0.02 eosinophils. Urine specific gravity is 1.030, pH 7. Urine is normal. Serum sodium is 139 mmol/liter, potassium 4.1, chloride 107, carbon dioxide 24, urea nitrogen 4.3, calcium 2.20, phosphorus 1.58, cholesterol 5.87, and glucose 5.9. Creatinine is 40 µmol/liter, uric acid 140, total bilirubin 3, and direct bilirubin 0. Total protein is 66 g/liter, albumin 42. Alkaline phosphatase is 328 U/liter, LDH 206, and SGOT 25.

CT scan after injection of contrast medium into lateral ventricle shows dilated lateral ventricles and forward displacement of compressed third ventricle by cyst that does not contain contrast medium (Figure 19-1).

At craniotomy, a cyst with clear liquid is in the middle cranial fossa under internal carotid arteries and optic chiasm.

Wall of the cyst is pale tan. Microscopic examination shows dense collagen.

Diagnosis: Arachnoid cyst, middle cranial fossa.

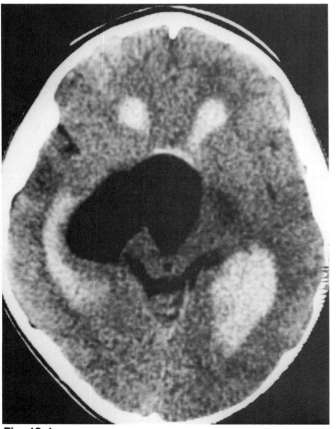

Fig. 19-1

Case 20

A 5-year-old boy is growing too fast. He has had body odor for 6 months, pubic hair for 4 months.

Pregnancy of mother was normal, birth weight 3.3 kg, length 51 cm.

Mother, father, sister (13 years old), and brother (9 years old) are well. Members of father's family have had brain, lung, and stomach cancer.

Temperature at 5 years is 36°C, heart rate 104, respiratory rate 16, blood pressure 86/48 mm Hg, height 125 cm, and weight 32 kg. He has small pubic hairs. Volume of each testis is 5 cm³. The rest of the physical findings are normal.

Hematocrit is 0.40. White cell count is 6.7 × 10⁹/liter with 0.41 polymorphonuclear cells, 0.01 bands, 0.49 lymphocytes, 0.06 monocytes, and 0.03 eosinophils. Platelet count is 303 × 10⁹/liter. Urine specific gravity is 1.019, pH 7. Urine is nor-

mal. Serum sodium is 139 mmol/liter, potassium 4.5, chloride 110, urea nitrogen 6.1, and glucose 5.6. Serum FSH is <2 U/liter (normal: 1–3), LH 6 (normal: 1–5). Serum testosterone is 8.47 nmol/liter (normal: <0.35). CSF has 2 × 10⁶/liter white cells, <1 × 10⁶/liter red cells, 3.6 mmol/liter glucose, and 0.24 g/liter protein.

Dorsum sellae is partly eroded; pneumatization of sphenoid sinus is advanced in Figure 20-1. CT scan in Figure 20-2 shows a spherical mass in interpeduncular cistern.

At operation, retraction of right frontal and temporal lobes exposes a tan mass behind optic chiasm.

Microscopic examination shows astrocytes, neurons, glial nodules, and small blood vessels.

Diagnosis: Neuroglial hamartoma.

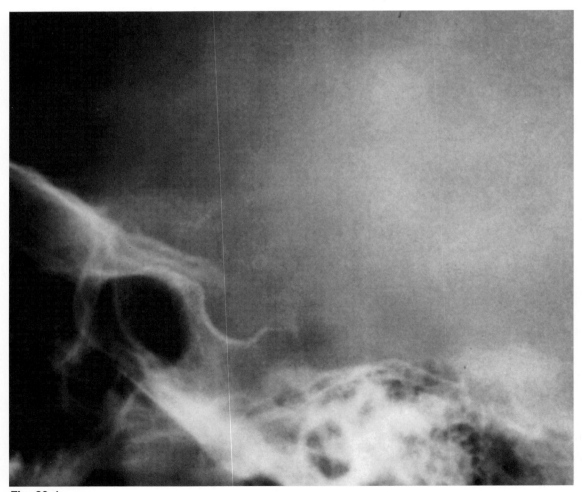

Fig. 20-1

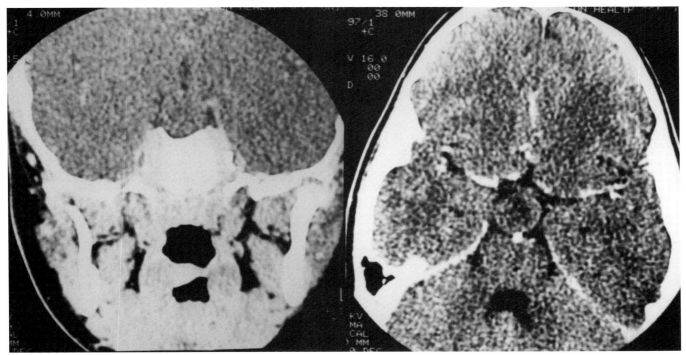

Fig. 20-2

Case 21

A 4-year-old girl is nearly blind, has headaches, and just lies around.

At 3 years, she began to bump into things. She stopped watching TV and looking at picture books. She held things close to her eyes.

Birth weight was 2.7 kg. She began to walk at 9 months. She has had otitis media several times.

Mother has epilepsy and asthma. Sister (2 years old) wheezes. A maternal aunt was born with a cataract and is weak.

Temperature at 4 years is 36.4°C, heart rate 116, respiratory rate 24, blood pressure 106/86 mm Hg, height 102 cm, and weight 16 kg. She cries when left eye is covered. She has horizontal nystagmus. Right optic disc is pale. Fluid is present behind the ear drums. Left side of face sags. Tongue deviates to left when she sticks it out. The rest of the physical findings are normal.

Hematocrit is 0.42. White cell count is 14.3×10^9/liter with 0.70 polymorphonuclear cells, 0.22 lymphocytes, 0.02 basophils, and 0.06 monocytes. Platelet count is 697×10^9/liter. ESR is 5 mm/hr. Urine specific gravity is 1.029, pH 6. Urine is normal. Serum osmolality is 0.284 mmol/kg. Serum sodium is 0.138 mmol/liter, potassium 4.8, chloride 105, carbon dioxide 20, urea nitrogen 5.4, calcium 2.39, phosphorus 1.61, cholesterol 4.97, and glucose 4.6. Creatinine is 40 μmol/liter, uric acid 170, total bilirubin 7, and direct bilirubin 0. Total protein is 65 g/liter, albumin 41. Alkaline phosphatase is 154 U/liter, LDH 350, and SGOT 19. T_4 is 127 nmol/liter (normal: 51–142), cortisol 830 at 8:00 AM (normal: 110–520) and 340 at 4:00 PM (normal: 50–410 at 6:00 PM). CSF has 2×10^6/liter white cells, 252×10^6/liter red cells, 5.5 mmol/liter glucose, and 0.11 g/liter protein.

Sutures are widened front to back in diminishing degree; dorsum sellae is eroded (Figure 21-1). Plaques of calcium density are above the sella turcica. CT scan after IV injection of contrast medium shows dilated lateral ventricles and a round mass with enhanced rim in middle cranial fossa (Figure 21-2).

At operation, a tumor is found under optic chiasm and between optic nerves.

The tumor is brown and contains brown liquid. Microscopic examination shows anastomosing cords of plump elongated cells with basophilic, hyperchromatic nuclei, scattered foci of stellate stroma, focal squamous metaplasia, and deposits of calcium.

Diagnosis: Craniopharyngioma.

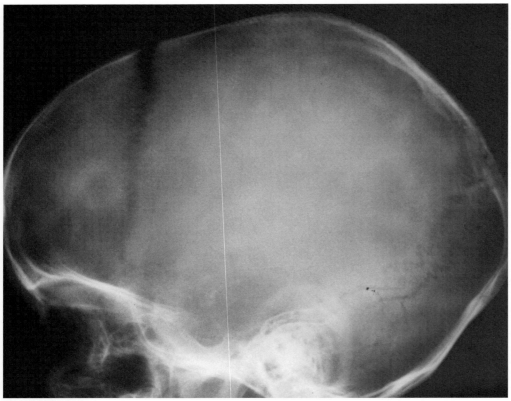

Fig. 21-1

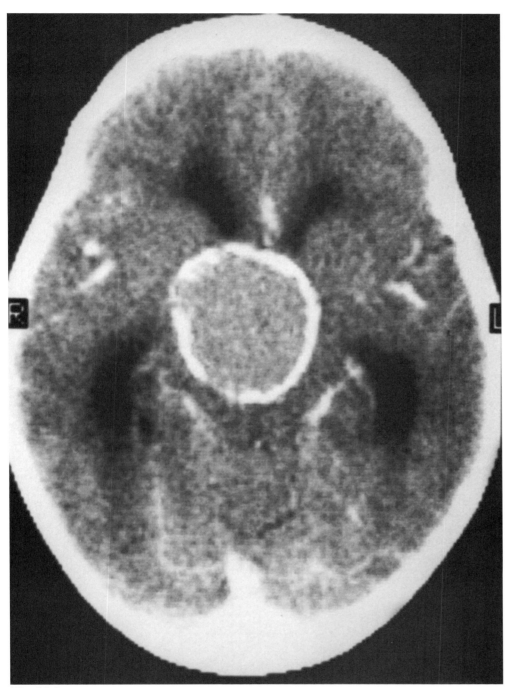

Fig. 21-2

Case 22

A 15-year-old girl has frontal headaches.

Headaches began at 12 years, often lasting 24 hours. They were several months apart when they started; they are now 2 weeks apart. She used to be happy and outgoing; she has been grouchy and moody for 3 years. During the past year she has had boils that took weeks to heal. She has not begun to menstruate.

Paternal grandmother and maternal grandfather are hypertensive. A cousin has diabetes mellitus.

Temperature at 15 years is 37.4°C, heart rate 52, respiratory rate 16, blood pressure 112/88 mm Hg, weight 60.4 kg, and height 144 cm. She is short and fat. Cheeks are fat. Chin is pimpled. Sparse, dark hair is on cheeks, chin, and limbs. Pads of fat are above clavicles. Breast areolae are raised and have fine black hairs. Belly is fat. Striae are on thighs, upper arms, and around umbilicus. External genitalia are mature. Pubis is hairy. A draining sore is on coccyx. Limbs are thin. Knuckles are dark. The rest of the physical findings are normal.

Hematocrit is 0.45. White cell count is 8.9×10^9/liter with 0.64 polymorphonuclear cells, 0.03 bands, 0.21 lymphocytes, 0.09 monocytes, 0.02 eosinophils, and 0.01 atypical lymphocytes. Platelet count is 277×10^9/liter. Urine specific gravity is 1.020, pH 5. Urine has urobilinogen, leukocyte esterase, mucus, amorphous phosphates, 3–6 white cells/HPF and few squamous epithelial cells/HPF. Serum sodium is 147 mmol/liter, potassium 4.4, chloride 103, carbon dioxide 29, urea nitrogen 5.7, calcium 2.35, phosphorus 1.16, cholesterol 4.84, and glucose 5.2. Creatinine is 80 μmol/liter, uric acid 400, total bilirubin 10, and direct bilirubin 2. Total protein is 75 g/liter, albumin 49. Alkaline phosphatase is 53 U/liter,

LDH 446, and SGOT 52. Plasma corticotropin is 20 pmol/liter (normal: 4–22). Serum cortisol is 970 nmol/liter in early morning (normal: 110–520), 860 in evening (normal: 50–410), and, after injection of 1.8 mg dexamethasone every 6 hours for 2 days, it is 480. Urine free cortisol is 1,320, 1,420, and 1,660 nmol/day (normal: 30–300). Urine 17-hydroxycorticosteroids, six determinations, range from 28.7 to 64.0 μmol/day (normal: 5.5–22.1). Urine 17-ketosteroids, six determinations, range from 36 to 59 μmol/day (normal: 17–42). Serum cortisol increases from basal level of 710 to maximum 1,050 nmol/liter 30 minutes after IV injection of 100 μg corticotropin-releasing factor. Free T_4 is 23 pmol/liter (normal: 10–36), prolactin <0.2 nmol/liter (normal: 0.08–0.60). Culture of drainage from sore on coccyx grows coagulase-negative staphylococcus, *Propionibacterium* species, *Corynebacterium* species, and *Bacteroides melaninogenicus*.

Pituitary fossa is enlarged in Figure 22-1. MRI in Figure 22-2A shows mass with enhancing rim in pituitary fossa. Top of mass is separate from optic chiasm in Figure 22-2.

At transsphenoidal operation, cottage cheese–like matter and clotted blood are released when tense dura in pituitary fossa is incised. Posterior lobe of pituitary gland is displaced upward and backward, anterior lobe forward.

Microscopic examination of the material removed shows proteinaceous material, blood, connective tissue, normal pituitary gland, aggregates of chromophobe cells with high nucleus-to-cytoplasm ratio, and basophils intermixed with normal pituitary tissue.

Diagnosis: Pituitary adenoma, Cushing's disease.

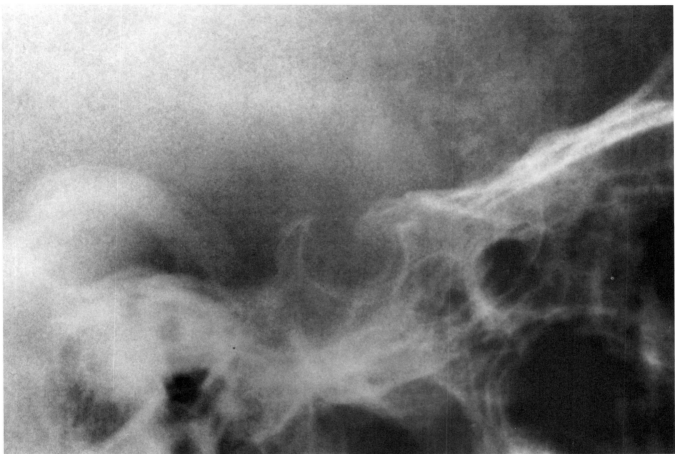

Fig. 22-1

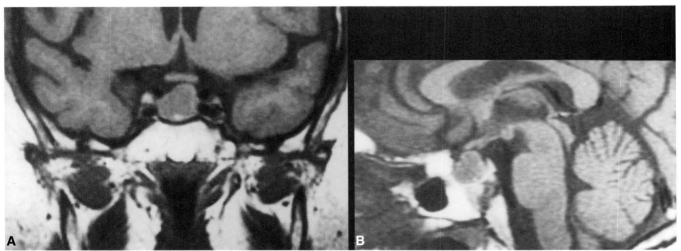

A   B

Fig. 22-2

Case 23

A 10½-year-old boy, who eats little, skips dinner, and sleeps 12–14 hours a day, is hoarse, constipated, and "lazy."

Parents began to worry when he stopped outgrowing his clothes at 8 years. Skin was dry and scaly at 10 years. Sores were slow to heal. School grades are good except for physical education.

Pregnancy of mother was normal, birth weight 3.2 kg. He was so active until 4 years that mother said, "If this were our first child, we would never have had any more." Height at 5 years was at fiftieth percentile, tenth percentile at 8 years, and below third percentile at 9½ years.

Mother (43 years old) has idiopathic pancytopenia and began treatment for hypothyroidism 8 years ago. Father (45 years old), three sisters (22, 14, and 7 years old), and brother (17 years old) are well. Paternal grandmother had pernicious anemia; a maternal uncle who had diabetes mellitus died at age 20. Paternal grandmother, grandfather, and uncle had cancer.

Weight at 10½ years is 32 kg, height 122 cm, temperature 35.9°C, heart rate 68, respiratory rate 16, and blood pressure 108/70 mm Hg. He is stocky and alert. Hair is coarse, sparse, and brittle; skin is dry, scaly, and cool, and tongue is large.

Mucous membranes are pale. Deep tendons react briskly and relax slowly. The rest of the physical findings are normal.

Hematocrit is 0.32. White cell count is 5.3×10^9/liter with 0.35 polymorphonuclear cells, 0.13 bands, 0.39 lymphocytes, 0.07 monocytes, 0.05 eosinophils, and 0.01 basophils. Platelet estimate is adequate. ESR is 6 mm/hr. Urine specific gravity is 1.019, pH 6. Urine has occasional white cells/HPF. Serum sodium is 139 mmol/liter, potassium 4.7, chloride 105, carbon dioxide 25, urea nitrogen 8.2, cholesterol 7.43, triglycerides 1.41, and glucose 4.7.

Pituitary fossa is enlarged and groove of a normal sphenoparietal sinus is prominent between coronal suture and pituitary fossa (Figure 23-1A). Bone age in left hand is about 6 years, 4–5 SDs below the mean (Figure 23-1B).

Serum T_3 resin uptake is 22 AU (normal: 24–32), total T_4 10 nmol/liter (normal: 83–172), TSH >120 mU/liter (normal: <10), thyroglobulin antibodies 1:100, and thyroid microsomal antibodies 1:1,600.

Diagnosis: Primary hypothyroidism; secondary pituitary hyperplasia.

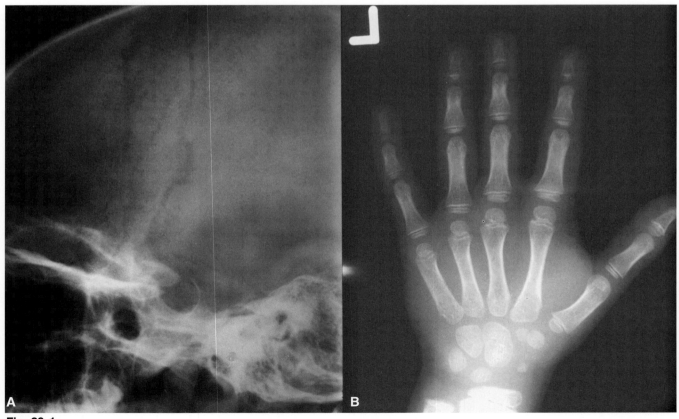

A

B

Fig. 23-1

Case 24

A 4-year-old boy has headaches and sleeps, drinks, and urinates a lot.

Mother noticed that left eye "jumped" when right eye was covered 6 months ago. He has vomited several times in the last month when he got out of bed in the morning.

Pregnancy of mother was normal, birth weight 4.1 kg. He broke his left arm several months ago.

Mother and brother (2 years old) are well. Father has high blood pressure. Some members of father's family have diabetes mellitus.

Temperature at 4 years is 36.1°C, heart rate 108, respiratory rate 16, blood pressure 100/50 mm Hg, weight 22 kg, and head circumference 53 cm. He is jumpy and inattentive. Left eye is blind. Left pupil constricts more with light in right eye than in left eye (Marcus Gunn pupil). The rest of the physical findings are normal.

Hematocrit is 0.39. White cell count is 9.4×10^9/liter with 0.51 polymorphonuclear cells, 0.02 bands, 0.43 lymphocytes, 0.03 monocytes, and 0.01 basophils. Platelet count is 422×10^9/liter. Urine specific gravity is 1.008, pH 7. Urine has occasional squamous epithelial cells/HPF. Serum osmolality is 284 mmol/kg, urine osmolality 247. Serum sodium is 136 mmol/liter, potassium 4.5, chloride 101, carbon dioxide 23, urea nitrogen 5.4, calcium 2.54, phosphorus 2.00, cholesterol 7.24, and glucose 4.4. Creatinine is 40 μmol/liter, uric acid 290, total bilirubin 7, and direct bilirubin 2. Total protein is 74 g/liter, albumin 47. Alkaline phosphatase is 199 U/liter, LDH 262, and SGOT 29. Free T_4 is 24 pmol/liter (normal: 10–36), TSH is 2 mU/liter (normal: 2–11), and cortisol is 330 nmol/liter (normal: 50–410).

Figure 24-1 shows protruding brow, widened coronal suture, a crescent of calcium density in anterior cranial fossa, enlarged pituitary fossa, eroded dorsum sellae, and depressed chiasmatic groove. CT scan in Figure 24-2 shows bilobed mass with calcium in its wall in anterior and middle cranial fossas that enhances after IV injection of contrast medium.

At operation, a vascular tumor of optic chiasm thins optic nerves and tracts.

The red to tan-brown tumor contains (1) moderately pleomorphic cells with indistinct cytoplasm and large nuclei with vesiculation and variably prominent nucleoli; (2) bands of eosinophilic fibers; and (3) myxomatous deposits with focal PAS-positive degeneration, prominent Rosenthal fibers, and venous channels.

A café au lait spot is on abdomen 10 months later.

Diagnosis: Optic glioma.

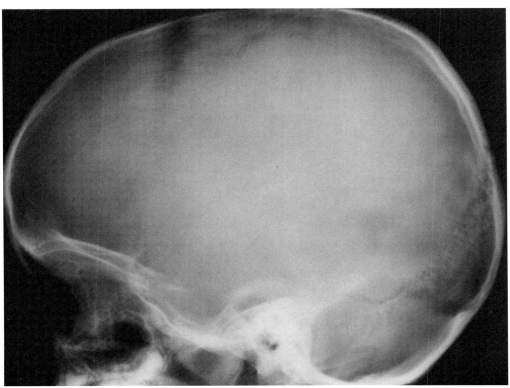

Fig. 24-1

(Continued)

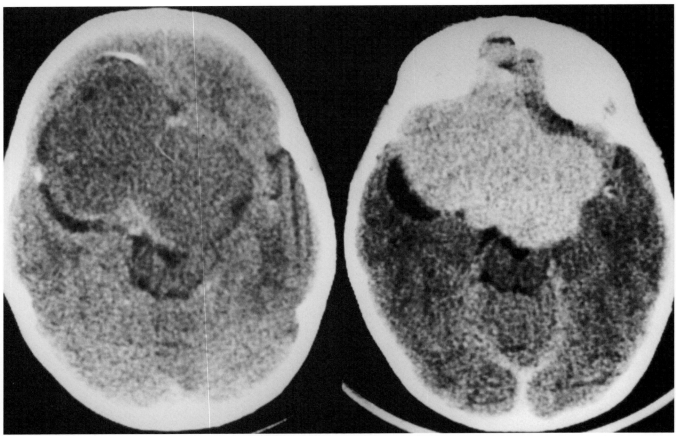

Fig. 24-2

Case 25

A 6-month-old girl's eyes are downcast. She used to roll over and sit up but stopped 3 weeks ago. She has been cranky for 2 weeks.

Mother (24 years old) is well. Pregnancy was normal, birth weight 3.9 kg, head circumference 35 cm, Apgar score 5/8 at 1 and 5 minutes, and heart rate 220. She was given digoxin for supraventricular tachycardia.

Temperature at 6 months is 36°C, heart rate 140, respiratory rate 50, blood pressure 114/70 mm Hg, weight 6.7 kg, and head circumference 45 cm. Eyes are downcast when she cries and go no higher than midline. She turns to noise and light. Anterior fontanel bulges. She scissors legs when held erect. Babinski's sign is in feet. The rest of the physical findings are normal.

Hematocrit is 0.44. White cell count is 11.9×10^9/liter with 0.26 polymorphonuclear cells, 0.04 bands, 0.66 lymphocytes, 0.02 monocytes, and 0.02 eosinophils. Platelet count is 621×10^9/liter. ESR is 5 mm/hr. Urine specific gravity is 1.001, pH 6. Urine is normal. Serum sodium is 144 mmol/liter, potassium 5.0, chloride 109, carbon dioxide 20, urea nitrogen 1.8, calcium 2.90, phosphorus 2.39, cholesterol 3.54, and glucose 4.8. Creatinine is 40 μmol/liter, uric acid 150, total bilirubin 2, and direct bilirubin 0. Total protein is 61 g/liter, albumin 46. Alkaline phosphatase is 383 U/liter, LDH 263, and SGOT 38. CSF has 2×10^6/liter white cells, 9.0 mmol/liter glucose, and 0.26 g/liter protein.

Lateral and third ventricles are dilated in Figure 25-1A. A mass with enhancing rim after IV injection of contrast medium is in back part of third ventricle (Figure 25-1B).

At right occipital craniotomy, milky arachnoid is found over a pineal tumor.

Microscopic examination of the firm, dark gray–brown tumor shows closely packed cells with little cytoplasm and round-to-oval nuclei divided into pseudolobules by blood vessels, mitoses, microcysts, necrosis, and gliotic hypercellular tissue along part of edge.

Diagnosis: Pineoblastoma.

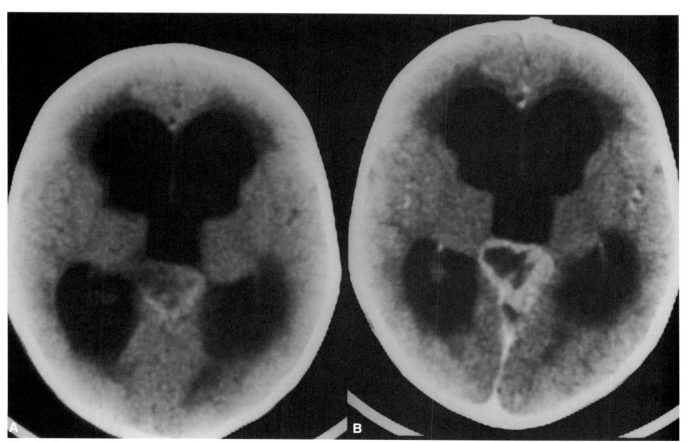

Fig. 25-1

Case 26

A 6-year-old boy will not eat. Appetite went from "bad to terrible" 8 months ago. He has had frontal headaches for 6 months.

Pregnancy of mother was normal, birth weight 4 kg, Apgar score 9/9 at 1 and 5 minutes. He weighed 11 kg at 2 years, 11.4 kg at 3½ years, when findings in small bowel biopsy were normal. Parents keep him at meal table for as long as 2 hours. He vomits sometimes when they make him eat. He used to cling to his mother but has been the "school jokester" this year.

Mother and brother (7 years old), the biggest boy in his class, are well. Father is nervous and has headaches and eczema.

Temperature at 6 years is 36°C, heart rate 88, respiratory rate 20, blood pressure 84/50 mm Hg, weight 13.7 kg, height 108 cm, and head circumference 52 cm. He is playful, alert, and cachectic. Margins of optic discs are indistinct. The rest of the physical findings are normal.

Hematocrit is 0.41. White cell count is 7.7×10^9/liter with 0.36 polymorphonuclear cells, 0.50 lymphocytes, 0.11 monocytes, 0.02 eosinophils, and 0.01 atypical lymphocytes. Platelet count is 438×10^9/liter. Urine specific gravity is 1.025, pH 6. Urine is normal. Serum sodium is 147 mmol/liter, potassium 4.2, chloride 105, carbon dioxide 19, urea nitrogen 6.4, calcium 2.50, phosphorus 1.00, cholesterol 3.23, and glucose 8.0. Creatinine is 60 µmol/liter, uric acid 200, total bilirubin 3, and direct bilirubin 0. Total protein is 68 g/liter, albumin 47. Alkaline phosphatase is 174 U/liter, LDH 260, and SGOT 22. Growth hormone is 1.5 µg/liter before exercise, 3.5 after exercise (normal: >10.5); TSH is 2 mU/liter (normal: 2–11); T_4 is 112 nmol/liter (normal: 51–142), prolactin is 16 µg/liter (normal: <20); and cortisol is 45 nmol/liter (normal: 50–410).

T1-weighted MRI in Figure 26-1 shows suprasellar mass of mixed signal intensity in hypothalamus and cerebral peduncles and dilation of lateral and third ventricles.

At transsphenoidal operation, part of jugum of sphenoid bone is thin or absent. A thick, white capsule is around tumor above jugum.

Microscopic examination shows moderately cellular tumor that contains Rosenthal fibers and many small blood vessels.

Diagnosis: Juvenile pilocytic astrocytoma, grade 1; diencephalic syndrome of infancy.

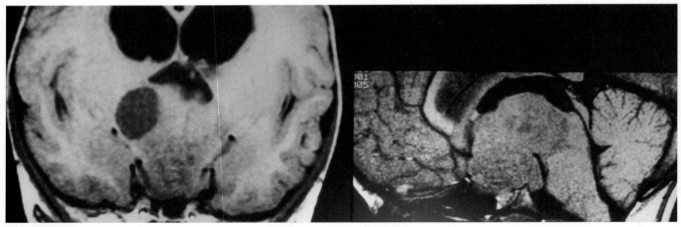

Fig. 26-1

Case 27

A 4-year-old boy is clumsy and has walked pigeon-toed for 2 months. He runs and rides his bicycle but falls more often now. Eyes do not move together. He had a headache a month ago. He has been sleeping more the past week. Appetite is good, speech normal.

Pregnancy of mother was normal, birth weight 3.3 kg, and Apgar score 8/9 at 1 and 5 minutes. He had three febrile convulsions at 2 years. He has had otitis media several times.

Parents and two younger siblings are well.

Temperature at 4 years is 35.9°C, heart rate 120, respiratory rate 18, blood pressure 90/52 mm Hg, and weight 13.7 kg.

Left eye turns inward; right eye does not abduct. He walks on his toes, feet far apart, and falls to left. The rest of the physical findings are normal.

T1-weighted sagittal MRI in Figure 27-1A shows a low-signal mass in pons and medulla that compresses cerebellum and fourth ventricle. T2-weighted axial image in Figure 27-1B shows a high-signal mass that surrounds basilar artery.

Diagnosis: Pontine glioma.

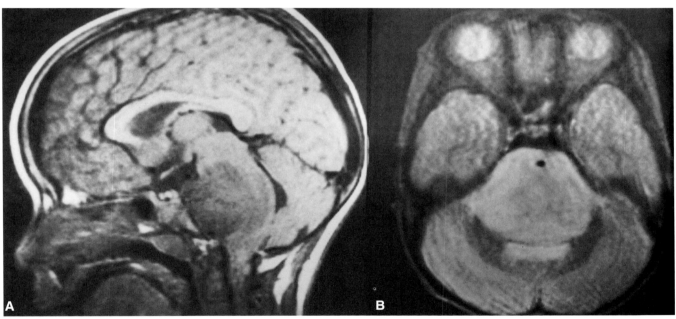

Fig. 27-1

Case 28

A 4-year-old girl has a protruding left eyeball.

Morning swelling and redness of left lids appeared 3 months ago and subsided during the day until 1 month ago. Left eyeball has protruded for 2 weeks. Vision has been blurred, left eye turned outward for a week.

Parents and four siblings are well.

Weight at 4 years is 13.2 kg, height 94 cm, temperature 37.7°C, heart rate 112, respiratory rate 24, and blood pressure 100/52 mm Hg. Left lids, swollen and red, can close over protruding eye. Eyes move normally. She sees light with left eye but does not follow objects. A systolic heart murmur is present. The rest of the physical findings are normal.

Hematocrit is 0.43. White cell count is 11.1×10^9/liter. Platelet count is 545×10^9/liter. Urine specific gravity is 1.038, pH 7. Urine has occasional squamous epithelial cells and 0–1 white cell/HPF. Serum osmolality is 275 mmol/kg, urine osmolality 1,240 mmol/kg. Serum sodium is 137 mmol/liter, potassium 4.0, chloride 102, carbon dioxide 21, urea nitrogen 4.3, calcium 2.42, phosphorus 1.65, cholesterol 5.17, and glucose 7.2. Creatinine is 50 µmol/liter, uric acid 180, total bilirubin 14, and direct bilirubin 2. Total protein is 70 g/liter, albumin 44. Alkaline phosphatase is 205 U/liter, LDH 244, and SGOT 31. Free T_4 is 15 pmol/liter (normal: 10–36), TSH is 3 mU/liter (normal: 2–11), cortisol is 220 nmol/liter (normal: 50–410), and prolactin is 6 µg/liter (normal: <20).

Left optic canal is enlarged in Figure 28-1. CT scan after IV injection of contrast medium shows enhancing mass in left orbit and middle cranial fossa (Figure 28-2).

At operation, a gray tumor extends along the base of skull from junction of left temporal and frontal lobes into left orbit, where is it indistinguishable from optic nerve.

Microscopic examination shows compact fibrils, loose cystic zones, myxomatous tissue, stellate-to-oval cells, and elongated eosinophilic fibers that suggest Rosenthal fibers.

Diagnosis: Juvenile pilocytic astrocytoma.

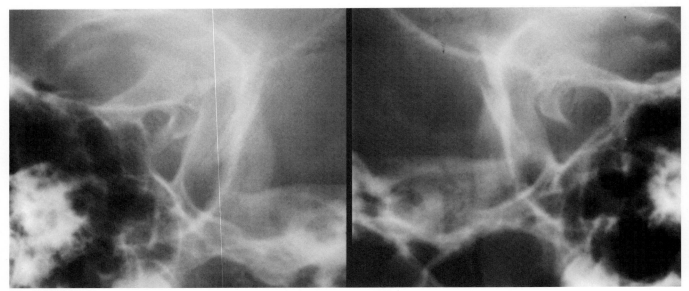

Fig. 28-1

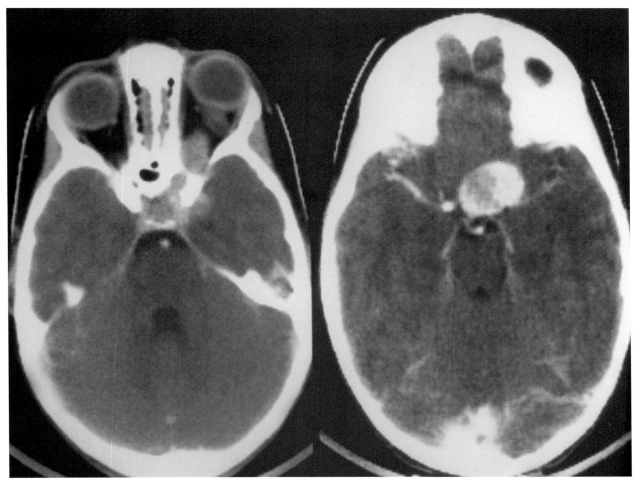

Fig. 28-2

Case 29

A 15-year-old boy says, "If I go to do an errand, I forget before I get there."

He had a convulsion at 9 years. At 13 years, he began to have blackout spells with eyes open and hands opening and closing, for as long as a minute several times a week. For the last year, these spells have occurred on a daily basis. He had a second generalized convulsion at 14 years. Vision is sometimes blurred or double until he blinks. School work has deteriorated.

Father and seven siblings are well. One sibling has asthma.

Temperature at 15 years is 37.7°C, heart rate 76, respiratory rate 18, blood pressure 130/92 mm Hg, and weight 63 kg. Finger tapping is slow. Pain perception is diminished in left arm and left leg. The rest of the physical findings are normal.

Hematocrit is 0.40. White cell count is 4.8×10^9/liter with 0.43 polymorphonuclear cells, 0.43 lymphocytes, 0.10 monocytes, and 0.04 eosinophils. Platelet count is 395×10^9/liter. Serum sodium is 145 mmol/liter, potassium 4.0, chloride 103, carbon dioxide 33, urea nitrogen 1.8, calcium 2.32, phosphorus 1.36, cholesterol 5.12, and glucose 5.6. Creatinine is 90

µmol/liter, uric acid 230, total bilirubin 3, and direct bilirubin 0. Total protein is 70 g/liter, albumin 44. Alkaline phosphatase is 187 U/liter, LDH 153, and SGOT 20. CSF has 1×10^6/liter white cells, 0.70 lymphocytes, 0.30 monocytes, 15×10^6/liter red cells, 4.3 mmol/liter glucose, and 0.19 g/liter protein.

EEG shows frequent left temporal spikes and generalized slowing.

MRI shows low-signal mass in left temporal lobe in T1-weighted image (Figure 29-1A) and high-signal mass in T2-weighted image (Figure 29-1B).

At left temporofrontal craniotomy, a soft gray tumor is in amygdala and hippocampus of left temporal lobe and extends along brain stem and left internal carotid artery.

Microscopic examination shows a cellular tumor with uniform nuclei and fibrillary extensions of cytoplasm and prominent capillaries.

Diagnosis: Fibrillary astrocytoma (medium-grade glioma).

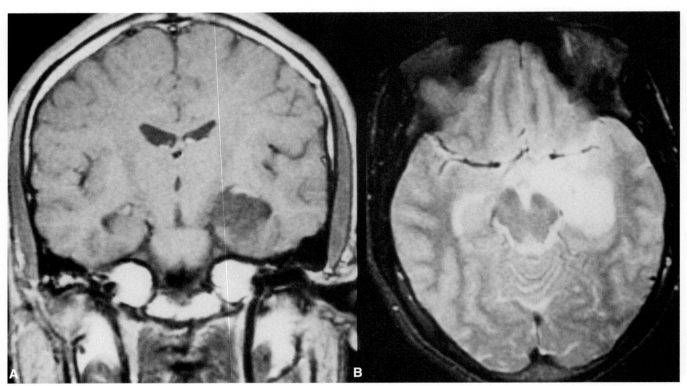

Fig. 29-1

Case 30

A 3-month-old boy cannot hold his head up. Mother has seen whites of his eyes above iris for several weeks. He eats well.

Mother (19 years old) was hypertensive during pregnancy and bled from vagina at the end. Birth weight was 3.1 kg, length 53 cm, head circumference 36 cm, and Apgar score 8/9 at 1 and 5 minutes. He had acrocyanosis and right cephalohematoma. The rest of the physical findings were normal. Total bilirubin was 160 μmol/liter at 3 days.

Temperature at 3 months is 36.3°C, heart rate 136, respiratory rate 40, systolic blood pressure 104 mm Hg, weight 7.4 kg, and head circumference 47 cm. Anterior fontanel bulges. Eyes turn inward. White sclera is visible above irises. He does not follow a light. Pupils are equal and react to light. Discs are normal. He smiles but not in response to external cues. Hearing seems normal. The rest of the physical findings are normal.

Hematocrit is 0.34. White cell count is 15.1 × 10⁹/liter with 0.22 polymorphonuclear cells, 0.01 bands, 0.69 lymphocytes, 0.04 monocytes, 0.03 eosinophils, and 0.01 basophils. Platelet count is 702 × 10⁹/liter. Urine specific gravity is 1.021, pH 5. Urine has rare epithelial cells/HPF, rare red cells/HPF, and rare white cells/HPF, uric acid crystals, calcium oxalate crystals, and bacteria. Serum sodium is 143 mmol/liter, potassium 4.8, chloride 106, carbon dioxide 16, urea nitrogen 1.8, calcium 2.67, phosphorus 2.07, triglycerides 0.99, cholesterol 4.50, and glucose 5.9. Creatinine is 50 μmol/liter, uric acid 380, total bilirubin 3, and direct bilirubin 0. Total protein is 57 g/liter, albumin 43. Alkaline phosphatase is 423 U/liter, LDH 221, SGOT 39, and GGT 25.

Lateral ventricles and suprapineal recess of third ventricle are dilated. Rim of cyst in middle cranial fossa enhances after IV injection of contrast medium (Figure 30-1).

At occipital craniotomy, a cyst under tentorium cerebelli is attached to colliculi.

Microscopic examination of translucent wall of the resected cyst shows fibrillar astrocytes with intensely eosinophilic cytoplasm, slightly pleomorphic nuclei, and no arachnoid elements.

Diagnosis: Cystic low-grade astrocytoma of quadrigeminal (tectal) lamina.

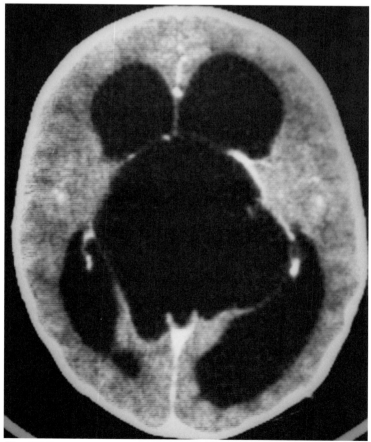

Fig. 30-1

Case 31

An 8-year-old girl is vomiting.

Frontal headaches, blurred vision, stumbling, and vomiting began 2 months ago. She has vomited "all day long" four times in the past 2 months and is vomiting everything today. She remembers neither stumbling nor vomiting.

Parents and two brothers are well.

Temperature is 37.4°C, heart rate 100, respiratory rate 18, blood pressure 110/64 mm Hg, height 133 cm, and weight 27 kg. Head is tilted to right. She does not swing right arm when she walks. Disc margins are indistinct, retinal vessels slightly enlarged. Blind spot is larger in right eye than in left. The rest of the physical findings are normal.

Hematocrit is 0.39. White cell count is 6.5×10^9/liter with 0.55 polymorphonuclear cells, 0.37 lymphocytes, 0.04 monocytes, and 0.04 eosinophils. Urine specific gravity is 1.025, pH 6.5. Urine is normal. Serum sodium is 141 mmol/liter, potassium 3.8, chloride 101, carbon dioxide 23, urea nitrogen 4.3, and glucose 5.0.

Sagittal MRI in Figure 31-1A shows low-signal mass in cerebellum and fourth ventricle and depression of pons at the level of vagal and hypoglossal trigones and facial colliculus. The midline cerebellar mass enhances with gadolinium in coronal section (Figure 31-1B).

At suboccipital craniotomy, an encapsulated tumor of soft gray tissue and white fibrous tissue is found in vermis of cerebellum. Microscopic examination shows cells with little cytoplasm, many mitoses, and intersecting bands of fibrous tissue.

Diagnosis: Medulloblastoma.

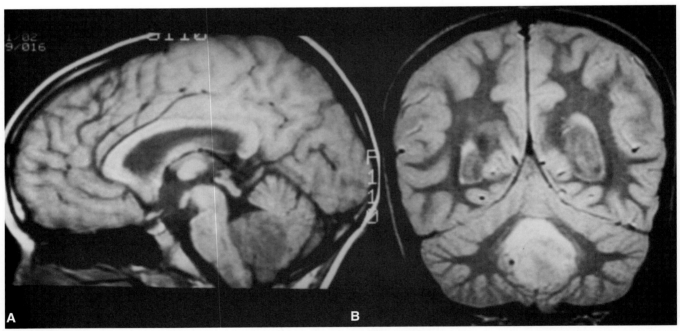

Fig. 31-1

Case 32

A 12-year-old boy has a headache and stiff neck.

He vomited for 2½ days, and then felt better 8 days ago and went to school, although still weak and not eating much. Head and neck pain woke him up in the middle of the night before last. He vomited several hours later and then ate a little but could not sit because of headache and stiff neck. He has vomited again and does not feel like eating.

Pregnancy of mother was normal, birth weight 3.7 kg. Appetite has been bad for a year, and he has gained little weight.

Parents, half sister (18 years old), and brother (14 years old) are well. Maternal grandmother had leukemia; paternal grandmother had diabetes mellitus.

Temperature at 12 years is 37.6°C, heart rate 60, respiratory rate 16, blood pressure 100/70 mm Hg, weight 29 kg, and height 142 cm. He grimaces when lights are turned on and whimpers at other times. Neck is stiff. He cannot lift legs straight off bed. The rest of the physical findings are normal.

Hematocrit is 0.45. White cell count is 8.8×10^9/liter with 0.68 polymorphonuclear cells, 0.01 bands, 0.23 lymphocytes, 0.06 monocytes, and 0.02 eosinophils. Platelet count is 302×10^9/liter. Urine specific gravity is 1.025, pH 6. Urine has trace ketones. Serum sodium is 137 mmol/liter, potassium 4.0, chloride 102, carbon dioxide 31, urea nitrogen 2.1, calcium 2.27, phosphorus 1.55, cholesterol 2.97, triglycerides 1.00, and glucose 5.6. Creatinine is 60 μmol/liter, uric acid 180, total bilirubin 9, and direct bilirubin 0. Total protein is 58 g/liter, albumin 35. Alkaline phosphatase is 98 U/liter, LDH 135, and SGOT 18. CSF has 2.6 mmol/liter glucose, 0.86 g/liter protein, 20×10^9/liter red cells, 0.5×10^9/liter white cells, 0.94 polymorphonuclear cells, and 0.06 lymphocytes.

T1-weighted MRI after IV gadolinium shows mass with increased signal in dilated fourth ventricle and between cerebellar hemispheres (Figure 32-1A) and mixed signal where mass goes over medulla and through foramen magnum (Figure 32-1B).

At craniotomy from inion to foramen magnum and C1 laminectomy, a gray tumor is found between cerebellar hemispheres and cerebellar tonsils and medulla, down over cervical cord, and up into lower half of fourth ventricle, where it is fixed at obex. Tumor in fourth ventricle is gelatinous and avascular. Old hemorrhage is in tumor. Encapsulated extraventricular tumor is resected. Intraventricular tumor is shaved almost flush with floor of the fourth ventricle.

He has distended abdomen and many loose green stools 10 days after operation while receiving aminoglycoside antibiotic. Colonoscopy shows pseudomembrane and superficial erosions in rectum and sigmoid. Stool toxin assay is positive for *Clostridium difficile*.

He is treated for residual tumor with chemotherapy and irradiation. At 14 years, free T_4 is 9 pmol/liter (normal: 10–36), TSH 27 mU/liter (normal: 2–11). He has more energy after he begins to take levothyroxine. At 15 years, weight is 41 kg, height 155 cm. He participates normally in school activities. He has endpoint nystagmus in all directions. Right side of tongue is weak and curves right when stuck out. Extension of neck is slightly restricted. Gait is slightly broad based. He tends to lose balance when doing deep knee bends.

Microscopic diagnosis: Ependymoma; antibiotic-associated pseudomembranous colitis.

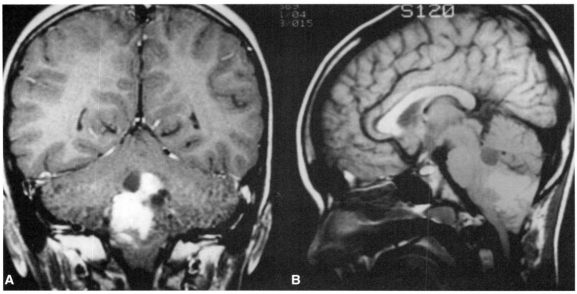

Fig. 32-1

Case 33

A 13-year-old boy has a headache and "funny vision" in right eye.

Chest roentgenogram at 12 years for cough, weight loss, tiredness, and dysphagia showed mediastinal tumor, which compressed left main bronchus at bronchoscopy. Biopsy of left paratracheal mass and lymph node showed a monoclonal B-cell malignant lymphoma, immunologic phenotype IgG-κ. He had a generalized tonic-clonic seizure after chemotherapy was begun and has been treated with phenobarbital. Bitemporal headaches that began 2 months ago are worse. Vision in the right eye is blurred after he looks at bright lights.

Temperature is 36.7°C, heart rate 62, respiratory rate 12, blood pressure 94/68 mm Hg, weight 35 kg, and height 147 cm. A surgical scar is on neck. The rest of the physical findings are normal.

Hematocrit is 0.41. White cell count is 4.4×10^9/liter with 0.64 polymorphonuclear cells, 0.01 bands, 0.15 lymphocytes, 0.09 monocytes, 0.02 basophils, and 0.09 eosinophils. Platelet count is 374×10^9/liter. Serum sodium is 141 mmol/liter, potassium 4.0, chloride 99, carbon dioxide 25, urea nitrogen 6.8, calcium 2.45, phosphorus 1.61, cholesterol 4.65, and glucose 5.2. Creatinine is 70 μmol/liter, uric acid 270, total bilirubin 7, and direct bilirubin 0. Total protein is 73 g/liter, albumin 48. Alkaline phosphatase 258 U/liter, LDH 116, and SGOT 12. CSF is clear and colorless and has 3×10^6/liter red cells, 138×10^6/liter white cells, 0.11 pia-arachnoid cells, 0.75 lymphocytes, 0.01 eosinophils, and 0.13 atypical lymphocytes with surface markers for T lymphocytes and no monoclonal B lymphocytes, glucose 2.7 mmol/liter, and protein 1.02 g/liter, diagnosis reactive lymphocytic pleocytosis.

CT scan after IV injection of contrast medium shows enhancement of pulvinar of right thalamus and ependyma of frontal horns of lateral ventricles (Figure 33-1A). At lower level, Figure 33-1B shows left hypothalamus, basal cisterns, and a focus in hypodense left temporoparietal lobes.

CT guided-needle biopsy specimen of right temporoparietal region shows perivascular proliferation of atypical lymphoid-like cells whose immunologic phenotype consists of large cell monoclonal B-cell population identical to mediastinal large cell lymphoma. At necropsy 4 months later, diffuse lymphoma is in CNS, subarachnoid and subependymal space, superficial cortical layers, hippocampus, and optic chiasm.

Diagnosis: B-cell lymphoma in mediastinum and CNS.

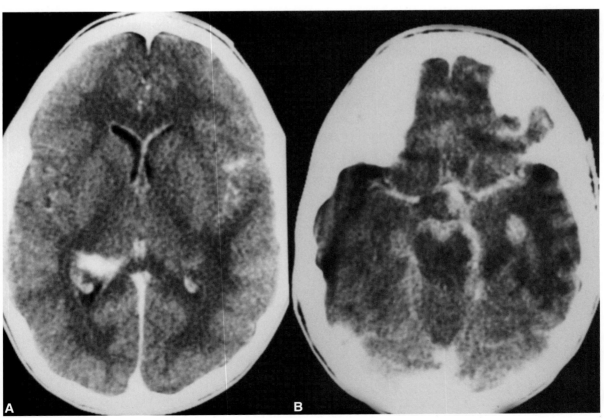

Fig. 33-1

Eye

Case 1

A 9-month-old boy has left "white eye." He has had several ear infections.

Paternal grandmother has been blind in one eye since infancy.

Temperature is 37°C, heart rate 132, respiratory rate 44, systolic blood pressure 110 mm Hg, and weight 9.3 kg. Fundus of left eye is white. Left eardrum is dull and retracted. The rest of the physical findings are normal.

Hematocrit is 0.34. White cell count is 12.5×10^9/liter. Platelet count is 172×10^9/liter. CSF is clear and has $<1 \times 10^6$/liter red cells and $<1 \times 10^6$/liter white cells.

CT scan in Figure 1-1 shows a mass of high attenuation in left eye.

At operation, a tumor in left eye detaches much of retina and obscures optic nerve and macula. Three small tumors are found in right eye. Left eye and part of left optic nerve are removed.

Microscopic examination shows mass in back of left eye that is made up of (1) dark-staining small cells, some in rosettes; (2) foci of necrosis; (3) tumor cells and blood cells in blood spaces that are not lined by endothelium; and (4) tumor cells on iris and suspensory ligament of lens. No calcifications are in tumor.

Diagnosis: Bilateral retinoblastoma. (Funduscopic examination of grandmother does not show sign of regressed retinoblastoma.)

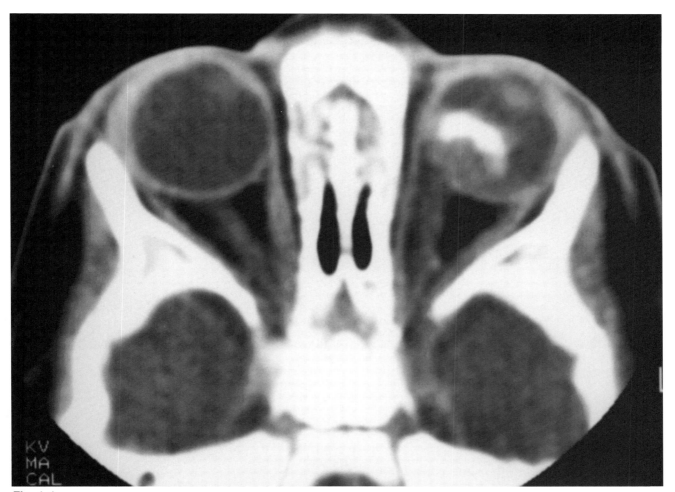

Fig. 1-1

Case 2

A 7-year-old girl is nearly blind in the left eye.

She has had an itchy, red rash for 4 months and frontal headaches for several weeks. Vision was normal in school examination 4 weeks ago. Left pupil has been small for 2 weeks; left iris is green and not its original brown. Left lower lid was cut when she was hit in eye at 2 years. Vision was normal after injury.

Mother, stepfather, and three brothers are well. The family has a dog, cat, and rabbit.

Weight at 7 years is 20.7 kg, height 120 cm. Red macules and papules are on body. Left pupil is keyhole shaped and nonreactive to light. A white mass is in left eye. A scar is on left lower lid. The rest of the physical findings are normal.

Hematocrit is 0.37. White cell count is 15.4×10^9/liter with 0.58 polymorphonuclear cells, 0.22 lymphocytes, 0.04 monocytes, 0.01 basophils, and 0.15 eosinophils. Platelet count is 255×10^9/liter. Serum sodium is 139 mmol/liter, potassium 4.4, chloride 105, carbon dioxide 20, urea nitrogen 5.0, calcium 2.52, phosphorus 1.84, cholesterol 4.40, and glucose 3.9. Creatinine is 50 μmol/liter, uric acid 140, total bilirubin 3, and direct bilirubin 2. Total protein is 68 g/liter, albumin 46. Alkaline phosphatase is 223 U/liter, LDH 232, and SGOT 29. *Hymenolepis nana* eggs are found in stool.

CT scan in Figure 2-1 shows irregular shadows of increased density in left eyeball. Ultrasound examination shows "possible total retinal detachment with massive . . . exudate or hemorrhage, left," according to examining ophthalmologist.

Serologic titer is 1:128 for *Toxocara canis* in enzyme immunoassay (diagnostic enzyme immunoassay titer 1:32).

Blind left eye is enucleated because of pain at 12 years. Visual acuity in right eye is 20/15–1.

Diagnosis: Ocular toxocariasis.

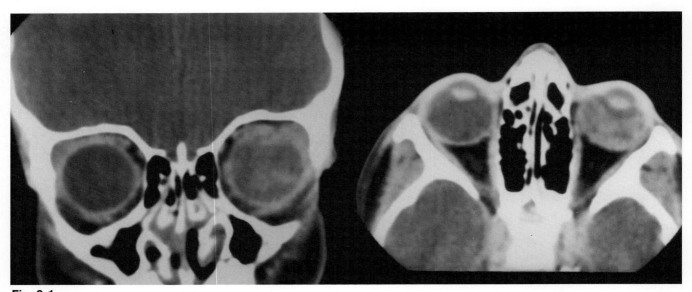

Fig. 2-1

Case 3

A 9-year-old boy has a black, swollen right eye. He was hit in the face by a baseball 2 hours ago. He bled from right side of the nose and then vomited.

Temperature is 36°C, heart rate 68, respiratory rate 20, and blood pressure 108/60 mm Hg. Right upward gaze is painful and limited. Dried blood is in mouth and right side of nose. The rest of the physical findings are normal.

Mucosa of right maxillary and ethmoid sinuses is thickened. A piece of dislodged bone in floor of right orbit presses against inferior rectus muscle (Figure 3-1).

At operation, orbital soft tissue is caught in a displaced, longitudinal fracture of orbital surface of right maxilla.

Diagnosis: Blowout fracture, right orbit.

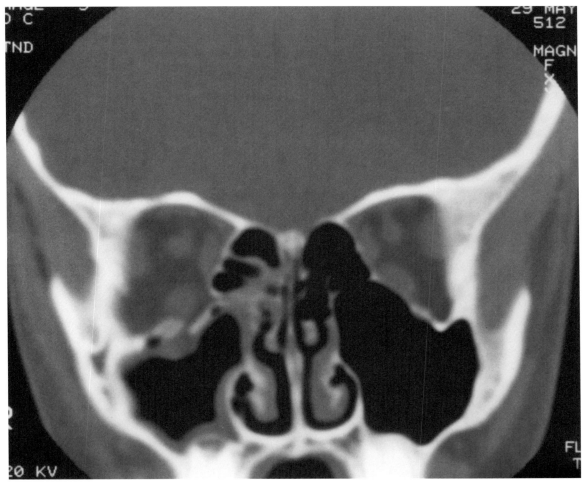

Fig. 3-1

Case 4

A 12-year-old girl has swollen, teary eyes. She has had headache and fever and has been vomiting for 2 days.

Temperature is 38.9°C, heart rate 60, respiratory rate 22, blood pressure 105/55 mm Hg, and weight 46.3 kg. Upper eyelids, scalp of forehead and right temple, and cheeks are swollen. Right eye is closed. Mucopus is present in nose and pharynx. Pharynx is injected. A systolic heart murmur is present. The rest of the physical findings are normal.

Hematocrit is 0.39. White cell count is 16.8×10^9/liter with 0.67 polymorphonuclear cells, 0.22 bands, 0.09 lymphocytes, and 0.02 monocytes. Culture of contents of left maxillary sinus obtained at washout through nose grows α streptococci and gram-positive anaerobes. Blood culture grows *Bacteroides melaninogenicus*.

CT scan after nasal washout shows liquid in ethmoidal air cells, more in left, and swelling of eyelids and right side of face (Figure 4-1).

She remains febrile despite treatment. An abscess of left eyelid is incised 5 days after treatment is begun. Two days after incision, she has a convulsion that starts with word repetition, followed by jerking of right arm and leg for 5 minutes and then alertness.

CT scan at start of treatment shows normal findings (Figure 4-2A). After convulsion and IV injection of contrast medium, CT scan shows liquid between frontal bone and dura and in interhemispheric fissure and enhancement of wall around the liquid (Figure 4-2B).

At craniotomy, yellow pus is found between frontal bone and dura as well as in interhemispheric fissure. Culture of pus grows coagulase-positive staphylococci.

Diagnosis: Sinusitis, periorbital cellulitis, epidural (frontal) and subdural (interhemispheric) empyema.

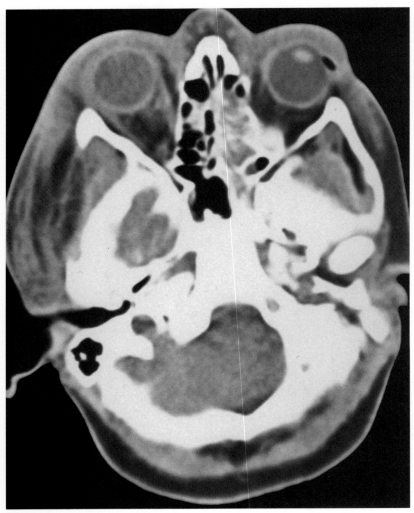

Fig. 4-1

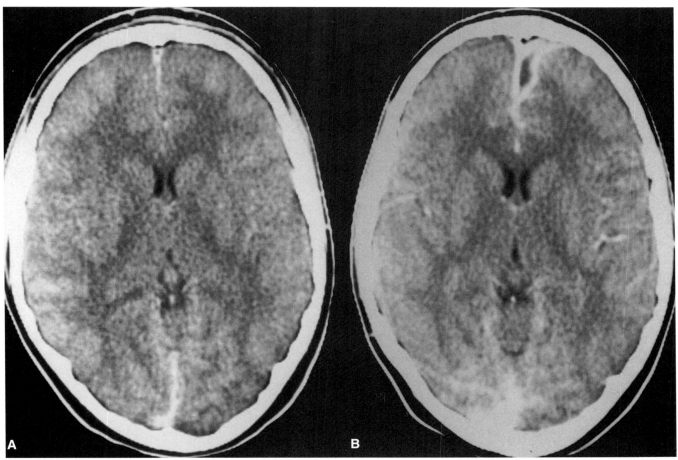

Fig. 4-2

Case 5

A 16-year-old boy has a bulging left eye that he has been aware of for 3 months.

A photograph at 8 years shows protrusion of left eye. Examination at 10 years for a thick nasal discharge that he had had for several years showed normal findings. Night vision has been impaired for 1 year. Vision is blurred when he reads.

He fractured his skull at 5 and 7 years. Tonsils and adenoids have been removed.

Mother has asthma. Father, three brothers, and one sister are well.

Temperature at 16 years is 36.7°C, heart rate 70, respiratory rate 16, and blood pressure 130/68 mm Hg. A tender mass, softer than bone around it, is present under the orbital surface of the left side of frontal bone. The rest of the physical findings are normal.

Hematocrit is 0.42. White cell count is 9.3×10^9/liter. Serum sodium is 143 mmol/liter, potassium 4.2, chloride 105, carbon dioxide 27, calcium 2.52, phosphorus 1.42, urea nitrogen 4.3, cholesterol 3.20, and glucose 3.7. Creatinine is 70 μmol/liter, uric acid 310, total bilirubin 5, and direct bilirubin 0. Total protein is 75 g/liter, albumin 47. Alkaline phosphatase is 178 U/liter, LDH 200, and SGOT 23.

Figure 5-1 shows a mass of bone density in left side of nose and in medial and upper part of left orbit.

At operation, a tumor in nose fills left middle meatus, pushes middle nasal concha against septum, pushes orbital plate of ethmoid bone into left orbit, and obstructs left nasofrontal duct. Mucus is in obstructed frontal sinus.

Microscopic examination of tumor shows broad trabeculae of mature bone in irregular pattern, foci of resorption and formation, and dense fibrous tissue around spicules of bone.

Diagnosis: Osteoma and fibrous dysplasia.

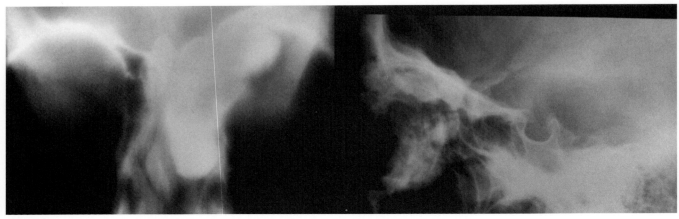

Fig. 5-1

Ear

Case 1

A 14-month-old boy has a small deformed left auricle, left conductive deafness, and no left external acoustic meatus. The rest of the physical findings are normal.

Parents are well. A brother has similar ear deformity.

CT scan in Figure 1-1 shows malformation, perhaps fusion, of left malleus and incus. Right ear and left inner ear are normal (see Figure 1-1).

Diagnosis: Left microtia-atresia and dysplasia of left middle ear (derivative of first branchial arch, including Meckel's cartilage, anlage of malleus and incus).

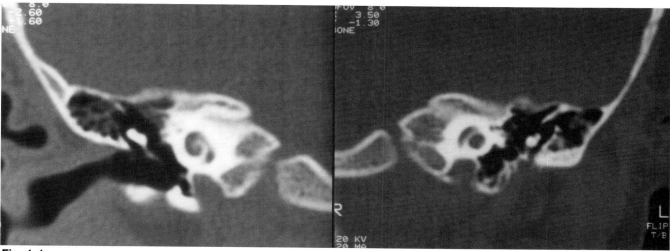

Fig. 1-1

Case 2

A 13-year-old boy, who was found in school examination at 7 years to be deaf in right ear, cannot hear well in left ear.

Physical findings are normal.

Audiogram shows conductive and sensorineural deafness in right ear and slight conductive deafness in left ear.

Axial CT scan shows absence of right cochlea at level of internal ear (Figure 2-1), and enlargement of right vestibule into region of lateral semicircular canal at higher level (Figure 2-2). Coronal scan in Figure 2-3 shows scutum tym-

panicum at bottom of epitympanic recess, in recess malleus, and in incus, on both sides, lateral to medial. In left inner ear (Figure 2-3B), but not in right medial pointing spur of bone, the crista transversa (falciformis), which separates the facial nerve and most of the vestibular nerve above from cochlear nerve below in internal acoustic meatus are shown. In Figure 2-3B, stapes and oval window above bulge of cochlear promontory are better seen in right ear (on reader's left).

Diagnosis: Aplasia of right cochlea.

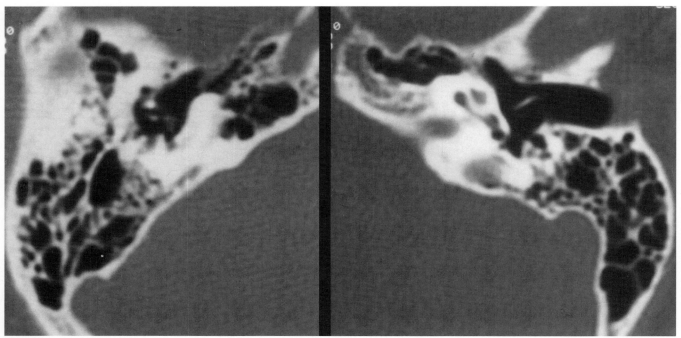

Fig. 2-1

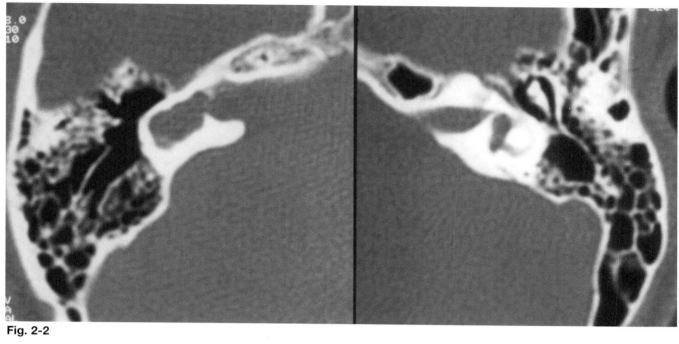

Fig. 2-2

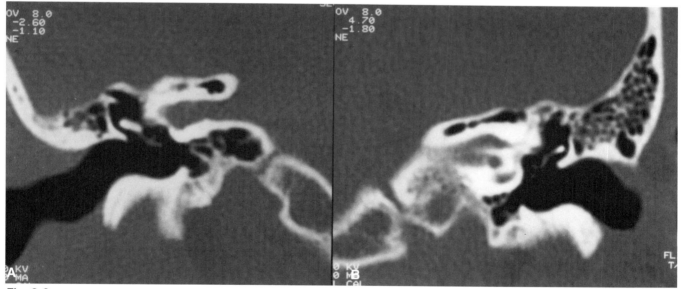

Fig. 2-3

Case 3

A 17-year-old girl has "swooshing" and pain in right ear and temporomandibular joint that began as discomfort years ago and have recently gotten worse.

Temperature is 37°C, heart rate 76, respiratory rate 24, blood pressure 116/74 mm Hg, weight 81 kg, and height 157 cm. A blue mass that blanches with positive pneumatic pressure is behind right eardrum. The rest of the physical findings are normal.

Hematocrit is 0.39. White cell count is 12.2×10^9/liter. Platelet count is 296×10^9/liter.

Bony margin of right carotid canal is thin or absent (Figure 3-1). Right internal carotid artery protrudes into right tympanic cavity just below oval window in coronal CT scan (Figure 3-2).

Diagnosis: Aberrant right internal carotid artery.

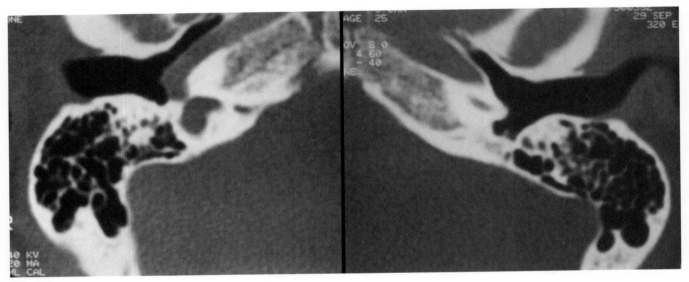

Fig. 3-1

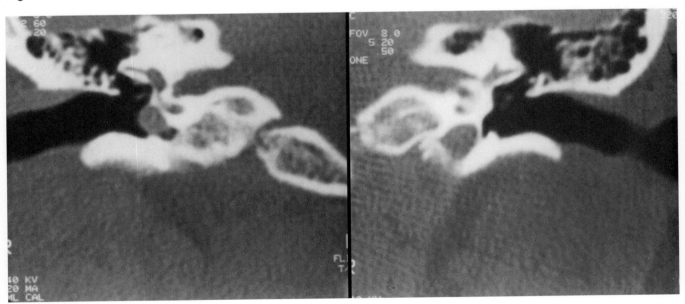

Fig. 3-2

Case 4

A 14-year-old boy has right earache.

For several years he has felt "something bouncing" in his right ear when he jumps up and down. He is sometimes unsteady.

He was born prematurely and had a high white cell count "like leukemia" for a while. Tonsils and adenoids were removed and tubes put in his ears at 4 years. He broke his arm recently.

Parents and brother (12 years old) are well. Paternal grandfather had lung cancer.

Temperature at 14 years is 36.4°C, heart rate 76, respiratory rate 12, blood pressure 120/68 mm Hg, weight 63 kg, and height 181 cm. A red-blue mass is behind lower part of right eardrum. The rest of the physical findings are normal.

Hematocrit is 0.45. White cell count is 5.9×10^9/liter with 0.42 polymorphonuclear cells, 0.01 bands, 0.42 lymphocytes, 0.07 monocytes, 0.06 eosinophils, and 0.02 basophils. Platelet count is 355×10^9/liter.

A mass of soft tissue extends into right tympanic cavity from jugular fossa of petrous part of temporal bone in axial CT scan (Figure 4-1), just below oval window in coronal CT scan (Figure 4-2).

At operation, superior bulb of right internal jugular vein is at incudostapedial joint and lower part of ear drum.

Diagnosis: Herniation of superior bulb of internal jugular vein into right tympanic cavity.

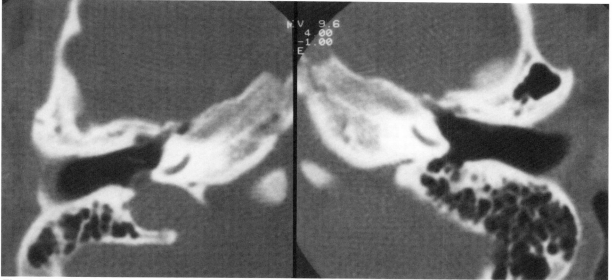

Fig. 4-1

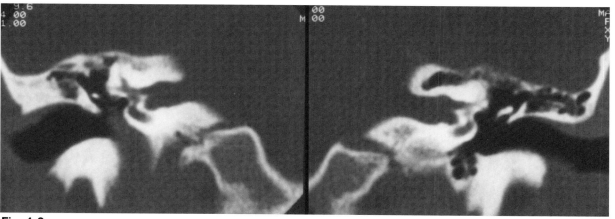

Fig. 4-2

Case 5

A 5-year-old boy is hard of hearing in the right ear.

He has had bilateral otitis media, myringotomies, and ear tubes. Audiogram shows 20-dB loss in right ear.

Right eardrum is red, thick, retracted, and immobile. A tube is in left drum. The rest of the physical findings are normal.

Hematocrit is 0.34. White cell count is 9.4×10^9/liter with 0.64 polymorphonuclear cells, 0.04 bands, 0.25 lymphocytes, 0.04 monocytes, 0.01 basophils, and 0.02 atypical lymphocytes. Platelet count is 372×10^9/liter.

A defect is in petrous part of right temporal bone in brow-down view (Figure 5-1) and in lateral-oblique view (Figure 5-2). Air cells in left temporal bone are normal (see Figures 5-1 and 5-2).

Examination 10 months later shows right eardrum retracted against promontory and auditory (eustachian) tube. Lower part of drum is red. Fluid is behind it. Audiogram shows 35–40 dB conductive loss and normal bone conduction in right ear.

At operation, serous liquid is in right tympanic antrum, and friable, vascular tissue is around ossicles, on facial nerve, and in epitympanic recess and mastoid bone.

Microscopic examination of the lacy, tan-pink to gray-white tissue shows dense fibrous connective tissue, stratified squamous epithelium, keratin, mononuclear inflammatory cells, and focal calcification.

Diagnosis: Cholesteatoma, right middle ear and temporal bone.

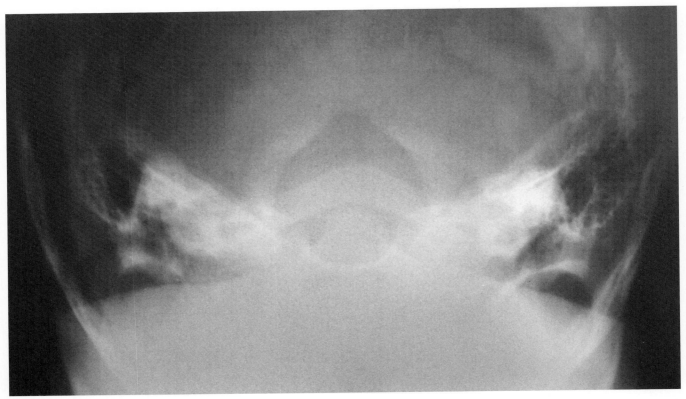

Fig. 5-1

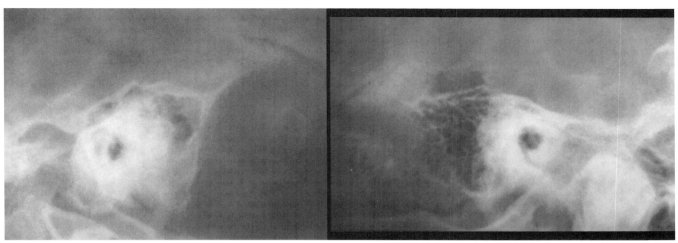

Fig. 5-2

Case 6

A 24-month-old boy is fussy.

Pregnancy of mother was normal, birth weight 3.5 kg. He had night cough, hoarseness, noisy breathing, and normal physical findings at 14 months. Eardrums were normal. He had a cold at 19 months. Eardrums were dull and inflamed. He has been fussy for 3 days at 24 months.

Weight at 24 months is 15 kg, height 95 cm. A white mass is in lower part of left tympanic cavity. A café au lait spot is on left forearm. The rest of the physical findings are normal.

No laboratory data are available.

Axial CT scan (Figure 6-1) and coronal CT scan (Figure 6-2) show a spherical mass in left tympanic cavity between ossicles and promontory of cochlea.

At operation, a soft, gray-white mass about the same size as seen in CT scan is removed.

Microscopic examination shows squamous epithelium and keratin.

Diagnosis: Questionable congenital cholesteatoma, left tympanic cavity.

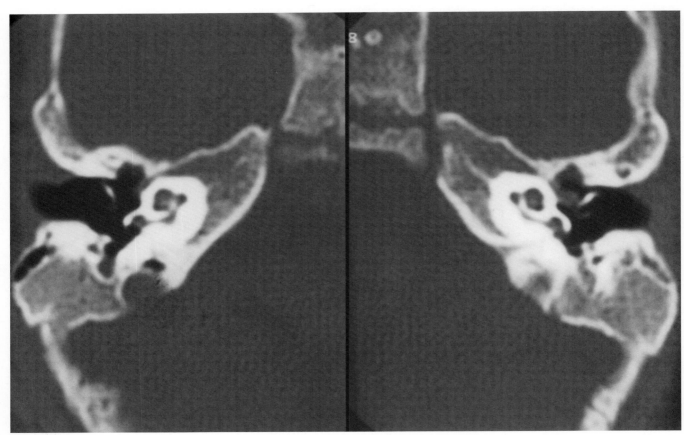

Fig. 6-1

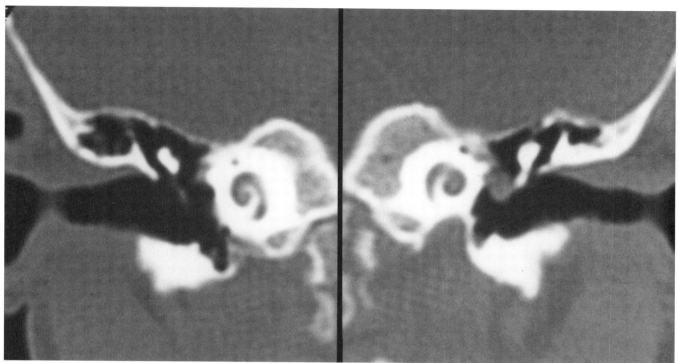

Fig. 6-2

Case 7

A 19-month-old girl has Down syndrome and ear infections.

Pregnancy of mother was normal, birth weight 4 kg. Chromosomes in cord blood were 47,XX,+21. A heart murmur at 3 months was ascribed to pulmonic stenosis after echocardiography. She had croup at 10 months; more respiratory infections and pink, immobile eardrums at 13 months; ear effusions at 14 months; right otitis media at 15 months; and left otitis media at 16 months. Examinations at 17 and 18 months showed a round, white mass, "like a pearl through isinglass," in upper front quadrant of each middle ear.

Mother and father (both 49 years old) and 10 siblings are well.

Temperature at 19 months is 37.2°C, heart rate 112, respiratory rate 20, blood pressure 78/42 mm Hg, and weight 11 kg. Nose is runny. External acoustic meatuses are small. Mouth is small, and tongue seems large. A systolic heart murmur is present. The rest of the physical findings are normal.

Hematocrit is 0.38. White cell count is 4.4×10^9/liter with 0.54 polymorphonuclear cells, 0.30 lymphocytes, 0.13 monocytes, and 0.03 eosinophils. Platelet count is 212×10^9/liter.

Figure 7-1 show a mass of soft tissue along medial side of malleus in tympanic cavities.

At exploration of right middle ear, a yellow mass (0.5 cm) medial to neck of malleus extends from opening of auditory tube to oval window.

Microscopic examination of the mass shows mixture of (1) large, clear, polygonal cells with flattened peripheral nuclei and (2) smaller, less angular cells with grainy cytoplasm and central, round nuclei.

Diagnosis: Fatty mass (white and brown fat) in right middle ear and at operation at 20 months in left middle ear.

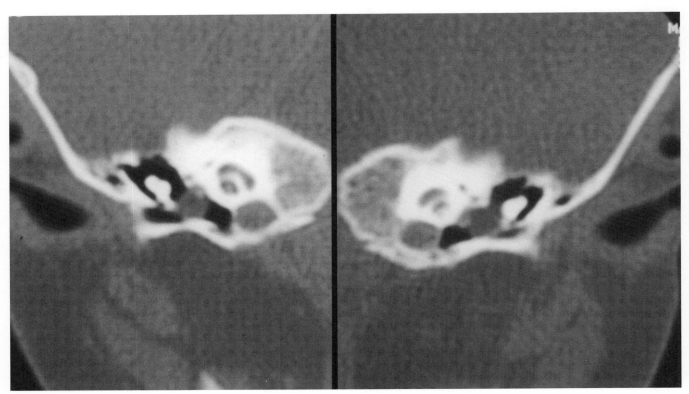

Fig. 7-1

Nose and Nasopharynx

Case 1

A 12-year-old boy has left nasal discharge and has not been able to breathe or smell through the left side of his nose for as long as his mother can remember.

Sometimes when he says "Buy baby a bib," it sounds hypernasal like "My mamy a mim." When he has a cold, words sound hyponasal: *banana* like *badada*, *mama* like *baba*, *singing a song* like *sigging a sog*. He had slight left hearing impairment when he started school. He has frequent colds. He had bilateral inguinal hernia repair as an infant.

Back of hard palate is notched. Soft palate pulls to left. The rest of the physical findings are normal. Deficit in left ear is 25 dB at 250 Hz.

CT scan in Figure 1-1 shows meeting of outcurving vomer and incurving perpendicular plate of left palatine bone at choana, matter in left side of nose, and focal thickening of mucosa of maxillary sinuses.

Diagnosis: Unilateral choanal atresia, (hyponasality), weakness of right side of soft palate (hypernasality).

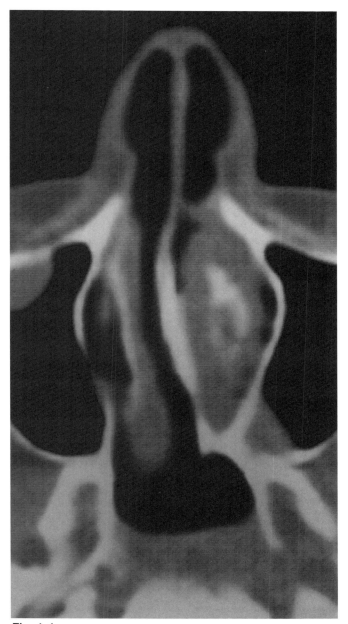

Fig. 1-1

Case 2

A 5-year-old boy with cystic fibrosis has nasal obstruction and nasal speech despite adenoidectomy.

Birth weight was 3.3 kg. Cough began at 6 weeks, frequent rectal prolapse at 18 months despite soft stools and painless bowel movement.

Parents and 2 brothers (8 and 11 years old) are well.

Temperature at 5 years is 35.5°C, heart rate 126, respiratory rate 28, blood pressure 98/60 mm Hg, weight 17.3 kg, and height 109 cm. Bridge of nose is flat. The rest of the physical findings are normal.

Hematocrit is 0.37. White cell count is 8.9×10^9/liter with 0.66 polymorphonuclear cells, 0.02 bands, 0.26 lymphocytes, 0.01 monocytes, 0.01 eosinophils, and 0.04 atypical lymphocytes. Platelet count is 368×10^9/liter.

Left side of nose is obstructed by mass that goes through choana into nasopharynx; right side is obstructed by mass that ends at choana (Figure 2-1). Roentgenogram of the chest at 3 years shows mucous plugs in left lower lobe and an aortic "nipple" at the arch (Figure 2-2A); roentgenogram of the chest of another boy (5 years old) shows cause of aortic "nipple" (Figure 2-2B). A catheter is in left highest intercostal vein; contrast medium injected through catheter is in accessory hemiazygos vein (see Figure 2-2B).

At operation, tissue is removed from both sides of the nose, ethmoid sinuses, and opening of left maxillary sinus. Thick, yellow-green mucopus is drained from maxillary sinuses. Culture grows β-hemolytic streptococci.

Resected tissue consists of translucent, gelatinous, white-to-yellow cysts and pink-tan to red-brown fragments.

Diagnosis: Cystic fibrosis, nasal polyps, aortic "nipple."

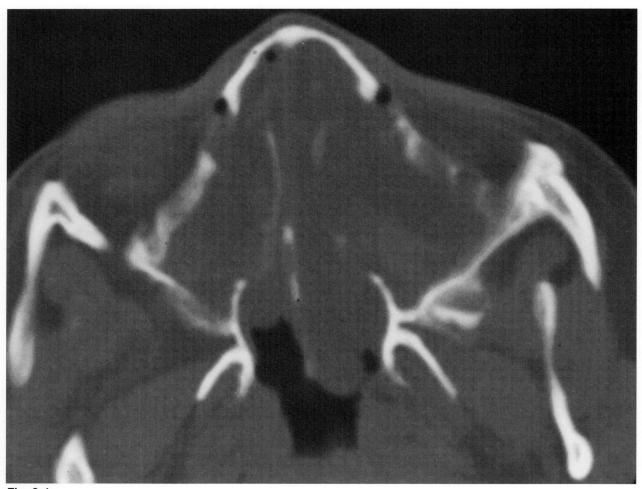

Fig. 2-1

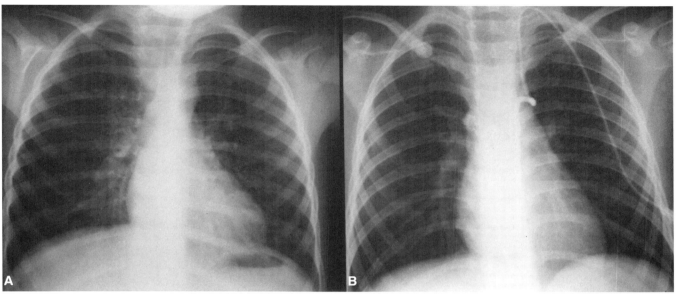

Fig. 2-2

Case 3

A 9-month-old boy has cough and runny nose. He vomits often.

Parents and sister (4 years old) are well.

Birth weight was 2.7 kg.

Weight at 9 months is 6.8 kg. He is thin and pale. The rest of the physical findings are normal.

Hematocrit is 0.34. White cell count is 7.6×10^9/liter with 0.20 polymorphonuclear cells, 0.05 bands, 0.67 lymphocytes, and 0.08 monocytes. Platelet estimate is adequate. Urine specific gravity is 1.006, pH 6. Urine has few epithelial cells/HPF and 3–4 white cells/HPF. Serum sodium is 137 mmol/liter, potassium 4.1, chloride 103, carbon dioxide 23, urea nitrogen 4.3, calcium 2.17, phosphorus 2.42, cholesterol 2.92, and glucose 5.2. Creatinine is 40 µmol/liter, uric acid 300, total bilirubin 3, and direct bilirubin 0. Total protein is 55 g/liter, albumin 35. Alkaline phosphatase is 341 U/liter, LDH 369, SGOT 53, and CK 193.

Ethmoidal and maxillary sinuses are opaque (Figure 3-1).

Sweat chloride is 114 mmol/liter.

Diagnosis: Opaque paranasal sinuses in infant with cystic fibrosis.

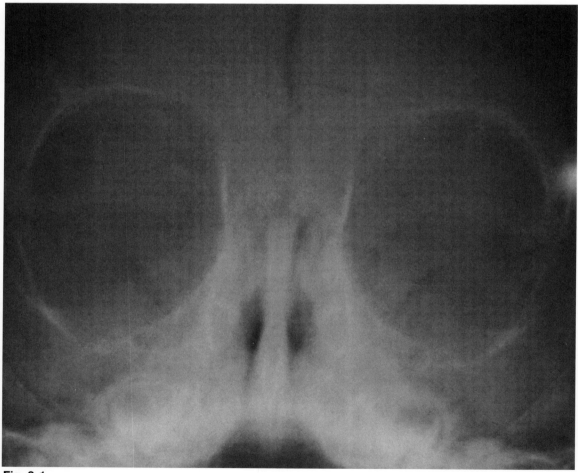

Fig. 3-1

Case 4

A 20-year-old man has cystic fibrosis.

He has been hospitalized 15 times, first time at 3 months when diagnosis was made. He cannot hold a job because he is sick so often. He watches TV "all day."

Weight at 20 years is 43.5 kg, height 156 cm. Throat is injected. Chest is barrel shaped. Fingers are clubbed. The rest of the physical findings are normal.

Hematocrit is 0.39. White cell count is 5.5×10^9/liter with 0.47 polymorphonuclear cells, 0.01 bands, 0.42 lymphocytes, 0.08 monocytes, and 0.02 basophils. Urine specific gravity is 1.018, pH 5. Urine has uric acid crystals, urates, and few epithelial cells/HPF. Sweat chloride is 106 mmol/liter.

Maxillary and ethmoidal sinuses are partly opaque, frontal and sphenoidal sinuses absent (Figure 4-1). Temporal air cells are normal.

Diagnosis: Opaque and immature paranasal sinuses in adult with cystic fibrosis.

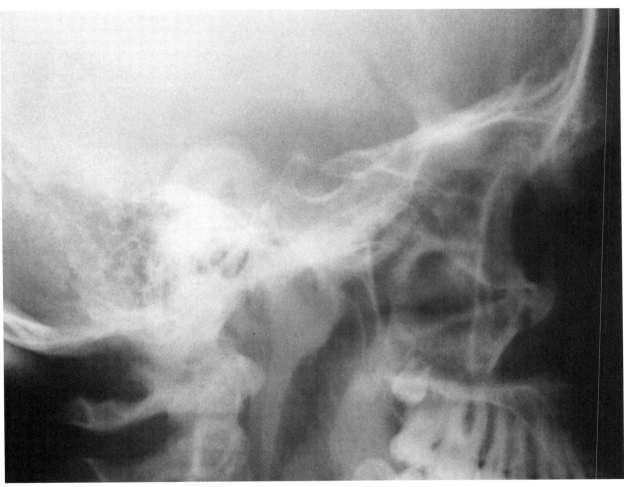

Fig. 4-1

Case 5

A 12-year-old boy cannot move his left arm and leg.

He had headache, runny nose, and fever 3 weeks ago. He felt bad and had worse headache 5 days ago, blew pus out of nose 4 days ago, and was weak in left arm and left leg 3 days ago.

Father died with kidney disease.

Temperature is 38.4°C, heart rate 86, blood pressure 150/90 mm Hg, and weight 50 kg. He is drowsy. Left side of face droops; left side of mouth drools. Nasal septum deviates left. White plaque is in dry mouth. Neck is stiff. Systolic heart murmur is present. Deep tendon reflexes are absent. Babinski's sign is in left foot. The rest of the physical findings are normal.

Hematocrit is 0.35. White cell count is 17.8×10^9/liter with 0.66 polymorphonuclear cells, 0.11 bands, 0.16 lymphocytes, and 0.07 monocytes. Urine has 1–3 white cells/HPF and 1–3 red cells/HPF. Serum sodium is 138 mmol/liter, potassium 4.0, chloride 98, urea nitrogen 3.2, and glucose 6.3. Creatinine is 60 µmol/liter, total bilirubin 7, and direct bilirubin 0. Alkaline phosphatase is 165 U/liter, LDH 218, and SGOT 12.

CT scan in Figure 5-1A shows convexity of falx cerebri to left and displacement of right frontal lobe from inner table, membrane between inner table and right frontal lobe that enhances after IV injection of contrast medium (Figure 5-1B), and left displacement of right lateral ventricle. Opaque right paranasal sinuses are also found but not shown.

At operation, 10 ml of creamy white pus is obtained through right frontal bur hole. Pus and granulation tissue are found in right ethmoidal, right sphenoidal, and both frontal sinuses.

Culture of pus from head and sinuses grows *Streptococcus viridans*; pus from head and blood grows coagulase-negative staphylococcus.

Diagnosis: Right frontal epidural abscess, right subdural empyema, sinusitis.

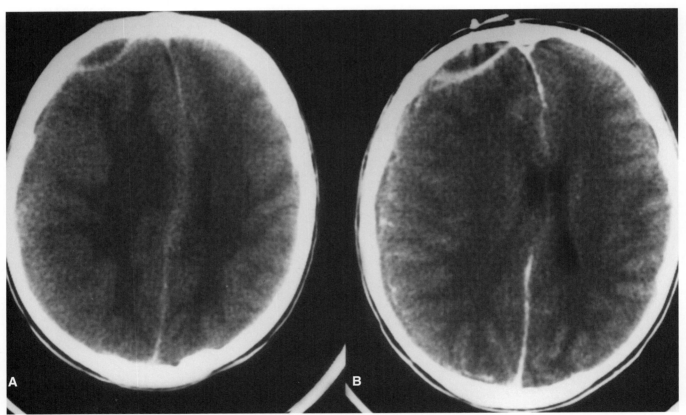

Fig. 5-1

Case 6

A newborn girl's breathing sounds like air being blown through pursed lips. She feeds well from right breast but not from left.

Parents and sister (3 years old) are well.

Pregnancy of mother was normal. Birth weight is 3.4 kg, respiratory rate 32.

A mass is behind left side of soft palate. The rest of the physical findings are normal.

A spherical mass is behind soft palate, attached to left lateral wall of nasopharynx in CT scan (Figure 6-1).

For the next 3 months, she breathes easily in prone position but not in supine position. She has trouble feeding. She often takes her thumb out of her mouth to breathe.

Weight at 3 months is 5.4 kg, length 58 cm, head circumference 40 cm, temperature 36.1°C, heart rate 140, respiratory rate 40, and systolic blood pressure 100 mm Hg. The mass behind soft palate protrudes into mouth. The rest of the physical findings are normal.

Hematocrit is 0.32. White cell count is 8.0×10^9/liter. Platelet count is 488×10^9/liter.

The tan, soft, slightly lobulated mass (2.5 × 1.5 cm) is removed from its attachment to soft palate and nasopharynx.

Microscopic examination shows keratinized, stratified squamous epithelium, sebaceous glands, dermal collagen, hair follicles, mature adipose tissue, skeletal muscle, and, in one section, mixed salivary gland tissue.

Diagnosis: Trepopnea, nasopharyngeal dermoid tumor.

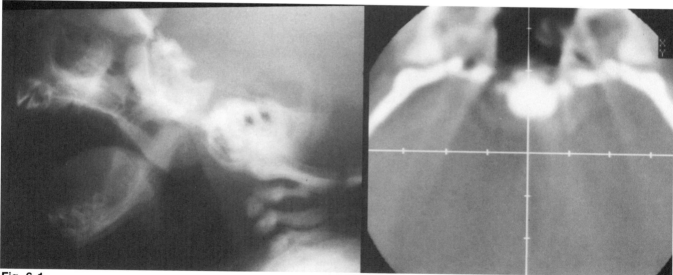

Fig. 6-1

Case 7

A 15-year-old boy has had frequent nosebleeds for 2–3 months.

Left side of nose has been blocked for 6 months. He has had left serous otitis media for 2 months despite myringotomy. He bled from left side of nose for 30 minutes a week ago. Right side of nose is partly blocked now. His voice sounds nasal to him but not to his parents.

Temperature is 36.5°C, heart rate 72, respiratory rate 16, blood pressure 134/72 mm Hg, height 172 cm, and weight 83 kg. A myringotomy tube is in left ear. Mucosa in left side of nose is pale. An irregular red-blue mass is present in left side of nasopharynx. The rest of the physical findings are normal.

Hematocrit is 0.42. White cell count is 7.9×10^9/liter, with 0.60 polymorphonuclear cells, 0.28 lymphocytes, 0.01 basophils, 0.09 monocytes, and 0.02 eosinophils. Platelet count is 334×10^9/liter. Urine specific gravity is 1.024, pH 7. Urine is normal. Serum sodium is 140 mmol/liter, potassium 5.1, chloride 107, carbon dioxide 29, urea nitrogen 3.2, calcium 2.37, and glucose 5.8. Creatinine is 60 µmol/liter.

CT scan in Figure 7-1 shows a mass in nasopharynx, oropharynx, and left pterygoid fossa, where it thins and spreads the medial and lateral plates of the left pterygoid process of the sphenoid bone and blocks or extends into left paranasal sinuses. Mass also extends into sphenoidal sinuses. Angiogram in Figure 7-2 shows branches of left maxillary artery in the mass.

At operation, a firm, lobed tumor is dissected from nasopharynx, base of sphenoid bone, sphenoid sinus, and scaphoid and pterygoid fossae of left pterygoid process.

Microscopic examination shows dense, hypocellular fibrous tissue and blood vessels, some wide with muscle in the wall, others narrow with prominent endothelial cells and pericytes.

Diagnosis: Angiofibroma.

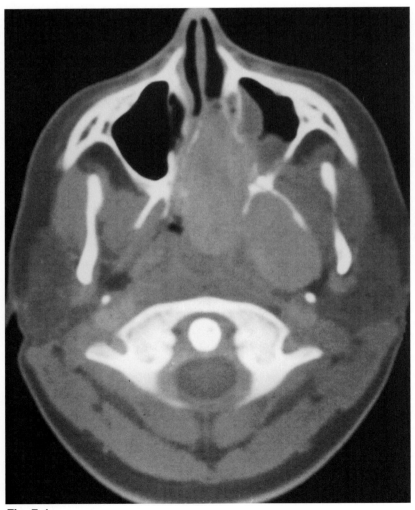

Fig. 7-1

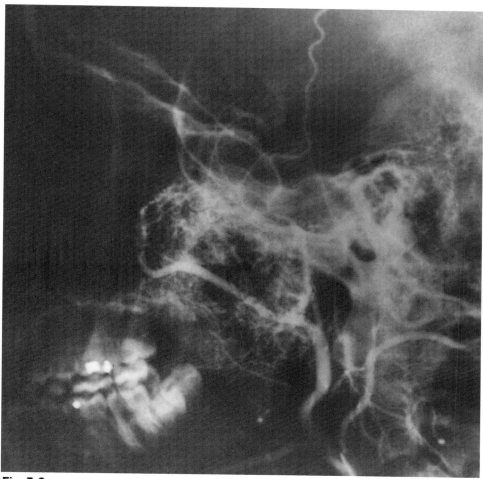

Fig. 7-2

Case 8

A 14½-year-old girl has pain over right eye.

She hit her head in a car accident 11 months ago. She had pain over right eye, fever, and frontal sinusitis 1½ weeks later. Pain recurs whenever she stops taking tetracycline.

She had meningococcal meningitis with purpura at 5 years and then impaired hearing until a year ago. Tonsils and adenoids were removed at 5 years; appendix was removed at 13 years. She has a "nervous stomach."

Parents and two brothers are well.

Weight at 14½ years is 54.5 kg, height 168 cm, temperature 37°C, heart rate 104, respiratory rate 24, and blood pressure 110/88 mm Hg. Right eyeball protrudes slightly. The rest of the physical findings are normal.

Hematocrit is 0.44. White cell count is 7.6×10^9/liter with 0.42 polymorphonuclear cells, 0.06 bands, 0.45 lymphocytes, 0.04 monocytes, 0.02 eosinophils, and 0.01 basophils. Platelet estimate is adequate. Urine specific gravity is 1.019, pH 5. Urine has hemoglobin, mucus, >100 red cells/HPF, and occasional white cells/HPF.

Figure 8-1 shows (1) one or two triangular shadows of air density with rim of bone in line of nasopharynx, (2) normal aeration of paranasal sinuses, and (3) small or absent adenoids.

Diagnosis: Recurrent right frontal sinusitis, normal aeration of sphenoid bone including pterygoid processes.

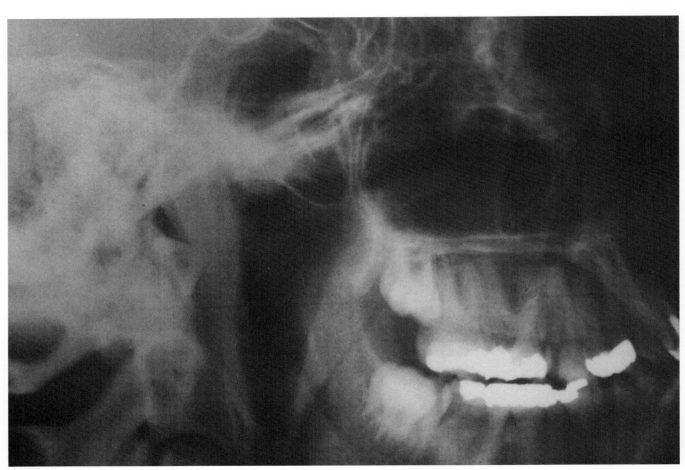

Fig. 8-1

Case 9

A 12-year-old girl has cough, runny nose, and fever. She wheezed and slept sitting up last night.

She had a similar illness a year ago. Tonsils were removed at 10 years. She had infectious mononucleosis 3 months later.

Temperature at 12 years is 36.6°C, weight 55 kg, and height 154 cm. She has rhonchi and wheezes. The rest of the physical findings are normal.

Roentgenograms at 11 and 12 years show adenoids and movement of velum of palate, down against back of tongue in first examination (Figure 9-1A), up against adenoids in second (Figure 9-1B).

Diagnosis: Normal velopharyngeal closure in girl with adenoids.

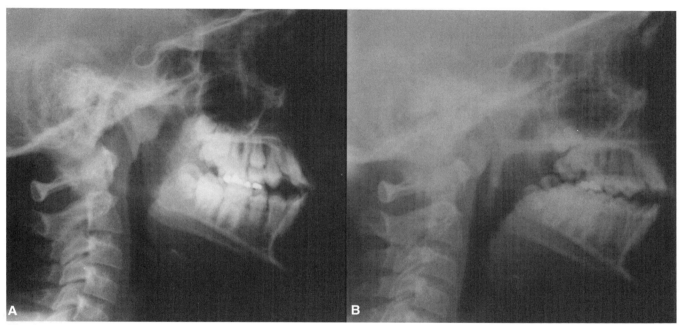

Fig. 9-1

Case 10

A 17-year-old boy is tired, hoarse, and achy.

Acute lymphoblastic leukemia was diagnosed 2½ years ago when he had pinpoint red rash, bruises, and sternal tenderness. Lymphoblasts were found in CSF a year ago when he had headache, vomiting, double vision, and slurred speech.

Temperature at 17 years is 37.5°C, heart rate 60, respiratory rate 16, blood pressure 138/96 mm Hg, weight 75 kg, and height 176 cm. He has right facial palsy. Left external acoustic meatus is injected. Left eye turns in. Sternum is tender. Deep tendon reflexes are depressed. The rest of the physical findings are normal.

Hematocrit is 0.38. White cell count is 36.7×10^9/liter with 0.52 polymorphonuclear cells, 0.13 bands, 0.08 lymphocytes, 0.04 monocytes, 0.04 eosinophils, 0.02 myelocytes, and 0.17 lymphoblasts. Platelet count is 295×10^9/liter. CSF has 28×10^6/liter white cells, 0.96 lymphoblasts, 4.6 mmol/liter glucose, and 0.42 g/liter protein. Marrow contains lymphoblasts. Chromosomes of 2 of 11 are 47,XY,6q⁻,+6q⁻.

Roentgenograms in Figure 10-1 show absence of adenoids and movement of velum of palate, down against back of tongue, up against retropharyngeal soft tissues.

Diagnosis: Normal velopharyngeal closure in boy with leukemia and no adenoids.

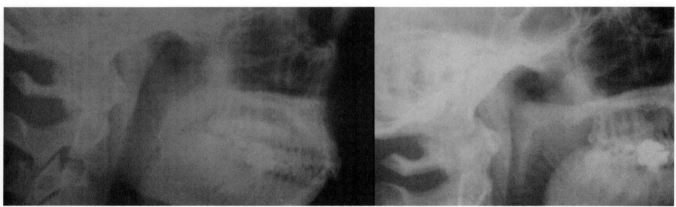

Fig. 10-1

Case 11

A 4-year-old boy is vomiting and febrile.

Pregnancy of mother was normal, birth weight 3.1 kg. Petechiae were on head. He had pneumonia at 4 months, boils at 5 months, weeping eczema at 6 months, severe chickenpox at 11 months, nosebleeds at 14 months, and "always colds." Petechiae were on head, neck, trunk, and limbs at 19 months.

Hematocrit at 19 months was 0.32. White cell count was 19.1×10^9/liter with 0.49 polymorphonuclear cells, 0.23 lymphocytes, 0.16 monocytes, 0.11 eosinophils, and 0.01 basophils. No platelets were present in blood smear, and platelet count 3 days later was 4×10^9/liter. He bled into left side of scrotum at 2½ years, into right side of face at 3 years. He had ankle and wrist pain and purpuric swelling of dorsa of hands and feet at 3 years. Lymph nodes were large in all regions. At 3 years, biopsy of left supraclavicular node (3×2 cm) showed a light tan, glistening capsule; normal architecture; depletion of paracortical lymphocytes and their replacement by histiocytes and plasma cells; lymphoblasts in germinal centers; aggregates of epithelioid cells, focal necrosis, plasma cells, and lymphocytes in cortex; and plasma cells, histiocytes, and mitoses in medulla.

Mother (24 years old), father (29 years old), and two sisters (1 and 5 years old) are well. No one else in mother's or father's family has had blood disease.

Temperature at 4 years is 38.9°C, heart rate 172, respiratory rate 32, weight 14.8 kg, and height 100 cm. Hair is red. Lymph nodes are large. Eczema is behind ears, on neck, in axillas, in groin, in front of elbows, and behind knees. The rest of the physical findings are normal.

Adenoids are absent, maxillary and ethmoidal sinuses opaque (Figure 11-1). Confluent shadows of water density and air bronchograms are in lungs the day of death 4 weeks later (Figure 11-2).

Culture of tracheal aspirate shows pure growth of *Candida*.

Diagnosis: Wiskott-Aldrich syndrome.

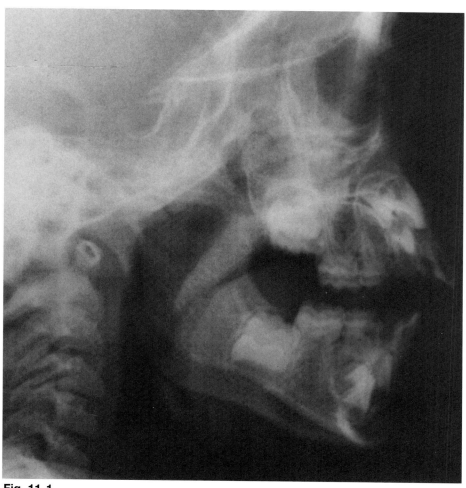

Fig. 11-1

(Continued)

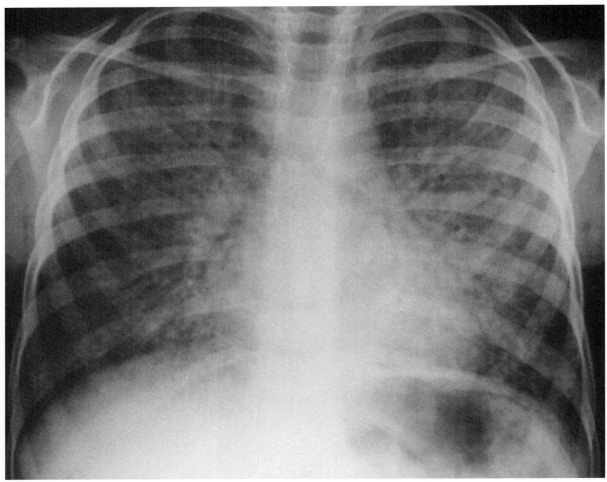

Fig. 11-2

Case 12

A newborn girl who is breathing hard has bubbly noises in the throat and turns blue when she cries. Breathing is easier with neck extended.

Mother (21 years old) had polyhydramnios and high blood pressure during pregnancy. Father (23 years old) is well. The girl is their only child.

Birth weight is 3.4 kg, Apgar score 9/10 at 1 and 5 minutes. A thin-walled cyst several centimeters in diameter is present in the pharynx. Suprasternal soft tissues retract during inspiration. The rest of the physical findings are normal.

Diaphragm is low and sternum bulges during inspiration (Figure 12-1A). Radiolucent coronal strips are between some ossified vertebral bodies and neural arches (see Figure 12-1A). A curved mass is in pharynx, a defect in clivus and sella turcica (Figure 12-1B).

She breathes easily after the cyst is incised. Cyst wall contains pseudostratified epithelium, ciliated in places, and fibrous tissue.

At 3 days, she is irritable, stiff, and twitching. Cry is high pitched. Temperature is 38.9°C. CSF has 175×10^9/liter red cells, 32×10^9/liter white cells, and 0.3 mmol/liter glucose when blood glucose is 7.3 mmol/liter. Stain shows gram-negative intracellular diplococci. Culture is sterile.

Diagnosis: Nasopharyngeal encephalocele, meningitis. (A brother born later has an encephalocele.)

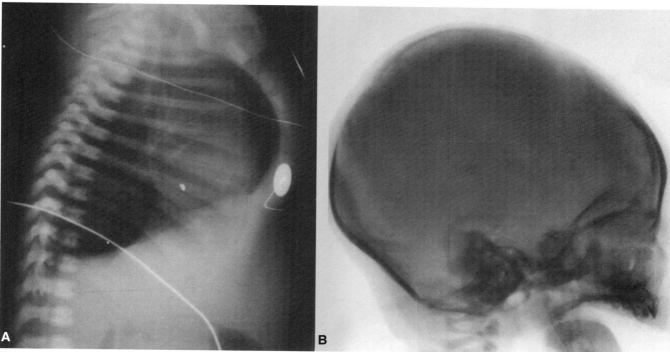

Fig. 12-1

Case 13

A 3½-year-old girl breathes noisily.

She has not been well for several weeks. Throat has been sore, voice muffled for 5 days. Breathing has been noisy, swallowing difficult for 3 days. She slept little last night.

Pregnancy of mother was normal, birth weight 3.7 kg. She has had thrush, iron deficiency anemia, otitis media, colds, and gastroenteritis.

Temperature at 3½ years is 38.7°C, heart rate 120, respiratory rate 30, systolic blood pressure 112 mm Hg, and weight 15 kg. She breathes through open mouth. Nose is blocked and runny. Supraclavicular and substernal soft tissues retract during inspiration, slight retraction at first but marked 7 hours later, when she is intubated. Tonsils are large, pus covered, and meet in midline. Lymph nodes (1 × 1 cm) are in neck. The rest of the physical findings are normal.

Hematocrit is 0.33. White cell count is 10.1×10^9/liter with 0.39 polymorphonuclear cells, 0.06 bands, 0.36 lymphocytes, 0.12 monocytes, and 0.07 atypical lymphocytes. Urine specific gravity is 1.024, pH 6. Urine has 1+ ketones, occasional squamous epithelial cells/HPF, 2–4 white cells/HPF, and amorphous urates. Arterial blood pH is 7.42 when FIO_2 = 0.20. PCO_2 is 35 mm Hg, PO_2 77.

Mouth is open, tongue elevated. Nasopharynx and oropharynx are filled with soft tissues, tonsils below, adenoids above, and superimposed earlobe in front of anterior arch of C1 (Figure 13-1).

Laryngoscopy shows beefy, red tonsils and normal larynx, epiglottis, and cervical esophagus.

Monospot test and screening test for heterophile antibody are positive.

Tonsils are removed 2 days later. Uncut surface is rough and hemorrhagic, cut surface is white-to-yellow with small hemorrhages. Microscopic examination shows lymphoid hyperplasia, ulceration, and acute inflammation.

Diagnosis: Infectious mononucleosis.

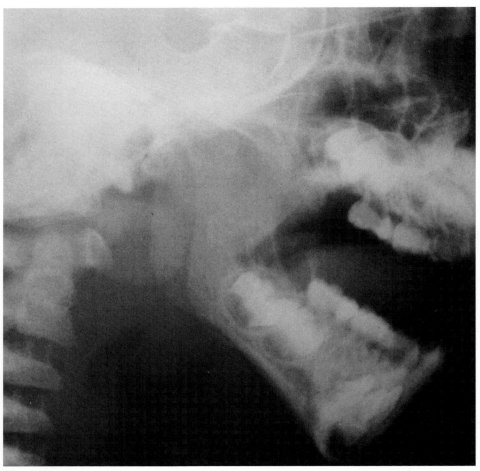

Fig. 13-1

Case 14

A 17-month-old boy who was grunting, retracting, and cyanotic this morning is now relaxed and sucking on a nipple.

Birth weight was 2.2 kg. Mother says, "He has never been right. He has snored since he was born." He sleeps sitting up. Sometimes no air moves while chest and abdomen rock up and down, and then he gasps, cries, and falls asleep until the cycle begins again. He does not cough. He vomits at night. He had an ear infection at 16 months. He has been sleeping more during the day for several weeks. He walks and eats table food.

Mother (34 years old) and father (37 years old), both smokers; two half brothers; and brother (6 days old) are well. Paternal grandmother died with amyotrophic lateral sclerosis.

Weight at 17 months is 8.4 kg, height 74 cm, head circumference 48 cm, temperature 37°C, heart rate 112, respiratory rate 26, and blood pressure 132/88 mm Hg. Limbs are thin. A hemangioma (0.5 cm) is on right shoulder. S_2 is loud. Abdomen is protuberant. Liver edge is at umbilicus. Diaper area is red. A hydrocele is in right side of scrotum. The rest of the physical findings are normal.

He becomes agitated and is given chloral hydrate. Stridor, grunting, retracting, and pulling of shoulders appear. Father says, "This is what he does at home." Blood oxygen saturation goes from 0.30 to 0.80 when he is propped up.

Hematocrit is 0.42. White cell count is 15.3×10^9/liter with 0.48 polymorphonuclear cells, 0.03 bands, 0.35 lymphocytes, 0.07 monocytes, and 0.07 atypical lymphocytes. Platelet count is 387×10^9/liter. Serum sodium is 139 mmol/liter, potassium 4.2, chloride 99, carbon dioxide 27, and glucose 5.1. Creatinine is 30 µmol/liter.

An orotracheal tube is put in.

Excess liquid is in lungs, pericardiocardiac is large (Figure 14-1A). Adenoids are prominent; orotracheal tube and enteric tube are in place in lateral examination of nasopharynx (Figure 14-1B).

ECG shows hypertrophy of right ventricle and right atrium. Echocardiogram shows enlargement and hypertrophy of right ventricle and tricuspid regurgitation.

At operation, mucopus is in pharynx. Adenoids block small choanae. Tonsils are large.

Microscopic examination of resected tonsils and adenoids shows reactive hyperplasia.

He has episodes of airway obstruction for as long as a minute, 5 nights later. A tracheostomy tube is put in place and left there until 3½ years, when his weight is 16 kg, height 102 cm, and blood pressure 130/70 mm Hg.

Diagnosis: Obstructive sleep apnea, cor pulmonale.

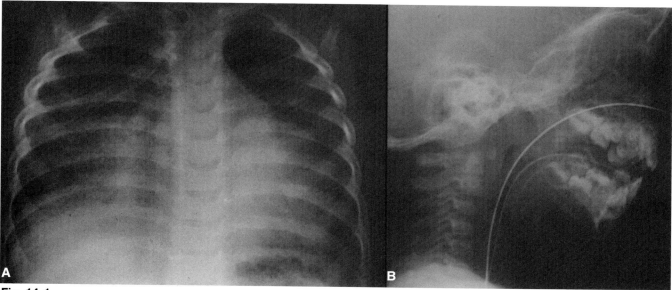

Fig. 14-1

Oropharynx

Case 1

A 3-year-old girl "talks like Donald Duck." She chokes on milk and water and sometimes vomits. Mother saw a mass "pop up" in back of throat when girl said, "Aah."

Temperature is 36.9°C, heart rate 88, respiratory rate 24, blood pressure 94/68 mm Hg, and weight 14 kg. She is hoarse. The rest of the physical findings are normal.

Hematocrit is 0.37. White cell count is 10.3 × 10⁹/liter. Platelet count is 473 × 10⁹/liter.

Retropharyngeal soft tissues bulge in Figure 1-1A. White ring of normal lamina dura in mandible is around unerupted permanent first molar teeth (sixth-year molars) in Figure 1-1A. Bulge disappears when she swallows barium (Figure 1-1B).

Endoscopy shows fullness of right vocal fold (true cord) and focal erythema near junction of vocal folds.

Diagnosis: Normal retropharyngeal soft tissues.

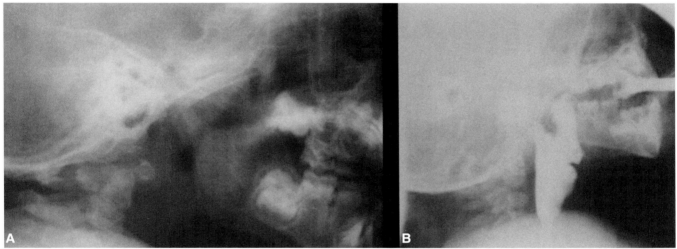

Fig. 1-1

Pharynx

Case 1

A 2-month-old girl fights for air, gasps, and coughs during nipple feedings.

Birth weight was 3.4 kg. She fed well the first 2 weeks but had trouble breathing. Bruises were on thighs when she was brought in for 6 week check-up.

Parents are well. She is their only child.

Temperature at 2 months is 37.3°C, heart rate 144, respiratory rate 48, systolic blood pressure 90 mm Hg, weight 3.7 kg, length 57 cm, and head circumference 38 cm. A continuous heart murmur is near left clavicle. Limbs are slightly hypertonic. The rest of the physical findings are normal.

Hematocrit is 0.35. White cell count is 6.8×10^9/liter with 0.43 polymorphonuclear cells, 0.02 bands, 0.38 lymphocytes, 0.11 monocytes, 0.05 eosinophils, and 0.01 basophils. Platelet count is 385×10^9/liter. Urine specific gravity is 1.014, pH 8. Urine has occasional squamous epithelial cells/HPF, 2–3 white cells/HPF, mucus, and bacteria. Serum sodium is 139 mmol/liter, potassium 5.4, chloride 102, carbon dioxide 23, urea nitrogen 3.6, calcium 2.52, phosphorus 1.94, cholesterol 4.01, triglycerides 1.14, and glucose 6.0. Creatinine is 40 μmol/liter, uric acid 160, total bilirubin 5, and direct bilirubin 2. Total protein is 53 g/liter, albumin 40. Alkaline phosphatase is 197 U/liter, LDH 606, SGOT 74, and CK 81.

Barium is in nipple, mouth, and nose in esophagram at 12 days; barium and air are in pharynx and esophagus; and constriction is in back half of the pharynx at level of C4 (Figure 7-1).

Endoscopic findings are normal at 2 months.

She takes her feedings well and "needs to stop for breath" every now and then while in hospital.

Diagnosis: Normal nasal regurgitation; normal constriction of pharynx at C4, the junction of insertion of middle and inferior pharyngeal constrictor muscles about two vertebral bodies above the cricoid cartilage, the cricopharyngeal part of the inferior pharyngeal constrictor muscle, and the level of origin of the esophagus; ductus arteriosus; unexplained bruises at 6 weeks.

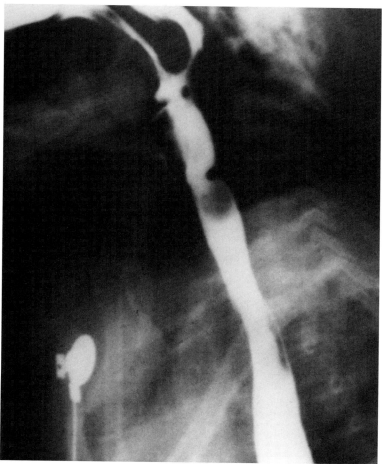

Fig. 7-1

Larynx

Case 1

A 14-year-old boy born with meningomyelocele comes in a wheelchair for a follow-up examination.

Birth weight was 3.1 kg, length 48 cm. Lumbosacral meningomyelocele was repaired, ventriculoatrial shunt placed for hydrocephalus, ileal loop diversion performed for neurogenic bladder, Harrington rod placed for scoliosis, calcaneal tendon lengthened for clubfeet, and triple arthrodesis later performed for feet.

Parents and three siblings are well.

Weight at 14 years is 41.3 kg, head circumference 55 cm, heart rate 120, respiratory rate 14, and blood pressure 124/80 mm Hg. One eye or the other turns out. Scars are on back and feet, ileal stoma and bag in right lower quadrant of abdomen, and flexion contractures at hips and knees. Legs are immobile, feet deformed. Motor and sensory level is at L4. The rest of the physical findings are normal.

Hematocrit is 0.42. White cell count is 8.9×10^9/liter. Urine specific gravity is 1.030, pH 7.5. Urine has 1+ protein, triple phosphates, amorphous phosphates, bacteria, and 7–8 white cells/HPF. Serum sodium is 145 mmol/liter, potassium 4.0, chloride 108, carbon dioxide 24, urea nitrogen 5.0, calcium 2.50, phosphorus 1.10, cholesterol 4.14, and glucose 6.8. Creatinine is 60 µmol/liter, uric acid 330, total bilirubin 5, and direct bilirubin 2. Total protein is 79 g/liter, albumin 49. Alkaline phosphatase is 272 U/liter, LDH 326, and SGOT 22.

Paired air sacs are on each side of larynx; a shunt tube is in right side of neck (Figure 1-1).

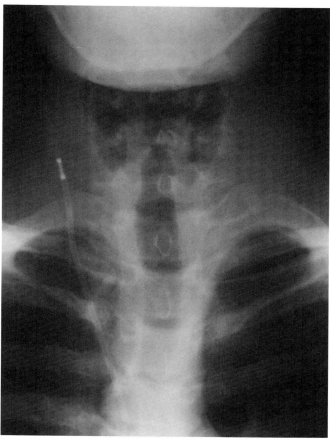

Fig. 1-1

He does not have a sore throat and is not hoarse. He is a high school junior at 18 years. IQ is 76. At 30 years, weight is 58 kg, head circumference 57 cm, heart rate 84, and blood pressure 154/89 mm Hg. Serum urea nitrogen is 5.7 mmol/liter. Creatinine is 90 µmol/liter. At 32 years, he lives alone, works in an auto body shop and an adult disabilities center and uses hand controls to drive his pickup truck.

Diagnosis: Internal laryngoceles from appendix of laryngeal ventricles, confined by thyroid cartilage; external laryngoceles, beyond them and higher, the result of herniation of internal laryngoceles through foramen in thyrohyoid membrane for superior laryngeal vessels and internal branch of superior laryngeal nerve.

Face

Case 1

A newborn boy breathes hard when crying in supine position and chokes when feeding.

Mother (28 years old), father (33 years old), sister (5 years old), and brother (3 years old) are well. Paternal grandmother and paternal uncle have diabetes mellitus.

Pregnancy of mother was normal. Birth weight is 2.9 kg, length 52 cm, head circumference 34 cm, Apgar score 7/8 at 1 and 5 minutes, temperature 36.6°C, heart rate 125, and respiratory rate 50. Right upper eyelid droops. Ear lobes are fleshy, external acoustic meatuses narrow and angled. Mandible is recessed. Soft palate is short. Thumbs are long. The rest of the physical findings are normal.

Chromosomes are 46,XY.

He is gavage-fed for 10 months because he refuses a nipple or chokes and regurgitates through nose when he accepts it. Hearing is impaired at 10 months. Thick wax and epithelial debris are present in external acoustic meatuses; seromucoid liquid is present in middle ears. Myringotomies and tube placement are performed at 10, 28, and 42 months under mask anesthesia. He can open his mouth only 0.5 in. at 42 months. Weight is 13.7 kg at 4 years, height 97 cm. Hearing is normal. He does not pronounce air pressure consonants such as *t*, *d*, *k*, and *g* well unless nose is pinched. He has dental caries and supernumerary upper lateral incisors. Antimongoloid slant of eyes; bilateral upper lid ptosis (right more than left); mandibular retrognathia; and short, immobile soft palate are observed at 5 years.

CT scan at 5 years (Figure 1-1A) shows absence of maxillary sinuses, coronoid processes of mandibles larger and higher than condyles, and almost no zygomatic process of temporal bones or temporal process of zygomatic bones. External acoustic meatus angles back more than normal. Three-dimensional reconstruction in Figure 1-1B shows mandibular condyle forward at articular tubercle of temporal bone, absence of mandibular fossa behind tubercle, and mandibular angle more oblique than normal.

Diagnosis: Mandibulofacial dysostosis (Treacher Collins syndrome).

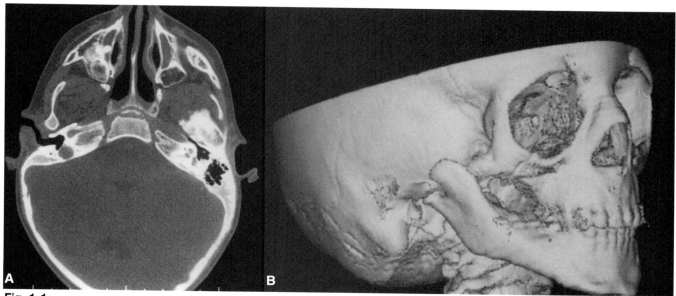

Fig. 1-1

Case 2

A 2½-week-old girl has swelling of left side of face.

Birth weight was 3.9 kg. A pea-sized lump on left alveolar process of left maxilla at birth is larger now.

Parents and sister (3 years old) are well.

Temperature is 37.6°C, heart rate 152, respiratory rate 52, systolic blood pressure 100 mm Hg, weight 3.9 kg, length 56 cm, and head circumference 38 cm. Left cheek and left side of upper lip are swollen. A soft, brown-purple, nontender, nonblanching mass (3.0 × 1.5 cm) is on alveolar process of left maxilla. The rest of the physical findings are normal.

Hematocrit is 0.45. White cell count is 11.7×10^9/liter with 0.28 polymorphonuclear cells, 0.04 bands, 0.58 lymphocytes, 0.08 monocytes, 0.01 eosinophils, and 0.01 basophils. Urine specific gravity is 1.002, pH 7. Urine has occasional epithelial cells/HPF, occasional white cells/HPF, and few bacteria. Serum chloride is 99 mmol/liter, carbon dioxide 16, urea nitrogen 3.2, calcium 2.37, phosphorus 1.97, cholesterol 3.44, and glucose 4.8. Uric acid is 180 μmol/liter, total bilirubin 9, and direct bilirubin 5. Total protein is 57 g/liter, albumin 33. Alkaline phosphatase is 261 U/liter, LDH 467, and SGOT 55.

Left maxilla is sclerotic and bulges into mouth (Figure 2-1).

At operation, a tumor that involves almost the whole left maxilla is removed.

The tumor (23.5 g) is streaked black and white. Microscopic examination shows small monomorphic cells that stain positive for melanin; prominent, evenly distributed nuclear chromatin; rare mitoses; and matrix of immature fibrous tissue.

Diagnosis: Pigmented neuroectodermal tumor of infancy (melanoameloblastoma).

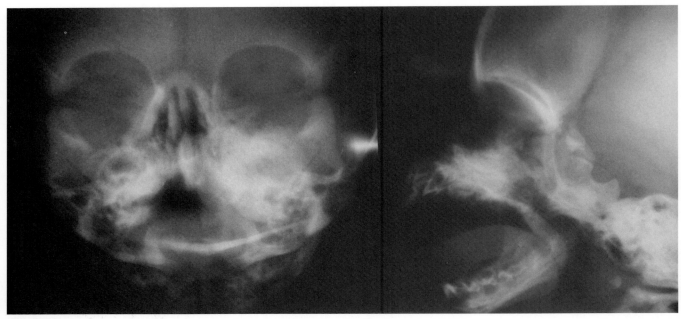

Fig. 2-1

Mouth

Case 1

A 13-year-old girl has swelling of left side of face.

She has had a hum in left ear for several years, loudest when she lies on her left side. Pulsations were below and in front of left ear lobe when she had left earache 2 months ago. She says that her teeth do not line up properly.

Parents are well. She is their only child.

Temperature at 13 years is 37.7°C, heart rate 75, and blood pressure 120/60 mm Hg. Left soft tissues from mandible to superior horn of thyroid cartilage are full and have thrill and bruit that diminish when left external carotid artery is compressed. Left lower canine, premolars, and molars are displaced into mouth. Superficial blood vessels are prominent in left lower gum and left side of nasopharynx. A venous hum is in neck and left side of chest. The rest of the physical findings are normal.

Hematocrit is 0.36. White cell count is 6.2×10^9/liter. Platelet estimate is adequate.

Left side of mandible is cystic and expanded, its cortex thinned, its third molar displaced (Figure 1-1). Selective left external carotid angiogram shows a cluster of small arteries supplied by facial artery and inferior alveolar branch of maxillary artery (Figure 1-2).

Diagnosis: Vascular malformation in mandible.

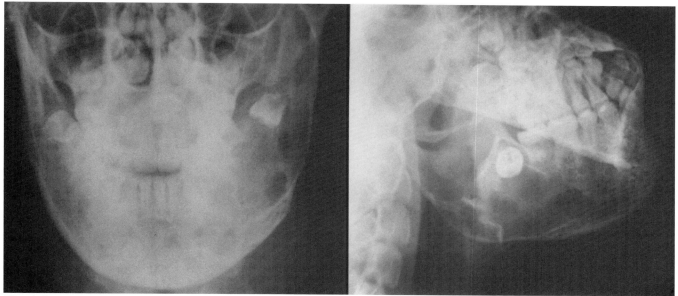

Fig. 1-1

(Continued)

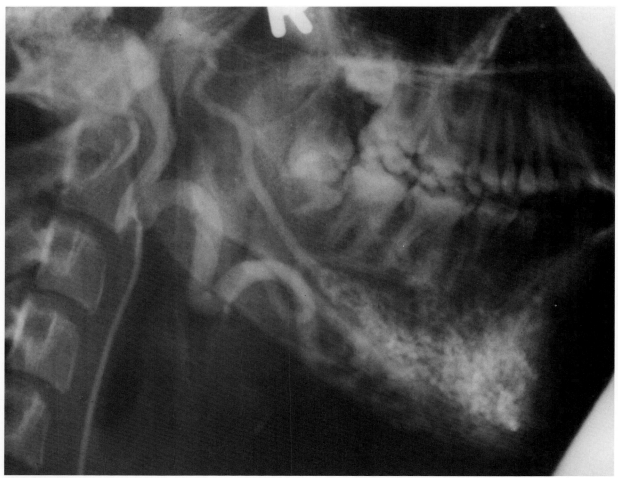

Fig. 1-2

Case 2

An 11-year-old boy has jaw cysts discovered in roentgenographic examination.

Mother (34 years old) and sister (12 years old) are well. Father (34 years old) has skin nevi. Sister (8 years old) has pits in her hands. Paternal grandfather, two paternal uncles, and paternal aunt have skin nevi.

Birth weight was 4.5 kg. He was given iron for anemia in infancy.

Weight at 11 years is 34.6 kg, height 141 cm, temperature 37.2°C, heart rate 84, respiratory rate 24, and blood pressure 118/72 mm Hg. Dark freckles are on back and forearms. A small, raised, light nevus is in right axilla. Right maxilla is thickened in cheek and mouth. Canine region of mandible is thickened on both sides. Teeth are missing. A small pit is in right palm. The rest of the physical findings are normal.

Hematocrit is 0.40. White cell count is 6.6×10^9/liter with 0.39 polymorphonuclear cells, 0.42 lymphocytes, 0.09 monocytes, 0.08 eosinophils, and 0.02 atypical lymphocytes. Urine specific gravity is 1.004, pH 6. Urine has rare squamous epithelial cells/HPF. Serum sodium is 140 mmol/liter, potassium 4.3, chloride 103, carbon dioxide 26, urea nitrogen 5.0, calcium 2.47, phosphorus 1.23, and glucose 6.8. Creatinine is 80 μmol/liter, uric acid 300, total bilirubin 3, and direct bilirubin 2. Total protein is 70 g/liter, albumin 47. Alkaline phosphatase is 449 U/liter, LDH 244, and SGOT 18.

A cyst is in mandible under left first premolar (Figure 2-1).

At operation, three cysts are in maxilla, two in mandible. Cyst walls are tan and semitranslucent; contents are white, cheesy matter and deciduous and permanent teeth.

Microscopic examination shows (1) cyst lining of thin, stratified squamous epithelium with varying amounts of keratin; (2) tall, cuboid, plump basal cells with darkly staining nuclei; (3) fibrous tissue; (4) abundant ground substance; (5) focal inflammation with lymphocytes, plasma cells, macrophages, and polymorphonuclear cells; (6) daughter cysts; and (7) islands of odontogenic epithelium, keratin, and cellular debris.

Diagnosis: Odontogenic keratocysts, basal cell nevus syndrome.

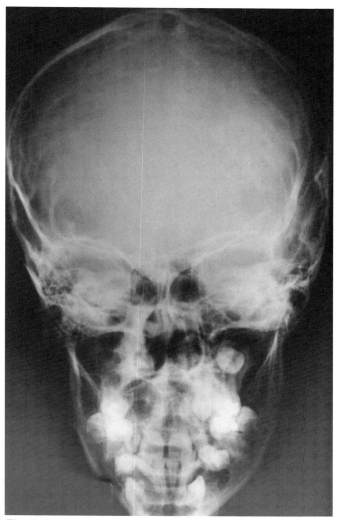

Fig. 2-1

Case 3

A 3½-year-old girl has a swollen jaw.

She hit her chin when she fell 4 months ago and hit her chin again and fractured the mandible when she knocked over a birdbath 3 months ago. A large bruise and swelling under mandible have subsided. She eats and plays normally.

Parents are well. She is their only child.

Temperature is 37.2°C, heart rate 120, respiratory rate 20, systolic blood pressure 100 mm Hg, weight 13.8 kg, and height 91 cm. Body of mandible is thick and firm; mandibular mucous membrane is stretched back to second molars. Occlusion is normal. Teeth are firm to palpation. The rest of the physical findings are normal.

Hematocrit is 0.36. White cell count is 18.7×10^9/liter with 0.53 polymorphonuclear cells, 0.05 bands, 0.39 lymphocytes, and 0.03 monocytes. Urine specific gravity is 1.027, pH 7. Urine has occasional squamous and nonsquamous epithelial cells/HPF, 1–3 white cells/HPF, and mucus. Serum sodium is 144 mmol/liter, potassium 4.7, chloride 108, carbon dioxide 21, urea nitrogen 4.6, calcium 2.54, phosphorus 1.32, cholesterol 4.34, and glucose 5.4. Creatinine is 80 μmol/liter, uric acid 320, total bilirubin 4, and direct bilirubin 2. Total protein is 72 g/liter, albumin 44. Alkaline phosphatase is 215 U/liter, LDH 409, and SGOT 36.

Random strands of bone are in body of expanded, radiolucent mandible (Figure 3-1).

At operation, granular pink-and-tan tissue is found in a cyst into which venous blood oozes.

Microscopic examination shows (1) dense clumps of multinucleated giant cells with as many as 20 nuclei in no particular intracellular location and (2) a cellular stroma in which cells have indistinct cytoplasmic margins and small round nuclei that resemble the giant cell nuclei. Giant cells are sparse in few places, and stroma is more fibrocytic.

Diagnosis: Giant cell reparative granuloma.

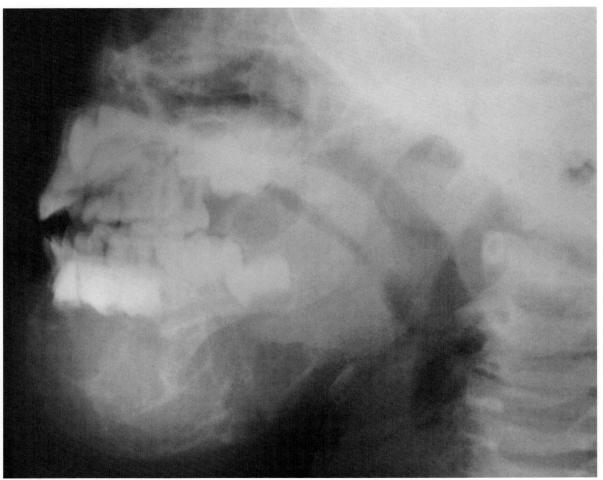

Fig. 3-1

Case 4

A 2½-year-old boy has loose teeth.

Scalp and ears have been red and scaly for 6 months. He began to drink and urinate a lot 2 months ago. Three loose teeth were removed from right side of mandible 5 days ago. A large soft spot was felt on back of head 3 days ago.

Pregnancy of mother was normal, birth weight 3.8 kg. He walked at 1 year. He often has runny nose and ear infection.

Temperature at 2½ years is 37.7°C, heart rate 164, respiratory rate 28, systolic blood pressure 136 mm Hg, weight 11.5 kg, and height 88 cm. Scalp and ears are red and covered with scabs. Cheeks are red and puffy. Chin recedes. Mandible deviates to right. Three teeth are missing. Liver edge is 2 cm below costal margin. A scaly rash covers buttocks and thighs. The rest of the physical findings are normal.

Hematocrit is 0.34. White cell count is 10.0×10^9/liter with 0.44 polymorphonuclear cells, 0.10 bands, 0.39 lymphocytes, and 0.07 monocytes. Urine specific gravity is 1.002, pH 7. Urine has occasional squamous epithelial cells/HPF. Serum sodium is 142 mmol/liter, potassium 5.5, chloride 98, carbon dioxide 25, urea nitrogen 1.4, calcium 2.47, phosphorus 1.42, cholesterol 4.27, and glucose 3.4. Creatinine is 30 μmol/liter, uric acid 250, total bilirubin 5, and direct bilirubin 0. Total protein is 61 g/liter, albumin 39. Alkaline phosphatase is 195 U/liter, LDH 319, SGOT 39, and CK 393. IgG is 6.64 g/liter (normal: 4.2–12.0), IgA 0.98 (normal: 0.18–1.50), IgM 0.77 (normal: 0.45–2.00), C3 1.77 (normal: 1.41 ± 0.15), and C4 0.79 (normal: 0.15–0.45).

Skin tests are negative for *Trichophyton*, *Candida*, streptokinase-streptodornase, and tuberculosis.

Defects are in skull and mandible (as well as in left humerus and left tenth rib); temporal bones are sclerotic (Figure 4-1). Roentgenogram of abdomen 6 months later shows normal tenth rib and toy motorcycle that the boy slipped under himself when he lay on x-ray table (Figure 4-2).

Examination of two molars that fall out at 3½ years shows infiltration of inter-radicular tissue by syncytia of histiocytes that are mostly fat-containing macrophages, scattered eosinophils, and focal destruction of roots.

Diagnosis: Langerhans' cell histiocytosis.

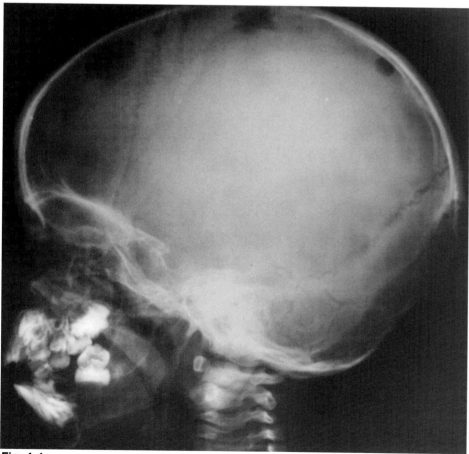

Fig. 4-1

(Continued)

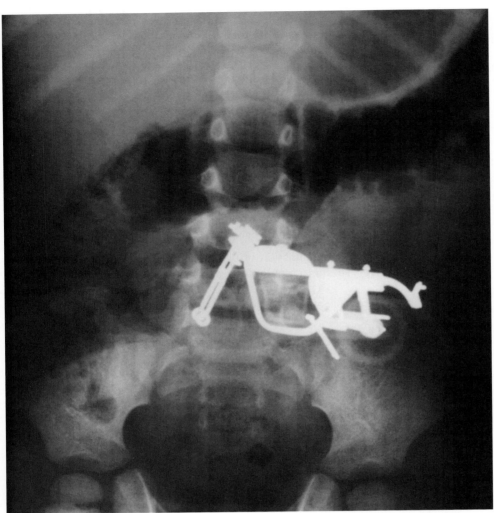

Fig. 4-2

Case 5

A 6-year-old girl has a swelling of the face that was noticed 6 months ago and has caused no symptoms.

Pregnancy was normal. She had tonsillitis 1 year ago.

Parents and two siblings are well.

Weight at 6 years is 25 kg, height 120 cm, heart rate 120, respiratory rate 24, and blood pressure 100/70 mm Hg. A bony, nontender swelling (5 × 5 cm) is in right side of face. Gum bulges over right side of mandible. Left side of mandible has three molars, right side two. The rest of the physical findings are normal.

Hematocrit is 0.38. White cell count is 10.1×10^9/liter.

Right side of mandible is expanded, cortex thinned, mineralization not uniform (Figure 5-1).

Biopsy of fleshy, pink tissue from right side of mandible shows (1) mesenchymal stroma of pale, eosinophilic material with many small fibers; (2) many small cells with round-to-oval nuclei and little eosinophilic cytoplasm in dendritic processes radiating from nuclei; (3) low cuboidal epithelium; (4) microcysts with papillomatous epithelial growths; (5) epithelial nests with peripheral row of low columnar cells, central cuboidal cells, and intervening layer of stellate cells; (6) deeply basophilic calcific material; and (7) spaces filled with epithelial cells of squamous appearance.

Diagnosis: Ameloblastic odontoma.

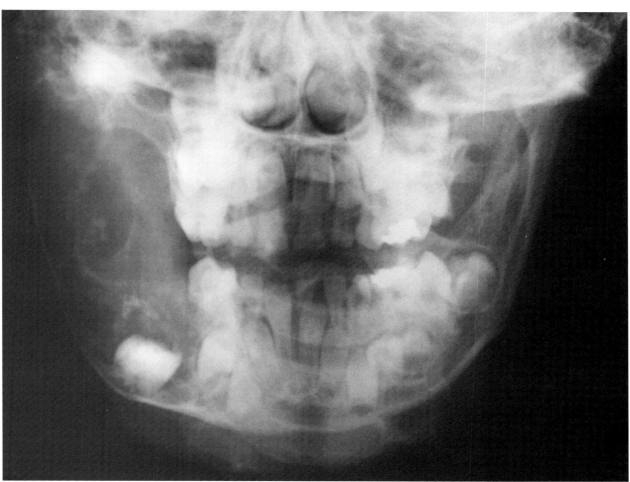

Fig. 5-1

Case 6

A 16-year-old boy, who does not like hot weather, is seen for a routine check-up.

Hair was sparse and fine at 16 months. His only teeth at 16 months were two upper, cone-shaped, widely separated central incisors. Skin was scaly and dry with eczema on arms, scabs on back of hands, and peeling palms and soles. Skin was dry at 7 years. He often had stuffy nose. Nose was swollen and scabbed at 7 years. Sores surrounded mouth. He has asthma.

Toenails of mother and maternal grandmother have longitudinal ridges.

Teeth are few at 7 years (Figure 6-1).

Weight at 16 years is 70 kg. Hair is fine and sparse. Skin is dry. He has false teeth. The rest of the physical findings are normal.

Diagnosis: Anhidrotic ectodermal dysplasia.

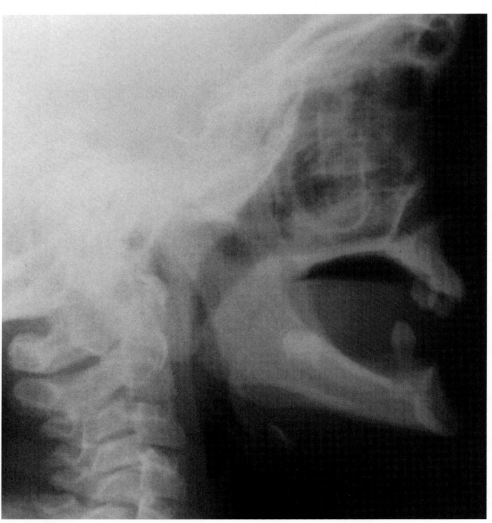

Fig. 6-1

Case 7

A 4-year-old boy has loose teeth. Mandibular central incisors erupted at 11 months and fell out at 24 months. Maxillary central incisors are loose.

Pregnancy of mother was normal, birth weight 3 kg. He sat at 5 months and walked at 10 months.

Parents (both 32 years old) and sister (6 years old) are well.

Weight at 4 years is 13.4 kg, height 99 cm, and head circumference 52 cm. Maxillary central incisors are discolored. The rest of the physical findings are normal.

Hematocrit is 0.37. White cell count is 9.8×10^9/liter. Platelet count is 489×10^9/liter. Serum sodium is 140 mmol/liter, potassium 4.5, chloride 108, carbon dioxide 22, urea nitrogen 4.0, calcium 2.42, phosphorus 1.91, cholesterol 4.22, and glucose 4.7. Creatinine is 40 µmol/liter, uric acid 210, total bilirubin 5, and direct bilirubin 2. Alkaline phosphatase is 63 and 56 U/liter (mother's: 33 U/liter), LDH 287, and SGOT 32. Urinary phosphoethanolamine is 913 µmol/g creatinine and, 2 years later, 808 (normal: 140–540).

Left ulnar metaphysis and left fibular metaphysis are undermineralized in Figure 7-1. Findings in rest of skeleton are normal.

Bone mineral analysis by photon densitometry at 4 years shows low value for cortical bone density and higher-than-normal ratio of trabecular to cortical bone.

Weight at 6½ years is 18.8 kg, height 117 cm, and head circumference 54 cm. According to examining physician, "Head and neck exam reveals absent teeth and bilateral submandibular nodes that are not tender." The rest of the physical findings are normal. Feet hurt at 7½ years when he walks a lot or runs. Feet are flat. The rest of the physical findings in the legs are normal.

Diagnosis: Hypophosphatasia.

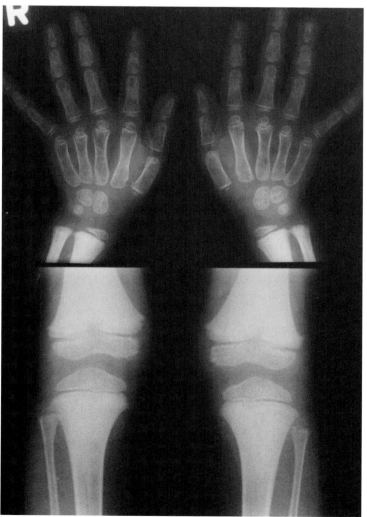

Fig. 7-1

Case 8

A 12-year-old boy has a crooked nose and crowded upper teeth.

He hit his face on the dashboard in a car crash 4 years ago. A swelling of upper jaw has been getting larger for 2 years.

Parents and two sisters are well.

Temperature at 12 years is 37°C, heart rate 80, respiratory rate 14, blood pressure 118/50 mm Hg, weight 39 kg, and height 151 cm. Right side of face bulges over swelling (3 × 3 cm) that crowds upper right lateral incisor and canine, bulges into hard palate, and pushes right inferior nasal concha medially. The rest of the physical findings are normal.

Hematocrit is 0.36. White cell count is 6.5×10^9/liter with 0.44 polymorphonuclear cells, 0.07 bands, 0.36 lymphocytes, 0.07 monocytes, 0.05 eosinophils, and 0.01 basophils. Platelet estimate is adequate. Urine specific gravity is 1.017, pH 6.5. Urine has few squamous epithelial cells/HPF and amorphous phosphates. Serum sodium is 137 mmol/liter,

potassium 4.6, chloride 100, carbon dioxide 24, urea nitrogen 5.7, and glucose 5.0.

Waters' view shows cystic mass in nose and lateral displacement of upper right lateral incisor (Figure 8-1A). Lateral view shows thin, curved rim of bone in front of mass in maxilla, top of rim where anterior nasal spine of maxilla should be (Figure 8-1B).

At intraoral operation, a blue cyst with thin bony wall involves maxillary sinus and roots of upper right lateral incisor and canine teeth.

Microscopic examination of cyst shows (1) rim of membranous bone around fibrous wall; (2) stratified, nonkeratinizing squamous epithelium; (3) acute and chronic inflammatory tissue; and (4) a red-black cavity.

Diagnosis: Globulomaxillary cyst.

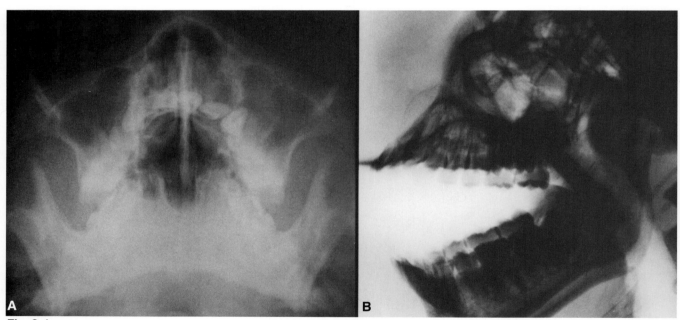

Fig. 8-1

Neck

Case 1

A 1-year-old boy has wet cough, noisy breathing, and a cyst in left side of neck.

Cough and stridor began 10 days ago. Left side of neck was swollen 9 days ago. Breathing has been noisier and swelling larger for 3 days. He has been cranky, lethargic, and anorectic for 2 days. He vomited yesterday.

Birth weight was 3.5 kg, length 53 cm. He had croup at 3 months. He was scratched by a cat on right side of neck 1 month ago.

Mother (19 years old) and father (30 years old) are well. He is their only child.

Temperature at 1 year is 36.4°C, heart rate 140, respiratory rate 40, blood pressure 100/56 mm Hg, weight 9.3 kg, and height 76 cm. Sternum retracts during inspiration. A fluctuant, nontender cyst (6 × 4 cm) is in neck beneath left angle of mandible and deep to sternocleidomastoid muscle. Uvula is displaced to right. Left palatine tonsil and semilunar fold are displaced into oropharynx. Breathing is noisy in upper airway. The rest of the physical findings are normal.

Hematocrit is 0.43. White cell count is 24.9 × 10⁹/liter with 0.60 polymorphonuclear cells, 0.10 bands, 0.23 lymphocytes, 0.03 monocytes, and 0.04 eosinophils. Platelet count is 751 × 10⁹/liter. Serum sodium is 133 mmol/liter, potassium 4.4, and chloride 95.

Retropharyngeal swelling displaces trachea forward (Figure 1-1) and to the right.

At direct laryngoscopy, a cyst in left side of neck compresses airway, mainly subglottic part. Aspiration of 15 ml serous liquid from cyst partly relieves obstruction. At operation, the following are removed: (1) a cyst deep to platysma; (2) part of stalk, which goes between carotid bifurcation and above hypoglossal nerve; and (3) some lymph nodes, which show follicular hyperplasia on microscopic examination.

Culture of aspirate grows *Streptococcus viridans*.

Diagnosis: Second pharyngeal pouch cyst.

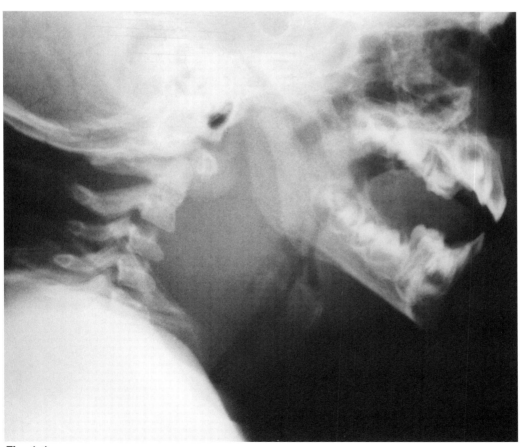

Fig. 1-1

Case 2

A 5-day-old girl breathes noisily and has a cyst in neck.

Mother (22 years old) had gestational diabetes. Birth weight was 3.5 kg, Apgar score 7/9 at 1 and 5 minutes.

Parents, sister (3 years old), and brother (1 year old) are well.

Temperature is 38°C, heart rate 140, respiratory rate 25, and blood pressure 70/50 mm Hg. She is pink and breathes quietly until disturbed. She is dusky when she cries and has inspiratory stridor and sternal retraction. When she cries, the cyst in left side of neck is firmer and bulges more. Liver edge is 1 cm below costal margin. The rest of the physical findings are normal.

Hematocrit is 0.60. White cell count is 23.7×10^9/liter with 0.60 polymorphonuclear cells, 0.12 bands, 0.19 lymphocytes, 0.05 monocytes, and 0.04 eosinophils. Platelet count is 311×10^9/liter. Serum sodium is 142 mmol/liter, potassium 5.2, chloride 112, calcium 2.42, and glucose 5.1. Total bilirubin is 183 µmol/liter.

In Figure 2-1, air and liquid are in cyst in left side of neck. Barium swallow shows compression of laryngopharynx and displacement to right (Figure 2-2A) and forward (Figure 2-2B). A drop of barium at level of piriform recess goes into cyst (see Figure 2-2B).

At laryngoscopy, left piriform recess bulges. At operation, a stalk from a retropharyngeal cyst deep to left sternocleido-mastoid muscle goes into left piriform recess. The cyst contains cheesy, tan-yellow matter.

The cyst ($3 \times 2 \times 2$ cm) has a thin, tan-purple wall. Microscopic examination shows granulation tissue, inflammatory cells, and foci of thyroid and parathyroid tissue.

Diagnosis: Left third pharyngeal pouch cyst.

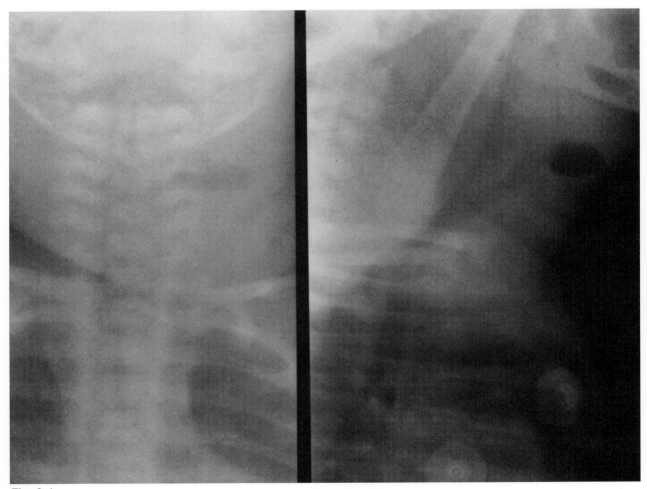

Fig. 2-1

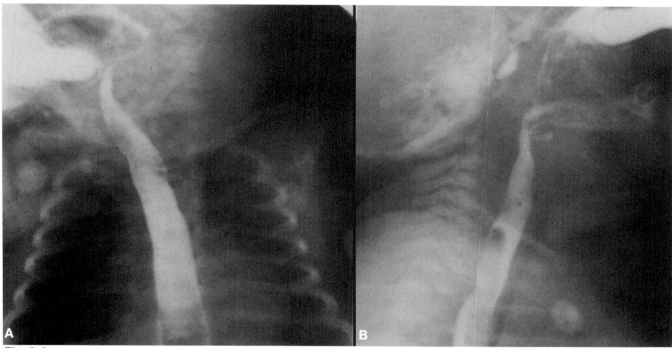

Fig. 2-2

Case 3

A newborn boy cannot breathe until intubation because of neck mass.

Mother (21 years old) and father (23 years old) are well.

Pregnancy of mother was normal. Birth weight is 3.6 kg, temperature 36.7°C, heart rate 140, and systolic blood pressure 60 mm Hg. Neck mass and systolic heart murmur are present. The rest of the physical findings are normal.

Roentgenogram at 1½ hours shows mass with plaques of calcium density in front of neck (Figure 3-1). An oropharyngeal tube ends at about level of epiglottis.

At operation at 3 hours, a cystic, multiloculated mass extends from mediastinum to posterior cervical triangles and adheres to trachea from cricoid cartilage to bifurcation. Two brown bodies (0.75 cm), thought to be parathyroid glands, are freed from lower edge of mass and are not removed from neck. Another similar body at upper edge above hyoid bone is thought to be the thyroid gland.

Resected mass (12 × 10 cm) is brown, irregular, and gritty when cut. Microscopic examination shows bone trabeculae, cartilage, respiratory epithelium, squamous epithelium, gastrointestinal epithelium, fibroblastic connective tissue, mature fibrous connective tissue, myxoid connective tissue,

CNS-like connective tissue with fibrillar ground substance, isolated neuronlike cells, peripheral nerve fibers, thyroid acini, and normal thyroid tissue at upper pole and at another knobby protuberance of capsule.

He loses an estimated 45 ml of blood during operation and is given 40 ml. Hematocrit after operation is 0.54. Serum sodium is 129 mmol/liter, potassium 4.2, chloride 92, urea nitrogen 6.8, calcium 2.47, and phosphorus 1.16. Alkaline phosphatase is 24 U/liter.

Endotracheal tube is removed at 5 days. Tracheotomy is performed for respiratory distress at 8 days. At laryngoscopy at 8 months, right vocal fold is flaccid, bowed, and fixed in midline. He sits at 7 months, walks at 14 months. Tracheostomy tube is removed at 14 months. He cries, gasps, vomits, and turns blue 4 days later. Granulation tissue around the stoma is removed at laryngoscopy, and another tube put in. The tube is removed at 3 years. Mucus comes out of stoma until fistula is excised at 4 years. Weight at 16 years is 69 kg, height 176 cm, and blood pressure 114/70 mm Hg. He is a member of his high school's wrestling team.

Diagnosis: Thyroid teratoma.

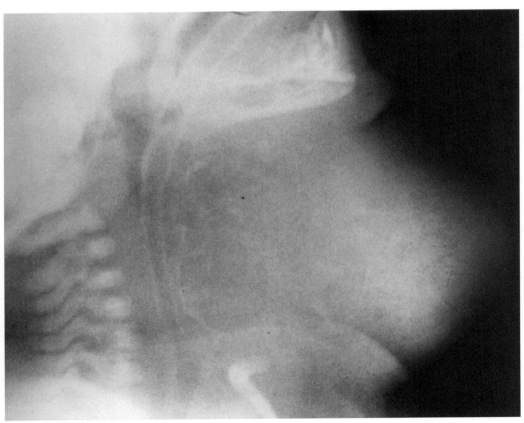

Fig. 3-1

Case 4

A newborn boy, who needs to be awakened for feedings and then will not suck, fusses, cries, sneezes, and drools. He passes meconium the first day but does not urinate until the third day.

Mother (25 years old) smoked, drank, and used cocaine during pregnancy. Chlamydial infection was diagnosed 19 days before delivery, vaginal discharge present 14 days before delivery. Birth weight is 2.7 kg, Apgar score 9/9 at 1 and 5 minutes. Temperature is 37.5°C at 3 days, heart rate 170, respiratory rate 40–52, and blood pressure 58/38 mm Hg. Nose is stuffy. Muscles are hypotonic, deep tendon reflexes normal. The rest of the physical findings are normal.

Hematocrit is 0.43. White cell count is 21.3×10^9/liter with 0.66 polymorphonuclear cells, 0.17 bands, 0.12 lymphocytes,

0.04 monocytes, and 0.01 eosinophils. Platelet count is 421×10^9/liter. T_4 is 107 nmol/liter at 3 days (normal: 152–292). TSH is >210 mU/liter (normal: 1.0–10.9). Total bilirubin at 4 days is 168 µmol/liter. Urine screen is positive the third day for cocaine and ecgonine.

Barium swallow at 12 days shows thickening of prevertebral tissues (Figure 4-1).

Diagnosis: Prevertebral myxedema, congenital hypothyroidism. (Treatment with levothyroxine is begun at 12 days.)

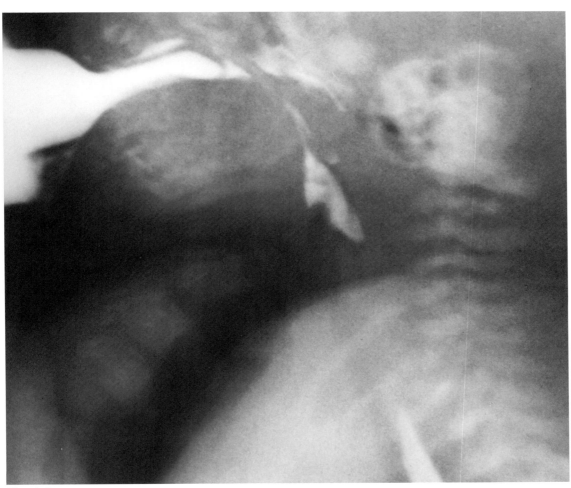

Fig. 4-1

Case 5

A 9-year-old girl has a painful lump in neck.

She vomited for 3 days 2½ weeks ago. Lump appeared 1½ weeks ago, along with right earache, fever, nausea, and dysphagia. She has lost 1 kg. Neck has been red for 1 day.

Parents and sister (10 years old) are well.

Temperature is 38.4°C, heart rate 108, respiratory rate 30, blood pressure 100/80 mm Hg, weight 26 kg, and height 133 cm. She will not turn her head. An indurated, fluctuant, tender mass (6-cm diameter) that does not move when she swallows is in front of neck. The rest of the physical findings are normal.

Laboratory data are not obtained.

Ultrasound examination in Figure 5-1A shows a midline mass with mixed echoes. Technetium 99m scan in Figure 5-1B

shows lateral displacement of lobes of thyroid with total uptake 3.9% at 20 minutes (normal: 2–5%).

Incision and drainage yields 50 ml yellow-green pus that contains gram-positive cocci and gram-negative rods. Culture grows γ streptococcus, *Eikenella corrodens*, *Bacteroides melaninogenicus*, and *Staphylococcus aureus*.

At operation one month later, a scarred track from thyroid isthmus to hyoid bone and middle third of hyoid bone are excised.

Diagnosis: Infected thyroglossal duct cyst.

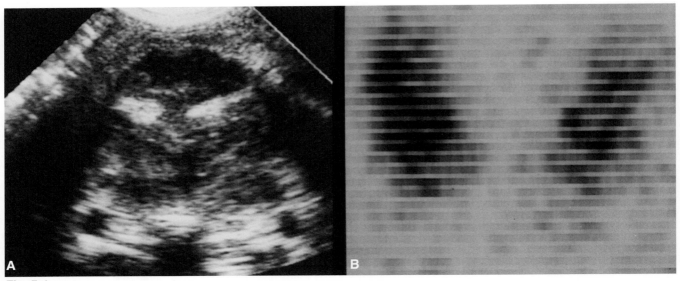

Fig. 5-1

Case 6

A 14¾-year-old girl is "hyper one minute, dead the next."

She has had headaches for the past few months. She cannot fall asleep at night. She does not feel like getting up in the morning. Heart beats fast with little exertion. Menarche was at 12 years. Periods have been more frequent during the last 2 months, separated by 2½-week intervals. She had a cold a few weeks ago and found a lump when she rubbed her neck.

Tubes were put in ears when she was an infant.

Weight is 56 kg, height 167 cm, temperature 37.5°C, heart rate 108, respiratory rate 20, and blood pressure 110/78 mm Hg. Outstretched hands are tremulous. A smooth, nontender mass in left side of neck moves up when she swallows. Deep tendon reflexes are brisk. The rest of the physical findings are normal.

Hematocrit is 0.39. White cell count is 10.3×10^9/liter with 0.51 polymorphonuclear cells, 0.43 lymphocytes, 0.04 monocytes, and 0.02 eosinophils. Platelet count is 328×10^9/liter. Serum calcium is 2.25 mmol/liter.

Ultrasound examination shows normal right lobe of thyroid gland and thin isthmus (Figure 6-1A) and mixed echoes in enlarged left lobe (Figure 6-1B).

Serum free T_4 is 34.8 pmol/liter (normal: 10.3–29.7). Total T_3 is 4.91 nmol/liter (normal: 1.28–3.28). TSH is 0.1 mU/liter (normal: 0.4–5.3).

At operation, a dark green mass is in left lobe of thyroid gland.

The resected mass (4.5 × 3.3 cm) contains papillary tissue and hemorrhagic foci inside a rim of normal thyroid tissue.

She is treated with daily levothyroxine after operation to prevent recurrence. Results of tests of thyroid function at 16 years are normal.

Diagnosis: Follicular adenoma with hemorrhage and cyst in left lobe of thyroid gland.

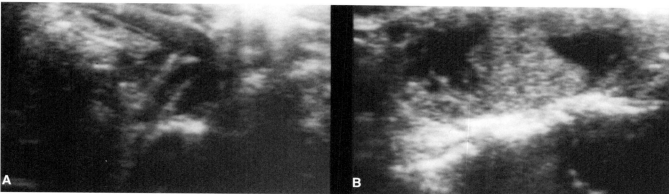

Fig. 6-1

Case 7

A 2-year-old girl has swelling on nape and right side of neck.

Pregnancy was normal, birth weight 2.8 kg. Swelling with red-brown spots was present at birth. She began to talk at 1 year and walk at 15 months.

Mother (34 years old), father (36 years old), and brother (14 years old) are well. A paternal aunt has café au lait spots.

Weight is 10 kg, height 84 cm. Café au lait spots are on chest and thighs, and the largest on nape of neck. Mass under the spot is smooth and nontender. The rest of the physical findings are normal.

Right side of neck is swollen at 7 years, trachea displaced to left, and spinal canal shallow front to back. Upper cervical vertebrae are dysplastic (Figure 7-1).

More café au lait spots appear during next several years. The mass—lumpy, irregular, boggy, and larger under red-brown skin—is resected at 13 years. Its light yellow to dark brown surface is coarsely granular and soft with scattered firm nodules. Microscopic examination of mass shows small foci of nerve tissue and cells that are scattered, whorled, and in cords. Cells have faintly fibrillar, eosinophilic cytoplasm and round-to-stellate basophilic nuclei.

Diagnosis: Neurofibromatosis, plexiform neuroma.

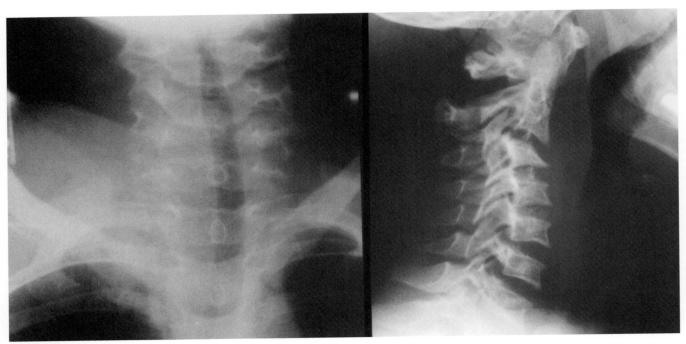

Fig. 7-1

Case 8

A 7-year-old girl has pain in the neck.

Nose began to run in early spring, a month ago. Eyes have been teary and itchy for a week. She began to cough 2 days ago, coughed and wheezed yesterday, and woke up this morning coughing hard and complaining of neck pain.

Parents are well. Sister (9 years old) and paternal uncle have allergies.

Temperature is 37.7°C, heart rate 180, respiratory rate 40, blood pressure 110/56 mm Hg, weight 30 kg, and height 122 cm. Eyes are red. Nose is runny. Crepitus is in neck. Prolonged expiration and inspiratory and expiratory wheezes are present. The rest of the physical findings are normal.

In Figure 8-1, air is in retropharyngeal soft tissues, mucosa of maxillary sinuses is thickened, and an earlobe is superimposed on anterior arch of C1 behind adenoids.

Diagnosis: Asthma, retropharyngeal dissection of mediastinal air.

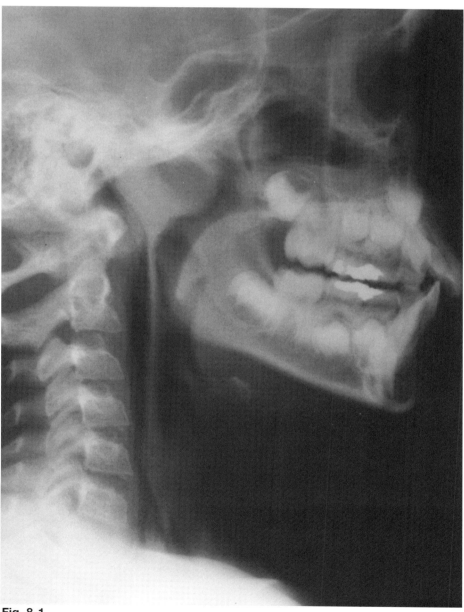

Fig. 8-1

Upper Airway

Case 1

A 5-month-old girl is drooling and breathing hard and noisily.

Pus drained from left ear yesterday. She ate lunch today, then became fussy and febrile, and began to breathe hard less than 2 hours ago. She has not coughed.

Pregnancy of mother was normal, birth weight 3.9 kg.

Temperature is 38.3°C, heart rate 180, respiratory rate 40, systolic blood pressure 110 mm Hg, and weight 6.3 kg. She is pink, alert, and retracting. Nose is runny. Pus is in left external acoustic meatus, left eardrum red and bulging. Epiglottis is red and swollen. Coarse rhonchi are in chest. The rest of the physical findings are normal.

Hemoglobin is 112 g/liter. White cell count is 23.6×10^9/liter with 0.70 polymorphonuclear cells, 0.05 bands, 0.22 lymphocytes, and 0.03 monocytes.

Mouth is open; supraglottic tissues are swollen (Figure 1-1).

Culture of pus in left ear grows *Haemophilus influenzae* type B and pneumococci.

Diagnosis: Epiglottitis (supraglottitis), *H. influenzae* type B infection.

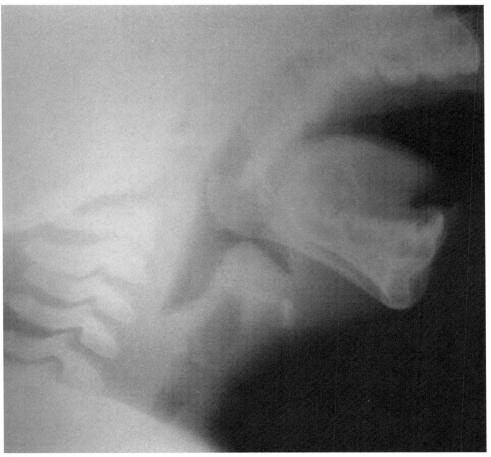

Fig. 1-1

Case 2

A 4-year-old boy drools, spits blood, and breathes noisily. Parents believe someone gave him a piece of hard candy.

Temperature is 37.5°C, heart rate 130, respiratory rate 20, blood pressure 110/50 mm Hg, and weight 15 kg. Nits are in hair. Petechiae are on face, eyelids, neck, and chest. Lips and gums are red and swollen. Tongue is eroded, soft palate swollen. A bruise is on a buttock. The rest of the physical findings are normal.

Hematocrit is 0.35. White cell count is 22.9 × 10⁹/liter. Platelet count is 378 × 10⁹/liter. Serum sodium is 141 mmol/liter, potassium 3.7, chloride 112, carbon dioxide 19, urea nitrogen 3.2, calcium 2.45, phosphorus 1.22, cholesterol 4.00, and glucose 8.6. Creatinine is 50 µmol/liter. Total protein is 71 g/liter, albumin 43.

Supraglottic tissues are swollen in Figure 2-1.

Endoscopy after endotracheal intubation shows burns in esophagus.

Diagnosis: Ingestion of caustic substance (found to be Drano), laryngeal edema, esophageal burns.

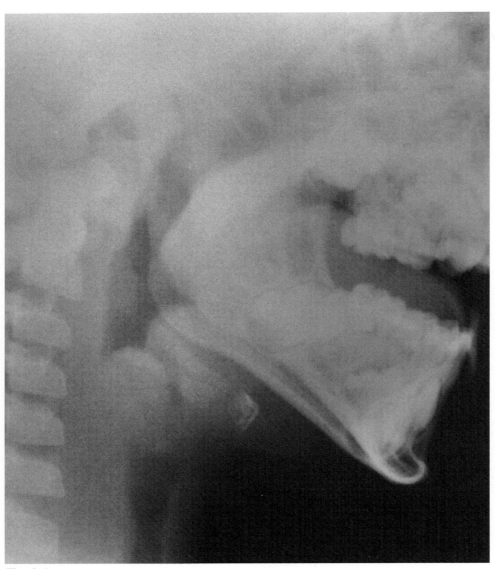

Fig. 2-1

Case 3

A 14-month-old boy cries noiselessly.

He suddenly began to cough and drool 6 days ago while eating chicken and spaghetti. He coughed all night, breathed noisily, wheezed, and then had fever. He has been drinking but not eating. He vomited today.

Parents and six siblings are well. A brother has fever and vomited today. The family has two cats.

Temperature is 39.5°C, heart rate 140, respiratory rate 40, blood pressure 120/70 mm Hg, weight 10.7 kg, and length 84 cm. He is listless and weak. Color changes from pale pink to dusky when he is agitated. Breathing is noisy with inspiratory retraction and prolonged expiration. Right eardrum is pink. A small capillary hemangioma is on left buttock, a depigmented spot on left side of chest. Left testicle is not palpable. The rest of the physical findings are normal.

Hematocrit is 0.42. White cell count is 16.1×10^9/liter with 0.56 polymorphonuclear cells, 0.26 bands, 0.13 lymphocytes, 0.03 monocytes, and 0.02 atypical lymphocytes. Serum sodium is 140 mmol/liter, potassium 5.2, chloride 102, urea nitrogen 2.0, and glucose 5.7. Arterial blood pH is 7.41 when FIO_2 = 0.20. PCO_2 is 49 mm Hg, PO_2 95.

An angular object, point down, is at glottis; epiglottis and aryepiglottic folds at level of body and greater horns of hyoid bone are normal (Figure 3-1).

At bronchoscopy, a foreign body is found in vascular granulation tissue just below vocal folds.

Diagnosis: Piece of chicken bone near glottis.

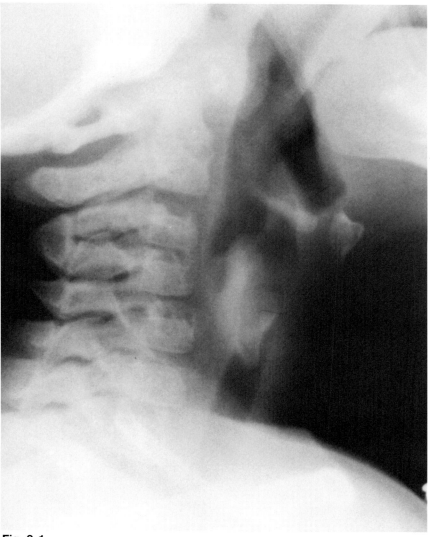

Fig. 3-1

Case 4

A 23-month-old girl is hoarse.

She had cough and noisy breathing 2 months ago and has been hoarse since then. Laryngoscopy was performed a month ago. She had a tracheostomy for 5 days.

Mother (24 years old), father (23 years old), and two sisters are well.

Temperature at 23 months is 36.7°C, heart rate 124, respiratory rate 20, and systolic blood pressure 80 mm Hg. She has inspiratory and expiratory stridor. A small growth is on left tonsil. A scar is on neck. The rest of the physical findings are normal.

Hematocrit is 0.36. White cell count is 9.5×10^9/liter with 0.43 polymorphonuclear cells, 0.05 bands, 0.46 lymphocytes, and 0.06 monocytes.

A mass of water density is at level of glottis (Figure 4-1).

At microlaryngoscopy, papillomas are found on left ventricular and vocal folds (false and true vocal cords), on right vocal fold, below left vocal fold, on left tonsil, and in left vallecula.

Microscopic examination of light tan tissue that is removed shows squamous papillomas.

Diagnosis: Laryngotracheal (and oropharyngeal) papillomatosis.

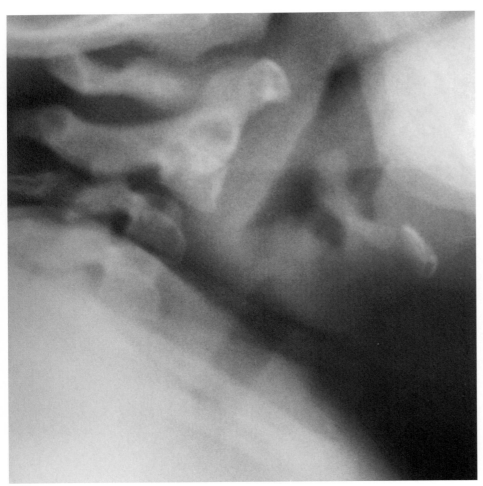

Fig. 4-1

Case 5

A 16-month-old boy breathes hard.

Mother had a seizure during the fifth month of pregnancy and has taken daily phenobarbital since then. Birth weight was 3.1 kg, length 50 cm. Breathing was hard at birth. He was given oxygen continuously at several weeks and is given oxygen now when excessively tired or after crying, when he sometimes turns blue, gasps, loses consciousness, and twitches without oxygen.

Mother (30 years old) and father (29 years old) are well. He is their only child.

Heart rate at 16 months is 140, respiratory rate 32, weight 6.3 kg, length 72 cm, and head circumference 46 cm. He is small, weak, and pale around lips. Nasal bridge is low. Grooves are alongside small alae nasi. Nasal spine of maxilla and alar cartilage are hypoplastic. Nasal septal cartilage is absent. He wheezes, and depressed sternum retracts during inspiration. The rest of the physical findings are normal.

Tracheal cartilage is calcified at 3 weeks (Figure 5-1A). Calcification is less at 16 months. At 16 months, deposits of calcium are in triradiate cartilage of innominate bones (Figure 5-1B) and lateral to transverse processes of lumbar vertebrae.

Diagnosis: Chondrodysplasia punctata.

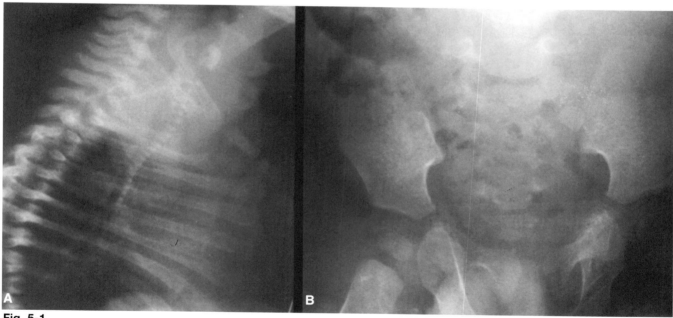

Fig. 5-1

Cervical Spine

Case 1

A 13-year-old girl walks stiffly, tilts head to right, and wears hearing aids.

Pregnancy of mother was normal, birth weight 3.2 kg. She did not react to noise at 6 weeks. Bulging anterior fontanel and bilateral papilledema at 3 months, associated with CSF pressure of 50 mm H_2O and right lateral ventricular pressure of 300 mm Hg, were treated by left nephrectomy and lumbar–left ureteral shunt. She walked at 1 year. Audiogram at 6 years showed bilateral sensorineural deficit. Weakness in limbs that changed from time to time and side to side appeared at 6 years. She wet her pants for the first time at 7 years. Left Horner's syndrome, bilateral Babinski's sign, and weak deep tendon reflexes appeared. At 9 years, she awoke one morning unable to move her left arm and unaware of its position. Deep tendon reflexes were brisk.

Parents and three siblings are well.

Weight at 13 years is 28 kg, height 126 cm, temperature 37.1°C, heart rate 82, respiratory rate 20, and blood pressure 110/60 mm Hg. Speech is slow and nasal. Gag reflex and tongue thrust are weak. Right shoulder is lower than left. Left scapula is winged. Thoracic spine is convex left, lumbar spine convex right. Left limbs are smaller than right. Arms are weak. Position sense in left leg is diminished. A midline scar is on back at L1, an oblique scar in left groin. The rest of the physical findings are normal.

Hematocrit is 0.37. White cell count is 5.2×10^9/liter with 0.20 polymorphonuclear cells, 0.25 bands, 0.49 lymphocytes, 0.04 monocytes, 0.01 eosinophils, and 0.01 basophils. Platelet count is 400×10^9/liter. ESR is 8 mm/hr.

Spinal canal is elongated at C1 and C2, and posterior arch of C1 and laminae of C2 are thin (Figure 1-1A). Right internal carotid arteriogram shows posterior inferior cerebellar artery originating from persistent trigeminal artery and going below foramen magnum (Figure 1-1B).

At operation, left cerebellar tonsil is at C2, right tonsil at C3, and lower part of fourth ventricle, the obex, at C2.

Diagnosis: Arnold-Chiari malformation, type 1.

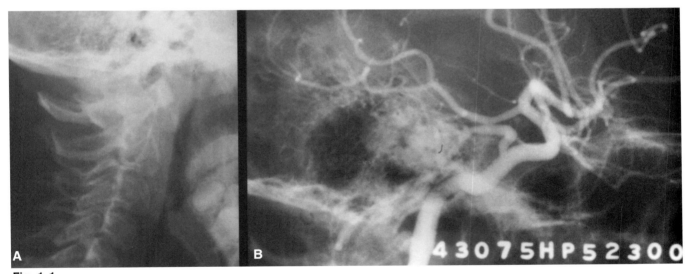

Fig. 1-1

Case 2

A 15-year-old boy has a cough and runny nose.

Weight is 60 kg, temperature 36.6°C, heart rate 60, and blood pressure 128/84 mm Hg. Conjunctivae are inflamed. Cervical lymph nodes are prominent. The rest of the physical findings are normal.

Stylohyoid ligaments and bottom edge of posterior atlanto-occipital membrane are ossified (Figure 2-1).

Diagnosis: Normal ossification of stylohyoid ligament and free border of posterior atlanto-occipital membrane over vertebral artery and suboccipital nerve (dorsal ramus of C1).

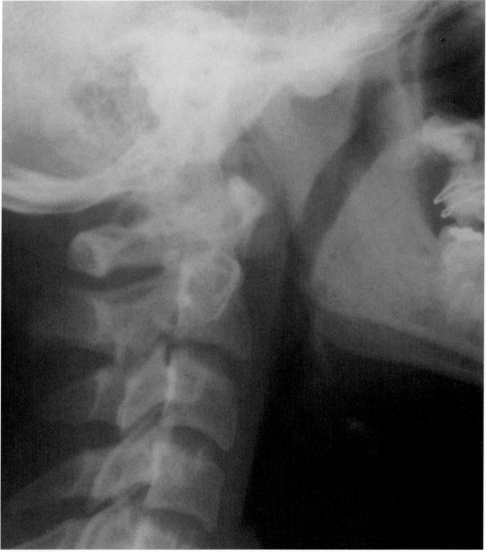

Fig. 2-1

Case 3

A 10-year-old boy has a spongy lump behind the right ear that has regrown after two attempts to remove it at 2 and 8 years.

He has had mumps, chickenpox, and ear infections. Tonsils and adenoids were removed at 3 years. Tubes were put in ears at 8 years.

Father (29 years old) is well. Mother (29 years old), sister (4 years old), and brother (8 years old) have neurofibromatosis. Maternal grandmother is only one of 14 siblings thought to have neurofibromatosis.

Temperature at 10 years is 37°C, heart rate 76, respiratory rate 18, blood pressure 118/68 mm Hg, weight 31 kg, and height 132 cm. The lump that feels "like a bag of worms" pushes right auricle out, narrows right external acoustic meatus, and extends down neck. Nodules (0.5 cm) are present along the left greater auricular nerve. Café au lait spots are on chest and abdomen. He has slight conduction hearing loss, right side more than left. The rest of the physical findings are normal.

Hematocrit is 0.41. White cell count is 7.6 × 10⁹/liter with 0.49 polymorphonuclear cells, 0.04 bands, 0.36 lymphocytes, 0.03 monocytes, 0.06 eosinophils, and 0.02 basophils.

Platelet estimate is adequate. Urine specific gravity is 1.019, pH 6. Urine has 0–1 white cell/HPF. Serum sodium is 141 mmol/liter, potassium 4.6, chloride 104, carbon dioxide 22, urea nitrogen 4.3, and glucose 4.3.

In Figure 3-1A, lower cervical and upper thoracic vertebrae and second and third ribs on the two sides are not symmetric. In Figure 3-1B, spinal canal is shallow at C1, hypoplastic odontoid articulates with bone spur from occipital bone, and a defect is in occipital bone.

At operation, a tumor behind right ear goes from dermis to periosteum, forward to lateral canthus, along external acoustic meatus, along facial nerve, and under sternocleidomastoid muscle.

Gelatinous cysts are in gray-tan fragments of cut tumor. Microscopic examination shows nodules of uniform cells with oblong, deeply basophilic nuclei and tapering eosinophilic cytoplasm; loose, edematous stroma; and myxoid foci.

Diagnosis: Neurofibromatosis, plexiform neuroma, hypoplastic dens, large occipital condyles.

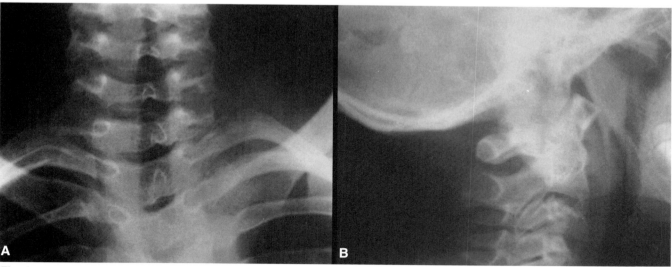

Fig. 3-1

Case 4

A 9½-month-old boy cannot turn head all the way to right and has high right shoulder.

Pregnancy of mother was normal, birth weight 3.3 kg. At 3 months, he was thought to have wry neck. He sat at 6 months. He cruises around furniture.

Mother (24 years old) and father (27 years old) are well. He is their only child. Paternal grandparents are first cousins. A paternal aunt has hearing defect and bicornuate uterus.

Weight at 9½ months is 8.5 kg, length 73 cm, and head circumference 50 cm. Head is tipped down and to right. Right scapula is high. Right side of chest is small and without breath sounds. The rest of the physical findings are normal.

Neck is short and has fewer than seven dysplastic vertebrae (Figure 4-1A). Upper thoracic vertebrae and upper right ribs are dysplastic; heart is in radio-opaque right side of chest (Figure 4-1B). Excretory urogram performed at 1¼ years because of skeletal abnormality shows dilated left renal pelvis and calyces, redundant left ureter, normal bladder, and no right kidney (Figure 4-2).

Diagnosis: Klippel-Feil deformity of neck, other skeletal abnormalities, congenital absence of right lung and probably right kidney.

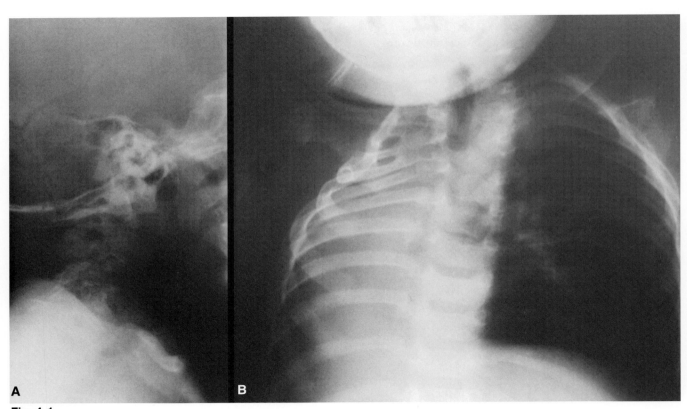

Fig. 4-1

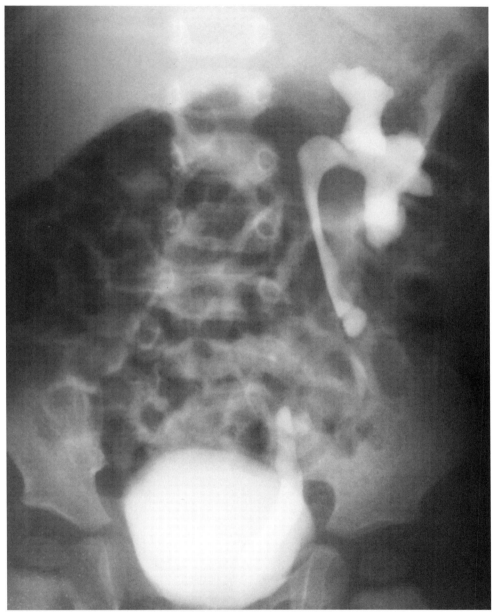

Fig. 4-2

Case 5

An 8-year-old girl has a slight hearing deficit.

She has had several ear infections since the first one at 1 year, when she had measles. Adenoids were removed 6 months ago.

Weight at 8 years is 27 kg, height 127 cm, and temperature 36.8°C. Eardrums are slightly retracted. The rest of the physical findings are normal.

Posterior arch of atlas, visible in foramen magnum in Towne's view (Figure 5-1A), is not completely ossified (Figure 5-1). Adenoids are small or absent (Figure 5-1B).

She is pregnant at 19 years. Physical findings are normal.

Diagnosis: Incomplete ossification of posterior arch of atlas in 8-year-old girl.

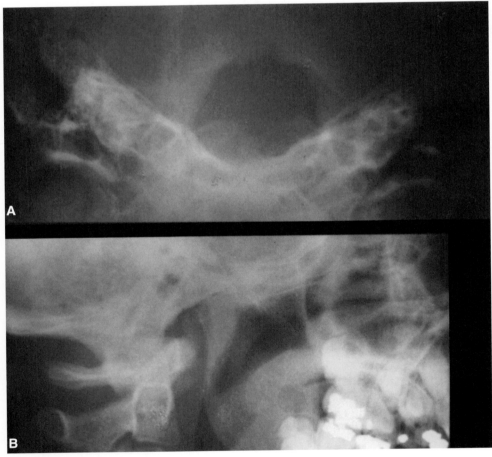

Fig. 5-1

Case 6

A 17-year-old boy has jaw and neck pain. One hour ago he was in a car crash; he sat in the front passenger's seat, wearing no seatbelt. He does not remember the accident.

Temperature is 36.8°C, heart rate 80, respiratory rate 18, blood pressure 124/40 mm Hg, and weight 68 kg. Bruises and cuts are on face, abrasions on right elbow, right knee, and left shank. Left side of face is weak. Neck is tender and hurts with flexion. The rest of the physical findings are normal.

Hematocrit is 0.39. White cell count is 7.9×10^9/liter. Platelet count is 230×10^9/liter.

Roentgenogram in Figure 6-1A shows asymmetry of relation of atlas to axis. CT scan in Figure 6-1B shows posterior arch fractures and fracture of right side of anterior arch of C1. Roentgenograms show hypoplasia of dens (Figures 6-1A and 6-2), back movement of anterior tubercle of C1 on dens when neck is extended (Figure 6-2A), prominent occipital condyles, and fractures of posterior arch of C1 (Figure 6-2).

Diagnosis: Hypoplasia of dens, Jefferson's fracture.

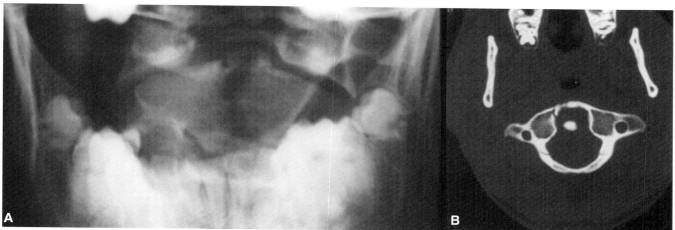

Fig. 6-1

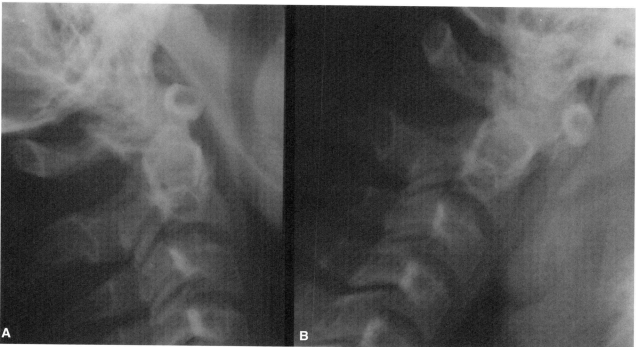

Fig. 6-2

Case 7

After falling from his bicycle onto a gravel road, a 6-year-old boy is sleeping soundly until disturbed.

Temperature is 37.4°C, heart rate 88, respiratory rate 20, and blood pressure 112/62 mm Hg. He opens his eyes when roused. Head is bruised and cut. Left eyelids are bruised, swollen, and soon black. Right cheek and left shoulder are scraped. Blood is in left external acoustic meatus and right side of nose. The rest of the physical findings are normal.

Hematocrit is 0.40. White cell count is 8.5×10^9/liter with 0.46 polymorphonuclear cells, 0.01 bands, 0.44 lymphocytes, and 0.09 monocytes. Platelet count is 264×10^9/liter.

A separate bone is between odontoid and occiput (Figure 7-1).

He is alert the next day and complains of pain in left eye.

Diagnosis: Os odontoideum.

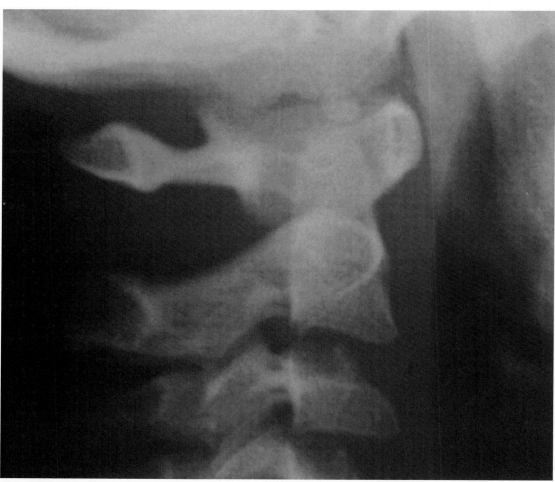

Fig. 7-1

Case 8

An 8-year-old boy is hit by a car and knocked out for 1 minute.

Heart rate is 100, respiratory rate 20, and blood pressure 142/90 mm Hg. He recognizes his family. Left side of forehead is scraped and swollen. Right leg is scraped. The rest of the physical findings are normal.

Hematocrit is 0.35. White cell count is 10.6×10^9/liter. Platelet count is 240×10^9/liter. Urine specific gravity is 1.020, pH 6. Urine is normal.

A bone spur projects back from superior articular facet of atlas for occipital condyle (Figure 8-1). Each vertebra moves forward on the next lower one when neck is flexed, and the angle between the spinous processes increases (Figure 8-1B).

Diagnosis: Normal movement of cervical vertebrae, normal cervical spine.

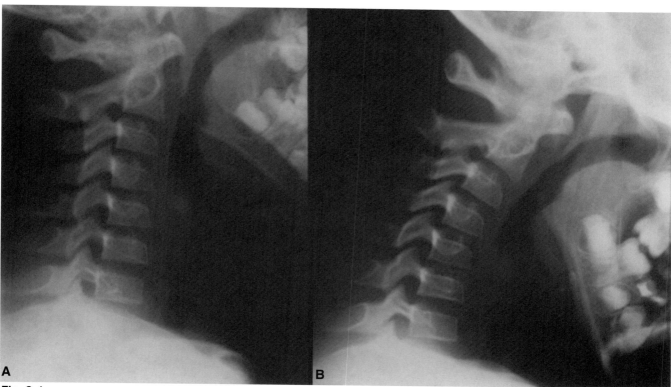

Fig. 8-1

Case 9

A 13-year-old girl who has Down syndrome has been wheelchair bound for 3 years.

She was able to play at home until 3 years ago when she fell back against a couch. She was able to walk for several hours but fell again and since then has been weak in arms and legs, weaker on left side. She can move legs but not walk. She feeds herself clumsily with right hand. She has had many ear infections. Tonsils and adenoids were removed at 4 years.

Mother (49 years old), father (51 years old), and sister (20 years old) are well.

Weight at 13 years is 21.3 kg, height 127 cm, head circumference 49 cm, temperature 36.8°C, heart rate 132, respiratory rate 24, and systolic blood pressure 100 mm Hg. Tongue is big for mouth. Muscle tone in limbs is increased. Right patella is dislocated. Feet are plantar flexed. Clonus is at ankles, Babinski's sign in feet. The rest of the physical findings are normal.

Hematocrit is 0.39. White cell count is 8.2×10^9/liter with 0.63 polymorphonuclear cells, 0.16 bands, 0.12 lymphocytes, 0.06 monocytes, 0.01 eosinophils, and 0.02 basophils. Platelet estimate is adequate. Serum calcium is 1.90 mmol/liter, phosphorus 1.26.

Occiput is displaced back on atlas before (Figure 9-1A) but not after (Figure 9-1B) operation. Posterior arch of C1 is not completely ossified.

At operation, posterior arch of atlas is at level of foramen magnum. Neck is fixed with wire and bone fragments from right ilium.

She does not breathe on her own and dies 1 month after operation.

Diagnosis: Down syndrome, occipitoatlantal subluxation.

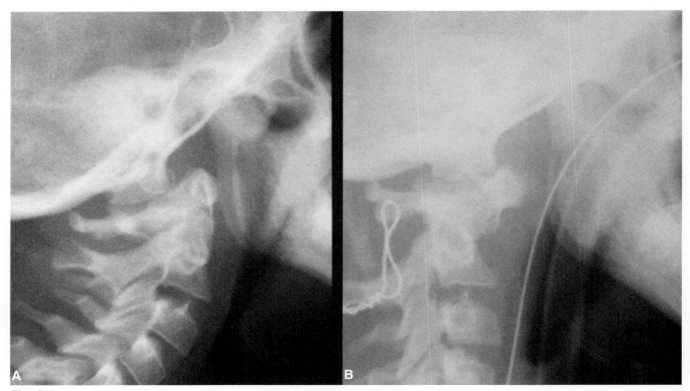

Fig. 9-1

Case 10

A 6-year-old girl who has Down syndrome will not move head or lift arms above chest. She hit back of head on floor when she fell 2 days ago. She was "floppy and blue" for a short time. She complains of pain in left side of neck and will not lie down on her left side.

Mother (23 years old), father (26 years old), and sister (3 years old) are well.

Temperature is 35.9°C, heart rate 100, respiratory rate 22, blood pressure 98/50 mm Hg, weight 14 kg, and height 97 cm. A systolic murmur is present. The rest of the physical findings are normal.

Hematocrit is 0.45. White cell count is 5.7×10^9/liter with 0.41 polymorphonuclear cells, 0.04 bands, 0.41 lymphocytes, 0.09 monocytes, 0.03 eosinophils, and 0.02 basophils. Platelet count is 514×10^9/liter.

C1 is 6 mm forward on C2, 2–3 mm more than normal in flexed neck of a child; posterior arch of C1 is not completely ossified (Figure 10-1).

At operation, occiput, atlas, and axis move independently. C1 posterior arch, cartilaginous in back, is removed. C2 is wired and fixed by autologous iliac bone to occiput.

She is alert, oriented, speaks clearly, and walks freely at 17 years.

Diagnosis: Down syndrome, atlantoaxial subluxation.

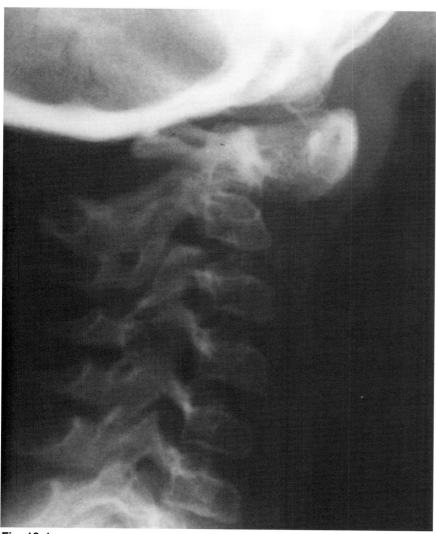

Fig. 10-1

Case 11

A 16-year-old boy who was driving without a seat belt is found in a car that has gone off the road and landed on its roof. He is curled upside down, head against roof, neck flexed. He complains of dirt in his eyes and says, "I only had a couple of beers tonight." A passenger is dead.

Temperature is 37.3°C, heart rate 86, respiratory rate 20, and blood pressure 136/82 mm Hg. Cuts are on left side of head, around left eye, and on right shoulder and left hand. Left eye and shins are bruised. Dirt is in eyes. Conjunctivae and sclerae are injected. Left cornea is scratched. Right flank is tender. The rest of the physical findings are normal.

Hematocrit is 0.44. White cell count is 20.8×10^9/liter with 0.64 polymorphonuclear cells, 0.07 bands, 0.23 lymphocytes, 0.05 monocytes, and 0.01 eosinophils. Platelet count is 256×10^9/liter. Urine specific gravity is 1.020, pH 7. Urine has moderate blood, 0.2 urobilinogen, 50–60 red cells/HPF, and occasional nonsquamous epithelial cells/HPF. Serum sodium is 145 mmol/liter, potassium 3.8, chloride 109, carbon dioxide 24, urea nitrogen 4.3, alcohol 28.0 (intoxicated: >2.2; comatose: ~65.1), and glucose 6.8. Creatinine is 90 μmol/liter.

He has pain in head, neck, and back the next day and is tender at C3–C4.

An inferior articular facet of C3 is in front of a superior articular facet of C4; C4 facet is bent back (Figure 11-1). Roentgenographic examination also shows wedging of left side of body of T9 and paraspinal swelling. CT scan shows left dislocation and also fracture of left lamina and left pedicle of C3 and left transverse process of C4.

At operation C3–C4 interspinous ligament is found to be torn. Open reduction and internal fixation with wire and with bone from right iliac crest are done.

Neurologic findings are normal at discharge 3 days after operation.

Diagnosis: Unilateral jumped facet, C3–C4.

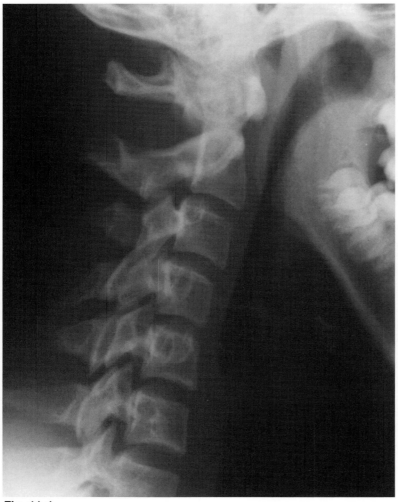

Fig. 11-1

Case 12

A 3-month-old boy vomits a lot and cries all night.

Pregnancy of mother was normal, delivery by cesarean section for irregular fetal heart rate. Birth weight was 2.2 kg, Apgar score 8/9 at 1 and 5 minutes. An umbilical arterial catheter was inserted at 6 hours and left in place for 4 days. He had spells of apnea and bradycardia. A toe on left foot was red at 7 days, left foot red and swollen at 9 days. He coughed at 6 weeks and had spells in which he cried until his face turned blue and heart rate slowed to 50–60. Mouth was full of frothy mucus. Breathing was fast and labored. He was better in a few days. He began to vomit and fuss again 1 week ago.

Mother (30 years old), father (42 years old), sister (12 years old), and brother (10 years old) are well.

Temperature at 3 months is 37.2°C, heart rate 164, respiratory rate 48, systolic blood pressure 102 mm Hg, weight 3.6 kg, length 54 cm, and head circumference 37 cm. A flame nevus is on forehead, a small hemangioma on back, a small hernia at umbilicus, and clonus at ankles. Liver edge is 1–2 cm below costal margin. Legs scissor occasionally. Their muscle tone is increased. The rest of the physical findings are normal.

Hematocrit is 0.26. Hemoglobin is 94 g/liter. Red blood cell count is 3.9×10^{12}/liter. MCV is 67 fl. MCH is 24 pg. MCHC is 360 g/liter. White cell count is 10.3×10^9/liter with 0.33 polymorphonuclear cells, 0.10 bands, 0.53 lymphocytes, 0.03 monocytes, and 0.01 eosinophils. Platelet estimate is increased. Urine specific gravity is 1.005, pH 7.5. Urine is normal. Serum sodium is 134 mmol/liter, potassium 5.6, chloride 105, carbon dioxide 21, urea nitrogen 2.1, calcium 2.50, phosphorus 1.74, cholesterol 3.15, triglycerides 1.48, and glucose 6.2. Creatinine is 40 μmol/liter, uric acid 140, and total bilirubin 2. Total protein is 62 g/liter, albumin 36. Alkaline phosphatase is 164 U/liter, LDH >600.

An upper mediastinal mass pushes trachea and esophagus forward and obscures adjacent vertebrae (Figure 12-1). Femoral cortices are thickened (Figure 12-2).

Laminae are thin at C7–T4 laminectomy. A rind of vascular gray tissue is around the dura. At later right thoracotomy an abscess is drained. Culture of wall and pus grows coagulase-positive *Staphylococcus aureus*. C6–T4 fusion with bone from his right ilium is performed at 9 months. Movement at right hip is limited at 5 years. Right leg is smaller than left. Deep tendon reflexes are increased in legs. Clonus is at right ankle, Babinski's sign in right foot. He cannot flex his knees enough to pedal a bicycle at 6 years. Clonus is at both ankles at 8 years. He fractures right femur at 9 years. Right hip is dysplastic in roentgenogram. At 13½ years, he returns for distal left femoral epiphysiodesis to slow growth in longer left leg. Neck is short. Babinski's sign and diminished vibratory and position sensation are in feet.

MRI at 13½ years shows deformity of cervicothoracic vertebrae, cord compression, and cervical syrinx (Figure 12-3).

Diagnosis: Disseminated neonatal staphylococcal infection with osteomyelitis, arthritis, spondylitis, cord compression, and syringomyelia.

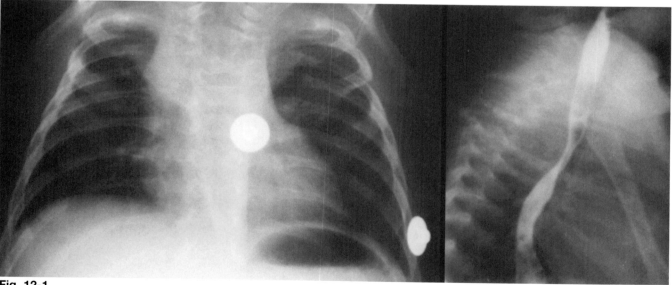

Fig. 12-1

(Continued)

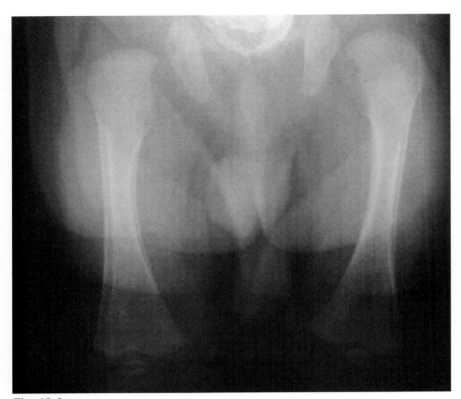

Fig. 12-2

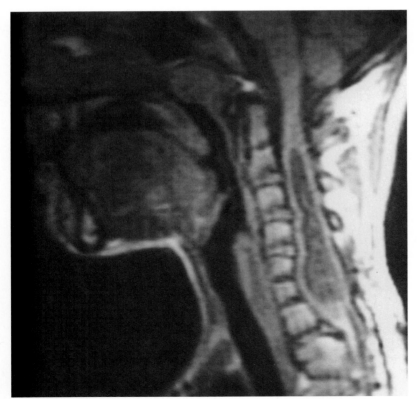

Fig. 12-3

Neck and Shoulders

Case 1

A newborn girl, delivered by cesarean section for fetal distress, has a delayed, weak cry. Heart rate slows to 50. She is intubated.

Apgar score is 3/3 at 1 and 5 minutes, weight 1.6 kg, length 40 cm, head circumference 29 cm, temperature 36.5°C. After intubation and oxygen, heart rate is 170, respiratory rate 60, and blood pressure 40/25 mm Hg. She is floppy. Eyes do not move together at times. The rest of the physical findings are normal.

Hematocrit is 0.42. White cell count is 16.1×10^9/liter with 0.34 polymorphonuclear cells, 0.05 bands, 0.53 lymphocytes, and 0.06 monocytes. Platelet count is 247×10^9/liter. Blood glucose is 5.0 mmol/liter. At 2 days, serum sodium is 140 mmol/liter, potassium 5.2, chloride 108, carbon dioxide 20, urea nitrogen 5.7, calcium 2.47, phosphorus 1.84, cholesterol 1.00, and glucose 7.9. Creatinine is 110 μmol/liter, uric acid 450, total bilirubin 48, and direct bilirubin 7. Total protein is 48 g/liter, albumin 35. Alkaline phosphatase is 159 U/liter, LDH 1,608, and SGOT 108. On the third day, urine specific gravity is 1.007, pH 6.0. Urine has 2+ hemoglobin/myoglobin, occasional nonsquamous epithelial cells/HPF, 12–15 red cells/HPF, and 3–5 white cells/HPF.

She is extubated at 17 days. Neck is short at 24 days. Left forearm is flaccid. Stool has occult blood at 1 month. Stools are watery green at 1½ months. She has rectal prolapse. Abdomen is distended. Left limbs are smaller than right. Muscle tone is increased. Deep tendon reflexes are active, right more than left. At 8 weeks, weight is 1.5 kg. A central venous catheter is put in for IV feeding. Stools are watery with osmolality of 280 mmol/kg. At 2½ months, head and neck are edematous.

Left first rib is slightly out of position at 4 days (Figure 1-1A). At 1½ months, left first and second ribs are poorly defined and soft tissues of left side of neck are prominent (Figure 1-1B). CT scan after IV injection of contrast medium shows a mass that may contain calcium in left side of neck and chest at 2½ months. Barium enema with reflux into small bowel shows narrow caliber and diffuse nodularity at 3 months (Figure 1-2).

She dies at 3½ months.

At necropsy, a mass is found in left side of chest and neck. Yellow-white, firm nodules are in muscle, on pleural surface of diaphragm, in right atrium, on undersurface of liver, on urinary bladder, in vertebrae, and in femur. Mucosa of small and large intestine is seeded with firm, yellow-white nodules (3-mm diameter). Microscopic examination of mass shows clumps of plump and spindle-shaped cells with abundant eosinophilic cytoplasm, large nuclei with finely dispersed chromatin and one or more eccentric nucleoli, dense fibrous tissue, necrosis, and calcification. Submucosa of small and large intestine is fibrotic. Pancreas is fibrotic. Nodules (8–10 cells thick) are in lungs. Bands of tumor cells are in spleen. The cells infiltrate ribs and muscle and encircle spinal cord.

Diagnosis: Multicentric infantile myofibromatosis.

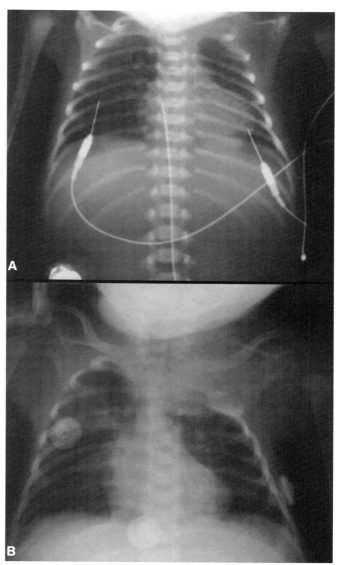

Fig. 1-1

(Continued)

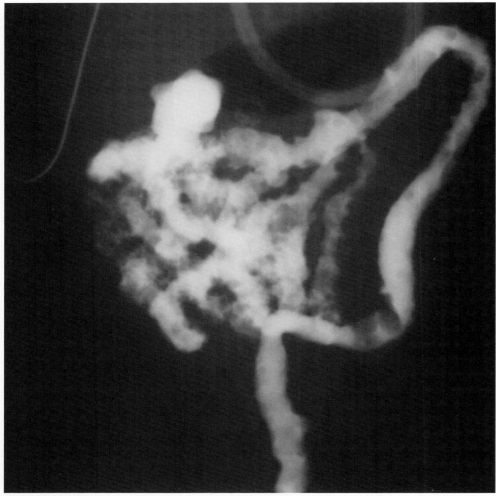

Fig. 1-2

Case 2

A 5-year-old boy has a hard lump above medial aspect of left scapula.

Mother had preeclampsia and gestational diabetes. The boy was the second of monochorionic diamniotic twins. Birth weight was 2.2 kg. Mother noticed "left shoulder blade was out of place" when the boy was 2½ weeks old.

Mother (25 years old), father (36 years old), and twin brother are well. Members of mother's family have heart disease; members of father's family have high blood pressure.

Weight is 16 kg, height 99 cm. A bony lump is above left scapula. Left scapula is higher than right. Movement at left shoulder and the rest of the physical findings are normal.

A bone that was above medial aspect of left scapula at 4 months is larger at 5 years; left scapula is higher than right and slightly winged (Figure 2-1).

At operation at 7 years, a bone 4–5 cm long with jointlike cartilaginous attachment to left scapula is removed. Resected tissue consists of trabeculated bone, articular cartilage, and synovium.

Diagnosis: Sprengel's deformity with omovertebral bone.

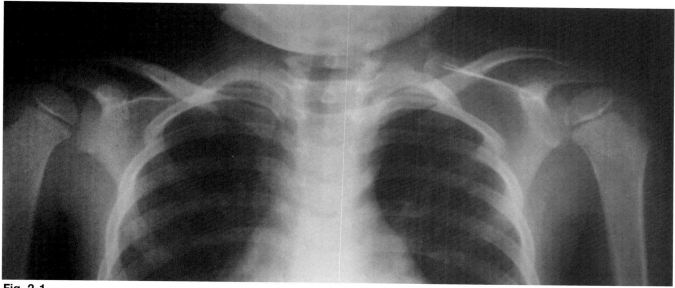

Fig. 2-1

Case 3

A newborn girl does not move her left arm.

Mother (18 years old) had high blood pressure during pregnancy. Membranes ruptured spontaneously 6 hours before delivery. Amniotic fluid looked like pea soup. Delivery was by low forceps because of left shoulder dystocia.

Apgar score is 2/8 at 1 and 5 minutes, weight 3.5 kg, length 47 cm, head circumference 34 cm, temperature 36.3°C, heart rate 120, and respiratory rate 50. Head is molded and has forceps marks. Moro's reflex is absent on left. Left arm is extended, adducted, and internally rotated. Left grasp is weak. The rest of the physical findings are normal.

Hematocrit is 0.53. White cell count is 27.3×10^9/liter with 0.66 polymorphonuclear cells, 0.13 bands, 0.08 lymphocytes, and 0.13 monocytes. Platelet count is 164×10^9/liter.

Left scapula is winged at 2½ hours; left side of diaphragm is higher than right (Figure 3-1).

Weight at 14 days is 3.7 kg, length 54 cm. Movement is almost normal at left shoulder and is normal at left elbow, left wrist, and left hand. Moro's reflex is normal.

Diagnosis: Erb's palsy (left), phrenic palsy (left).

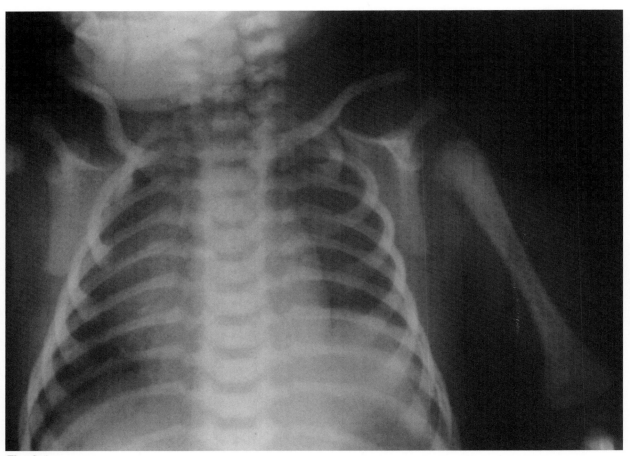

Fig. 3-1

Case 4

A 16-year-old boy is weak.

At 8 years, he was clumsy, fell often when he ran, and could not close his eyes tightly or smile broadly. At 9 years, he was round-backed and could not whistle, but at 14 years he played the flute in his high school band. He can walk 4 miles.

Similar weakness has afflicted mother since she was 14 years old. She is now in a wheelchair. It also affects older brother and sister.

Weight at 14 years is 44 kg, height 173 cm, heart rate 82, and blood pressure 110/78 mm Hg. Muscles of shoulders, upper arms, and thighs are atrophied. He flings his arm to raise it overhead. Shoulders dislocate and relocate. Back is round, sternum depressed, belly protuberant. Supination is weak. Feet are cavus. Deep tendon reflexes are absent. The rest of the physical findings are normal.

Scapulas are normally placed at 12 years (Figure 4-1A), winged at 16 years (Figure 4-1B).

Diagnosis: Facioscapulohumeral muscular dystrophy (Landouzy-Dejerine muscular dystrophy).

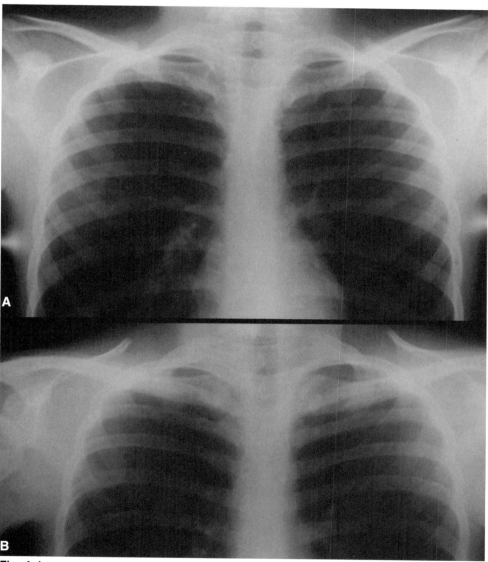

Fig. 4-1

Case 5

A 13-year-old boy's right scapula sticks out.

He often wrestles with an older brother. He quit judo class 1 year ago because of pain in right shoulder and right arm. Scapula was sticking out 7 months ago.

Weight is 47 kg, height 163 cm. Right deltoid, trapezius, triceps, biceps, and wrist extensor muscles are weak. Right grip is weak. Right scapula sticks out more when he extends right arm. The rest of the physical findings are normal.

Winged right scapula thickens subcutaneous tissues of upper part of right side of back (Figure 5-1).

EMG findings are compatible with denervation of right serratus anterior and right triceps muscles. Normal motor conduction velocity and sensory action potentials of ulnar and median nerves suggest lesion proximal to dorsal root ganglion.

Diagnosis: Winged right scapula due to denervation of serratus anterior and triceps muscles.

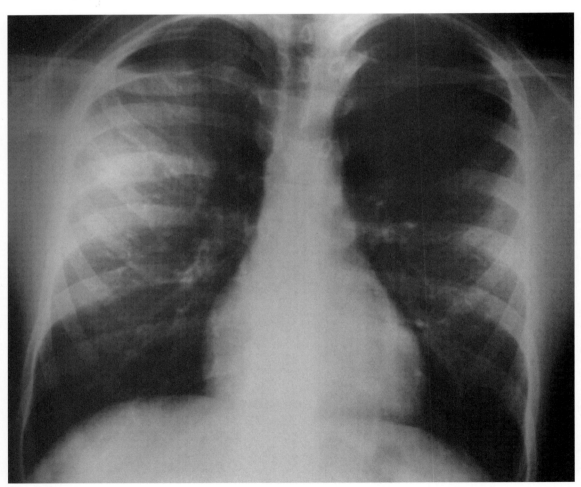

Fig. 5-1

Case 6

A 14-year-old boy has pain in right shoulder. He was thrown onto right shoulder in a wrestling match last night. Now he feels "grinding" pain in front of right shoulder when he moves it forward.

Soft tissues over lateral end of right clavicle are slightly edematous. Movement at right shoulder is slightly limited in all directions. Point tenderness is at right acromioclavicular joint 4 days later, and right shoulder abduction is limited 5–10 degrees.

He recovers enough to wrestle but is thrown onto right shoulder again 3½ weeks after the first injury. Right shoulder hurts 4 days later.

Lateral end of right clavicle is prominent 4 days after reinjury without bruise, tenderness, or limitation of movement at right shoulder.

Roentgenographic findings at the shoulder are normal the day after first injury (Figure 6-1A). A gap that contains a piece of bone separates right clavicle and acromion 4 days after reinjury (Figure 6-1B). Acromion, coracoid, proximal humeral, and medial clavicular growth plates are present in Figure 6-1.

All physical findings, including movement and strength of arms, are normal 6 months later.

Diagnosis: First degree acromioclavicular separation; 3½ weeks later, third degree acromioclavicular separation, normal growth plates.

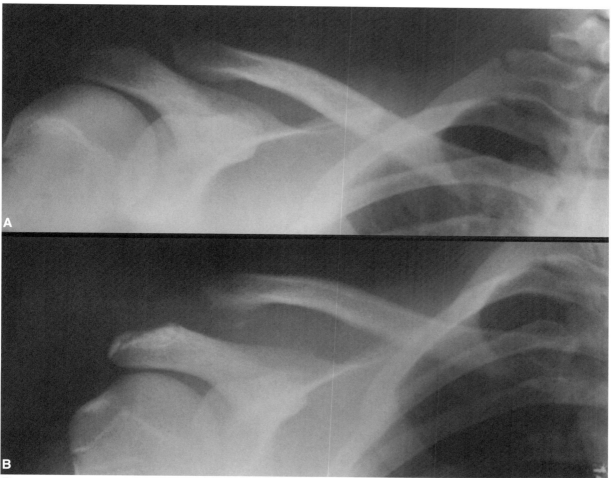

Fig. 6-1

Case 7

A 13-month-old girl has swollen left shoulder and does not use left arm.

Pregnancy was normal, birth weight 4 kg. She had several respiratory infections in the first 5 months and a rash on back and perineum. Swelling of left scapula that appeared 2 months ago is larger.

Parents and three siblings are well.

Temperature at 13 months is 36.4°C, heart rate 144, respiratory rate 40, blood pressure 130/80 mm Hg, and weight 10.3 kg. A scattered rash of greasy plaques on red base is on scalp, behind ears, and on upper back. Right external acoustic meatus is red and focally granular. Occipital, cervical, and axillary lymph nodes are palpable. A tender swelling approximately 2 cm in diameter is at left scapula. Spleen edge is 1 cm below costal margin. The rest of the physical findings are normal.

Hematocrit is 0.26. White cell count is 13.3×10^9/liter with 0.80 polymorphonuclear cells, 0.08 bands, 0.08 lymphocytes, 0.02 monocytes, and 0.02 eosinophils. Platelet count is 644×10^9/liter. Urine specific gravity is 1.015, pH 7. Urine has 0.30 g/liter protein, bacteria, amorphous phosphates, few squamous epithelial cells/HPF, and 10–12 white cells/HPF. Serum sodium is 141 mmol/liter, potassium 3.9, chloride 108, carbon dioxide 19, urea nitrogen 4.3, calcium 2.45, phosphorus 1.78, cholesterol 3.26, and glucose 7.3. Creatinine is 40 μmol/liter, uric acid 390, total bilirubin 7, and direct bilirubin 2. Total protein is 66 g/liter, albumin 34. Alkaline phosphatase is 132 U/liter, LDH 306, and SGOT 22.

Left scapula is expanded and radiolucent; a similar lesion is near axillary part of right eighth rib and a mass of water density is at level of hilum of left lung (Figure 7-1).

Biopsy of brown fragments removed from left scapula shows histiocytes with finely vesicular and some lobulated nuclei and eosinophilic cytoplasm, giant cells, eosinophils, neutrophils, necrosis, and bone spicules. Biopsy of thymus at 14 months shows fibrosis, few lymphocytes, and inconspicuous Hassall's corpuscles. Biopsy also shows histiocytes with abundant eosinophilic cytoplasm, folded delicate nuclear membranes, and finely dispersed chromatin; eosinophils; and Langerhans' giant cells. Biopsy of a cervical node shows similar cells but few eosinophils.

Diagnosis: Langerhans' cell histiocytosis.

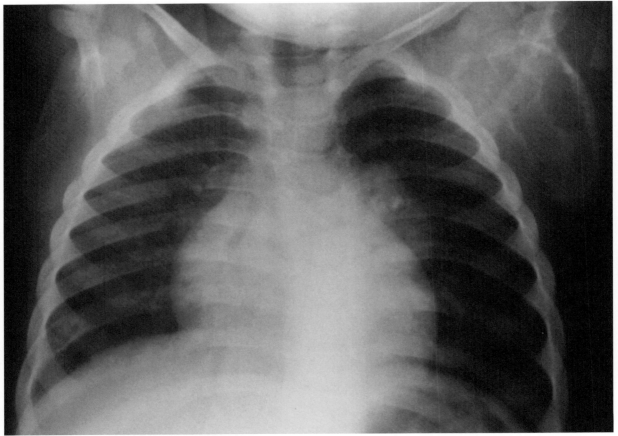

Fig. 7-1

Case 8

A 12-year-old girl has pain near her left shoulder.

She hurt her left shoulder 10 months ago while playing volleyball. It ached 2 months ago and again when she was hit there 2 weeks ago.

An inguinal node that was removed at 7 years showed "reactive" changes, according to pathologist.

Parents and two siblings (8 and 13 years old) are well.

Temperature at 12 years is 36.6°C, heart rate 100, respiratory rate 20, blood pressure 98/78 mm Hg, weight 53 kg, and height 155 cm. A lump is behind left scapula. The rest of the physical findings are normal.

Hematocrit is 0.41. White cell count is 11.5×10^9/liter with 0.65 polymorphonuclear cells, 0.13 bands, 0.17 lymphocytes, and 0.05 monocytes. Platelet count is 398×10^9/liter. Urine specific gravity is 1.016, pH 6. Urine has occasional squamous epithelial cells/HPF. Serum sodium is 142 mmol/liter, potassium 4.3, chloride 107, carbon dioxide 20, urea nitrogen 3.6, calcium 2.52, phosphorus 1.61, cholesterol 4.42, and glu-

cose 4.4. Creatinine is 60 μmol/liter, uric acid 280, total bilirubin 7, and direct bilirubin 0. Total protein is 74 g/liter, albumin 50. Alkaline phosphatase is 304 U/liter, LDH 162, and SGOT 15.

Soft tissues behind left scapula are swollen and left scapula is eroded (Figure 8-1).

At operation, liquefied red and gray matter is under pressure in left supraspinatus fossa.

Histochemical stain of resected tissue is vimentin positive, neuron-specific enolase weakly positive, actin negative, desmin negative, and common leukocyte antigen negative and confirms microscopic diagnosis.

She is treated with autologous bone marrow transplantation at 18 years. Six months later she is chronically ill with Fanconi-like kidney disease, hypokalemia, hypophosphatemia, and hypoproteinemia.

Diagnosis: Ewing's sarcoma.

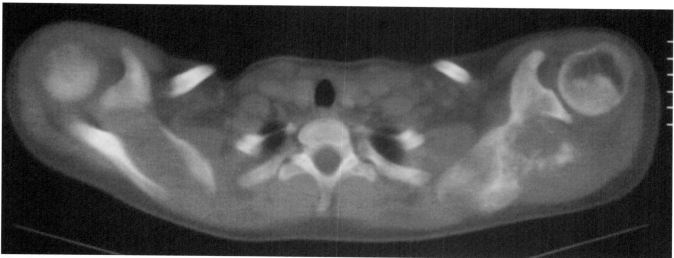

Fig. 8-1

Thorax

Case 1

A newborn boy has circumoral cyanosis when feeding at 12 hours. A systolic heart murmur is present a few hours later.

Mother (30 years old), father (32 years old), two brothers (8 and 10 years old), and sister (2 years old) are well.

Pregnancy was normal. Birth weight is 2.7 kg, Apgar score 9/9 at 1 and 5 minutes, temperature 37.2°C. At 1 hour, heart rate is 148, respiratory rate 42. The rest of the physical findings are normal.

At 6 weeks, he is more blue and has a spell of crying hard, breathing fast, and becoming limp.

Weight at 2 months is 3.1 kg, temperature 37.1°C, heart rate 138, respiratory rate 40, and systolic blood pressure 110 mm Hg. He is pale and becomes more blue when he cries. A systolic heart murmur is present. Liver edge is 1 cm below costal margin. The rest of the physical findings are normal.

Hematocrit is 0.37 at 2 months.

At cardiac catheterization, oxygen saturation is <0.20 in superior vena cava, right atrium, and right ventricle, and 0.50 in aorta. Pressure is 54/3 mm Hg in right ventricle and 75/40 mm Hg in the aorta. Mean pressure is 1 mm Hg in superior vena cava. Angiocardiogram shows high ventricular septal defect, overriding aorta, infundibular pulmonic stenosis or atresia, small main pulmonary artery, and ductus arteriosus.

Roentgenograms at 3 days (Figure 1-1A) and 2 months (Figure 1-1B) show separation of right clavicle into two parts, normal-sized heart, and, in Figure 1-1B (after creation of shunt between back of aorta and front of right pulmonary artery), endotracheal tube in right main bronchus and right chest tube.

At second operation at 18 months, in which subvalvar pulmonary atresia is found, defects are corrected and Waterston shunt closed. He is small and healthy at 14¾ years. Weight is 28 kg, height 135 cm, and blood pressure 100/60 mm Hg. A systolic and diastolic murmur are present.

Diagnosis: Cyanotic congenital heart disease, congenital pseudoarthrosis of right clavicle.

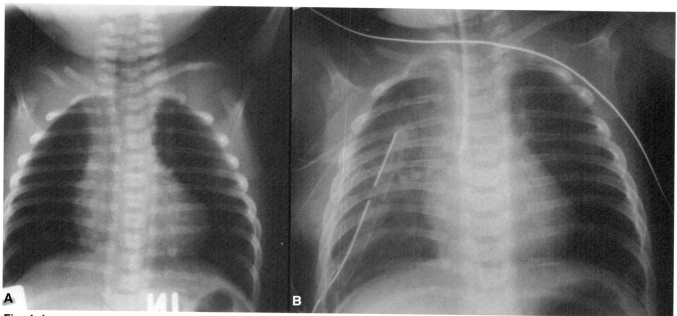

Fig. 1-1

Case 2

A newborn boy is grunting, blue, and flaccid.

Mother (35 years old) smoked during pregnancy. Delivery was slowed by shoulder dystocia. Birth weight is 3.2 kg, Apgar score 2/6 at 1 and 5 minutes, length 46 cm, head circumference 33 cm, temperature 38.4°C, heart rate 174, respiratory rate 60, blood pressure 85/55 mm Hg, and capillary blood glucose 3.1 mmol/liter. Head is molded. Bruises are on scalp, right forearm, and groin; petechiae are on chest. Left clavicle is fractured. A systolic heart murmur is present. Liver edge is 3 cm below costal margin. Muscle tone is slightly diminished. He moves legs more than arms. The rest of the physical findings are normal. Cry is soon lusty, color pink.

Hematocrit is 0.56. White cell count is 25.5×10^9/liter with 0.37 polymorphonuclear cells, 0.06 bands, 0.51 lymphocytes, 0.05 monocytes, and 0.01 eosinophils. Urine specific gravity is 1.028, pH 5. Urine has 4+ occult blood, 0–1 epithelial cell/HPF, and amorphous urates. Serum sodium is 135 mmol/liter, potassium 4.5, chloride 105, and calcium 2.14. Total bilirubin is 80 μmol/liter.

At 24 hours, roentgenogram (Figure 2-1A) shows fracture of clavicles and high right side of diaphragm. At 6 days, chest fluoroscopy shows that right side of diaphragm moves up during inspiration, left side down.

At 10 days, capillary blood pH when $FIO_2 = 0.39$ is 7.36. PCO_2 is 53 mm Hg, PO_2 56. Right side of diaphragm is plicated.

At 12 days, ossified callus around left clavicular fracture is first clearly visible; right sixth rib is displaced downward (Figure 2-1B).

Diagnosis: Healing fracture of clavicles in newborn infant; right phrenic palsy; paradoxic movement of right side of diaphragm.

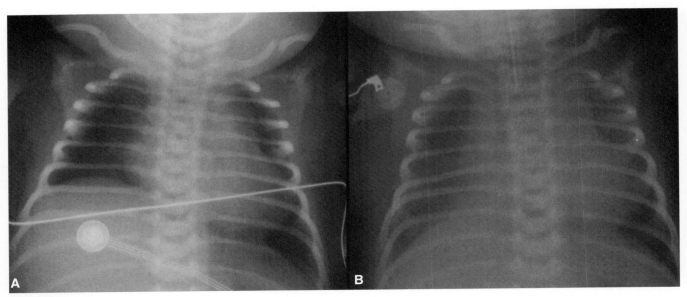

Fig. 2-1

Case 3

A 2¾-year-old girl will not use her right arm after a fall on steps.

Weight is 13.7 kg, height 92 cm. Right shoulder is tender. Any motion of right arm hurts. A systolic heart murmur is present. The rest of the physical findings are normal.

Right clavicle is bent upward at about junction of lateral and middle thirds (Figure 3-1).

Diagnosis: Fracture of right clavicle in usual location at medial attachment of coracoclavicular ligament at conoid tubercle below; medial origin of deltoid muscle above, in front, and below; and medial insertion of superior fibers of trapezius muscle above and behind.

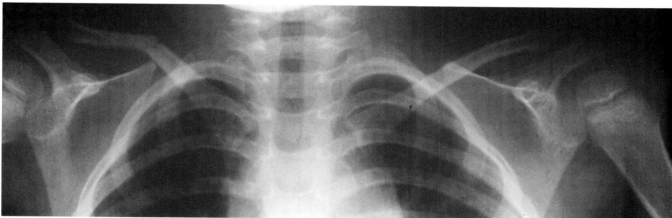

Fig. 3-1

Case 4

A 10-year-old girl has pain at left shoulder.

Pain began soon after she had flu 6 months ago. A swelling that is getting larger appeared in upper part of left side of chest 4 months ago. Tubes were put in ears for otitis media 3 months ago. The family has dogs and cats.

Temperature at 10 years is 37.4°C, heart rate 80, respiratory rate 14, blood pressure 108/74 mm Hg, weight 38 kg, and height 140 cm. Swelling and tenderness are present along medial third of left clavicle. The rest of the physical findings are normal.

Hematocrit is 0.42. White cell count is 13.1 × 10⁹/liter with 0.69 polymorphonuclear cells, 0.05 bands, 0.16 lymphocytes, 0.08 monocytes, and 0.02 atypical lymphocytes. Platelet count is 320 × 10⁹/liter. ESR is 48 mm/hr. Serum sodium is 140 mmol/liter, potassium 3.9, chloride 98, carbon dioxide 27, urea nitrogen 4.6, calcium 2.57, phosphorus 1.52, cholesterol 5.48, and glucose 5.6. Creatinine is 60 μmol/liter, uric acid 240, total bilirubin 5, and direct bilirubin 0. Total protein is 79 g/liter, albumin 49. Alkaline phosphatase is 220 U/liter, LDH 179, and SGOT 18.

Medial part of left clavicle is expanded; cortex of left first rib is thickened (Figure 4-1).

At operation, thick, vascular soft tissue is around left clavicle. Periosteum comes off easily. Bone is soft and contains gray material.

Microscopic examination of tan, rubbery fragments shows fibrous tissue, acute inflammation in muscle and lymphoid tissue, and acute and chronic inflammation in reactive bone. Cultures are sterile.

Diagnosis: Questionable osteomyelitis of left clavicle.

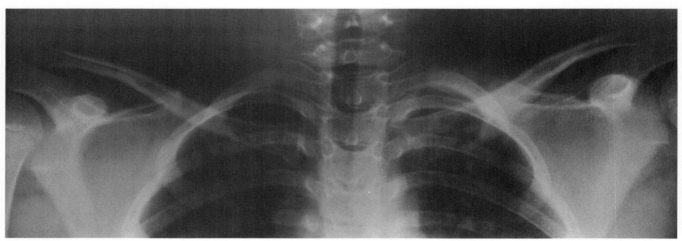

Fig. 4-1

Case 5

Two newborn girls are joined from jugular (suprasternal) notch to omphalocele.

Pregnancy of mother (18 years old) was normal, delivery by cesarean section. Combined weight is 5.7 kg. Girl A (on reader's left) cries spontaneously. Girl A's length is 46 cm, head circumference 34 cm, Apgar score 3/7 at 1 and 10 minutes, temperature 36.4°C, respiratory rate 40, systolic blood pressure 40 mm Hg, and heart rate 136–140, synchronous with that of girl B. Liver is palpable in omphalocele between them, gut visible. Spleen and two kidneys are palpable in girl A's abdomen. Girl B does not cry spontaneously. Girl B's length is 44 cm, Apgar score 2/7 at 1 and 10 minutes, temperature 36.9°C, respiratory rate 60, systolic blood pressure 46 mm Hg, and heart rate 136–140, synchronous with that of girl A. Spleen and two kidneys are palpable in girl B's abdomen. Heads, external genitalia, and limbs are normal.

Roentgenogram in Figure 5-1 shows ventral fusion. Angiocardiogram in Figure 5-2 shows heart in girl A and an aorta in each.

They die the day after birth. Necropsy shows (1) single pericardium investing two aortas up to two thymus glands;

(2) one heart (in girl A); (3) aortas in front of hypoplastic pulmonary arteries, each aorta with ductus arteriosus; (4) atretic pulmonary valve in girl A; (5) stenotic pulmonary valve in girl B; (6) two ventricles, each with atrioventricular valve, aorta, pulmonary artery, and ridges of tissue between the valves; (7) girl A's atrium receiving girl A's superior and inferior vena cava and opening into girl A's ventricle; (8) an enlarged vein, thought to be a persistent left duct of Cuvier and to be girl B's atrium, receiving girl B's vena cava, girl A's left internal jugular vein, and communicating with girl A's atrium through a defect and with girl B's ventricle; (9) another atrial chamber that receives hypoplastic pulmonary veins from both girls and ends blindly; (10) an isthmus (6 × 4 cm in cross section) through narrowest part connecting the two livers; (11) a single gall bladder (in girl A) with single bile duct to point 4 cm beyond pylorus, where duodenums become single, common proximal small bowel, separate distal small bowel, appendix, colon, and rectum; and (12) common umbilical cord with a hepatic artery and urachus from each girl and a single umbilical vein.

Diagnosis: Thoracopagus (conjoined twins).

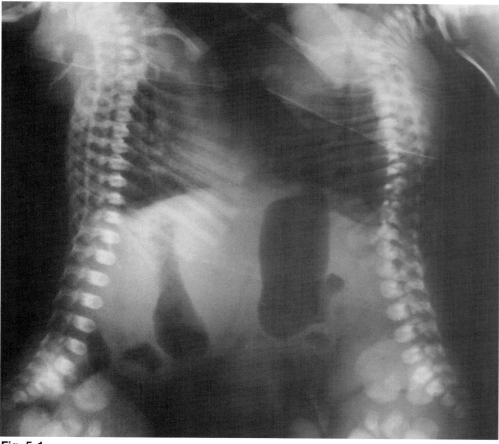

Fig. 5-1

(Continued)

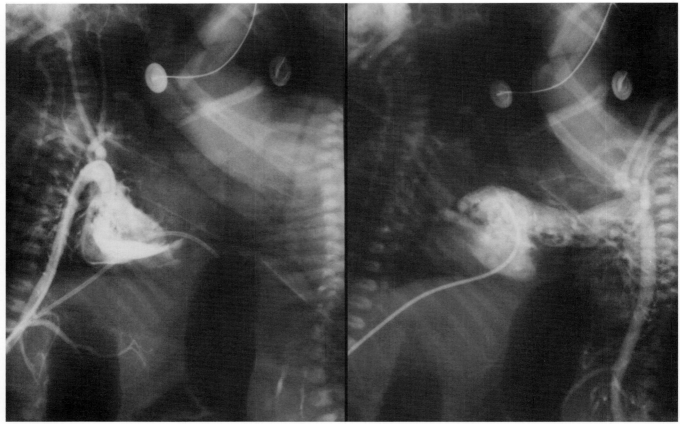

Fig. 5-2

Case 6

A newborn girl is delivered by cesarean section because of polyhydramnios, hydrops, and other abnormalities found today in prenatal ultrasound examination.

Mother (21 years old) has gained 5 kg in the last week. Birth weight is 2.9 kg, Apgar score 4 at 1 minute. She is intubated and given oxygen. Heart rate goes from 70 to 100. Temperature is 36°C, systolic blood pressure 95 mm Hg, length 48 cm, and head circumference 36 cm. Heart is outside chest near right nipple, apex up. Sternum is absent. Amnion covers 4 cm-wide chest defect and omphalocele. Gut is in left side of chest. Forty-five ml clear yellow liquid is obtained by right thoracentesis. The rest of the physical findings are normal.

Arterial blood pH is 7.09. P_{CO_2} is 101 mm Hg, P_{O_2} 31. Hematocrit is 0.44. White cell count is 15.4×10^9/liter with 0.59 polymorphonuclear cells, 0.03 bands, 0.26 lymphocytes, 0.10 monocytes, and 0.02 eosinophils. Platelet count is 320×10^9/liter. Serum sodium is 145 mmol/liter, potassium 3.9, chloride 110, and calcium 2.25.

Ultrasound examination shortly before delivery shows polyhydramnios, hydrops, ectopia cordis, and right pleural liquid (Figure 6-1). Roentgenogram shows heart at right shoulder, gut in left side of chest, umbilical venous catheter in ductus venosus that is displaced upward and to the left, and end of umbilical arterial catheter at level of L1 (Figure 6-2).

At operation, intestine, stomach, spleen, and left lobe of liver are herniated into left side of chest through a defect (4.5 × 2.5 cm) in ventral part of diaphragm formed by septum transversum. She dies during operation when air appears in coronary arteries and frothy blood in ventricles.

At necropsy, left lung consists of only lower lobe and is rotated top down and forward at hilum. Heart has ventricular septal defect and no pulmonary artery.

Diagnosis: Pentad of Cantrell (Cantrell-Haller-Ravitch syndrome).

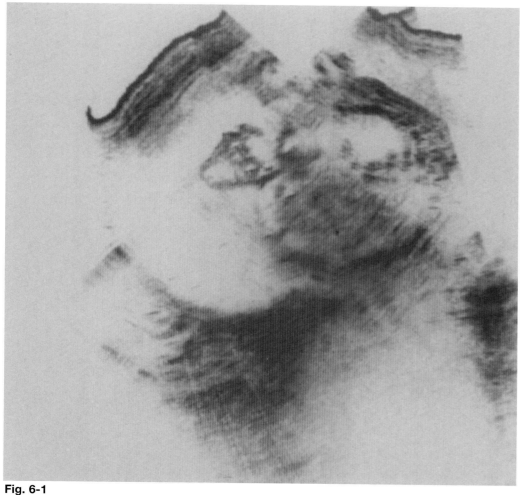

Fig. 6-1

(Continued)

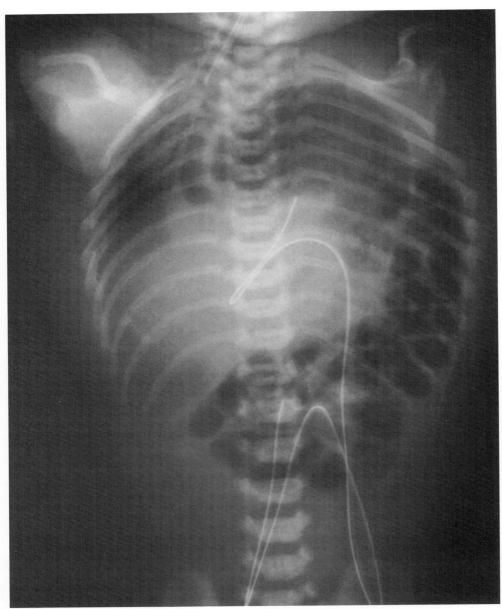

Fig. 6-2

Case 7

A newborn boy is floppy. He was "fairly active" during pregnancy, which was marred by polyhydramnios.

Mother (24 years old) and a sibling had cleft palate. Father (29 years old) and brother (2 years old) are well. Paternal grandfather has diabetes mellitus; maternal grandmother and maternal great-grandmother have thyroid trouble.

Birth weight is 2.5 kg, length 48 cm, head circumference 34 cm, and Apgar score 3/5 at 1 and 5 minutes, when limbs are flexed and respirations slow and irregular. At 1 hour, temperature is 35.6°C, heart rate 140, and respiratory rate 40. He is floppy, grunting, and retracting. Alae nasi flare. Rales are in lungs. Testes are not palpable. He does not cry during lumbar puncture at 2 hours. He is "very floppy" at 12 hours. Tips of fingers and toes are blue at 14 hours. At 15 hours, respiratory rate is 70, systolic blood pressure 50 mm Hg. Liver edge is 1–2 cm below costal margin. The rest of the physical findings are normal.

Hematocrit is 0.60 at 1¼ hours. White cell count is 3.2 × 10^9/liter with 0.08 polymorphonuclear cells, 0.91 lymphocytes, and 0.01 eosinophils. At 2 hours, white cell count is 14.5 × 10^9/liter with 0.43 polymorphonuclear cells, 0.01 bands, 0.51 lymphocytes, 0.02 monocytes, and 0.03 eosinophils. Blood glucose is 4.4 mmol/liter, CSF glucose 3.6.

Roentgenogram at 22 hours shows thin ribs and right umbilical arterial catheter that ends in descending aorta (Figure 7-1).

At 2 days, he has spells of apnea and bradycardia, a mouth full of mucus, and swollen feet. He is fed by nasojejunal tube because of gastric residuals. He is dusky at 7 days. At 9 days, he is floppier and swallows weakly. Cultures of blood and CSF are sterile. EMG at 13 days shows abnormal fibrillation and positive sharp waves. He dies at 6 weeks.

A specimen of thigh muscle obtained by needle at 14 days shows muscle fibers of uniformly small diameter that have red crystalline inclusions in trichrome preparation. Parents' EMGs are normal.

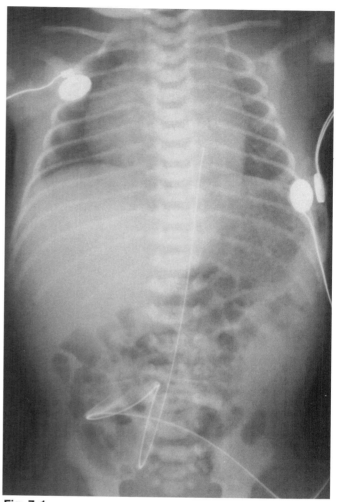

Fig. 7-1

Diagnosis: Nemaline myopathy.

Case 8

A 16-year-old girl has had a lump in left breast for 1 month.

Temperature is 37.5°C, heart rate 68, respiratory rate 20, blood pressure 130/86 mm Hg, weight 71.5 kg, and height 171 cm. A smooth, firm, mobile mass is in medial part of left breast. The rest of the physical findings are normal.

Hematocrit is 0.33. White cell count is 5.7×10^9/liter. Platelet count is 247×10^9/liter.

Ultrasound examination in Figure 8-1 shows solid mass. Mammography finds mass with distinct margin.

At operation, a smooth, rubbery mass is removed.

The oval mass ($9.0 \times 6.0 \times 2.5$ cm) is yellow to light red, its cut surface glistening. Microscopic examination shows fibrous connective tissue and compressed ducts.

Diagnosis: Fibroadenoma of breast.

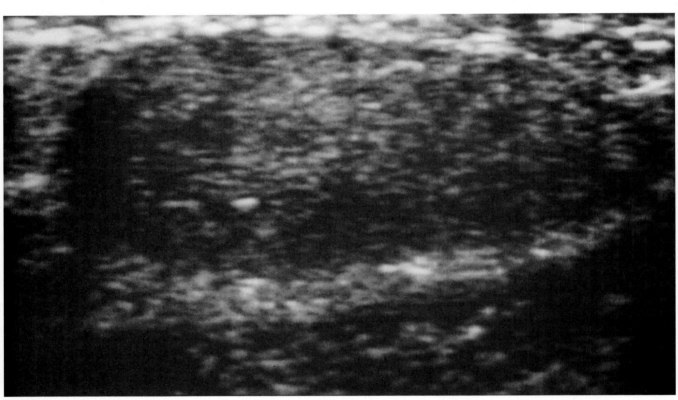

Fig. 8-1

Case 9

A 4-month-old girl breathes fast, sweats a lot, and does not gain weight.

Treatment with digitalis for heart failure was begun at 1 month. Cardiac catheterization at 3 months showed atrioventricular canal and ductus arteriosus.

Weight was 3.1 kg at birth. Weight at 4 months is 4.1 kg, length 62 cm, head circumference 39 cm, temperature 36°C, heart rate 120, respiratory rate 40, and blood pressure 80/56 mm Hg. She has Down syndrome. She is pale. Systolic and diastolic murmurs are present. Liver edge is 2 cm below costal margin. The rest of the physical findings are normal.

Hematocrit is 0.39. White cell count is 8.1×10^9/liter with 0.13 polymorphonuclear cells, 0.02 bands, 0.81 lymphocytes, 0.02 monocytes, 0.01 eosinophils, and 0.01 basophils. Platelet count is 325×10^9/liter. Urine specific gravity is 1.010, pH 8. Urine has trace leukocyte esterase and 0–1 hyaline cast/LPF.

Heart is larger than normal, diaphragm depressed; 11 ossified ribs are on each side (Figure 9-1A). Manubrium in lateral view is bifid, and T12 and L1 vertebral bodies are square and not rectangular (Figure 9-1B).

Diagnosis: Down syndrome.

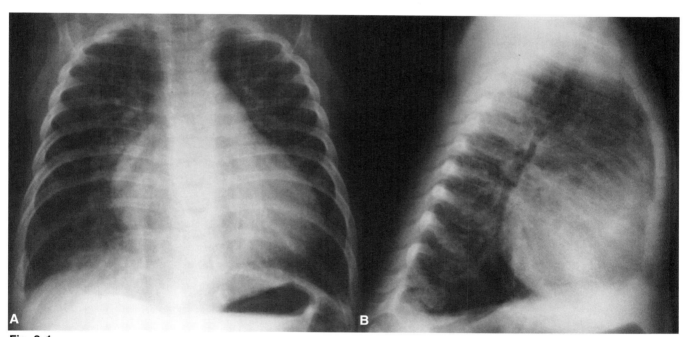

Fig. 9-1

Case 10

An 11-year-old boy has had a cough after hard activity for 6 weeks, sometimes with white phlegm. He was operated on at 6 months for an unspecified abnormality.

Temperature at 11 years is 37.6°C, heart rate 70, respiratory rate 18, blood pressure 100/60 mm Hg, weight 38 kg, and height 140 cm. He has infrequent wet cough. Inconstant rhonchi are in upper left side of back. A scar is on abdomen. The rest of the physical findings are normal.

Hematocrit is 0.42. White cell count is 6.6×10^9/liter with 0.52 polymorphonuclear cells, 0.01 bands, 0.37 lymphocytes, 0.09 monocytes, and 0.01 eosinophils. Platelet count is 321×10^9/liter. Urine specific gravity is 1.019, pH 6. Urine is normal. Pulmonary function test results are normal.

An extra shadow in left side of chest (Figure 10-1) is shown in CT scan (Figure 10-2) to be of bone density at level of T2 and T3, thinning to soft tissue density farther down.

Diagnosis: Intrathoracic rib.

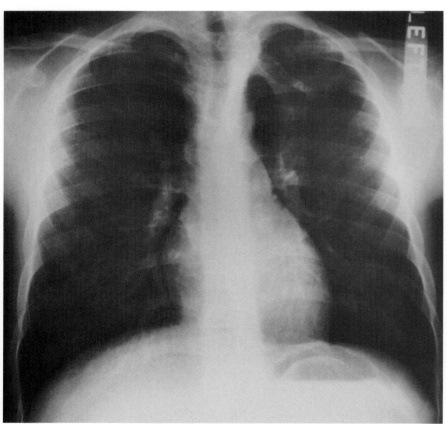

Fig. 10-1

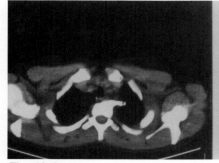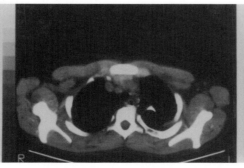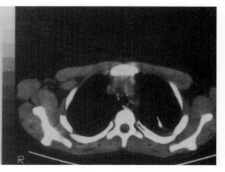

Fig. 10-2

Case 11

A newborn dwarf boy has small thorax, short limbs, and subcutaneous edema.

Pregnancy of mother (17 years old) was marred by polyhydramnios.

Apgar score is 8/8 at 1 and 5 minutes. Temperature at 20 minutes is 36.7°C, heart rate 173, respiratory rate 40, weight 2.1 kg, length 40 cm, and head circumference 34 cm. Liver edge is 2 cm below costal margin, spleen edge 3 cm. Umbilical cord is edematous. The rest of the physical findings are normal. Blood glucose is 5.0 mmol/liter.

Ultrasound examination 2 days before birth shows polyhydramnios, small chest between normal skull (on reader's right) (Figure 11-1), and distended abdomen. Roentgenogram minutes after birth shows short ribs, short bones, expanded metaphyses, flat vertebral bodies, square ilia, edematous umbilical cord, and subcutaneous edema (Figure 11-2).

At 50 minutes, arterial blood pH is 7.12 when FIO_2 = 0.80 by hood. PCO_2 is 77 mm Hg, PO_2 46. He is then intubated. At 4 hours, hematocrit is 0.54. White cell count is 9.8×10^9/liter with 0.39 polymorphonuclear cells, 0.05 bands, 0.46 lymphocytes, 0.07 monocytes, 0.01 eosinophils, 0.01 basophils, and 0.01 metamyelocytes. Platelet count is 145×10^9/liter. Calculated oxygen saturation in arterial blood is 0.13 when FIO_2 = 0.60 at 50 hours.

Ventilation is stopped at 75 hours. He dies 15 minutes later.

Diagnosis: Thanatophoric dwarf.

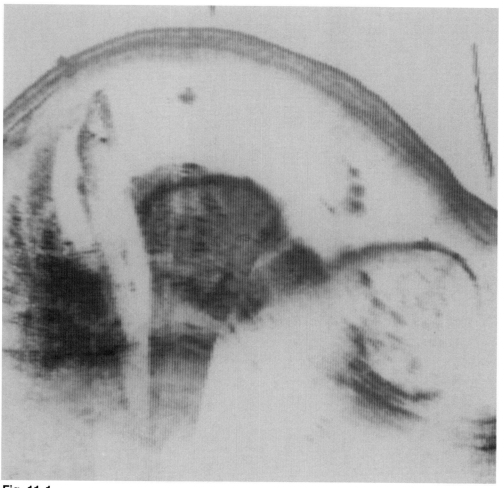

Fig. 11-1

(Continued)

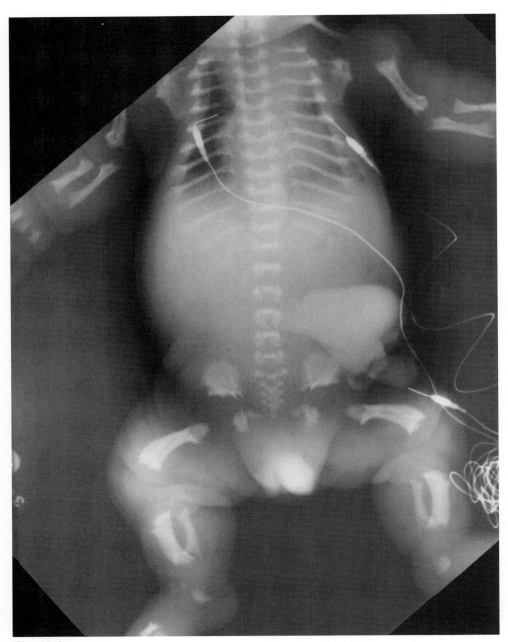

Fig. 11-2

Case 12

An 8-month-old girl is too small. She breast-feeds for 20–40 minutes every 3 hours.

Birth weight was 3.0 kg, length 48 cm. She has had several colds and has 5–8 mushy stools a day.

Weight at 8 months is 5.3 kg, length 61 cm, head circumference 42 cm, temperature 37.6°C, heart rate 125, respiratory rate 35, and blood pressure 80/58 mm Hg. Chest is smaller than abdomen. Lower ribs flare. Ribs bulge at costochondral junctions. Abdomen is distended. Liver edge and spleen edge are 4 cm below costal margin. Petechiae are on legs. The rest of the physical findings are normal.

Hematocrit is 0.38. White cell count is 10.6×10^9/liter with 0.29 polymorphonuclear cells, 0.67 lymphocytes, and 0.04 monocytes. Platelet count is 402×10^9/liter. PT is 13.2 seconds, activated PTT 35.9. Urine specific gravity is 1.002, pH 6. Urine has occasional nonsquamous epithelial cells/HPF and 0–1 white cell/HPF. Serum sodium is 140 mmol/liter, potassium 4.8, chloride 108, carbon dioxide 20, urea nitrogen 1.4, calcium 2.67, phosphorus 1.60, cholesterol 1.94, and glucose 4.7. Creatinine is 20 µmol/liter, uric acid 490, total bilirubin 10, and direct bilirubin 2. Total protein is 68 g/liter, albumin 41, and α_1-antitrypsin 3.4 (normal: 1.5–3.5). Alkaline phosphatase is 289 U/liter (and 361 U with elevated bone isoenzyme), LDH 412, SGOT 137, and GGT 38 (normal: 0–30). Sweat chloride is 6 mmol/liter. Fecal fat is 22 mmol/day (normal: 7–21). Serum 25-OH-cholecalciferol is 15 and 22 nmol/liter (normal: 25–150). Parathormone, C-terminal (serum calcium 2.59 mmol/liter) is 82 µEq/ml (normal: 40–100). Urine phosphoethanolamine is <0.48 mol/mg$_{\text{creatinine}}$ (normal).

Ribs are short, metaphyses flared (Figure 12-1). Metaphyses in rest of skeleton are normal.

She has pneumonia and ear infections. At 2½ years, she eats until "she is so full she can't breathe" and still wants more. She has 4–6 stools per day that contain undigested food. She bruises easily, even from mosquito bites. She has frequent nosebleeds for 2 weeks, mostly from left side, that start when she cries and stop when she stops. Breath smells bad. A "rotting discharge" comes from left side of nose.

Weight at 2½ years is 8.9 kg, length 79 cm, temperature 37.2°C, heart rate 90, respiratory rate 20, and blood pressure 90/60 mm Hg. Blood is in left side of nose. Teeth are decayed. Abdomen is large, chest small. Liver edge is 6 cm below costal margin. Serum beta carotene is 0.2 µmol/liter (normal: 0.9–4.6). IgG is 13.3 g/liter (normal: 4.0–12.0), IgA 0.77 (normal: 0.18–1.50), and IgM 0.80 (normal: 0.45–2.00). IgD is <10 mg/liter (normal: 0–150). IgE is 14 µg/liter (normal: 1–24). Complement C3 is 0.7 g/liter (normal: 0.7–1.6). Sweat chloride is 8 mmol/liter. Duodenal aspirate has no trypsin activity at 1:5 dilution.

"Rotting" nasal discharge and bad breath clear when a piece of rubber (2 × 1 cm) is removed from left side of nose. Fecal fat decreases from 74 to 21 µmol/day when she is given pancreatic enzymes. Ear infections continue. At 4 years, weight is 14.5 kg, height 90 cm. Teeth are decayed or capped. Legs are bowed. At 5 years, skin is dry. Openings of parotid ducts cannot be seen; openings of submandibular ducts are hypoplastic. Mouth is dry.

Bones of legs are normal at 2½ years; legs are bowed, metaphyses frayed at 4½ years (Figure 12-2).

Diagnosis: Shwachman syndrome.

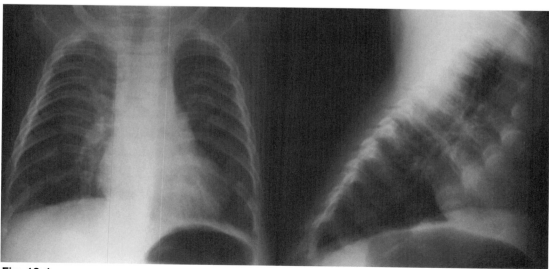

Fig. 12-1

(Continued)

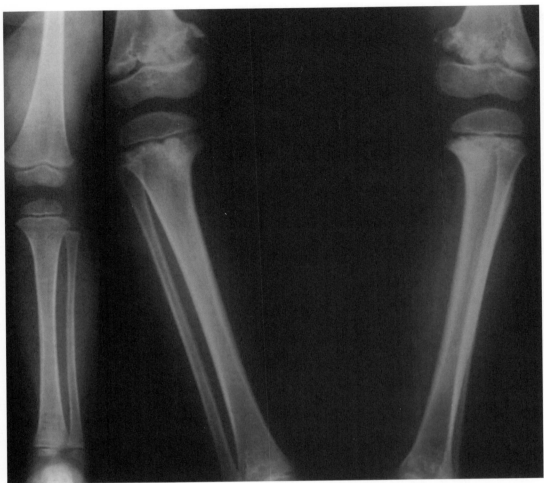

Fig. 12-2

Case 13

A 3-year-old girl has a heart murmur.

Pregnancy of mother was normal, birth weight 4.7 kg. She was blue at birth and had a heart murmur. A systolic heart murmur was present at 15 months, no murmur at 2 years, and a diastolic murmur at 3 years. At 9 months, she broke a leg. Tubes have been put in her ears twice.

Mother and father (both 31 years old) are well. A sister (2 years old) was treated for dislocation at a hip. Maternal grandmother has high blood pressure, maternal grandfather had intracranial aneurysm, and maternal great-grandfather died of a heart attack. Father and members of his family have chest deformity.

Weight at 3 years is 14.5 kg, height 97 cm, temperature 37.1°C, heart rate 140, respiratory rate 40, and blood pressure 94/60 mm Hg. She has a tube in each ear, chest deformity, and systolic heart murmur. The rest of the physical findings are normal.

Hematocrit is 0.38. White cell count is 4.9×10^9/liter with 0.40 polymorphonuclear cells, 0.02 bands, 0.41 lymphocytes, 0.14 monocytes, 0.01 eosinophils, 0.01 basophils, and 0.01 atypical lymphocytes. Urine specific gravity is 1.005, pH 7. Urine has 0–1 white cell/HPF.

ECG shows right ventricular conduction delay to one interpreter, normal findings to another. Findings at cardiac catheterization and angiocardiography are normal.

Her twin brother has frequent ear infections, runny nose, systolic heart murmur, diastolic murmur, widely split S_2, and chest deformity. Birth weight was 4.8 kg, length 57 cm. His weight at 6 years is 24 kg, height 124 cm, and blood pressure 80/40 mm Hg. He has no murmur. ECG findings are normal.

Roentgenographic examinations of the chests of the twins at 3 years (Figures 13-1 and 13-2) show sternal depression. Air in depression in boy's chest casts a radiolucent shadow in front of the heart (see Figure 13-2).

Father, paternal grandmother, paternal great-grandfather, paternal great-uncle, and paternal cousin have pectus excavatum.

Diagnosis: Familial pectus excavatum.

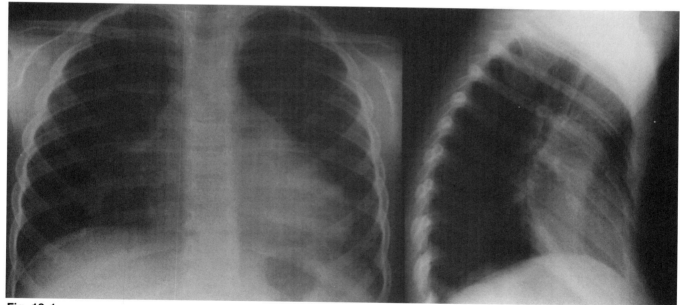

Fig. 13-1

(Continued)

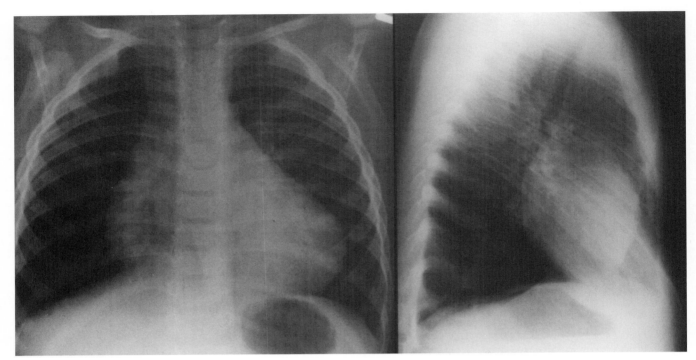

Fig. 13-2

Case 14

A 13-year-old girl stands slumped forward. She has had asthma since 3 years that is now "almost continuous" despite oral and IV medicine. No more clinical information is available.

Chest is deep front to back; sternum is convex forward, and a strip of atelectasis is behind lower part of sternum (Figure 14-1).

Impression: Pectus carinatum because of emphysema.

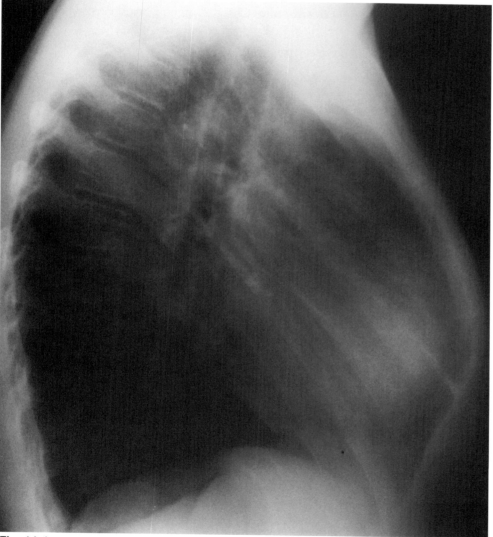

Fig. 14-1

Case 15

A 14-year-old girl has asymmetry of chest (left side smaller than right) that she has been aware of since 10 years and no one else has noticed.

Parents and two older brothers are well.

Birth weight was 2.3 kg, length 44 cm, and Apgar score 8/10 at 1 and at 5 minutes. Neck was short. At 8 months, dorsa of hands and feet were puffy. Chest was broad. Eyebrows met. Mandible was small. Muscle tone was poor. Excretory urography at 3 years and isotope scan at 4 years showed that she did not have a functioning right kidney. Neck was broad, hairline low in back at 4 years. Back had right hump when she bent forward at 6 years. She had astigmatism at 8 years.

Weight at 14 years is 40 kg, height 155 cm. Chromosomes are 46,XX.

A shadow of water density is parallel to front of chest from apex to left side of diaphragm; upper ribs of right side protrude farther back than those of left (Figure 15-1).

Diagnosis: Chest asymmetry, Noonan's syndrome.

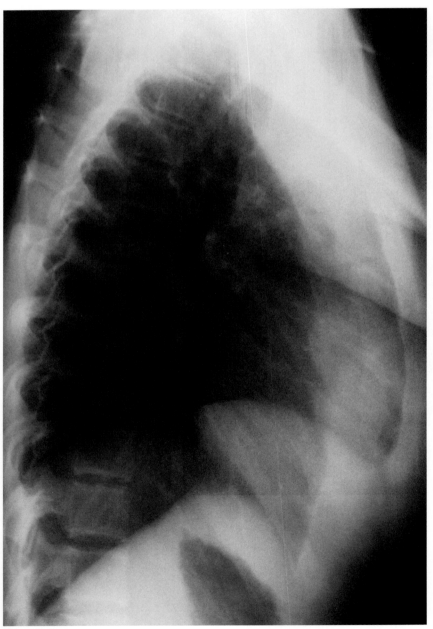

Fig. 15-1

Case 16

A 3-month-old boy spits up blood, the first time at 1 month, next at 2 months, and now every 2–3 days. He does not cough or vomit. Blood is on sheet near his face when he wakes. A stool was black several weeks ago. He has bled from penis four times. He goes to sleep unbruised and awakes bruised. His left leg was broken 3 weeks ago when his cousin fell on it.

Birth weight was 3.8 kg. He vomited a lot the first few weeks. He smiled at 1 month and now holds onto objects placed in his hand.

Mother and father are well. He is their only child. Father is unemployed.

Weight at 3 months is 5.5 kg with cast on left leg, length 60 cm, head circumference 43 cm, temperature 37°C, heart rate 128, respiratory rate 30, and systolic blood pressure 120 mm Hg in arm and leg. Small bruises are on face, back, and right knee. Nose is stuffy. Liver edge is 5 cm below costal margin, spleen edge 3 cm. A sore is at urethral meatus. The rest of the physical findings are normal.

Hematocrit is 0.39. White cell count is 9.9×10^9/liter with 0.22 polymorphonuclear cells, 0.08 bands, 0.57 lymphocytes, 0.07 monocytes, 0.05 eosinophils, and 0.01 myelocytes. Platelet count is 486×10^9/liter. Urine specific gravity is 1.002, pH 6.5. Urine has 0–2 nonsquamous epithelial cells/HPF, occasional squamous epithelial cells/HPF, 2–4 white cells/HPF, and bacteria. Serum urea nitrogen is 8.9 mmol/liter, glucose 5.3. Creatinine is 40 μmol/liter, total bilirubin 12. Total protein is 53 g/liter. SGOT is 58 U/liter.

Older and newer fractures are in back part of some ribs and healing fractures near axillary part of right third and fifth ribs, right first rib is not normal (Figure 16-1).

Diagnosis: Older and newer rib fractures, battered child.

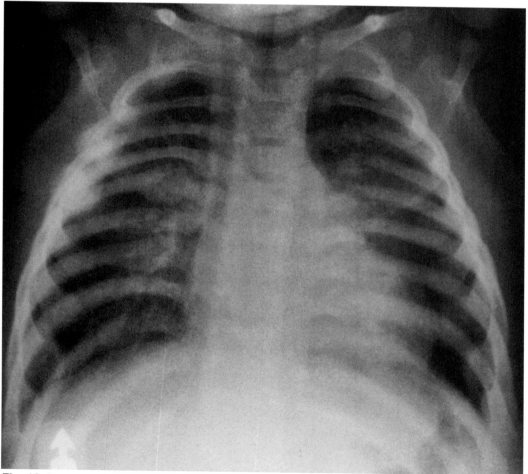

Fig. 16-1

Diaphragm

Case 1

A 2½-month-old girl has tight legs.

Pregnancy of mother (17 years old) was normal, presentation breech, delivery by cesarean section. Birth weight was 2.8 kg, length 51 cm, and Apgar score 8 at 1 minute.

Weight at 2½ months is 4 kg, length 55 cm, head circumference 39 cm, temperature 37.2°C, heart rate 120, respiratory rate 36, and systolic blood pressure 106 mm Hg. Hips are tight, some fingers flexed. Right foot is rocker-bottom. The rest of the physical findings are normal.

Hematocrit is 0.31. White cell count is 4.8×10^9/liter with 0.08 polymorphonuclear cells, 0.06 bands, 0.75 lymphocytes, 0.09 monocytes, and 0.02 eosinophils. Platelet estimate is adequate. Urine specific gravity is 1.004, pH 7. Urine has few squamous epithelial cells/HPF, occasional nonsquamous epithelial cells/HPF, and bacteria.

EMG findings in right gastrocnemius and left biceps muscles are normal.

A round shadow of water density is along right side of heart (Figure 1-1).

Diagnosis: Normal chest, normal anteromedial bulge of right side of diaphragm.

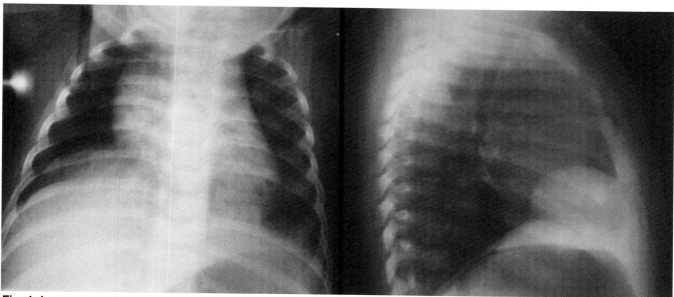

Fig. 1-1

Case 2

A 1-year-old boy vomits often.

Vaginal bleeding occurred during first trimester. Birth weight was 2.8 kg. He "would forget to breathe," his heart rate "was too slow at times," and he gagged with feedings. At 2 months, weight was 3.1 kg. Head was large, occiput prominent, face narrow, nose broad with longitudinal midline crease, mouth small, and palate high. He had epicanthi, simple low auricles, an extra ulnar finger on each hand, and inguinal hernias. The rest of the physical findings were normal. Initially, vomiting was several times a week. Now it is several times a day, unrelated to his feeding or being awake or asleep.

Mother (23 years old) and father (27 years old) are well. He is their only child.

Weight at 1 year is 6 kg, length 65 cm, head circumference 48 cm, temperature 37.1°C, heart rate 144, respiratory rate 36, and systolic blood pressure 52 mm Hg. Head is large, body small and pale. Physical findings match those at two months.

Hematocrit is 0.43. White cell count is 19.1×10^9/liter with 0.23 polymorphonuclear cells, 0.04 bands, 0.52 lymphocytes, 0.15 monocytes, 0.01 eosinophils, 0.01 basophils, and 0.04 atypical lymphocytes. Platelet count is 364×10^9/liter. Urine specific gravity is 1.033, pH 6. Urine has 2+ ketones, few squamous epithelial cells/HPF, occasional red cells/HPF, and occasional white cells/HPF. Serum sodium is 141 mmol/liter, potassium 5.1, chloride 99, carbon dioxide 24, urea nitrogen 6.4, calcium 2.74, phosphorus 1.39, cholesterol 4.01, and glucose 4.7. Creatinine is 50 μmol/liter, uric acid 310, total bilirubin 7, and direct bilirubin 2. Total protein is 73 g/liter, albumin 49. Alkaline phosphatase is 442 U/liter, LDH 396. Arterial blood pH is 7.32. P_{CO_2} is 57 mm Hg, P_{O_2} 24. Chromosomes are 46,XY,5q+, the result of interstitial deletion of material from a parental chromosome 2q32.2→2q23 and insertion into chromosome 5q.

Esophagus and stomach are dilated with gas (Figure 2-1A). Back of diaphragm is elevated on both sides (Figure 2-1B). At chest fluoroscopy, back of diaphragm moves up when he breathes in, rest of diaphragm moves down.

Diagnosis: Paradoxic movement of diaphragm in boy with chromosome 5q+.

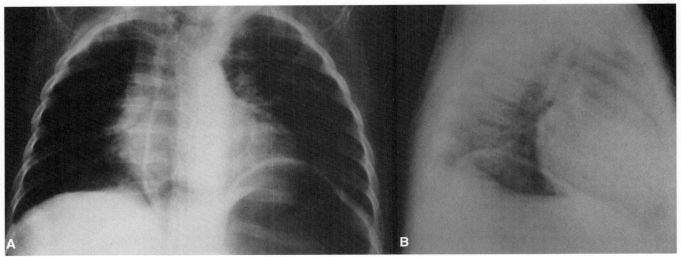

Fig. 2-1

Case 3

A 2½-year-old boy has a heart murmur. He has occasional colds. Mother is tuberculin positive and has been taking antituberculous drugs for a year.

Weight is 11.6 kg. A holosystolic heart murmur is present. The rest of the physical findings are normal.

Hematocrit is 0.40. White cell count is 10.2×10^9/liter with 0.19 polymorphonuclear cells, 0.03 bands, 0.66 lymphocytes, 0.10 monocytes, 0.01 eosinophils, and 0.01 basophils. Platelet count is 463×10^9/liter. Serum sodium is 144 mmol/liter, potassium 4.3, chloride 109, carbon dioxide 19, urea nitrogen 5.4, calcium 2.52, phosphorus 1.58, cholesterol 4.71, and glucose 5.4. Creatinine is 40 µmol/liter, uric acid not determined, total bilirubin 3, and direct bilirubin 2. Total protein is 73 g/liter, albumin 46. Alkaline phosphatase is 244 U/liter, LDH 342, and SGOT 50.

Roentgenograms show an ill-defined shadow of water density in mid–right lung, displacement of heart to right (Figure 3-1A), and, in lateral view (Figure 3-1B), a strip of water density behind sternum.

He is able to run and kick normally at 3 years, despite a cut on right knee. Weight is 12.3 kg, height 86 cm.

Diagnosis: Small ventricular septal defect, accessory right side of diaphragm.

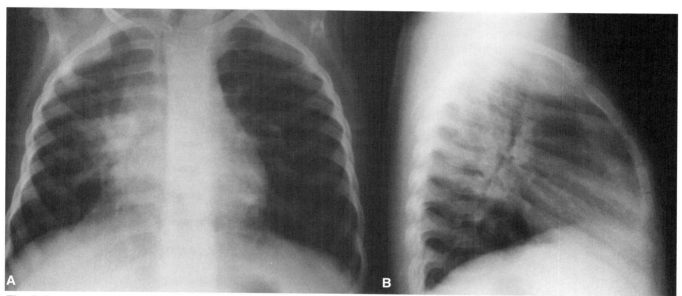

Fig. 3-1

Case 4

A newborn girl is cyanotic. Respirations have just changed from easy to labored. She was delivered by cesarean section for failure to progress.

Weight is 3.9 kg, length 56 cm, and Apgar score 8/7 at 1 and 5 minutes. At 45 minutes, temperature is 36.7°C, heart rate 200, respiratory rate 60, and systolic blood pressure 50 mm Hg. Heart sounds are louder in right side of chest. Breath sounds are poor in both sides. The rest of the physical findings are normal.

Hematocrit is 0.51. White cell count is 32.0×10^9/liter with 0.44 polymorphonuclear cells, 0.02 bands, 0.35 lymphocytes, 0.15 monocytes, 0.01 eosinophils, 0.01 basophils, and 0.02 myelocytes. At 1¼ hours, arterial blood pH when $FIO_2 = 1.0$ is 7.00. PCO_2 is 64 mm Hg, PO_2 46.

At 1 hour, left side of chest and most of right side are radioopaque; a curved, tubular shadow of mixed air and water density, the dilated esophagus, is in right side of chest; and no gas is in abdomen (Figure 4-1).

At operation, tip of left lobe of liver, spleen, stomach, and intestine are herniated into left side of chest through a large posterolateral defect in left side of diaphragm.

She dies soon after operation. Combined lung weight is 20 g (normal: 65 g). Diameter of left lung is 2 cm. Enlarged, cartilaginous bronchi are near edge of left lung.

Diagnosis: Left Bochdalek's hernia, hypoplasia of lungs.

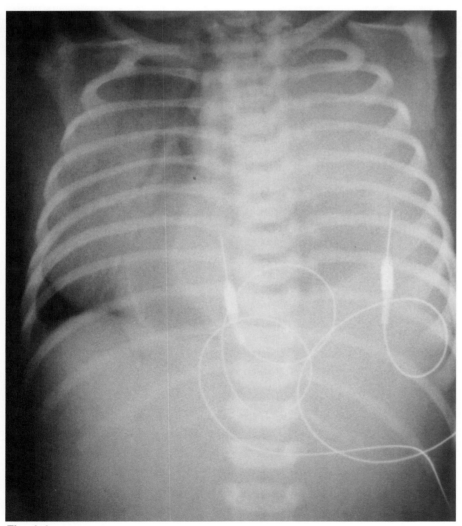

Fig. 4-1

Case 5

A newborn girl is blue and not breathing. After she is intubated and given oxygen, breath sounds are present only in left side of chest.

Apgar score is 2/1 at 1 and 5 minutes, weight 3.5 kg. Temperature at 4 hours is 37.2°C, heart rate 170, respiratory rate 100, and systolic blood pressure 80 mm Hg. The rest of the physical findings are normal.

Hematocrit is 0.56. Serum sodium is 132 mmol/liter, potassium 3.8, chloride 102, carbon dioxide 8, calcium 2.52, and glucose 4.4. Creatinine is 100 μmol/liter. Arterial blood pH is 7.28 when $FIO_2 = 1.0$. PCO_2 is 54 mm Hg, PO_2 37.

At 15 minutes, a faint tubular shadow of air density in left side of chest curves toward midline at level of diaphragm; shadows of air density are in right side of chest (Figure 5-1A). At 2 hours, shadows of air density are increased when diaphragm is continuous across midline, air is in subcutaneous tissues of neck and right axilla, and gas is in abdomen (Figure 5-1B).

At right thoracotomy, hemorrhagic lung and peritoneal sac with liver and much of small bowel are in right side of chest, and a defect is in posterolateral part of right side of diaphragm.

Diagnosis: Right Bochdalek's hernia, pneumomediastinum (continuous diaphragm sign).

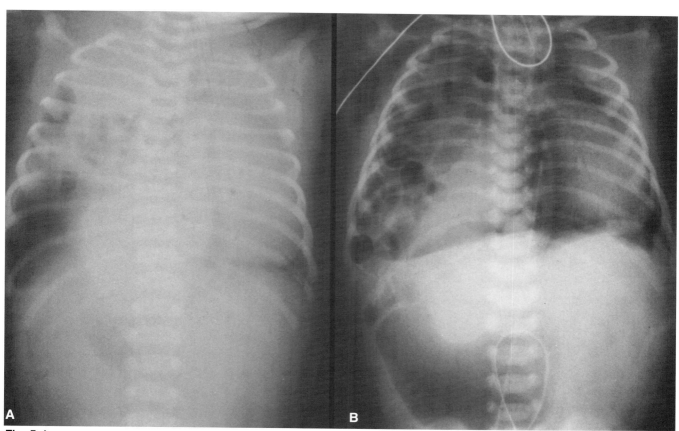

Fig. 5-1

Case 6

A 2-month-old girl vomits right after one breast-feeding or before next, gurgles and whimpers during feeding, and feeds hungrily.

She has been spitting up a little for several weeks. Vomiting began 3 days ago. Vomit was tinged pink with stringy brown matter 2 nights ago. Stool was brown-black 3 days ago.

Pregnancy of mother was normal, birth weight 3.5 kg. She lifts her head, smiles, follows with her eyes, and rolls over.

Mother (32 years old) is well. Father (37 years old) had allergies in childhood and has had pneumothorax. (He dies at 40 years during operation for aortic aneurysm.) Paternal grandfather, who was 183 cm tall, had pectus excavatum and heart failure and died with aortic dissection at 50 years.

Weight at 2 months is 4 kg, length 59 cm, head circumference 39 cm, temperature 37.7°C, heart rate 136, respiratory rate 40, and systolic blood pressure 70 mm Hg. A pink spot is on forehead, a small brown birthmark is on right calf. Xiphoid process protrudes. Fingers and toes are long. The rest of the physical findings are normal.

Hematocrit is 0.36. White cell count is 11.7×10^9/liter with 0.03 polymorphonuclear cells, 0.02 bands, and 0.95 lympho-cytes. Urine specific gravity is 1.017, pH 7. Urine has bacteria, 15–20 white cells/HPF, and occasional squamous and nonsquamous epithelial cells/HPF. Serum sodium is 138 mmol/liter, potassium 5.3, chloride 94, urea nitrogen 1.4, and glucose 4.6.

Barium shows stomach behind heart (Figure 6-1).

At operation, stomach that is herniated into left side of chest through a dilated esophageal hiatus is easily put into abdomen.

She walks at 9 months and feeds herself at 1 year. Ophthalmologic findings are normal at 3 years. Weight at 5 years is 19 kg, height 117 cm. She has a holosystolic heart murmur, echocardiographic prolapse of mitral valve, and flat feet. At 10 years, she is operated on for left second hammer toe. At 12 years, she wears glasses for myopia and astigmatism and has recurrent dislocation of patellas. At 20 years, weight is 68 kg, height 175 cm, heart rate 87, and blood pressure 129/86 mm Hg. She has midsystolic click and no murmur. Ultrasound examination shows diameter of aorta is 40 mm at sinuses of Valsalva, 24 mm at arch.

Diagnosis: Esophageal hiatal hernia, Marfan syndrome.

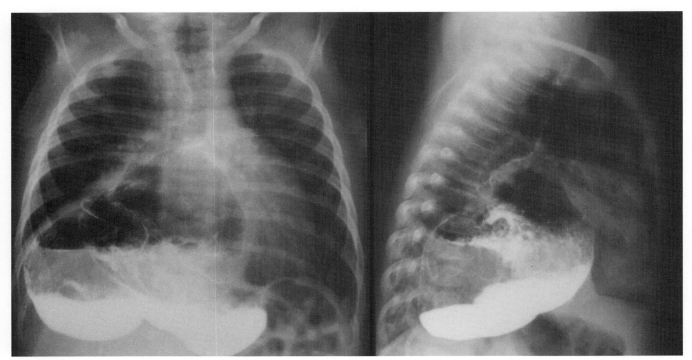

Fig. 6-1

Case 7

A 2-month-old boy has right pleural liquid.

Pregnancy of mother was normal, birth weight 3.8 kg. He vomited often the first month. At 5 weeks, he had a "whistling" cough, two blue spells, and intercostal and substernal retractions. In right side of chest at 5 weeks, he had dullness; diminished breath sounds; and sterile, clear amber pleural liquid.

Mother (23 years old), father, and three siblings are well.

Temperature at 2 months is 36.1°C, heart rate 135, respiratory rate 60, systolic blood pressure 80 mm Hg, weight 4.5 kg, length 56 cm, and head circumference 39 cm. White plaque is inside left cheek. A tube is in right side of chest with 30 ml clear yellow liquid in the drainage bottle. Breath sounds are diminished in right side. A hydrocele is in each side of scrotum. The rest of the physical findings are normal.

Hematocrit is 0.37. White cell count is 11.3×10^9/liter with 0.41 polymorphonuclear cells, 0.17 bands, 0.35 lymphocytes,

0.02 monocytes, and 0.05 eosinophils. Platelet estimate is adequate. Specific gravity of pleural liquid is 1.010 with 47×10^6/liter white cells, 0.48 polymorphonuclear cells, 0.52 lymphocytes, and 11.5 g/liter protein.

At 5 weeks, lower part of right side of chest is opaque, and gas-containing gut is high in right side of abdomen (Figure 7-1).

At 9 weeks, isotope scan shows a waistlike band of decreased uptake in liver at level of diaphragm. At 11 weeks, he cries for 15 minutes and then is pale, sweaty, and retracting. Respiratory rate is 50–90.

At 11 weeks, gas liquid–containing gut is in right side of chest (Figure 7-2).

At right thoracotomy, liver and small bowel are herniated into right side of chest through a posterolateral defect in diaphragm.

Diagnosis: Delayed appearance of right Bochdalek's hernia.

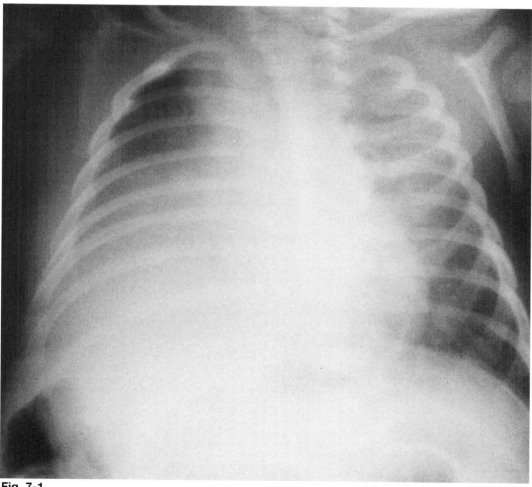

Fig. 7-1

(Continued)

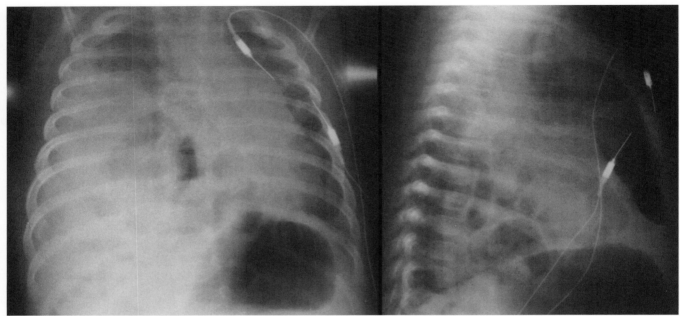

Fig. 7-2

Case 8

A 2½-month-old boy is coughing and vomiting. Stools are loose.

Pregnancy of mother was normal, birth weight 3.3 kg, and Apgar score 8/9 at 1 and 5 minutes. He breathed hard and was fussy first night and had two spells the second day, during which he stopped breathing for 15 seconds and became dusky. Respiratory pauses and slowing of heart occur several times a week.

Mother (20 years old), father (23 years old), and brother (3 years old) are well. They had colds 2 weeks ago.

Temperature at 2½ months is 36.8°C, heart rate 174, respiratory rate 48, systolic blood pressure 60–80 mm Hg, weight 5.0 kg, length 57 cm, and head circumference 40 cm. He is pale and grunting. Breath sounds are diminished at left base. The rest of the physical findings are normal.

Hematocrit is 0.31. White cell count is 13.6×10^9/liter with 0.64 polymorphonuclear cells, 0.07 bands, 0.18 lymphocytes, 0.09 monocytes, and 0.2 atypical lymphocytes. Platelet count is 811×10^9/liter. Capillary blood pH is 7.30 when $FIO_2 = 0.20$. PCO_2 is 45 mm Hg, PO_2 37. Serum sodium is 138 mmol/liter, potassium 4.7, chloride 107, and carbon dioxide 22.

At 3 days, the findings are normal (Figure 8-1). At 2½ months, gut is in left side of chest (Figure 8-2).

At operation, half the small bowel without a sac is herniated into left side of chest through a posterolateral defect in diaphragm.

Diagnosis: Delayed appearance of left Bochdalek's hernia.

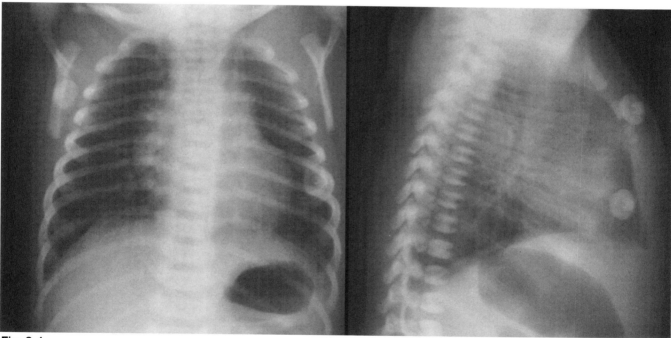

Fig. 8-1

(Continued)

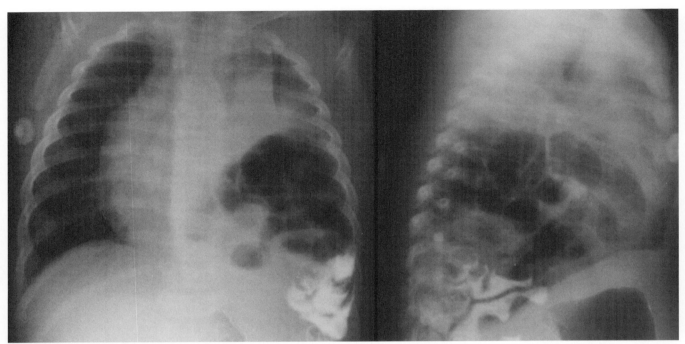

Fig. 8-2

Case 9

A 2½-year-old boy with Down syndrome has watery stools and will not eat.

Diarrhea began 3 weeks ago. He has had water, caffeine-free soda, and almost no food for a week. He has not vomited. He has had many colds.

Temperature is 36.2°C, heart rate 156, respiratory rate 32, blood pressure 114/70 mm Hg, weight 10 kg, and height 83 cm. Eyes are sunken. Mouth is dry. Left side of chest is tympanitic. Heart sounds are distant. Gurgly, tinkly bowel sounds are in left side of chest. Bowel sounds are increased in abdomen. Liver edge is 4 cm below costal margin. Muscle tone is poor. The rest of the physical findings are normal.

Hematocrit is 0.45. White cell count is 13.8×10^9/liter with 0.14 polymorphonuclear cells, 0.63 bands, 0.21 lymphocytes, 0.01 monocytes, and 0.01 eosinophils. Platelet estimate is adequate. Urine specific gravity is 1.002 (IV fluids), pH 5.5. Urine has 4–5 granular casts/LPF, 0–2 white cells/HPF, rare red cells/HPF, and occasional epithelial cells/HPF. Serum sodium is 120 mmol/liter, potassium 3.4, chloride 94, urea nitrogen 5.0, and glucose 3.9. Chromosomes are 47,XY,21+.

Dilated gut is in front of heart and in left side of chest (Figure 9-1).

At operation, transverse colon, omentum, and part of liver are herniated into pericardium through a 5-cm defect in diaphragm just to right of midline and behind sternum. Liver is large and pale. Cecum and appendix are in upper right quadrant of abdomen.

Biopsy of excised piece of liver shows distended, vacuolated hepatocytes throughout the lobules, fibrosis in and between portal triads, as many as four bile ducts in triads, and a few lymphocytes and polymorphonuclear cells in triads.

Diagnosis: Retrosternal herniation of abdominal viscera into pericardium, malrotation of gut, and fatty change and early cirrhosis in liver.

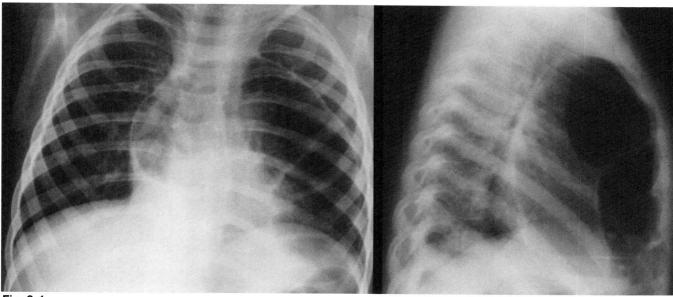

Fig. 9-1

Case 10

A 4-day-old girl vomits and is hard to burp.

Birth weight was 4.3 kg, Apgar score 7/7 at 1 and 5 minutes. Appetite was poor. Respirations were fast and grunting. She fed slowly at 2 days, vomited formula at 3 days, and curds most of her feeding at 4 days.

Mother (26 years old), father (30 years old), and sister (2 years old) are well.

Weight at 4 days is 3.9 kg, length 55 cm, head circumference 37 cm, temperature 37.1°C, heart rate 148, respiratory rate 56, and systolic blood pressure 70 mm Hg. Heart sounds are loud in right side of chest. The rest of the physical findings are normal.

Hematocrit is 0.49. Serum sodium is 143 mmol/liter, potassium 6.1, and chloride 106. Venous blood pH is 7.41. P_{CO_2} is 33 mm Hg, P_{O_2} 43.

Figure 10-1 shows a shadow of mixed water and gas density in left side of chest; heart is displaced to right. Barium shows esophagus in normal place and much of stomach in left side of chest (Figure 10-2).

At operation, a membrane covers stomach, small bowel, colon, spleen, and left lobe of liver, which are herniated into chest through a large central defect in left side of diaphragm. Cecum and appendix are in lower right quadrant of abdomen, midgut is normally rotated, and Ladd's bands are not present.

Diagnosis: Central left diaphragmatic hernia.

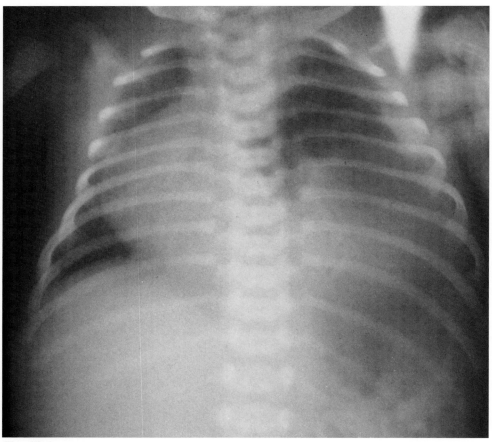

Fig. 10-1

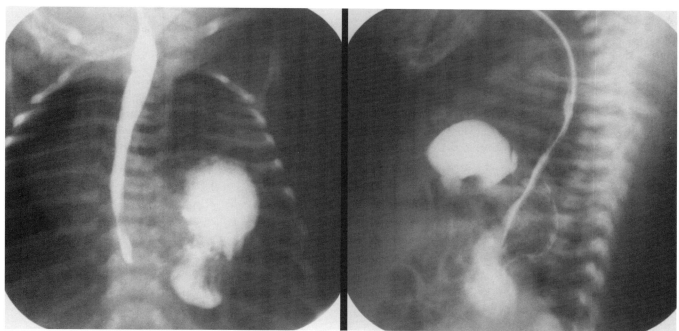

Fig. 10-2

Case 11

A newborn boy is cyanotic and breathing hard.

Mother (24 years old) had genital sores in midpregnancy. Herpes simplex virus was cultured from cervix at 36 weeks. Birth weight is 3.0 kg, Apgar score 4/8 at 1 and 5 minutes, length 52 cm, head circumference 36 cm, heart rate 160, and systolic blood pressure 60 mm Hg. He is intubated and given oxygen. Heart sounds and coarse breath sounds are in right side of chest. Abdomen is scaphoid. The rest of the physical findings are normal.

Hematocrit is 0.55. White cell count is 16.0×10^9/liter. Arterial blood pH is 7.05 when $F_{IO_2} = 1.0$. P_{CO_2} is 68 mm Hg, P_{O_2} 61. Serum sodium is 140 mmol/liter, potassium 3.9, chloride 104, calcium 2.25, and urea nitrogen 1.8. Creatinine is 100 μmol/liter.

Gas-containing gut fills left side of chest, extends into right side, and pushes heart, endotracheal tube, and aortic catheter to right (Figure 11-1).

At operation, stomach, spleen, part of liver, most of small bowel, and ascending and transverse colon are herniated into left side of chest through a defect in diaphragm.

He is hypoxic the next day. Heart rate slows to <100; blood pressure decreases from 55 to 40 mm Hg.

Soon after operation, heart is near midline, air is in left side of chest, and tubes and catheters are in place (Figure 11-2A). Heart is in left side of chest in roentgenogram made after heart rate slows and blood pressure falls (Figure 11-2B). Two thin, curved strips of water density, one pericardium visible because of pericardial air, one visceral pleura visible because of pleural air are just to right of T8 and T9 (see Figure 11-2B).

He dies 10 minutes after second roentgenogram.

At necropsy, left half of pericardium is absent. Left medial parietal pleura has a hole. Heart is herniated through the pericardial defect, and right atrium and inferior vena cava are compressed at edge of defect. Left lung is hypoplastic.

Diagnosis: Left Bochdalek's hernia, herniation of heart through pericardial defect.

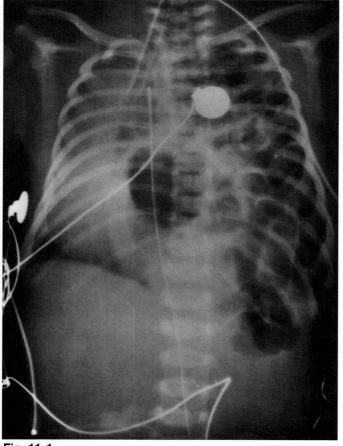

Fig. 11-1

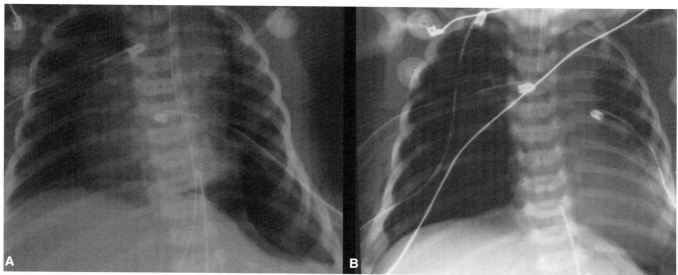

Fig. 11-2

Case 12

A 7-year-old girl, who was run over by school bus, is pale and mumbling 1½ hours after the accident and comatose a few minutes later. Heart rate is 160, respiratory rate 32, and systolic blood pressure 120 mm Hg. Blood pressure falls to 86/70 mm Hg and then is unobtainable. Breath sounds are diminished in left side of chest. Left humerus is fractured.

Hematocrit is 0.22. Hemoglobin is 75 g/liter. Urine is bloody.

Left side of diaphragm is disrupted (Figure 12-1). Roentgenographic examination also shows fracture of both pubic bones.

At operation, both sides of diaphragm are ruptured. Spleen, left side of colon, and some of small bowel are in left side of chest. Right kidney and right adrenal gland are lacerated and surrounded by blood. Blood is in retroperitoneum behind duodenum; subcapsular blood is around liver.

Serum amylase is 365 U/liter 4 days after operation and above normal (i.e., 0–130) for 2 months. Ninety days after operation, right pleural liquid is cloudy and has 86 g/liter protein, 3.9 mmol/liter glucose, 4.20 triglycerides, and 2.22 cholesterol. Two and a half months after operation, SGOT is 576 U/liter. Serum is nonreactive for HBsAg and does not contain HBsAb or HBcAb. Needle biopsy of liver shows swollen hepatocytes, acidophil bodies, chronic inflammatory cells, and periportal necrosis. Hair falls out. Angles of mouth are cracked, fingertips blistered. Perianal skin is blistered and then macerated. Serum zinc is 4.4 µmol/liter (normal: 11.5–18.5).

Diagnosis: Rupture of both sides of diaphragm, ruptured viscera, fractures, pancreatitis, chylothorax, viral hepatitis (questionable hepatitis C), and acrodermatitis enteropathica.

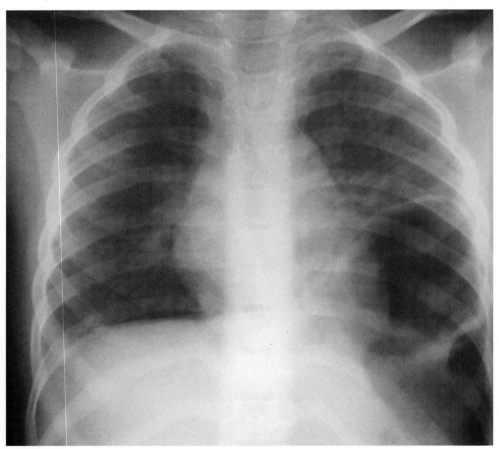

Fig. 12-1

Pleura

Case 1

A newborn boy is grunting and blue at 1 hour when FIO_2 = 0.30.

Pregnancy of mother (24 years old) was normal. Birth weight is 3.4 kg, length 50 cm, head circumference 36 cm, and Apgar score 9/9 at 1 and 5 minutes.

Temperature at 1 hour is 36.3°C, heart rate 142, respiratory rate 50, and systolic blood pressure 54 mm Hg. Subcostal tissues retract. Heart sounds are distant. Liver edge is 1–2 cm below costal margin. A skin tag is on left little finger. The rest of the physical findings are normal.

Hematocrit is 0.63. Serum sodium is 140 mmol/liter, potassium 4.6, chloride 108, and carbon dioxide 20. At 6 days, peak bilirubin is 209 μmol/liter.

At 1 hour, air is in both pleural spaces; lungs lack air (Figure 1-1A). At 3 hours he looks well and, without thoracentesis, has less pleural air. Thymus is large (Figure 1-1B). At 24 hours, roentgenographic findings are normal.

Diagnosis: Normal newborn boy.

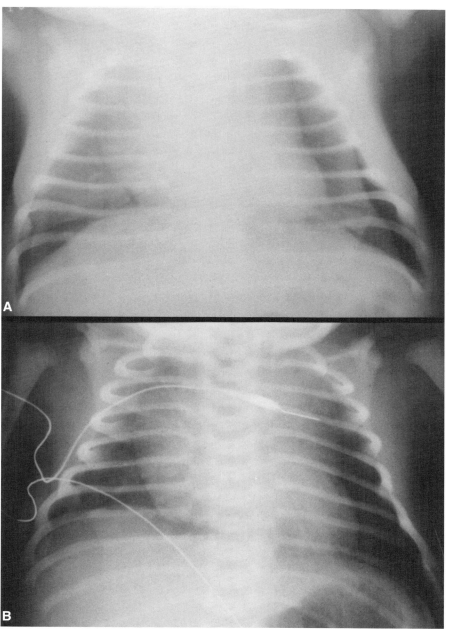

Fig. 1-1

Case 2

A newborn boy is grunting and breathing hard.

Mother (29 years old) bled from vagina 1 day before delivery. Delivery is vaginal, birth weight 2.1 kg, length 45 cm, Apgar score 7/8 at 1 and 5 minutes, temperature 37.3°C, heart rate 172, respiratory rate 52, and blood pressure 64/38 mm Hg. He is pale and sometimes mottled. Breath sounds are noisy. The rest of the physical findings are normal.

Hematocrit is 0.44. White cell count is 7.2×10^9/liter with 0.41 polymorphonuclear cells, 0.02 bands, 0.43 lymphocytes, 0.12 monocytes, 0.01 basophils, and 0.01 atypical lymphocytes. Platelet count is 259×10^9/liter. At 1 day, serum sodium is 140 mmol/liter, potassium 4.6, chloride 105, carbon dioxide 23, urea nitrogen 5.0, calcium 1.95, phosphorus 1.68, cholesterol 1.94, and glucose 4.9. Creatinine is 80 μmol/liter, uric acid 390, total bilirubin 96, and direct bilirubin 7. Total protein is 42 g/liter, albumin 31. Alkaline phosphatase is 258 U/liter, LDH 850, and SGOT 58. Blood oxygen saturation is 0.86 when FIO_2 = 0.63 by nasal continuous positive airway pressure at 24 hours, 0.72 when FIO_2 = 0.99 at 31 hours when he is agitated, crying, and pulling hard and then intubated.

At approximately 31 hours, pleural air compresses right lung and stretches slips of attachment of costal part of diaphragm at right eighth and ninth costochondral junctions (Figure 2-1). Endotracheal tube ends at level of C7–T1, umbilical arterial catheter at T8–T9 in Figure 2-1.

Diagnosis: Right tension pneumothorax.

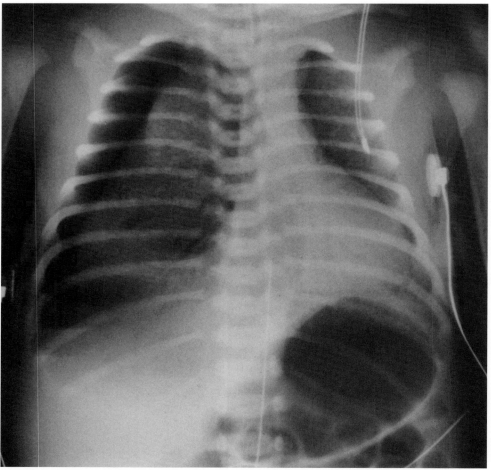

Fig. 2-1

Case 3

A 2½-year-old boy is coughing, wheezing, and febrile.

He had a runny nose 2 days ago, a cough that night, and wheezing and fast breathing yesterday. He did not eat much yesterday, drank only a few ounces of milk, and vomited once.

Birth weight was 3.1 kg. At 3 months, he wheezed and had a runny nose and has had several mild attacks since then. He gets hives from eating eggs and is allergic to cows' milk and possibly root beer.

Mother and father have hay fever. He is their only child.

Temperature at 2½ years is 38.9°C, heart rate 122, respiratory rate 64, blood pressure 100/60 mm Hg, weight 13.1 kg, and height 93 cm. Dry phlegm is in nose. Lips are dry. Thick white phlegm is in throat. Trachea deviates to right. Soft tissues retract during inspiration. Right side of chest expands less than left. Upper part of right side of chest is hyper-resonant. Breath sounds are diminished in right side. Liver edge is 1 cm below costal margin. The rest of the physical findings are normal.

Hematocrit is 0.40. White cell count is 10.4×10^9/liter with 0.70 polymorphonuclear cells, 0.02 bands, 0.24 lymphocytes, and 0.04 monocytes. Platelet estimate is adequate. Urine specific gravity is 1.030, pH 5. Urine has 4+ acetone, occasional epithelial cells/HPF, and occasional white cells/HPF. Serum sodium is 140 mmol/liter, potassium 5.9, chloride 105, carbon dioxide 18, and urea nitrogen 5.4.

Right upper lobe is atelectatic, pleural air is around its apex, and trachea is displaced to right (Figure 3-1).

For the next 3 days, he is comfortable, afebrile, and playful. Respiratory rate is 30–43. Right upper lobe is still atelectatic after 3 days. Bronchoscopy shows edema and inflammation of trachea and main bronchi. A mucous cast is removed from right upper lobe bronchus 3 days after first roentgenogram.

Diagnosis: Asthma, right upper lobe atelectasis, pleural air cap.

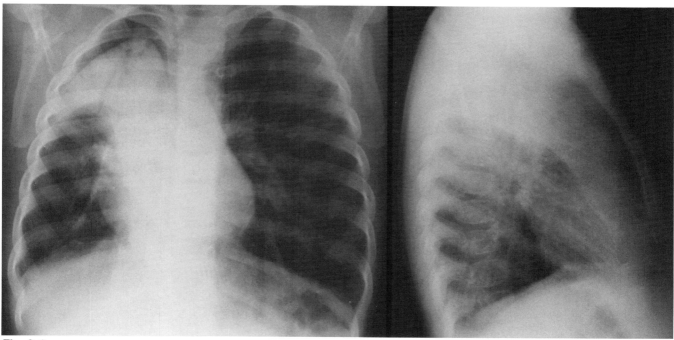

Fig. 3-1

Case 4

A 3-year-old girl cries for her mother after being run over by a car.

Heart rate is 100, respiratory rate 20, and systolic blood pressure 120 mm Hg. She moves arms and legs. Right side of face, right shoulder, and right arm are scraped. Breath sounds are diminished in right side. A deep laceration from vulva to anus is in left side of perineum. Babinski's sign is in left foot. The rest of the physical findings are normal.

Hematocrit is 0.35. White cell count is 16.1×10^9/liter with 0.71 polymorphonuclear cells, 0.13 bands, 0.11 lymphocytes, and 0.05 monocytes. Platelet count is 414×10^9/liter. Urine specific gravity is 1.035, pH 5. Urine has 0.30 g/liter protein, 13.9 mmol/liter glucose, and 2+ hemoglobin/myoglobin.

First roentgenogram shows right tension pneumothorax (Figure 4-1A). Fifteen hours after insertion of chest tube, endotracheal tube, and enteric tube, and after abdominal operation (at which pelvic hematoma was found), roentgenogram shows right tension pneumothorax (Figure 4-1B).

At bronchoscopy, tears are in right main bronchus and right upper lobe bronchus. The tears are closed at thoracotomy.

Diagnosis: Bronchopleural fistula.

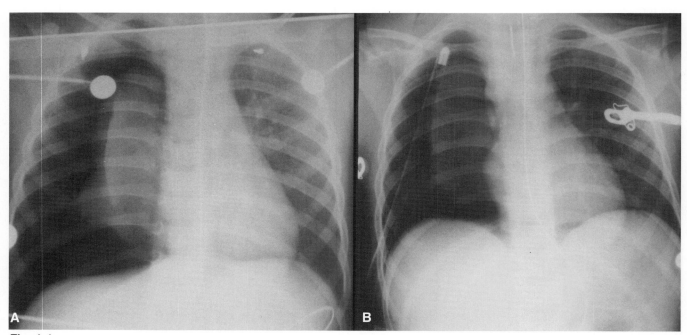

Fig. 4-1

Case 5

A 6-year-old boy has taut skin, distended abdomen, bruises on right eyelids and legs, swollen penis, and pitting edema of legs.

He was swollen and tired 5 months ago and pale 3 months ago, when systolic heart murmur was present and liver edge was 3 cm below costal margin. Treatment was begun with IV albumin and prednisone until he got chickenpox. He now takes prednisone.

Mother died of liver disease at 30 years.

Weight at 6 years is 34 kg (3 months ago: 22 kg), height 118 cm, heart rate 72, respiratory rate 36, and blood pressure 130/90 mm Hg (3 months ago: 90/56 mm Hg). The rest of the physical findings are normal.

Three months ago, hematocrit was 0.52. White cell count was 11.6×10^9/liter with 0.65 polymorphonuclear cells, 0.32 lymphocytes, and 0.03 eosinophils. Serum urea nitrogen was 9.6 mmol/liter, calcium 2.15, phosphorus 1.84, and glucose 5.4. Uric acid was 330 μmol/liter, total bilirubin 3, and direct bilirubin 0. Total protein was 41 g/liter, albumin 11. Alkaline phosphatase was 170 U/liter, LDH 430, and SGOT 80. Cholesterol was too high to measure.

Today, urine specific gravity is 1.051, pH 6.5. Urine has 4+ albumin, amorphous urates, oval fat bodies, 3–10 epithelial cells/HPF, 1–2 white cells/HPF, 1–2 red cells/HPF, 3–5 hyaline casts/LPF, and 0–4 granular casts/LPF. ESR is 116 mm/hr.

In Figure 5-1A, heart is small and subcutaneous and pleural liquid is present. In Figure 5-1B, peritoneal liquid is present.

At 6½ years, he has early posterior subcapsular cataracts, and, at 7½ years, he is cushingoid and has distended abdomen, pitting edema, and transverse lines in toenails.

Excretory urogram at 7½ years shows crossed ectopy of kidneys (Figure 5-2A) and ureters in front of ectopic kidney (Figure 5-2B) and displaced medially in pelvis, presumably by steroid-induced fat (see Figure 5-2A). A normal bulge of early ossification is at left ischiopubic synchondrosis in Figure 5-2A.

At 7½ years, biopsy of kidney shows normal microscopic findings. Electron microscopy shows scattered electron-dense deposits in mesangium, subepithelial dense deposits, fusion of foot processes, red cell rouleaux in capillaries, collapsed capillaries, thickening of capillary basement membrane, and fibrillation of mesangial matrix. Fluorescent microscopy shows granular and diffuse deposits of IgG, IgA, and IgM in basement membrane and mesangium of glomeruli; C3 and debris in tubules; and debris in apices of epithelial cells.

Diagnosis: Nephrotic syndrome, immune complex nephritis, and crossed ectopy of kidneys.

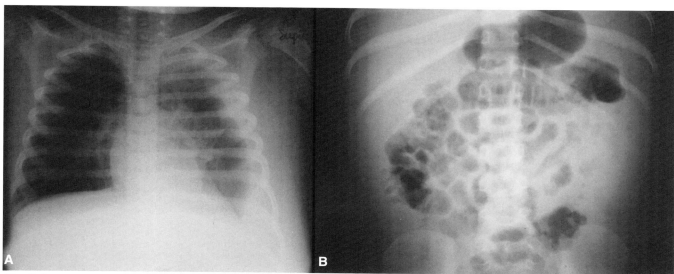

Fig. 5-1

(Continued)

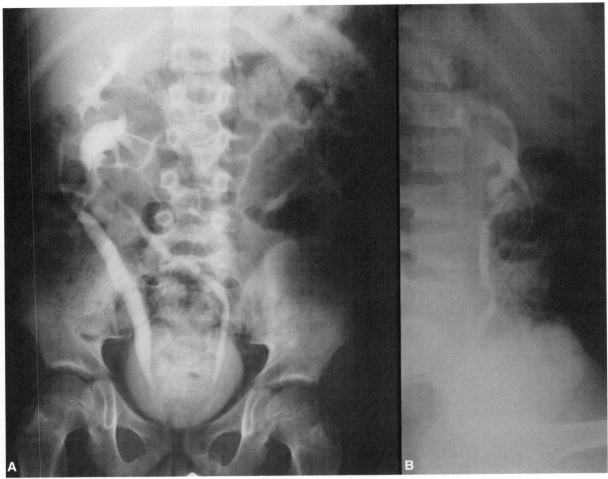

Fig. 5-2

Case 6

A 2-week-old boy, one of twins, has been breathing quickly for 2 days.

Mother and father (both 35 years old), twin sister, and older siblings are well.

Temperature is 36.8°C, heart rate 160, respiratory rate 82, weight 3.2 kg (birth weight: 3.1 kg), and length 52 cm. The rest of the physical findings are normal.

Hematocrit is 0.41. White cell count is 16.5×10^9/liter with 0.64 polymorphonuclear cells, 0.08 bands, 0.24 lymphocytes, 0.02 monocytes, and 0.02 eosinophils.

Liquid is in lower left side of mediastinum and in right pleural space (Figure 6-1).

At right thoracentesis, 190 ml of milky liquid that has 14.0×10^9/liter white cells (all lymphocytes), 54 g/liter protein, and 4.3 mmol/liter glucose is obtained. Gram's stain is negative, culture sterile.

Lymphangiogram in a 46-year-old man with Hodgkin's disease shows thoracic duct and opacified lymph node above left clavicle, perhaps at end of thoracic duct at angle of junction of left subclavian and left internal jugular veins (Figure 6-2).

Diagnosis: Chylothorax, rupture of mediastinal chyloma, rupture of thoracic duct.

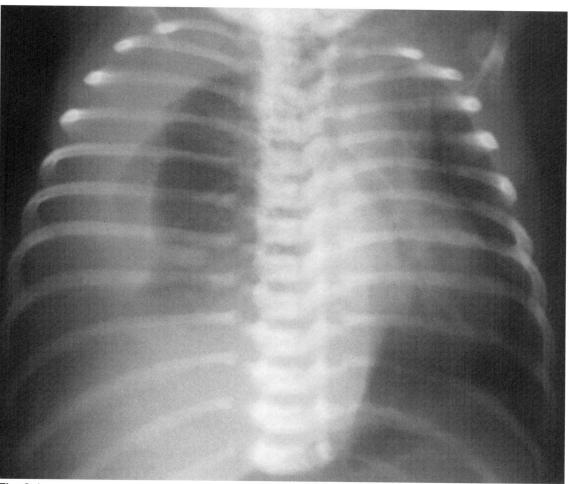

Fig. 6-1

(Continued)

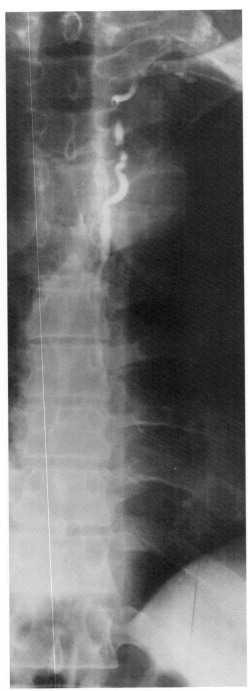

Fig. 6-2

Case 7

A 1-year-old boy has spells in which he pants, turns blue, and "stiffens up."

Pregnancy of mother was normal. Fetal heart rate slowed during labor. A heart murmur was present at 1 day. Lips and nailbeds were blue when he ate at 2 weeks. He tires easily. He had a cold and fever a month ago. He crawled at 9 months and now walks with help.

Mother (24 years old), father (25 years old), brother (6 years old), and sister (3 years old) are well. Paternal grandfather has diabetes mellitus.

Weight at 1 year is 7.3 kg, length 73 cm, head circumference 46 cm, temperature 36.9°C, heart rate 150, respiratory rate 40, and blood pressure 70/40 mm Hg. Limbs are thin, nails blue. A systolic heart murmur is present. The rest of the physical findings are normal.

Hematocrit is 0.56. White cell count is 18.8×10^9/liter with 0.20 polymorphonuclear cells, 0.03 bands, 0.76 lymphocytes, and 0.01 monocytes. Platelet estimate is adequate. Urine specific gravity is 1.012, pH 6.5. Urine has few bacteria. Serum sodium is 140 mmol/liter, potassium 4.2, chloride 106, urea nitrogen 5.4, and glucose 4.3.

ECG shows right ventricular hypertrophy. Angiocardiogram shows ventricular septal defect with right-to-left shunt and pulmonary infundibular and valvar stenosis.

At operation, pulmonary infundibulum is resected, valvotomy performed at bicuspid pulmonary valve, septal defect closed with patch, and patch placed along pulmonary infundibulum and valve.

Five days after operation, a flat band of dullness to percussion is in the back just above right side of diaphragm. He is sitting up and bright eyed, smiling, and eating well with heart rate 125, respiratory rate 48.

Preoperative roentgenographic findings are normal. On the third day after operation, a strip of water density is present in lateral part of right side of chest when boy is in a supine position (Figure 7-1A). On the fifth day after operation, right side of diaphragm is obscured by hump of water density when the boy is sitting up (Figure 7-1B).

Chest roentgenographic findings are normal 7 weeks after operation. He is well at 17 years. Weight is 52 kg, height 168 cm.

Diagnosis: Fallot's tetrad, total correction; postoperative chylothorax.

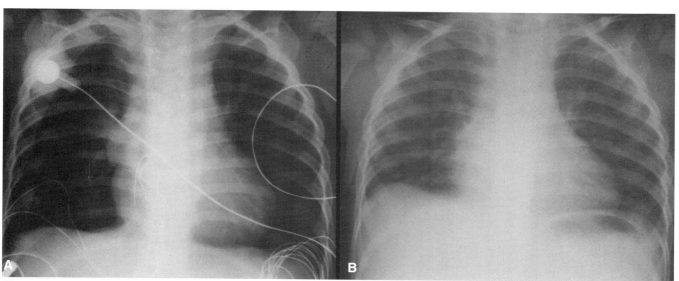

Fig. 7-1

Case 8

A 1½-year-old girl has been fussy and febrile for 2 weeks. She is being given an antibiotic for otitis media.

Temperature is 38.9°C, heart rate 154, respiratory rate 46, systolic blood pressure 90 mm Hg, and weight 10.5 kg. Right ear drum is dull and injected. Breath sounds in right side of chest are diminished. The rest of the physical findings are normal.

Hematocrit is 0.31. White cell count is 21.1 × 10⁹/liter with 0.70 polymorphonuclear cells, 0.03 bands, 0.22 lymphocytes, 0.04 monocytes, and 0.01 basophils. Platelet count is 572 × 10⁹/liter. Urine specific gravity is 1.025, pH 6. Urine has trace protein, 0.80 g/liter ketones, mucus, occasional squamous epithelial cells/HPF, and 2–4 white cells/HPF. Serum sodium is 136 mmol/liter, potassium 3.9, chloride 100, carbon dioxide 25, urea nitrogen 1.8, calcium 2.15, phosphorus 1.32,

cholesterol 3.50, and glucose 5.4. Creatinine is 30 μmol/liter, uric acid 120, total bilirubin 5, and direct bilirubin 2. Total protein is 61 g/liter, albumin 29. Alkaline phosphatase is 190 U/liter, LDH 288, and SGOT 16.

A shadow of water density is in right side of chest (Figure 8-1).

No liquid is obtained at right thoracentesis. Blood culture grows *Haemophilus influenzae* type B, β-lactamase negative.

She is comfortable and afebrile in the hospital. Chest roentgenographic findings 7 months later are normal except for slight right pleural thickening.

Diagnosis: Right pleural exudate, questionable *H. influenzae* type B infection.

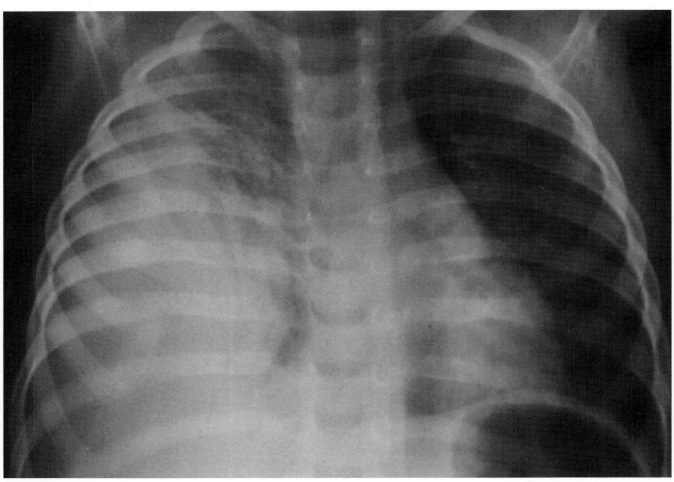

Fig. 8-1

Case 9

A 10-year-old boy, who fainted at school, comes home, vomits, and says head, chest, and belly hurt. He is breathing fast 2 days later. Three days later, he is coughing and has bilateral flank pain, bloody urine, and temperature of 39.5°C.

Birth weight was 2.8 kg. He walked at 1 year. He had measles and chickenpox at 5 and mumps at 9 years. He had pinkeye 10 months ago, abdominal pain and cloudy urine 6 months ago and again 5 months ago, when normal appendix was removed.

Parents and sister (8 years old) are well. Both grandfathers died with heart disease and high blood pressure. Maternal aunt has heart and kidney disease.

Temperature at 10 years is 37.3°C, heart rate 70, respiratory rate 35, blood pressure 120/80 mm Hg, weight 28.9 kg, and height 137 cm. He is thin and pale. Dullness and diminished breath sounds are in left side of chest. A systolic heart murmur is present. A surgical scar is on abdomen. Liver edge is 1 cm below costal margin. The rest of the physical findings are normal.

Hematocrit is 0.34. White cell count is 30.2×10^9/liter with 0.61 polymorphonuclear cells, 0.24 bands, 0.14 lymphocytes, and 0.01 eosinophils. Platelet estimate is increased. ESR is 106 mm/hr. Serum is negative for C-reactive protein. Urine specific gravity is 1.015, pH 5.5. Urine has clumps of white cells, 8–10 red cells/HPF, 0–1 epithelial cell/HPF, 2+ albumin, occasional granular casts/LPF, 1+ uric acid crystals, amorphous urates, and bacteria. Twenty four–hour urine volume is 630 ml with 3 mmol/liter sodium, 40 potassium, and 0.2 glucose. Serum sodium is 128 mmol/liter, potassium 4.3, chloride 91, carbon dioxide 28, urea nitrogen 18.6 (10 days later: 5.7), and glucose 8.5. Creatinine is 50 μmol/liter.

Much of left side of chest is opaque in first examination (Figure 9-1A). Two and a half months later, when he feels well, a small amount of pleural liquid or thickened pleura is on left side (Figure 9-1B).

Small amounts of blood-tinged liquid are obtained at three thoracenteses on left side after first roentgenogram. Cultures of chest aspirates, gastric aspirates, blood, and urine show no growth. Skin test for tuberculosis is negative. During the next year, serum C3 ranges from 0.1 to 0.2 g/liter (normal: 0.7–1.6) in three determinations.

When he returns for roentgenogram of chest (which shows slight left pleural thickening) at 12½ years, physical findings are normal, weight 38 kg, and blood pressure 110/80 mm Hg. Roentgenograms of knees in Figure 9-2 show postarrest growth lines in femurs. Growth lines are easier to see and closer to growth plates in tibias.

Renal biopsy at 12½ and 14 years shows that almost all glomeruli have large cellular tufts; prominent mesangium with increase in cells; split, irregularly nodular basement membrane; occasional eosinophilic material in Bowman's capsule and in second specimen PAS-positive extracellular deposits; and chronic inflammatory cells in interstitium.

Electron microscopy of second specimen shows increased laminar electron density in much of glomerular basement membrane, mesangial interposition between endothelium and epithelium, mesangial cell proliferation, increase in mesangial matrix, and focal fusion of foot processes.

He needs hemodialysis for kidney failure at 25 years and dies at 27 years.

Diagnosis: Sterile pleural effusion in boy who has membranoproliferative glomerulonephritis.

(Continued)

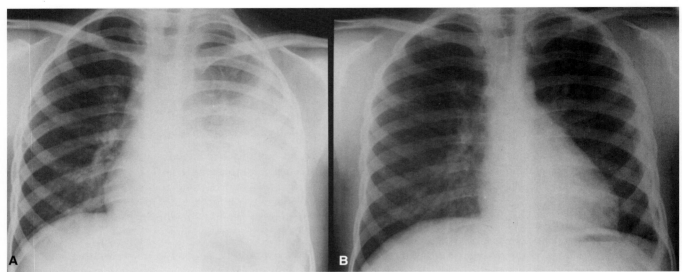

Fig. 9-1

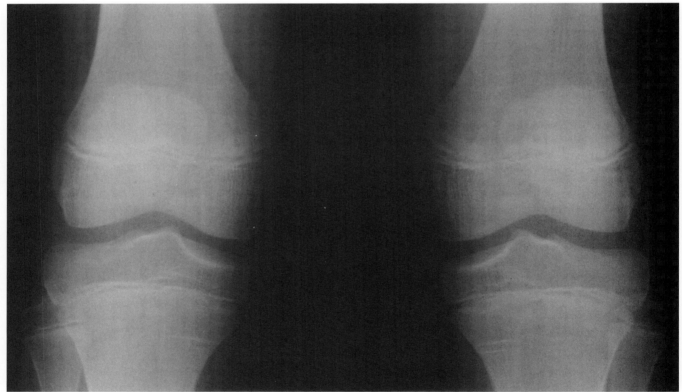

Fig. 9-2

Lungs

Case 1

A 2-month-old girl is blue and breathing fast.

Birth weight was 3.7 kg. At 10 days, hands and feet were blue, and lips were blue when she cried. She has been grunting, blue, and breathing fast for 4 days.

Weight is 4.3 kg, temperature 37°C, heart rate 186, respiratory rate 64, and blood pressure 100/50 mm Hg. Lips and nailbeds are blue. A systolic heart murmur is present. Liver edge is 2 cm below costal margin. The rest of the physical findings are normal.

Hematocrit is 0.63. White cell count is 10.7×10^9/liter with 0.48 polymorphonuclear cells, 0.02 bands, 0.46 lymphocytes, and 0.04 monocytes. Platelet count is 61×10^9/liter. Capillary blood pH is 7.21. PCO_2 is 35 mm Hg, PO_2 18.

Echocardiogram shows tricuspid atresia, hypoplastic right ventricle, atrial septal defect, ventricular septal defect, and pulmonic stenosis.

At left thoracotomy, a Gore-Tex (Artex Sportswear, Scarborough, Ontario) graft is placed between left subclavian artery and left pulmonary artery.

Shadows of water density in upper lobes 5 hours after operation (Figure 1-1A) are partly gone 38 hours after operation (Figure 1-1B). A thin, curved strip of water density with bulge at bottom is now in upper part of right lung (see Figure 1-1B).

Diagnosis: Postoperative atelectasis, azygous lobe and apicoposterior segment of left upper lobe.

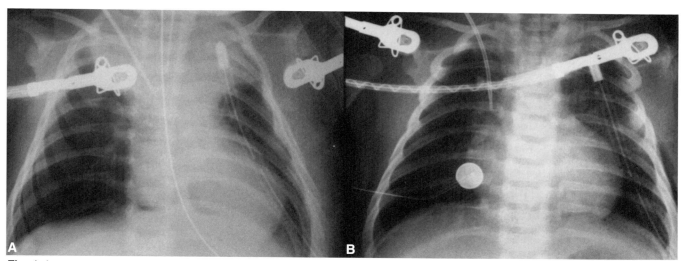

Fig. 1-1

Case 2

A 12-year-old girl with Down syndrome has had a cough and fever for 2 days.

Pregnancy of mother was normal until premature spontaneous rupture of membranes. Birth weight was 1.2 kg. She sat at 8 months, walked at 14 months. She had many respiratory infections until tonsils and adenoids were removed at 3 years.

Temperature at 12 years is 39.2°C, heart rate 90, respiratory rate 30, blood pressure 85/60 mm Hg, and weight 59 kg. She has epicanthi, speckled irises, clinodactyly of little fingers, flat feet, gap between first and second toes, blue nailbeds, percussion dullness at lung bases, and coarse breath sounds. The rest of the physical findings are normal.

Hematocrit is 0.41. White cell count is 9.3×10^9/liter with 0.22 polymorphonuclear cells, 0.62 bands, 0.13 lymphocytes, and 0.03 monocytes. Urine specific gravity is 1.019, pH 5. Urine has 2+ protein, 2+ hemoglobin/myoglobin, 7–10 squamous epithelial cells/HPF, 5–7 white cells/HPF, and 2+ amorphous matter. Serum sodium is 142 mmol/liter, potassium 3.9, chloride 107, carbon dioxide 24, urea nitrogen 8.0, and glucose 9.6.

In Figure 2-1, lungs are expanded with normal markings; a thin, curved strip of water density is in base of right lung; and size of heart is normal.

Diagnosis: Accessory fissure between medial basal and anterior basal segments of right lower lobe.

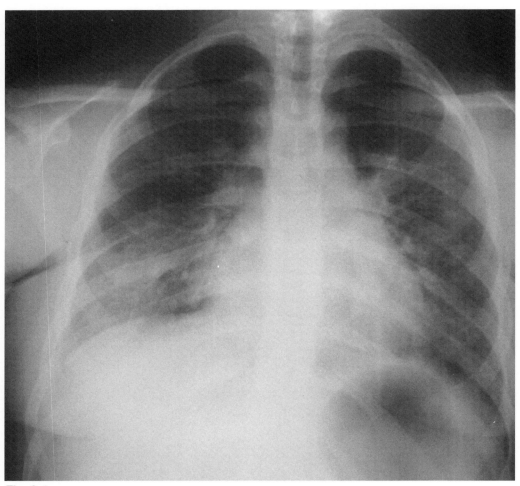

Fig. 2-1

Case 3

A 4-year-old girl, who choked on a chicken bone 30 minutes ago, is coughing and red in the face.

She was dusky at birth. She runs less and breathes harder than her playmates and tires when she walks a block or two. She wheezes with colds and exercise.

Parents and one sibling are well.

Temperature is 36.8°C, weight 19 kg. Physical findings are normal.

In Figure 3-1, heart is displaced to right; a longitudinal, slightly oblique strip of water density in lower right side of chest is joined at lung base by a smaller strip; an oblique line of water density is in lower part of left side of chest; left lung is herniated across midline above heart; and an extra bronchus in right side of chest below left main bronchus curves to left at level of T6.

Diagnosis: Hypoplasia of right lung, scimitar syndrome, horseshoe lung (pleural line in lower part of left side of chest and extra left bronchus at level of T6).

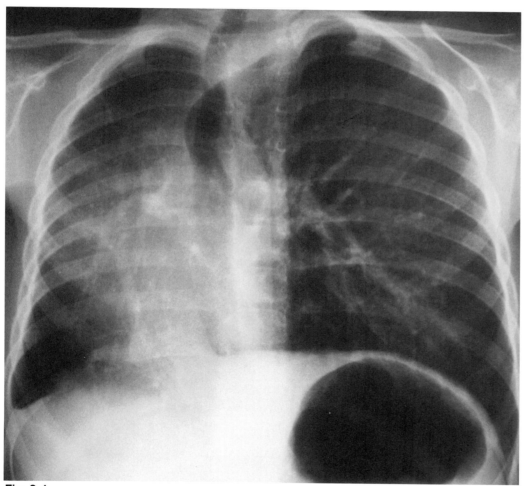

Fig. 3-1

Case 4

A 14-month-old girl has frequent respiratory and ear infections. Breathing is always noisy. Pneumonia was diagnosed 2 months ago.

Mother (29 years old), father (37 years old), and two siblings are well. Maternal grandmother has asthma.

Weight is 10.6 kg, temperature 36.7°C, heart rate 148, respiratory rate 44, and blood pressure 80/50 mm Hg. Noisy breath sounds and expiratory wheeze are present. Apical impulse of heart is at sternum. The rest of the physical findings are normal.

Hematocrit is 0.38. White cell count is 13.9×10^9/liter with 0.35 polymorphonuclear cells, 0.03 bands, 0.56 lymphocytes, and 0.06 monocytes. Platelet count is 464×10^9/liter.

In Figure 4-1, heart is displaced to right, and right first and second ribs are fused. Two bronchi, a smaller upper bronchus and a larger lower one, go to left lung (Figure 4-1A), and a thin, curved shadow of water density is on right side at level of T5–T7 (Figure 4-1B). Barium powder bronchography shows accessory bronchi and lobes (Figure 4-2).

Diagnosis: Accessory pulmonary lobes.

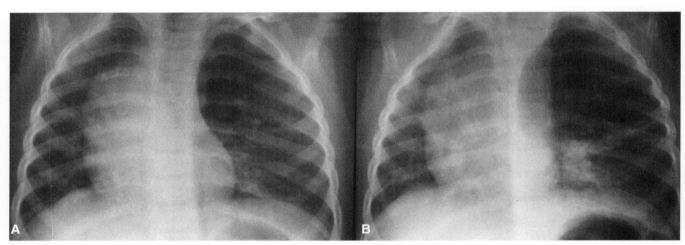

Fig. 4-1

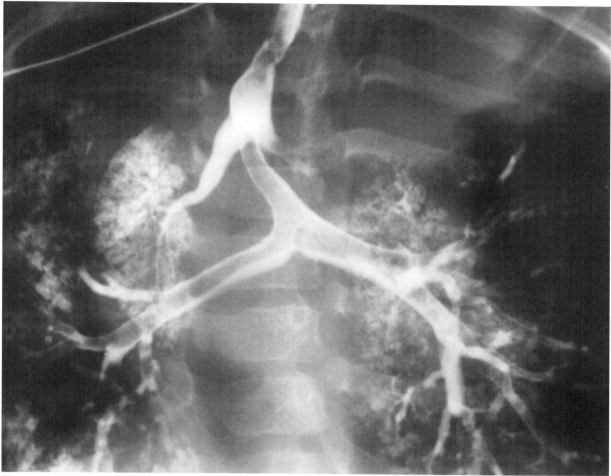

Fig. 4-2

Case 5

An 8-month-old girl wheezes when awake but not when asleep. The expiratory wheeze is louder when she is excited.

Birth weight was 1.9 kg, Apgar score 3/9 at 1 and 10 minutes.

Mother (33 years old) is well. The girl is her only child.

Weight is 8.5 kg, temperature 37.2°C, heart rate 134, respiratory rate 44, and blood pressure 117/86 mm Hg. Physical findings are normal.

Left lung is emphysematous in Figure 5-1. At fluoroscopy, heart moves to left during inspiration and to right during expiration.

At bronchoscopy, left main bronchus dilates during inspiration and collapses during expiration. Trachea and right main bronchus are normal.

Diagnosis: Left bronchomalacia (Williams-Campbell syndrome).

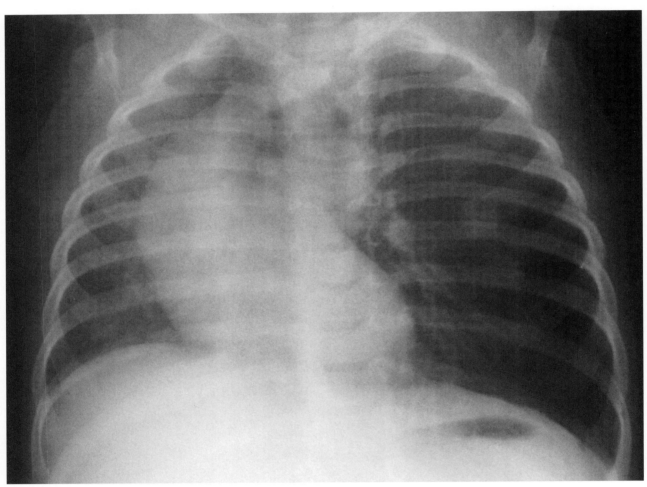

Fig. 5-1

Case 6

A 7-week-old boy who has Down syndrome has had a cough and runny nose for 2 days, and fever and vomiting today.

Pregnancy of mother was normal, birth weight 3.4 kg, and Apgar score 5/9 at 1 and 5 minutes.

Mother (26 years old), father (33 years old), and sister (4 years old) are well.

Temperature is 36.7°C, heart rate 150, respiratory rate 40, and systolic blood pressure 120 mm Hg. He is dusky, grunting, and retracting when FIO_2 = 0.35. Breath sounds are diminished on left, heart sounds are louder on right. Liver edge is 1 cm below costal margin. The rest of the physical findings are normal.

ECG findings are normal.

Hematocrit is 0.40. White cell count is 18.0×10^9/liter with 0.77 polymorphonuclear cells, 0.22 lymphocytes. Platelet count is 629×10^9/liter.

In Figure 6-1A, lungs, especially left lung, are emphysematous; left upper lobe is herniated across midline; and heart is displaced to right. In Figure 6-1B, sternum protrudes and diaphragm is depressed.

Left lung is removed.

Left upper lobe is emphysematous and has a large cyst in apex. A basal segment of left lower lobe is emphysematous. Microscopic examination of left lung shows distended interstitial spaces lined by hyalinized, fibrotic tissue; giant cells; and compressed and expanded alveoli.

Diagnosis: Interstitial infantile lobar emphysema.

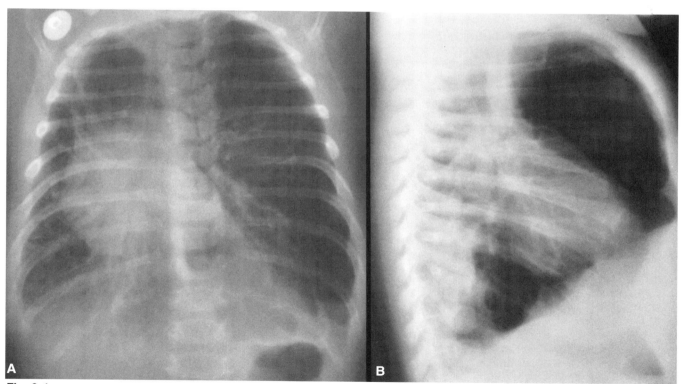

Fig. 6-1

Case 7

A 4-month-old boy breathes fast when feeding and sleeps a lot.

Pregnancy of mother was normal, birth weight 4.5 kg. He is breast-fed.

Parents and sister (21 months old) are well.

Weight is 6.8 kg, length 64 cm, head circumference 43 cm, temperature 37°C, heart rate 128, respiratory rate 64, and systolic blood pressure 82 mm Hg. Breath sounds are absent in right side of chest. The rest of the physical findings are normal.

Hematocrit is 0.37. White cell count is 11.4×10^9/liter with 0.47 polymorphonuclear cells, 0.44 lymphocytes, 0.05 monocytes, 0.03 eosinophils, and 0.01 basophils. Platelet count is 677×10^9/liter. Urine specific gravity is 1.003, pH 7. Urine has occasional epithelial cells/HPF and 0–1 white cell/HPF.

In Figure 7-1, a large shadow of air density distends right side of chest, and markings in left lung are normal.

At operation, right lung is compressed and pushed up by an adherent purple sac. Sac and stalklike connection to right lower lobe bronchus are removed.

Examination of sac shows slightly wrinkled outer surface and inner surface crisscrossed with fibrous bands.

Diagnosis: Bronchogenic cyst. (Right lung looks normal in postoperative roentgenographic examination.)

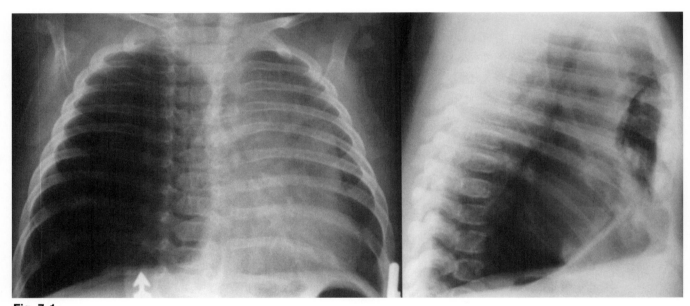

Fig. 7-1

Case 8

A newborn girl is grunting and retracting.

Pregnancy of mother (19 years old) was normal. Ultrasound examination at 27 weeks showed fetal lung cysts. Labor was induced.

Apgar score is 7/8 at 1 and 5 minutes, temperature 36.5°C, heart rate 185, respiratory rate 48, and blood pressure 65/44 mm Hg. Breath sounds are normal in right side of chest, absent in left. The rest of the physical findings are normal.

Hematocrit is 0.49. Arterial blood pH is 7.27. P_{CO_2} is 40 mm Hg, P_{O_2} 176. Bicarbonate is 18 mmol/liter.

Prenatal ultrasound examination in Figure 8-1 shows lung cysts. Roentgenogram the day of birth, after intubation and oxygen, shows air in lower left lung, less air in rest of lungs, displacement of heart to right, and gas in normally placed gut

below diaphragm (Figure 8-2A). Roentgenogram 1 day after operation and hours before death shows peritoneal air around falciform ligament and catheterized umbilical vein (which—in a healthy infant—would later become round ligament, the ligamentum teres of the liver) (Figure 8-2B).

At operation, cysts are in left upper lobe. Left lower lobe is compressed and airless.

Pleura of resected left upper lobe is smooth and glistening. Creamy, white matter is in bronchi. Many cysts (0.3–0.6 cm) that contain yellow-white mucus or clear liquid are in lung and separated by compact, airless tissue.

Diagnosis: Congenital cystic adenomatoid malformation.

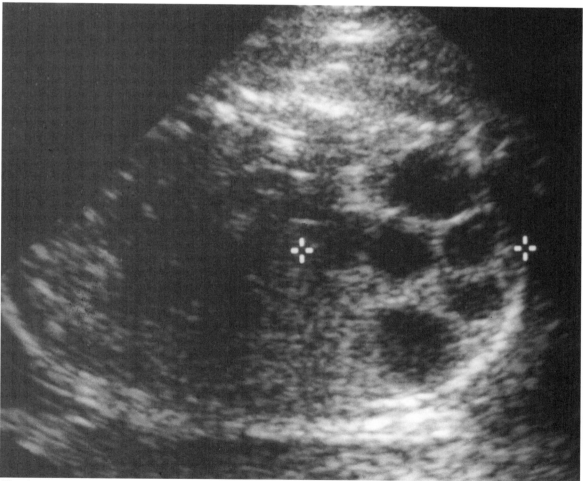

Fig. 8-1

(Continued)

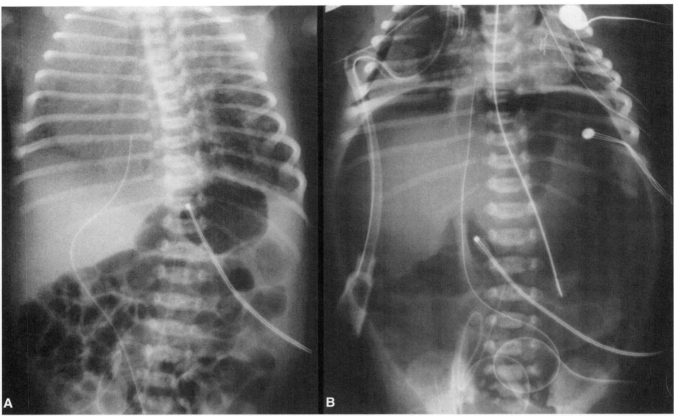

Fig. 8-2

Case 9

An 8-year-old girl examined for hyperactivity has a heart murmur.

Birth weight was 3 kg. She had a bladder infection at 2 years.

Temperature is 37.2°C, heart rate 100, respiratory rate 20, blood pressure 110/70 mm Hg, weight 22.5 kg, and height 118 cm. A holosystolic murmur is present. The rest of the physical findings are normal.

Hematocrit is 0.44. White cell count is 4.2×10^9/liter with 0.58 polymorphonuclear cells, 0.35 lymphocytes, 0.01 monocytes, 0.05 eosinophils, and 0.01 basophils.

ECG shows right ventricular hypertrophy and right axis deviation.

A curved shadow of water density, thicker in lower part, is in right side of chest (Figure 9-1A). A shadow of water density is behind heart just above diaphragm in lateral view (Figure 9-1B).

At catheterization, oxygen saturation is 0.96 in left atrium, 0.65 in superior vena cava, 0.87 in right pulmonary artery, 0.87 in right ventricle, 0.90 in right atrium, 0.73 in inferior vena cava 2 cm below diaphragm, and 0.86 in inferior vena cava at diaphragm.

At operation, a small secundum atrial septal defect is closed. Pulmonary veins from right upper lobe and two small veins from right lower lobe enter left atrium. A vein (1.5-cm diameter) from right lower lobe goes through diaphragm.

Diagnosis: Atrial septal defect, scimitar syndrome.

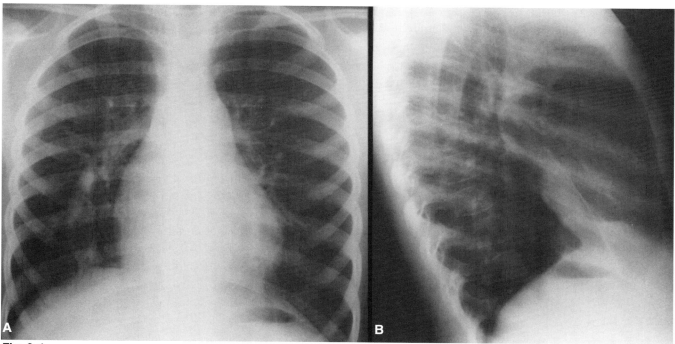

Fig. 9-1

Case 10

A 2-day-old girl is breathing fast.

Pregnancy of mother was normal, birth weight 2.9 kg, length 52 cm, head circumference 34 cm, Apgar score 8/9 at 1 and 5 minutes, heart rate 138, and respiratory rate 46. At 21 hours, she was stuffy and wheezy. Respiratory rate was 60. Hematocrit was 0.43. White cell count was 9.0×10^9/liter with 0.49 polymorphonuclear cells, 0.09 bands, 0.37 lymphocytes, and 0.05 eosinophils.

Mother (28 years old) and father (31 years old) are well. Maternal great-grandmother and maternal grandmother have asthma.

Temperature at 2 days is 36.4°C, heart rate 150, respiratory rate 70 (soon down to 50), and systolic blood pressure 64 mm Hg. Point of maximal impulse of heart is in right side of chest, liver edge at left costal margin. The rest of the physical findings are normal.

Hematocrit is 0.46. Urine specific gravity is 1.005. Serum sodium is 140 mmol/liter, potassium 2.7, chloride 103, calcium 2.42, and glucose 4.2.

Situs inversus is present in Figure 10-1. An ill-defined shadow of water density in left lung obscures lower part of contiguous edge of heart at 2 days (see Figure 10-1). Roentgenographic findings in chest are similar at 1½ years (Figure 10-2). Paranasal sinuses are varyingly opaque at 1½ years, temporal air cells undeveloped (Figure 10-3).

At 3 months, she has a runny nose and middle ear fluid. Bilateral myringotomy and tube placement are both performed at 16 and 30 months. At 30 months, ear drums are thick and dull. Thick mucus is in middle ears. Nasal mucosa is "mildly hypertrophied," according to ear, nose, and throat specialist. Mucosa from an inferior turbinate does not contain ciliated epithelium at biopsy. At 8 years, she coughs frequently. Nose is runny. Eardrums are scarred. Weight is 25 kg, height 128 cm. Forced vital capacity is 0.81 predicted in pulmonary function tests, FEV 0.85, and maximal midexpiratory flow rate 0.94. At 10 years, she has runny nose, right ear discharge, rales, and end-expiratory wheezes. Her brother, 4 years younger, has situs inversus, runny nose, and persistent middle ear fluid.

Diagnosis: Kartagener's syndrome.

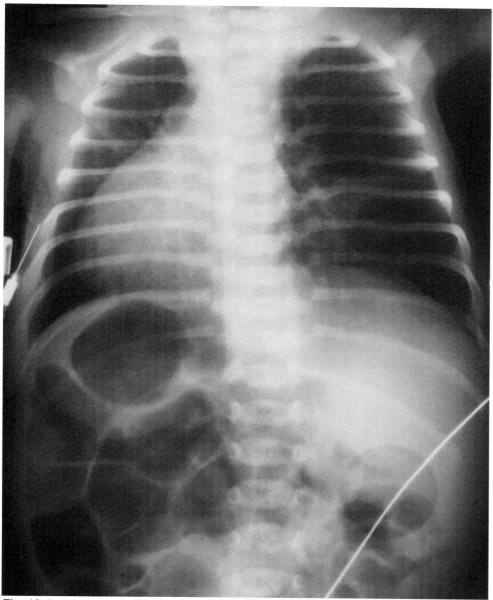

Fig. 10-1

(Continued)

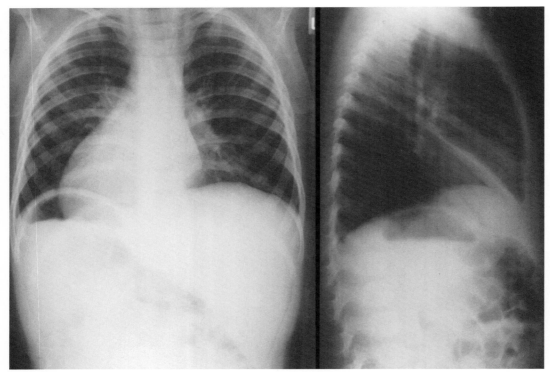

Fig. 10-2

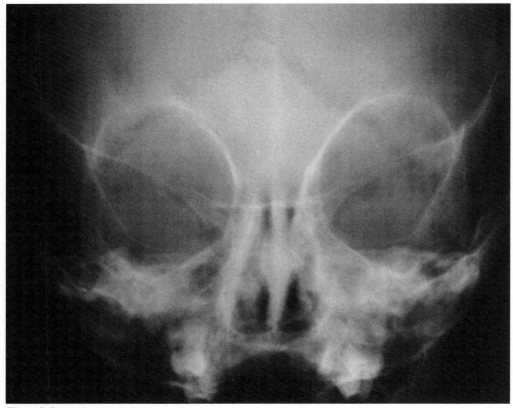

Fig. 10-3

Case 11

A newborn girl is delivered by cesarean section when scalp electrode shows pH decline from 7.42 to 7.26 during slow labor.

Mother (23 years old) had splenectomy at 9 years for hereditary spherocytic anemia. Mother's mother, grandmother, and great-grandmother had spherocytic anemia; mother's mother also had splenectomy and cholecystectomy.

Pregnancy was normal. Birth weight is 3.5 kg, Apgar score 3/6 at 1 and 5 minutes. Temperature at 30 minutes is 36.5°C, heart rate 155, respiratory rate 70, and blood pressure 57/33 mm Hg. A small bruise and slight meconium stain are on head. Rhonchi are in lungs. The rest of the physical findings are normal.

Umbilical arterial blood pH is 7.22 at 12 minutes when hood FIO_2 = 0.80. PCO_2 is 57 mm Hg, PO_2 22. At 20 minutes, hematocrit is 0.42. White cell count is 33.0×10^9/liter with 0.47 polymorphonuclear cells, 0.11 bands, 0.30 lymphocytes, 0.08 monocytes, 0.02 metamyelocytes, and 0.02 myelocytes. Platelet count is 327×10^9/liter. At 2½ hours, pH is 7.35. PCO_2 is 40 mm Hg, PO_2 65.

At 9 hours, she is pink and breathing easily. Chest vibration and patting result in appearance of small amounts of cloudy white secretions in mouth.

Liquid is in much of right lung at 3 hours (Figure 11-1A). Liquid is decreased at 26½ hours. Roentgenographic findings in chest are normal at 48 hours (Figure 11-1B).

Weight at 2 years is 12.5 kg, height 87 cm. Physical findings are normal. Hematocrit is 0.30. Red-blood-cell distribution width is 20.5% (normal: 11.5–15.0). Smear shows moderate spherocytosis.

Impression: Normal newborn lungs with gradual complete aeration, hereditary spherocytosis.

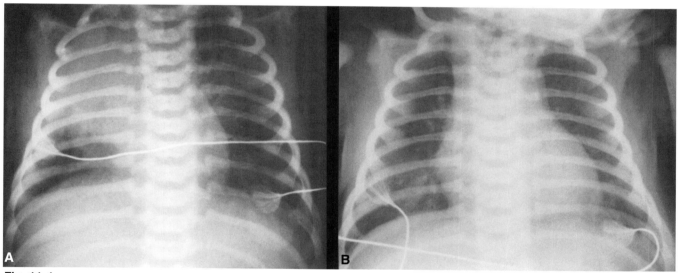

Fig. 11-1

Case 12

A newborn girl is breathing fast and has acrocyanosis. Labor was induced with oxytocin (Pitocin) 2 weeks after expected date of birth.

Amniotic fluid and baby are meconium stained. Apgar score is 7/9 at 1 and 5 minutes, weight 3.7 kg, length 51 cm, head circumference 33 cm, temperature 35.8°C, heart rate 170, and respiratory rate 80. She retracts slightly. The rest of the physical findings are normal. At 16 hours, color is good, respiratory rate 50.

Hematocrit is 0.73 at 5 hours, 0.60 at 7 hours.

Ill-defined shadows of water density are in lungs at 4½ hours (Figure 12-1A) and absent the next day (Figure 12-1B).

Diagnosis: Normal baby, transient tachypnea of newborn.

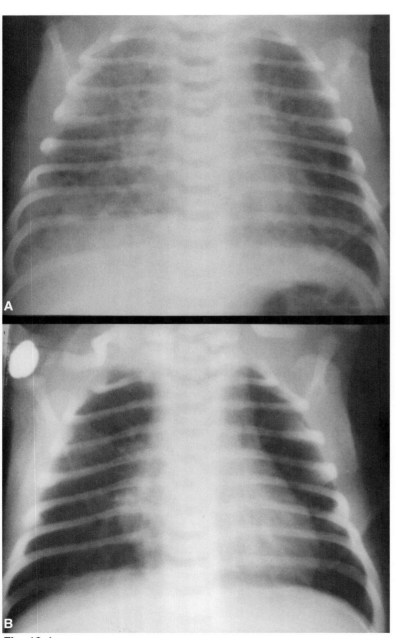

Fig. 12-1

Case 13

A newborn boy is blue, tachypneic, and meconium stained.

Mother (31 years old) and father are well.

Pregnancy was normal, delivery by cesarean section after 22-hour labor. Apgar score is 4/4 at 1 and 5 minutes, birth weight 4.2 kg, length 54 cm, and head circumference 36 cm. At 3 hours, temperature is 37.6°C, heart rate 150, respiratory rate 160, and systolic blood pressure 58 mm Hg. Skin is dry, wrinkled, and dusky. Respirations are shallow. Rales are in lungs. The rest of the physical findings are normal.

At 31 hours, umbilical venous blood pH when hood FIO_2 = 0.40 is 7.32. PCO_2 is 40 mm Hg, PO_2 54. Serum sodium is 140 mmol/liter, potassium 3.1, chloride 105, carbon dioxide 20,

urea nitrogen 1.4, calcium 1.85, and glucose 6.3. Total bilirubin is 50 μmol/liter.

Roentgenogram at 29 hours shows coarse, stringy markings in lungs (Figure 13-1). Roentgenogram at 8 days shows normal markings.

At 2 days, he is agitated, gasping, and sweating. Venous blood pH is 7.16 when hood FIO_2 = 0.60. PCO_2 is 63 mm Hg, PO_2 30. He is intubated for 5 days. He is alert at 9 days. Physical findings are normal at 11 days.

Diagnosis: Meconium aspiration.

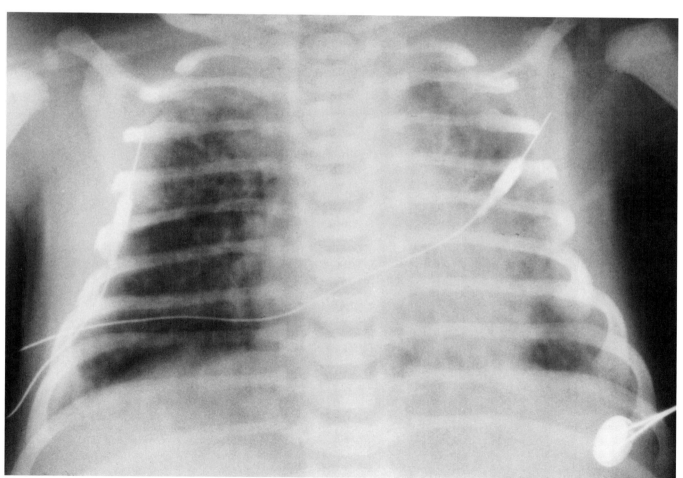

Fig. 13-1

Case 14

A newborn boy, delivered by cesarean section because of placenta previa, 40% abruption, and slowed heart rate in utero, is flaccid and cries weakly. He is given oxygen by bag and then by tube.

Birth weight is 1.7 kg, Apgar score 4/7 at 1 and 5 minutes, length 40 cm, and head circumference 29 cm. At 1 hour, heart rate is 145, respiratory rate 80, and blood pressure 54/35 mm Hg. Crackles are in lungs. The rest of the physical findings are normal.

Hematocrit is 0.52. Blood sugar is 5.0 mmol/liter. Umbilical arterial blood pH is 7.12 when $FIO_2 = 1.00$. PCO_2 is 63 mm Hg, PO_2 53.

He is on ventilator at 10 days. Oral feeding is begun at 11 days. At 35 days, respiratory rate is 60. Crackles are in right lung.

Roentgenogram at 2 hours shows almost airless lungs (Figure 14-1A). At 35 days, more air is in left lung than in right lung (Figure 14-1B).

At 4 months, he begins to vomit. Pyloromyotomy is performed for pyloric stenosis, and right inguinal hernia is repaired. At 9 months, left inguinal hernia is repaired.

Bronchoscopy at 3 and 9 months shows minimal collapse of left lower lobe bronchus. Bronchography at 3 years shows normal findings.

At 5 years, he is well. Weight is 15.2 kg, height 107 cm. Left side of chest is larger than right and has diminished breath sounds.

Left lung is overaerated at 5 years (Figure 14-2).

Ophthalmologic findings are normal at 7 years.

Diagnosis: Prematurity, respirator lungs.

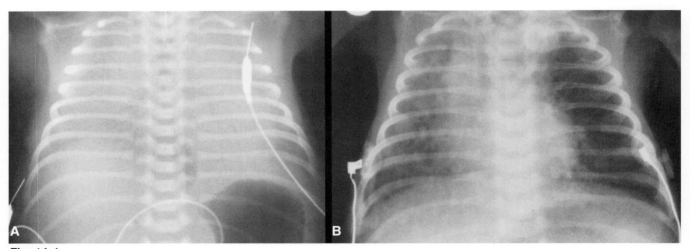

Fig. 14-1

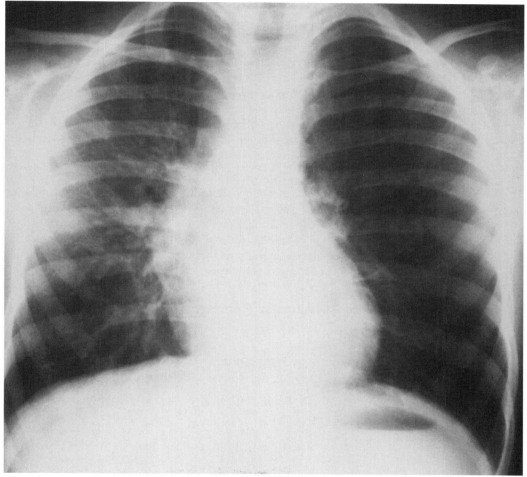

Fig. 14-2

Case 15

At 1 hour, a newborn girl is acrocyanotic and grunts when she breathes.

Mother is 19 years old. Birth weight is 1.4 kg, length 43 cm, head circumference 28 cm, and Apgar score 8 at 1 minute. At 1 hour, umbilical venous blood pH is 7.28. P_{CO_2} is 48 mm Hg, P_{O_2} 45. At 7 hours, temperature is 37.2°C, heart rate 160, respiratory rate 60 while she breathes 0.50 oxygen by hood, and systolic blood pressure 36 mm Hg. She is red, retracting, and grunting. Lanugo hair is on scalp and torso. Auricles are soft. A hematoma is on right side of head. Breast areolae are flat. Limbs slightly resist passive movement. The rest of the physical findings are normal.

Serum sodium is 136 mmol/liter, potassium 4.2, chloride 100, carbon dioxide 30, and calcium 1.82. Total bilirubin is 68 µmol/liter.

At 10 hours, she is dusky. Respiratory rate is 70. She is intubated and ventilated with 0.80 oxygen at positive end-expiratory pressure 5 cm water (next day: 0.60 and 12 cm). She is jaundiced at 33 hours. At 36 hours, she is mottled and blue when heart rate is 80–100. At 37 hours, a tube is put into right side of chest for pneumothorax; then into left side at 38 hours for same reason. At 48 hours, she is edematous. She dies at 104 hours.

Lungs lack air at 8 hours (Figure 15-1A). In Figure 15-1B, at 100 hours, (1) heart is small; (2) air is under tension in left pleural space and between parietal pleura and left side of diaphragm; (3) medial base of left lung is retained in mediastinum by pulmonary ligament; (4) nodules and strips of water density are in distended lungs; and (5) endotracheal tube, chest tubes, and skin needles are in place.

Necropsy shows 0.1 cm subcutaneous fat, a small amount of blood under temporal lobes, autolysis of brain, ductus arteriosus, probe patent foramen ovale, and lungs that sink in water. Microscopic examination shows hematopoiesis in liver, congestion of kidneys, ulceration of trachea, and thick alveolar walls in lungs, diffuse emphysema, focal atelectasis, mild edema, and, according to pathologist, "minimal hyaline membranes."

Diagnosis: Prematurity, respiratory distress.

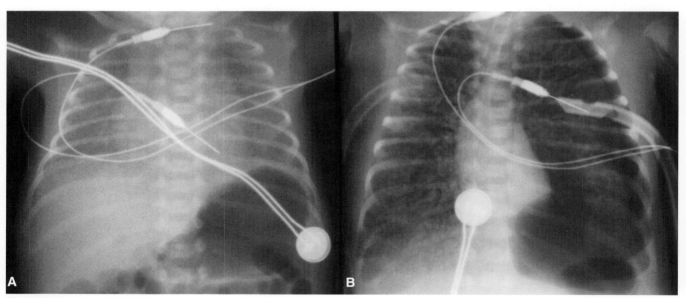

Fig. 15-1

Case 16

A newborn girl, pink at birth and soon crying loudly, has acrocyanosis at 20 minutes.

Pregnancy of mother (23 years old) was normal. Apgar score is 8/10 at 1 and 5 minutes, birth weight 3 kg, length 48 cm, and temperature 36.3°C. At 20 minutes, respiratory rate is 64 with grunting and alar flare. At 2 hours, heart rate is 150, respiratory rate 75, systolic blood pressure 65 mm Hg, and liver edge 3 cm below costal margin. Hands and feet are blue. Muscles are hypotonic. The rest of the physical findings are normal.

At 5 hours, ill-defined shadows of water density are almost confluent in lungs (Figure 16-1).

At 7 hours, capillary blood pH is 7.20 when F_{IO_2} = 0.80 by mask. P_{CO_2} is 62 mm Hg, P_{O_2} 26. Glucose is 3.1 mmol/liter.

She dies at 18 hours.

At necropsy, ductus arteriosus is large. Lungs vary from light pink to dark red to almost black along lobular septa. Microscopic examination shows widespread hemorrhage, red blood cells in bronchi, and a few spotty open alveoli surrounded by engorged capillaries.

Diagnosis: Atelectasis; interlobular and intra-alveolar hemorrhage.

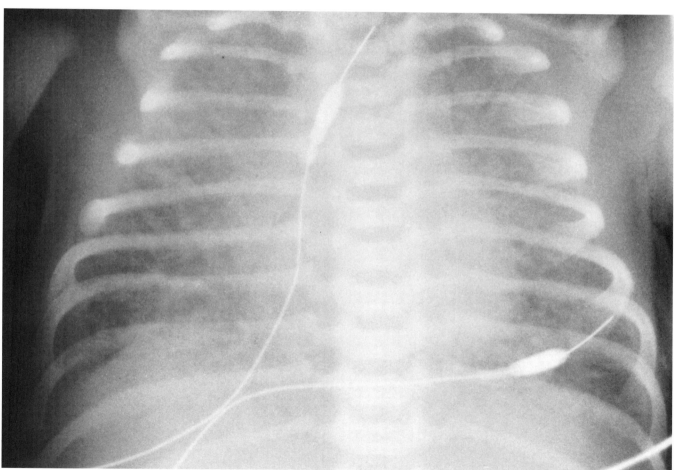

Fig. 16-1

Case 17

A newborn girl is apneic at 2½ hours.

Membranes ruptured spontaneously 14 hours before birth. Birth weight is 2.7 kg, Apgar score 9/9 at 1 and 5 minutes, length 50 cm, and head circumference 33 cm. She breastfeeds at 2 hours, then is soon blue, apneic, intubated, and mechanically ventilated with supplemental oxygen. White cell count is 1.6×10^9/liter. Umbilical arterial blood pH is 7.29. P_{CO_2} is 33 mm Hg, P_{O_2} 384.

Temperature at 12 hours is 36.5°C, heart rate 200, systolic blood pressure 40 mm Hg, and respiratory rate on ventilator 30. Rales are in lungs. Liver edge is 3 cm below costal margin. Limbs are blue. The rest of the physical findings are normal.

Hematocrit is 0.28. White cell count is 6.9×10^9/liter with 0.15 polymorphonuclear cells, 0.09 bands, 0.70 lymphocytes, 0.01 eosinophils, 0.03 metamyelocytes, and 0.02 myelocytes. Platelet count is 105×10^9/liter. Serum sodium is 195 mmol/liter, potassium 6.4, chloride 120, and calcium 3.27.

In Figure 17-1 at 12 hours, excess liquid is in lungs, in pleural spaces, and in and around gut; heart is small; umbilical arterial catheter ends at approximately level of L4; and umbilical venous catheter loops at ductus venosus, its loop in right branch of portal vein, its end in left lobe of liver.

She dies at 16 hours.

Necropsy shows polymorphonuclear cells, macrophages, and gram-positive cocci in lungs; hemorrhage in enlarged adrenals, in renal medullas, and in gastrointestinal mucosa.

Impression: Group B β-hemolytic streptococcal (*Streptococcus agalactiae*) infection. (Cultures were obtained, but results were not entered in chart so specific bacterial diagnosis is not made.)

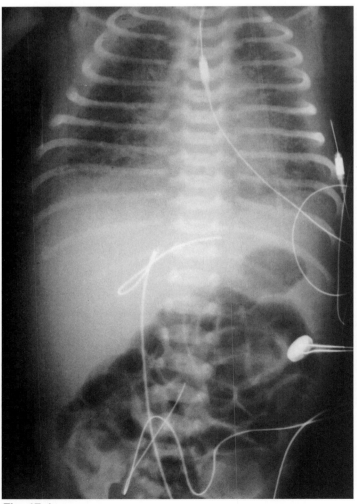

Fig. 17-1

Case 18

A newborn girl is breathing fast and retracting.

Mother (19 years old) was treated for chlamydial infection during pregnancy. Birth weight is 4.1 kg, length 50 cm, head circumference 36 cm, and Apgar score 4/8 at 1 and 5 minutes. At 13 hours, temperature is 36.7°C, heart rate 150, respiratory rate 80–100, and blood pressure 60/40 mm Hg. The rest of the physical findings are normal.

On the second day, she has pinpoint red spots on thorax and upper arms. Respiratory rate is 75–140, arterial blood oxygen saturation is 0.92 when F_{IO_2} = 0.40. Respiratory rate decreases to 50 during the next 2 weeks.

Hematocrit at 13 hours is 0.49. White cell count is 31.3 × 10^9/liter with 0.70 polymorphonuclear cells, 0.08 bands, 0.16 lymphocytes, and 0.06 monocytes. Platelet count is 242 × 10^9/liter. Urine specific gravity is 1.025, pH 5.5. Urine has nitrite, 2+ reducing substances, 0.30 g/liter protein, amorphous crystals, and moderate red cells/HPF. Capillary blood pH is 7.27. P_{CO_2} is 56 mm Hg, P_{O_2} 28. Serum IgM is 0.61 g/liter (normal: <0.25). Serum is negative for HBsAg, toxoplasmosis IgM antibody, rubella IgM antibody, HIV antibody, rapid plasma reagin, rheumatoid factor, and antinuclear antibody. Nasopharyngeal swab and conjunctival scraping are negative for *Chlamydia trachomatis* by direct fluorescent antibody test. No virus is isolated from nasopharynx, CSF, or urine. Mycoplasma pneumoniae and ureaplasma urealyticum are not isolated from tracheal aspirate. Nasopharyngeal aspirate is negative for respiratory syncytial virus antigen at 8 days but positive at 22 days. Sweat chloride is 20 mmol/liter.

Findings are questionably normal at 13 hours (Figure 18-1A). Lungs are distended and underaerated at 2 weeks (Figure 18-1B).

At 16 days, middle lobe biopsy shows slight interstitial pneumonia, predominantly lymphocytic, no fibrosis, and no acid-fast bacilli on fluorochrome stain.

At 5½ months, weight is 7.6 kg, length 68 cm. Physical and roentgenographic findings are normal except for scar on right side of chest and metal sutures in middle lobe.

Diagnosis: Lymphocytic interstitial pneumonia.

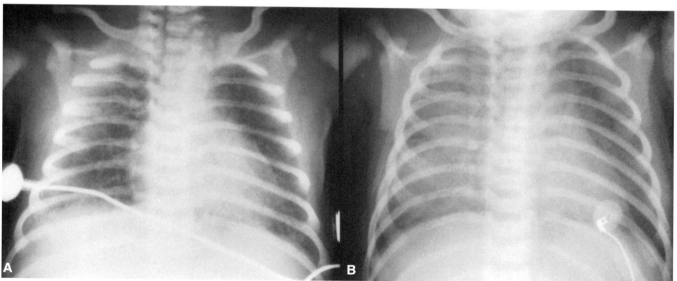

Fig. 18-1

Case 19

A 1-year-old girl has a cough, runny nose, and fever.

She had bronchitis at 4 and 10 months. Birth weight was 2.9 kg. She was breast-fed for 7 months. Appetite is good.

Mother is well; father is allergic to house dust. Maternal grandfather had diabetes mellitus, emphysema, and cancer.

Temperature at 1 year is 39.1°C, weight 7.3 kg. She has slightly red throat, diminished breath sounds on right side, pot belly, and thin muscles. She tastes salty. The rest of the physical findings are normal. Sweat chloride is 97 and 136 mmol/liter. Treatment with enzymes by mouth is begun.

She coughs more at 20 months. Appetite is good. Weight is 8.9 kg, temperature 37.8°C. Fine rales are in chest. Rhonchi clear when she coughs. Hematocrit is 0.36.

At 2 years, she is active and has a good appetite. Weight is 9.2 kg. Ears and throat are slightly red. Chest is normal, abdomen protuberant. Hematocrit is 0.38. White cell count is 18.5 × 10⁹/liter with 0.14 polymorphonuclear cells, 0.20 bands, 0.64 lymphocytes, and 0.02 monocytes. Sputum contains *Streptococcus viridans*, γ streptococcus, *Neisseria,* and other gram-negative bacteria. Sputum earlier had *S. viridans, Pseudomonas aeruginosa, Neisseria,* and *Haemophilus aphrophilus.*

Diaphragm is low at 12 months (Figure 19-1), 20 months (Figure 19-2A), and 24 months (Figure 19-2B). Streaks and nodules of water density appear in lungs (see Figure 19-2A). Heart gets smaller, and bulge appears along upper left margin (Figure 19-2).

Diagnosis: Cystic fibrosis; microcardia and bulge of main pulmonary artery because of hypoxic increase in pulmonary vascular resistance.

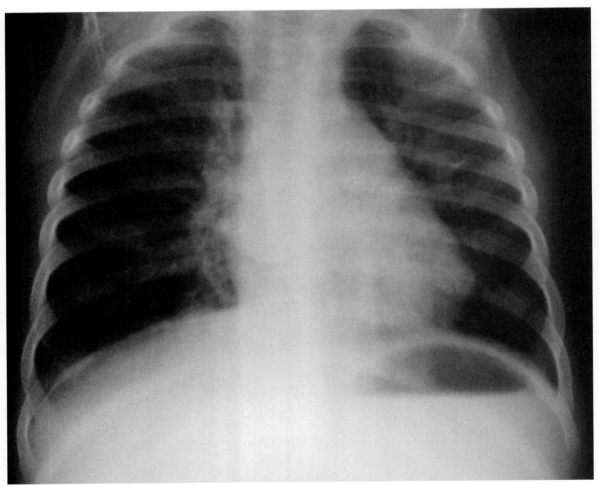

Fig. 19-1

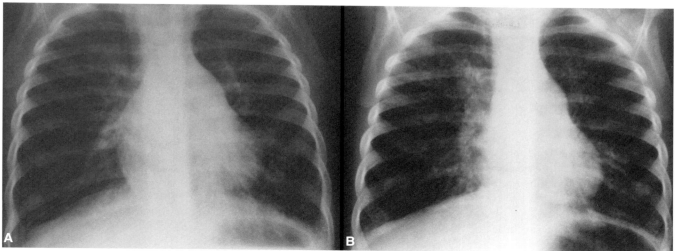

Fig. 19-2

Case 20

A 6-year-old girl has puffy face and ankles.

Mother (32 years old) and father (43 years old) are well. Brother (13 years old), who has cystic fibrosis, plays on school basketball team.

Pregnancy of mother was normal, birth weight 2.6 kg. She began to cough, often vomiting feedings, at 4 weeks. At 2 months, sweat chloride was 105 mmol/liter. At 3 years, she was thin, pale, and potbellied. Fingers were dusky and clubbed. Cough got worse 1 month ago. She had night sweats. Knees hurt. Head, chest, and abdomen ached and nose sometimes bled during coughing spells. Weight 1 month ago was 12.6 kg, liver edge 2 cm below costal margin. Face was puffy when she woke up 10 days ago. Ankles have been swollen the last three evenings. She eats little and sleeps most of the day.

Weight at 6 years is 13.5 kg, temperature 37.4°C, heart rate 136, respiratory rate 42, and blood pressure 100/70 mm Hg. Face is ashen. Lips are blue. White patches are on tongue and buccal mucosa. Neck veins are distended. Alae nasi flare and soft tissues retract during inspiration. Rales are in chest. Second heart sound is loud. Liver edge is 4 cm below costal margin. Limbs are thin, fingers and toes clubbed.

Hematocrit is 0.38. White cell count is 12.7×10^9/liter with 0.05 polymorphonuclear cells, 0.61 bands, 0.24 lymphocytes, 0.07 monocytes, and 0.03 metamyelocytes. Serum sodium is 136 mmol/liter, potassium 3.8, chloride 86, carbon dioxide 31, urea nitrogen 3.9, calcium 2.07, phosphorus 1.07, cholesterol 1.81, triglycerides 0.69, and glucose 5.3. Creatinine is 40 μmol/liter, uric acid 640, total bilirubin 15, and direct bilirubin 7. Total protein is 76 g/liter, albumin 33. Alkaline phosphatase is 296 U/liter, LDH 773, SGOT 525, and CK 295. Sputum culture grows *Pseudomonas aeruginosa* and *Haemophilus influenzae*.

She answers questions inappropriately the next day, does not react to venipuncture the second day, and dies the third day.

Roentgenogram of chest at 6 years, 12 weeks shows small heart in erect film, low diaphragm, large hilar shadows, rings and parallel strips of water density, which are thickened bronchial walls and thickened tissues around them, and mucous plugs (Figure 20-1A). Last roentgenogram at 6 years, 15 weeks (3 days before she dies) shows enlarged heart in supine film (Figure 20-1B).

Diagnosis: Cystic fibrosis, chronic and acute cor pulmonale.

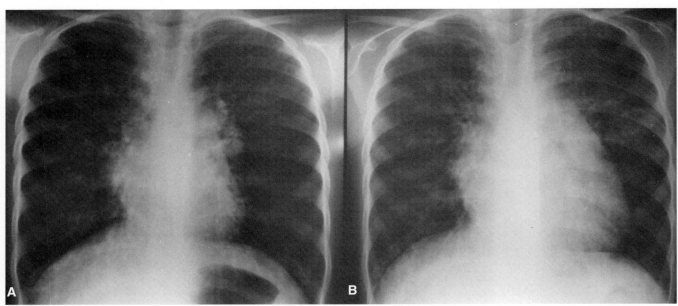

Fig. 20-1

Case 21

A 14-year-old boy is tired and watches television a lot.

Frequent cough and 6–8 stools a day led to diagnosis of cystic fibrosis at 6 months.

Weight is 30 kg, height 149 cm. He is pale. Breath sounds are diminished in right side of chest. Fingers are clubbed and mildly blue. The rest of the physical findings are normal.

Hematocrit is 0.41. White cell count is 11.6×10^9/liter with 0.71 polymorphonuclear cells, 0.06 bands, 0.16 lymphocytes, and 0.07 monocytes.

Pleural air is on right side; heart is small (Figure 21-1).

Diagnosis: Cystic fibrosis, tension pneumothorax.

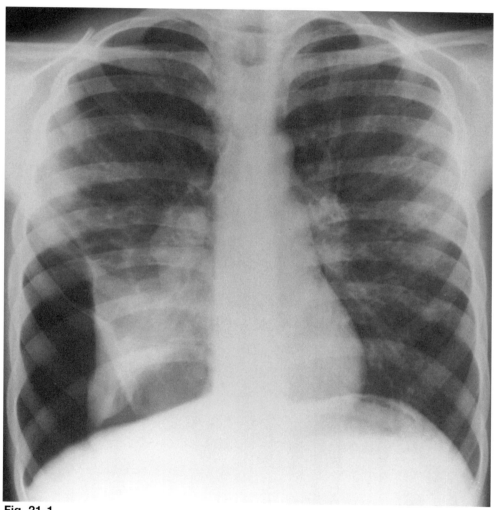

Fig. 21-1

Case 22

A 15-year-old girl with cystic fibrosis coughs up ¼ cup thick, white-green sputum a day. Cough is worse during the several colds she has each year. Climbing stairs and running half a block make her cough and short of breath. Menarche was at 12 years.

Sister (17 years old) has cystic fibrosis.

Weight is 47 kg, height 156 cm, heart rate 56, respiratory rate 16, and blood pressure 126/86 mm Hg. She coughs up thick, green sputum during examination. Voice is nasal. Rhonchi are in chest. The rest of the physical findings are normal.

Hematocrit is 0.40. White cell count is 6.5×10^9/liter with 0.40 polymorphonuclear cells, 0.06 bands, 0.48 lymphocytes, and 0.06 monocytes.

In Figure 22-1A at 15 years, rings and parallel strips of water density, the thickened walls of bronchi and the thickened tissues around them, are in the lungs. Also in Figure 22-1A, a collection of fingerlike shadows of water density, broader distally, is in left lower lobe behind the heart. At 17 years, the branched shadow is in left lower lobe, lateral to right parietal pleura, which is visible as a curved shadow of water density just to left of T9–T11 (Figure 22-1B). Trachea is convex left in Figure 22-1B. At 21 years, left lower lobe is collapsed, trachea convex farther left, and right lung expanded farther across midline (Figure 22-2).

Diagnosis: Cystic fibrosis, mucous plug in bronchi of left lower lobe, gradual collapse of left lower lobe (as interalveolar fenestrae and bronchoalveolar canals of Lambert are closed by inflammation).

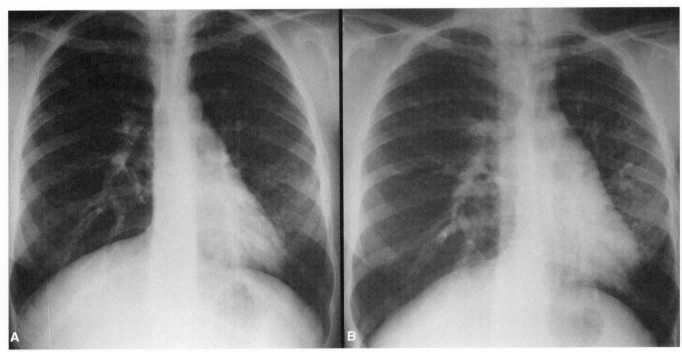

Fig. 22-1

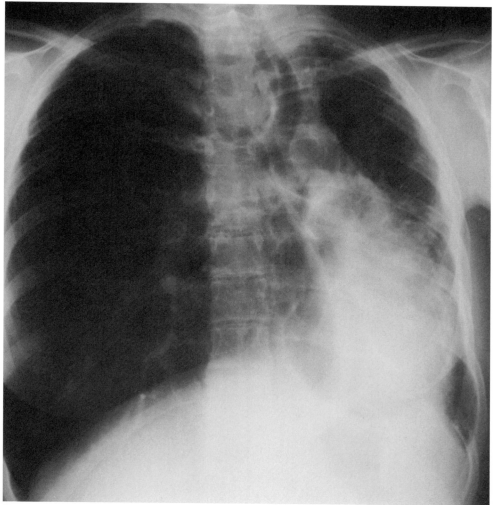

Fig. 22-2

Case 23

A 13-year-old girl with cystic fibrosis, who has occasionally coughed up blood-streaked sputum for almost 3 years, coughs up blood for 20 minutes tonight and has gurgles in left side of chest. She is receiving IV antibiotics.

Parents and five siblings are well.

Temperature is 36.5°C, heart rate 105, respiratory rate 24, blood pressure 98/54 mm Hg, and weight 29.4 kg. Rales are in lungs, most in left upper lobe. Fingers are clubbed. The rest of the physical findings are normal.

Hematocrit is 0.37. White cell count is 17.8×10^9/liter with 0.69 polymorphonuclear cells, 0.02 bands, 0.16 lymphocytes, 0.05 monocytes, 0.04 eosinophils, and 0.04 basophils. Platelet count is 579×10^9/liter. Serum sodium is 137 mmol/liter, potassium 3.8, chloride 99, carbon dioxide 30, urea nitrogen 6.4, calcium 2.30, phosphorus 1.39, cholesterol 2.20, and glucose 5.6. Creatinine is 50 μmol/liter, uric acid 260, total bilirubin 5, and direct bilirubin 0. Total protein is 73 g/liter, albumin 41. Alkaline phosphatase is 275 U/liter, LDH 188, and SGOT 22. Culture of sputum grows *Burkholderia cepacia*.

At bronchoscopy, blood is coming from left upper-lobe bronchus. Small amounts of mucopus are in other bronchi.

In Figure 23-1, a central venous catheter is in place and contrast medium is in superior left bronchial artery. After embolization, wire coils are in superior left bronchial artery.

Diagnosis: Cystic fibrosis, embolization of bleeding superior left bronchial artery.

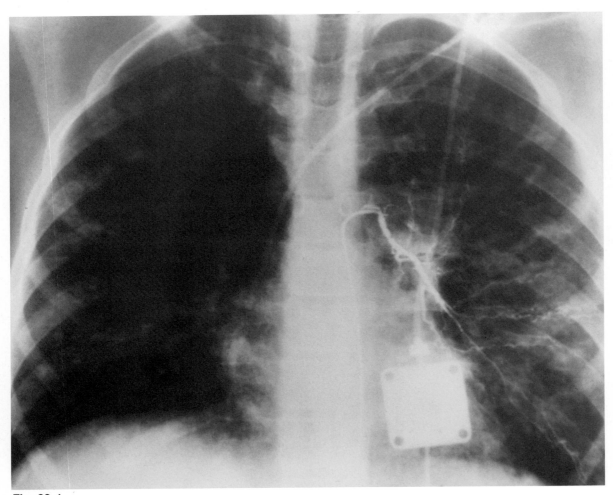

Fig. 23-1

Case 24

An 8-week-old girl is coughing and vomiting.

Mother had glycosuria and bacterial and monilial vaginitis during pregnancy and smoked five cigarettes a day. Apgar score was 8/9 at 1 and 5 minutes, birth weight 3.7 kg. She vomited frequently. At 2 weeks, weight was 4 kg. At 6 weeks, she began to cough and take only 2–3 oz at a feeding. She has bursts of wet coughs and vomits part of her feedings.

Weight at 8 weeks is 4 kg, length 57 cm, head circumference 37 cm, temperature 37.4°C, heart rate 140, respiratory rate 44, and systolic blood pressure 122 mm Hg. Eyelids are puffy. Stringy mucus is on injected conjunctivae. Nose is runny. Rales are in lungs. The rest of the physical findings are normal.

Hematocrit is 0.41. White cell count is 12.8×10^9/liter with 0.30 polymorphonuclear cells, 0.08 bands, 0.44 lymphocytes, 0.05 monocytes, and 0.13 eosinophils (absolute: 1.7×10^9/liter). Urine specific gravity is 1.004, pH 6. Urine has many squamous epithelial cells/HPF, >100 white cells/HPF,

and moderate bacteria. Serum sodium is 138 mmol/liter, potassium 6.2, chloride 104, carbon dioxide 21, urea nitrogen 2.1, calcium 2.59, phosphorus 2.03, cholesterol 2.97, and glucose 5.2. Creatinine is 50 μmol/liter, uric acid 250, total bilirubin 7, and direct bilirubin 3. Total protein is 75 g/liter, albumin 39. Alkaline phosphatase is 222 U/liter, LDH 140, and SGOT 44.

Nodules of water density are in lungs (Figure 24-1). The curved shadow of water density near left apex may be focal atelectasis or small thymus made visible because of mediastinal air (see Figure 24-1).

Microscopic examination of conjunctival scrapings shows vacuolar cytoplasmic inclusions in epithelial cells.

Diagnosis: *Chlamydia trachomatis* conjunctivitis and pneumonia.

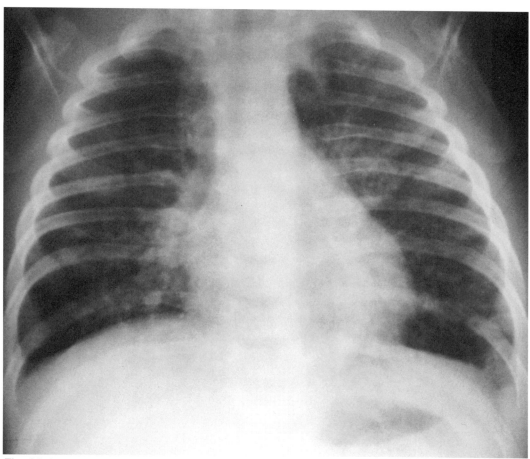

Fig. 24-1

Case 25

An 8-week-old boy has a cough and fever.

Cough began 4 days ago. Two days ago, temperature was 38.3°C. Stools were watery yesterday. He has vomited three times today after coughing spells.

Mother (22 years old) is well. A 2-year-old child she baby-sits is in hospital with pneumonia. Father and an uncle who lives with family had colds recently.

Pregnancy of mother was normal. Weight at birth on January 4 was 3.6 kg. He has had one dose of oral (attenuated) poliovirus vaccine. He had a yeast diaper rash at 6 weeks.

Temperature at 8 weeks is 38°C, heart rate 150, respiratory rate 44, systolic blood pressure 90 mm Hg, and weight 4.8 kg. He is fussy when prone. Anterior fontanel is depressed. Eardrums are pink. Nose is runny. He retracts, grunts, and has bilateral rales. The rest of the physical findings are normal.

Hematocrit is 0.30. White cell count is 16.5×10^9/liter with 0.07 polymorphonuclear cells, 0.20 bands, 0.50 lymphocytes, 0.22 monocytes, and 0.01 metamyelocytes. Platelet count is 631×10^9/liter. Urine specific gravity is 1.019, pH 6. Urine has trace protein and trace reducing substance. Serum sodium is 136 mmol/liter, potassium 4.7, chloride 102, and urea nitrogen 2.5. Creatinine is 40 μmol/liter.

Anterior segment of right upper lobe is atelectatic, chest deep front to back, and diaphragm so depressed that its slips of costochondral attachment show at right costophrenic angle (Figure 25-1).

He has a seizure 4 hours after chest roentgenogram. He is intubated and given oxygen and IV fluids. Two hours after intubation, CSF has 2×10^6/liter white cells, 0.51 pia-arachnoid cells, 0.49 lymphocytes, 10.9 mmol/liter glucose, and 0.93 g/liter protein.

Diagnosis: Respiratory syncytial virus pneumonia. (Result of examination of nasopharyngeal swab with monoclonal fluorescent antibody to respiratory syncytial viral antigen is positive.)

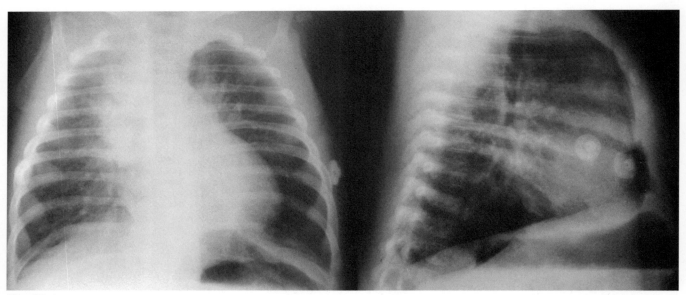

Fig. 25-1

Case 26

A 2-month-old girl has been coughing for 6 days.

Pregnancy of mother was normal, birth weight 3.5 kg, and length 52 cm.

Mother (26 years old) and three siblings (3, 6, and 9 years old) are well. Father (27 years old) has allergies.

Temperature is 36.9°C, heart rate 186, respiratory rate 70–80, systolic blood pressure 84 mm Hg, weight 4.1 kg, length 55 cm, and head circumference 38 cm. She is alert and pink. Breath sounds are noisy. The rest of the physical findings are normal.

Hematocrit is 0.34. White cell count is 7.9×10^9/liter. Sweat chloride is 11 mmol/liter.

Strips of water density are in lungs (Figure 26-1). Diaphragm is so depressed that its slips of costochondral attachment are apparent in costophrenic angles (Figure 26-1A).

In the next 6 days, she is without fever or respiratory distress, feeds well, and gains 100 g.

Six days after first examination, diaphragm is higher (Figure 26-2A). Middle lobe is atelectatic except for front part of medial segment (Figure 26-2B).

Diagnosis: Bronchiolitis.

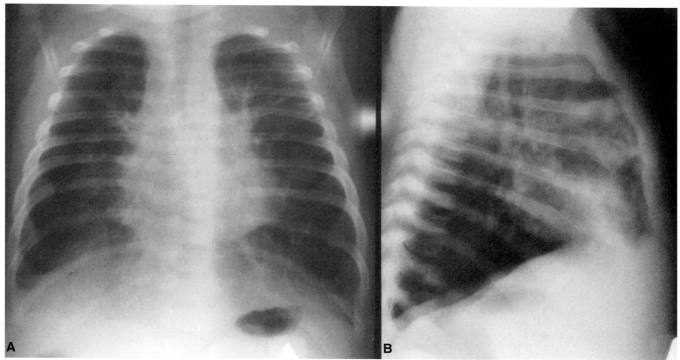

Fig. 26-1

(Continued)

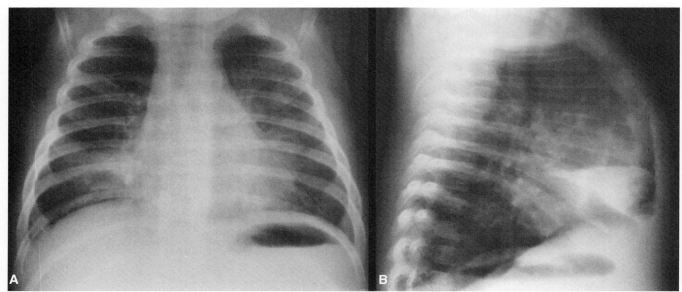

Fig. 26-2

Case 27

A 6-year-old boy has had chickenpox for 6 days. He has not walked for 5 days because of knee pain. He vomited and was drowsy yesterday. He is taking acetaminophen for itching.

Parents and sister (4 years old) are well.

Temperature is 37.1°C, heart rate 132, respiratory rate 28, blood pressure 110/80 mm Hg, and weight 21.1 kg. He is alert. Papules and vesicles are on body, limbs, face, and head. Eyelids are crusted. Mouth is sticky. The rest of the physical findings are normal.

Hematocrit is 0.44. White cell count is 20.8×10^9/liter with 0.53 polymorphonuclear cells, 0.18 bands, 0.07 lymphocytes, 0.11 monocytes, 0.10 atypical lymphocytes, and 0.01 myelocytes. Serum sodium is 131 mmol/liter, potassium 4.1, chloride 97, carbon dioxide 25, urea nitrogen 15.4, calcium 1.92, phosphorus 1.26, cholesterol 3.08, and glucose 10.8 (IV fluids). Creatinine is 90 μmol/liter, uric acid 640, total bilirubin 3, and direct bilirubin 2. Total protein is 52 g/liter, albumin 34. Alkaline phosphatase is 148 U/liter, LDH 4,160. Capillary blood pH is 7.44. P_{CO_2} is 33 mm Hg, P_{O_2} 57. CSF has 1×10^6/liter white cells, 4.8 mmol/liter glucose, and 0.18 g/liter protein. Twelve hours ago, blood ammonia was 26 μmol/liter (normal: 10–80).

He gets dusky and breathes harder. He is disoriented and combative, speaks gibberish, and then is unresponsive.

Ill-defined shadows of water density are in lungs (Figure 27-1), pox marks in skin above clavicles.

He dies 13 hours after roentgenogram and 7 days after appearance of chickenpox.

Buffy coat and CSF cultures are negative for cytomegalovirus and varicella zoster virus 3 weeks later.

Diagnosis: Chickenpox, encephalitis, pneumonia.

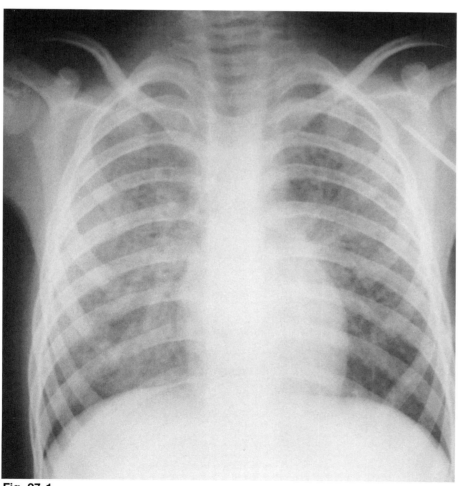

Fig. 27-1

Case 28

A 6-month-old girl has had a cough and runny nose for 5 days and temperature up to 38°C.

Weight is 7.3 kg, temperature 37°C, heart rate 100, and respiratory rate 42. Nose is runny. Percussion note and breath sounds are diminished over left lower lobe. The rest of the physical findings are normal.

Hematocrit is 0.31. White cell count is 19.5×10^9/liter with 0.38 polymorphonuclear cells, 0.14 bands, 0.45 lymphocytes, and 0.03 monocytes. *Staphylococcus aureus* is cultured from trachea.

A shadow of water density in left lower lobe includes cyst with air-liquid interface (Figure 28-1).

She remains afebrile. Cough and runny nose stop.

Six days later, left lower lobe is almost normally aerated (Figure 28-2).

Diagnosis: Viral infection, postinflammatory seropneumatocele in lung.

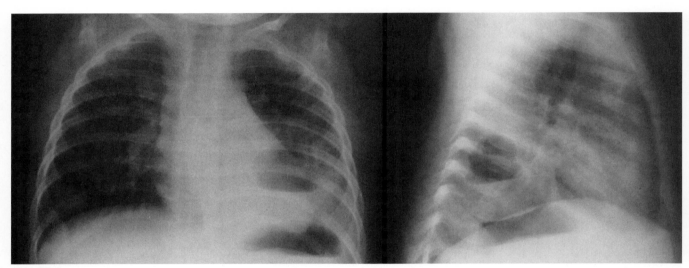

Fig. 28-1

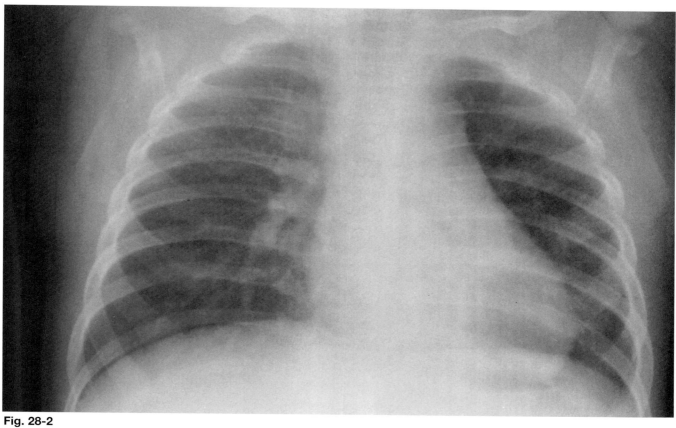

Fig. 28-2

Case 29

A 17-year-old boy, who has smoked cigarettes for several years, has an abnormality in roentgenographic examination.

He was born with intestinal obstruction and operated on right after birth. He has had pneumonia six times since he was 5 years old. Sweat chloride is normal.

Weight at 17 years is 58 kg, height 78 cm. Breath sounds are diminished in left side of chest. A transverse scar and a small scar in left upper quadrant are on abdomen. The rest of the physical findings are normal.

Vital capacity is 3.71 liters (0.72 of predicted amount), FEV_1 3.09 liters (0.71 of predicted amount), mean forced expiratory flow during the middle of vital capacity 1.53 liters (0.56 of pre-

dicted amount), and peak expiratory flow 495 liters/min (0.90 of predicted amount), values interpreted as showing mild restrictive defect.

A shadow of water density in lingula and superior part of left upper lobe at 7 years (Figure 29-1A) is replaced by a cyst with an air-liquid level and sparse lung markings above it 6 months (Figure 29-1B) and 10 years later (Figure 29-2), when cyst is slightly larger.

Diagnosis: Postinflammatory seropneumatocele in lung, questionable focal bronchiolitis obliterans.

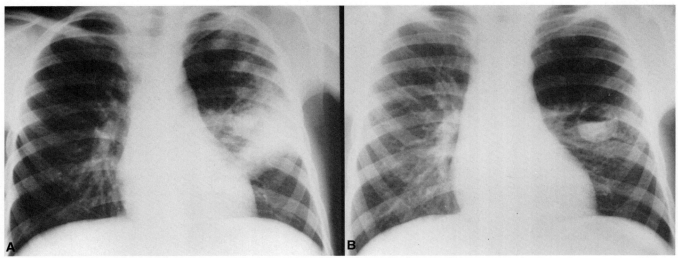

Fig. 29-1

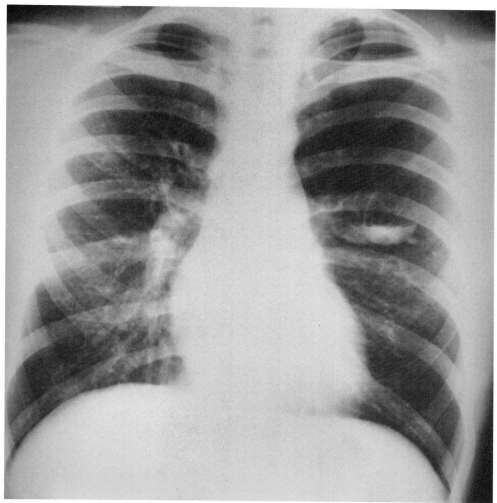

Fig. 29-2

Case 30

An 8-year-old girl has had a cough and runny nose for 3 weeks. When she had a similar illness at 3 years, she had iron deficiency anemia and diminished breath sounds in left upper lobe.

Temperature is 37.6°C, heart rate 130, respiratory rate 20, and blood pressure 90/60 mm Hg. Physical findings are normal. Tuberculin skin test is negative.

Hematocrit is 0.35. White cell count is 9.8×10^9/liter with 0.36 polymorphonuclear cells, 0.09 bands, 0.54 lymphocytes, and 0.01 eosinophils. Platelet count is 277×10^9/liter. ESR is 10 mm/hr. Urine specific gravity is 1.025, pH 6. Urine has 2–4 epithelial cells/HPF, 15–20 white cells/HPF, 0–2 red cells/HPF, bacteria, and mucus. Urine homovanillic acid is 28 µmol/day (normal: <45), vanillylmandelic acid 6 (normal: <35). Serum calcium is 2.20 mmol/liter, phosphorus 1.45, urea nitrogen 3.6, cholesterol 3.23, and glucose 4.4. Uric acid is 200 µmol/liter, total bilirubin 7. Total protein is 70 g/liter, albumin 41. Alkaline phosphatase is 230 U/liter, LDH 315, and SGOT 58.

A roughly spherical mass of water density is in left upper lobe at 3 years (Figure 30-1A) and in an examination at 8 years (Figure 30-1B) because of earlier abnormality.

At left thoracotomy, adhesions between left upper lobe and mediastinum are lysed and left upper lobe is resected.

Pleura over cyst (2.5 × 1.8 cm) is thick and hemorrhagic, normal elsewhere. Cyst wall—which is white to pink, granular, and trabeculated in gross examination—consists of respiratory epithelium, fibrous tissue, smooth muscle, cartilage, and submucous glands in microscopic examination. Small, dilated bronchial spaces lined by respiratory epithelium are adjacent to a small part of cyst wall, compressed alveoli with extravasated red cells and neutrophils, and thickened septa around cyst wall. Cyst contains purulent material that is sterile in aerobic and anaerobic culture. A parabronchial node has tertiary reaction centers in cortex.

Diagnosis: Sterile pyocele in lung, questionable postinflammatory bronchial atresia.

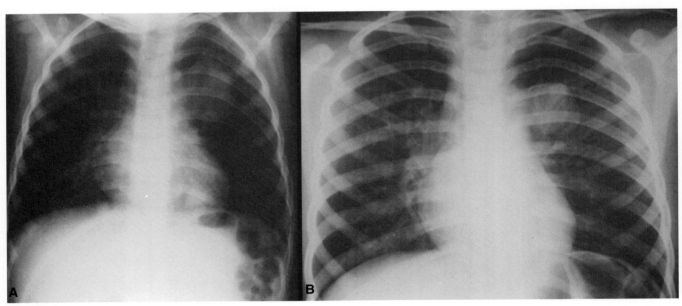

Fig. 30-1

Case 31

A 6½-year-old girl has chest abnormality in preschool examination.

She sat at 6 months, walked at 1 year. She had chickenpox at 5 months and measles at 2½ years. She did not begin eating normally or gaining weight until 1 month after measles. She coughed while eating peanuts 1–2 weeks after measles but has coughed little since then.

Mother (28 years old), father (29 years old), and three brothers (4, 8, and 10 years old) are well.

Temperature at 6½ years is 37.6°C, heart rate 100, respiratory rate 24, blood pressure 100/70 mm Hg, weight 20 kg, and height 116 cm. Nose is runny, left eardrum perforated. Teeth are decayed. Sternum moves in during inspiration. Tactile fremitus is increased over left lower lobe, percussion note is dull, and breath sounds are diminished. A systolic heart murmur is present. The rest of the physical findings are normal.

Hemoglobin is 150 g/liter. White cell count is 9.8×10^9/liter with 0.42 polymorphonuclear cells, 0.01 bands, 0.47 lymphocytes, 0.01 monocytes, 0.01 eosinophils, and 0.08 disintegrated cells. ESR is 11 mm/45 minutes. Urine specific gravity is 1.028, reaction acid. Urine has acetone, white cells, epithelial cells, occasional red cells/HPF, and mucus.

Plain film shows air in dilated bronchi in atelectatic left lower lobe and displacement of heart to left (Figure 31-1A). Bronchography shows dilated bronchi in both lobes of left lung (Figure 31-1B) and undilated bronchi in right lung.

At 10 years, she coughs up ½ cup of yellow sputum per day.

At left thoracotomy, pleural adhesions are thick, especially along diaphragm. A large artery extends from descending aorta to left lung. Left lower lobe is small. Large lymph nodes are along aorta and in left hilum.

Resected left lung is rubbery and covered by shaggy, fibrous tissue. Bronchi contain mucopus and seem glued together by fibrous tissue. They are lined with pink-tan mucosa and dilated outward to pleural surface. Bronchopulmonary nodes are large. Microscopic examination shows (1) mucosal folds in bronchi; (2) submucosal lymphocytes, few eosinophils and polymorphonuclear cells, fibrosis, and many capillaries; (3) thick fibrous tissue; (4) atelectasis; (5) collections of lymphocytes, few multinucleated foreign body and Langerhans' giant cells; (6) loose vascular fibrous tissue instead of pleura; and (7) no doubly refractile foreign bodies.

Diagnosis: Bronchiectasis, atelectasis, fibrosis, and chronic suppurative bronchitis of left lung.

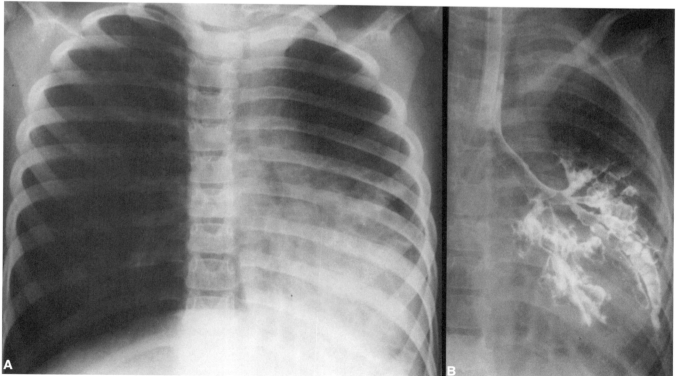

Fig. 31-1

Case 32

A 7-year-old boy, who has had cough and sometimes fever frequently since he was 2 years old, is coughing again.

Parents and two brothers are well.

Temperature is 37°C, heart rate 104, respiratory rate 24, blood pressure 70/40 mm Hg, and weight 21.2 kg. Percussion note is dull, and breath sounds and vocal fremitus are diminished over left lower lobe. A systolic heart murmur is present. The rest of the physical findings are normal.

Hematocrit is 0.37. White cell count is 15.0×10^9/liter with 0.78 polymorphonuclear cells, 0.05 bands, 0.16 lymphocytes, and 0.01 eosinophils. ESR is 16 mm/hr. Urine specific gravity is 1.021, pH 7. Urine has 0–1 epithelial cell/HPF, 0–1 white cell/HPF, and amorphous sediment. Serum urea nitrogen is 5.7 mmol/liter, calcium 2.35, phosphorus 1.55, cholesterol 3.23, and glucose 4.4. Uric acid is 230 µmol/liter, total bilirubin 5. Total protein is 63 g/liter, albumin 41. Alkaline phosphatase is 170 U/liter, LDH 230, and SGOT 25.

A shadow of water density in posterior basal segment and part of lateral basal segment of left lower lobe (Figure 32-1) has blood supply from aorta (Figure 32-2).

Bronchoscopy shows inflammation and narrowing of bronchial orifices to left lower lobe and increased distance between them. Culture grows normal flora.

At operation, an oval mass is adherent to left lower lobe and supplied by three arteries from aorta.

The mass (7.1 × 5.5 × 1.3 cm), red to purple-gray to yellow, contains yellow exudate. Microscopic examination shows fat and granulation tissue in bronchioles, inflammation and fibrosis in parenchyma, focal occlusions in small vessels, dystrophic calcification in lymphoid follicles, and hyperplasia in lymph nodes. Cultures are sterile.

Diagnosis: Intralobar (acquired) bronchopulmonary sequestration.

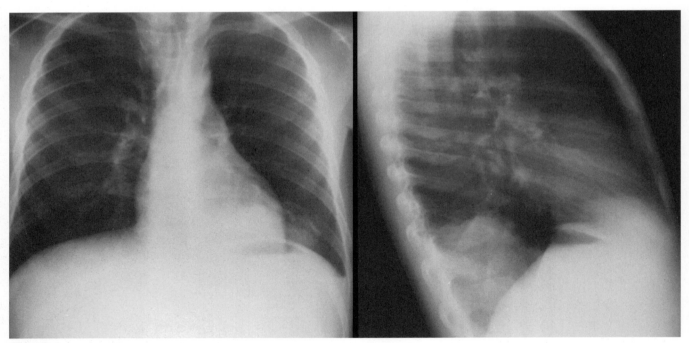

Fig. 32-1

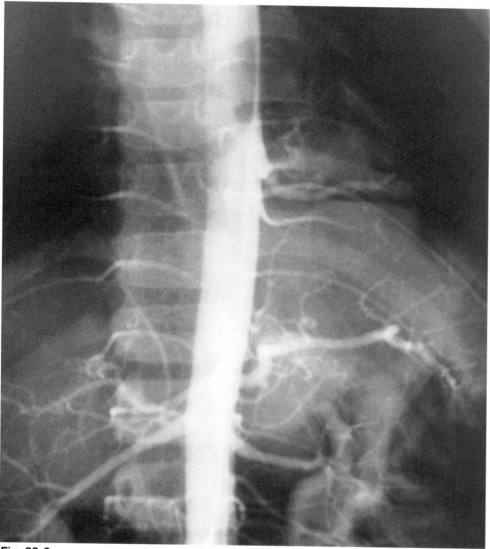

Fig. 32-2

Case 33

A 7½-year-old girl has swollen lips, a rash, and fever.

Cough and fever began 2 weeks ago. She has been taking acetaminophen and cough syrup. Swelling of lips and rash appeared 2 nights ago. Temperature was 40.6°C. She stopped eating and drinking. Eye discharge appeared this morning.

Parents and four siblings are well.

Temperature is 39°C, heart rate 145, respiratory rate 36, blood pressure 100/70 mm Hg, and weight 15.2 kg. Body is covered with small red spots and bumps, some with central pustule or blister, some scratched raw. Palms and soles are free of rash. Lids are swollen, lower lids coated with white mucus, palpebral conjunctivae injected. Lips are swollen, crusted yellow, and have small, white blisters inside. Nasal alae flare and subcostal tissues retract during inspiration. Inspiratory and expiratory wheezes are present. The rest of the physical findings are normal.

Hematocrit is 0.34. White cell count is 10.4 × 10⁹/liter with 0.39 polymorphonuclear cells, 0.34 bands, 0.19 lymphocytes, 0.03 monocytes, and 0.05 eosinophils. Platelet count is 338 × 10⁹/liter. ESR is 40 mm/hr. Serum sodium is 139 mmol/liter, potassium 4.1, chloride 103, carbon dioxide 14, urea nitrogen 3.6, calcium 2.22, phosphorus 1.07, cholesterol 3.26, and glucose 8.5 (IV fluids). Creatinine is 40 µmol/liter, uric acid 330, total bilirubin 3, and direct bilirubin 0. Total protein is 65 g/liter, albumin 36. Alkaline phosphatase is 67 U/liter, LDH 375, and SGOT 30. Two days later, urine specific gravity is 1.026, pH 5.5. Urine has 0.30 g/liter protein, 0.2 AU urobilinogen, 0–2 white cells/HPF, 10 red cells/HPF, 15 nonsquamous epithelial cells/HPF, and bacteria.

Two days after appearance of rash, strips of water density are in lower left lobe (Figure 33-1). Left lower lobe is partly atelectatic, and left upper lobe is overexpanded 10 months after illness (Figure 33-2A) and to a lesser degree 5 years after illness (Figure 33-2B).

Culture of eye discharge grows *Staphylococcus aureus*; sputum grows normal flora. Stool has ova of *Ascaris lumbricoides*. One day after appearance of rash, serum complement fixation titer for *Mycoplasma pneumoniae* is <1:8. Three days after appearance of rash, sputum DNA probe for *M. pneumoniae* is negative. Tzanck smear at edge of deroofed blister is negative.

Two weeks after appearance of rash, the rash is fading, scabs are branny, and lips are still ulcerated and crusted. She begins to eat at day 18 and still has sores in mouth 3½ weeks later. At 13 years, weight is 39.8 kg, height 154 cm. She coughs up yellow sputum. Breath sounds are decreased at left base; crackles are at left apex. The rest of the physical findings are normal.

Diagnosis: Stevens-Johnson syndrome.

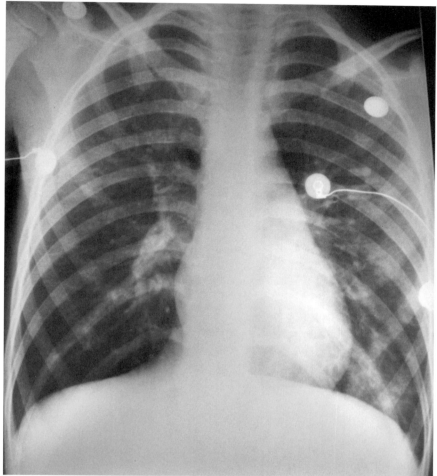

Fig. 33-1

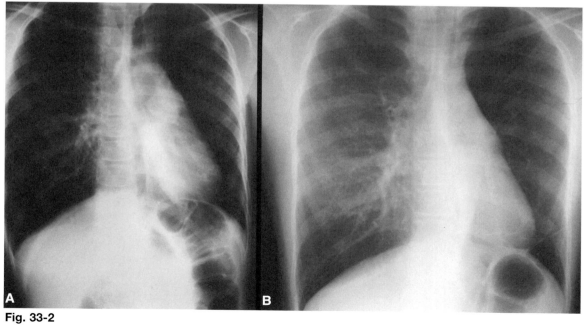

A   B

Fig. 33-2

Case 34

A 6-year-old girl has a cough and fever. She had a headache and temperature of 39.4°C 2 days ago and then began to cough.

Birth weight was 3.3 kg.

Mother (30 years old), father (32 years old), and three brothers (4, 9, and 11 years old) are well. Father and paternal grandparents have allergies.

Temperature is 39.7°C, heart rate 120, respiratory rate 30, blood pressure 120/70 mm Hg, and weight 21.5 kg. She has a raspy, barking cough that is almost continuous at times. Breathing is shallow, with occasional retractions. Rales are in both sides of chest. The rest of the physical findings are normal.

Hematocrit is 0.40. White cell count is 7.2×10^9/liter with 0.73 polymorphonuclear cells, 0.07 bands, 0.17 lymphocytes, 0.02 monocytes, and 0.01 eosinophils. ESR is 36 mm/hr. Urine specific gravity is 1.011, pH 6.5. Urine has rare white cells/HPF.

Left upper lobe is partly atelectatic. Strips of water density are in lower lobes (Figure 34-1).

Daily or twice-daily fevers of 39.4–40.0°C occur for the next week. Adventitious breath sounds remain. On the ninth day, spleen edge and liver edge are 3 cm below costal margin. Tuberculin skin test is negative. Serum sodium is 137 mmol/liter, potassium 4.7, chloride 100, carbon dioxide 26, urea nitrogen 2.1, calcium 2.42, phosphorus 1.29, triglycerides 0.60, cholesterol 2.10, and glucose 6.0. Creatinine is 40 μmol/liter, uric acid 120, total bilirubin 7, and direct bilirubin 0. Total protein is 71 g/liter, albumin 39. Alkaline phosphatase is 137 U/liter, LDH 616, SGOT 21, and CK 38. On the tenth day, tetracycline treatment is begun. She is afebrile days 10–13. Liver and spleen are not palpable. On the fourteenth day, red spots are on face and chest and confluent on back of hands. Temperature is 39.4°C. Liver edge is 3–4 cm below costal margin. Tetracycline is stopped. Fever gradually subsides during next few days, and rash fades. She looks and feels well after 3 weeks.

Serum cold agglutinin titer is <1:8 on day 7, 1:2,048 on day 21, and 1:128 at month 3. Serum complement fixation titer for *Mycoplasma pneumoniae* is 1:32 on day 9, 1:256 on day 21, and 1:64 at month 3.

Diagnosis: Mycoplasma pneumonia, questionable allergic reaction to tetracycline.

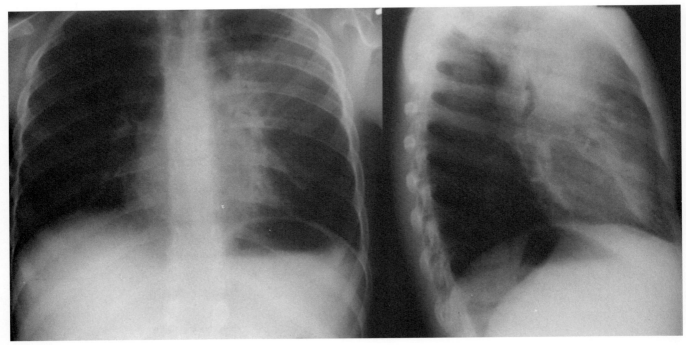

Fig. 34-1

Case 35

An 11-year-old boy is coughing and has inspiratory pain in right side of chest. He had fever 2 days ago. He vomited and had ringing in his ears yesterday.

Temperature is 40.7°C, blood pressure 100/60 mm Hg, weight 49 kg, and height 160 cm. Physical findings are normal.

Hematocrit is 0.41. White cell count is 21.3×10^9/liter with 0.71 polymorphonuclear cells, 0.13 bands, 0.08 lymphocytes, and 0.08 monocytes. Platelet count is 322×10^9/liter.

A shadow of water density is in right posterior segment of right upper lobe (Figure 35-1).

He is treated with penicillin and is afebrile the next day.

Impression: Pneumococcal pneumonia.

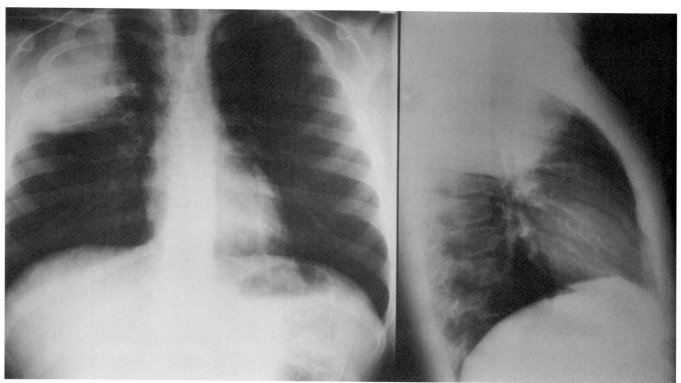

Fig. 35-1

Case 36

An 8-year-old girl has a 17-mm skin reaction to tuberculin in routine school test. Treatment with isoniazid, rifampin, ethambutol, and pyrazinamide is begun.

Parents and three siblings are well and tuberculin negative.

Three months after treatment is begun, temperature is 37.5°C, heart rate 96, respiratory rate 20, blood pressure 96/50 mm Hg, weight 23 kg, and height 125 cm. Physical findings are normal.

Twenty-one days after treatment is begun, hematocrit is 0.39. White cell count is 8.9×10^9/liter with 0.59 polymorphonuclear cells, 0.39 lymphocytes, 0.01 monocytes, and 0.01 basophils. Serum sodium is 141 mmol/liter, potassium 3.9, chloride 103, carbon dioxide 29, urea nitrogen 2.9, calcium 2.25, phosphorus 1.71, cholesterol 3.93, and glucose 5.1. Creatinine is 50 μmol/liter, uric acid 230, total bilirubin 3, and direct bilirubin 0. Total protein is 77 g/liter, albumin 39. Alkaline phosphatase is 153 U/liter, LDH 187, and SGOT 28. Sputum smears and cultures are negative for *Mycobacterium tuberculosis*.

Twenty-one days after treatment is begun, a shadow of water density in lateral basal segment of right lower lobe (Figure 36-1A), between heart and spine in lateral view (Figure 36-1B), is associated with thickened pleura or pleural liquid. CT scan 3 months after treatment shows the shadow of water density contiguous to oblique fissure.

At operation, right pleural space and oblique fissure are scarred. Right lower lobe is resected. A tan-brown capsule (5.0 × 3.0 × 1.5 cm) is around pale yellow, granular matter. Microscopic examination of capsule shows caseous granulomas, surrounded by an inner rim of histiocytes and giant cells, a middle rim of lymphocytes and plasma cells, and an outer rim of new vessels and scar with calcification.

Culture grows coagulase-negative staphylococci. Stain shows acid-fast bacilli.

Diagnosis: Primary tuberculosis.

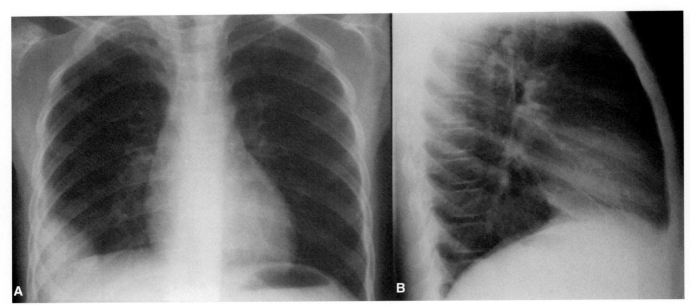

Fig. 36-1

Case 37

A 1½-year-old girl has had a fever, pus in ears, and loose stools for 4 days. She has been cranky for 2 months.

Birth weight was 2 kg. She crawled at 8 months but does not walk.

Mother (18 years old), father (21 years old), and brother (3 months old) are well. Maternal grandfather has tuberculosis.

Temperature at 1½ years is 38.3°C, heart rate 150, respiratory rate 50, weight 6.6 kg, length 66 cm, and head circumference 43 cm. She is pale. Yellow-white pus is in external acoustic meatus, mucus in nose. Cervical, axillary, and inguinal nodes are palpable. Breath sounds are diminished in left side of chest. Liver edge and spleen edge are 2 cm below costal margin. The rest of the physical findings are normal.

Hematocrit is 0.36. White cell count is 14.7×10^9/liter with 0.28 polymorphonuclear cells, 0.02 bands, 0.64 lymphocytes, and 0.06 monocytes. ESR is 28 mm/45 minutes. Urine specific gravity is 1.020, pH 5. Urine is normal. Serum sodium is 125 mmol/liter, potassium 5.3, chloride 90, and carbon dioxide 18. CSF is clear and colorless with 16×10^6/liter white cells, 0.85 lymphocytes, 0.15 polymorphonuclear cells, 1.2 mmol/liter glucose, and 0.90 g/liter protein.

A shadow of water density in left lower lobe is associated with pleural liquid or thickened pleura and displacement of trachea to right (Figure 37-1).

Tuberculin skin test causes 1.5-cm induration. Acid-fast bacilli are in gastric aspirate. CSF (nine specimens) is sterile. Culture of urine, kept for 8 weeks, grows micrococcus, *Streptococcus faecalis*, *Escherichia coli*, and no other organisms.

Diagnosis: Tuberculosis, Ghon tubercle in left lower lobe, *Mycobacterium tuberculosis* also beyond left bronchopulmonary (hilar) nodes, which with Ghon tubercle would form primary complex, beyond inferior tracheobronchial (carinal) nodes, and (continuing normal lymph drainage from left lower lobe) beyond right superior tracheobronchial nodes, in enlarged right tracheal (paratracheal) nodes, and perhaps, via blood, in brain.

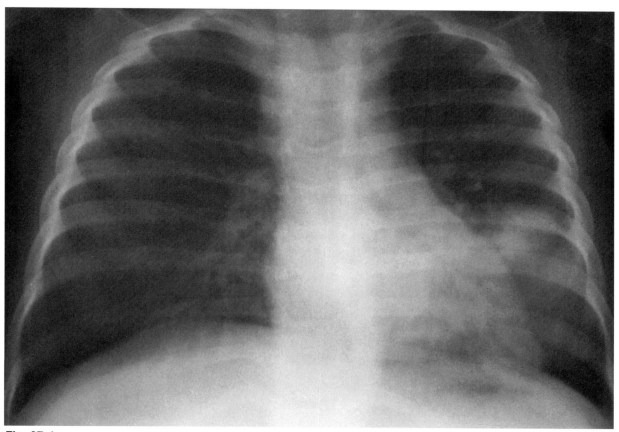

Fig. 37-1

Case 38

A 1-year-old girl has had a fever for 2 days and raspy breathing for a week. She has not been "her bubbly self" for 3 months.

Mother (31 years old) and three older half brothers are well. Father (61 years old) smokes 10 cigars a day and has been coughing for 6 months.

Temperature is 37.2°C, heart rate 140, respiratory rate 44, blood pressure 90/60 mm Hg, weight 9.9 kg, and height 79 cm. Cervical nodes are palpable. Eardrums are injected. Nose is runny. Pharynx is injected. Diminished percussion note, tubular breath sounds, and rales are in left side of chest. Liver edge is 1 cm below costal margin. The rest of the physical findings are normal.

Hematocrit is 0.32. White cell count is 12.9×10^9/liter with 0.64 polymorphonuclear cells, 0.34 lymphocytes, and 0.02 monocytes. Urine specific gravity is 1.005, pH 6. Urine has occasional epithelial cells/HPF and mucus. CSF has no cells, 4.3 mmol/liter glucose, and 0.14 g/liter protein. Throat culture grows α streptococci and *Haemophilus influenzae*.

Left upper lobe is distended with liquid in Figure 38-1.

She has 12-mm skin induration 2 days after skin test with PPD. Gastric aspirate has *Mycobacterium tuberculosis*.

Diagnosis: Primary tuberculosis (epituberculosis).

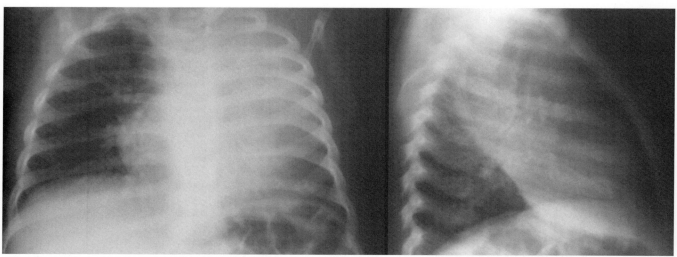

Fig. 38-1

Case 39

A 3-year-old boy is "more tired lately." He has been wheezing for 5 days.

Birth weight was 4.7 kg. He had six seizures at 4 months during which he became pale, eyes rolled back, mouth opened, and body and limbs jerked for 1–2 minutes.

A baby-sitter is being treated for tuberculosis.

Temperature is 36.7°C, heart rate 144, respiratory rate 40, blood pressure 116/76 mm Hg, and weight 19 kg. He wheezes during inspiration and expiration. Breath sounds are diminished on left side. The rest of the physical findings are normal.

Hematocrit is 0.35. White cell count is 15.0×10^9/liter with 0.52 polymorphonuclear cells, 0.36 bands, 0.06 lymphocytes, 0.03 monocytes, 0.01 eosinophils, 0.01 basophils, and 0.01 atypical lymphocytes. Platelet count is 556×10^9/liter. ESR is 15 mm/hr. Serum sodium is 142 mmol/liter, potassium 4.6, chloride 111, carbon dioxide 17, urea nitrogen 4.3, calcium 2.62, phosphorus 1.52, cholesterol 4.26, and glucose 4.7. Creatinine is 50 μmol/liter, uric acid 240, total bilirubin 3, and direct bilirubin 2. Total protein is 76 g/liter, albumin 49. Alkaline phosphatase is 242 U/liter, LDH 258, and SGOT 30.

Left lung is overaerated in Figure 39-1A. In Figure 39-1B, a mass of water density above heart is prominent, and barium is in esophagus and stomach. CT scan in Figure 39-2 shows masses of soft tissue density along ascending aorta, arch of aorta, left pulmonary artery, and left main bronchus.

At bronchoscopy, left main bronchus is compressed, its mucosa pale. Biopsy shows chronic inflammation. Culture grows normal flora.

Skin test with intermediate strength PPD causes 2-cm swelling.

Diagnosis: Primary tuberculosis.

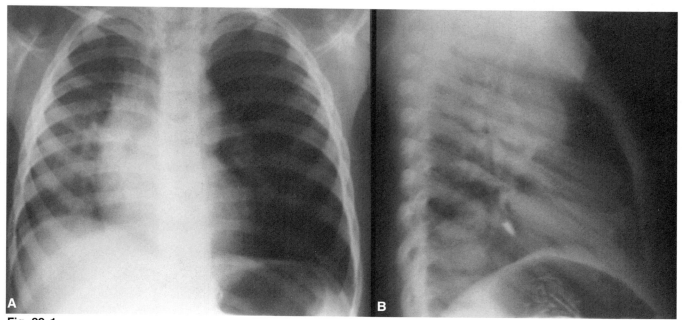

Fig. 39-1

(Continued)

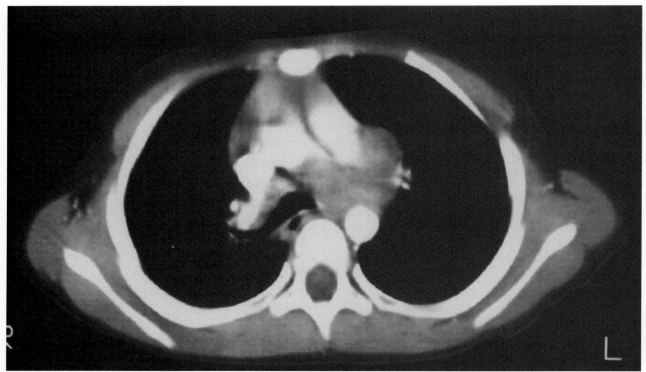

Fig. 39-2

Case 40

An 11-year-old girl is tired and not eating much.

Two weeks ago, she was sent home from school because she was tired. She coughs occasionally during the day. Right side of chest hurts when she breathes in.

Grandfather, who was being treated for tuberculosis, stayed with the family 5 months ago.

Temperature is 37.4°C, heart rate 100, respiratory rate 20, blood pressure 120/60 mm Hg, weight 31 kg, and height 140 cm. A small, firm lymph node is in left axilla. Breath sounds are diminished on right side. The rest of the physical findings are normal.

Hematocrit is 0.36. White cell count is 5.4×10^9/liter. Urine specific gravity is 1.010, pH 7.5. Urine has 2–4 white cells/HPF. Serum sodium is 141 mmol/liter, potassium 5.4, chloride 98, carbon dioxide 28, urea nitrogen 4.3, calcium 2.49, phosphorus 1.71, cholesterol 4.97, and glucose 4.5. Creatinine is 60 µmol/liter, uric acid 230, total bilirubin 3, and direct bilirubin 2. Total protein is 73 g/liter, albumin 39. Alkaline phosphatase is 245 U/liter, LDH 335, SGOT 30, and CK 26.

A small amount of liquid is in right pleural space in roentgenogram taken 10 days ago; an oval shadow of water density, presumably enlarged lymph nodes, is in left hilum (Figure 40-1A). More liquid is in the right pleural space today (Figure 40-1B).

A skin test for tuberculosis the next day shows a red, firm swelling (1.5 × 1.0 cm). Pleural liquid and two gastric aspirates are negative for *Mycobacterium tuberculosis* at eighth week.

Diagnosis: Primary tuberculosis.

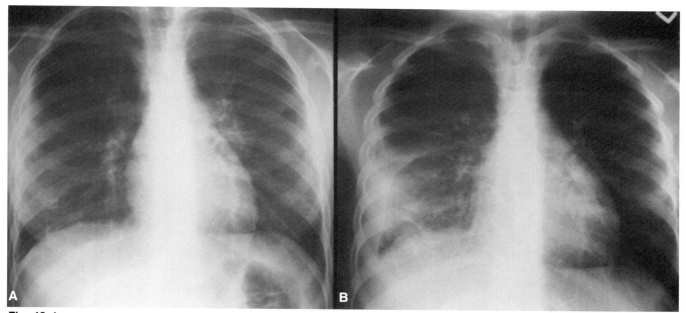

Fig. 40-1

Case 41

A 6-week-old boy has been coughing for 2 weeks.

Pregnancy was normal, birth weight 2.7 kg, and Apgar score 9/10 at 1 and 5 minutes.

Mother (23 years old) had a fever after he was born. He has been home with his mother for 3 weeks. A brother (2 years old) is well. Maternal grandmother and two maternal aunts were treated for tuberculosis 20 years ago.

Weight is 3 kg, length 48 cm, temperature 37.8°C, heart rate 180, respiratory rate 32, and systolic blood pressure 85 mm Hg. He is thin. The rest of the physical findings are normal.

Hematocrit is 0.31. White cell count is 21.1 × 10^9/liter with 0.30 polymorphonuclear cells, 0.59 bands, 0.09 lymphocytes, and 0.02 monocytes. Platelet number is slightly increased. Urine specific gravity is 1.008, pH 6. Urine has 0–1 cast/LPF, 1–2 white cells/HPF, rare red cells/HPF, 1–2 epithelial cells/HPF, and bacteria. On third day, serum sodium is 131 mmol/liter, potassium 4.6, and chloride 84. Creatinine is 60 µmol/liter. Total protein is 57 g/liter.

Shadows of water density are in lungs. Paratracheal soft tissues are thickened (Figure 41-1).

Mother began to have daily fever to 38.7°C the day after delivery. Culture of lochia grew *Escherichia coli* and coagulase-negative staphylococci. Six days after delivery, uterus was tender. Urine and blood cultures were negative. Two to 3 weeks after delivery, she began to cough up small amounts of white sputum, have chills, sweats, and headaches, and still had brown vaginal discharge.

Five weeks after delivery, mother's temperature is 38.7°C, heart rate 110, respiratory rate 20, and blood pressure 105/70 mm Hg. She is flushed and crying. Teeth are carious. Tongue is white. Percussion note and breath sounds are diminished in chest. Rales are in lungs. A systolic murmur is present. Uterus is enlarged. Uterus and adnexa are tender. The rest of the physical findings are normal.

Mother's hematocrit is 0.34. White cell count is 11.1 × 10^9/liter with 0.63 polymorphonuclear cells, 0.32 bands, 0.02 lymphocytes, and 0.03 monocytes. Platelet estimate is increased. Urine specific gravity is 1.020, pH 5.5. Urine has 3 casts/LPF, 20–30 white cells/HPF, occasional epithelial cells/HPF, and bacteria. Serum sodium is 135 mmol/liter, potassium 4.0, chloride 103, carbon dioxide 18, urea nitrogen 4.3, and glucose 4.6.

Roentgenogram of mother's chest 1 month before delivery shows normal findings (Figure 41-2A). One month after delivery, nodules of water density are in both lungs (Figure 41-2B).

Mother's skin test with intermediate strength PPD is negative. At 48 hours, son has slight redness at site of injection of PPD.

Mycobacterium tuberculosis is cultured from boy's tracheal and gastric aspirate and from mother's lung washing, CSF, urine, and cervix, but not from boy's urine or CSF.

Diagnosis: Primary tuberculosis in son, miliary tuberculosis in mother.

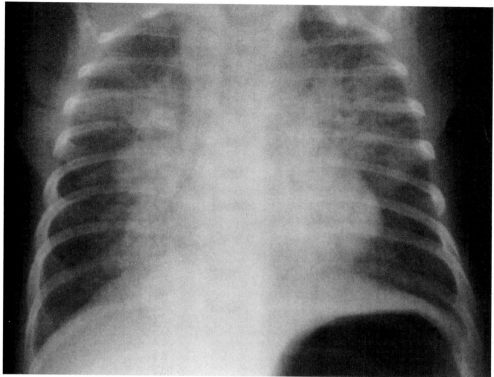

Fig. 41-1

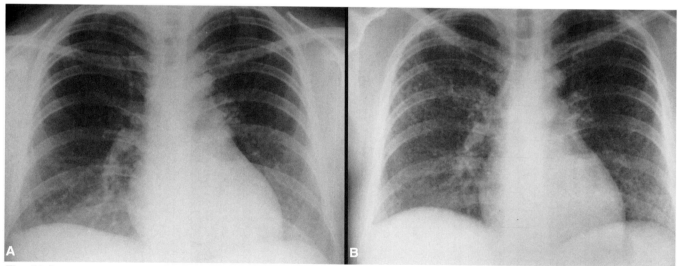

Fig. 41-2

Case 42

An 11-year-old girl has a swollen right thumb.

Right thigh was sore for a week several months ago. She has coughed occasionally for 2 months. She and some schoolmates tested tuberculin positive 2 months ago.

Parents and four siblings are well. Her mother works in a veterans' hospital.

Temperature is 37.8°C, heart rate 90, respiratory rate 24, blood pressure 100/60 mm Hg, weight 34 kg, and height 142 cm. Right first metacarpophalangeal joint is swollen. Liver edge is 2 cm below costal margin. The rest of the physical findings are normal.

Hemoglobin is 111 g/liter. White cell count is 9.9×10^9/liter with 0.42 polymorphonuclear cells, 0.21 bands, 0.17 lymphocytes, 0.10 monocytes, 0.03 eosinophils, 0.01 basophils, and 0.06 disintegrated cells. ESR is 26 mm/45 minutes. Urine specific gravity is 1.010, reaction acid. Urine has occasional white cells/HPF, occasional red cells/HPF, 3+ epithelial cells/HPF, bacteria, and amorphous urates.

Two weeks later, she complains of a stiff neck. Findings in physical examination of neck are normal. CSF has 173 × 10^6/liter white cells, 0.85 lymphocytes, 0.15 polymorphonuclear cells, 4.1 mmol/liter glucose, and 0.44 g/liter protein.

In Figure 42-1, heart size is normal; faint nodules of water density are in lungs; and supracardiac shadow is widened at level of hilum of right lung. Lateral soft tissues at right first metacarpophalangeal joint are thickened (Figure 42-2).

Skin test for tuberculosis is positive. Sixteen smears and cultures of throat, gastric fluid, CSF, urine, and pus from soft tissues at right first metacarpophalangeal joint are negative for *Mycobacterium tuberculosis*.

At operation on right thumb, 3 ml of thick, yellow-brown pus is obtained. A mass (1.5-cm diameter) of yellow-brown fatty granulation tissue is contiguous to metacarpophalangeal joint. Joint capsule is thickened. Microscopic examination shows muscle, fibrous connective tissue, and granulomatous inflammation with many giant cells around a core of caseation.

Diagnosis: Tuberculosis with right mediastinal lymph node enlargement (residuum of primary complex) and miliary and appendicular tuberculosis (hematogenous dissemination).

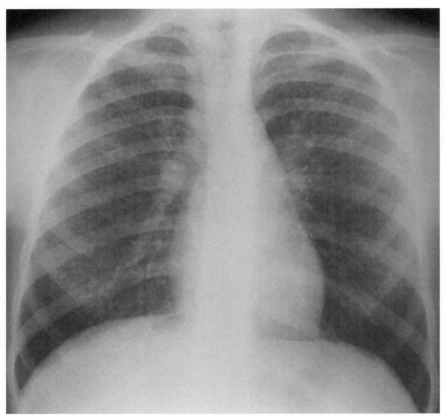

Fig. 42-1

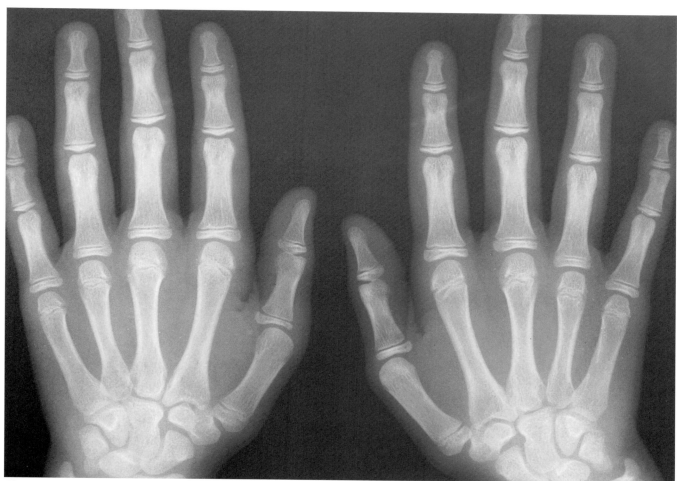

Fig. 42-2

Case 43

A 5½-year-old boy, who was treated for pneumonia 6 months ago when he had a cough, runny nose, and temperature of 40.6°C, is still coughing and febrile to 39.4–40.0°C. He has lost 3 kg. Three weeks ago, he began to sleep propped up on three pillows. Nose bled three times last week.

Mother had epilepsy. Birth weight was >4 kg. He has lived with maternal aunt and her husband, who have no children of their own, since he was 5 days old. He walked at 13 months. He has had chickenpox and, at 2 years, tonsillectomy and adenoidectomy. An uncle and his son, who lived with the family for several months 2 years ago, were found to have tuberculosis.

Temperature at 5½ years is 37.3°C, heart rate 128, respiratory rate 72, blood pressure 100/60 mm Hg, weight 12.5 kg, and height 103 cm. He is pale, cranky, and skinny. Bones stick out. He coughs up thick, yellow sputum and stains tissue with blood. He is barrel-chested. Respirations are shallow, rales in lungs. Liver edge is 7 cm below costal margin. Right kidney is palpable. The rest of the physical findings are normal.

Hematocrit is 0.37. White cell count is 16.8×10^9/liter with 0.80 polymorphonuclear cells, 0.02 bands, 0.16 lymphocytes, 0.01 eosinophils, and 0.01 disintegrated cells. ESR is 27 mm/45 minutes. Urine is cloudy yellow with specific gravity 1.015, pH 5.5, trace albumin, few bacteria, 1–3 red cells/HPF, and 20–30 white cells/HPF.

ECG findings are normal.

He has a bellyache and vomits breakfast 1 month after treatment is begun. He is tired, refuses lunch, and is then sweaty, pale, and coughing. He screams with bellyache in early afternoon, flexes legs on belly, and vomits mucus.

The new finding a month after first roentgenogram is right pneumothorax (Figure 43-1A). Excretory urogram 12 days after treatment is begun shows normal left calyces and pelvis at 12 minutes, faintly opacified right calyces, and normal bladder (Figure 43-1B).

Cultures of sputum, gastric aspirate, and urine grow *Mycobacterium tuberculosis*. Skin tests for tuberculosis, histoplasmosis, coccidioidomycosis, and blastomycosis are negative. Tuberculosis test becomes positive 2½ months after treatment is begun. At 9 years, he is cheerful and well. Weight is 24 kg.

Diaphragm is low at 11½ years, strips of water density are in lungs, and supracardiac shadow is slightly widened at level of hila (Figure 43-2).

Diagnosis: Miliary and renal tuberculosis.

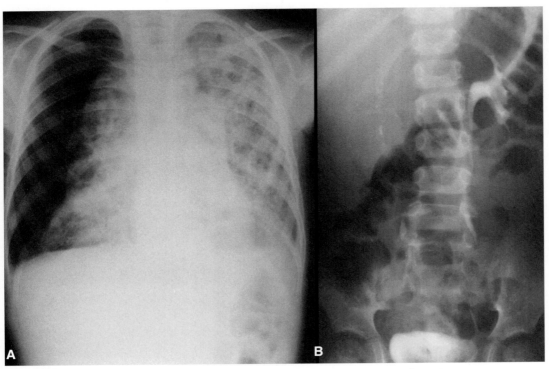

Fig. 43-1

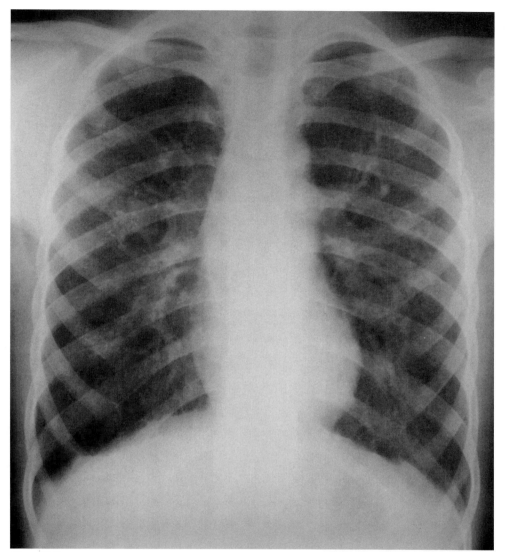

Fig. 43-2

Case 44

An 8-year-old girl is partially deaf in right ear.

She has had several painless ear infections with drainage from right ear for 2 years, usually after a cold. Left knee was operated on for tuberculosis at 2½ years.

Temperature at 8 years is 36.7°C, heart rate 90, respiratory rate 15, blood pressure 126/70 mm Hg, weight 26 kg, and height 146 cm. Left eardrum is red, right eardrum retracted around a central perforation. Tonsils are large. A systolic heart murmur is at apex. A scar is on left knee. The rest of the physical findings are normal.

Hematocrit is 0.39. White cell count is 5.8×10^9/liter with 0.45 polymorphonuclear cells, 0.04 bands, 0.45 lymphocytes, 0.05 monocytes, and 0.01 eosinophils. Urine specific gravity is 1.012, pH 5. Urine has occasional white cells/HPF.

In Figure 44-1, small spherical shadows of calcium density are in right lower lobe, several in apical segment, two in base. Shadows of calcium density are in hilum of right lung and in azygous node (see Figure 44-1).

Diagnosis: Calcified granulomas and lymph nodes, residua of primary tuberculosis.

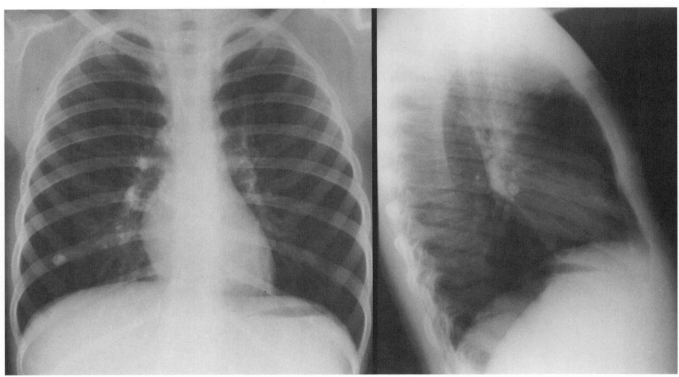

Fig. 44-1

Case 45

A 3-year-old girl, who has been tired for 2 weeks, is febrile now and sleeping much of the day.

She has had colds and ear infections. Tonsils and adenoids were removed and ear tubes put in several months ago.

Mother (27 years old), father (29 years old), and two sisters (4 and 6 years old) are well.

Temperature is 39.1°C, heart rate 164, respiratory rate 20, blood pressure 112/68 mm Hg, weight 16.3 kg, and height 86 cm. She is pale. Nose is runny. A tube is in each external acoustic meatus. Breath sounds are decreased on right. Liver edge is 4 cm below costal margin. The rest of the physical findings are normal.

Hematocrit is 0.26. White cell count is 43.9×10^9/liter with 0.60 polymorphonuclear cells, 0.06 bands, 0.17 lymphocytes, 0.08 monocytes, 0.06 eosinophils, 0.02 basophils, and 0.01 myelocytes. Platelet count is 728×10^9/liter. Urine specific gravity is 1.019, pH 8. Urine has few squamous epithelial cells/HPF, 1–3 white cells/HPF, and mucus. Serum sodium is 137 mmol/liter, potassium 4.3, chloride 100, carbon dioxide 24, urea nitrogen 2.0, calcium 2.35, phosphorus not determined, cholesterol 3.28, and glucose 4.9. Creatinine is 40 µmol/liter, uric acid 150, total bilirubin 5, and direct bilirubin 5. Total protein is 70 g/liter, albumin 29. Alkaline phosphatase is 376 U/liter, LDH 211, and SGOT 21.

In Figure 45-1A, a shadow of water density is in lateral segment of middle lobe, a less well-defined shadow is in medial part of superior segment of right lower lobe, and right side of supracardiac shadow is widened. In Figure 45-1B, pleura is slightly thickened at level of posterior midthorax in lateral view.

Skin tests for mumps, *Candida*, and tuberculosis are negative.

Acid-fast bacilli in gastric aspirate are found to belong to *Mycobacterium avium-intracellulare* complex.

Her response to antituberculous drugs waxes and wanes. Her peripheral lymphocytes show below normal response to concanavalin A and, in later test, below normal response to phytohemagglutinin and low-normal response to concanavalin A and pokeweed mitogen, when surface marker analysis shows decreased T helper and inducer cells (CD4+) and increased activator and memory T cells.

At right pneumonectomy at 8 years, pleura and pericardium are thickened. Adhesions are at hilum. Mediastinal nodes are large. She dies at 9 years.

Examination of both lungs shows that they are consolidated and crossed by firm tan-white fibrous bands. Bronchi are compressed, peribronchial lymph nodes firm with 1.0–1.5-cm diameter. Microscopic examination shows intra-alveolar foamy histiocytes with intracytoplasmic clusters of acid-fast bacilli, lymphocytes, neutrophils, few giant cells, no well-formed granulomas, and no caseation.

Diagnosis: Disseminated atypical mycobacterial infection.

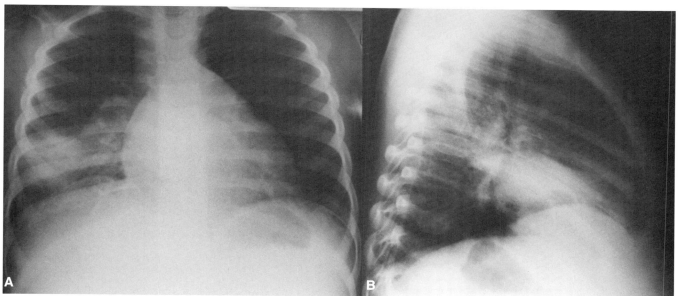

Fig. 45-1

Case 46

An 8-year-old boy, who went to Bakersfield, California, for 2 days 1 month ago with his father and jogged at his side, has had a cough, fever, and abdominal pain for 1 week. His father has had a cough and fever to 40°C for approximately 2 weeks.

No more clinical information is available.

An ill-defined shadow of water density is in anterior segment of right upper lobe of boy in examination on August 23, 1978, the year of dust storms in California (Figure 46-1) and in left upper lobe of father in examination on August 17, 1978 (Figure 46-2).

Both are sick for approximately 3 weeks.

Clinical Diagnosis: Coccidioidomycosis (Valley fever).

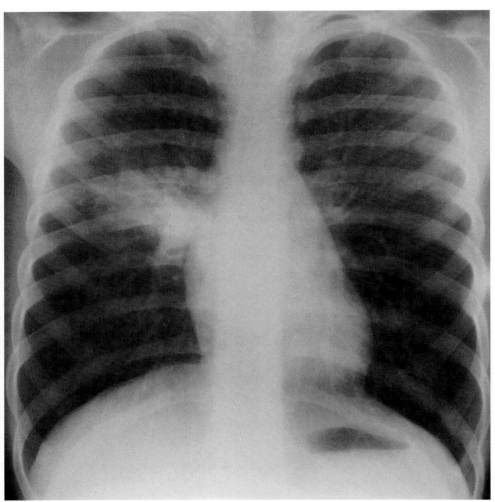

Fig. 46-1

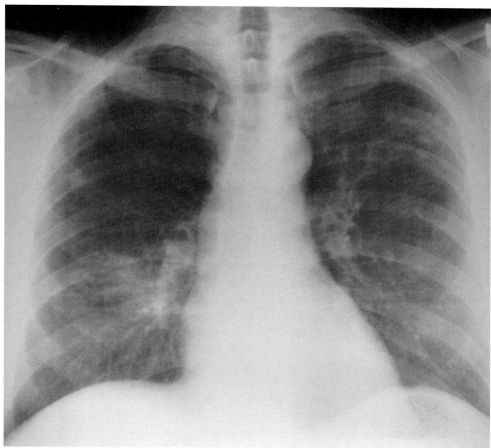

Fig. 46-2

Case 47

An 11-year-old girl has abdominal pain.

She had periumbilical pain and dry heaves 2 days ago, fever 1 day ago, and now has pain in lower abdomen that is worse when she stands or bends.

She lived in Bakersfield, California, until 8 months ago. She had pneumonia at 5 years, operation for right esotropia at 7 years.

Temperature at 11 years is 38°C, heart rate 136, respiratory rate 28, and blood pressure 120/80 mm Hg. Abdomen is full, lower half tender with guarding. Bowel sounds are diminished. Rectal examination hurts. The rest of the physical findings are normal.

Hematocrit is 0.40. White cell count is 8.9×10^9/liter with 0.14 polymorphonuclear cells, 0.69 bands, 0.13 lymphocytes, 0.03 monocytes, and 0.01 basophils. Urine specific gravity is 1.023, pH 5.5. Urine has 1+ glucose, 4+ acetone, 0–1 white cell/HPF, rare epithelial cells/HPF, and amorphous sediment.

A calcified granuloma is in mid–right lung (Figure 47-1).

At operation, perforated appendix and slightly cloudy, yellow peritoneal liquid are found.

Skin tests with intermediate strength PPD and histoplasmin are negative. Coccidioidin causes induration of 1.7 × 1.8 cm.

Diagnosis: Appendicitis with perforation, calcified granuloma in lung from coccidioidomycosis.

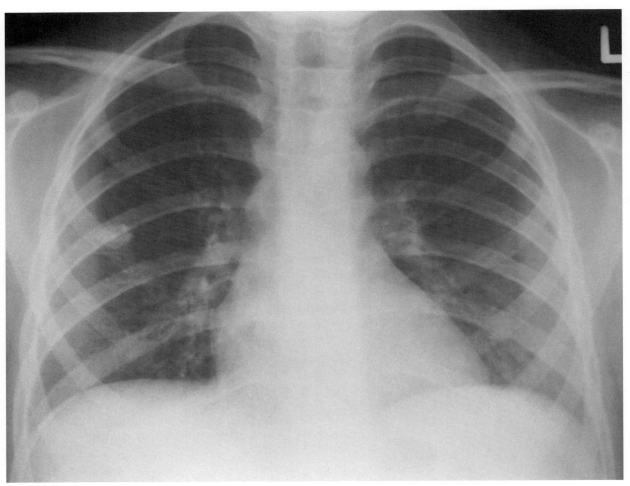

Fig. 47-1

Case 48

A 15-year-old Laotian boy has an abnormal finding in screening roentgenogram of the chest.

He had chest pain and coughed up blood at 4 years and had chest pain again 1 year ago, during forced march from Cambodia to Thailand.

Weight at 15 years is 34.5 kg, height 136 cm, temperature 37.7°C, heart rate 72, respiratory rate 20, and blood pressure 110/50 mm Hg. Physical findings are normal.

Hematocrit is 0.41. White cell count is 9.7×10^9/liter with 0.54 polymorphonuclear cells, 0.02 bands, 0.21 lymphocytes, 0.08 monocytes, and 0.15 eosinophils. ESR is 24 mm/hr. Urine specific gravity is 1.018, pH 6. Urine has 0–1 white cell/HPF. Serum sodium is 143 mmol/liter, potassium 3.1, chloride 107, carbon dioxide 23, urea nitrogen 4.6, calcium 2.54, phosphorus 1.65, cholesterol 3.70, and glucose 5.6. Creatinine is 30 µmol/liter, uric acid 390, total bilirubin 5, and direct bilirubin 0. Total protein is 83 g/liter, albumin 43. Alkaline phosphatase is 553 U/liter, LDH 309, and SGOT 19. Stool has rare *Trichostrongylus* ova. Three PPD skin tests are negative.

An ill-defined shadow of water density with thickened pleura or pleural liquid is in left upper lobe 7 months ago (Figure 48-1A). Cysts are also there now (Figure 48-1B).

At left thoracotomy, peribronchial lymph nodes are large. Thick pleura around left upper lobe contains many 3–5-mm foci of necrosis that smell bad when ruptured. Interconnected cysts (about 1-cm diameter) are in lung. A larger cyst contains lumpy, gray-yellow matter; another contains a smooth, elliptical, gray-brown mass ($1.0 \times 0.3 \times 0.1$ cm), in which smooth muscle, ovary, and vitellarium are present. Other cysts contain debris and birefringent, refractile eggs (some of them operculated) 100 µm long. Cyst walls of thick, sparsely cellular fibrous tissue and multinucleated giant cells are surrounded by cellular fibrous tissue, hemorrhage, dense infiltrates of eosinophils, lymphocytes, plasma cells, and compressed lung. Blood and inflammatory cells are in thickened interlobular septa. Yeast and fungi are not isolated during 4 weeks. Culture shows no growth.

Diagnosis: Paragonimiasis. (Serum titer for *Paragonimus westermani* is 1:128.)

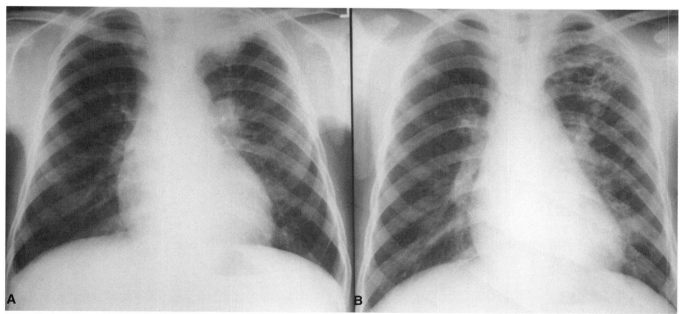

Fig. 48-1

Case 49

An 8-month-old girl has up to eight watery stools a day.

Right ear has drained for 3 months. Diarrhea began 2 weeks ago. She has been vomiting for 2 days.

Weight is 10.6 kg, length 72 cm, temperature 37.3°C, heart rate 156, respiratory rate 40, and systolic blood pressure 150 mm Hg. Mucous membranes are dry. Neck is stiff. Right eardrum is dull. She is edematous. The rest of the physical findings are normal.

Hematocrit is 0.42. White cell count is 47.4×10^9/liter with 0.77 polymorphonuclear cells, 0.16 bands, and 0.06 lymphocytes. Urine specific gravity is 1.006. Urine has 3–5 white cells/HPF, 12–15 epithelial cells/HPF. Serum sodium is 130 mmol/liter, potassium 5.5, chloride 104, and carbon dioxide 19. Total protein is 24 g/liter, albumin 8, IgG 0.25 (normal: 2.2–9.0), IgA 0.16 (normal: 0.08–0.80), and IgM 0.07 (normal: 0.35–1.25). CSF has 2×10^6/liter lymphocytes, 0.12 g/liter protein, 3.9 mmol/liter glucose, and is sterile. *Streptococcus pneumoniae* grows in blood culture.

Diarrhea persists. She is edematous despite IV infusions of albumin. Two weeks later, respiratory rate is 80, systolic blood pressure 110 mm Hg, and liver edge 2 cm below costal margin. Serum total protein is 50 g/liter, albumin 38.

Shadows of water density are in lungs (Figure 49-1).

Twenty hours after roentgenogram, capillary blood pH is 7.02 when $FIO_2 = 0.6$. PCO_2 is 59 mm Hg, PO_2 48. She is intubated. Her lymphocyte transformation test shows stimulation index with phytohemagglutinin 8.5 (normal: >130), concanavalin A 2.7 (normal: >40), pokeweed mitogen 2.9 (normal: >20), and no specific stimulation with *Candida albicans*, tetanus toxoid, PPD, or streptolysin.

Biopsy of lingula 1 week after roentgenogram shows alveolar cuboidal cell metaplasia, interstitial edema, fibroblast proliferation, atelectatic alveoli, macrophages in open alveoli, and occasional cells with large nuclei and intranuclear inclusions with clear halo.

Cytomegalovirus is isolated from lung and urine.

She dies at 9½ months. Necropsy shows (1) no primary or secondary follicles and no distinguishable cortical, paracortical, and medullary regions in lymph nodes; (2) round spaces (2.2 g) with amorphous to slightly granular, pale, eosinophilic material; scattered small lymphocytes; and no Hassall's corpuscles in thymus; (3) little white pulp and no lymph follicles in spleen; (4) no germinal centers in appendix; and (5) cytomegalovirus in lungs and pancreatic exocrine cells.

Diagnosis: Severe combined immune deficiency, cytomegalovirus infection.

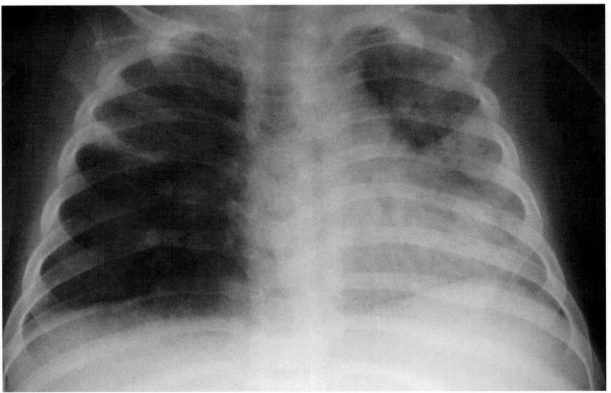

Fig 49-1

Case 50

A 6-year-old boy has a fever.

Birth weight was 3.1 kg, Apgar score 8/9 at 1 and 5 minutes. He had pneumococcal meningitis at 4 and 22 months and bloody urine at 4 years. In light microscopy, biopsy of right kidney showed mesangial expansion, segmental subepithelial and subendothelial irregularity, holes in mesangial matrix, and segmental thickening of glomerular basement membrane. In immunofluorescence microscopy, biopsy showed granular deposits of IgG in mesangium and glomerular capillary walls. In electron microscopy, biopsy showed electron-dense deposits in mesangium, segmental thickening, nodularity, and irregularity of basement membrane, and collapse of epithelial foot processes.

At 22 months, his C3 titer, assessed by hemolytic activity, is 0.01 normal, mother's 0.49, father's 0.59, two sisters' 0.62 and 0.37, and brother's, who is not of family haplotype, 2.00.

Parents, two sisters, and one brother are well. Paternal uncle has frequent infections.

Temperature at 6 years is 38.9°C, heart rate 136, respiratory rate 22, blood pressure 108/72 mm Hg, and weight 22.4 kg. Face is flushed. Hyperpigmented macules are on trunk and limbs. A systolic heart murmur is present. A scar is on right flank. The rest of the physical findings are normal.

Hematocrit is 0.44. White cell count is 25.0×10^9/liter with 0.57 polymorphonuclear cells, 0.19 bands, 0.17 lymphocytes, 0.03 monocytes, 0.02 eosinophils, and 0.02 basophils. Urine specific gravity is 1.022, pH 7. Urine has 1+ hemoglobin/myoglobin, 3–6 red cells/HPF, and 1–2 white cells/HPF. Serum sodium is 137 mmol/liter, potassium 5.1, and chloride 102. Creatinine is 40 μmol/liter. Total hemolytic complement is 7 and 61 kU/liter (normal: 75–160). Urine volume is 1,055 ml/day, creatinine 4.1 mmol/day, and creatinine clearance 1.10 ml/sec (normal: 1.24–2.08).

A shadow of water density is in middle lobe (Figure 50-1A) (contiguous to horizontal fissure in lateral view).

He is treated and afebrile the next day. At 8½ years, he has fever, headache, and red throat and, with treatment, is afebrile the next day.

A shadow of water density is in superior segment of lingula (Figure 50-1B).

Diagnosis: Meningitis, pneumonia, mesangiopathic glomerulonephritis in boy who has complement component 3 deficiency.

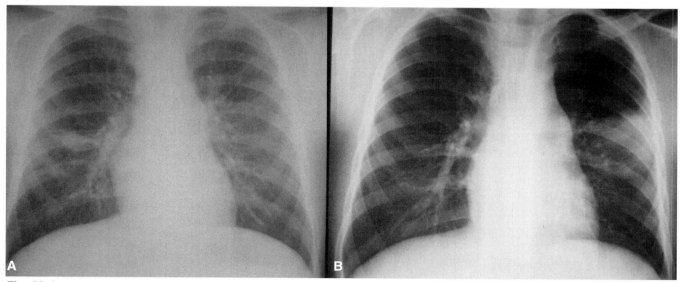

Fig. 50-1

Case 51

A 3½-year-old boy has had a fever and cough for 9 days.

Pregnancy of mother was normal, birth weight 3.3 kg. He had fever, hepatosplenomegaly, and microcytic anemia at 2½ years. At 3 years, he had a fever to 40.6°C for 2 weeks, a convulsion, perianal warts, and salmonella in urine. Stimulated nitroblue tetrazolium reduction test showed no strongly positive neutrophils in his blood, 0.51 strongly positive cells in mother's blood, and 0.24 strongly positive cells in half sister's blood. Oxygen consumption by his neutrophils was 0.26 mol/hr/10^8 cells (normal: 7.0–12.0).

Mother (29 years old), father (39 years old), and half sister (9 years old) are well.

Temperature at 3½ years is 38.5°C, heart rate 140, respiratory rate 62, blood pressure 120/60 mm Hg, and weight 13.7 kg. Throat is red. Rhonchi are in left lung. A systolic murmur is present. Liver edge is 7 cm below costal margin, spleen edge 3 cm. Papules and vesicles are on buttocks and thighs. Fingers are clubbed. The rest of the physical findings are normal.

Hematocrit is 0.32. Hemoglobin is 109 g/liter. Red blood cell count is 4.0×10^{12}/liter. MCV is 80 fl. MCH is 27 pg. MCHC is 340 g/liter. White cell count is 27.2×10^9/liter with 0.61 polymorphonuclear cells, 0.14 bands, 0.20 lymphocytes, 0.04 monocytes, and 0.01 eosinophils. Platelet count is 472×10^9/liter. Urine specific gravity is 1.028, pH 6. Urine has bacteria. Serum sodium is 141 mmol/liter, potassium 4.9, chloride 104, carbon dioxide 22, urea nitrogen 1.0, calcium 2.30, phosphorus 1.52, cholesterol 3.08, and glucose 6.7. Creatinine is 50 µmol/liter, uric acid 190, total bilirubin 3, and direct bilirubin 0. Total protein is 67 g/liter, albumin 34. Alkaline phosphatase is 183 U/liter, LDH 431, and SGOT 19. IgG is 7.0

g/liter (normal: approximately 4.6–12.4), IgA 0.16 (normal: 0.25–1.60), and IgM 0.88 (normal: 0.45–2.00). PT is 11 seconds (control: 10.2), activated PTT 42.7 (control: 34.8).

Biopsy of lingula at 3½ years shows firm, yellow-tan lung, much of it granulomas with epithelial cells, multinucleated giant cells, neutrophils, eosinophils, and few hyphae, one of them septate. Culture grows *Aspergillus fumigatus*.

At 3½ years, ill-defined nodules and strips of water density are in lungs. A curved shadow of water density is prominent at level of azygous node (Figure 51-1A). Upper part of left side of chest is opaque at 12½ years, left third rib expanded (Figure 51-1B). Metal sutures are in lungs near costophrenic angles after biopsy (see Figure 51-1B). CT scan at 12½ years shows left upper lobe mass and erosion of left third rib (Figure 51-2). Angiogram shows many small, irregular arteries in the mass (Figure 51-3).

At 6½ years, he does not play much. Liver and spleen are not palpable. At 12½ years, he is out of breath sooner than his friends. He hurts his left shoulder wrestling. Weight is 30 kg, height 137 cm. Tender left shoulder, left pleural rub, left diminished breath sounds, and surgical scars are present. ECG shows probable right ventricular hypertrophy; pulmonary function test shows mild restriction without response to bronchodilator.

At 13 years, he has an abscess on left side of chest from which *A. nidulans* is cultured. At 14 years, he has a fever, chills, headache, 4-kg weight loss in 1 month, and *Staphylococcus epidermidis* in blood.

Diagnosis: Chronic granulomatous disease.

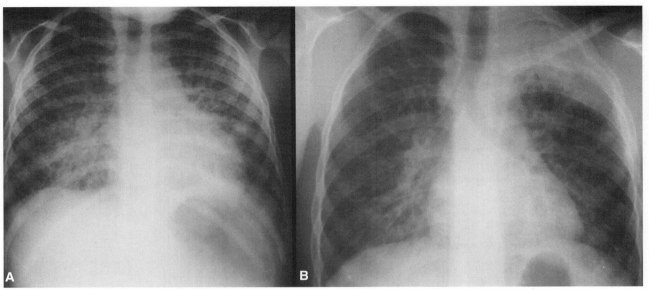

Fig. 51-1

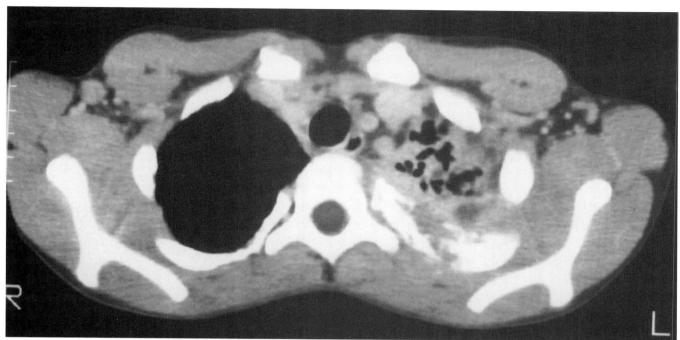

Fig. 51-2

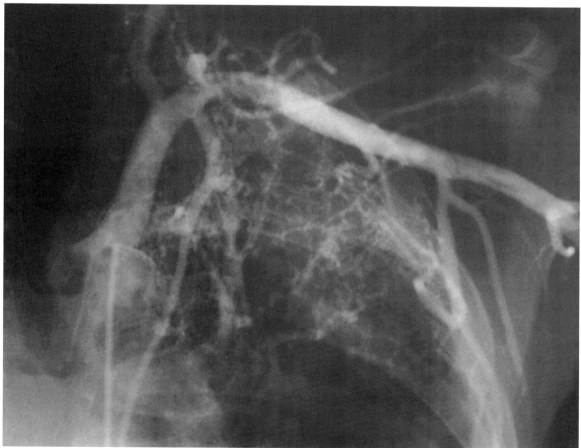

Fig. 51-3

Case 52

A 5-year-old girl has a cough and fever. She is being treated for acute lymphoblastic leukemia that was diagnosed 8 months ago.

Temperature is 40.8°C, heart rate 160, respiratory rate 28, blood pressure 100/60 mm Hg, weight 14.4 kg, and height 104 cm. She is pale. Rales are in lungs. Liver edge and spleen edge are 1 cm below costal margin. A paronychia is on right index finger. The rest of the physical findings are normal.

Hematocrit is 0.22. Hemoglobin is 77 g/liter. White cell count is 0.6×10^9/liter with 8 lymphocytes, 1 monocyte, and 1 eosinophil in 10 cells counted. Platelet count is 71 × 10^9/liter. Urine specific gravity is 1.021, pH 8. Urine has 2+ protein, 0–1 epithelial cell/HPF, rare white cells/HPF, rare red cells/HPF, and bacteria.

Ill-defined shadows of water density are in lower lobes, more in left lower lobe (Figure 52-1).

Needle aspirate of left lower lobe contains *Pneumocystis carinii*.

Diagnosis: Treated acute lymphoblastic leukemia; *P. carinii* pneumonia.

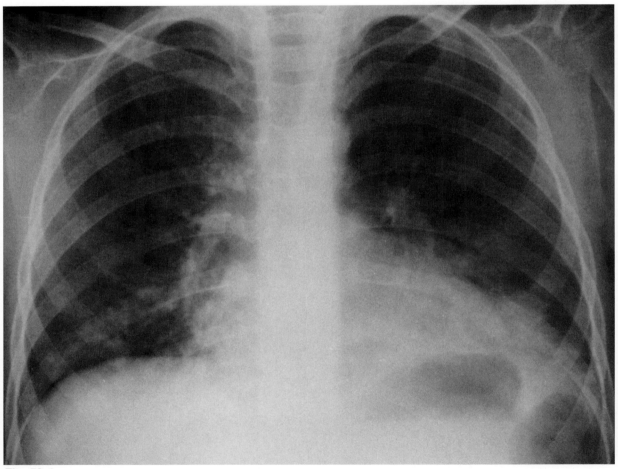

Fig. 52-1

Case 53

A 5½-month-old boy breathes noisily, retracts slightly, wheezes occasionally, and wakes up sometimes with coughing spells.

Birth weight was 4.0 kg, length 54 cm. He was fed only breast milk for 10 weeks. He had cough and runny nose at 2 months, ear infection and wheeze at 4 months. He still coughs and wheezes. He takes formula and eats rice and bananas. He is in day care during the week.

Mother (29 years old), father (32 years old), and sister (4 years old) are well.

Temperature is 37.6°C, heart rate 152, respiratory rate 40, systolic blood pressure 85 mm Hg, weight 9.4 kg, and length 69 cm. Subcostal tissues retract. Expiration is prolonged and sometimes wheezing. Liver edge is 1 cm below costal margin. The rest of the physical findings are normal.

Hematocrit is 0.36. White cell count is 11.8×10^9/liter with 0.26 polymorphonuclear cells, 0.13 bands, 0.41 lymphocytes, 0.14 monocytes, 0.02 eosinophils, 0.04 atypical lymphocytes, and 0.3×10^9/liter eosinophils. Platelet count is 549 ×

10^9/liter. Urine specific gravity is 1.003, pH 7. Urine has occasional squamous epithelial cells/HPF. Sweat chloride is 19 mmol/liter. Serum IgG is 2.3 g/liter (normal: 2.0–7.0), IgA 0.24 (normal: 0.04–0.80), IgM 0.37 (normal: 0.25–1.00). IgE is 55 μg/liter (normal: 1–24). Capillary blood pH is 7.40 when $F_{IO_2} = 0.20$. P_{CO_2} is 28 mm Hg, P_{O_2} 101.

Laryngoscopy and bronchoscopy show mild erythema along back wall of trachea and into main bronchi.

At 5½ months, roentgenogram of chest shows a segment of atelectasis in mid–right lung. At 6½ months, a roentgenogram, performed because he has respiratory infection and is breathing harder and coughing more, shows depressed diaphragm and chest deep front to back because of diffuse small airway obstruction (Figure 53-1). Left upper lobe is atelectatic 7 days later (Figure 53-2). Findings are normal on the tenth day.

Diagnosis: Reactive airway disease.

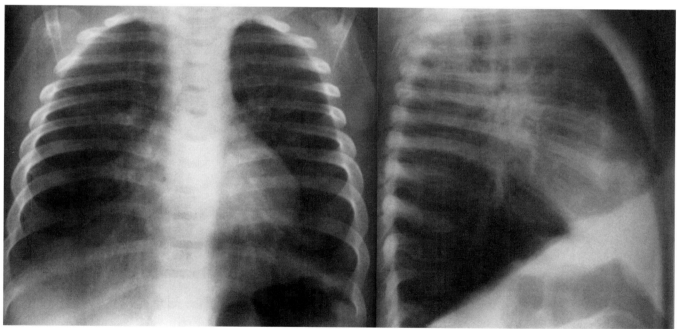

Fig. 53-1

(Continued)

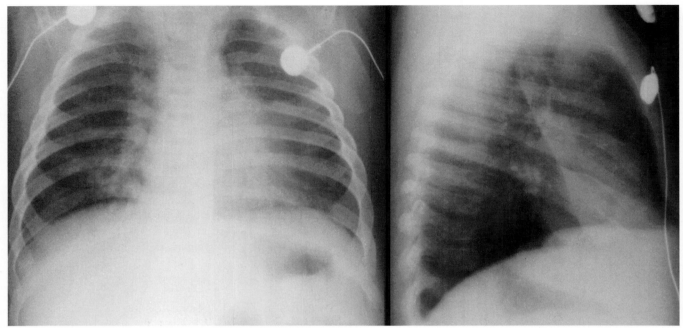

Fig. 53-2

Case 54

An 8-year-old boy has chest pain. He has been coughing and wheezing for 3 days and has gotten worse for several hours.

Pregnancy of mother was normal, birth weight 3.9 kg. He had cradle cap and eczema at 4 months, asthma at 2 years. He was operated on for cross-eyes at 2 years. He had fever, headache, abdominal pain, and knee pain 5 months ago and was weak for the next 3 months.

Father and two siblings have asthma.

Temperature at 8 years is 37.9°C, heart rate 104, respiratory rate 28, blood pressure 114/72 mm Hg, weight 24.4 kg, and height 125 cm. Skin of antecubital fossas, buttocks, and shins is red, scratched, and pustular. Dark circles are around eyes. Bridge of nose is creased. Breath sounds are diminished on right side. Rhonchi and expiratory wheezes are present. The rest of the physical findings are normal.

Hematocrit is 0.37. White cell count is 7.9×10^9/liter with 0.82 polymorphonuclear cells, 0.05 bands, 0.06 lymphocytes,

and 0.07 monocytes. Platelet count is 279×10^9/liter. Sweat chloride is 9 mmol/liter.

Heart moves to right, left lung is blacker, and left side of diaphragm is lower than right during inspiration (Figure 54-1A). Heart moves to midline, right lung is blacker than left, and left side of diaphragm is almost as high as right during expiration (Figure 54-1B).

At bronchoscopy, thick gray-brown mucus is sucked out of intermediate and right lower lobe bronchi. Culture of mucus grows coagulase-negative staphylococcus, *Neisseria* species, *Corynebacterium* species, and *Streptococcus viridans*.

Diagnosis: Asthma, eczema, and mucous plugs in intermediate and lower lobe bronchi of right lung.

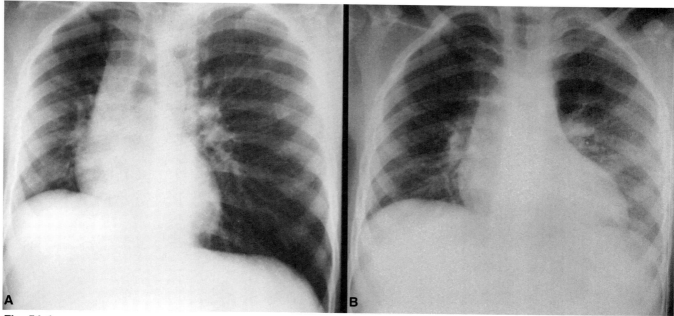

Fig. 54-1

Case 55

A 14-month-old boy is breathing irregularly after swallowing lighter fluid the night before Halloween. He choked, coughed, and foamed at the mouth. Eyes rolled back. Face flushed. The lighter fluid is 98% paraffin and 2% other hydrocarbons.

He sat at 9 months, walked at 13 months, and explores "enthusiastically."

Weight is 10.1 kg, temperature 35.7°C, heart rate 150–160, and blood pressure 114/60 mm Hg. Pupils are dilated. Mouth is blue. Limbs are floppy. The rest of the physical findings are normal. He is given vecuronium bromide, intubated, and given oxygen after heart rate oximetry shows oxygen saturation 0.76.

Hematocrit is 0.37. White cell count is 26.7×10^9/liter with 0.22 polymorphonuclear cells, 0.03 bands, 0.68 lymphocytes, 0.05 monocytes, 0.01 eosinophils, and 0.01 atypical lymphocytes. Platelet count is 531×10^9/liter. Serum sodium is 141 mmol/liter, potassium 3.7, chloride 112, carbon dioxide 21, urea nitrogen 8.6, and glucose 8.8. Creatinine is 40 µmol/liter.

Roentgenogram 1½ hours after ingestion and after placement of endotracheal and enteric tubes shows ill-defined shadows of water density in lungs and small heart (Figure 55-1A). Twelve hours later, shadows in lungs are larger (Figure 55-1B).

Diagnosis: Hydrocarbon pneumonia.

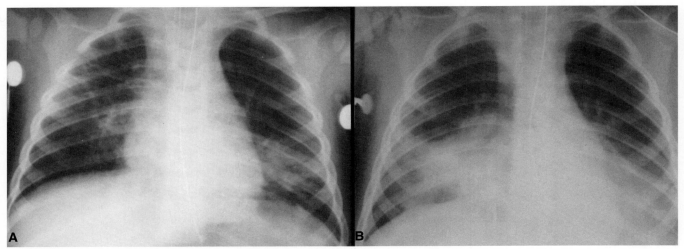

Fig. 55-1

Case 56

A 13-month-old girl is coughing and wheezing.

Cough started 6 months ago and became worse 3 months ago, when she began to "wheeze and rattle." Mother noticed 3 months ago that a broken piece of plastic ring from a toy could not be found.

Mother (25 years old) and father (30 years old) are well.

Pregnancy of mother was normal, birth weight 4 kg.

Temperature at 13 months is 36.4°C, heart rate 126, respiratory rate 30, systolic blood pressure 100 mm Hg, and weight 10.2 kg. Eardrums are dull. Throat is injected. Rhonchi are in lungs. Liver edge is 2 cm below costal margin. The rest of the physical findings are normal.

Hematocrit is 0.44. White cell count is 24.3×10^9/liter with 0.50 polymorphonuclear cells, 0.01 bands, 0.39 lymphocytes, 0.07 monocytes, and 0.03 basophils.

Right lung is blacker than left; thickened pleura or pleural liquid is on right (Figure 56-1). At fluoroscopy, heart moves to right during inspiration as volume of left lung increases, to left during expiration as volume of left lung decreases, while volume of right lung changes little.

At bronchoscopy, a curved piece of black plastic ($1.7 \times 0.5 \times 0.2$ cm) is removed from right main bronchus.

Diagnosis: Foreign body in right main bronchus.

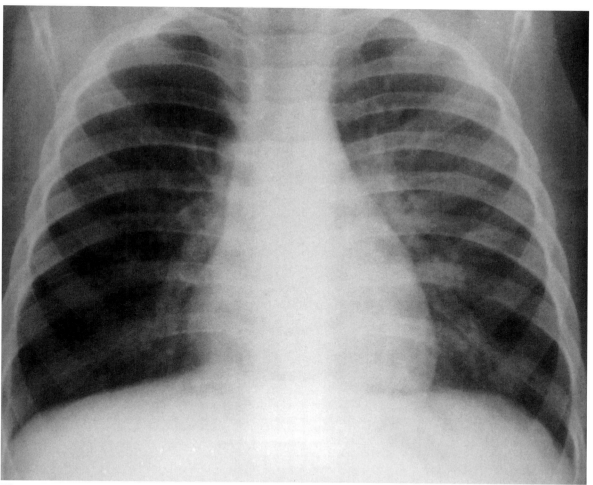

Fig. 56-1

Case 57

A 1-year-old boy is coughing and wheezing and has a stuffy nose.

Six days ago, he choked on a sunflower seed and spit the seed out after grandmother stuck her finger down his throat. He has coughed and had a fever for 5 days.

Parents have colds. Father has asthma. Members of mother's family have allergies and diabetes mellitus.

Temperature is 38.7°C, heart rate 160, respiratory rate 48, systolic blood pressure 120 mm Hg, weight 8.6 kg, and height 75 cm. Slight intercostal retractions and bilateral rhonchi and wheezes are in chest. The rest of the physical findings are normal.

Hematocrit is 0.34. White cell count is 8.6×10^9/liter with 0.30 polymorphonuclear cells, 0.29 bands, 0.36 lymphocytes, and 0.05 monocytes. ESR is 53 mm/hr. Urine specific gravity is 1.003, pH 8.5. Urine has occasional epithelial cells/HPF, triple phosphate crystals, and bacteria.

Right lung, unlike left, stays black and its markings do not change whether he lies right side down (Figure 57-1A) (gas bubble lateral in fundus of stomach) or left side down (Figure 57-1B) (bubble medial). Arrows point in direction of up side. Left side of diaphragm moves up >1 interspace when he is turned left side down; right side of diaphragm stays at level of tenth rib with either side down.

At bronchoscopy, firm, yellow fragments (aggregate size 1.0 × 1.0 × 0.2 cm) are removed from intermediate bronchus.

Diagnosis: Foreign body in intermediate bronchus of right lung.

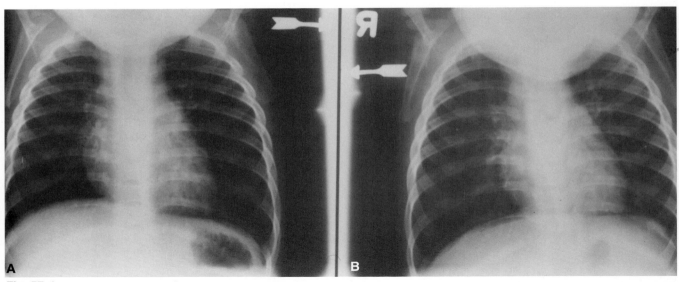

Fig. 57-1

Case 58

A 6½-year-old boy has had a cough for 1 year, sometimes with stuffy nose, sometimes with pink eardrum, sometimes with expiratory wheeze, sometimes with large cervical nodes, and sometimes with fever. Pulmonary function test shows mild obstructive defect.

Weight is 22 kg, height 117 cm, temperature 36.9°C, heart rate 100, respiratory rate 24, and blood pressure 104/78 mm Hg. Right eardrum is pink. Expiration is prolonged with wheezes on forced expiration. The rest of the physical findings are normal.

At 6 years, 2 months, hematocrit is 0.37. White cell count is 6.5 × 10⁹/liter with 0.59 polymorphonuclear cells, 0.02 bands, 0.33 lymphocytes, 0.03 monocytes, and 0.03 basophils. Platelet count is 394 × 10⁹/liter. Serum sodium is 138 mmol/liter, potassium 5.1, chloride 101, carbon dioxide 23, urea nitrogen 2.9, calcium 2.54, phosphorus 1.65, cholesterol 3.57, triglycerides 0.68, and glucose 4.7. Creatinine is 50 μmol/liter, uric acid 360, total bilirubin 7, and direct bilirubin 2. Total protein is 69 g/liter, albumin 42, IgG 10.8 (normal: 6.5–16.0), IgA 1.74 (normal: 0.35–2.00), and IgM 2.08 (normal: 0.45–2.00). Sweat chloride is 20 mmol/liter.

Findings are normal when he begins to cough at 5½ years (Figure 58-1A). Right upper lobe is atelectatic at 6 years, 2 months (Figure 58-1B), partly aerated at 6 years, 2½ months (Figure 58-2A), and atelectatic at 6½ years (Figure 58-2B).

At bronchoscopy, a flap of granulation tissue and soft, yellow matter obstruct right upper-lobe bronchus (eparterial bronchus).

Microscopic examination shows granulation tissue, squamous epithelium, and red-tan vegetable matter (1.0 × 0.5 × 0.5 cm).

At 6 years, 7½ months, bronchoscopy shows a small amount of granulation tissue at origin of right upper-lobe bronchus. Cough is gone. Physical findings are normal at 6 years, 9 months.

Diagnosis: Foreign body in right upper-lobe bronchus.

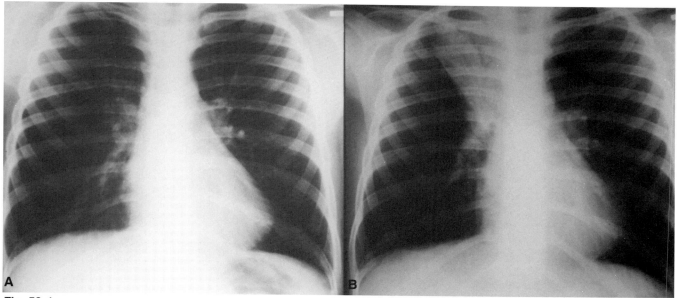

Fig. 58-1

(Continued)

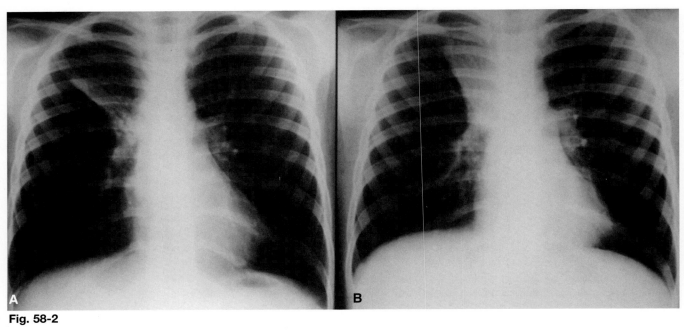

Fig. 58-2

Case 59

A 26-month-old boy drinks and urinates a lot.

Birth weight was 2.2 kg. Mother gave up breast-feeding because he pushed the nipple out when he tried to suck. He sweated a lot. His temperature went quickly from normal to 41°C. Hands and feet blanched. At 14 months, he drank liquids from a cup and ate only pureed foods, choked when he ate, had pneumonia, and spoke no words. Level of motor function was 11 months. He did not cry when he fell. No tears came when he did cry. Deep tendon reflexes were diminished. A scratch test with histamine and intradermal injection of histamine caused a weal without flare. During his second year, he had pneumonia once and otitis media three times. At 2 years, weight was 10.4 kg, length 74 cm, and head circumference 47 cm. A shifting, reticulated pattern of red and white was on body. Ulcers were on buttocks and perineum.

Mother (32 years old), father (29 years old), and sister (3 years old) are well. Parents are Ashkenazi Jews. Paternal grandfather has diabetes mellitus.

Temperature at 26 months is 37°C, heart rate 130, respiratory rate 24, and blood pressure 90/60 mm Hg. Tip of tongue is smooth. White plaques are on tongue. Rales are at lung bases. Muscles are thin. Deep tendon reflexes are absent in legs. The rest of the physical findings are normal.

Hematocrit is 0.34. White cell count is 8.4×10^9/liter with 0.66 polymorphonuclear cells, 0.19 bands, 0.11 lymphocytes, and 0.04 monocytes. Platelet count is 305×10^9/liter. Urine specific gravity is 1.001, pH 7. Urine is normal. Serum sodium is 154 mmol/liter (2 days later: 148), potassium 4.0, chloride 111, carbon dioxide 23, urea nitrogen 1.8, calcium 2.40, phosphorus 1.07, cholesterol 2.38, and glucose 5.5. Creatinine is 50 µmol/liter, uric acid 560, total bilirubin 7, and direct bilirubin 0. Total protein is 67 g/liter, albumin 35. Alkaline phosphatase is 232 U/liter, LDH 327, and SGOT 40. Plasma epinephrine is 2,724 pmol/liter in morning, 6,844 in evening (normal: ≤480). Norepinephrine is 8.5 nmol/liter in morning, 7.56 in evening (normal: 0.61–3.24), dopamine 0.21 in morning, 0.18 in evening (normal: ≤0.21). Plasma renin, when eating normal diet and lying supine, is 12.9 µg/hr/liter angiotensin 1 (normal: 1.7–11.2).

Ill-defined shadows of water density are confluent in much of lungs (Figure 59-1).

Diagnosis: Familial dysautonomia (Riley-Day syndrome), questionable aspiration, central diabetes insipidus. (Intranasal 1-deamino-8-D-arginine vasopressin mitigates his polyuria and polydipsia.)

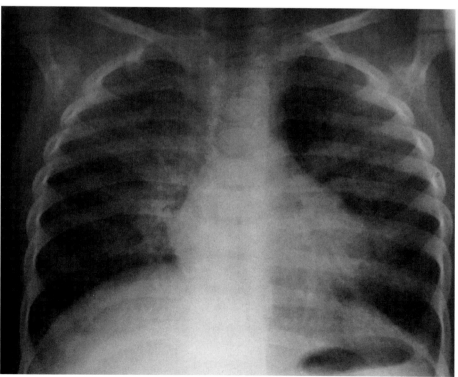

Fig. 59-1

Case 60

A 5-year-old boy, who saw double while watching television this morning, is choking on a graham cracker.

Back of knees began to ache 2 weeks ago. One and one-half weeks ago, he had a fever to 39.4°C that lasted 2 days. Five days ago, left upper lid and left side of mouth drooped. Voice was changed, gait "weaving." Elbows ache today.

Pregnancy of mother was normal, birth weight 3.7 kg, and Apgar score 8/8 at 1 and 5 minutes. He began to walk at 14 months. Immunizations are complete.

Mother (26 years old) had rheumatic fever; father (35 years old) has heart disease. Sister (9 years old) is well.

Temperature is 37.2°C, heart rate 108, respiratory rate 30, blood pressure 120/86 mm Hg, weight 15.9 kg, and height 102 cm. Pale blotches are on cheeks. He has to be helped to stand from sitting and cannot hop. Liver edge is 1 cm below costal margin. Deep tendon reflexes are absent at knees and ankles. Babinski's sign is in feet. The rest of the physical findings are normal.

Hematocrit is 0.39. White cell count is 10.9×10^9/liter with 0.23 polymorphonuclear cells, 0.63 lymphocytes, 0.10 mono-cytes, 0.02 eosinophils, and 0.02 atypical lymphocytes. Platelet count is 469×10^9/liter. Urine specific gravity is 1.026, pH 6. Urine has 1–2 white cells/HPF and mucus. Serum sodium is 137 mmol/liter, potassium 4.8, chloride 104, and urea nitrogen 5.4. Creatinine is 60 μmol/liter. CSF is clear and colorless and has 4×10^6/liter white cells, 2×10^6/liter red cells, 1.28 g/liter protein, and 3.3 mmol/liter glucose.

On fourth day, he chokes on soda and sees "two of everything." He cannot lift head the fifth day. He is itchy the sixth day. Blood pressure is 150/110 mm Hg. Breathing is noisy and hard the eighth day, easier the ninth day. On the tenth day, he is hungry and moves his arms. He is not choking when he drinks on the eleventh day. On the thirteenth day, soft tissues retract and alae nasi flare when he breathes.

Posterior basal segment of left lower lobe is atelectatic on the thirteenth day (Figure 60-1).

On the eighteenth day, cough is strong. After 1 month, he walks 15 meters with knees hyperextended and without support. At 11 years, neurologic findings are normal.

Diagnosis: Aspiration, Guillain-Barré syndrome.

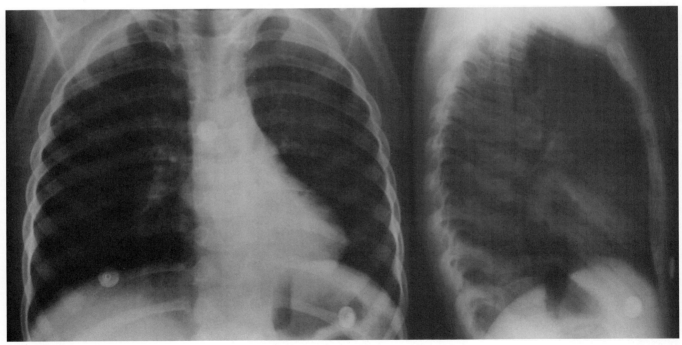

Fig. 60-1

Case 61

A 15-year-old boy is comatose.

His brother hit him on left side of face with his fist tonight in a fight that started over the noise from a radio. The boy fell to the floor, got up, said he had a headache, walked to a couch, and lapsed into coma. An ambulance was called, and a nasotracheal tube inserted.

Heart rate is 80, blood pressure 140/80 mm Hg. He is thin, pale, flaccid, and motionless except for breathing. Left side of face is bruised. Pink, frothy mucus comes out of tube. Diameter of left pupil is 5 mm; it reacts slowly to light. Right pupil is pinpoint. Breath sounds are coarse. No reflexes, including dilation of pupil when neck is scratched (ciliospinal), can be elicited. The rest of the physical findings are normal.

Hematocrit is 0.39. White cell count is 20.9×10^9/liter with 0.61 polymorphonuclear cells, 0.11 bands, 0.21 lymphocytes, and 0.07 monocytes. Venous blood pH is 7.24. P_{CO_2} is 45 mm Hg, P_{O_2} 29. Serum sodium is 126 mmol/liter, potassium 3.3, chloride 94, urea nitrogen 6.1, and glucose (after a bolus of IV 50% glucose) 17.9. PT is 11.5 seconds (control: 9.9), activated PTT 31.5 (control: 33.4).

CT scan in Figure 61-1 shows an elliptical shadow of increased density in left side of head, obliteration of left lateral ventricle, and swelling of left subcutaneous tissues. In Figure 61-2, excess liquid is in lungs (before IV fluids are given).

At left craniotomy, blood is in temporalis muscle, and blood oozes from temporal bone, which is fractured in front of left ear. An epidural hematoma (estimated volume 300 ml) displaces brain to right from in front of coronal suture to lambdoidal suture. Bleeding from middle meningeal artery stops with ligation after clot is removed.

Diagnosis: Skull fracture, torn middle meningeal artery, and epidural hematoma; pulmonary edema from increased systemic blood pressure in response to increased intracranial pressure (Cushing's phenomenon).

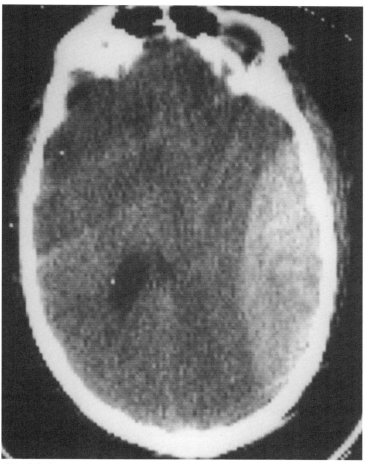

Fig. 61-1

(Continued)

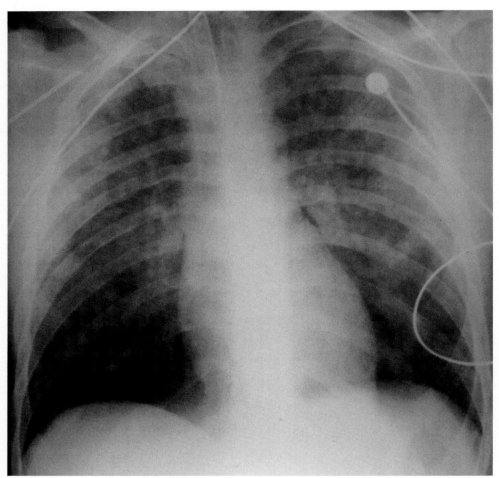

Fig. 61-2

Case 62

A 6-month-old boy has runny nose, large liver, and large spleen.

Birth weight was 3.6 kg. He can sit up.

Parents are well. He is their only child. Maternal grandmother has diabetes mellitus.

Temperature is 36.7°C, heart rate 140, respiratory rate 60, systolic blood pressure 100 mm Hg, weight 7.3 kg, length 69 cm, and head circumference 42 cm. Liver edge is 5 cm below costal margin, spleen edge 2–3 cm. The rest of the physical findings are normal.

Hematocrit is 0.36. Hemoglobin is 102 g/liter. Red blood cell count is 4.2×10^{12}/liter. MCV is 84 fl. MCH is 24 pg. MCHC is 290 g/liter. Reticulocyte fraction is 16×10^{-3}, white cell count 16.5×10^9/liter with 0.24 polymorphonuclear cells, 0.04 bands, 0.68 lymphocytes, 0.03 monocytes, and 0.01 eosinophils. Platelet count is 375×10^9/liter. Urine specific gravity is 1.010, pH 8. Urine is normal. Serum sodium is 141 mmol/liter, potassium 5.7, chloride 105, carbon dioxide 19, urea nitrogen 5.0, calcium 2.84, phosphorus 1.81, cholesterol 5.02, and glucose 5.9. Creatinine is 30 µmol/liter, uric acid 260, total bilirubin 9, and direct bilirubin 5. Total protein is 71 g/liter, albumin 51. Alkaline phosphatase is 318 U/liter, LDH 403, and SGOT 322. Marrow biopsy shows large histiocyte-like cells that, in electron microscopy, have pleomorphic lamellae-containing vacuoles with a ring around them and similar rings and lamellae in them. At 9 months, sphingomyelin activity of skin fibroblasts is 19 U (normal: 164). At 28 months, light microscopy of bone marrow shows storage cells with compact, round, central nuclei and pale, foamy cytoplasm.

Ophthalmologic findings are normal at 16 months. Edges of liver and spleen meet in right groin at 28 months. Nosebleeds occur between 28 months and 4 years. Fingers and toes are clubbed at 5 years. At 6 years, a systolic heart murmur is heard. Serum total bilirubin is 38 µmol/liter, direct bilirubin 14. PT is 14.5 seconds, activated PTT 69.6. Echocardiogram shows dilation of all heart chambers. At 9½ years, he has osteomyelitis of right foot caused by coagulase-positive staphylococci. At 11 years, he has left upper quadrant pain, tender spleen, and *Staphylococcus aureus* in blood culture.

At 28 months, nodules of water density are in lungs (Figure 62-1). Flanks bulge. Lungs are normal in roentgenogram at 6 months. At 6 years, femurs are flask-shaped and have postarrest growth lines (Figure 62-2). In CT scan at 11 years (Figure 62-3), liver is large and spleen larger; both contain foci of calcium density. Cysts are in spleen, liquid is lateral to spleen, and retroperitoneal lymph nodes are large in Figure 62-3.

At 11 years, spleen and wedge of liver are removed. Foamy macrophages are in both; necrosis is in spleen, fibrosis in liver. Electron-dense lamellar inclusions are in hepatocyte lysosomes.

He dies at 13 years with hyperkalemia, hypoalbuminemia, and anasarca.

Diagnosis: Niemann-Pick disease.

(Continued)

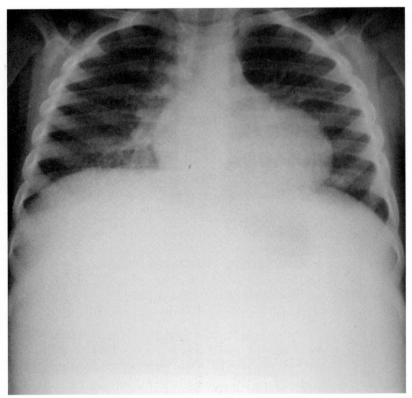

Fig. 62-1

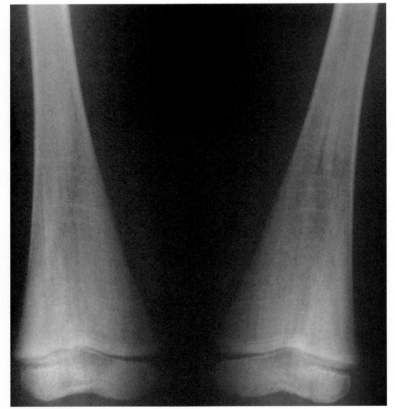

Fig. 62-2

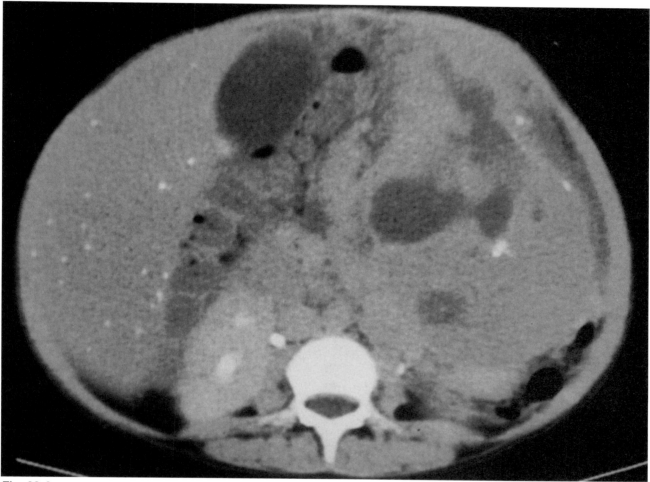

Fig. 62-3

Case 63

A 2-year-, 4-month-old girl is too weak to feed herself.

She and two siblings had a cough and fever 2 months ago. They recovered; she did not. She sleeps a lot. She vomited three times yesterday.

Father and two siblings are well. Mother has been treated for tuberculosis and anemia. Members of mother's family have asthma. Paternal grandmother has allergies.

Temperature is 38.4°C, heart rate 180, respiratory rate 46, blood pressure 95/60 mm Hg, weight 9.4 kg, and height 83 cm. She is pale. Sclerae are white. Gallop rhythm and systolic murmur are present. Liver edge is at umbilicus. The rest of the physical findings are normal.

Hematocrit is 0.09. Hemoglobin is 15 g/liter. MCV is 60 fl. MCH is 10 pg. MCHC is 120 g/liter. Reticulocyte fraction is 77×10^{-3}. White cell count is 12.0×10^9/liter. Platelet count is 783×10^9/liter. Red cells are Coombs' negative. Urine specific gravity is 1.009, pH 8.5. Urine has 2–4 white cells/HPF. Serum sodium is 132 mmol/liter, potassium 5.4, and urea nitrogen 5.4. Total bilirubin is 7 μmol/liter. Stool contains *Giardia lamblia*, *Entamoeba coli*, and *E. histolytica*.

Treatment with iron is begun. She is pale and has cough at 2 years, 8 months. At 3 years, 10 months, she has pain in left side of chest. Hematocrit is 0.30. Reticulocyte fraction is 30×10^{-3}. At 4 years, she coughs up blood. Bronchographic findings are normal. At 5 years, 10 months, she has fever, periumbilical pain, retractions, and rales. She stops drinking milk. At 11 years, she drinks a cup of milk and wheezes all night. Menarche is at 13 years. Physical findings are normal at 14 years.

At 3 years, 10 months, shadows of water density are in left lower lobe and right upper lobe (Figure 63-1A). Interstitial markings in lungs are excessive at 8½ years (Figure 63-1B), almost 3 years after she stops drinking milk.

Diagnosis: Pulmonary hemosiderosis, milk allergy (Heiner's syndrome).

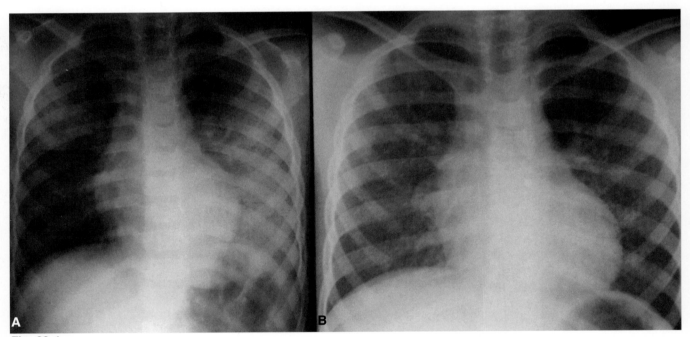

Fig. 63-1

Case 64

A 13-month-old girl is jaundiced.

Pregnancy of mother was normal, birth weight 3.7 kg. She had the first of six or seven ear infections at 3 months, chickenpox at 6 months, and roseola at 9 months. At 11 months, she scratched a diaper rash bloody. At 11 months, fever to 38.8°C and jaundice appeared. She has had three blood-streaked stools. She has had a runny nose and has eaten and played little for a week.

Mother (35 years old) and sister (6 years old) are well. Father (33 years old) had shingles and meningitis.

Temperature at 13 months is 37.8°C, heart rate 160, respiratory rate 36, systolic blood pressure 88 mm Hg, weight 8 kg, and length 71 cm. Sclerae and skin are yellow green. Yellow papules, scaly and bloody, are on scalp. External acoustic meatuses are blocked by wax. Spider angiomas are on trunk. A systolic murmur is present. Distended abdomen has an umbilical hernia. Liver edge is 6 cm below costal margin, spleen edge 2 cm. Large lymph nodes are in neck and groin. Skin of thighs is loose. The rest of the physical findings are normal.

Hematocrit is 0.29. White cell count is 32.8×10^9/liter with 0.70 polymorphonuclear cells, 0.03 bands, 0.24 lymphocytes, 0.02 monocytes, and 0.01 eosinophils. Platelet count is 865×10^9/liter. Urine is amber, with specific gravity 1.024, pH 6. Urine has 30.0 g/liter protein, 50 mg/liter ketones, trace reducing substances, 2–4 white cells/HPF, few bacteria, and mucus. Serum sodium is 133 mmol/liter, potassium 4.1, chloride 97, carbon dioxide 18, urea nitrogen 0.7, calcium 2.17, phosphorus 0.93, cholesterol 7.16, and glucose 5.9. Creatinine is 20 µmol/liter, uric acid 110, total bilirubin 239, direct bilirubin 132, and ammonia 46 (normal: 5–50). Total protein is 56 g/liter, albumin 25. Alkaline phosphatase is 976 U/liter, LDH 209, and SGOT 86. PT is 46 seconds, activated PTT 111.

Nodules and strands of water density are in lungs. Mediastinal image is widened on right. Gas-containing gut is displaced downward by large liver and large spleen (Figure 64-1).

Punch biopsy of scalp papule shows central loss of epidermis; peripheral parakeratosis and spongiosis; cells with eosinophilic cytoplasm and large, hyperchromatic nuclei, some bean-shaped; and poor dermal-epidermal demarcation. At 17 months, biopsy of large, firm, yellow-brown liver shows well-formed bile ducts, inflammatory cells, and varying amounts of fibrous tissue and biliary epithelium in enlarged portal triads, centrilobular bile in dilated canaliculi, and coarsely clumped PAS-positive material in Kupffer's cells.

At endoscopic retrograde cholecystopancreatography at 2½ years, intrahepatic ducts are attenuated as if by cirrhosis or infiltrative disease.

Diagnosis: Langerhans' cell histiocytosis, sclerosing cholangiolitis.

(Continued)

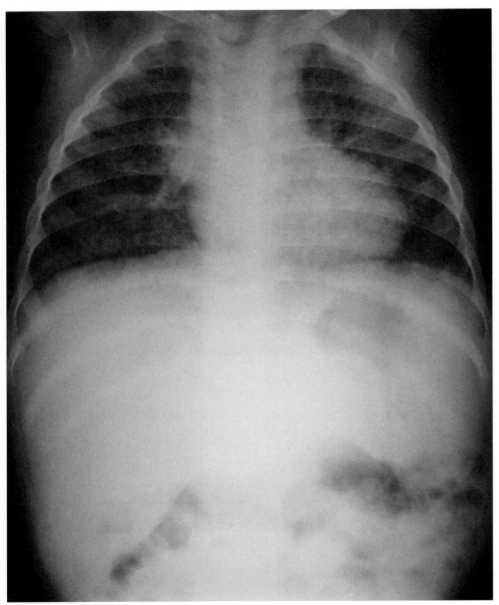

Fig. 64-1

Case 65

A 12-year-old boy has cough and fever. He is tired and eats little. He has felt sick for several weeks.

Pregnancy of mother was normal, birth weight 3.5 kg. At 9 years, he began to have one to two seizures per month in which he was conscious and "shook all over" for 15–25 minutes. At 10 years, he stumbled, "talked out of his head," and objected to noises.

Mother (33 years old), father (36 years old), and five siblings are well.

Temperature at 12 years is 37.6°C, heart rate 72, respiratory rate 18, blood pressure 120/68 mm Hg, weight 33.4 kg, and height 145 cm. Firm, nontender nodes (0.5–3.0 cm) are in neck, behind ears, above left clavicle, and in axillas and groins. The rest of the physical findings are normal.

Hemoglobin is 111 g/liter. White cell count is 4.5×10^9/liter with 0.44 polymorphonuclear cells, 0.40 lymphocytes, 0.07 monocytes, 0.07 eosinophils, and 0.02 basophils. Urine specific gravity is 1.012, reaction acid. Urine is normal. Serum calcium is 3.07 mmol/liter (in July), phosphorus 1.91. Total protein is 86 g/liter, albumin 45. Alkaline phosphatase is 80 U/liter.

In Figure 65-1, large shadows of water density are in lung hila, stringy markings in lungs and thickened pleura or pleural liquid is on right side. At 12 years, radiolucent defects are in proximal phalanx of left second digit and middle phalanx of fifth digit (Figure 65-2A). They are larger and the fingers are swollen at 15 years (Figure 65-2B).

A lymph node ($1.8 \times 1.0 \times 1.0$ cm), removed from right side of neck at 12 years, has firm, gray cut surface with follicles (<1-mm diameter). Microscopic examination shows replacement of node and salivary gland tissue near hilum by granulomas consisting of discrete clusters of epithelioid cells, some granulomas with central pink foci in which are few chronic inflammatory cells, mainly lymphocytes, scattered giant cells with peripheral nuclei, and many peripheral lymphocytes.

Hoarseness at 14 years is caused by white thickening of left ventricular fold and left laryngeal ventricle by aggregates of histiocytes, macrophages, and plasma cells. At 23 years, he cries in pain with headache. Speech is slurred and "crazy." CSF opening pressure is 280 mm Hg. CSF has 1×10^6/liter red cells, 47×10^6/liter white cells, 0.72 polymorphonuclear cells, 0.28 small lymphocytes, 2.1 mmol/liter glucose, and 9.12 g/liter protein. Cultures are sterile. Findings in cerebral angiogram are normal 1 month later. At 25 years, he has bilateral retinal detachment from uveitis and vitreal traction bands.

Diagnosis: Sarcoidosis with peripheral and pulmonary lymphadenopathy, skeletal defects, laryngitis, meningitis, uveitis, retinopathy, and hypercalcemia.

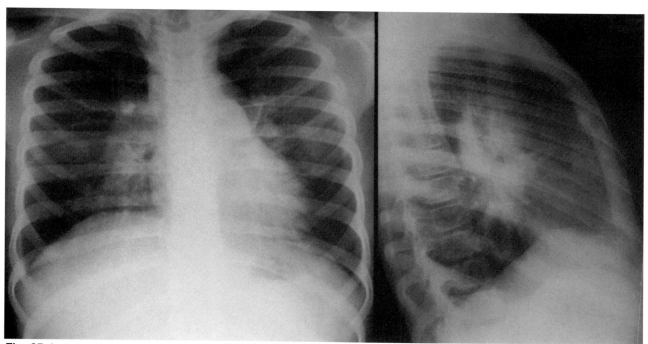

Fig. 65-1

(Continued)

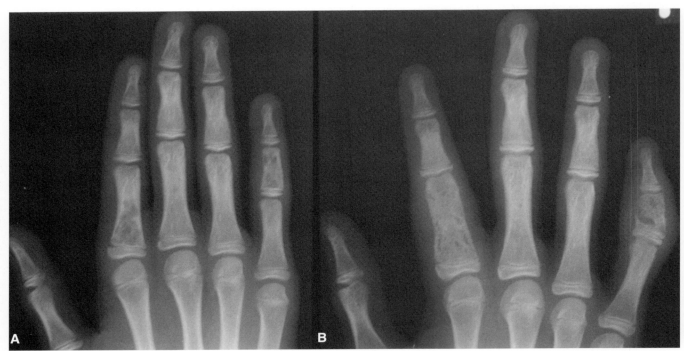

Fig. 65-2

Case 66

A 13-year-old boy is coughing and has pain in right side of chest.

He has had recurrences of cough and fever for 8 months. Cough is worse with exercise, cold air, and recumbency. He has lost 3 kg in the last month. At 6 years, tonsils and adenoids were removed and ear tubes placed.

Temperature at 13 years is 36.4°C, heart rate 88, respiratory rate 20, blood pressure 120/60 mm Hg, and weight 45 kg. Dullness to percussion, diminished breath sounds, and rales are at base of right lung. The rest of the physical findings are normal.

Hematocrit is 0.38. White cell count is 8.2×10^9/liter with 0.56 polymorphonuclear cells, 0.34 lymphocytes, and 0.10 monocytes. Platelet count is 240×10^9/liter. Arterial blood pH is 7.39 while he breathes room air. P_{CO_2} is 39 mm Hg, P_{O_2} 104. Bicarbonate is 23 mmol/liter, total carbon dioxide 24, and oxygen saturation 0.97.

A shadow of water density is in middle lobe, more in medial than lateral segment (Figure 66-1). Findings are similar in roentgenogram 8 months earlier.

Bronchoscopy shows a lobed white tumor surrounded by granular mucosa in middle-lobe bronchus. Microscopic examination shows respiratory mucosa; clusters of cells with uniform basophilic nuclei and moderate amounts of pale eosinophilic cytoplasm, indistinct margins, and fine fibrovascular septa; and no mitoses. Electron microscopy shows cells that have abundant mitochondria; well-developed Golgi complexes and rough endoplasmic reticulum; and neurosecretory-like granules with round, electron-dense cores, electron-lucent halos, and limiting membranes. Tumor cells stain with antibody to neuron-specific enolase.

Thick, vascular pleural adhesions and friable vessels are at thoracotomy. Visceral pleura is rough and gray, middle lobe consolidated, middle lobe bronchus obstructed by yellow-tan tumor that infiltrates lung, and red-brown fibrinous matter beyond tumor. Acute and chronic inflammation, abscesses, peribronchiolar lymphoid hyperplasia, and dense fibrosis are in middle lobe. Tumor is in peribronchial lymph nodes.

Diagnosis: Carcinoid tumor.

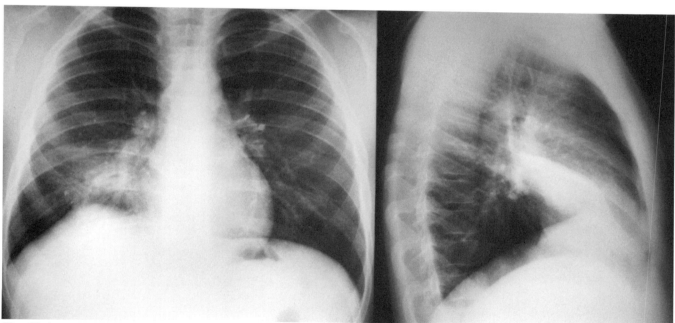

Fig. 66-1

Case 67

A 19-year-old man with laryngotracheal papillomatosis has fever, cough, and pain in the left side of the chest.

He skied 2 weeks ago but was short of breath. His voice got weaker. He began to have fever, chills, and night sweats. He coughed more, especially at night, and brought up green sputum, sometimes with pieces of tissue. Left side of chest hurts when he coughs. He has lost 2 kg.

His earliest words were whispered. He breathed hard at 2½ years. He "passed out" while playing. Mother learned that an early sign of trouble was suprasternal retraction. At 3 years, laryngoscopy showed papillomas in larynx and on undersurface of epiglottis. Tracheotomy was performed. Papillomas have been resected, later excised with lasers, 4–10 times per year. Microscopic examination has shown fibrous stalks covered by normally maturing squamous cells. Papillomas were mostly parastomal in trachea from 4–16 years, then from subglottis to openings of main bronchi. Tracheostomy tube was removed 1½ years ago.

Parents (both 47 years old) and two sisters (22 and 28 years old) are well.

Temperature at 19 years is 38.4°C, heart rate 90, respiratory rate 16, blood pressure 124/70 mm Hg, weight 57 kg, and height 173 cm. A scar is in neck. Percussion dullness, tactile fremitus, bronchophony, egophony, and diminished breath sounds are beneath left scapula. The rest of the physical findings are normal.

Hematocrit is 0.28 (2 months ago: 0.38). White cell count is 16.1×10^9/liter with 0.67 polymorphonuclear cells, 0.20 bands, 0.04 lymphocytes, 0.06 monocytes, and 0.03 eosinophils. Platelet count is 636×10^9/liter. Reticulocyte fraction is 11×10^{-3}. Serum sodium is 134 mmol/liter, potassium 4.4, chloride 100, carbon dioxide 26, urea nitrogen 3.9, calcium 2.54, phosphorus 1.23, cholesterol 2.17, and glucose 6.1. Creatinine is 50 µmol/liter, uric acid 290, total bilirubin 10, direct bilirubin 2, iron 1 (normal: 14–32), and iron-binding capacity 33 (normal: 45–82). Ferritin is 187 µg/liter (normal: 18–300). Total protein is 90 g/liter, albumin 32. Alkaline phosphatase is 148 U/liter, LDH 147, and SGOT 28.

A shadow of water density, distended in upper part, is in left lower lobe (Figure 67-1). CT scan shows pleural liquid and a mass of varying density in left side of chest (Figure 67-2).

At bronchoscopy, papillomas are in trachea and main bronchi, and pus is in left main bronchus. Firm, gray-white tissue is removed from left main bronchus.

Microscopic examination shows single and groups of atypical squamous cells beyond basement membrane and in underlying stroma, focal absence of elastic lamina propria, and abnormal mitoses. Tumor cells are large with pleomorphic nuclei and prominent nucleoli. Culture of pus grows *Neisseria, Streptococcus viridans,* Corynebacterium, *Eikenella corrodens, Haemophilus parainfluenzae,* and *Chaetomium* fungus.

Diagnosis: Laryngotracheal papillomatosus, squamous cell carcinoma.

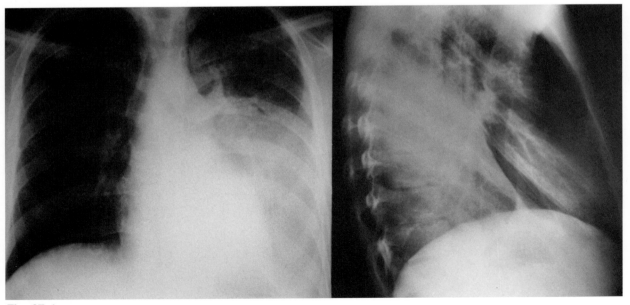

Fig. 67-1

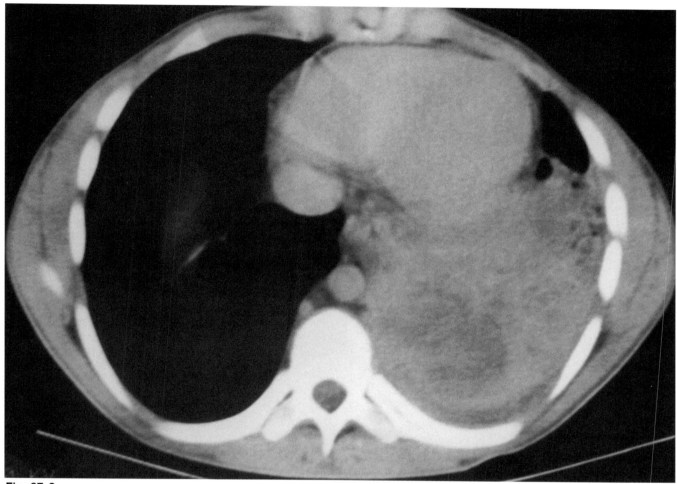

Fig. 67-2

Case 68

For 2 months, an 11-year-old girl has had chest pain when she runs or gets excited.

Mother thinks that she may have had roentgenogram during pregnancy. Family lived in Bakersfield, California, until girl was 2 years old.

Mother and maternal grandmother took thyroid pills for years. Paternal grandmother had breast cancer, paternal uncle has a brain tumor, and paternal cousin has leukemia. Maternal grandfather has diabetes mellitus.

Weight is 26 kg, height 132 cm. Cervical nodes are slightly enlarged and nontender. A systolic murmur is present. The rest of the physical findings are normal.

Hemoglobin is 133 g/liter. White cell count is 3.7×10^9/liter with 0.50 polymorphonuclear cells, 0.37 lymphocytes, 0.11 monocytes, 0.01 eosinophils, and 0.01 basophils. ESR is 7 mm/hr. IgE is 43 µg/liter (normal: 12–240). Sweat chloride is 19 mmol/liter. Angiotensin-converting enzyme is 70 U/liter (normal: <40). Coccidioidin skin test is negative.

At 13 years, cervical nodes are mobile, nontender, and 2 cm. Breasts are developing. Pubic hair is present. Serum sodium is 142 mmol/liter, potassium 4.5, chloride 104, carbon dioxide 19, urea nitrogen 4.3, calcium 2.57, phosphorus 1.03, cholesterol 4.03, and glucose 2.3. Creatinine is 80 µmol/liter, uric acid 170, total bilirubin 5, and direct bilirubin 0. Total protein is 74 g/liter, albumin 44. Alkaline phosphatase is 244 U/liter, LDH 226, and SGOT 19.

At 15 years, weight is 42 kg, temperature 37°C, heart rate 88, respiratory rate 16, and blood pressure 100/60 mm Hg. Cervical nodes are small. A systolic murmur is present. The rest of the physical findings are normal. Bronchoscopic findings are normal. Microscopic examination of transbronchial specimens shows macrophages in alveoli and slight interstitial fibrosis.

At 17 years, cervical nodes are 4–5 cm, firm, and mobile.

Nodules of water density are in lungs at 11 years (Figure 68-1A). At 17 years, the nodules have increased in number and size (Figure 68-1B), a month after excision of a piece of middle lobe.

At operation a month before second roentgenogram, two large cervical nodes, a piece of right lung, and thyroid gland are removed. Right lobe of thyroid gland is irregular. Tumor is in sternothyroid muscle. Adjacent tissues are fibrosed and vascular.

Microscopic examination of thyroid gland, lymph node, and lung shows cells with uniform, round nuclei and homogeneous chromatin; aggregates of cells around eosinophilic colloid; and scattered psammoma bodies. Size of lung nodules vary; some are smaller than ½ HPF.

She is clinically euthyroid 1 month after operation. Thyroid scan shows 60% uptake at 14 hours, 13% in lungs, rest in neck.

Diagnosis: Metastatic papillary adenocarcinoma of thyroid gland.

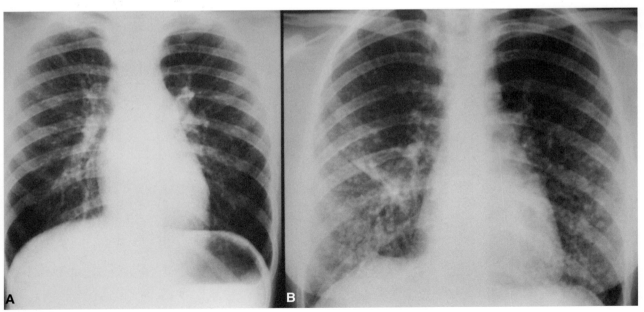

Fig. 68-1

Case 69

A 9-year-old girl is coughing, sweating, and short of breath.

She has lost 4.5 kg in 2 months. She has been waking at night with shoulder pain for several weeks, weak and pale for 2 weeks, and coughing a lot and sweating for several days.

Birth weight was 3.3 kg. She was operated on at 3 and 4 years for juvenile aponeurotic fibroma of left palm. She broke right forearm at 7 and 8 years.

Mother (28 years old) had hysterectomy for fibroids 2 years ago. Father (30 years old) and two sisters (7 and 11 years old) are well. Maternal grandfather had lipoma. Maternal great-aunt had uterine cancer and another maternal great-aunt benign tumors of breast, back, and throat. Maternal great-great-aunt had cervical cancer. Maternal great-great-uncle had kidney cancer and another maternal great-great-uncle had lung cancer. Maternal great-great-grandmother had colon cancer. Maternal great-great-grandfather had skin tumors.

Weight at 9 years is 30.5 kg, height 131 cm, temperature 37.5°C, heart rate 110, respiratory rate 20, and blood pressure 110/70 mm Hg. Right shoulder is higher than left. Small lymph nodes are in neck and groin. Pleural rub, diminished tactile fremitus, and diminished breath sounds are in right side of chest. The rest of the physical findings are normal.

Hematocrit is 0.36. White cell count is 9.2×10^9/liter with 0.57 polymorphonuclear cells, 0.01 bands, 0.31 lymphocytes, 0.07 monocytes, 0.01 eosinophils, and 0.03 atypical lympho-cytes. Platelet count is 494×10^9/liter. ESR is 102 mm/hr. Serum sodium is 133 mmol/liter, potassium 4.1, chloride 102, carbon dioxide 20, urea nitrogen 2.5, calcium 2.45, phosphorus 1.32, cholesterol 3.57, and glucose 6.3. Creatinine is 50 μmol/liter, uric acid 120, total bilirubin 3, and direct bilirubin 0. Total protein is 72 g/liter, albumin 38. Alkaline phosphatase is 180 U/liter, LDH 281, and SGOT 20.

Masses of water density are in right side of chest and in superior and medial part of posterior basal segment of left lower lobe, just left of T10 (Figure 69-1). Radiolucent defects are in metaphyses at knees (Figure 69-2A). A smaller radiolucent defect is in proximal metaphysis of humeri, distal part of shaft of left radius, and a parietal bone. Middle phalanges of second and fifth digits, distal phalanges of thumbs, and fifth metacarpals (and left first metatarsal) are shorter than normal (Figure 69-2B).

At right thoracotomy, cream-colored tumor is on pleura, in lung, and in mediastinal lymph nodes.

Microscopic examination shows parallel fascicles of large spindle cells with abundant eosinophilic cytoplasm and large, spindle to oval nuclei with coarsely clumped chromatin, intercellular edema, focal hemorrhage and necrosis, and 1 mitosis/HPF. She dies 4 months later.

Diagnosis: Fibrosarcoma, brachydactyly, family tumors; juvenile aponeurotic fibroma.

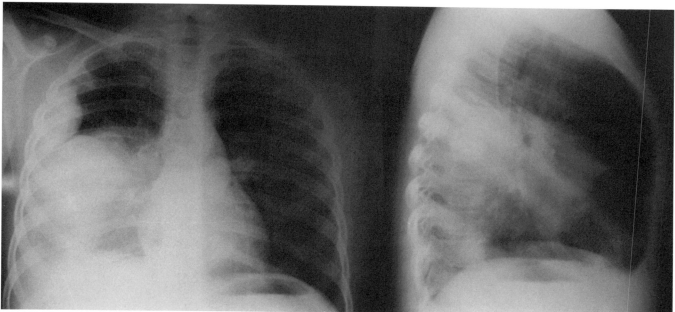

Fig 69-1

(Continued)

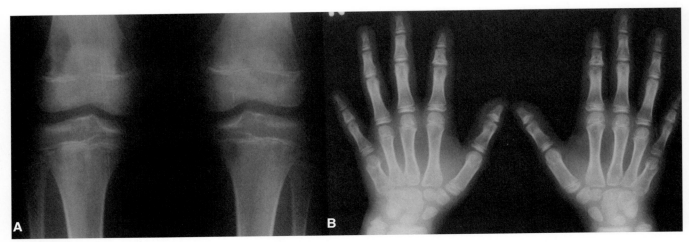

Fig. 69-2

Case 70

A 4-year-old boy has a murmur that was heard during examination for respiratory infection 2 weeks ago.

Pregnancy of mother was normal, birth weight 2.7 kg. He sat at 9 months, walked at 22 months, and is "extremely active."

Mother (34 years old), father (34 years old), two brothers (6 and 10 years old), and sister (8 years old) are well.

Temperature is 37.7°C, heart rate 140, respiratory rate 24, blood pressure 100/56 mm Hg, weight 12 kg, and height 101 cm. Right eardrum is scarred. Teeth are carious. Systolic murmur is widely transmitted. The rest of the physical findings are normal.

Hematocrit is 0.34. White cell count is 9.4×10^9/liter with 0.44 polymorphonuclear cells, 0.46 lymphocytes, 0.06 monocytes, and 0.04 eosinophils. Platelet estimate is adequate. Urine specific gravity is 1.014, pH 6. Urine has 0–1 white cell/HPF and bacteria.

ECG shows right axis deviation and right ventricular hypertrophy.

Roentgenogram of chest in Figure 70-1A shows normal findings.

At cardiac catheterization, right atrial mean pressure is 2 mm Hg, right ventricular pressure 95/7, main pulmonary artery mean pressure 48, left pulmonary artery mean pressure 15, and distal left pulmonary artery mean pressure 4. No shunt is present.

Right ventricular angiocardiogram in Figure 70-1B shows stenoses at origins of lobar pulmonary arteries.

At 20 years, he has no symptoms. Weight is 52 kg, height 169 cm. A systolic murmur is present. The rest of the physical findings and ECG and echocardiographic findings are normal.

Diagnosis: Peripheral pulmonic stenosis.

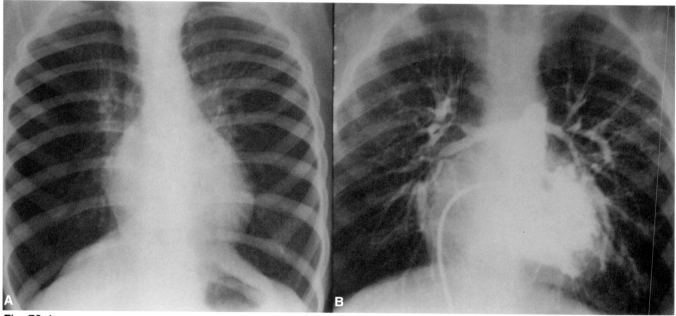

Fig. 70-1

Case 71

A 12-year-old girl has been "winded, out of breath" for 6 weeks. She feels her heart pounding when she walks fast and has pain in left side of chest.

Brother (14 years old) became short of breath 1 year ago, began to cough and vomit 6 months ago when his FEV and forced vital capacity were 60% of predicted level, and died 5 months ago. Parents are well.

Temperature is 36.7°C, heart rate 60, respiratory rate 28, blood pressure 112/64 mm Hg, weight 43 kg, and height 157 cm. Precordial impulse is hyperdynamic; S_2 is narrowly split and loud. The rest of the physical findings are normal.

Examination of brother's chest 2 weeks before his death shows large heart, ill-defined streaks of water density in lungs, and thickened pleura or pleural liquid (Figure 71-1A). Roentgenogram of girl's chest 2½ months ago (1 month before her symptoms began) shows less marked, but similar findings (Figure 71-1B).

ECG shows right axis deviation. Echocardiogram shows enlargement of right ventricle. At cardiac catheterization, pulmonary artery pressure is 70/37 mm Hg, mean 50, unresponsive to oxygen and vasodilators. Mean pulmonary artery wedge pressure is 5 mm Hg. Pulmonary function testing shows moderately severe restrictive impairment with lung volume 0.40 of predicted value.

Three weeks later, hematocrit is 0.41. White cell count is 13.7×10^9/liter with 0.67 polymorphonuclear cells, 0.03 bands, 0.14 lymphocytes, 0.04 monocytes, 0.09 eosinophils, and 0.03 basophils. Platelet count is 306×10^9/liter. Serum sodium is 140 mmol/liter, potassium 3.9, chloride 106, carbon dioxide 23, urea nitrogen 3.9, calcium 2.42, phosphorus 1.42, cholesterol 3.88, and glucose 3.9. Creatinine is 80 μmol/liter, uric acid 330, total bilirubin 22, and direct bilirubin not determined. Total protein is 74 g/liter, albumin 40. Alkaline phosphatase is 180 U/liter, LDH 306, and SGOT 28.

She dies 6 months after roentgenogram.

Diagnosis: Pulmonary veno-occlusive disease in sister and brother.*

*Necropsy findings were reported by P Davis, L Reid. Pulmonary veno-occlusive disease in siblings: case report and morphometric study. Hum Pathol 13:911, 1982.

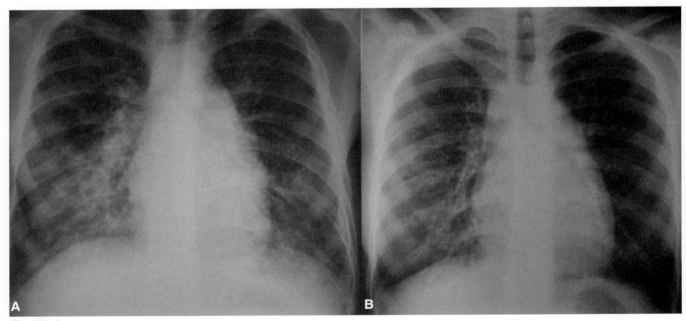

Fig. 71-1

Case 72

A 14-year-old girl slurs words and cannot name common objects.

She fainted twice 7 months ago. She has felt lightheaded and had headaches for several months. She was lying on the stairs at home this morning. She did not know where she was. Right side of face and left side of body were weak.

Birth weight was 3.6 kg. At 9 months, she had a febrile convulsion. She had ear infections. She broke left arm at 12 years. Pus was in left ear at 13 years.

Mother (43 years old), father (49 years old), brother (18 years old), and sister (11 years old) are well.

Temperature is 37.3°C, heart rate 76, respiratory rate 20, blood pressure 128/88 mm Hg, weight 55 kg, and height 163 cm. She is groggy. She has right facial palsy. Lips pucker when tapped (*snout reflex*). Babinski's sign is in left foot. The rest of the physical findings are normal.

Hematocrit is 0.43. White cell count is 9.2×10^9/liter with 0.82 polymorphonuclear cells, 0.03 bands, 0.13 lymphocytes, and 0.02 monocytes. Urine specific gravity is 1.020, pH 7. Urine has hemoglobin/myoglobin, bacteria, occasional squa-

mous epithelial cells/HPF, and 0–1 red cell/HPF. Serum sodium is 141 mmol/liter, potassium 4.3, chloride 106, carbon dioxide 24, urea nitrogen 3.2, calcium 2.54, phosphorus 1.13, cholesterol 4.84, and glucose 6.0. Creatinine is 60 μmol/liter, uric acid 180, total bilirubin 10, and direct bilirubin 2. Total protein is 84 g/liter, albumin 51. Alkaline phosphatase is 87 U/liter, LDH 217, and SGOT 21.

A curved shadow of water density is in left upper lobe (Figure 72-1). Left pulmonary angiogram shows contrast medium in normal arteries (Figure 72-2A) and later in curved tube that drains into left atrium (Figure 72-2B).

At operation, an abnormal vessel (largest diameter: 2 cm) with turbulent flow is on medial surface of left upper lobe just in front of pulmonary artery.

Examination of resected left upper lobe shows many thin-walled vessels (0.3–2.5-cm diameter).

Diagnosis: Pulmonary venous malformation, embolic stroke.

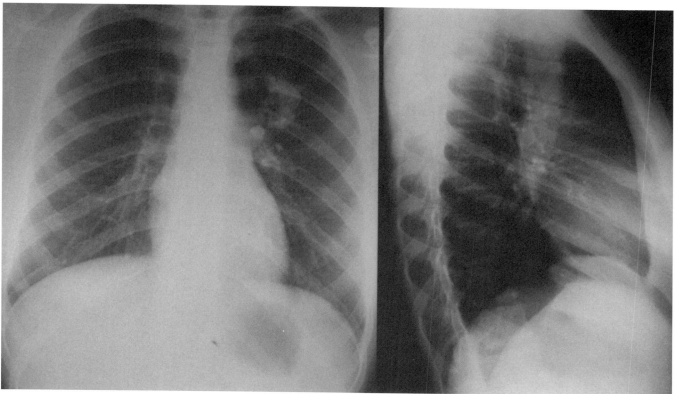

Fig. 72-1

(Continued)

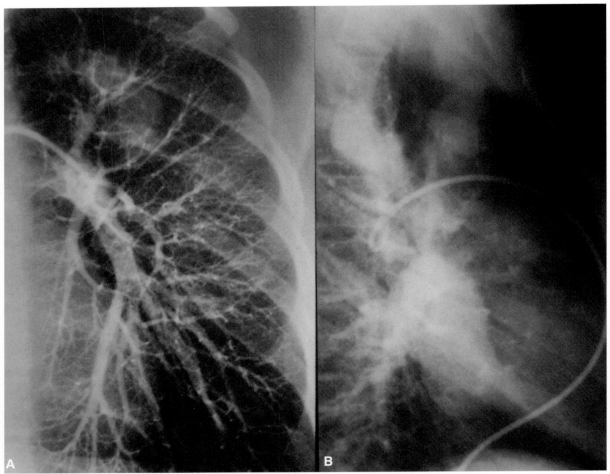

Fig. 72-2

Case 73

A newborn boy is cyanotic.

Mother (24 years old), father (25 years old), and brother (15 months old) are well.

Pregnancy was normal. Birth weight is 3.5 kg, Apgar score 8/8 at 1 and 5 minutes, length 50 cm, head circumference 34 cm, temperature 37.1°C, heart rate 136, respiratory rate 60, and blood pressure 72/44 mm Hg. The rest of the physical findings are normal.

Hematocrit is 0.53, blood sugar 2.8 mmol/liter. Capillary blood pH is 7.24 when F_{IO_2} = 1.0. P_{CO_2} is 42 mm Hg, P_{O_2} 20.

Balloon septostomy is performed for transposition of great arteries. At 11 months, a Mustard operation is performed and results in complete heart block and placement of a pacemaker.

At 3 years, weight is 16 kg, height 105 cm, temperature 36.3°C, heart rate 116, respiratory rate 32, and blood pressure 84/54 mm Hg. A continuous murmur is in right side of chest, front and back. A scar is over sternum. A pacemaker is in subcutaneous tissues of left lower quadrant of abdomen. The rest of the physical findings are normal.

Size of heart is normal at birth; vascular markings in medial part of right lung are excessive for a newborn infant (Figure 73-1A). Heart is larger than normal at 4 years. Vascular markings in medial part of right lung are excessive. Pacemaker lead is in place. Aortogram at 4 years shows large artery in right lung (Figure 73-1B), which is then occluded by placement of wire coils.

Diagnosis: Systemic pulmonary arterial collateral.

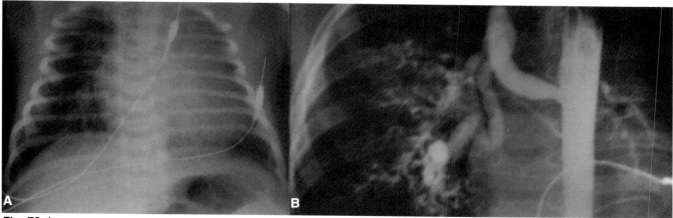

Fig. 73-1

Case 74

A 14-year-old girl is cyanotic. She is always last to finish a race with classmates. She gets short of breath, but muscles do not feel tired. Menarche was at 13 years.

Mother died at 31 years with subarachnoid hemorrhage; father died at 39 years with cirrhosis of liver. A brother (12 years old) is well.

Temperature is 36.1°C, heart rate 82, respiratory rate 20, blood pressure 90/68 mm Hg, weight 47 kg, and height 157 cm. Lips and nailbeds of hands and feet are blue, fingers clubbed. An inspiratory bruit is in right axilla. A few dark spots are on abdomen. The rest of the physical findings are normal.

Hemoglobin is 190 g/liter. Hematocrit is 0.55. Red blood cell count is 6.2×10^{12}/liter. MCV is 88 fl. MCH is 31 pg. MCHC is 350 g/liter. Reticulocyte fraction is 7×10^{-3}. White cell count is 7.4×10^9/liter with 0.45 polymorphonuclear cells, 0.03 bands, 0.27 lymphocytes, 0.03 monocytes, 0.06 eosinophils, 0.03 basophils, and 0.13 atypical lymphocytes. Platelet count is 203×10^9/liter. Serum sodium is 153 mmol/liter, potassium 4.7, chloride 120, carbon dioxide 16,

urea nitrogen 6.8, calcium 2.54, phosphorus 1.49, cholesterol 4.27, and glucose 7.8. Creatinine is 70 µmol/liter, uric acid 390, total bilirubin 12, and direct bilirubin 2. Total protein is 74 g/liter, albumin 44. Alkaline phosphatase is 124 U/liter, LDH 307, SGOT 30, and CK 59. Venous blood pH is 7.39. P_{CO_2} is 25 mm Hg, P_{O_2} 43.

ECG findings are normal.

Plain films (Figure 74-1) and pulmonary arteriogram (Figure 74-2) show a two-branch shadow that makes a hairpin turn in middle lobe.

At operation, thin-walled, dilated vessels are on visceral pleural surface of middle lobe. Microscopic examination of resected middle lobe shows, adjacent to cartilage-containing bronchi and atelectasis, distended vascular channels whose walls are thicker than those of normal veins and contain elastic fibers and are thickened in places by sclerotic eosinophilic deposits. Arteries enter distended veins.

Diagnosis: Pulmonary arteriovenous malformation.

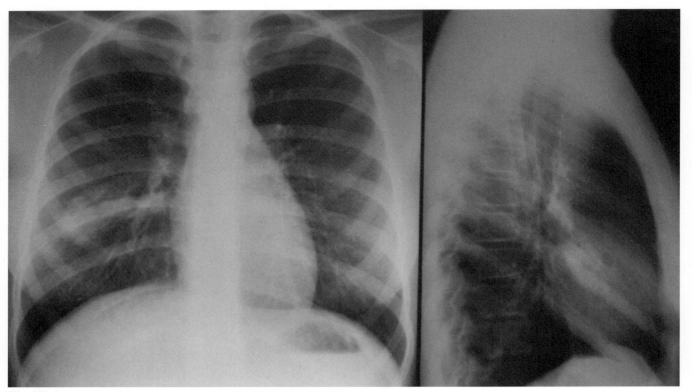

Fig. 74-1

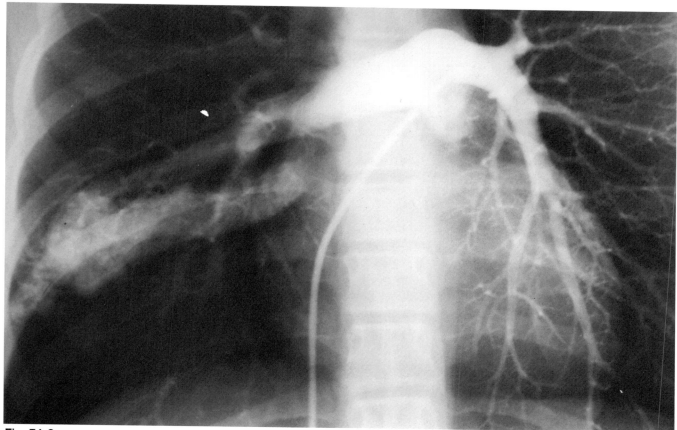

Fig. 74-2

Thymus

Case 1

A 2-week-old boy has a heart murmur.

Pregnancy of mother (28 years old) was normal, birth weight 4 kg, and Apgar score 9/9 at 1 and 5 minutes. A systolic heart murmur was present.

Weight is 4.6 kg, length 54 cm. A systolic murmur is present. The rest of the physical findings are normal.

Left side of supracardiac shadow is a ripple, right side a "sail." A healing fracture is in left clavicle (Figure 1-1).

ECG findings are normal.

Diagnosis: Normal thymus, ripple front part of thymus contiguous to ribs and interspaces, sail back part in mediastinum, healing fracture of clavicle. (He is thought to be normal at 6 weeks.)

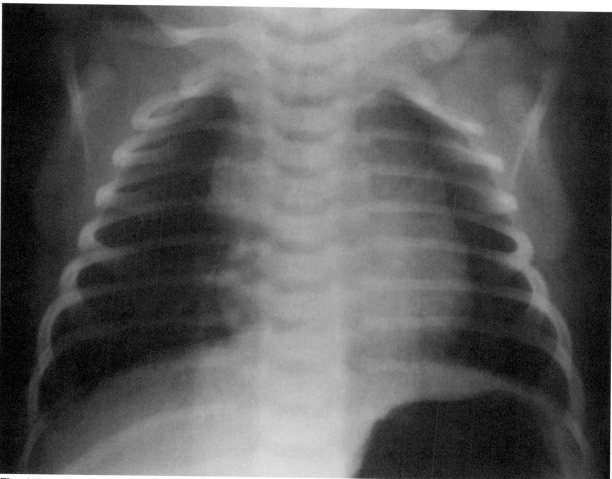

Fig. 1-1

Case 2

A newborn boy has a swollen scrotum.

Pregnancy of mother was normal, birth weight 3.5 kg, and Apgar score 9/9 at 1 and 5 minutes. At 17 minutes, temperature is 37.1°C, heart rate 172, and respiratory rate 68. At start of operation, systolic blood pressure is 60 mm Hg. Right side of head is swollen. Right side of scrotum is dark, tense, and larger than left side. The rest of the physical findings are normal.

Cord hematocrit is 0.38.

At operation at 5 hours, right testis and epididymis are dark blue, and tunica vaginalis and distal spermatic cord are thickened. Microscopic examination of resected right testis shows hemorrhage inside a rim of thickened fibrous tissue.

Respiratory rate is 85 at 10 hours. He grunts. Alae nasi flare. At 18 hours, he is pink and active. Cry is strong. He is hungry and seems well at 42 hours.

Heart is small, diaphragm low at 10½ hours (Figure 2-1A). Supracardiac shadow is widened on both sides at 2 months (Figure 2-1B).

At 2 months, weight is 5.6 kg, length 60 cm, and head circumference 41 cm. A systolic murmur is present. Scrotum is healed. The rest of the physical findings are normal.

Diagnosis: Intrauterine testicular torsion, normal thymus at 2 months.

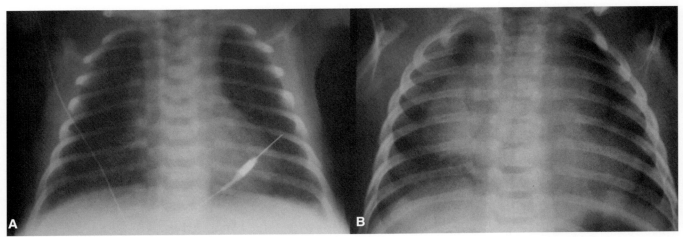

Fig. 2-1

Case 3

An 11-year-old girl coughs and sometimes vomits after coughing.

Mother had proteinuria and high blood pressure during pregnancy. Birth weight was 1.8 kg. Mandible was small. Muscles were lax, fingers were long and stiff, and feet were clubbed. At 3 years, she had ear infections and placement of tubes in her ears.

Mother (32 years old), 150 cm tall, has narrow face, small mandible, limitation of pronation and supination at elbows, scoliosis, stiff fingers, thin muscles, and normal findings in muscle biopsy. Sister (10 years old) has long, stiff fingers and stiff elbows and knees. Maternal grandfather has stiff fingers, elbows, and knees; diabetes mellitus; and poor vision because of corneal deterioration. All have limited eye movement and deep posterior iliac dimples. Father (34 years old), 191 cm tall, is normal.

Weight at 11 years is 22 kg, height 130 cm, temperature 37.6°C, heart rate 80–100, respiratory rate 24, and blood pressure 90/47 mm Hg. She cannot make a fist. Spleen edge is 2 cm below costal margin. The rest of the physical findings are normal.

Hematocrit is 0.33. White cell count is 14.1×10^9/liter with 0.73 polymorphonuclear cells, 0.03 bands, 0.19 lymphocytes, and 0.05 monocytes. Urine specific gravity is 1.015, pH 5. Urine has 0–2 white cells/HPF. Serum sodium is 141 mmol/liter, potassium 4.3, chloride 104, carbon dioxide 27, urea nitrogen 4.3, calcium 2.30, phosphorus 1.16, cholesterol 3.13, and glucose 5.2. Creatinine is 50 µmol/liter, uric acid 230, total bilirubin 7, and direct bilirubin 2. Total protein is 68 g/liter, albumin 35. Alkaline phosphatase is 293 U/liter, LDH 267, and SGOT 19.

Right side of supracardiac shadow is widened in examination at 7 years for scoliosis and in examination at 11 years (Figure 3-1). CT scan at 11 years shows mass of soft tissue just behind junction of brachiocephalic veins and similar mass in front of left brachiocephalic vein (Figure 3-2).

Diagnosis: Dwarfism with stiff joints (Moore-Federman syndrome), normal retrocaval thymus.

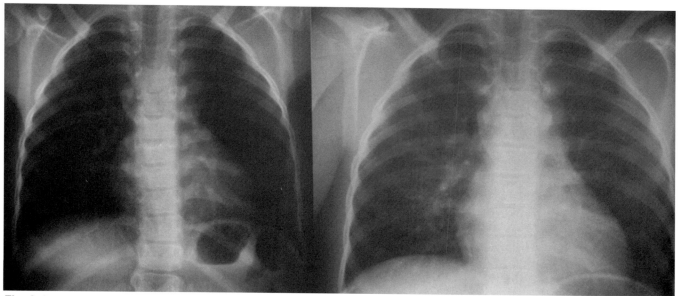

Fig. 3-1

(Continued)

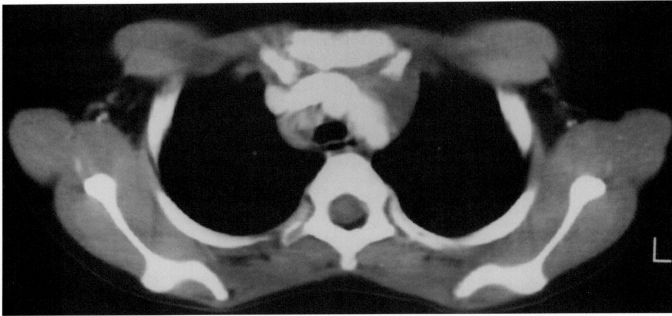

Fig. 3-2

Case 4

A newborn boy is breathing fast.

Delivery was by cesarean section for placenta previa in prenatal ultrasound examination of mother (25 years old). Birth weight is 3 kg, Apgar score 1/8 at 1 and 5 minutes, temperature 37.2°C, heart rate 134, systolic blood pressure 56 mm Hg, length 50 cm, and head circumference 33 cm. Respiratory rate is 116 when hood FIO_2 = 0.65. Infant grunts and retracts. Alae nasi flare. Skin is mottled. The rest of the physical findings are normal.

Hematocrit is 0.37. White cell count is 6.5×10^9/liter.

Findings are normal 20 minutes after delivery (Figure 4-1A). Wedges of water density are in upper part of chest at 21 hours (Figure 4-1B).

Diagnosis: Dissection of left lobe and right lobe of thymus from surface of pericardium by mediastinal air (pneumomediastinum).

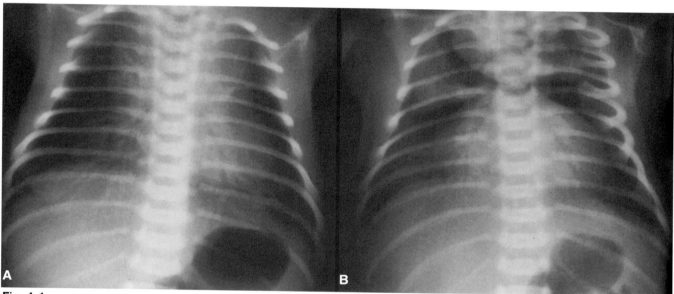

Fig. 4-1

Case 5

A 16-year-old girl has chest pain front and back that began yesterday during a calculus class. She had to sleep sitting up last night.

Physical findings are normal.

A thin, curved strip of water density is lateral to apex of heart in frontal view (Figure 5-1). A mass with lower inward bulge is between sternum and front of heart in lateral view (Figure 5-2A).

Pain has subsided the next day.

Findings are normal 3 weeks later (Figure 5-2B).

Diagnosis: Pneumopericardium and pneumo-mediastinum with air between thymus and heart in first lateral examination.

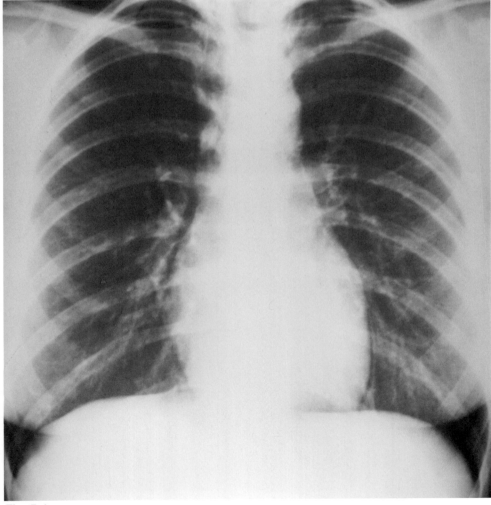

Fig. 5-1

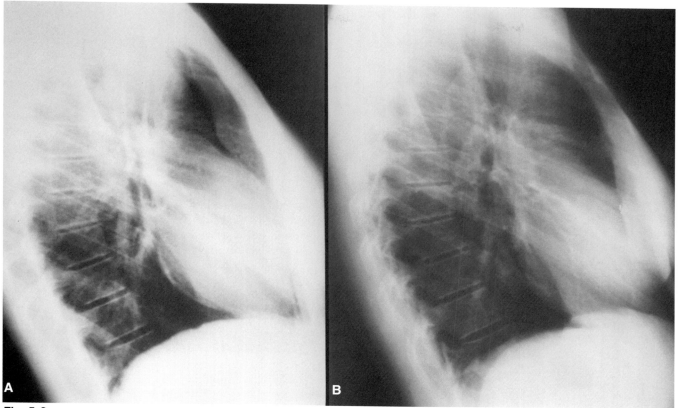

Fig. 5-2

Case 6

A 19-month-old girl, who was well until this afternoon, is convulsing with limbs jerking and, 30 minutes later, back arched. She has had three watery stools in the hour since the convulsion began.

Temperature is 39.8°C, heart rate 150, respiratory rate 48, blood pressure 110/50 mm Hg, and weight 10.7 kg. She is unresponsive. She has doll's eye reflex. Pupils are 2 mm. Respirations are noisy. She retracts with inspiration. Liver edge is 2 cm below costal margin. Back is arched. Limbs are extended. Babinski's sign is in feet. The rest of the physical findings are normal.

She reacts to annoyance 3 hours after convulsion begins. She tenses abdomen and grunts at start of each expiration. Arms are flexed, legs extended. She is alert 12 hours after convulsion begins.

One hour after convulsion begins, hematocrit is 0.35. White cell count is 10.3 × 10⁹/liter with 0.54 polymorphonuclear cells, 0.32 bands, and 0.14 lymphocytes (1.4 × 10⁹/liter lym-

phocytes). Four and one-half hours after convulsion begins, hematocrit is 0.38. White cell count is 23.8 × 10⁹/liter with 0.43 polymorphonuclear cells, 0.28 bands, 0.17 lymphocytes (4.0 × 10⁹/liter lymphocytes), and 0.12 monocytes. Serum sodium is 135 mmol/liter before IV glucose, potassium 3.0, chloride 101, calcium 2.17, and glucose 20.5. SGOT is 45 U/liter. CSF is clear, colorless, and has 3 × 10⁶/liter white cells, 2 × 10⁶/liter red cells, 0.25 g/liter protein, and 7.9 mmol/liter glucose. Urine specific gravity is 1.020 after IV glucose, pH 6. Urine has few squamous epithelial cells/HPF, 2–4 white cells/HPF, and many urate crystals. Stool has normal flora. Blood is sterile.

Supracardiac shadow is widened on left 1½ hours after convulsion begins (Figure 6-1A), not widened 6½ hours after convulsion begins (Figure 6-1B). Right fist is superimposed on chest in later examination.

Diagnosis: Febrile convulsion, shrinkage of thymus.

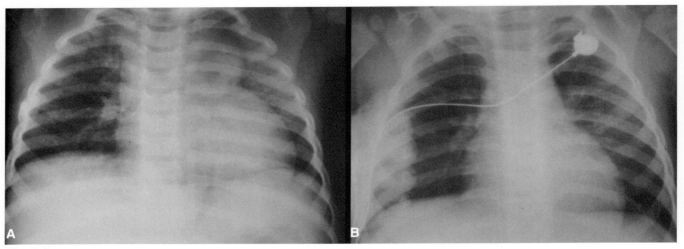

Fig. 6-1

Case 7

An 18-year-old man has an abnormality that was discovered in roentgenogram of the chest 16 days ago, performed for induction into the U.S. Navy.

For the past 3 months, he has become short of breath when swimming or walking uphill. He was hit in the chest 2½ months ago and had sharp pain there several days later for 1½ weeks. Pain was worse with cough, laughter, or movement. He had pneumonia 4½ months ago.

Parents and 10 siblings are well.

Temperature is 36.4°C, heart rate 70, respiratory rate 16, blood pressure 106/70 mm Hg, and weight 57 kg. Physical findings are normal.

Hematocrit is 0.47. White cell count is 9.9 × 10⁹/liter with 0.70 polymorphonuclear cells, 0.23 lymphocytes, 0.05 monocytes, and 0.02 eosinophils. Platelet estimate is normal. Urine specific gravity is 1.022, pH 7. Urine has 1+ protein, bacteria, and occasional squamous epithelial cells/HPF. Serum sodium is 142 mmol/liter, potassium 4.0, chloride 103, carbon dioxide 24, urea nitrogen 4.6, calcium 2.60, phosphorus 1.03, cholesterol 3.41, and glucose 4.7. Creatinine is 90 μmol/liter, uric acid 430, total bilirubin 14, and direct bilirubin 2. Total protein is 72 g/liter, albumin 51. Alkaline phosphatase is 109 U/liter, LDH 158, and SGOT 33.

Findings are normal in roentgenogram examination 4½ months ago (Figure 7-1). Supracardiac shadow is now widened on both sides by an anterior mediastinal mass of water density (Figure 7-2). CT scan after IV injection of contrast medium shows nonvascular mass in front and on both sides of great arteries and slight compression of ascending aorta along lateral aspect (Figure 7-3).

At operation, a mediastinal cyst (14 × 10 × 5 cm) is, according to surgeon, "bilobed to some degree" and contains yellow-brown liquid.

Cross-section of resected mass reveals several cysts with trabeculated inner walls. Deposits are in walls of cysts; some are soft and look like fat, some are firm and look like keratotic debris, and others have a cartilage-like consistency when cut across. Microscopic examination shows (1) thin walls of loose, vascular fibrous tissue in which are infiltrates of lymphocytes with germinal centers, plasma cells, a few eosinophils; (2) cholesterol granulomas with hemosiderin and foreign body giant cells; and (3) plaques of calcium. Cyst lining is a single layer of epithelial cells that vary from squamous to cuboid to columnar. Old blood, necrotic matter, and cholesterol spicules are in the cyst liquid. Normal thymus is attached to one side of the cyst.

Diagnosis: Thymic cyst.

(Continued)

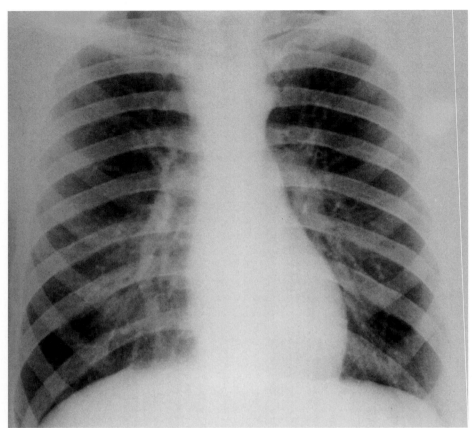

Fig. 7-1

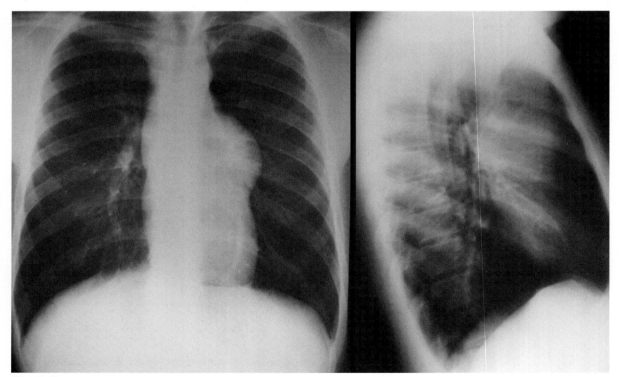

Fig. 7-2

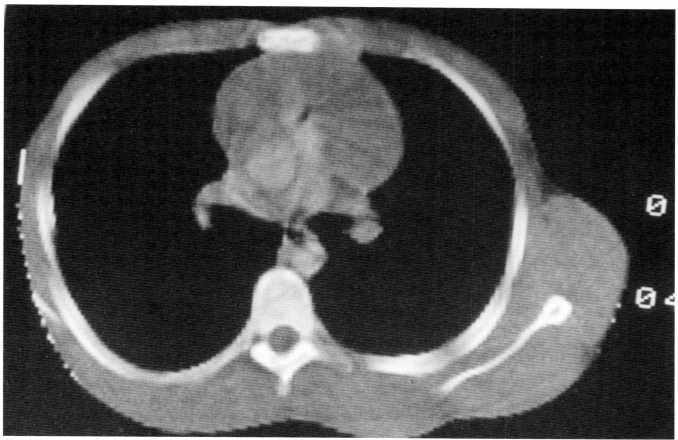

Fig. 7-3

Case 8

A 20-month-old girl and an older sister are coughing and wheezing.

Pregnancy of mother was normal, birth weight 3.6 kg, and Apgar score 9/9 at 1 and 5 minutes. She had a cold and red eardrums 7 weeks ago.

Temperature is 37.2°C. Nose is clear. She is better a week later but roentgenogram of chest is performed because she has "rare wheezes."

Supracardiac shadow is widened on left side by an anterior mediastinal mass that contains calcium (Figure 8-1).

Six days after roentgenogram, temperature is 36.9°C, heart rate 120, respiratory rate 24, systolic blood pressure 100 mm Hg, and weight 10.5 kg. Physical findings and ECG findings are normal.

Six days after roentgenogram, hematocrit is 0.37. White cell count is 7.7×10^9/liter with 0.27 polymorphonuclear cells, 0.02 bands, 0.61 lymphocytes, 0.06 monocytes, 0.03 eosinophils, and 0.01 atypical lymphocytes. Platelet count is 524×10^9/liter. Urine specific gravity is 1.023, pH 7. Urine has occasional squamous epithelial cells and 0–1 white cell/HPF. Serum sodium is 138 mmol/liter, potassium 5.2, chloride 109, carbon dioxide 22, urea nitrogen 4.6, calcium 2.50, phosphorus 1.94, cholesterol 3.78, and glucose 3.1. Creatinine is 20 μmol/liter, uric acid 290, total bilirubin 7,

and direct bilirubin 2. Total protein is 62 g/liter, albumin 42. Alkaline phosphatase is 217 U/liter, LDH 300, and SGOT 30. Carcinoma embryonic antigen is <4 μg/liter (normal: <5), α_1-fetoprotein <10 (normal: <20).

CT scan just below bifurcation of trachea with and without IV contrast medium shows displacement of left pulmonary artery to right by an avascular mass of varying density including fat and calcium in left side of chest (Figure 8-2).

At left thoracotomy, a pear-shaped, pink-tan mass (8.0 × 5.5 × 3.6 cm) is removed. Smaller part is hard, larger part is rubbery.

Some of surface in cross section is smooth, yellow, and glistening. Translucent white-gray fragments and bone fragments are near one end. Cysts of different size with clear liquid and inner translucent gray-white folded lining and other cysts with thicker, green-black liquid are near middle; fibroadipose tissue is elsewhere.

Microscopic examination shows thymus, bone marrow with three cell lines, cancellous bone, cartilage, colonic wall including Auerbach's plexus, keratinized squamous epithelium with adnexa and inflammation, and neural epithelium and stroma.

Diagnosis: Benign teratoma.

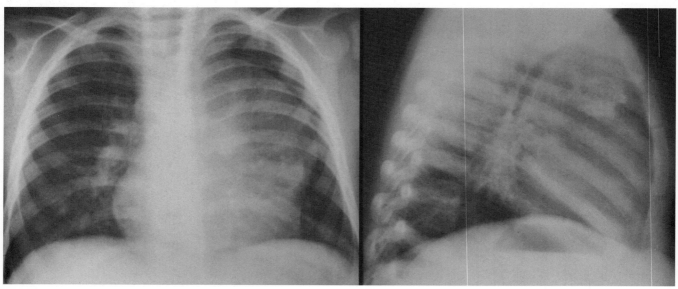

Fig. 8-1

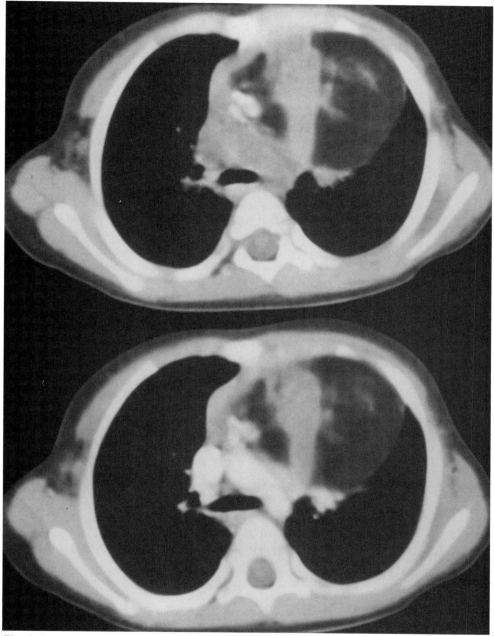

Fig. 8-2

Case 9

A 10-year-old boy is "changing too fast." Voice has been deep for 2–3 years. He has had pains in lower right side of chest for several weeks when he runs fast.

Weight at 10 years is 37.1 kg, height 142 cm, temperature 37.5°C, heart rate 96, respiratory rate 28, and blood pressure 105/60 mm Hg. He is muscular and has facial hair and pimples. Right side of chest bulges slightly and has dullness and diminished breath sounds. Heart is displaced left. Liver edge is 1 cm below costal margin. He has pubic hair, adult penis, and small testes (volume of each: 3–4 cm³). The rest of the physical findings are normal.

Hematocrit is 0.34. White cell count is 10.7×10^9/liter with 0.68 polymorphonuclear cells, 0.19 lymphocytes, 0.07 monocytes, and 0.06 eosinophils. Platelet count is 561×10^9/liter. Serum sodium is 129 mmol/liter, potassium 4.5, chloride 94, carbon dioxide 25, urea nitrogen 3.2, calcium 2.22, phosphorus 1.65, cholesterol 2.07, and glucose 7.9. Creatinine is 60 μmol/liter, uric acid 230, total bilirubin 7, and direct bilirubin 2. Total protein is 57 g/liter, albumin 32. Alkaline phosphatase is 281 U/liter, LDH 244, and SGOT 21. Testosterone is 65.6 nmol/liter (normal man: 10.4–41.6), 17-hydroxyprogesterone 11.3 (normal: 1.5–6.0). HCG is 114 IU/liter (normal: <5). α_1-Fetoprotein is 1,470 μg/liter (normal: 2–16).

A mass is along right side of heart in Figure 9-1.

Cytogenetic analysis of 20 blood cells shows 13 with 46 chromosomes and seven with 47 chromosomes (karyotype in three of these cells is 47,XXY/46,XY).

At operation, an encapsulated mass, partly cystic, partly solid, is removed from right side of chest.

Mass ($14.5 \times 10.0 \times 8.0$ cm) is orange-to-tan and bumpy on outside, pink-to-tan on inside with fibrosis, soft spots, cysts (0.2–2.0 cm), some with shiny lining and clear liquid, others with rough, white lining; white-to-green thick liquid; and small hemorrhages. Microscopic examination shows (1) fibrous stroma, cystic and solid; (2) disorganized mature and immature derivatives of ectoderm, endoderm, and mesoderm; (3) clusters of cells with little cytoplasm and large, irregular nuclei with clumped chromatin and prominent nucleoli; (4) rare Schiller-Duval microcysts with glomeruli and fibrovascular core; and (5) a focus of extracellular eosinophilic globules. Tumor cells consist of one cell line with extra chromosome 21, one cell line with extra chromosomes 17 and 21, and all but one cell line with extra chromosome X.

Diagnosis: Klinefelter's syndrome, malignant teratoma with yolk sac elements, sexual precocity.

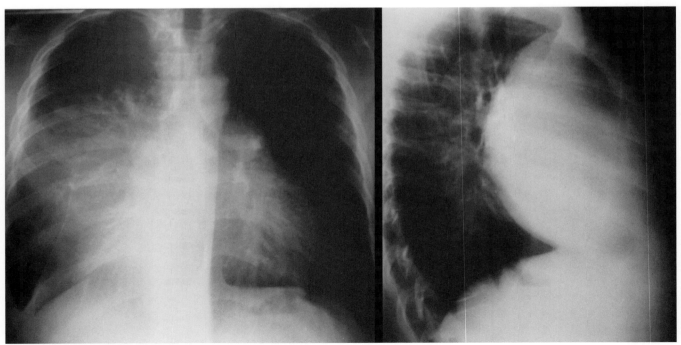

Fig. 9-1

Case 10

A 7-year-old boy has been coughing and making gurgly noises at night for 1½ weeks. He could not catch his breath 2 days ago. He had a headache and bellyache yesterday.

Temperature is 37.9°C, heart rate 122, respiratory rate 28, blood pressure 102/68 mm Hg, weight 19.5 kg, and height 109 cm. Breathing is rattled when he lies supine, breathing out noisier than breathing in. Cervical and inguinal lymph nodes are palpable. A larger node (1.0 × 0.5 cm) is above right clavicle. A systolic heart murmur is present. The rest of the physical findings are normal.

Hematocrit is 0.35. White cell count is 9.5 × 10⁹/liter with 0.41 polymorphonuclear cells, 0.10 bands, 0.31 lymphocytes, 0.16 monocytes, 0.01 eosinophils, and 0.01 basophils. Platelet count is 570 × 10⁹/liter. Urine specific gravity is 1.021, pH 7. Urine has 1+ ketones. Serum sodium is 138 mmol/liter, potassium 4.2, chloride 100, carbon dioxide 24, urea nitrogen 4.3, calcium 2.42, phosphorus 1.29, cholesterol 4.37, and glucose 5.9. Creatinine is 50 μmol/liter, uric acid 100, total bilirubin 5, and direct bilirubin 3. Total protein is 72 g/liter, albumin 40. Alkaline phosphatase is 172 U/liter, LDH 407, and SGOT 27.

Chest is deep front to back, diaphragm low. A mass of water density widens supracardiac shadow, more on right side (Figure 10-1). Lateral tomographic view shows compression of trachea (Figure 10-2).

At operation firm, gray tumor is in front of trachea.

Tumor is pearly white in cut section. Microscopic examination shows diffuse proliferation of lymphocytoid cells in nodal and extranodal tissue and in surrounding fibrous tissue and 1–2 mitoses/HPF. Cells have indistinct borders; little eosinophilic cytoplasm; round to oval pleomorphic nuclei, some cleaved; convoluted nuclear membranes; and small nucleoli. Electron microscopy shows smooth cell membranes, few intracytoplasmic organelles, vacuoles in few nuclei, and nucleoli in the most immature cells.

Diagnosis: Lymphoblastic lymphoma in thymus.

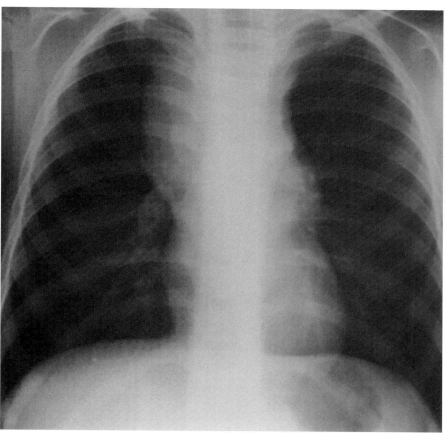

Fig. 10-1

(Continued)

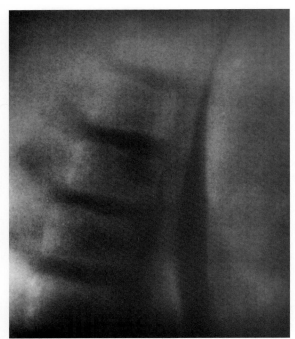

Fig. 10-2

Mediastinum

Case 1

A 10-year-old boy who has sometimes coughed all day and night for 1½ years now skips meals because he is not hungry.

Pregnancy of mother was normal, birth weight 3.4 kg.

Mother (51 years old), father (57 years old), and seven siblings are well.

Weight is 25 kg, height 131 cm, temperature 36.9°C, heart rate 60, respiratory rate 16, and blood pressure 104/60 mm Hg. Physical findings are normal.

In roentgenograms at 10 years, a mass is in hilum of right lung, and findings in skeleton are normal. Bronchoscopic findings are normal. Examination of a cervical lymph node shows distention of sinuses by histiocytes with small collections of polymorphonuclear cells.

At 12 years, cough is worse and fingers are clubbed.

Roentgenogram of chest at 11 years shows widening of supracardiac shadow, apparently thymus, and a spherical mass in hilum of right lung (Figure 1-1). Masses are larger in examination at 12 years, and a new mass is in each lower lobe, one in left at level of dome of diaphragm, one in right below medial part of dome of diaphragm (Figure 1-2A). Cortex of ulnas (also humeri, femurs, tibias, and fibulas) is thickened (Figure 1-2B).

Hematocrit at 12 years is 0.31. White cell count is 11.4 × 10⁹/liter with 0.69 polymorphonuclear cells, 0.04 bands, 0.20 lymphocytes, 0.03 monocytes, and 0.04 eosinophils. Platelet count is 540 × 10⁹/liter. ESR is 137 mm/hr. Serum sodium is 141 mmol/liter, potassium 4.1, chloride 102, carbon dioxide 23, urea nitrogen 5.0, calcium 2.10, phosphorus 1.13, cholesterol 5.38, and glucose 6.1. Creatinine is 60 µmol/liter, uric acid 190, total bilirubin 5, and direct bilirubin 2. Total protein is 80 g/liter, albumin 29. Alkaline phosphatase is 223 U/liter, LDH 368, and SGOT 10.

Biopsy of a left infraclavicular lymph node 1 month later shows sclerotic bands of collagen around nodules of lymphoid tissue that contain cells with hyperlobated nuclei in lacunar-like spaces, prominent nucleoli in some lacunar cells that appear to be Reed-Sternberg cell variants, and focal aggregates of atypical pleomorphic cells around necrotic foci.

Weight at 19 years is 62 kg, height 169 cm, and blood pressure 120/82 mm Hg. Physical findings are normal in examination for the U.S. Army.

Diagnosis: Nodular sclerosing Hodgkin's disease, hypertrophic osteoarthropathy.

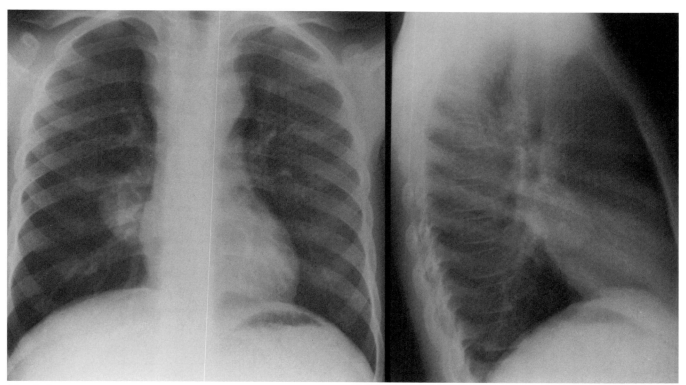

Fig. 1-1

(Continued)

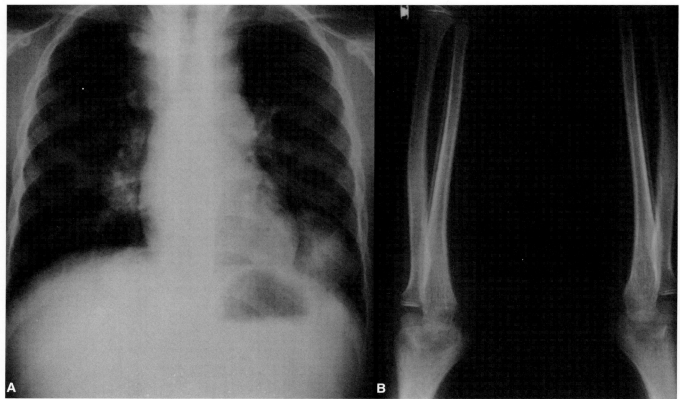

Fig. 1-2

Case 2

A 14-year-old boy has headache and heart murmur.

He has had headache, numbness in legs, right arm, and tongue, and a wavy line in right eye three times in 15 months.

Temperature is 36.3°C, heart rate 72, respiratory rate 16, blood pressure 100/60 mm Hg, and weight 51 kg. A systolic murmur is present. The rest of the physical findings are normal.

Hematocrit is 0.42. White cell count is 5.8 × 10⁹/liter with 0.49 polymorphonuclear cells, 0.33 lymphocytes, 0.14 monocytes, and 0.04 eosinophils. ESR is 7 mm/hr. Serum sodium is 142 mmol/liter, potassium 5.3, chloride 101, carbon dioxide 27, urea nitrogen 4.3, calcium 2.62, phosphorus 1.42, cholesterol 4.19, and glucose 5.5. Creatinine is 60 μmol/liter, uric acid 270, total bilirubin 5, and direct bilirubin 2. Total protein is 73 g/liter, albumin 44, IgG 9.00 (normal: 6.5–16.0),

IgA 1.65 (normal: 0.40–3.50), IgM 2.40 (normal: 0.50–3.00), and IgD 0.07 (normal: 0.00–0.08). Alkaline phosphatase is 400 U/liter, LDH 206, and SGOT 30.

In Figure 2-1, masses of water density are in lung hila and right paratracheal shadow is widened.

At mediastinoscopy, bits of right paratracheal lymph node and bits of thymus are removed.

Microscopic examination shows normal thymus and noncaseating granulomas with large central epithelioid cells and giant cells surrounded by chronic inflammatory cells in lymph node.

Chest roentgenogram findings are normal 1 year later.

Diagnosis: Sarcoidosis.

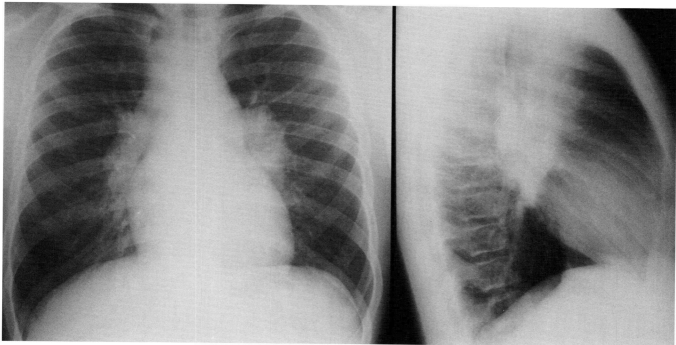

Fig. 2-1

Case 3

A 2½-month-old girl has had a barking cough since birth and sometimes cannot swallow even though she is hungry.

Pregnancy of mother was normal, birth weight 4.9 kg.

Parents smoke. Mother is allergic to dogs, cats, and dust. Sister (3 years old) is well. Father was hypothyroid in infancy.

Weight is 6.4 kg, length 62 cm, and heart rate 140. Cry is hoarse. The rest of the physical findings are normal.

Bifurcation of trachea is at level of T4–T5. Esophagus and trachea are separated just above bifurcation (Figure 3-1). Left pulmonary artery goes to right and then makes hairpin turn to left lung (Figure 3-2).

Diagnosis: Aberrant left pulmonary artery (pulmonary sling).

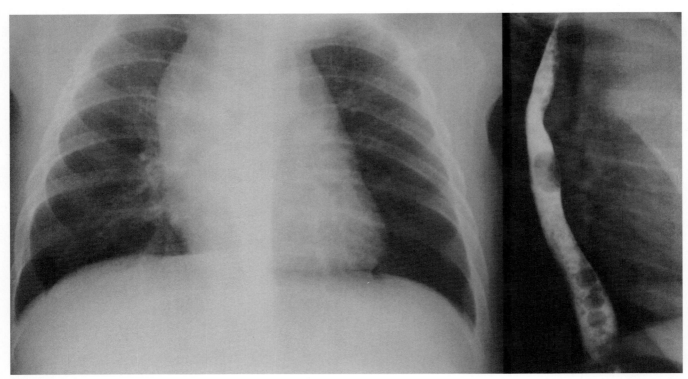

Fig. 3-1

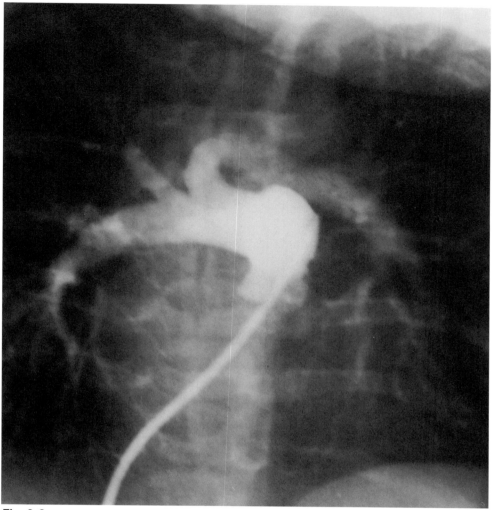

Fig. 3-2

Case 4

A 6-month-old boy has been breathing noisily since birth and often vomits when he eats. Expiration is noisier when he is supine than when sitting.

He had croup 5 weeks ago.

Temperature is 36.6°C, heart rate 140, respiratory rate 35, systolic blood pressure 98 mm Hg, weight 9 kg, and length 61 cm. A systolic murmur is present. Liver edge is 1 cm below costal margin. A hemangioma is on left calf. The rest of the physical findings are normal.

Hematocrit is 0.38. White cell count is 12.3×10^9/liter with 0.22 polymorphonuclear cells, 0.66 lymphocytes, 0.05 monocytes, 0.06 eosinophils, and 0.01 basophils. Platelet count is 524×10^9/liter.

Arch of aorta is on left side of trachea, trachea concave to right at same level (Figure 4-1A), and, in lateral view (Figure 4-1B), pushed forward. Esophagram shows forward displacement of esophagus at same level (Figure 4-2).

Bronchoscopy shows pulsating compression of right side of trachea just above bifurcation.

Angiographic findings (Figure 4-3) are similar to findings at operation: (1) double aortic arch around trachea and esophagus; (2) origin of right subclavian artery and right common carotid artery from right arch, and of left common carotid artery and left subclavian artery from left arch; and (3) junction of two arches behind esophagus to form descending aorta.

At operation, adhesions are between smaller right arch and trachea and esophagus.

Diagnosis: Vascular ring, double aortic arch.

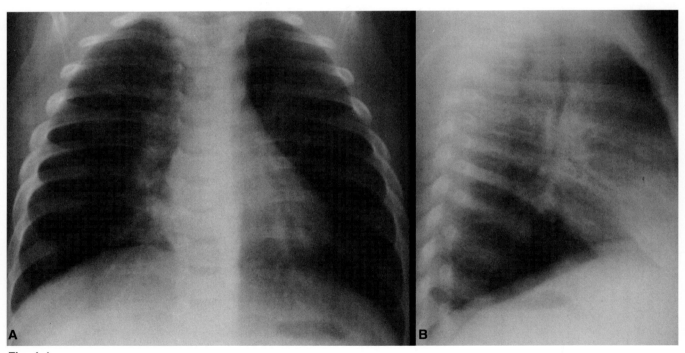

Fig. 4-1

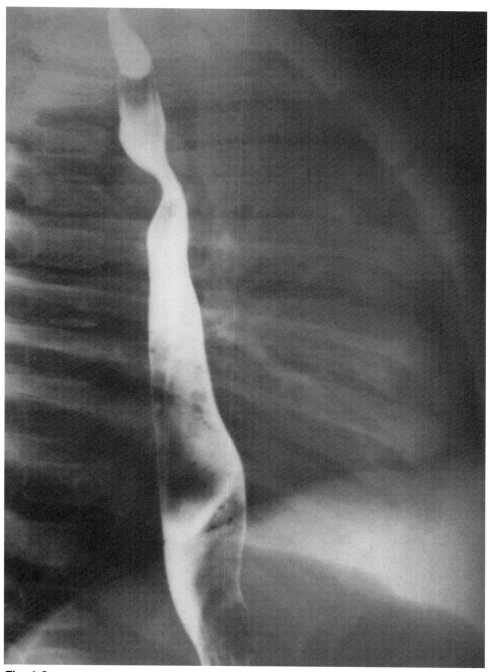

Fig. 4-2

(Continued)

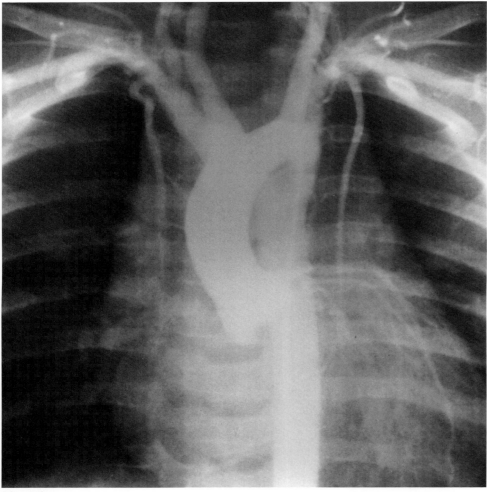

Fig. 4-3

Case 5

A 10-month-old boy who has Down syndrome wheezes loudly enough to be heard across the room. Wheezing began at 6 weeks.

Mother (18 years old) smoked one-half pack of cigarettes a day during pregnancy. Birth weight was 2.8 kg. He scoots on the floor. He eats well "if he can take his time."

Temperature is 36.5°C, heart rate 168, respiratory rate 20, systolic blood pressure 84 mm Hg, and weight 5.9 kg. Brushfield's spots are in irises. Rhonchi are in chest. Liver edge is 3 cm below costal margin. Right testicle is not in scrotum. A longitudinal plantar crease is between first and second toes. Muscle tone is diminished. The rest of the physical findings are normal.

Hematocrit is 0.32. White cell count is 20.8×10^9/liter with 0.24 polymorphonuclear cells, 0.58 bands, 0.06 lymphocytes, 0.11 monocytes, and 0.1 metamyelocytes. Platelet count is 141×10^9/liter. Urine specific gravity is 1.013, pH 6. Urine has 1+ hemoglobin/myoglobin, few squamous epithelial cells/HPF, 0–2 red cells/HPF, and 0–2 white cells/HPF. Serum sodium is 133 mmol/liter, potassium 5.0, chloride 99, carbon dioxide 26, urea nitrogen 3.9, calcium 1.95, phosphorus 1.49, cholesterol 2.30, and glucose 4.2. Creatinine is 50 μmol/liter, uric acid 290, total bilirubin 3, and direct bilirubin 0. Total protein is 48 g/liter, albumin 30. Alkaline phosphatase is 75 U/liter, LDH 1,230, and SGOT 143.

Trachea is concave right and back in Figure 5-1. Aortogram in Figure 5-2 shows right arch from which the following come in order: left common carotid artery, right common carotid artery, and right subclavian artery. Aortogram also shows a diverticulum behind esophagus, from which comes left subclavian artery (see Figure 5-2).

At bronchoscopy, trachea and main bronchi are flattened.

At thoracotomy, ligamentum arteriosum is divided, and ends are separated 0.5 cm.

He has frequent respiratory infections. He coughs and wheezes. He chokes on food.

Esophagram at 5½ years shows esophagus compressed from right and back (Figure 5-3).

At second thoracotomy, left subclavian artery is divided, aorta tacked back, and trachea tacked forward.

At 8 years, he breathes noisily, snores, stops breathing, wakes, starts breathing, and prefers to sleep prone or sitting up. He has ear infections.

At bronchoscopy at 9 years, the segment of trachea 1–4 cm above carina is collapsed. At operation, tonsils and large adenoids are removed.

Diagnosis: Vascular ring, right arch; large adenoids; sleep apnea.

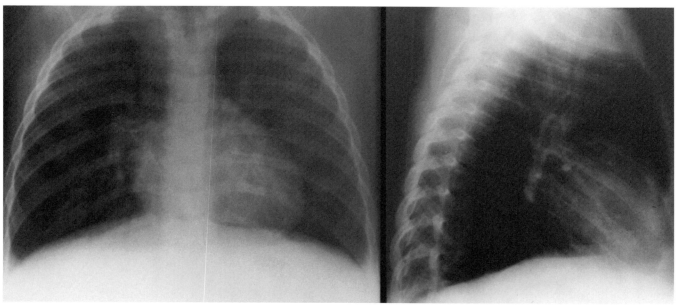

Fig. 5-1

(Continued)

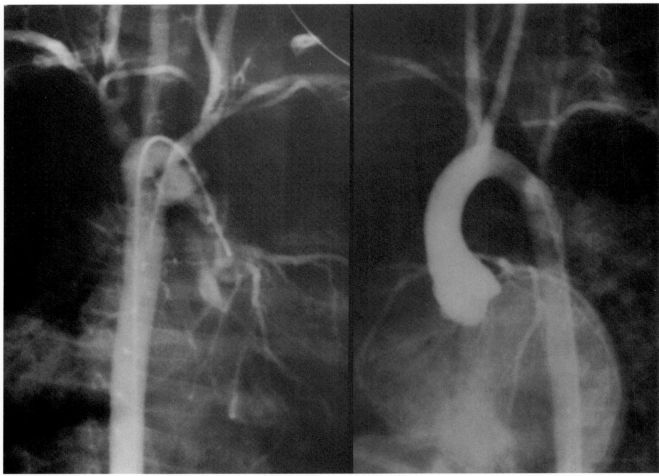

Fig. 5-2

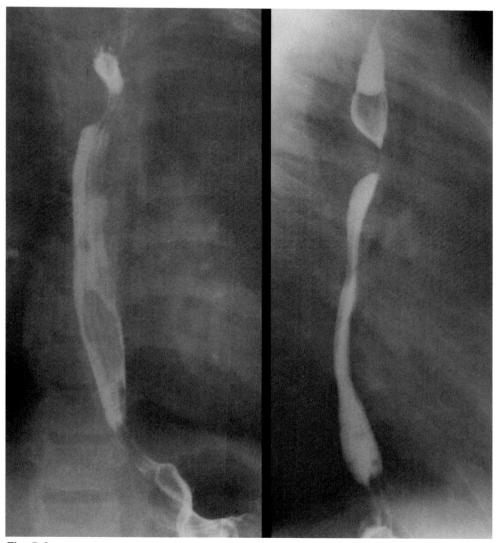

Fig. 5-3

Case 6

A 5-year-old boy vomits often.

He vomited in infancy. Vomiting gradually diminished but recurred 2 months ago. He has dry heaves before breakfast, vomits after breakfast, and begins to eat again. Although hungry, he eats little. He has lost 1 kg in the last 2 months. Birth weight was 4.2 kg. He has been hospitalized twice for bronchitis.

Temperature at 5 years is 37.2°C, heart rate 104, respiratory rate 24, weight 15 kg, and height 105 cm. Physical findings are normal.

Hematocrit is 0.39. White cell count is 10.3×10^9/liter with 0.47 polymorphonuclear cells, 0.01 bands, 0.47 lymphocytes, 0.02 monocytes, and 0.03 eosinophils. Platelet count is 337×10^9/liter. Urine specific gravity is 1.008, pH 7. Urine is normal. Serum sodium is 136 mmol/liter, potassium 4.8, chloride 104, carbon dioxide 19, urea nitrogen 8.6, calcium 2.37, phosphorus 1.42, cholesterol 4.55, and glucose 7.4. Creatinine is 60 μmol/liter, uric acid 140, total bilirubin 3, and direct bilirubin 0. Total protein is 67 g/liter, albumin 44. Alkaline phosphatase is 185 U/liter, LDH 366, and SGOT 36.

Esophagram shows barium, air bubbles, and an oblique defect at level of aortic arch in frontal view (Figure 6-1A) and for-ward displacement of esophagus at this level in lateral view (Figure 6-1B).

Esophagoscopy shows 1.5-cm pulsating compression at 17 cm and friable, red mucosa at gastroesophageal junction.

He is treated for gastroesophageal reflux. Vomiting continues.

Weight at 8 years is 19.8 kg, temperature 37.2°C, heart rate 76, respiratory rate 22, and blood pressure 90/58 mm Hg.

Aortogram at 8 years shows arch, right common carotid artery, left common carotid artery, left subclavian artery (Figure 6-2A), and, later, right subclavian artery originating at Kommerell's diverticulum (Figure 6-2B).

At operation, right subclavian artery begins at junction between arch and descending aorta and goes behind esophagus to apex of right side of chest. It is transferred to right common carotid artery.

Diagnosis: Aberrant right subclavian artery, questionable dysphagia lusoria.

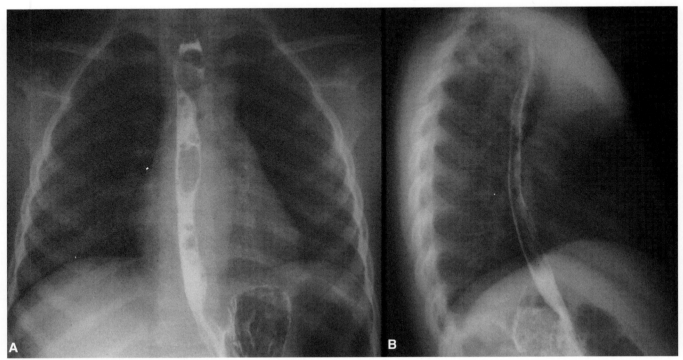

Fig. 6-1

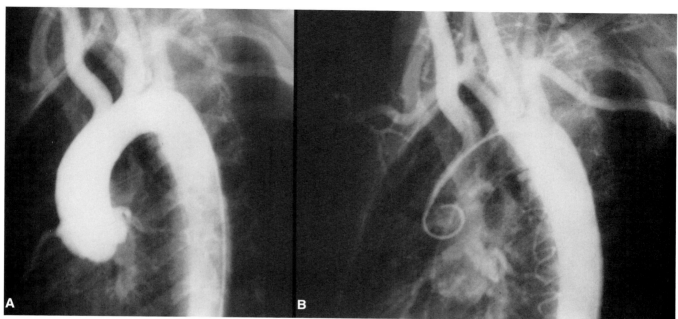

Fig. 6-2

Case 7

A 6-month-old girl "can't catch her breath and coughs a lot."

Pregnancy was normal, birth weight 4.1 kg, and Apgar score 8/9 at 1 and 5 minutes. At 8 hours, she was dusky when she cried. A systolic heart murmur was present. ECG showed rate 150, left ventricular hypertrophy, left axis deviation, and p pulmonale. Cardiac catheterization showed right ventricular hypoplasia, ventricular septal defect, atrial-septal defect, ductus arteriosus, and valvar and subvalvar pulmonic stenosis.

Mother (21 years old), father, and brother (20 months old) are well.

Weight at 6 months is 5 kg, length 61 cm, head circumference 43 cm, temperature 37.5°C, heart rate 144, respiratory rate 56, and blood pressure 86/54 mm Hg. She is blue. Systolic murmur and S_3 are present. The rest of the physical findings are normal.

Hematocrit is 0.45. White cell count is 9.5×10^9/liter with 0.38 polymorphonuclear cells, 0.23 bands, 0.20 lympho-cytes, 0.08 monocytes, 0.2 eosinophils, and 0.09 atypical lymphocytes. Platelet count is 342×10^9/liter. Urine specific gravity is 1.021, pH 5. Urine has trace hemoglobin/myoglobin. Serum sodium is 137 mmol/liter, potassium 4.4, chloride 106, carbon dioxide 24, urea nitrogen 4.6, calcium 2.29, phosphorus 0.94, cholesterol 2.90, and glucose 4.7. Creatinine is 40 μmol/liter, uric acid 130, total bilirubin 15, and direct bilirubin 2. Total protein is 60 g/liter, albumin 40. Alkaline phosphatase is 113 U/liter, LDH 268, and SGOT 48.

Trachea is concave right (Figure 7-1). Esophagram shows an oblique impression at level of aortic arch in frontal view (Figure 7-2A) and compression of esophagus from behind in lateral view (Figure 7-2B).

Diagnosis: Cyanotic heart disease with right aortic arch and aberrant left subclavian artery.

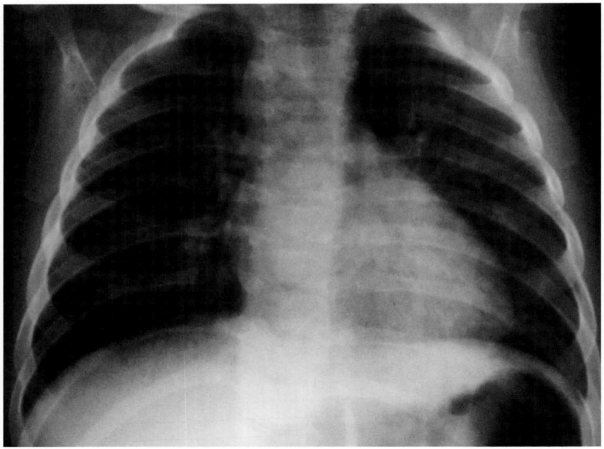

Fig. 7-1

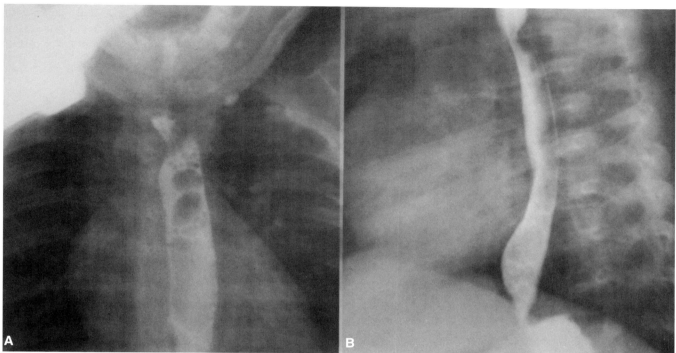

Fig. 7-2

Case 8

An 8-month-old boy has blue lips and breathes fast when he eats. Birth weight was 4.2 kg.

Temperature is 36.2°C, heart rate 144, respiratory rate 44, blood pressure 106/83 mm Hg, weight 6.8 kg, length 65 cm, and head circumference 43 cm. Cardiac impulse is in right side of chest. A systolic murmur at lower right sternal border radiates to back. S_2 is single. The rest of the physical findings are normal.

ECG shows right axis deviation, probable right ventricular hypertrophy, and inferior Q waves.

Hematocrit is 0.34. White cell count is 10.2×10^9/liter. Platelet count is 258×10^9/liter. Urine specific gravity is 1.005, pH 7. Urine has moderate blood and 0.2 AU urobilinogen. Serum sodium is 144 mmol/liter, potassium 4.2, chloride 109, carbon dioxide 19, urea nitrogen 2.9, calcium 2.12, phosphorus 1.49, cholesterol 2.25, and glucose 4.5. Creatinine is 40 μmol/liter, uric acid 290, total bilirubin 12, and direct bilirubin 2. Total protein is 53 g/liter, albumin 37. Alkaline phosphatase is 3,870 U/liter, LDH 357, and SGOT 49.

Enlarged heart is in right side of chest. Course of trachea suggests right aortic arch. Gas-containing gut, high in right side of abdomen, suggests horizontal liver. Gas and liquid are in dilated stomach in left side of abdomen (Figure 8-1). Esophagram shows vascular impression behind lower part of esophagus (Figure 8-2). 99m-Technetium sulfur colloid scintiscan shows horizontal liver and no spleen.

Cardiac catheterization, echocardiogram, and angiocardiogram show systemic arterial oxygen saturation 0.85, pulmonary hypertension, dextrocardia, AV canal septal defect, pulmonary atresia, ductus arteriosus, total anomalous pulmonary venous return to left vertical vein, D-transposition of great arteries, left superior vena cava, aorta to left and in front of atretic pulmonary annulus, and systemic-pulmonary arterial collateral to left lower lobe.

At right thoracotomy, right ductus arteriosus (diameter: 8 mm) is ligated. Left pulmonary artery is long and tortuous; main pulmonary artery and right pulmonary artery are not seen. A Taussig-Blalock shunt is placed.

Diagnosis: Cyanotic heart disease, aberrant bronchial artery behind esophagus.

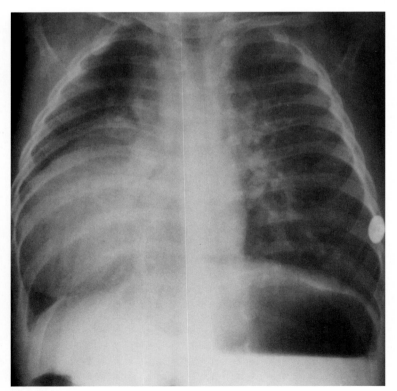

Fig. 8-1

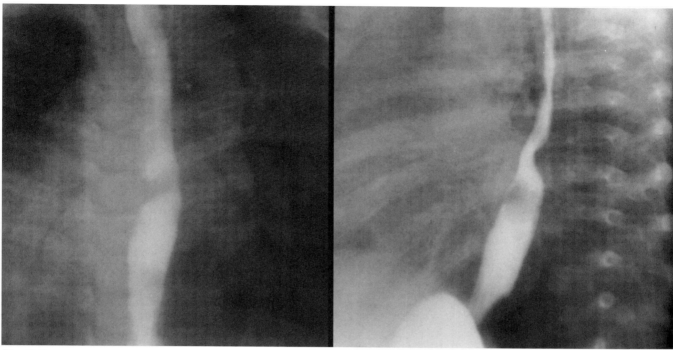

Fig. 8-2

Case 9

A 3-year-old boy vomits everything but liquids.

His mother and he had fever, vomiting, and diarrhea 3 months ago. She was well in 3 days. He continued to vomit a few minutes to 1–2 hours after he ate and has had abdominal pain with vomiting for several weeks. He is "hungry all the time." Two months ago, weight was 16 kg.

Mother and three older half sisters are well.

Weight is 14.3 kg, height 94 cm, temperature 36.2°C, heart rate 108, respiratory rate 30, and systolic blood pressure 110 mm Hg. Breath sounds are diminished on left side. The rest of the physical findings are normal.

Hematocrit is 0.30. White cell count is 7.9×10^9/liter with 0.38 polymorphonuclear cells, 0.04 bands, 0.53 lymphocytes, 0.03 monocytes, 0.01 basophils, and 0.01 atypical lymphocytes. Platelet count is 611×10^9/liter. Urine specific gravity is 1.019, pH 6. Urine has 0–2 white cells/HPF. Serum sodium is 135 mmol/liter, potassium 3.9, chloride 104, carbon dioxide 18, urea nitrogen 2.0, calcium 2.32, phosphorus 1.52,

cholesterol 3.15, and glucose 5.1. Creatinine is 40 μmol/liter, uric acid 270, total bilirubin 5, and direct bilirubin 0. Total protein is 81 g/liter, albumin 37. Alkaline phosphatase is 117 U/liter, LDH 234, and SGOT 21.

In Figure 9-1, an irregular shadow of air and water density is in left side of chest, and heart is displaced left. CT scan in Figure 9-2 shows pleural nodules and calcium in a mass that goes behind left lower lobe bronchus and around aorta and esophagus.

At thoracotomy, a rubbery mass is in lingula and left lower lobe, and nodules are on pleural surface.

Microscopic examination of white to pale yellow mass shows collagen, plasma cells, lymphocytes, bands of fibroblasts, fibrotic alveoli and septa infiltrated by plasma cells and lymphocytes, and hyperplastic type II pneumocytes lining alveoli.

Diagnosis: Plasma cell granuloma of lung with sclerosing mediastinitis.

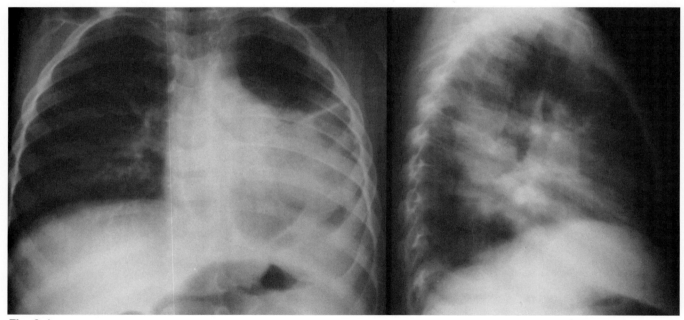

Fig. 9-1

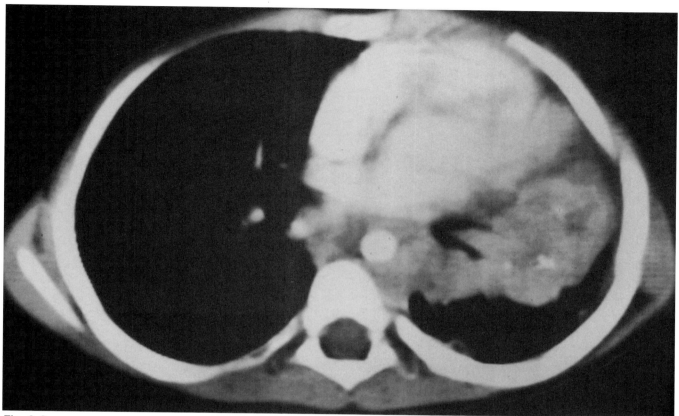

Fig. 9-2

Case 10

A 22-month-old girl has a chest tumor in roentgenographic examination performed yesterday because of a fever that began 2 days ago.

Birth weight was 1.4 kg, length 41 cm, head circumference 29 cm, Apgar score 3/7 at 1 and 5 minutes, and systolic blood pressure 48 mm Hg. She has had four watery stools per day for 4 months. Weight was 10.2 kg at 18 months.

Mother (33 years old), father (37 years old), and sister (3 years old) are well.

Weight at 22 months is 10.3 kg, height 85 cm, temperature 39.6°C, heart rate 180, respiratory rate 52, and blood pressure 136/74 mm Hg. Physical findings are normal.

Hematocrit is 0.38. White cell count is 4.6×10^9/liter with 0.43 polymorphonuclear cells, 0.08 bands, 0.39 lymphocytes, and 0.10 monocytes. Platelet count is 293×10^9/liter. Urine specific gravity is 1.028, pH 6. Urine has 1+ ketones, mucus, and 2–5 white cells/HPF. Serum sodium is 142 mmol/liter, potassium 3.3, chloride 107, carbon dioxide 19, urea nitrogen 3.2, and glucose 6.4. Creatinine is 40 µmol/liter. PT is 10.4 seconds, activated PTT 52.2 (control: 34.7).

A paraspinal mass of water density with a broad top and tapered base is in left side of chest from T3–T9. Excess liquid is in dilated gut (Figure 10-1).

At left thoracotomy, an encapsulated tumor, part yellow, part red and brown, is resected.

Microscopic examination shows (1) sheets of cells with little cytoplasm and oval basophilic nuclei, some with prominent nucleoli; (2) pale, eosinophilic, fibrillar trabeculae; (3) hemorrhage; (4) necrosis; and (5) calcification.

At 24 months, weight is 12 kg, blood pressure 100/45 mm Hg. At 31 months, parents are worried about her constipation. She has one stool every 1–3 days.

Diagnosis: Ganglioneuroblastoma (diarrhea from ectopic vasoactive intestinal polypeptide).

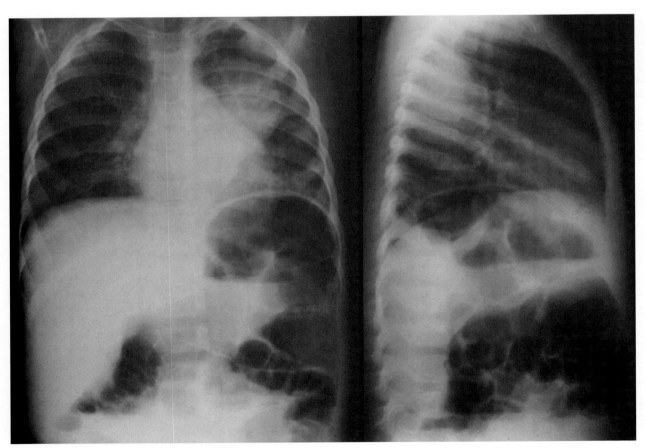

Fig. 10-1

Case 11

A 10-year-old girl is paraplegic.

Pregnancy of mother was normal, birth weight 3.7 kg. She did not move her legs at 4½ months and had a swelling along upper left side of back.

CT scan at 4½ months shows tumor that pushes bronchi forward and to right and contains calcium, including a calcified strip that goes through a neural foramen into spinal canal (Figure 11-1). Myelogram shows a block at T9.

At laminectomy at 4½ months, tumor is in subcutaneous tissue. Red-purple, meaty tumor, which is deep to spinous processes, laminae, and ligamentum flavum, compresses spinal cord to thickness of 2–3 mm from T5 to T9. Tumor is easily separated from dura underneath and removed. At left thoracotomy 2½ weeks later, tumor in left side of chest behind aorta extends into right side of chest and into left intervertebral foramina from T5 to T9. Most of tumor is removed.

Microscopic examination of tumor shows small-to-medium cells that have indistinct margins, variable amounts of eosinophilic cytoplasm, ovoid nuclei with finely granular chromatin, prominent nucleoli in some nuclei, occasional mitoses, rosettes, necrosis, calcification, and thin, irregular fibrous septa. Electron microscopy shows dense core secretory granules in tumor cell processes.

Thoracolumbar spinal left convexity is treated with Harrington rod at 2 years and anterior spinal fusion at 7 years. She is in fifth grade at 10 years. She catheterizes her bladder and gives herself a daily enema. Her legs sometimes shake. She wears a plastic body jacket and uses a wheelchair.

Weight at 10 years is 23 kg, height 114 cm, head circumference 51 cm, and blood pressure 88/60 mm Hg. She has a cough, which is ascribed to kinked trachea because of high thoracic gibbus. Operative scars are present. Legs are flaccid. Sensory level is at T5. The rest of the physical findings are normal.

Hematocrit is 0.41. White cell count is 8.6 × 10⁹/liter. Platelet count is 343 × 10⁹/liter. Serum sodium is 138 mmol/liter, potassium 3.9, chloride 99, carbon dioxide 29, urea nitrogen 5.0, calcium 2.47, phosphorus 1.49, cholesterol 3.90, and glucose 5.9. Creatinine is 40 μmol/liter, uric acid 210, total bilirubin 10, and direct bilirubin 0. Total protein is 76 g/liter, albumin 47. Alkaline phosphatase is 207 U/liter, LDH 289, and SGOT 29.

Diagnosis: Neuroblastoma.

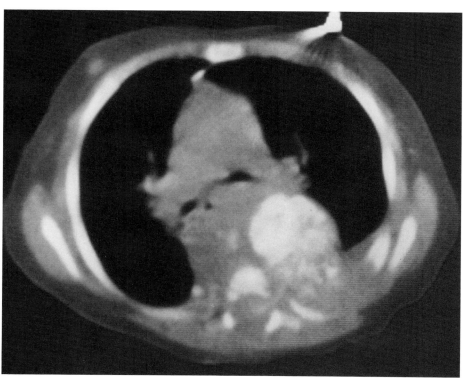

Fig. 11-1

Case 12

A 16-year-old boy, a defensive end on his high school football team, has high blood pressure that was discovered in examination for sore throat 2 weeks ago. He plays with usual energy and sweats a lot, but has not sweated on right side of face for last 2 years.

Parents and two brothers (13 and 19 years old) are well.

Temperature is 37.2°C, heart rate 76, respiratory rate 20, blood pressure 152/92 mm Hg, weight 81 kg, and height 180 cm. He sweats during examination. A systolic murmur is present. The rest of the physical findings are normal.

Hematocrit is 0.43. White cell count is 12.2×10^9/liter. Platelet count is 441×10^9/liter. Serum sodium is 141 mmol/liter, potassium 4.0, chloride 96, carbon dioxide 20, urea nitrogen 4.3, calcium 2.42, phosphorus 1.49, cholesterol 4.50, and glucose 5.2. Creatinine is 80 μmol/liter, uric acid 400, total bilirubin 3, and direct bilirubin 0. Total protein is 74 g/liter, albumin 45. Alkaline phosphatase is 97 U/liter, LDH 142, and SGOT 12. Urine vanillylmandelic acid by high-performance liquid chromatography is 135 μmol/day (normal: 9–36), homovanillic acid 38 (normal: 8–48).

A shadow of water density is alongside trachea in upper part of right side of chest in roentgenogram (Figure 12-1) and in unenhanced CT scan (Figure 12-2).

Blood pressure is 145/90 mm Hg at start of operation, >300/150 mm Hg when hand is on soft purple tumor, 90/50 mm Hg when hand is off. Tumor is fixed to apex of right lung and right second and third ribs, extends into intervertebral foramen and along theca, and is supplied by an artery along a main vein that drains into branch of azygous vein. Tumor is excised in two operations, first extraspinal, second intraspinal.

Extraspinal tumor (4.8 × 4.5 × 3.8 cm) is pink to tan to purple and bosselated on outside. In cut section, tumor is gray to dark red; is "like fish flesh," according to pathologist; and has whorls, lobules, and random red foci. Microscopic examination shows (1) collagenous bands of varying thickness around nests of large pleomorphic cells that have coarse, granular, eosinophilic cytoplasm; (2) round-to-oval, vacuolated, pleomorphic nuclei; (3) stellate processes that create a vacuolated appearance between cells; (4) many small blood vessels; (5) perivascular foci of plasma cells; and (6) frequent large, bizarre multinucleated cells. Electron microscopy shows many dense core secretory granules (diameter: 200–275 nm).

At 19 years, diameter of right pupil is 3 mm, left 5 mm. At 22 years, blood pressure is 146/66 mm Hg, pulse 54, weight 83 kg, and height 180 cm.

Diagnosis: Paraganglioma.

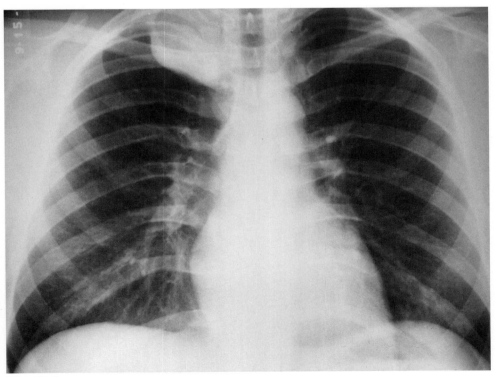

Fig. 12-1

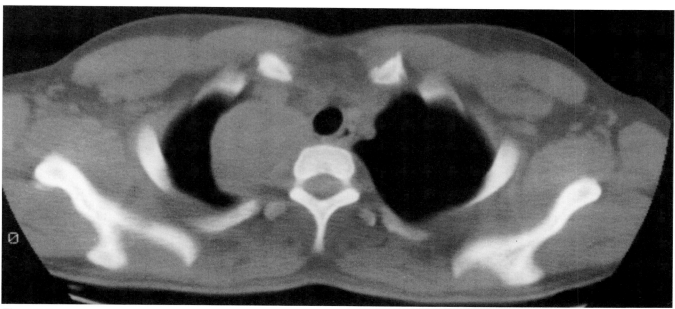

Fig. 12-2

Case 13

A 6-year-old boy has been orthopneic the last 2 nights. Wheezing began 1 month ago and persists despite bronchodilators. Appetite is bad. Chest hurts.

Temperature is 37°C, heart rate 120, respiratory rate 28, blood pressure 88/54 mm Hg, weight 19 kg, and height 117 cm. Breathing is noisy. Heart sounds are distant. Liver edge is 2 cm below costal margin. The rest of the physical findings are normal.

Hematocrit is 0.43. White cell count is 10.2×10^9/liter with 0.76 polymorphonuclear cells, 0.04 bands, 0.18 lymphocytes, and 0.02 monocytes. Platelet count is 354×10^9/liter. Serum sodium is 137 mmol/liter, potassium 5.0, chloride 100, carbon dioxide 25, urea nitrogen 4.3, calcium 2.35, phosphorus 1.52, cholesterol 3.49, and glucose 5.3. Creatinine is 40 μmol/liter, uric acid 180, total bilirubin 6, and direct bilirubin 0. Total protein is 74 g/liter, albumin 37. Alkaline phosphatase is 173 U/liter, LDH 942, and SGOT 58. Capillary blood pH is 7.30 when F_{IO_2} = 1.0 by mask. P_{CO_2} is 50 mm Hg, P_{O_2} 48. Bicarbonate is 24 mmol/liter.

In Figure 13-1, the pericardiocardiac image is large, left lower lobe compressed, and medial part of right clavicle rarefied.

The visual counterpart of Ewart's sign—that is, diminished percussion note and bronchial breath sounds—is below left scapula. The strip of water density in right lung is caused by liquid or thickened pleura in horizontal fissure or a strip of atelectasis (Figure 13-1).

Six hundred milliliters of pink, milky liquid obtained at pericardiocentesis has 10×10^9/liter white cells, 0.01 polymorphonuclear cells, 0.93 lymphocytes, 0.04 monocytes, 0.01 metamyelocytes, 0.01 myelocytes, clumped red cells, and is sterile. At right thoracotomy 2 days later because of recurrence, pericardium is tense, white, and thin around another 600 ml of sterile milky liquid. Parietal pleura is mildly hyperemic. Lungs are edematous. Pericardial liquid recurs. Pleural liquid accumulates on both sides. Right side of neck swells.

CT scan at 7 years shows rarefaction of right side of base of skull (Figure 13-2A), swelling of soft tissues of right side of neck (Figure 13-2B), and thinning of right side of posterior arch of atlas (see Figure 13-2B).

Diagnosis: Pericardial effusion, vanishing bones; lymphangiomatosis.

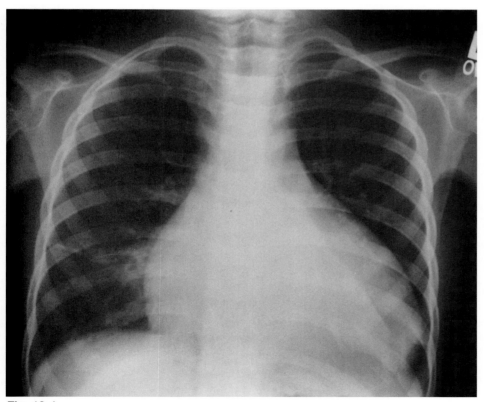

Fig. 13-1

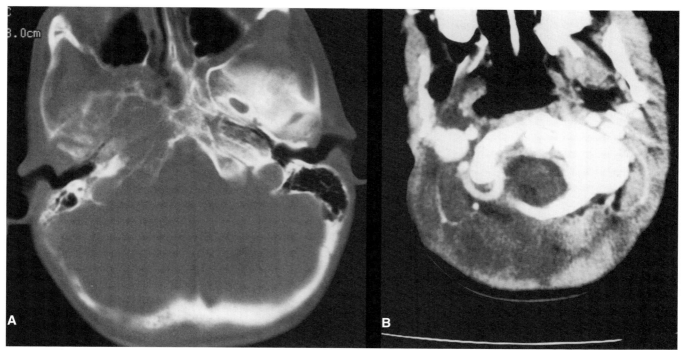

Fig. 13-2

Case 14

A 3-year-old girl has a heart murmur that was first heard at 8 months.

Pregnancy of mother was normal. She sat at 6 months, walked at 1 year. She had two ear infections during the first year. She broke a clavicle at 2 years, a forearm at 2½ years.

Mother (27 years old) and father (28 years old) are well.

Weight at 3 years is 13.4 kg, height 92 cm, temperature 36.6°C, heart rate 120, respiratory rate 32, and blood pressure 92/60 mm Hg. A systolic murmur and a diastolic murmur are present. S_2 is fixed and widely split. The rest of the physical findings are normal.

Hematocrit is 0.39. White cell count is 7.7×10^9/liter with 0.52 polymorphonuclear cells, 0.03 bands, 0.39 lymphocytes, 0.05 monocytes, and 0.01 eosinophils. Urine specific gravity is 1.014, pH 8. Urine has occasional squamous epithelial cells/HPF. Serum sodium is 139 mmol/liter, potassium 4.5, chloride 101, urea nitrogen 5.4, and glucose 3.7. Creatinine is 30 µmol/liter.

ECG findings are normal.

At cardiac catheterization, oxygen saturation in superior vena cava is 0.73, right atrium 0.74, right ventricle 0.80, pulmonary artery 0.79, left atrium 0.89, lower left pulmonary vein 0.92, and left ventricle 0.91. Pressure in right atrium is 4 mm Hg (mean), right ventricle 35/4, pulmonary artery 14 (mean), left atrium 6 (mean), and left ventricle 95/9. At angiocardiography, catheter goes through an atrial-septal defect.

At operation, sievelike defects up to 2 cm in atrial septum are closed with sutures.

Her 4½-year-old sister has a heart murmur that was first heard at 10 months.

Pregnancy of mother was normal, birth weight 3.6 kg. She sat at 5 months, walked at 10 months. She had pneumococcal meningitis at 10 months. ECG findings were normal. At cardiac catheterization at 1 year through azygous vein, oxygen saturation in superior vena cava was 0.60, right atrium 0.75, upper right pulmonary vein 0.92, left atrium 0.90, and left ventricle 0.90. Pressure in right atrium was 7 mm Hg (mean), right ventricle 36/8, pulmonary artery 20 (mean), and left ventricle 90/10.

Weight at 4½ years is 11.4 kg, height 95 cm, temperature 37.2°C, heart rate 80, respiratory rate 20, and blood pressure 100/70 mm Hg. Teeth are carious. A systolic murmur is present. The rest of the physical findings are normal.

Hematocrit is 0.36. White cell count is 7.1×10^9/liter with 0.61 polymorphonuclear cells, 0.02 bands, 0.28 lymphocytes, 0.08 monocytes, and 0.01 basophils. Platelet count is 390×10^9/liter. Urine specific gravity is 1.022, pH 7. Urine has occasional white cells/HPF and mucus. Serum sodium is 143 mmol/liter, potassium 5.0, chloride 109, carbon dioxide 23, urea nitrogen 5.0, calcium 2.72, phosphorus 1.36, cholesterol 3.72, and glucose 6.6. Creatinine is 20 µmol/liter, uric acid 240, total bilirubin 7, and direct bilirubin 3. Total protein is 76 g/liter, albumin 46. Alkaline phosphatase is 233 U/liter, LDH 297, and SGOT 34.

At operation on the same day as her 3-year-old sister, a secundum atrial-septal defect (2 cm) and a smaller one nearby are closed with sutures.

Preoperative findings in chest of 3-year-old girl are normal (Figure 14-1A). In preoperative examination of 4½-year-old sister, supracardiac shadow is widened on right side of trachea by a curved shadow of water density just above bifurcation (Figure 14-2A).

The 3-year-old girl is well 10 days after operation. She has a systolic murmur. The 4½-year-old girl is pale 10 days after operation, breathing fast, and has a systolic murmur, gallop rhythm, and liver edge palpable 5 cm below costal margin.

Pericardiocardiac image of 4½-year-old girl is large 10 days after operation (Figure 14-2B).

The 4½-year-old girl is better 24 days after operation. Liver edge is barely palpable. Her 3-year-old sister is well 24 days after operation and returns only because the 4½-year-old girl is to be examined. The 3-year-old girl has normal ECG findings and no murmur.

Pericardiocardiac image of 3-year-old girl is large 24 days after operation (Figure 14-1B).

Diagnosis: Sisters with atrial-septal defect and postpericardiotomy syndrome, azygous continuation of inferior vena cava in older sister.

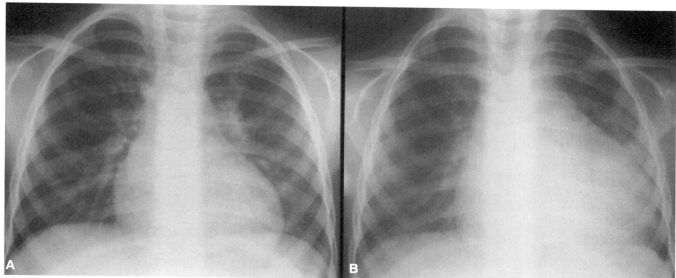

Fig. 14-1

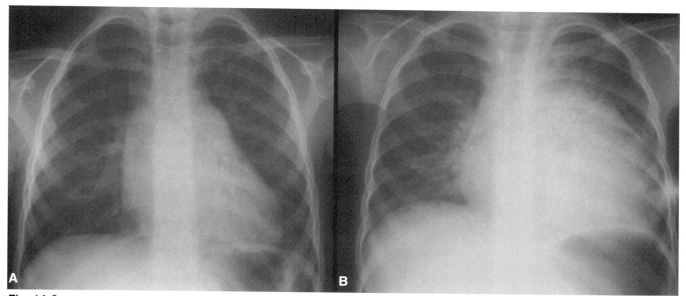

Fig. 14-2

Case 15

A 5½-month-old boy who used to sit will not lift his head, smile, or eat. He has fever, raspy breathing, and chest rash. Temperature has been up to 39.4°C for 3 weeks, breathing noisy for 1½ weeks, and rash present for 1 week.

He smiled at 2½ months, sat alone at 4½ months, and reaches for objects and transfers them.

Mother (26 years old) and father are well. He is their only child. Maternal grandmother had breast cancer, paternal grandmother high blood pressure.

Weight at 5½ months is 7.4 kg, height 73 cm, head circumference 44 cm, temperature 39.7°C, heart rate 146, respiratory rate 48, and blood pressure 98/60 mm Hg. A small red spot is on right upper lid. The rest of the physical findings are normal.

Hematocrit is 0.31. White cell count is 18.0×10^9/liter with 0.41 polymorphonuclear cells, 0.15 bands, 0.41 lymphocytes, 0.01 monocytes, and 0.02 eosinophils. Platelet count is 510×10^9/liter. ESR is 92 mm/hr. Urine specific gravity is 1.021, pH 5. Urine has 3–4 epithelial cells/HPF, 2–4 white cells/HPF, and 4+ amorphous matter. Serum sodium is 131 mmol/liter, potassium 4.8, chloride 95, urea nitrogen 1.8, calcium 2.32, phosphorus 1.42, cholesterol 6.33, and glucose 5.2. Creatinine is 20 µmol/liter, uric acid 200, total bilirubin 7, and direct bilirubin 2. Total protein is 78 g/liter, albumin 36. Alkaline phosphatase is 199 U/liter, LDH 1,071, and SGOT 295. CSF has 17×10^6/liter white cells, all lymphocytes, no red cells, 3.8 mmol/liter glucose, and 0.12 g/liter protein. Culture of blood and CSF is sterile. Bone marrow is hypercellular.

Chest rash is gone 3 days later. Pinpoint red rash is on head, body, and limbs the fourth day and gone later that day. Lymph nodes (2–5 mm) are in neck, axillas, and groins at 6 months. Spleen edge is 2 cm below costal margin, liver edge 3 cm. At 6½ months, he coughs, sneezes, vomits, sleeps little, and grunts with each breath.

At 6 and 6½ months, liquid is in each pleural space, more in right than in left (Figure 15-1A). Pericardiocardiac image is large at 6½ months (Figure 15-1B). "Sick child" lines are in distal femoral metaphyses at 6½ months (Figure 15-2).

Sixty-five milliliters of serous blood-tinged liquid are obtained by pericardiocentesis at 6½ months. Liquid has 10.6×10^9/liter red cells, 2.8×10^9/liter white cells, 0.96 polymorphonuclear cells, 0.02 lymphocytes, 0.01 basophils, and 0.01 mesothelial cells. Culture grows coagulase-negative staphylococci.

He is afebrile. He is given prednisone for 2 months. He is well until 18 months, when he refuses to stand or crawl. Ankles and knees are red and warm, and right ankle is swollen at 19 months. Treatment with steroids and IV gold is begun. He walks with hips and knees flexed and runs with fast shuffle at 2¾ years and climbs stairs at 3¼ years. Treatment with gold is stopped at 5 years. At 8 years, weight is 27 kg, height 130 cm, and blood pressure 90/70 mm Hg. Physical findings are normal.

Diagnosis: Juvenile rheumatoid arthritis (Still's disease).

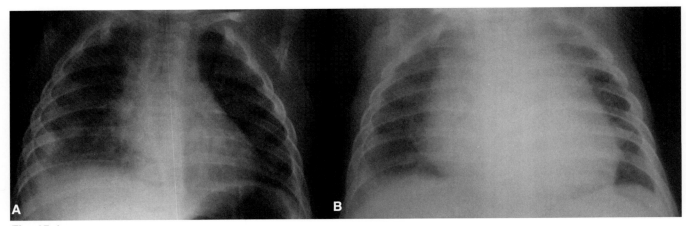

Fig. 15-1

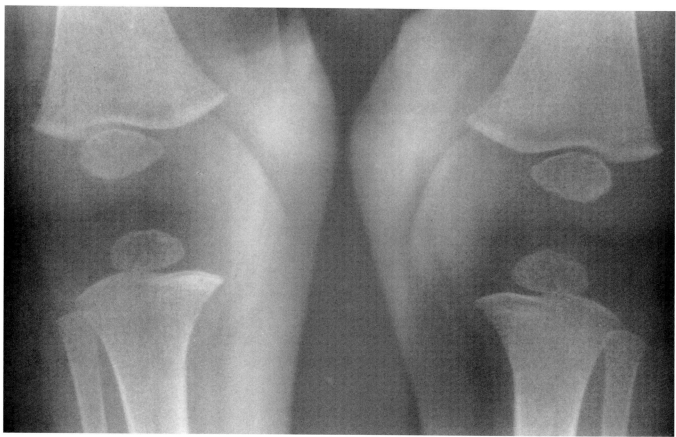

Fig. 15-2

Case 16

A 2-year-old girl is breathing hard.

Cough and fever began 1 month ago. She has been afebrile for 12 days. Milky liquid that contained 30 g/liter protein and 22.6×10^9/liter white cells, 0.80 lymphocytes, was obtained at right thoracentesis 10 days ago.

Birth weight was 3.4 kg. She was breast-fed for 3 months. She had fever and swelling in left side of neck at 4 months. Operation after treatment with antibiotics showed matted, partly fibrotic lymph nodes that contained lymphocytes, plasma cells, germinal centers, and polymorphonuclear cells.

Mother and two older siblings are well. Father has asthma. A sibling died at 3 days with hypoplastic heart. Maternal grandfather had stomach cancer. Paternal grandfather has emphysema.

Temperature at 2 years is 37.2°C, heart rate 140, respiratory rate 30, systolic blood pressure 90 mm Hg, weight 11.8 kg, and height 90 cm. A scar is on left side of neck. Breath sounds are diminished at right base. Heart sounds are muffled. Liver edge is below umbilicus. The rest of the physical findings are normal.

Hematocrit is 0.39. White cell count is 13.5×10^9/liter with 0.21 polymorphonuclear cells, 0.19 bands, 0.50 lymphocytes, and 0.10 monocytes. Platelet count is 402×10^9/liter. Urine specific gravity is 1.014, pH 5. Urine has 3–5 white cells/HPF and occasional red cells/HPF. Serum sodium is 140 mmol/liter, potassium 4.7, chloride 102, carbon dioxide 16, urea nitrogen 6.4, calcium 2.45, phosphorus 1.23, cholesterol 4.03, and glucose 6.0. Creatinine is 40 μmol/liter, uric acid

600, total bilirubin 10, and direct bilirubin 5. Total protein is 73 g/liter, albumin 36. Alkaline phosphatase is 216 U/liter, LDH 1,038, and SGOT 457. PT is 14.9 seconds (control: 10.1), activated PTT 33.6 (control: 32.2). Serum does not contain HBsAg or HBsAb. Blood cultures are sterile.

ECG shows inversion of left precordial T waves. Earlier ECG showed elevated ST segments. Echocardiogram shows a large, echodense pericardial space; dilated inferior vena cava; hyperdynamic ventricles; and early closure of aortic valve.

Roentgenogram from 3 weeks ago shows large pericardiocardiac image and excessive interstitial markings in lungs that blur heart edge (Figure 16-1A). Size of pericardiocardiac image is normal now. Pleural liquid is on both sides (Figure 16-1B).

Cardiac catheterization shows decreased ventricular compliance, almost equal diastolic pressure in the ventricles, and low cardiac index.

At operation, pericardium is thick. Cheesy, fibrinous exudate is between it and epicardium. Central venous pressure goes from 22 to 12 mm Hg when exudate is removed from around right atrium.

Pericardial sac (0.75 cm thick) is purple, rubbery, and contains yellow exudate and hemorrhagic foci. Microscopic examination shows fibrinoid necrosis and acute and chronic inflammatory cells. Stains for microorganisms are negative. Exudate is sterile.

Diagnosis: Constrictive pericarditis.

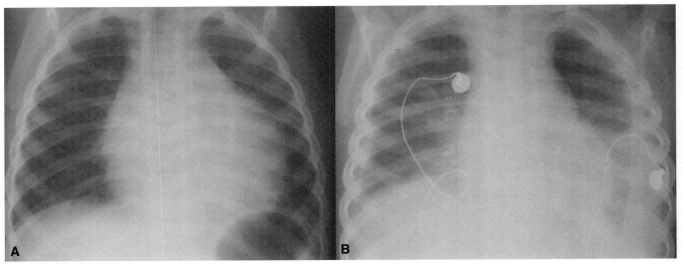

Fig. 16-1

Case 17

A 3-month-old boy has a heart murmur.

Mother (26 years old) drank beer during first trimester. Birth weight was 3.7 kg. He sucked weakly, vomited yellow mucus, and had two small stools the first day. Heart murmur and abdominal distension were present the second day. Colostomy for distal sigmoid Hirschsprung's disease was done. A gastrostomy tube was in place for 1½ weeks. He is slow and sweats during feeding. Chin becomes blue when he cries. He smiles, lifts head, and gazes at moving objects.

Weight at 3 months is 4.3 kg, length 54 cm, head circumference 40 cm, temperature 37.3°C, heart rate 152, respiratory rate 40, and systolic blood pressure 115 mm Hg. External acoustic meatus are narrow. Lower part of sternum is depressed. Holosystolic murmur and diastolic murmur are present. Liver edge is 1 cm below costal margin. A scar is on upper abdomen, colostomy in left lower quadrant. The rest of the physical findings are normal.

ECG shows left ventricular hypertrophy.

Hematocrit is 0.24. White cell count is 17.4×10^9/liter with 0.73 polymorphonuclear cells, 0.11 bands, 0.14 lymphocytes, and 0.02 eosinophils. Urine specific gravity is 1.020, pH 6. Urine has hemoglobin/myoglobin, bacteria, 1–2 white cells/HPF and moderate squamous epithelial cells/HPF.

Heart is displaced left, aortic arch high and prominent. Vascular markings in lungs are prominent in Figure 17-1.

At cardiac catheterization, oxygen saturation in superior vena cava is 0.65, right atrium 0.67, right ventricle 0.85, pulmonary artery 0.84, left atrium 0.91, and aorta 0.94. Pressure in right atrium is 5 mm Hg (mean), right ventricle 47/6, pulmonary artery 43/13, left atrium 9 (mean), left ventricle 145 (systolic), and aorta 120 (systolic). Angiocardiogram shows membranous ventricular septal defect.

At operation, much of left side of pericardium and part of left parietal pleura are absent. Atria are large. Foramen ovale is probe patent. A defect (0.7 cm) in membranous ventricular septum is repaired. At 2 years, colostomy is taken down and colon anastomosed. He has sinus arrhythmia at 6 years and sinus bradycardia at 7 years, when he is diagnosed as having sick sinus syndrome. At 10 years, school work is at first grade level. At 11 years, Holter monitor shows heart rate <35 and episodes of monomorphic ventricular tachycardia. School work improves after a pacemaker is implanted.

Diagnosis: Hirschsprung's disease, membranous ventricular septal defect, absence of left side of pericardium, and sick sinus syndrome.

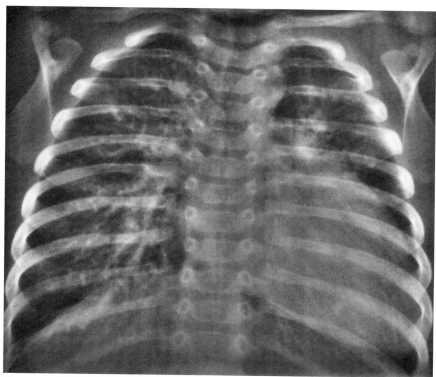

Fig. 17-1

Heart and Aorta

Case 1

A 17-year-old boy has a heart murmur that was first heard when he was examined for bronchitis at 4 years.

He plays on his school football team and works on a farm. He is "phenomenally fit," the best of 50–60 youths in exercise testing, and able to produce the energy to lift a car 1 m/min "for a long time" on a bicycle ergometer, according to the cardiologist.

Weight is 69 kg, height 186 cm, heart rate 45, and blood pressure 110/66 mm Hg. A high-pitched systolic heart murmur is present. The rest of the physical findings are normal.

ECG shows sinus bradycardia and notched P wave.

Roentgenogram at 16 years (Figure 1-1A), when heart rate was 50 and ECG showed predominant atrioventricular nodal rhythm with occasional sinus beats, shows smaller heart than in roentgenogram at 17 years (Figure 1-1B).

Weight at 19 years is 76 kg, height 188 cm. He has a systolic murmur. ECG shows sinus bradycardia and heart rate 50. Roentgenographic findings are like those at 17 years.

Diagnosis: Small ventricular septal defect, athlete's heart.

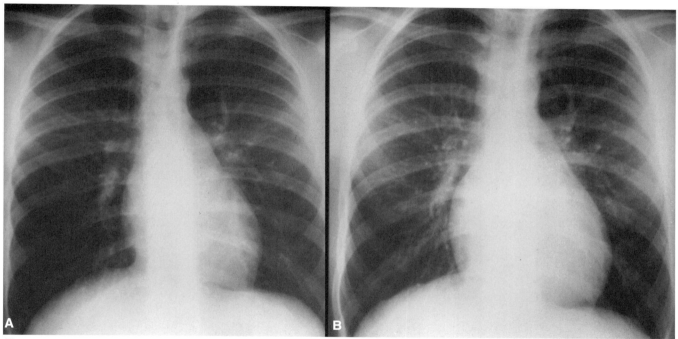

Fig. 1-1

Case 2

A 7-week-old girl barely responds to stimuli. Diaper was dry this morning. She slept a lot today and did not eat.

Birth weight was 4.1 kg, length 53 cm, head circumference 37 cm, and Apgar score 8/9 at 1 and 5 minutes. Physical findings were normal. Weight was 4.1 kg 1 week ago.

Weight at 7 weeks is 3.7 kg, length 57 cm, head circumference 38 cm, temperature 35.6°C, heart rate 45–60, respiratory rate 20, and blood pressure not obtainable. She does not move. Cry is weak. Skin turgor is poor. Anterior fontanel is depressed. Liver edge is 1 cm below costal margin. Clitoris is large. Labia majora are dark and wrinkled. Vagina is shallow. The rest of the physical findings are normal.

Hematocrit is 0.26. Serum sodium is 116 mmol/liter, potassium 8.5, chloride 81, urea nitrogen 26.0, and glucose 9.7.

Heart is small in Figure 2-1.

Chromosomes are 46,XX. Urine pregnanetriol is 21.4 μmol/day (normal: <0.6). Urine 17-ketosteroids are 21 μmol/day after IV steroids are begun and 5 μmol/day 1 week later (normal: <3).

Weight at 17½ years is 91 kg, height 162 cm.

Diagnosis: Steroid 21-hydroxylase deficiency of salt-losing variety (congenital adrenal hyperplasia).

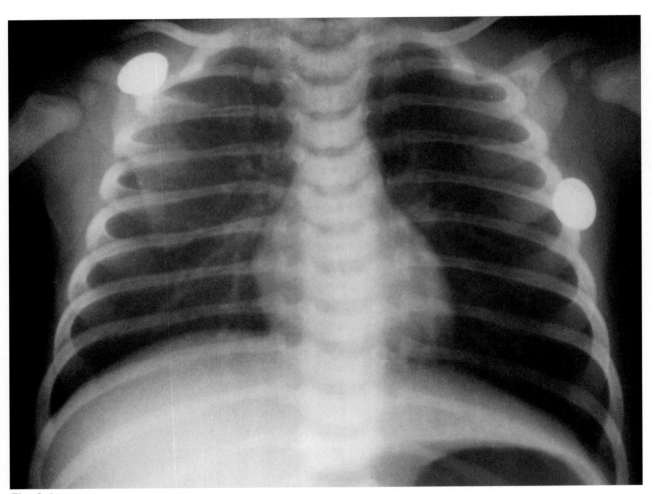

Fig. 2-1

Case 3

A newborn girl is "tomato-faced" and has a heart murmur.

Mother (43 years old) had gestational diabetes and 4–5 liters amniotic fluid at cesarean section for transverse lie. Birth weight is 4.3 kg, length 55 cm, head circumference 36 cm, Apgar score 6/7 at 1 and 5 minutes, temperature 36.7°C, heart rate 150, and respiratory rate 70. Retractions, systolic murmur, and acrocyanosis are present. Liver edge is 2 cm below costal margin. The rest of the physical findings are normal.

At 15 minutes, blood glucose is 2.5 mmol/liter. At 1½ hours, hematocrit is 0.50.

At 2 hours, she is cyanotic until given oxygen. She is pink at 18 hours. Blood glucose is 1.4 mmol/liter at 20 hours. At 53 hours, systolic blood pressure is 72 mm Hg. Systolic murmur and S_3 are present. Liver edge is 2 cm below costal margin.

At 56 hours, heart is large. Lungs lack air. Thick axillary soft tissues are streaked with fat (Figure 3-1).

ECG shows right ventricular hypertrophy and right atrial enlargement. Cardiac catheterization shows systolic pressure 70 mm Hg in right ventricle, pulmonary artery, and aorta. Angiocardiogram shows large right ventricle and tricuspid regurgitation.

She is well at 4 days. Physical findings are normal at 1 month.

Diagnosis: Transient cardiomyopathy in infant of mother with gestational diabetes.

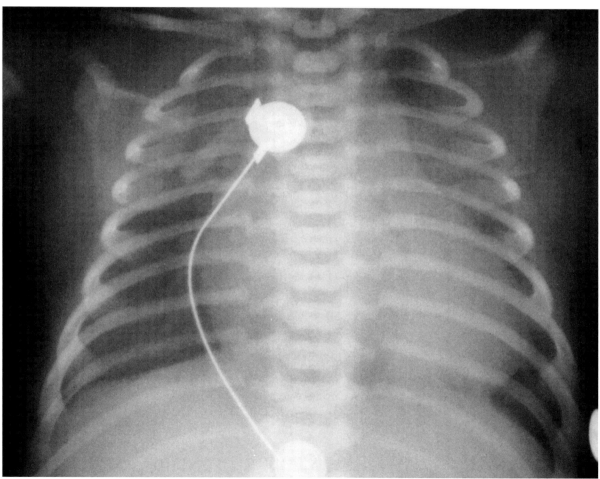

Fig. 3-1

Case 4

A 6-month-old girl has a fever, labored breathing, and a "peculiar, high-pitched cry."

Birth weight was 3.9 kg. Skin was blistered at birth. At 9 days, she had paroxysmal atrial tachycardia. Examination of a stained smear of material from the base of a blister showed multinucleated giant cells. Weight was 4.5 kg at 2 months; blisters were present. At 4 months, she was floppy and had blisters. Weight was 5.0 kg, length 67 cm, and head circumference 41 cm. At 5 months, she had gastroenteritis. Liver was not palpable.

At 6 months, she sometimes reaches for objects. Temperature is 39.4°C, heart rate 150, respiratory rate 60, systolic blood pressure 85 mm Hg, weight 5.5 kg, and length 67 cm. She is pale and floppy. Several sores less than 1 cm in diameter and some blisters are on abdomen. Eardrums are pink. Tongue is prominent. A systolic murmur is present. Liver edge is 3 cm below costal margin. The rest of the physical findings are normal.

Hematocrit is 0.41. White cell count is 18.9×10^9/liter with 0.59 polymorphonuclear cells, 0.12 bands, 0.15 lymphocytes, 0.13 monocytes, and 0.01 basophils. Platelet count is 286×10^9/liter. Urine specific gravity is 1.034, pH 5. Urine has 0.30 g/liter protein, reducing substances, and uric acid crystals. Serum sodium is 132 mmol/liter, potassium 5.7, chloride 100, carbon dioxide 22, urea nitrogen 4.6, calcium 2.42, phosphorus 0.94, cholesterol 3.13, and glucose 5.7. Creatinine is 60 μmol/liter, uric acid 380, total bilirubin 15, and direct bilirubin 2. Total protein is 56 g/liter, albumin 35. Alkaline phosphatase is 203 U/liter, LDH 1,380, and SGOT 136. Serum titer for herpesvirus by complement fixation is <1:8.

Heart is larger than normal; shape is similar at 9 days (Figure 4-1A) and 6 months (Figure 4-1B).

ECG shows PR interval 60–70 milliseconds, Wolff-Parkinson-White conduction, and left atrial and left and right ventricular hypertrophy. Echocardiogram shows thick-walled, dilated, and poorly contracting left ventricle.

Base of a blister is Tzanck test negative. Punch biopsy of skin and subcutaneous tissue shows subcorneal vesicle that has necrotic and acantholytic keratinocytes, lymphocytes, histiocytes, neutrophils, eosinophils, and nuclear debris and that overlies a lymphohistiocytic infiltrate.

Her leukocytes and fibroblasts show no α-1,4-glucosidase (acid maltase) activity.

She dies at 7 months. At necropsy, heart is large. Wall of left ventricle is 2 cm thick and waxy, light tan on cut section. Right ventricular wall is 0.5 cm thick. Liver is large and waxy, red-brown when cut. Microscopic examination shows vacuoles in heart, liver, and diaphragm, some of which are PAS positive with moderately decreased staining after diastase digestion. Clear, frothy cytoplasm is in some pancreatic acinar cells, in lymphocytes in white pulp of spleen, and in ovary.

Diagnosis: Glycogenosis IIA (Pompe's disease), questionable herpetic blisters.

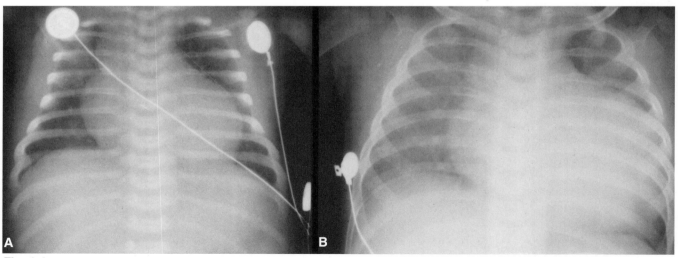

Fig. 4-1

Case 5

A 7-month-old girl will not eat.

Pregnancy of mother was marred by morning sickness, vaginal spotting, and oligohydramnios. Delivery was by cesarean section. Birth weight was 1.7 kg. She has always been floppy and has never eaten well. She smiled at 3 months, lifted her head at 6 months, and now reaches for objects. At 6 months, she had a holosystolic heart murmur, large liver, and thin, weak muscles. Plasma total carnitine was 12.4 µmol/liter (normal: 35–75). She was treated with digitalis, diuretic, and levocarnitine.

Mother (20 years old), father (23 years old), and brother (19 months old) are well.

Weight at 7 months is 4.6 kg, length 60 cm, head circumference 40 cm, heart rate 132, respiratory rate 48, and blood pressure 100/65 mm Hg. Muscle tone is poor. A systolic heart murmur is present. Liver edge is 1–2 cm below costal margin. The rest of the physical findings are normal.

Pericardiocardiac image is large (Figure 5-1).

ECG shows left ventricular hypertrophy and secondary ST-T wave abnormality. Echocardiogram shows dilation of heart chambers, bowing of atrial septum into right atrium, patent foramen ovale, and poor ventricular function.

She coughs and vomits for 2 days at 8 months. Weight is 5 kg, heart rate 134, and respiratory rate 60. Breathing is noisy. Systolic murmur and, occasionally, gallop rhythm are present. Liver edge is 3 cm below costal margin.

Hematocrit at 8 months is 0.36. White cell count is 13.4 × 10^9/liter with 0.35 polymorphonuclear cells, 0.01 bands, 0.48 lymphocytes, and 0.16 monocytes. Platelet count is 350 × 10^9/liter. Serum sodium is 144 mmol/liter, potassium 4.8, chloride 106, carbon dioxide 26, urea nitrogen 6.8, calcium 2.47, phosphorus 2.32, cholesterol 4.76, and glucose 3.9. Creatinine is 50 µmol/liter, uric acid 600, total bilirubin 3, and direct bilirubin 2. Total protein is 69 g/liter, albumin 47. Alkaline phosphatase is 149 U/liter, LDH 738, and SGOT 75.

Echocardiographic ejection fraction is 0.28.

At gastrostomy at 11 months, specimens of liver and muscle are normal in light and electron microscopy. She dies at 1 year. Heart, especially left ventricle, is hypertrophied and dilated at necropsy. Lungs, kidneys, and spleen are congested. Pigment-containing macrophages are in lung alveoli, petechiae in kidneys and adrenals.

Diagnosis: Dilated cardiomyopathy.

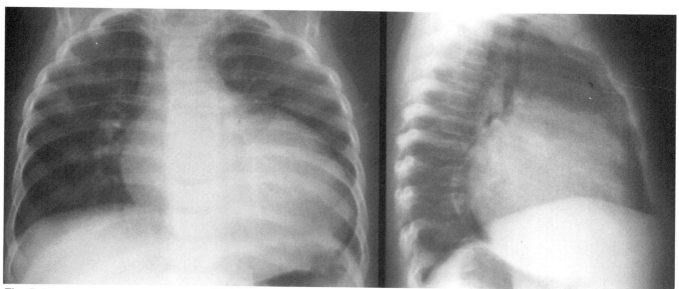

Fig. 5-1

Case 6

A 4½-year-old girl tires easily and has had chest pains and a cough for 4 months.

Pregnancy of mother was normal, birth weight 3.3 kg. She had café au lait spots and systolic murmur at 6 months. She has had colds and ear infections.

Mother (38 years old) has diabetes mellitus; father (46 years old) has neurofibromatosis. Half sister (14 years old) is well.

Weight is 17.7 kg, height 102 cm, heart rate 100, respiratory rate 25, and blood pressure 90/70 mm Hg. Café au lait spots are on trunk and legs. Systolic thrill; long, harsh systolic murmur; and questionable early diastolic murmur are present. A subcutaneous nodule is on abdomen and bottom of first toes. Peripheral pulses are weak. The rest of the physical findings are normal.

Hematocrit is 0.41. White cell count is 11.7×10^9/liter with 0.41 polymorphonuclear cells, 0.44 lymphocytes, 0.10 monocytes, 0.04 eosinophils, and 0.01 basophils. Platelet count is 313×10^9/liter. Urine specific gravity is 1.026, pH 7. Urine has 0–1 red cell/HPF, 0–1 white cell/HPF, bacteria, and amorphous urates. Serum sodium is 141 mmol/liter, potassium 4.4, chloride 108, urea nitrogen 7.5, and glucose 5.3. Creatinine is 40 μmol/liter, total bilirubin 7, and direct bilirubin 2.

ECG shows deep S waves in right precordium, tall R waves in left precordium, and sagging ST-T segments.

Roentgenographic findings are normal at 6 months. At 4½ years, heart is large, and its shape suggests dilation of left ventricle (Figure 6-1).

Echocardiogram shows concentric hypertrophy of left ventricle and asymmetric hypertrophy of ventricular septum.

At operation, ventricular septum is thickened, anterior cusp of mitral valve thickened and fibrotic.

Microscopic examination of core of pale, tan-white tissue and dark red, firm myocardium shows thickened fibrous endocardium on myocardium of subendothelial cells with small nuclei and deeper myocardial cells with larger nuclei.

One year later, gradient across left ventricular outflow track is 85 mm Hg. Septal myomectomy and myotomy are performed.

At 15 years, she becomes short of breath and tires easily. Weight is 58 kg, height 152 cm, heart rate 90, and blood pressure 122/53 mm Hg. At operation, mitral valve is replaced because thickened, calcified chordae tendineae of anterior (aortic) cusp obstruct left ventricular outflow track.

Diagnosis: Asymmetric septal hypertrophy (hypertrophic cardiomyopathy), neurofibromatosis.

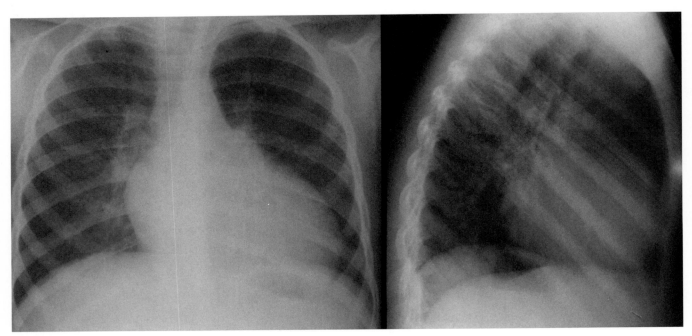

Fig. 6-1

Case 7

A 9-year-old girl has spells of "pounding in chest," weakness, faint voice, and sometimes nausea.

Pregnancy of mother was normal. The girl walked at 10 months, talked at 1 year, has been clumsy since 3 years, cannot steer her bike straight, and has tired easily since 7 years, when a heart murmur was first heard. She has had chicken-pox and ear infections, although none recently. She is in special education class.

Mother (33 years old), father (36 years old), and brother (13 years old) are well. Mother and others in her family have headaches.

Weight at 9 years is 27.2 kg, height 130 cm, temperature 37.3°C, heart rate 92, respiratory rate 20, and blood pressure 122/80 mm Hg. A systolic heart murmur is present. She sways when she walks and when she stands with eyes closed and feet together (Romberg's sign). Deep tendon reflexes in legs are diminished. Feet are cavus. The rest of the physical findings are normal.

Hematocrit is 0.42. White cell count is 9.4×10^9/liter, with 0.61 polymorphonuclear cells, 0.05 bands, 0.22 lymphocytes, 0.09 monocytes, 0.01 eosinophils, and 0.02 basophils. Platelet count is 321×10^9/liter. At 10 years, urine specific gravity is 1.015, pH 6. Urine has mucus, amorphous matter, 1–4 red cells/HPF, 3–6 white cells/HPF, and 0–3 squamous epithelial cells/HPF. Serum sodium is 141 mmol/liter, potassium 4.5, chloride 106, carbon dioxide 27, urea nitrogen 2.9, calcium 2.27, phosphorus 1.68, cholesterol 3.88, and glucose 5.1. Creatinine is 50 µmol/liter, uric acid 190, total bilirubin 9, and direct bilirubin 0. Total protein is 57 g/liter, albumin 38. Alkaline phosphatase is 186 U/liter, LDH 402, and SGOT 41.

ECG shows flattened T waves; echocardiogram shows concentric left ventricular hypertrophy.

Heart is large at 9 years (Figure 7-1A) and 11 years (Figure 7-1B). Spine is convex right, apex T8, at 11 years (see Figure 7-1B), and more convex right, apex T11, at 13 years. CT scan of brain shows normal findings.

Menarche is at 13 years. She is in a wheelchair and feels sick and dizzy if she gets up too quickly. Echocardiogram shows left ventricular outflow track obstruction (gradient: 46 mm Hg) due to systolic anterior movement of mitral valve. Brain stem auditory-evoked potentials are normal. She has supraventricular tachycardia at 16 years. At 20 years, weight is 61.3 kg, height 170 cm, and head circumference 57 cm. Menstruation is associated with day-long abdominal pain and vomiting.

Diagnosis: Friedreich's ataxia.

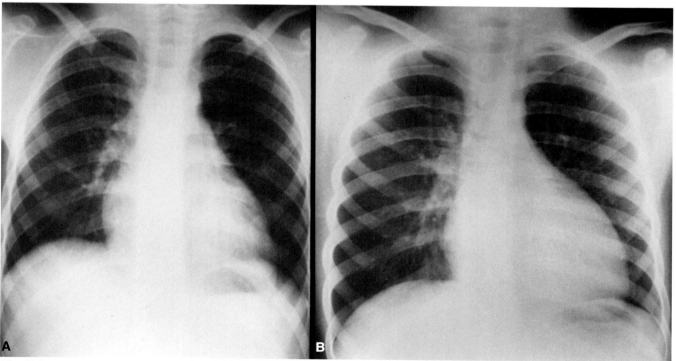

Fig. 7-1

Case 8

A 20-month-old boy has a choking, coughing spell. He has been cranky and febrile for 4 days. He had a rash on his cheeks last night.

Parents and two brothers (4 and 5 years old) are well. Two and a half years ago, a brother (5 months old) died suddenly.

Temperature is 37.5°C, heart rate 140, respiratory rate 50, blood pressure 99/77 mm Hg, and weight 11.9 kg. He is alternately lethargic and combative. Petechiae are on cheeks. Lips are dry and dusky. Acetone is on breath. Pharynx is injected. Rhonchi are in lungs. Liver edge is 4 cm below costal margin. The rest of the physical findings are normal.

Hematocrit is 0.42. White cell count is 11.0×10^9/liter with 0.40 polymorphonuclear cells, 0.50 lymphocytes, and 0.10 monocytes. Platelet count is 255×10^9/liter. Urine specific gravity is 1.012, pH 7. Urine has occasional squamous epithelial cells/HPF, 0–1 white cell/HPF, and 0–1 hyaline cast/LPF. Serum sodium is 143 mmol/liter, potassium 4.6, chloride 105, carbon dioxide 25, and glucose 5.9.

Heart is large, and its shape suggests left ventricular dilation (Figure 8-1). Excess liquid in lung parenchyma creates air bronchograms in upper lobes (see Figure 8-1).

ECG shows sinus rhythm, rate 121, and probable left ventricular hypertrophy. Echocardiogram shows dilated cardiomyopathy and decreased left ventricular function. Cardiac catheterization shows dilated cardiomyopathy and normal pulmonary vascular resistance.

He undergoes heart transplantation.

Heart weighs 107 g. Petechiae are on smooth, glistening epicardial surface. Atrial and left ventricular endocardium are thickened. Maximal diameter of left ventricular cavity is 5 cm, its lining white and fibrous, its wall 7–8 mm thick, and interventricular septum 6 mm thick. Pulmonary and mitral valve cusps are slightly thickened. Microscopic examination shows marked thickening of endocardium in left ventricle and atria with interlacing bundles of elastic fibers and myocytolysis of myocardium. A mural thrombus is in left ventricle.

Diagnosis: Endocardial fibroelastosis.

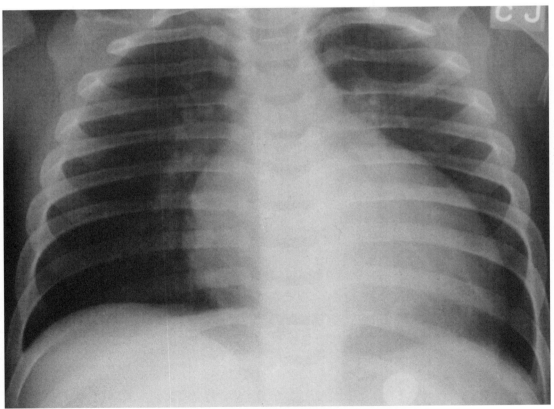

Fig. 8-1

Case 9

A 9-year-old boy is short of breath and cyanotic with exertion.

He has tired easily since a high fever at 3 years. Dyspnea got worse and cyanosis appeared 3 months ago.

Heart rate is 70, respiratory rate 20, blood pressure 90/75 mm Hg, height 123 cm, and weight 21.6 kg. A loud crescendo diastolic murmur is at cardiac apex and left axilla. Liver edge is 2 cm below costal margin. The rest of the physical findings are normal.

Hematocrit is 0.37. White cell count is 7.8×10^9/liter with 0.55 polymorphonuclear cells, 0.05 bands, 0.27 lymphocytes, 0.03 monocytes, 0.09 eosinophils, and 0.01 metamyelocytes. Urine specific gravity is 1.006, pH 5.5. Urine has 0–1 red cell/HPF. Stool contains rhabdoid larvae of *Strongyloides stercoralis*.

ECG shows right axis deviation and borderline right ventricular hypertrophy.

Heart is large and bulges midway along left margin, left main bronchus is narrow, and ill-defined strips of water density are in lungs (Figure 9-1).

At cardiac catheterization, pressure in right atrium is 4 mm Hg (mean), right ventricle 45/5, pulmonary artery 33 (mean), pulmonary capillary wedge 18, left ventricle 89/16, and aorta 80/51. Angiocardiography shows mitral stenosis, slight mitral regurgitation, and calculated mitral valve area of 0.69 cm².

At operation, heart is enlarged and diameter of main pulmonary artery is 1½ times that of aorta. Mitral valve cusps are thickened along edges and fused at commissures. Chordae tendineae are pliable.

Diagnosis: Rheumatic mitral stenosis.

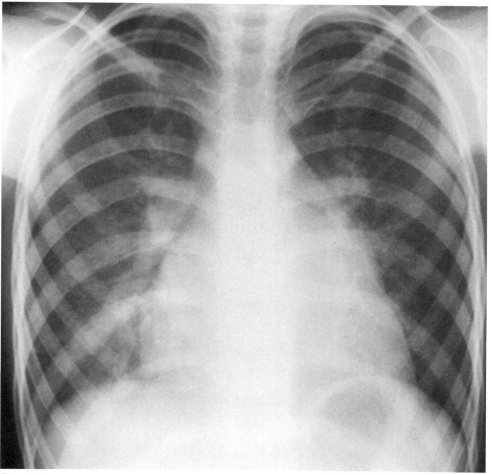

Fig. 9-1

Case 10

A 7-year-old girl, who has had a cardiac pacemaker for 5 years, has bradycardia.

Pregnancy of mother was normal, birth weight 2.8 kg, and heart rate 50–60. At 2 years, she collapsed and was unconscious. Heart rate was 60. She collapsed again the next day. Heart rate was 215. ECG showed complete heart block, premature ventricular contractions, and QT interval corrected for heart rate of 550–690 milliseconds (normal: approximately 450). A pacemaker with rate 90 was placed. Transtelephone monitoring shows heart rate 80.

Mother (29 years old) is well. Father (30 years old) has hypokalemic-type periodic paralysis. Brother (10 years old) and sister (5 years old) are well and have normal QT interval corrected for heart rate.

Temperature at 7 years is 36.9°C, heart rate 80, respiratory rate 20, blood pressure 113/55 mm Hg, weight 26 kg, and height 122 cm. Pacemaker pack is in subcutaneous tissues of left side of abdomen. The rest of the physical findings are normal.

Hematocrit is 0.42. White cell count is 8.4×10^9/liter. Platelet count is 243×10^9/liter. Serum sodium is 139 mmol/liter, potassium 3.9, and chloride 108.

Pacemaker battery is replaced. Heart rate after battery replacement is variable, usually 72.

Figure 10-1 shows new pacemaker battery in situ after second operation (Figure 10-1A) and after third operation (Figure 10-1B).

At third operation, the lead along right side of battery is loose. It is reinserted and screwed tightly. She no longer has bradycardia or skipped beats.

Diagnosis: Probable Ward-Romano syndrome, loose pacemaker lead.

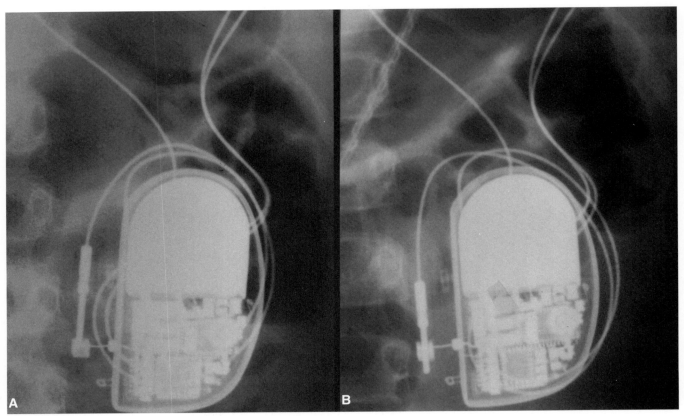

Fig. 10-1

Case 11

A 2½-year-old girl has a heart block that was diagnosed because of slow fetal heart rate. Birth weight was 2.4 kg, ventricular rate 44–52, atrial rate 120.

Father and brother (6 years old) are well. Mother has keratoconus.

Weight is 10.4 kg, height 81 cm, heart rate 46, respiratory rate 42, and systolic blood pressure 90 mm Hg. A loud systolic heart murmur is present. Liver edge is 4 cm below costal margin. The rest of the physical findings are normal.

Hematocrit is 0.45. White cell count is 7.7 × 10⁹/liter with 0.23 polymorphonuclear cells, 0.10 bands, 0.56 lymphocytes, and 0.11 monocytes. Urine specific gravity is 1.019, pH 6. Urine has trace protein, 0–1 epithelial cell/HPF, 3–4 red cells/HPF, and 1–2 white cells/HPF.

Heart is larger than normal and bulges in sector of main pulmonary artery (Figure 11-1).

At cardiac catheterization, pressure in right ventricle is 85/5 mm Hg with 55 mm gradient across pulmonary valve. A block between atrioventricular node and bundle of His is found with a tripolar electrode. At operation, commissures between partly fused pulmonary cusps are opened, and a pacemaker is placed.

Mother has dry eyes when girl is 8 years old. At 11 years, girl cannot keep up with her friends. She has blue nailbeds, systolic murmur, diastolic murmur, edematous feet, poor ventricular function, and diffuse membranous and mesangial glomerulosclerosis.

Mother's serum contains SS-B/La antibodies. Daughter's serum is negative for antinuclear antibodies for liver cells and positive for KB cells in a speckled pattern at a titer of 1:240.

Diagnosis: Congenital heart block, pulmonic stenosis, later cardiomyopathy and glomerulosclerosis in girl with Sjögren antibodies and whose mother has Sjögren's syndrome.

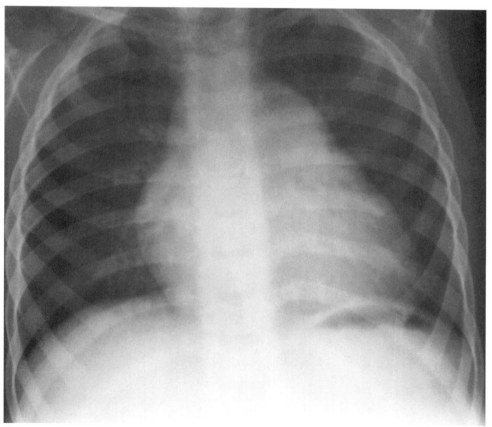

Fig. 11-1

Case 12

A newborn boy is breathing fast, grunting, and retracting.

Mother is well. Sibling (2 years old) has ventricular septal defect.

Mother smoked a half pack of cigarettes per day during pregnancy. Amniotic fluid was meconium stained. Birth weight is 4.5 kg, Apgar score 4/7 at 1 and 5 minutes, heart rate 105–115, respiratory rate 80, and temperature 36.7°C. Caput succedaneum and forceps marks are on head. Head is molded. Subconjunctival blood is in right eye. The rest of the physical findings are normal.

Hematocrit at 15 hours is 0.38. White cell count is 12.5 × 10⁹/liter with 0.16 polymorphonuclear cells, 0.10 bands, 0.55 lymphocytes, 0.13 monocytes, 0.02 eosinophils, 0.01 basophils, and 0.03 atypical lymphocytes. Platelet count is 235×10^9/liter.

In Figure 12-1A at 14 hours, air is in mediastinum and between diaphragm and right parietal pleura, heart is small, and strips of water density are in lungs. At 31 hours, physical findings are normal when respiratory rate is 60. In Figure 12-1B, a curved shadow of water density is on left side at level of T2 and T3.

Diagnosis: Ductus bump, likely related to functional closure of ductus arteriosus before anatomic obliteration, which usually starts at pulmonary end.

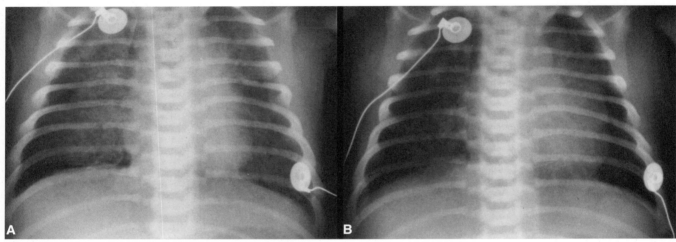

Fig. 12-1

Case 13

A newborn boy is slow to breathe.

Pregnancy of mother (29 years old) was marred by anemia, proteinuria, and edema. Birth weight is 2.9 kg. He breathes on his own at 6 minutes after mouth-to-mouth resuscitation and extra oxygen. At 6 hours, he is intubated because of cyanosis. At 11 hours, temperature is 35.9°C, heart rate 140–160, systolic blood pressure 58–65 mm Hg, length 47 cm, and head circumference 32 cm. Skin on back of neck is loose. Forehead recedes. Auricles are small. Right helix is misshapen. Nose is bulbous. Upper lip lacks philtrum. Point of maximal impulse of heart is midline. Umbilical cord has two vessels. Supernumerary fifth fingers are on hands. Prominence of heels suggests rocker-bottom feet. Testes are not in scrotum. The rest of the physical findings are normal.

His immobility is broken by seizures during which he becomes stiff and jittery and arches his back.

Hematocrit is 0.59. White cell count is 11.3×10^9/liter with 0.75 polymorphonuclear cells, 0.10 bands, 0.10 lymphocytes, and 0.05 monocytes. Platelet count is 153×10^9/liter. Blood glucose is 0.6 mmol/liter. Chromosomes are 47,XY,+13.

In Figure 13-1, heart is in right side of chest, pattern of intestinal gas suggests horizontal liver, umbilical venous catheter curves at high midline ductus venosus and goes into left-sided inferior vena cava, and 11 ossified ribs are on each side.

He dies 12 hours after mechanical ventilation is stopped.

Necropsy findings are (1) situs inversus, (2) membranous ventricular septal defect, (3) over-riding aorta, (4) all four heart valves bicuspid, (5) trilobed left lung with eparterial bronchus, (6) midline esophagus, (7) right-sided stomach, (8) nearly horizontal liver, (9) right-sided spleen, (10) malrotated intestine with ileocecal valve and appendix in left lower quadrant, (11) pelvic testicles, (12) right pyelocaliectasis, (13) small brain, (14) disproportionately small frontal lobes, and (15) absent olfactory bulbs.

Diagnosis: Trisomy 13, situs inversus.

(Continued)

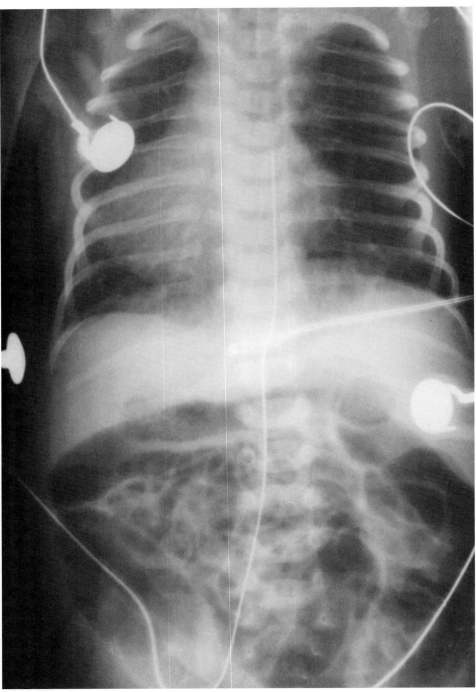

Fig. 13-1

Case 14

A 29-year-old woman, who works in a hardware store, is cyanotic and has clubbed fingers.

Weight is 53 kg, height 161 cm, heart rate 59, and blood pressure 122/90 mm Hg. Systolic heart murmur and diastolic heart murmur are present. The rest of the physical findings are normal.

Pregnancy of mother was normal, birth weight 4 kg. She had "strangling blue spells, never seemed to breathe right," and tired during feedings. She sat at 1 year, walked at 2 years, and ran vigorously at 3 years. She was in the first grade for 90 minutes per day at 6 years, too tired to stay longer. She attended second grade full time. Color improved. At 11 years, she kept up with friends. Lips were faintly blue. At 15 years, she again began to tire quickly. Fingers were clubbed. She later could climb two flights of stairs after a stop on the landing.

At 3 months, heart is large, diaphragm low (Figure 14-1).

Hematocrit at 3 months was 0.36. White cell count was 14.4 × 10⁹/liter. Hematocrit was 0.45 at 11 years. At cardiac cath-

eterization at 3 months, oxygen saturation in right ventricle was 0.46, right atrium 0.43, inferior vena cava 0.37, superior vena cava 0.38, left atrium 0.93, and left ventricle 0.76. Mean pressure in right atrium and left atrium was 4 mm Hg, pressure in left ventricle and right ventricle 80/4. At 3 years, pulmonary artery oxygen saturation was 0.84, pressure 83/38 mm Hg (mean: 50 mm Hg). Angiocardiogram at 3 years showed simultaneous opacification of aorta and pulmonary artery from a trabeculated ventricle, aorta to left and forming upper part of left side of heart margin in frontal view, aorta and pulmonary artery side by side in lateral view.

Heart and main pulmonary arteries are large at 11½ years (Figure 14-2A) and 29 years (Figure 14-2B). Heart bulges along upper left margin at 11½ years (see Figure 14-2A).

Diagnosis: Corrected (l–) transposition of great arteries, atrial septal defect, ventricular septal defect, bidirectional shunt, pulmonary hypertension; Eisenmenger's complex.

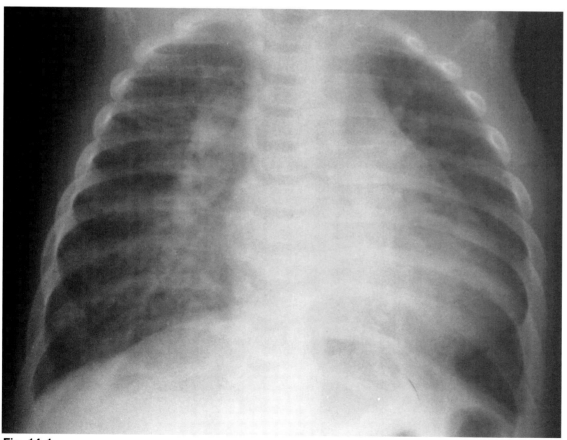

Fig. 14-1

(Continued)

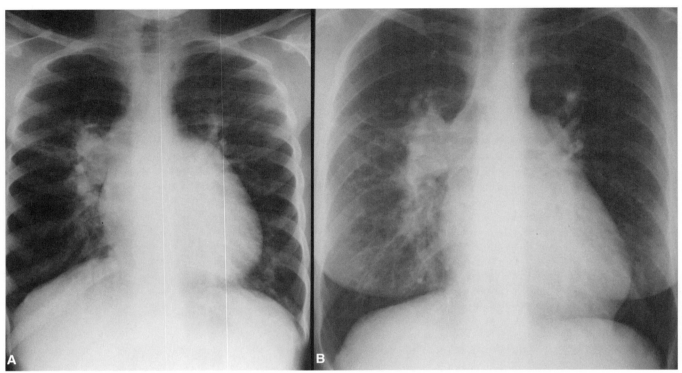

Fig. 14-2

Case 15

A newborn girl is cyanotic, more so when she cries.

Mother (33 years old), father, and three siblings are well.

Pregnancy of mother was normal. Birth weight is 3.3 kg, length 48 cm, head circumference 33 cm, Apgar score 7/8 at 1 and 5 minutes, temperature 36.5°C, heart rate 150, respiratory rate 60, and blood pressure 84/46 mm Hg. Neck is fat and short. Right side of mouth droops. S_2 is loud and single. A systolic heart murmur is present. Two vessels are in umbilical cord. Liver edge is 2 cm below costal margin. The rest of the physical findings are normal.

Hematocrit is 0.52. White cell count is 20.4 × 10⁹/liter with 0.74 polymorphonuclear cells, 0.04 bands, 0.13 lymphocytes, 0.08 monocytes, and 0.01 metamyelocytes. Platelet count is 202 × 10⁹/liter. Serum sodium is 142 mmol/liter, potassium 4.7, chloride 111, and urea nitrogen 6.4. Creatinine is 160 µmol/liter, uric acid 500, and total bilirubin 9. Arterial blood pH is 7.40 when FIO_2 = 0.20. PCO_2 is 33 mm Hg, PO_2 39. Chromosomes are 46,XX.

Roentgenographic findings are normal. Heart is egg shaped; longitudinal radiolucent clefts separate laminae of thoracic vertebrae (Figure 15-1).

Echocardiography shows ventricular septal defect beneath a single artery. Angiocardiography shows filling of left and right pulmonary arteries from ascending aorta, ventricular septal defect with left-to-right shunt, no outflow from right ventricle, and no ductus arteriosus.

Weight at 2½ months is 3.4 kg. She is cyanotic, grunting, and retracting. Loud single S_2, systolic murmur, and diastolic murmur are present. At operation, a valve conduit is placed between bifurcation of pulmonary arteries at back wall of truncus arteriosus and right ventricle, and ventricular septal defect is closed.

She has thrush from 6 to 14 months, monilial diaper rash, and frequent respiratory infections. Levels of serum calcium and immunoglobulins are normal. Number of B lymphocytes is normal. Total T-cell number and subset distribution by rosette formation and monoclonal antibodies are normal. T cells do not respond in vitro to *Candida*, tetanus, PPD, or streptolysin O.

Diagnosis: Truncus arteriosus, type 2; partial DiGeorge syndrome.

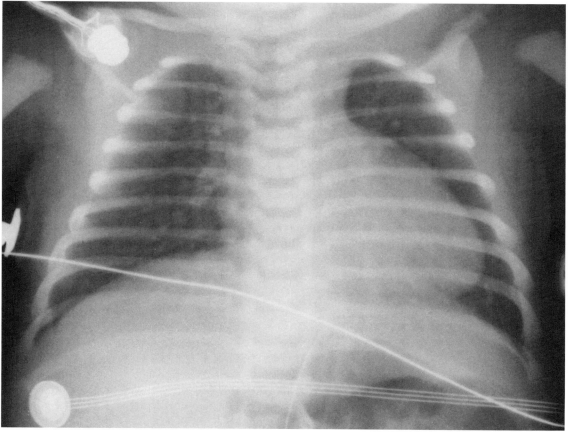

Fig. 15-1

Case 16

A 14-month-old girl with cyanotic heart disease is tachypne-ic. Cough and sniffles began yesterday. Breathing was shallow and fast this morning, temperature 40°C.

Birth weight was 2.5 kg. She was "mucousy" and cyanotic at birth. She has had pneumonia five times.

Mother (19 years old), father (23 years old), and brother (2 years old) are well.

Temperature is 38°C, heart rate 140, respiratory rate 64, systolic blood pressure 92 mm Hg, and weight 5.9 kg. She is dusky. Nailbeds are blue, fingers slightly clubbed. A continuous murmur is present. Liver edge is 3 cm below costal margin. The rest of the physical findings are normal.

Hematocrit is 0.48. White cell count is 25.4×10^9/liter with 0.43 polymorphonuclear cells, 0.20 bands, 0.31 lymphocytes, 0.05 monocytes, and 0.01 atypical lymphocytes. Urine specific gravity is 1.007, pH 5. Urine has 1–2 white cells/HPF and bacteria. Serum sodium is 133 mmol/liter, potassium 6.0, and chloride 104.

Heart is large, arch of aorta is on right side of trachea, and shadows of water density are in upper lobes (Figure 16-1).

ECG shows biventricular hypertrophy.

At cardiac catheterization at 6 weeks, oxygen saturation in right atrium is 0.61, right ventricle 0.71, left atrium and left ventricle 0.90, and aorta 0.82. Peak pressure in right atrium and left atrium is 25 mm Hg, right ventricle 85, left ventricle 90, and aorta 75. Angiocardiography shows ventricular septal defect, over-riding aorta, no pulmonary artery, and many bronchial arteries that opacify from aorta.

At left thoracotomy at 7 years, no suitable pulmonary artery for a shunt can be found. At midline thoracotomy 3 days later, a conduit is placed between aorta and a small artery to left upper lobe. At right thoracotomy at 9 years, three right bronchial arteries are united into one artery that is then anastomosed to descending aorta.

Menarche is at 16 years. Weight is 37.4 kg, height 149 cm. She is cyanotic.

Diagnosis: Truncus arteriosus, type 4, with ventricular septal defect, over-riding aorta, absent sixth (pulmonary) aortic arch derivatives, systemic to pulmonary collaterals.

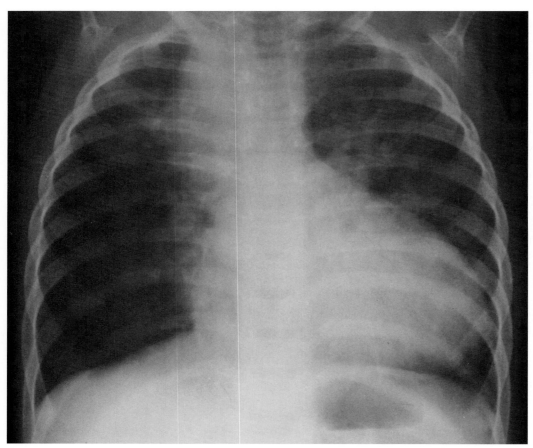

Fig. 16-1

Case 17

A 2½-month-old boy is cyanotic.

Pregnancy of mother was normal, birth weight 3.8 kg. He had a heart murmur at 2 weeks, duskiness at 3 weeks, which changed to cyanosis of lips, fingers, and toes when he cried. Breathing was sometimes fast when he was lying down, slower when he was picked up.

Mother (35 years old), father (29 years old), and three half siblings are well. Members of mother's family have asthma and heart disease.

Temperature at 2½ months is 37°C, heart rate 150, respiratory rate 42, systolic blood pressure 45 and 60 mm Hg in right arm, weight 5.7 kg, length 61 cm, and head circumference 40 cm. Liver edge is 2 cm below costal margin. Femoral pulses are diminished. The rest of the physical findings are normal.

Hematocrit is 0.61. Urine specific gravity is 1.009, pH 6.5. Urine has rare epithelial cells/HPF, rare red cells/HPF, rare white cells/HPF, and amorphous phosphates. Serum sodium is 139 mmol/liter, potassium 6.8, and chloride 104.

ECG shows sinus tachycardia, right atrial hypertrophy, and right ventricular hypertrophy.

Markings in right lung are excessive and diaphragm is low (Figure 17-1).

At cardiac catheterization, right atrial pressure is 3 mm Hg (mean), right ventricular pressure 75/4, and aortic pressure 70/50. Oxygen saturation in superior vena cava is 0.46 and 0.48, right atrium 0.63, right ventricle 0.69 and 0.73, and aorta 0.73. Catheter will not enter left heart chambers. Angiocardiogram shows high ventricular septal defect and displacement of aortic valve high and forward.

Findings at operation are hypoplasia of left ventricle, inability to pass probe through mitral valve, ventricular septal defect, and double-outlet right ventricle.

Diagnosis: Double-outlet right ventricle.

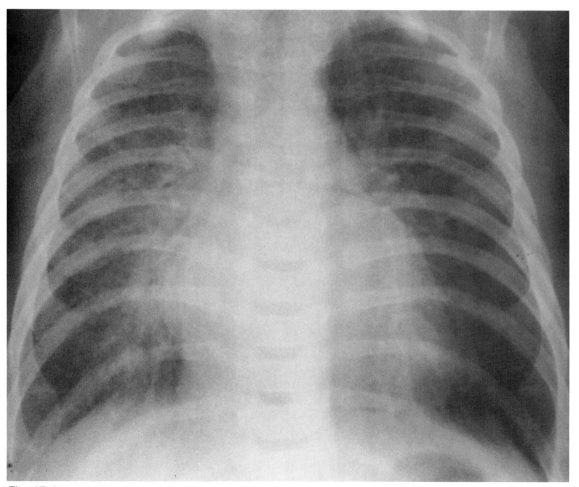

Fig. 17-1

Case 18

A 5-day-old girl is cyanotic.

Mother was hypertensive in last weeks of pregnancy. Birth weight was 3 kg, length 49 cm, and head circumference 34 cm. Until 2 days ago, she was dusky only when crying.

Mother (24 years old), father (24 years old), and brother (2 years old) are well.

Temperature is 37.2°C, heart rate 150, respiratory rate 60, and systolic blood pressure 70 mm Hg. Liver edge is 1 cm below costal margin. The rest of the physical findings are normal.

Hematocrit is 0.70. White cell count is 18.6×10^9/liter with 0.46 polymorphonuclear cells, 0.50 lymphocytes, 0.02 eosinophils, and 0.02 atypical lymphocytes. Capillary blood pH is 7.29 when FIO_2 = 0.40. PCO_2 is 35 mm Hg, PO_2 23. Urine specific gravity is 1.008, pH 6. Urine has bacteria, trace albumin, occasional white cells/HPF, rare red cells/HPF, and 20–25 epithelial cells/HPF. Serum sodium is 134 mmol/liter, potassium 4.4, chloride 88, carbon dioxide 13, and calcium 2. Total bilirubin is 7 µmol/liter.

ECG shows peaked P waves.

Roentgenographic findings are normal (Figure 18-1).

At angiocardiography, contrast medium goes from right atrium to left atrium and from left ventricle into aorta and right and left pulmonary arteries at level of ductus arteriosus.

At operation, a polytetrafluoroethylene tube graft is placed between aorta and right pulmonary artery. She dies at 10 days.

At necropsy, size and shape of heart are normal. An opening (0.5-cm diameter) is between right atrium and the 1.2-cm deep pouch that forms right ventricle. A probe can pass from right atrium to left atrium through foramen ovale. Right ventricle has no outflow track and no pulmonary valve. Pulmonary trunk is a thin cord. Right and left pulmonary arteries are normal. Upper and lower left pulmonary veins join before they reach left atrium. Left side of heart and aorta are normal. Ductus arteriosus is narrow.

Diagnosis: Variant tricuspid atresia with hypoplastic tricuspid valve, small right ventricle without outflow track or pulmonary valve, and rudimentary pulmonary trunk.

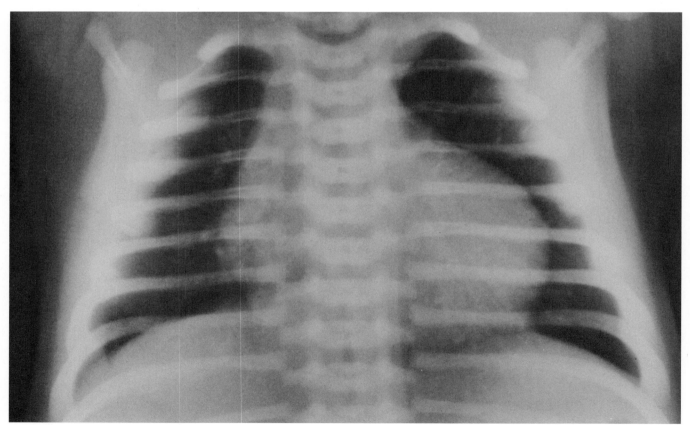

Fig. 18-1

Case 19

A 15-year-old girl with congenital heart disease likes to run and swim.

Mother took thyroid pills during first trimester.

The girl had circumoral cyanosis and acrocyanosis at birth and no heart murmur. At 2 weeks, she was blue during feedings and had systolic thrill and murmur. She was not blue at 3 months. At 6 years, she ran with playmates. At 10 years, she had systolic click, systolic murmur, and loud S_3. Menarche was at 14 years.

Parents and four siblings are well. Maternal grandmother has diabetes mellitus, paternal grandmother had stroke, and grandfathers died with strokes.

Temperature at 15 years is 35.9°C, heart rate 96, respiratory rate 28, blood pressure 110/70 mm Hg, weight 58 kg, and height 160 cm. Precordial thrill, systolic heart murmur, diastolic heart murmur, and questionable S_3 are present. The rest of the physical findings are normal.

Hematocrit is 0.45. White cell count is 9.1×10^9/liter with 0.71 polymorphonuclear cells, 0.03 bands, and 0.26 lymphocytes. Platelet count is 186×10^9/liter. Urine specific gravity is 1.007, pH 6. Urine is normal. Serum sodium is 139 mmol/liter, potassium 3.7, chloride 109, and glucose 4.4.

Pericardiocardiac image is large and its right margin prominent at 2 weeks (Figure 19-1) and 15 years, when it also bulges along mid–left margin (Figure 19-2).

ECG shows right ventricular conduction delay.

At cardiac catheterization, oxygen saturation in right atrium is 0.76, in right ventricle 0.70, in left atrium 0.95, and in aorta 0.94. Angiocardiogram shows large right atrium, abnormal location of tricuspid valve, and tricuspid regurgitation. Intracavitary ECG shows ventricular complexes at tricuspid valve, where pressure is atrial.

She is pregnant at 22 years. She has occasional pause in heartbeat at night that goes away when she gets out of bed and walks. She is short of breath with hard activity or big meals.

Diagnosis: Ebstein's malformation.

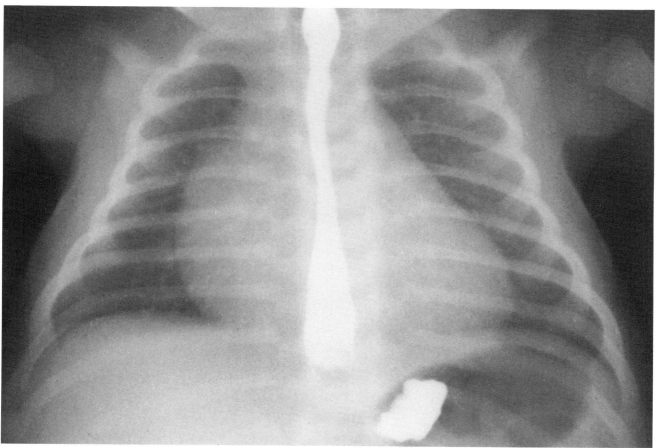

Fig. 19-1

(Continued)

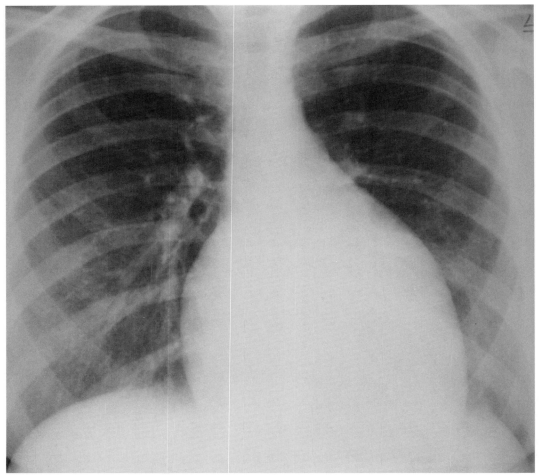

Fig. 19-2

Case 20

A newborn girl has a heart murmur.

Mother (29 years old), father (30 years old), two brothers (8 and 6 years old), and sister (7 years old) are well.

Pregnancy of mother was normal. Birth weight is 3.8 kg, length 52 cm, head circumference 34 cm, Apgar score 7/9 at 1 and 5 minutes, temperature 37.6°C, heart rate 144, and respiratory rate 56. At 4½ hours, systolic blood pressure in arms is 70–76 mm Hg, in legs 100–120. Lips are blue in room air, pink when FIO_2 = 0.40 by hood. A systolic to continuous murmur is present. Liver edge is 1 cm below costal margin. The rest of the physical findings are normal.

Hematocrit is 0.52. White cell count is 18.3×10^9/liter with 0.63 polymorphonuclear cells, 0.01 bands, 0.32 lymphocytes, 0.01 monocytes, and 0.03 eosinophils.

At 16 hours, heart is large, and markings in lungs are normal (Figure 20-1).

At cardiac catheterization, oxygen saturation in right atrium is 0.31, right ventricle 0.26, pulmonary vein 0.95, left atrium 0.52, left ventricle 0.48, and aorta 0.61. Pressure in right atrium is 5 mm Hg (mean), right ventricle 140/14, left atrium 3 (mean), left ventricle 70/8, and aorta 55/30. At angio-cardiography, main and branch pulmonary arteries fill from ductus arteriosus. Cavity of right ventricle is small. Contrast medium goes into pulmonary infundibulum but not into pulmonary artery.

At operation, closed pulmonary valvotomy (Brock's procedure) is performed. Ductus arteriosus is present. A defect is in atrial septum.

She begins to walk at 10 months. She turns blue when she cries hard. She has a systolic murmur.

At second operation at 17 months, the fibrotic, stenosed, rudimentary pulmonary valve is excised, pulmonary infundibular muscle removed, right ventricular outflow track widened with a polyester patch, and stretched foramen ovale closed.

At 10 years, she is healthy. Weight is 31 kg, height 135 cm, and blood pressure 106/60 mm Hg. Systolic murmur and diastolic murmur are present. Echocardiogram at 13 years shows right ventricular enlargement, paradoxic ventricular septal motion, and mild tricuspid and pulmonary regurgitation.

Diagnosis: Pulmonary atresia.

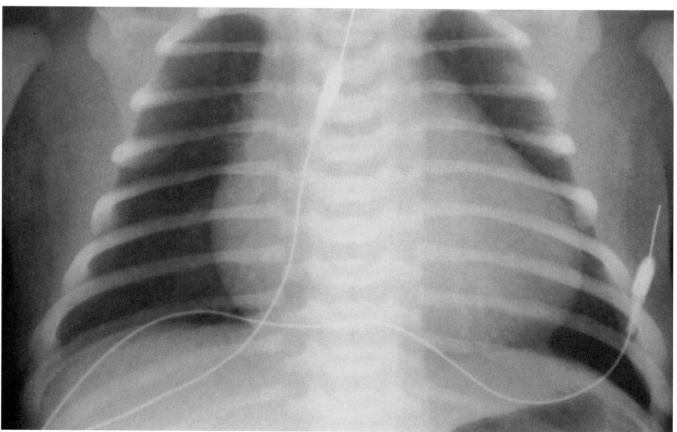

Fig. 20-1

Case 21

A 12-year-old girl, who was given epinephrine for asthma 9 days ago, when the only abnormality in physical examination was wheezing, now has a heart murmur in follow-up examination.

Mother (29 years old), father (37 years old), and brother (10 years old) are well. Maternal grandmother had rheumatic fever; maternal great-grandfather had cancer. Members of both families have asthma.

Pregnancy of mother was normal, birth weight 3.2 kg. She had ear infection, systolic murmur, and diastolic murmur at 1½ years; similar murmurs at 4 and 7 years; and no murmur at 8½ years. She had a cough and sore throat 3 months ago.

Three months ago, temperature was 38.6°C, heart rate 120, respiratory rate 40, blood pressure 120/70 mm Hg, weight 34 kg, and height 140 cm. Lymph nodes were palpable in neck. Expiratory wheezes were present. Rales were at right base. The rest of the physical findings were normal.

Three months ago, hematocrit was 0.38. White cell count was 8.8 × 10⁹/liter with 0.60 polymorphonuclear cells, 0.03 bands, 0.33 lymphocytes, 0.02 monocytes, and 0.02 eosinophils. Urine specific gravity was 1.011, pH 5. Urine had 10–12 epithelial cell/HPF.

Heart bulges in sector of main pulmonary artery (Figure 21-1).

At cardiac catheterization at 4 years, pressures in four heart chambers are normal and gradient across pulmonary valve is 5 mm Hg. At cardiac catheterization at 18 years, mean right atrial pressure is 3 mm Hg, right ventricular pressure 28/10 (mean: 3), pulmonary artery pressure 26/12 and 28/10, mean left atrial pressure 8, left ventricular pressure 91/10, and aortic pressure 103/75 (mean: 92). Oxygen saturation in superior vena cava is 0.71, right atrium 0.81, pulmonary artery 0.80, and left atrium 0.95.

Diagnosis: Normal heart, persistent foramen ovale.

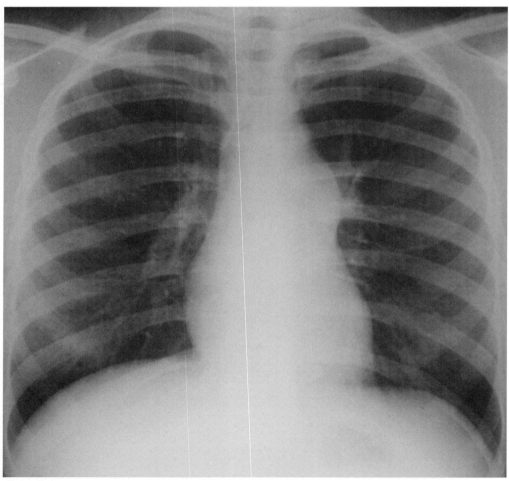

Fig. 21-1

Case 22

A 2-month-old boy has been cyanotic when crying during the last few days.

Mother (17 years old) and father (24 years old) are well. He is their only child.

Pregnancy of mother was normal, birth weight 3.2 kg. Physical findings were normal at birth and 3 weeks.

Weight at 2 months is 5.1 kg, length 59 cm, and head circumference 38 cm. S_2 is single. A systolic heart murmur at left sternal border radiates to back. The rest of the physical findings are normal.

ECG shows right ventricular hypertrophy and right axis deviation. Hematocrit is 0.35.

Findings at 2 months are normal in frontal (Figure 22-1A) and lateral (Figure 22-1B) views. Barium and belched air are in esophagus (see Figure 22-1).

Cyanosis at rest appears at 4 months, clubbing of fingers at 8 months. Hematocrit is 0.46 at 8 months.

At 1 year, weight is 8.6 kg, length 75 cm. Systolic murmur and single S_2 are present. The rest of the physical findings are normal. ECG shows right ventricular hypertrophy. Hematocrit is 0.48.

At 1 year, right concavity of trachea just above bifurcation is apparent and heart is somewhat concave along upper left margin (Figure 22-2).

Cardiac catheterization at 1½ years shows ventricular septal defect and infundibular pulmonic stenosis. Oxygen saturation is 0.73 in right ventricle, 0.87 in left ventricle, 0.80 in aorta, and 0.94 in left atrium. He is more cyanotic at 22 months. He squats for 5–10 minutes after he runs across a room. Physical findings are similar. Weight is 10.1 kg, height 75 cm, and hematocrit 0.58.

At start of operation at 22 months, systolic blood pressure is 60 mm Hg. Ventricular septal defect and infundibular pulmonic stenosis are repaired and ductus arteriosus is closed.

Diagnosis: Fallot's tetrad, right aortic arch.

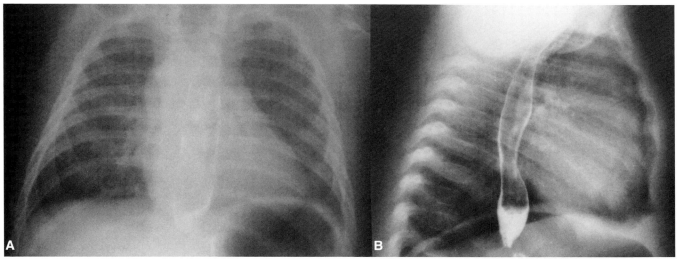

Fig. 22-1

(Continued)

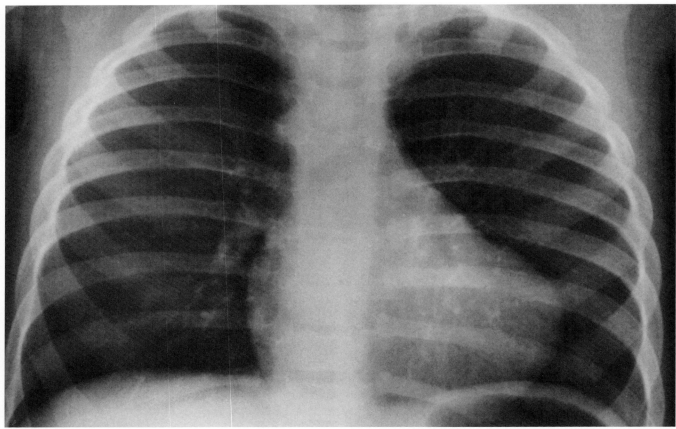

Fig. 22-2

Case 23

A 4-month-old boy sweats during feedings, sometimes turns blue around the mouth, and always seems tired. Sometimes he takes 5–6 oz of formula in 15 minutes, sometimes 1 oz in 30 minutes. Mother had albuminuria in last trimester of pregnancy. Birth weight was 3.8 kg.

Mother and father are well. He is their only child. Paternal grandfather died with heart disease, paternal grandmother has diabetes mellitus, and paternal uncle has heart disease.

Temperature is 37.9°C, heart rate 120, respiratory rate 30, systolic blood pressure 86 mm Hg, weight 6.7 kg, and length 65 cm. He is more blue when he cries. A systolic heart murmur is present. Liver edge is 2 cm below costal margin. The rest of the physical findings are normal.

Hematocrit is 0.43. Serum sodium is 135 mmol/liter, potassium 7.5, and chloride 112. Urine specific gravity is 1.025, pH 5. Urine has uric acid crystals.

ECG shows right axis deviation and right ventricular hypertrophy.

Cardiac catheterization and angiocardiography show right-to-left shunt at ventricular level, infundibular pulmonic stenosis, large aorta over-riding ventricular septal defect, and right ventricular pressure 104/20 mm Hg.

In Figure 23-1A, size of heart is normal, heart is concave in sector of main pulmonary artery, and an obliquely longitudinal shadow of water density widens left side of supracardiac shadow. In Figure 23-1B, a venous catheter is in sagittal plane of widened supracardiac shadow in left side of mediastinum 2 days after surgical correction of heart defects.

Diagnosis: Fallot's tetrad, left superior vena cava.

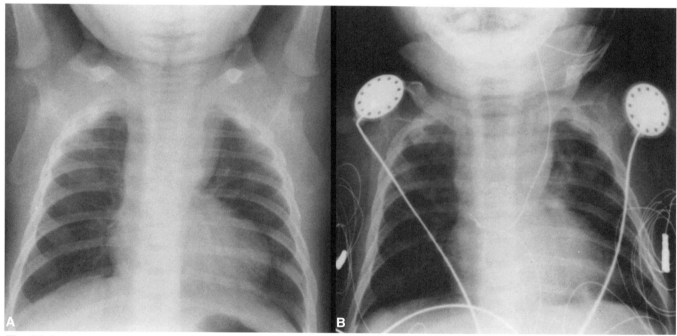

Fig. 23-1

Case 24

A newborn boy is dusky and has a heart murmur.

Mother (28 years old) had rheumatic fever. Father (30 years old) has heart "flutter." Two brothers (2 and 6 years old) are well. A sibling died at 2½ months with heart disease. Maternal grandfather had heart attack. Great-grandmothers had diabetes mellitus.

Pregnancy of mother was normal. Birth weight is 3.0 kg, length 48 cm, and head circumference 34 cm. Temperature at 5 days is 36.6°C, heart rate 180, and respiratory rate 44. Lips are dusky. Systolic murmur and diastolic murmur are present. Liver edge is 1 cm below costal margin. The rest of the physical findings are normal.

Hematocrit is 0.48. White cell count is 11.6×10^9/liter with 0.34 polymorphonuclear cells, 0.51 lymphocytes, 0.09 monocytes, 0.05 eosinophils, and 0.01 disintegrated cells. Platelet estimate is adequate. Urine specific gravity is 1.008, pH 5.5. Urine has trace protein, bacteria, and 1+ pus.

A large shadow of water density is in sector of pulmonary artery at 5 days (Figure 24-1) and 9 years (Figure 24-2), 2 months after heart operation. Heart is more enlarged in Figure 24-1 than in Figure 24-2.

He has many colds during infancy. He walks with help at 1 year. At 8 years, he plays baseball and wins a prize in a push-up contest. Heart rate is 100, respiratory rate 20, and blood pressure 105/70 mm Hg. Systolic murmur and single S_2 are present. The rest of the physical findings are normal.

At cardiac catheterization at 8 years, oxygen saturation in superior vena cava is 0.72, right atrium 0.74, right ventricle 0.88, pulmonary artery 0.79, brachial artery 0.95, and pulmonary vein 0.97. Pressure in right atrium is 3 mm Hg (mean), right ventricle 93/18, pulmonary artery 13 (mean), and left atrium 6 (mean). As catheter is withdrawn, pressure in pulmonary artery is 18/8 mm Hg, pulmonary infundibulum 73/5, and right ventricle 86/5. Angiocardiogram shows infundibular pulmonic stenosis; no pulmonary valve; aneurysm of main, left, and right pulmonary arteries; pulmonary regurgitation; and ventricular septal defect.

At operation at 9 years, right ventricle is large, its outflow track narrowed by hypertrophied muscle. A thick rim of intima and no cusps are at pulmonary valve. Pulmonary artery is dilated and thin walled. Ventricular septal defect is closed, pulmonary outflow track reconstructed.

At 15 years, he plays baseball in high school. Weight is 58 kg, height 166 cm.

Diagnosis: Fallot's tetrad; absence of pulmonary valve; aneurysm of main, left, and right pulmonary arteries.

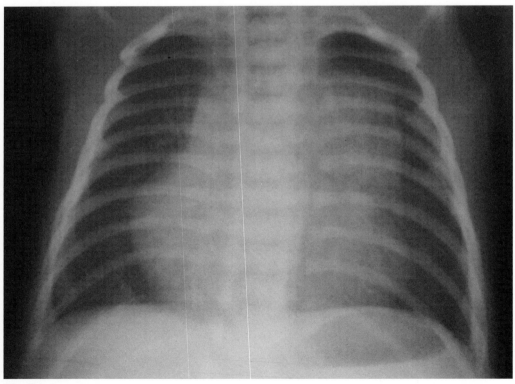

Fig. 24-1

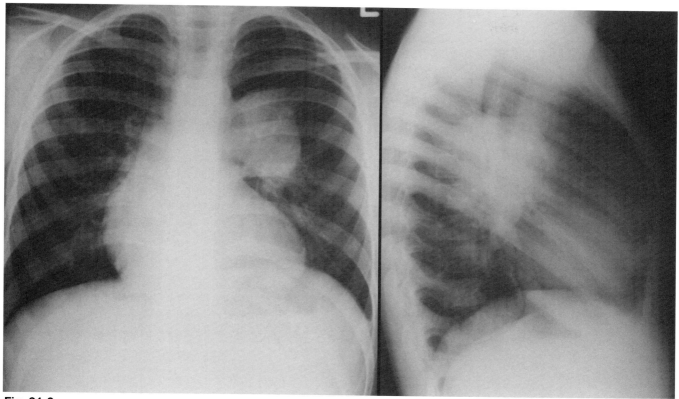

Fig. 24-2

Case 25

A newborn girl is cyanotic.

Pregnancy of mother (24 years old) was normal. Fetal heartbeat was irregular just before delivery. Birth weight is 3.4 kg, length 52 cm, head circumference 34 cm, and Apgar score 7 at 1 minute. She is pale pink in oxygen, blue in room air. At 20 minutes, temperature is 36.1°C, heart rate 148, and respiratory rate 36. Breath sounds are decreased on left side. A holosystolic murmur is present. At 2½ hours, systolic blood pressure is 85 mm Hg. Systolic murmur and diastolic murmur are present. Respiratory rate is 72 at 5 hours. Liver edge is 4 cm below costal margin at 9 hours. The rest of the physical findings are normal.

At 20 minutes, hematocrit is 0.59. White cell count is 18.9×10^9/liter. Blood glucose is 2.8 mmol/liter at 5 hours.

ECG shows right and left ventricular hypertrophy.

In Figure 25-1, a shadow of water density is in hilum of right lung, diaphragm is depressed, and right lung is overaerated.

At 8 hours, arterial blood pH is 7.27 when F_{IO_2} = 0.90. P_{CO_2} is 36 mm Hg, P_{O_2} 36. At cardiac catheterization, pressure in right atrium is 1 mm Hg (mean), right ventricle 80/3, pulmonary artery 24/2, and left atrium 5 (mean). Oxygen saturation in right atrium is 0.50, right ventricle 0.53, superior vena cava 0.48, left atrium 0.94, femoral artery 0.57, and pulmonary artery 0.52. At angiocardiography, contrast medium goes from right ventricle through ventricular septal defect to right aortic arch and from right ventricle to pulmonary artery and into aneurysm of right pulmonary artery but not into left pulmonary artery.

She dies during operation at 2 days. Necropsy shows (1) membranous ventricular septal defect; (2) left pulmonary artery from ascending aorta; (3) aneurysm of right pulmonary artery; (4) right aortic arch; (5) 2-mm pulmonary valve orifice composed of fibromyxoid connective tissue; (6) no pulmonary valve cusps; and (7) hemorrhage, alveolar collapse, and perivascular inflammation in lungs.

Diagnosis: Fallot's tetrad, absent pulmonary valve, aneurysm of right pulmonary artery, aberrant left pulmonary artery from aorta.

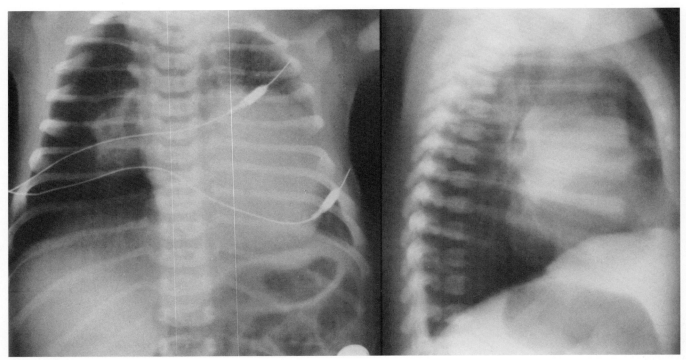

Fig. 25-1

Case 26

A 3-month-old girl has a murmur. Pregnancy of mother was normal, birth weight 3.5 kg.

Mother (21 years old) is well. Father (28 years old) has high blood pressure. Paternal uncle died at 32 years with high blood pressure and stroke. Maternal grandmother has high blood pressure; maternal grandfather has leukemia.

Weight is 5.5 kg, length 61 cm, head circumference 39 cm, respiratory rate 32, and systolic blood pressure 110 mm Hg in arm, 100 in leg. A thrill is along left sternal border. A continuous murmur is present. Liver edge is 2 cm below costal margin. Femoral pulses are strong. The rest of the physical findings are normal.

ECG shows left ventricular hypertrophy.

At 9 months, she walks. Weight is 7.7 kg, height 71 cm. Precordium bulges. A thrill is along upper left sternal border. A grinding, to-and-fro murmur is present. Peripheral pulses are strong. The rest of the physical findings are normal.

Hematocrit at 9 months is 0.34. White cell count is 9.6 × 10^9/liter with 0.29 polymorphonuclear cells, 0.05 bands, 0.58 lymphocytes, and 0.08 monocytes. Platelet estimate is adequate. Urine specific gravity is 1.019, pH 5. Urine has occasional squamous epithelial cells/HPF and 3–4 white cells/HPF. Serum sodium is 137 mmol/liter, potassium 4.8, chloride 100, urea nitrogen 10.4, and glucose 5.0.

ECG shows left atrial hypertrophy and borderline left ventricular hypertrophy.

Roentgenographic findings are normal at 3 months. At 9 months, cardiothymic image is large and vascular markings in lungs are excessive (Figure 26-1).

At operation, ductus arteriosus (1.5-cm diameter) is transected and closed.

Diagnosis: Ductus arteriosus.

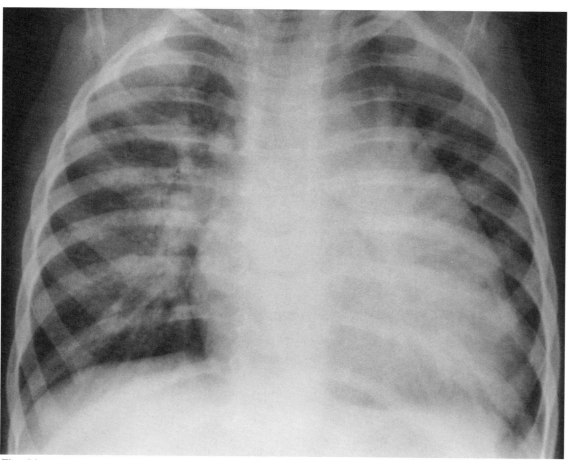

Fig. 26-1

Case 27

A 5-year-old girl is cyanotic but keeps up with her playmates.

Mother had worse nausea and vomiting during this pregnancy than during four earlier pregnancies and took pills to suppress her appetite. Birth weight was 3.1 kg, length 48 cm, and head circumference 34 cm. At 8 days, temperature was 36.6°C, heart rate 120, respiratory rate 60, and blood pressure 100/50 mm Hg. She was dusky around the mouth when she cried. Hands and nailbeds were blue. A skin tag was in front of left ear, another on left cheek near mouth. A holosystolic murmur was present. A dimple was in place of anus. Rectum emptied through a fistula to vestibular fossa of vagina. She had ear infections during first 2 years. She had chickenpox at 3 years. Teeth were carious. She had ptosis of left upper eyelid at 4 years. She tilted her head at times to see better. ECG at 4 years showed right axis deviation and right ventricular hypertrophy.

Mother (32 years old), father (35 years old), and four siblings (9, 11, 14, and 15 years old) are well. Maternal grandmother has heart disease; paternal great-grandmother had dropsy. Maternal uncle was born with one ear; paternal uncle has ear tags.

Weight at 5 years is 14.5 kg, height 108 cm, temperature 37.4°C, heart rate 100, respiratory rate 24, and blood pressure 100/60 mm Hg. Nailbeds are blue. A skin tag (1 cm broad and 1 cm high) is in front of left ear, a smaller one on left cheek. Left upper eyelid droops. Teeth are capped or missing. A systolic murmur is at left sternal border, a continuous murmur near mid–left clavicle. A rectovaginal fistula is present. The rest of the physical findings are normal. Ophthalmologic examination shows bilateral lateral rectus paresis, exotropia, anisocoria, and no pupillary constriction from far to near vision.

Hematocrit is 0.49. White cell count is 10.6×10^9/liter with 0.45 polymorphonuclear cells, 0.50 lymphocytes, 0.02 monocytes, and 0.03 eosinophils.

At 5 years, heart and supracardiac shadow form a figure 8 (Figure 27-1A). Cervical ribs are present. Contrast medium injected into main pulmonary artery is soon in pulmonary veins, a horizontal vein, left vertical vein, left brachiocephalic vein, and superior vena cava (Figure 27-1B).

At cardiac catheterization, mean right atrial pressure is 4 mm Hg, mean left atrial pressure 5, right ventricular pressure 75/5, and left ventricular pressure 80/7. Oxygen saturation in mid–left brachiocephalic vein is 0.92, superior vena cava and right atrium 0.85, left atrium 0.78, left ventricle 0.77, and left subclavian vein 0.72.

At 10 years, she tires quickly. Weight is 20 kg, height 132 cm. Fingers are clubbed. At operation, heart is large, aorta overrides high ventricular septal defect, pulmonic valve orifice is 3 mm, ostium secundum defect is in atrial septum, ductus arteriosus is present, and pulmonary venous return through a horizontal retrocardiac vein is the same as in pulmonary angiogram 5 years ago. The defects are corrected. At operation 4 days later for infarction of right side of colon, cecum is mobile on a long mesenteric pedicle, midgut is incompletely rotated, and transverse colon and descending colon pass behind inferior mesenteric vessels, descending colon turning right at splenic flexure.

Diagnosis: Congenital defects of face, skeleton (cervical ribs), heart (atrial-septal defect and Fallot's tetrad), pulmonary venous return (supracardiac), and gut.

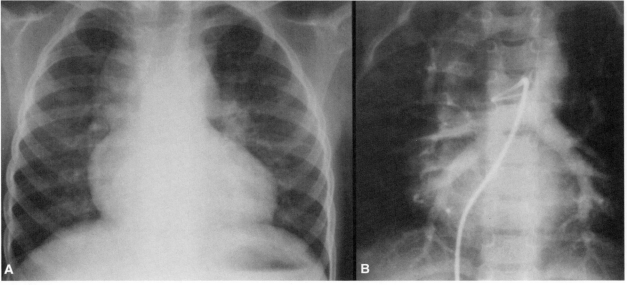

Fig. 27-1

Case 28

A newborn boy is pale and gray.

Pregnancy of mother (16 years old) was normal. Birth weight is 2.8 kg, length 48 cm, head circumference 32 cm, Apgar score 8/9 at 1 and 5 minutes, temperature 35.8°C, heart rate 140, respiratory rate 30–40, and blood pressure 63/36 mm Hg. Hands and feet are blue at 5 minutes in room air and when FIO_2 = 0.30 at 4 hours. A systolic murmur is present. Respiratory rate is 80–90 at 8 hours. At 11 hours, he continues to be periodically gray. The rest of the physical findings are normal.

At 11 hours, arterial blood pH is 7.42 when FIO_2 = 1.0. PCO_2 is 34 mm Hg, PO_2 55. Hematocrit is 0.49. White cell count is 16.2×10^9/liter with 0.40 polymorphonuclear cells, 0.33 bands, 0.22 lymphocytes, 0.01 monocytes, 0.03 eosinophils, and 0.01 metamyelocytes. Serum sodium is 130 mmol/liter, potassium 5.1, chloride 102, and calcium 2.02.

Findings in chest are normal at 21 hours (Figure 28-1).

Echocardiogram shows a vascular channel behind left atrium.

At cardiac catheterization and angiocardiography, oxygen saturation in high superior vena cava is 0.61, low superior vena cava 0.76, right atrium 0.71, left atrium 0.74, right ventricle 0.91, left ventricle 0.71, and aorta 0.86. Mean right atrial pressure is 4 mm Hg, left atrial pressure 3. Pressure in right ventricle is 47/4 mm Hg, left ventricle 54/4, and aorta 55/38. Contrast medium injected into right ventricle quickly opacifies coronary sinus and right atrium.

At operation, size of heart is normal. Ascending aorta is half the size of main pulmonary artery. A common pulmonary venous channel that enters a dilated coronary sinus is anastomosed to left atrium, and right atrial orifice of coronary sinus, ductus arteriosus, and patent foramen ovale are closed.

Diagnosis: Total anomalous venous return to coronary sinus (intracardiac anomalous pulmonary venous return).

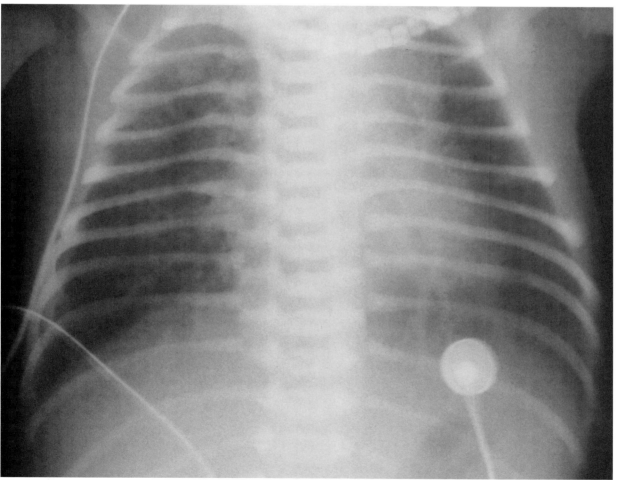

Fig. 28-1

Case 29

An 11-day-old boy is breathing fast and will not eat.

Pregnancy of mother was normal, birth weight 3.7 kg. He was blue at 10 hours; color improved with oxygen. He took 1.25 oz of formula every 3 hours. He vomited 2 days ago and began to breathe fast and have circumoral cyanosis. Today he refuses feeding.

Mother (26 years old), father (27 years old), and brother (20 months old) are well.

Temperature at 11 days is 35.7°C, heart rate 160, respiratory rate 80, systolic blood pressure 70 mm Hg in arms and 50 in legs, weight 3.6 kg, length 56 cm, and head circumference 36 cm. He is pale and dusky. Lips, mouth, tongue, hands, and feet are blue. He has thrush. Red papules are on neck and chest. Nose flares and sternum retracts during inspiration. Liver edge is 4 cm below costal margin. The rest of the physical findings are normal.

Hematocrit is 0.38. White cell count is 9.2×10^9/liter with 0.34 polymorphonuclear cells, 0.02 bands, 0.62 lymphocytes, 0.01 monocytes, and 0.01 eosinophils. Urine specific gravity is 1.010, pH 8. Urine has hemoglobin/myoglobin, few squamous epithelial cells/HPF, and occasional white cells/HPF. Serum sodium is 133 mmol/liter, potassium 6.2, chloride 100, and carbon dioxide 22. PT is 13.4 seconds (control: 10.2), activated PTT 43.5 (control: 31.3). Fibrinogen is 1.3 g/liter (normal: 2.0–4.0). Arterial blood P_{O_2} is 34 mm Hg while he breathes room air, 56 when $F_{IO_2} = 1.0$.

ECG findings are normal. Echocardiography shows paradoxic septal motion, large right ventricle, and small left atrium.

In Figure 29-1 at 14 days, heart is small, ill-defined nodules and strips of water density are in lungs, and liquid is in right pleural space.

At cardiac catheterization, right ventricular pressure is 85/7 mm Hg, pulmonary artery pressure 80/40. Angiocardiography shows atrial-septal defect and confluence of pulmonary veins behind left atrium into common vein that descends below diaphragm to porta hepatis, where flow of contrast medium is obstructed.

At operation, diameter of pulmonary artery is three times that of aorta. Right ventricle is large, left side of heart small. Pulmonary venous abnormality is corrected, patent foramen ovale closed.

He dies 24 hours after operation. Necropsy shows thickness of right ventricle to be 0.6 cm, left ventricle 0.5 cm. Lungs contain foci of interstitial and intra-alveolar hemorrhage and edema, coagulation necrosis and hyperplasia of endothelial cells, and possibly collagen in vessel walls. Sinusoids of spleen and interstitial vessels of kidneys are congested with red cells.

Diagnosis: Total anomalous pulmonary venous return to hepatic portal system (infracardiac) and patent foramen ovale.

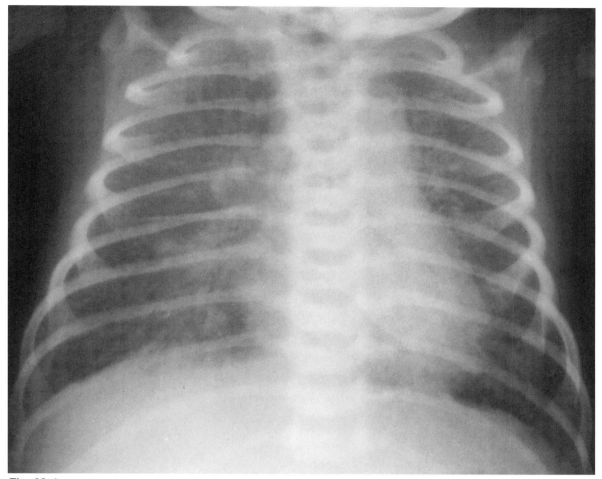

Fig. 29-1

Case 30

A 6-month-old girl is pale, less active, and eats half the amount she ate 1 month ago. She sweats, vomits, and is gassy and constipated.

Pregnancy of mother was normal, birth weight 2.8 kg.

Parents (both 30 years old) are well. Paternal grandfather had tuberculosis, and maternal great-aunt had diabetes mellitus.

Temperature is 36.8°C, heart rate 165, respiratory rate 45 with expiratory grunt, systolic blood pressure 110 mm Hg, weight 5 kg, length 66 cm, and head circumference 41 cm. A faint systolic murmur is present. Liver edge is 5 cm below costal margin. The rest of the physical findings are normal.

Hematocrit is 0.38. White cell count is 20.5×10^9/liter with 0.52 polymorphonuclear cells, 0.10 bands, and 0.37 lymphocytes. Urine specific gravity is 1.019, pH 6. Urine has 3–5 white cells/HPF, occasional red cells/HPF, occasional epithelial cells/HPF, urates, and bacteria.

ECG shows p pulmonale.

Heart is large and bulges along left margin and excess liquid is in lungs (Figure 30-1).

At cardiac catheterization, pressure in right atrium is 10 mm Hg (mean), right ventricle 120/15, and pulmonary artery 80–90 with mean wedge pressure of 25 mm Hg. Oxygen saturation in right atrium is 0.30, right ventricle 0.36, and pulmonary artery 0.34.

Angiocardiogram shows contrast medium in right ventricle and pulmonary artery (Figure 30-2A). Angiocardiogram shows contrast medium in left ventricle, aorta, and blocked in left atrium (Figure 30-2B).

At operation, right ventricle is large and hypertrophied, left atrium large. A white, rubbery membrane that looks like septal tissue is in left atrium.

Diagnosis: Cor triatriatum.

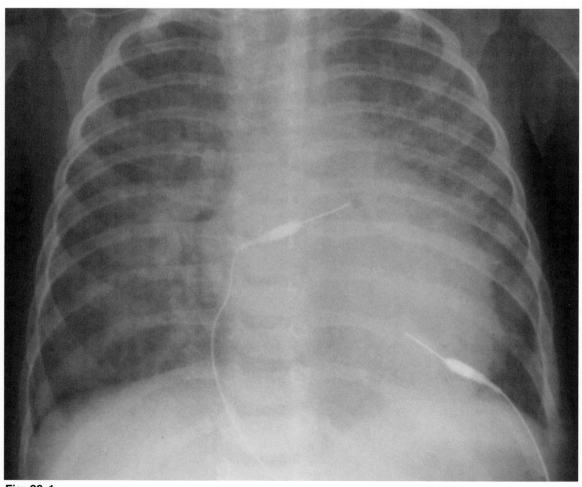

Fig. 30-1

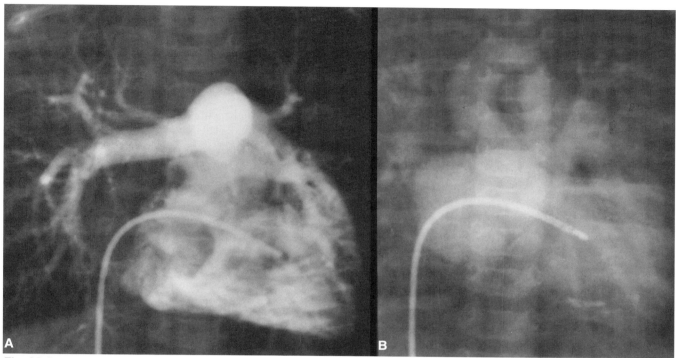

Fig. 30-2

Case 31

An 11-month-old boy will not eat and is "dwindling away."

Mother had a "viral" illness in early pregnancy. Birth weight was 3.0 kg, length 51 cm, and Apgar score 8/9 at 1 and 5 minutes. His breathing was fast at 3–4 weeks. He was cranky at 3–4 months. He has had an ear infection. He sweats a lot. He will not lie prone. He stands with support.

Parents are well. He is their only child.

Weight at 11 months is 6.6 kg, height 73 cm, head circumference 46 cm, temperature 37.4°C, heart rate 140, respiratory rate 76, and blood pressure 124/86 mm Hg (3 weeks ago: 92/50 mm Hg). He is sweaty. The rest of the physical findings are normal.

Hematocrit is 0.39. White cell count is 21.4×10^9/liter with 0.39 polymorphonuclear cells, 0.02 bands, 0.56 lymphocytes, and 0.03 monocytes. Platelet count is 322×10^9/liter. Urine specific gravity is 1.022, pH 6. Urine has 0.3 g/liter protein, occasional squamous epithelial cells/HPF, 0–1 red cell/HPF, 0–2 white cells/HPF, amorphous urates, and mucus. Serum sodium is 135 mmol/liter, potassium 6.0, chloride 104, carbon dioxide 19, urea nitrogen 5.7, calcium 2.57, phosphorus 1.97, cholesterol 2.90, and glucose 9.7. Creatinine is 40 µmol/liter, uric acid 300, total bilirubin 12, and direct bilirubin 2. Total protein is 60 g/liter, albumin 46. Alkaline phosphatase is 126 U/liter, LDH 464, and SGOT 49.

Heart is large, diaphragm is low, chest is deep front to back, and right upper lobe and left lung lack air (Figure 31-1).

He eats and sleeps little and is cyanotic during the next week. Heart has gallop rhythm. Liver edge is 4–5 cm below costal margin. Echocardiogram shows left atrial enlargement, little movement of mitral valve, left ventricular hypertrophy, and probable aortic stenosis.

At operation, pleura is edematous and bile stained. Lungs are atelectatic. A discrete juxtaductal coarctation of aorta is repaired. Biopsy of a piece of gray-brown left upper lobe shows (1) thickened pleura; (2) interstitial inflammation of polymorphonuclear cells, lymphocytes, monocytes, and macrophages; (3) many small vascular spaces; (4) larger vessels than normal in lung periphery; and (5) thickened alveolar walls.

He dies 3 days later during emergency operation in which pulmonary artery is large and tense, right side of heart dilated and thick, and left ventricle small. Mitral commissures are fused, chordae tendineae short, partly fused, and attached to a single posterior papillary muscle. Aortic valve is bicuspid and partly fused at commissures. Thickened septal tissue protrudes into left ventricular outflow track.

At necropsy, circumference of mitral valve is 3.5 cm, pulmonary valve 6 cm. Mitral cusps are warty. Partly fused chordae tendineae are attached to a left ventricular posterior papillary muscle of normal size. Short, fused chordae extend from small anterior papillary muscle to posterior cusp of mitral valve. Lungs are hyperemic and firm. Microscopic examination shows (1) decrease in alveolar sacs, alveoli, and septa; (2) thickened alveolar walls in right upper lobe; and (3) thickened, edematous alveolar walls, and hypercellular interstitial infiltrate in left lower lobe.

Diagnosis: Shone's anomaly with parachute mitral valve, subaortic stenosis, and coarctation of aorta; bicuspid aortic valve; hypoplasia of right upper lobe.

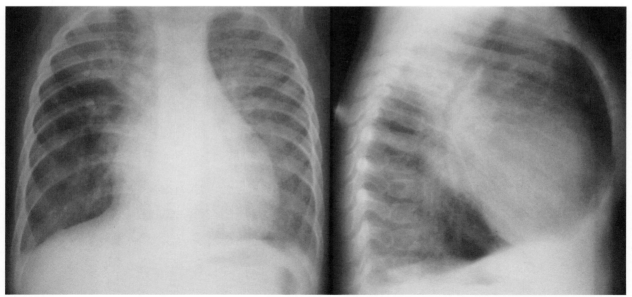

Fig. 31-1

Case 32

A 4-day-old girl is breathing fast.

Birth weight was 3.3 kg, Apgar score 5/8 at 1 and 5 minutes. Respiratory rate at 4 hours was 80 with substernal retractions. At 4 days, temperature is 36.4°C, heart rate 150, respiratory rate 80, blood pressure 75/45 mm Hg, weight 3.1 kg, length 52 cm, and head circumference 34 cm. She is jaundiced. A holosystolic heart murmur is present. The rest of the physical findings are normal.

Hematocrit is 0.52. White cell count is 9.6×10^9/liter with 0.29 polymorphonuclear cells, 0.68 lymphocytes, 0.02 monocytes, and 0.01 eosinophils. Platelet count is 257×10^9/liter. At 5 days, serum sodium is 149 mmol/liter, potassium 4.8, chloride 100, carbon dioxide 19, urea nitrogen 1.8, calcium 2.47, phosphorus 2.94, cholesterol 2.64, and glucose 4.2. Creatinine is 70 µmol/liter, uric acid 420, total bilirubin 101, and direct bilirubin 9. Total protein is 55 g/liter, albumin 35. Alkaline phosphatase is 77 U/liter, LDH 930, and SGOT 42. Capillary blood pH is 7.41 at $FIO_2 = 0.20$. PCO_2 is 35 mm Hg, PO_2 53.

Roentgenographic findings are normal at 1 day (Figure 32-1).

At cardiac catheterization at 5 days, oxygen saturation in superior vena cava is 0.65, right atrium 0.88, right ventricle 0.89, pulmonary artery 0.90, left atrium 0.90, pulmonary vein 0.95, and left ventricle 0.95. Pressure in right atrium is 5 mm Hg (mean), right ventricle 60/10, pulmonary artery 48/17, left ventricle 68/10, and descending aorta 68/50.

Angiocardiogram shows atrial-septal defect and ventricular septal defect.

She has gallop rhythm at 8 days. She is breathing fast at 2 weeks. Holosystolic murmur and diastolic murmur are present. Liver edge is 4 cm below costal margin. At operation at 17 days with temperature probes in esophagus and rectum, she is (1) surrounded with ice bags until temperature is 32°C, (2) put on cardiopulmonary bypass until temperature is 18°C, (3) exsanguinated, and (4) subjected to cardiac arrest while ventricular membranous septal defect is closed with a polyester patch and atrial-septal defect with sutures. Sternal wound is red at 19 days; a small amount of pus is in lower part. At 27 days, a tender, irregular band under dry, scaly skin is on each side of chest down to wound in each upper quadrant of abdomen that remains after removal of drainage tubes.

Biopsy of skin and subcutaneous tissue removed from left side of abdomen at 35 days shows necrotic, calcified subcutaneous fat lobules.

At 65 days, 48 days after operation, plaques of subcutaneous calcium are in legs (Figure 32-2). Roentgenogram at 42 days did not show subcutaneous calcification.

Diagnosis: Subcutaneous fat necrosis from hypothermia during closure of atrial and ventricular septal defects.

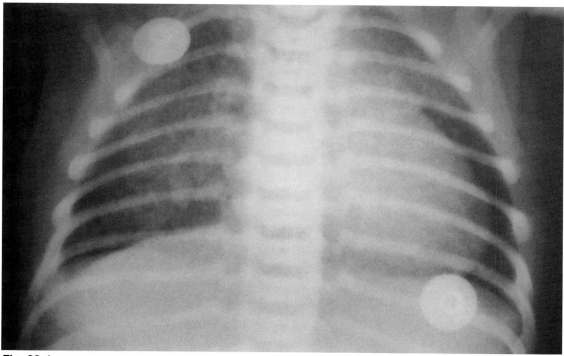

Fig. 32-1

(Continued)

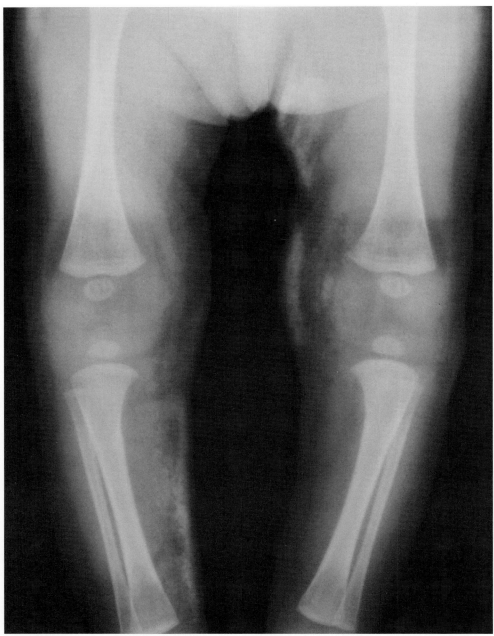

Fig. 32-2

Case 33

A 4-month-old boy has abnormal arms and hands.

Mother had hepatitis during sixth month of pregnancy. Birth weight was 2.7 kg, Apgar score 7/8 at 1 and 5 minutes.

Mother (24 years old) was operated on for atrial-septal defect at 13 years. Father (26 years old) is well. The boy is their only child. Maternal grandmother had cancer of uterus, maternal grandfather had heart disease, and paternal uncle had cancer.

Weight is 4.5 kg, length 61 cm, and head circumference 40 cm. Arms are short. Two fingers and long fingerlike thumb are on each hand. Systolic heart murmur and diastolic heart murmur are present. Liver edge is 1 cm below costal margin. The rest of the physical findings are normal.

In Figure 33-1, heart is large, although size is exaggerated by child's supine position, and humeri and bones of forearm are asymmetrically dysplastic. Mother's carpal bones and right thumb are abnormal, middle phalanges of fifth digits are short (Figure 33-2).

Weight at 5 years is 12 kg, height 96 cm, temperature 37°C, heart rate 88, respiratory rate 38, and systolic blood pressure 105 mm Hg. Systolic murmur and arm deformities are present. Hematocrit is 0.35. White cell count is 6.9 × 10⁹/liter with 0.27 polymorphonuclear cells, 0.04 bands, 0.53 lymphocytes, 0.11 monocytes, and 0.05 eosinophils. Platelet count is 320 × 10⁹/liter. Urine specific gravity is 1.024, pH 6.5. Urine is normal. Serum sodium is 136 mmol/liter, potassium 4.3, chloride 106, and urea nitrogen 6.8. ECG shows first-degree heart block and right ventricular hypertrophy. Cardiac catheterization and angiocardiogram show left-to-right shunt through secundum-type atrial-septal defect, which, at operation, is 2.5 × 2.0 cm and closed with sutures. At 10 years, Holter monitor shows periods of sinoatrial block, bradycardia, and junctional escape. A pacemaker is placed at 12 years. At 22 years, weight is 58 kg. He is studying to become a computer technologist.

Diagnosis: Atrial-septal defect and upper limb defects in mother and son.

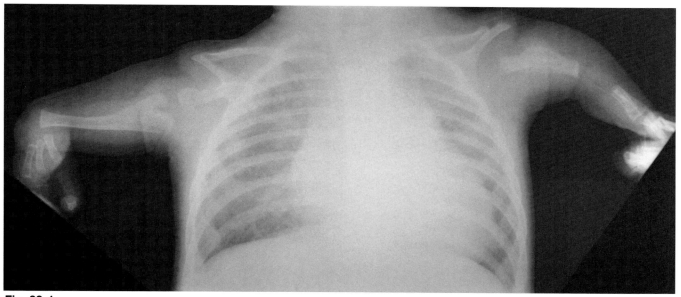

Fig. 33-1

(Continued)

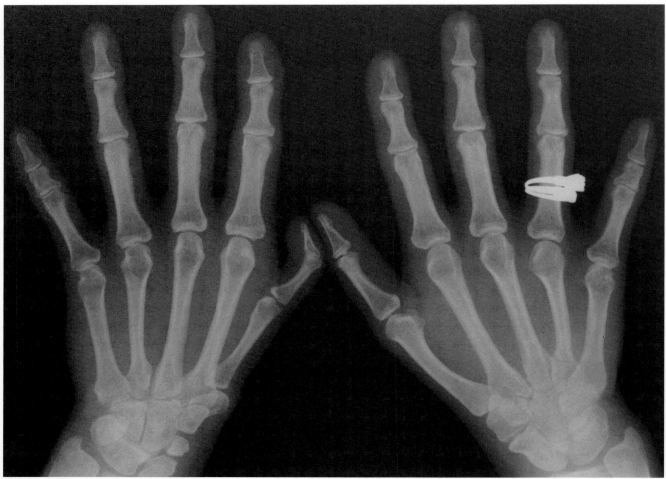

Fig. 33-2

Case 34

A newborn boy has a membrane-covered abdominal defect with umbilical cord at its apex.

Birth weight is 2.4 kg, Apgar score 5/7 at 1 and 5 minutes, temperature 34.8°C at 10 minutes, heart rate 152, systolic blood pressure 64 mm Hg, and respiratory rate 32 (at 3 hours: 70). Right parietal cephalohematoma is present. Right testis is not in scrotum. The rest of the physical findings are normal.

Blood sugar is 0.8 mmol/liter before IV glucose and 5.9 after. Hematocrit is 0.68. White cell count is 27.0 × 10⁹/liter with 0.40 polymorphonuclear cells, 0.24 bands, 0.24 lymphocytes, 0.06 monocytes, 0.04 eosinophils, and 0.02 atypical lymphocytes. Serum sodium is 135 mmol/liter, potassium 5.2, chloride 98, urea nitrogen 3.9, and calcium 2.50. Total bilirubin is 38 μmol/liter.

At operation, abdominal defect containing liver and small intestine is converted to a ventral hernia.

A systolic murmur is present at 2 weeks. At operation at 8 months, a defect (1.5 × 1.0 cm) in interventricular septum is closed and ductus arteriosus is ligated.

At 6 years, he is "quite social." Weight is 17.6 kg, height 116 cm. Scars are on chest and abdomen. The rest of the physical findings are normal.

Size of heart is in upper part of normal range at 6 years. First ribs are not symmetric. Disc between T11 and T12 is calcified in Figure 34-1. Review of earlier roentgenograms shows that disc was calcified at 6 months.

Diagnosis: Omphalocele, ventricular septal defect, persistent ductus arteriosus, and calcification of intervertebral disc. (He has never complained of backache.)

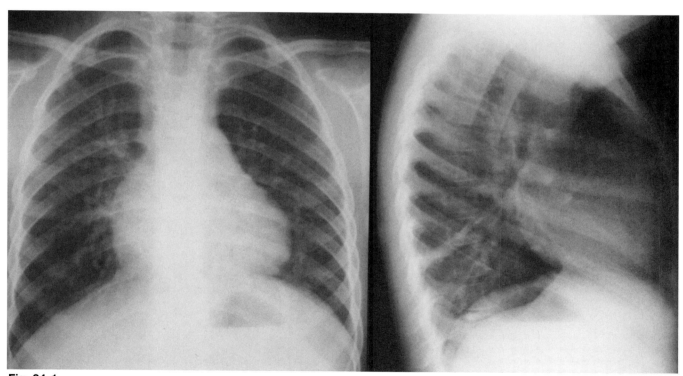

Fig. 34-1

Case 35

A 2-day-old boy is cyanotic and has a heart murmur.

Mother (27 years old) is well. Father (30 years old) has asthma. Grandfathers have heart disease, and two maternal aunts have diabetes mellitus.

Pregnancy of mother was normal, birth weight 3.5 kg, length 51 cm, head circumference 36 cm, Apgar score 8/9 at 1 and 5 minutes, and heart rate 148. He fed well at 8 hours, slowly at 16 hours. At 24 hours, he was pink. He spit up mucus and would not feed. At 30 hours, he was pink but lethargic. Temperature was 37.2°C, respiratory rate 48. At 31 hours, he was mottled blue. Heart rate was 240, respiratory rate 100. At 37 hours, he was flaccid. Heart rate was 140–220, respiratory rate 80. Respirations were labored. A murmur was present. At 39 hours, lips were blue, alae nasi flaring. Neck was extended. He vomited at 44 hours.

At 53 hours, he is pale and blue. Systolic blood pressure is 64 mm Hg. A systolic murmur is present. Liver edge is 4–5 cm below costal margin. The rest of the physical findings are normal.

Hematocrit is 0.43. White cell count is 14.6×10^9/liter. Platelet count is 385×10^9/liter. Serum sodium is 138 mmol/liter, potassium 4.7, chloride 102, urea nitrogen 10.0, calcium 2.32, and glucose 6.6 (IV fluids). Total bilirubin is 101 µmol/liter. Arterial blood pH is 7.35 while he breathes room air. PCO_2 is 19 mm Hg, PO_2 49. PO_2 is 92 mm Hg when $FIO_2 = 0.95$.

Diaphragm is low, size of heart is in upper part of normal range, and excess liquid is in gut (Figure 35-1).

ECG shows right and left ventricular hypertrophy and left ventricular strain.

Echocardiogram shows small left ventricle, small aorta, large right ventricle, and paradoxic septal motion.

At necropsy 3 days after birth, circumference of tricuspid valve is 5.5 cm, mitral valve 2.2, pulmonary valve 3, and aortic valve 1. Foramen ovale is patent. A 1-cm defect is in lower part of atrial septum. Aorta is smaller than pulmonary artery. Lungs and liver are congested.

Diagnosis: Hypoplastic left heart.

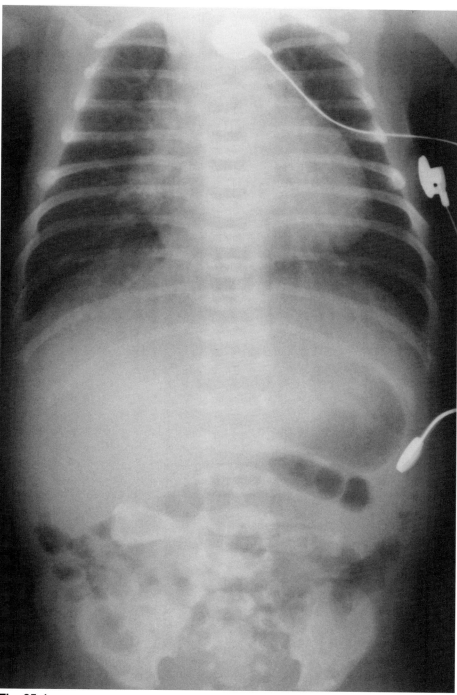

Fig. 35-1

Case 36

A 23-year-old man who does heavy labor and plays basketball has a heart murmur. A systolic murmur was present at 9 months.

He swam, played soccer, and walked 20 miles for the March of Dimes at 8 years. Systolic thrill in jugular (suprasternal) notch and systolic murmur that radiated into neck were present. ECG findings were normal. He played football, basketball, and softball at 15 years and was a distance runner at 16 years.

Weight at 23 years is 66 kg, height 181 cm, heart rate 80, and blood pressure 124/70 mm Hg. Precordial impulse is prominent. S_1 is normal, S_2 normally split. Early systolic click, systolic murmur, and diastolic murmur are present. The rest of the physical findings are normal.

ECG shows normal findings at 16 years, primary atrioventricular block at 18 years, and primary block and left ventricular hypertrophy at 20 years.

Roentgenographic findings in chest are normal at 6 years (Figure 36-1) and 23 years.

Cardiac catheterization at 8 years shows systolic pressure gradient of 10–15 mm Hg across aortic valve, at 17 years 43 mm Hg gradient at rest and during exercise and 30 mm Hg gradient after exercise. Supravalvar aortogram at 8 years shows bicuspid aortic valve and trace aortic regurgitation. Echocardiogram at 23 years shows slight left ventricular enlargement, slight thickening of aortic cusps, slight reduction of aortic cusp motion, and slight thickening of anterior cusp of mitral valve. Doppler ultrasound examination shows a gradient of at least 20 mm Hg across aortic valve, slight aortic regurgitation, and trace tricuspid regurgitation.

Diagnosis: Aortic stenosis, bicuspid aortic valve.

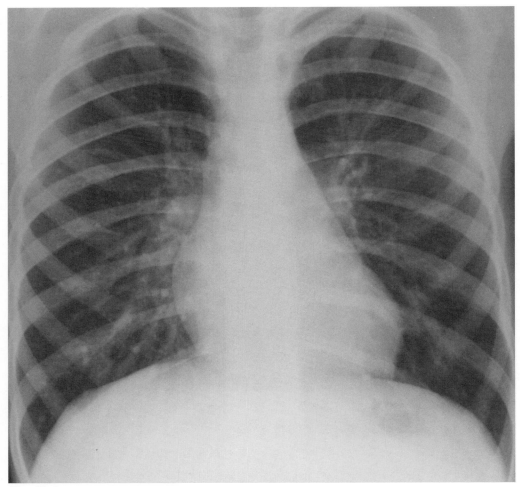

Fig. 36-1

Case 37

A 9-year-old boy cannot keep up with playmates. He rests 15 minutes every hour. Hands and feet sometimes tingle.

Birth weight was 3.3 kg. A heart murmur was present at 6 months. He sat at 10 months, walked at 16 months. He would sit while he played at 2½ years. Blood pressure was 104/50 mm Hg. Systolic and diastolic murmurs were present. ECG showed left ventricular hypertrophy. Tonsils were removed at 6 years. He had pneumonia at 7 years.

Mother (29 years old), father (36 years old), brother (11 years old), and sister (7 years old) are well.

Weight at 9 years is 27 kg, height 136 cm, temperature 37.2°C, heart rate 86, respiratory rate 20, and blood pressure 100/70 mm Hg. S_2 is single. Thrill, systolic murmur which goes to neck and back, and diastolic decrescendo murmur are present. The rest of the physical findings are normal.

Hematocrit is 0.37. White cell count is 6.2×10^9/liter with 0.39 polymorphonuclear cells, 0.06 bands, 0.42 lymphocytes, 0.08 monocytes, and 0.05 eosinophils. Platelet count is 267×10^9/liter.

Heart is large; its shape suggests dilation of left ventricle (Figure 37-1).

ECG at 2½ years shows left ventricular hypertrophy. Cardiac catheterization shows a systolic pressure gradient of 50 mm Hg across aortic valve. Angiocardiography shows slight aortic stenosis and moderate aortic regurgitation. Cardiac catheterization at 9 years shows left ventricular pressure 190 mm Hg, aortic pressure 90, and moderate aortic regurgitation.

At operation, heart is large. A systolic thrill is over ascending aorta, bounding pulse at arch and descending aorta. Right semilunar cusp of aortic valve is so small that valve consists of left semilunar cusp and posterior semilunar cusp, which are fused. A prosthetic valve is placed.

Diagnosis: Dysplastic aortic valve, aortic regurgitation, and aortic stenosis.

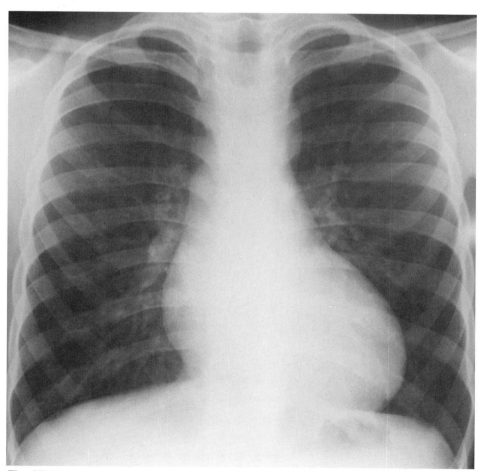

Fig. 37-1

Case 38

A 5-year-old boy has a murmur in his chest.

He runs with playmates. He has colds once in a while. One year ago, a cut on his foot was closed with 22 stitches.

Weight is 23.6 kg, height 116 cm, temperature 37.4°C, heart rate 96, respiratory rate 20, and blood pressure 98/68 mm Hg. Nose is runny. Legs are bruised. A to-and-fro murmur is loudest in left fourth and fifth interspaces next to sternum according to one examiner, at cardiac apex according to another. A scar is on right foot. The rest of the physical findings are normal.

Hematocrit is 0.35. White cell count is 6.5×10^9/liter with 0.39 polymorphonuclear cells, 0.06 bands, 0.48 lymphocytes, 0.06 monocytes, and 0.01 eosinophils. Urine specific gravity is 1.024, pH 6.5. Urine has occasional white cells/HPF and occasional epithelial cells/HPF. Serum sodium is 136 mmol/liter, potassium 4.4, chloride 96, urea nitrogen 4.6, and glucose 4.4.

Heart is slightly enlarged (Figure 38-1). Selective injection of contrast medium into a branch of left coronary artery shows a fistula near cardiac apex between an anomalous artery and right ventricle (Figure 38-2).

At operation, a fistula between circumflex branch and anterior interventricular branch (left anterior descending), 4.0 × 0.4 cm, is ligated.

Diagnosis: Coronary AV fistula (coronary artery–cameral shunt).

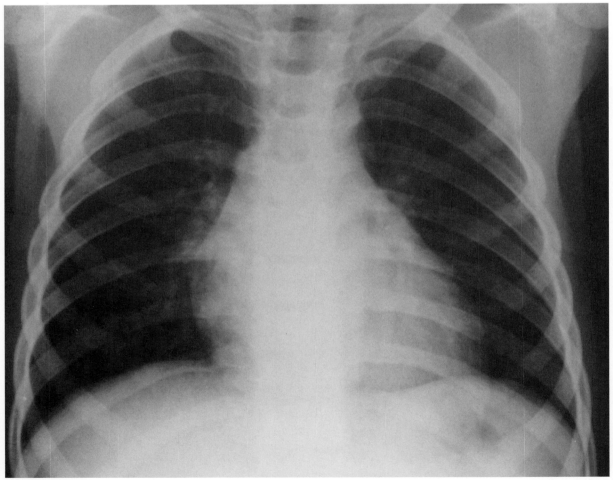

Fig. 38-1

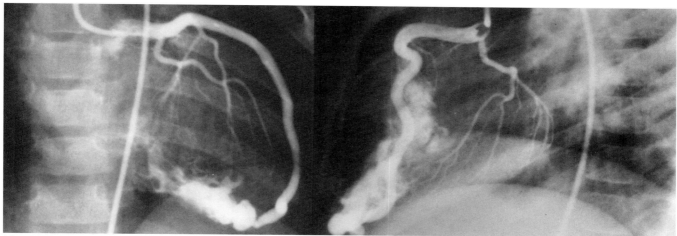

Fig. 38-2

Case 39

A 17-month-old boy has lumps in his arms.

Pregnancy of mother was normal, birth weight 4.2 kg, and Apgar score 5/8 at 1 and 5 minutes. At 10 months, he had a fever to 40.6°C and a rash that spread from trunk to limbs. Neck was swollen. Eyes and mouth were red, lips cracked and bloody. Fingers and toes peeled soon after. Mother noticed lumps in boy's arms 1 month ago.

Mother (23 years old) and father (43 years old) are well.

Temperature at 17 months is 35.7°C, heart rate 122, respiratory rate 32, blood pressure 100/60 mm Hg, weight 14.5 kg, and height 88 cm. A pulsating lump (2 cm) is in the inner side of each upper arm. The rest of the physical findings are normal.

Hematocrit is 0.36. White cell count is 10.1×10^9/liter with 0.73 polymorphonuclear cells, 0.24 lymphocytes, and 0.03 monocytes. Platelet count is 270×10^9/liter.

Echocardiogram shows aneurysms of right and left coronary arteries.

Plain film findings are normal. Angiocardiogram shows stenosis near origin of left anterior descending coronary artery and aneurysm beyond (Figure 39-1A); aneurysm, stenosis, and smaller distal aneurysm in right coronary artery (Figure 39-1B); and aneurysm in left brachial artery.

Lumps in arms are smaller 1 month later.

Diagnosis: Mucocutaneous lymph node syndrome (Kawasaki disease).

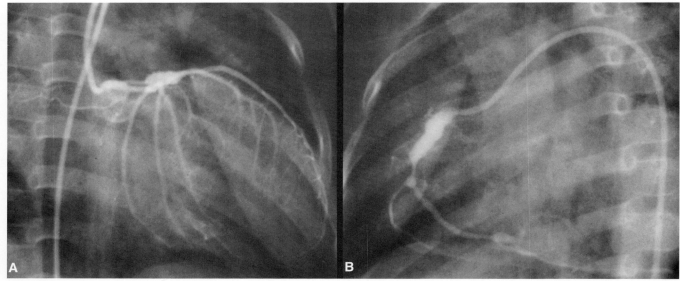

Fig. 39-1

Case 40

A 9-year-old girl has had a cough for 5 days.

Mother was treated for tuberculosis during the year before girl was born. Pregnancy was normal, birth weight 4 kg. At 3 months, the girl vomited and had fever to 40.5°C. Conjunctivae were red 2 days later. A red macular rash was on body the third day; red-purple macules were on palms and soles. Eyelids were puffy, eardrums pink. A systolic murmur was present. Heart rate was 184–210. On the thirteenth day, temperature was 38.9°C and physical findings were normal. At 16 months, weight was 12.5 kg, heart rate 80, and blood pressure 102/70 mm Hg. A 2-cm pulsatile, soft, mobile mass was in each axilla. Small lymph nodes were in right side of neck and left groin. A rash was in diaper area.

Hematocrit was 0.38. White cell count was 15.2×10^9/liter with 0.27 polymorphonuclear cells, 0.02 bands, 0.61 lymphocytes, 0.08 monocytes, 0.01 eosinophils, and 0.01 basophils. Platelet count was 352×10^9/liter. Urine specific gravity was 1.022, pH 7. Urine was normal. Serum VDRL test was nonreactive. Serum did not contain HBsAg or HBsAb. Pulses in arms were normal at 4½ years. Blood pressure in both arms was 90/50 mm Hg. She had head lice at 7½ years. Axillary masses were present. She was bitten on lower lip by a stray dog 2½ weeks ago and has been given rabies prophylaxis.

Weight at 9 years is 30 kg, height 138 cm, and blood pressure 90/70 mm Hg in right arm. Pulse is weak in left arm, blood pressure unobtainable. The rest of the physical findings are normal.

ECG findings are normal. Echocardiogram shows normal heart anatomy and function, normal proximal coronary arteries, and normal aorta.

Arteriogram at 16 months shows an aneurysm in left brachial artery (Figure 40-1). Aneurysm was also in right brachial artery. Calcium is in medial soft tissues of left arm at 9 years (Figure 40-2A). Round shadows of calcium density are in axial plane of upper part of heart in lateral roentgenogram at 9 years (Figure 40-2B).

Diagnosis: Calcified aneurysms, mucocutaneous lymph node syndrome (Kawasaki disease).

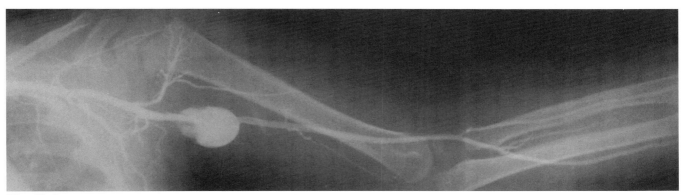

Fig. 40-1

(Continued)

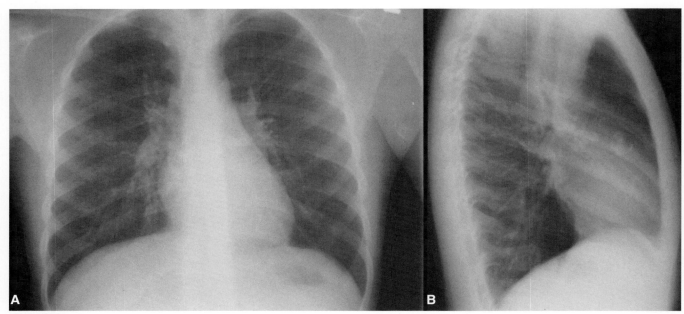

Fig. 40-2

Case 41

An 8-year-old boy has chest pain.

He had a fever 2½ weeks ago. Eyes were red, and neck was swollen 12 days ago. Throat was red 11 days ago. Fingertips began to peel 8 days ago. Eyes were still red. Throat culture grew group F β-hemolytic streptococci. He had inspiratory chest pain 7 days ago. He vomited, had loose stools, and still had fever 5 days ago. Three days ago, palms peeled. Fever was gone. Chest pain came during supper last night. He was sweating and breathing fast during the night. He vomited breakfast this morning and now complains of retrosternal pain and pain in jaw, left arm, and epigastrium.

He has had chickenpox and a broken right arm.

Temperature at 8 years is 37°C, heart rate 122, respiratory rate 24, blood pressure 88/42 mm Hg, weight 27 kg, and height 128 cm. Lips are bright red. Friction rub is at heart apex. Gallop rhythm is present. The rest of the physical findings are normal.

Three days ago, hematocrit was 0.35. White cell count was 6.2 × 10⁹/liter with 0.46 polymorphonuclear cells, 0.05 bands, 0.34 lymphocytes, 0.11 monocytes, and 0.04 basophils. Platelet count was 874 × 10⁹/liter. Urine specific gravity was 1.018, pH 7. Urine had 4–6 white cells/HPF. SGOT was 38.

Today, hematocrit is 0.44. White cell count is 31.9 × 10⁹/liter with 0.91 polymorphonuclear cells, 0.01 bands, 0.07 lympho-

cytes, and 0.01 basophils. Platelet count is 616 × 10⁹/liter. Serum sodium is 135 mmol/liter, potassium 4.6, chloride 102, carbon dioxide 18, urea nitrogen 4.3, calcium 2.27, phosphorus 1.81, cholesterol 5.25, and glucose 5.8. Creatinine is 60 μmol/liter, uric acid 60, total bilirubin 5, and direct bilirubin 2. Total protein is 74 g/liter, albumin 37. Alkaline phosphatase is 129 U/liter, LDH 1,000. CK was 38 U/liter 3 days ago; today it is 1,520 (normal: 0–150). CK isoenzyme, MB fraction, is 105 IU/liter, 0.07 of total CK activity (>0.05 in myocardial infarction).

In Figure 41-1A 3 days ago, size of heart is in upper part of normal range, its shape suggestive of dilation of left ventricle. In Figure 41-1B, pericardiocardiac image is larger than normal today.

ECG was normal 3 days ago. Today ECG shows Q waves and ST segment elevation in left precordial leads. Echocardiograms 3 days ago and today show aneurysms of left and right coronary arteries. Echocardiogram today also shows decreased septal and anterior wall motion.

Diagnosis: Inferior wall and anteroseptal myocardial infarction; mucocutaneous lymph node syndrome (Kawasaki disease).

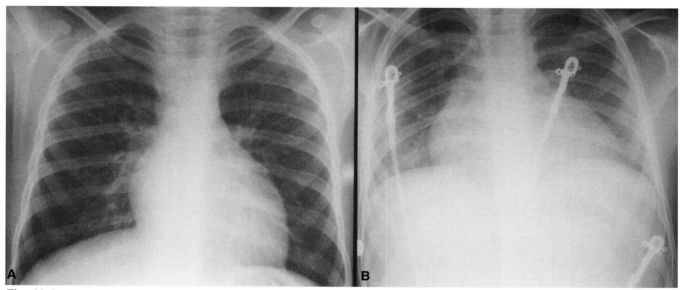

Fig. 41-1

Case 42

A 2⅓-year-old boy cruises around furniture, stumbles, falls, jabbers, and does not talk.

Pregnancy of mother was normal, birth weight 3.2 kg, length 53 cm. He ate poorly. Hands and feet were often blue. Ductus arteriosus was ligated at 11 months. He had otitis media 6 months ago, bronchitis 3 months ago. The noise of a blender makes him scream; noises of other children seem to scare him.

Mother (29 years old), father (27 years old), and sister (1 year old) are well.

Weight at 2⅓ years is 11.4 kg, height 81 cm. Eyes are oval with medial flare of eyebrows, epicanthi, and stellate irises. Forehead and cheeks are full. Bridge of nose is low, tip turned up. Philtrum is long. Lips are full. Systolic murmur and left chest scar are present. Fingers are short. Elbows are valgus. The rest of the physical findings are normal.

Hematocrit is 0.34. Chromosomes are 46,XY.

In Figure 42-1, left fourth rib is hypoplastic from operation, size of heart is normal, and markings in lungs are normal.

At 13 years, he is inactive and talks like a 4-year-old. Heart rate is 88, respiratory rate 24, and blood pressure 138/88 mm Hg. Systolic murmur is present. Hematocrit is 0.42. White cell count is 5.8×10^9/liter with 0.40 polymorphonuclear cells, 0.02 bands, 0.44 lymphocytes, 0.07 monocytes, 0.06 eosinophils, and 0.01 basophils. Platelet count is 308×10^9/liter. Urine specific gravity is 1.010, pH 5.5. Urine has urobilinogen, 0–5 white cells/HPF, 0–3 red cells/HPF, and 0–1 hyaline cast/LPF. Serum sodium is 140 mmol/liter, potassium 4.1, chloride 106, urea nitrogen 1.8, calcium 2.32, phosphorus 2.00, and glucose 6.1. Creatinine is 40 μmol/liter.

At cardiac catheterization at 13 years, pressure in left ventricle is 155/12–28 mm Hg, aortic root 156/69, and ascending aorta 100/70. Angiocardiogram shows supravalvar aortic stenosis.

At operation, a ridge (0.3 × 0.2 cm) and membrane in aorta just above openings of coronary arteries narrow lumen to 0.7 cm. Microscopic examination of the excised white tissue shows fibroblastic proliferation and myxoid change.

At 18 years, he is autistic, weighs 44 kg, is 145 cm tall, and has marked scoliosis.

Diagnosis: Williams syndrome.

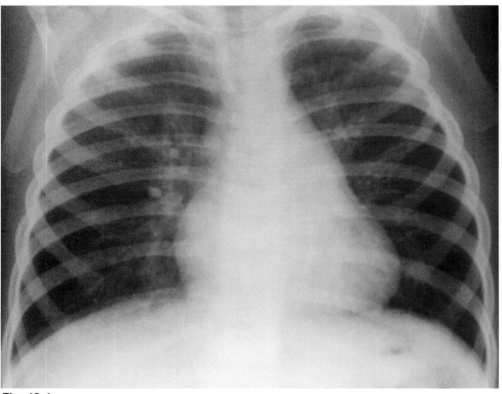

Fig. 42-1

Case 43

A 16-year-old boy has steady pain in right shoulder and chest that began 1 week ago and is now worse.

Pregnancy of mother was normal, birth weight 3.9 kg. He was dusky and tachypneic and had precordial thrill, systolic murmur, and diastolic murmur. ECG showed left ventricular hypertrophy and no right ventricular potentials. At operation at 3 days, sinuses of Valsalva were dilated and a fistula from an aneurysm of right sinus to right ventricle was closed. At 28 months, a fistula between right sinus and left ventricle and 1-cm foramen ovale were closed, and commissurotomies performed between thickened, slightly fused aortic cusps. At 8 years, knees had thin scars, shins were bruised. He was double jointed. Skin biopsy showed normal amount and fragmentation of elastic fibers. He was nearsighted at 11 years.

Mother (40 years old) has worn glasses for myopia since second grade. She bruises easily, has loose ears and skin, is double jointed, and can touch tongue to nose. Sister (13 years old) has similar skin, joints, ears, and tongue; brother, (11 years old) has epicanthi, similar skin, and slightly tighter joints. Maternal grandmother has thin skin, hyperextensible fingers, and can touch wrist with ipsilateral thumb. Maternal aunt, who was born with a blood clot on her brain, has similar skin, joints, and marked lumbar lordosis.

Weight at 16 years is 58 kg, height 173 cm, heart rate 110, respiratory rate 20, and blood pressure 130/70 mm Hg. Murmurs and scars are present. Femoral pulses, strong 5 months ago, are now weak.

Hematocrit is 0.33. Serum sodium is 128 mmol/liter, potassium 4.4, chloride 95, and glucose 7.4.

ECG shows left axis deviation, delayed interventricular conduction, ST segment convex upward, and T wave inversion.

Heart is large and ascending aorta dilated at 5 years (Figure 43-1) and 16 years (Figure 43-2). Roentgenographic findings in chest are similar in examination at 15 years.

Echocardiogram shows double wall in ascending aorta and two strips of tissue floating over valve.

At operation, a posterior dissection is in aorta, and aortic valve is bicuspid and regurgitant. Valve is replaced and ascending aorta is repaired with a conduit.

Pathologic examination shows mucoid degeneration of valve and cystic medial necrosis of aorta.

Anticoagulant treatment is begun. He has right flank pain and blood clots in urine 4 months later. Incisions are healed.

Cystogram in Figure 43-3 shows diverticulum on left side of bladder.

He has left indirect inguinal hernia at 21 years.

Diagnosis: Ehlers-Danlos syndrome.

(Continued)

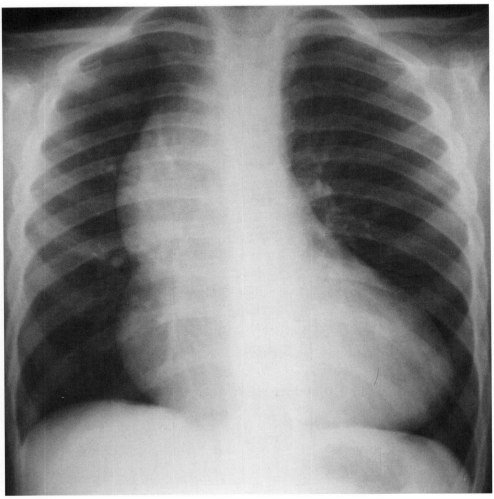

Fig. 43-1

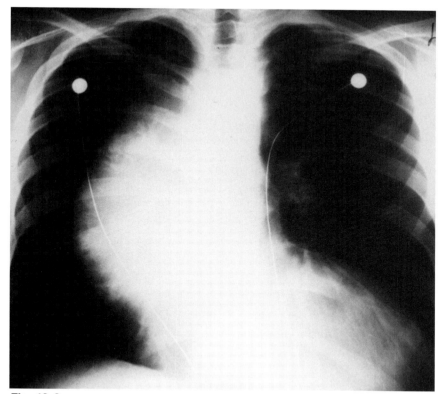

Fig. 43-2

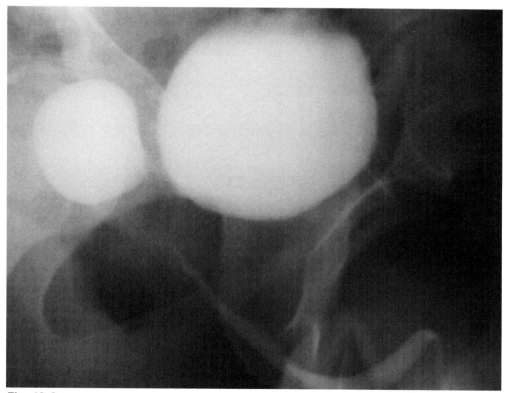

Fig. 43-3

Case 44

A 17-day-old boy is tachypneic.

Mother bled from vagina during first trimester. Birth weight was 3.3 kg. Cry was "squeaky." He was breathing fast soon after birth but seemed well. Tip of penis was blue 1 week ago. He was restless 4 days ago and took less breast milk. Cry was "soft, inward." Inspiration was noisy yesterday. He was blue and gasping in the emergency room last night. Breathing and heart stopped until chest was massaged and oxygen given by mask and then endotracheal tube.

Mother, father, and sister are well.

Temperature is 37°C, heart rate 168, and respiratory rate 72. Systolic blood pressure in arm is 80–90 mm Hg, in leg 40–50. Weight is 3.5 kg, length 53 cm, and head circumference 36 cm. Crepitant rales are in lungs. Point of maximal impulse of heart is in left midaxillary line. Liver edge is 4 cm below costal margin. Femoral pulses are weak. The rest of the physical findings are normal.

ECG shows right axis deviation and right ventricular hypertrophy.

Hematocrit is 0.44. White cell count is 19.6×10^9/liter with 0.68 polymorphonuclear cells, 0.06 bands, 0.17 lymphocytes, and 0.09 monocytes. Serum sodium is 140 mmol/liter, potassium 3.9, chloride 101, carbon dioxide 27, urea nitrogen 5.0, calcium 1.87, and glucose 29.0 (IV fluids). Creatinine is 60 µmol/liter.

Pericardiocardiac image is large, diaphragm is depressed, and excess liquid is in gut (Figure 44-1).

At cardiac catheterization, oxygen saturation in superior vena cava is 0.78, right atrium and right ventricle 0.89, pulmonary artery 0.91, left atrium 0.93, and left ventricle 0.94. Pressure in right atrium is 7 mm Hg (mean), right ventricle 60/10, pulmonary artery 60/25, left atrium 10 (mean), and left ventricle 92/16. Angiocardiogram shows coarctation of aorta distal to left subclavian artery.

At operation, coarctation 6 mm beyond left subclavian artery is repaired with a patch from left subclavian artery.

At 12½ years, weight is 51 kg, height 132 cm, and blood pressure 120/60 mm Hg.

Diagnosis: Coarctation of aorta.

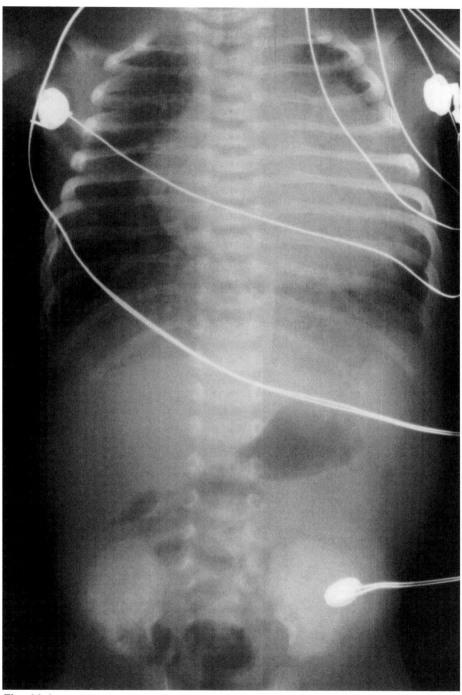

Fig. 44-1

Case 45

A 15-year-old boy has a murmur and high blood pressure in physical examination at summer camp. He wrestles and golfs.

Parents and seven siblings are well.

Temperature is 37.5°C, heart rate 62, respiratory rate 20, blood pressure 140/104 mm Hg, weight 45.4 kg, and height 152 cm. Left ventricular heave is palpable. Systolic ejection click is at cardiac apex and along left sternal border. Systolic murmur at apex is louder in back. Arterial pulsations are palpable below scapulas, along ribs, and at wrists but not in legs. Right dorsalis pedis systolic pressure is 100 mm Hg (Doppler). The rest of the physical findings are normal.

ECG findings are normal.

Hematocrit is 0.40. White cell count is 6.2×10^9/liter with 0.54 polymorphonuclear cells, 0.07 bands, 0.28 lymphocytes, 0.06 monocytes, 0.04 eosinophils, and 0.01 basophils. Platelet count is 252×10^9/liter. Urine specific gravity is 1.015, pH 6. Urine has occasional bacteria, occasional squamous epithelial cells/HPF, and 0–1 white cell/HPF. Serum sodium is 139 mmol/liter, potassium 3.8, chloride 105, carbon dioxide 26, urea nitrogen 4.6, calcium 2.40, phosphorus 1.65, cholesterol 3.23, and glucose 6.8. Creatinine is 70 μmol/liter, uric acid 380, total bilirubin 7, and direct bilirubin 2. Total protein is 69 g/liter, albumin 49. Alkaline phosphatase is 290 U/liter, LDH 144, and SGOT 41.

In Figure 45-1, size of heart is in upper part of normal range, its shape suggests dilation of left ventricle; aorta is dilated in ascending part, notched between arch and descending part, and dilated in descending part; and undersurface of left sixth rib is notched.

At operation, aorta tapers from 1.5 cm to a constriction just below the ligamentum arteriosum and dilates distally. Intercostal and bronchial arteries are large. Coarctation is repaired with a Gore-Tex (Artex Sportswear, Scarborough, Ontario) patch.

Microscopic examination of the pale yellow tissue that is removed shows elastic artery with cystic medial degeneration.

Diagnosis: Coarctation of aorta, bicuspid aortic valve.

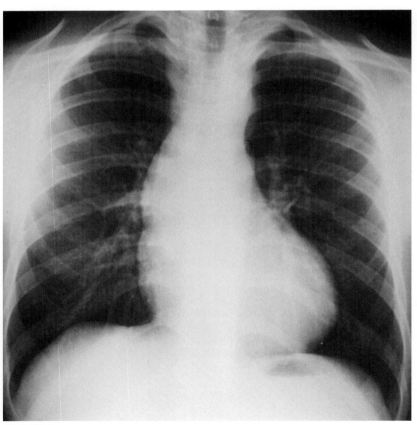

Fig. 45-1

Case 46

A 12-year-old boy has had headaches for 1 month. The most recent lasted 2 days. Legs "go to sleep."

Birth weight was 3.6 kg.

Parents and three younger siblings are well.

Temperature is 36.3°C, heart rate 84, respiratory rate 20, blood pressure in left arm 110/70 mm Hg, in one leg 80/60 mm Hg, weight 30.6 kg, and height 147 cm. Systolic heart murmur and early systolic ejection click are present. Femoral pulses are weak, distal leg pulses not palpable. The rest of the physical findings are normal.

Hematocrit is 0.39. White cell count is 7.7 × 10⁹/liter with 0.43 polymorphonuclear cells, 0.10 bands, 0.38 lymphocytes, 0.05 monocytes, and 0.04 eosinophils. Platelet estimate is adequate. Urine specific gravity is 1.012, pH 5. Urine has 1–2 white cells/HPF. Serum sodium is 139 mmol/liter, potassium 4.0, chloride 106, carbon dioxide 27, and urea nitrogen 6.8.

Roentgenographic findings in frontal view are normal (Figure 46-1A). Undulating shadows of water density are behind sternum in lateral view (Figure 46-1B).

At operation, a segment of aorta (length: 5.5 mm) just beyond ligamentum arteriosum is resected. Lumen is 1 cm in diameter on either side of central constriction (3.5 mm).

Diagnosis: Coarctation of aorta, bicuspid aortic valve, dilation of internal thoracic arteries.

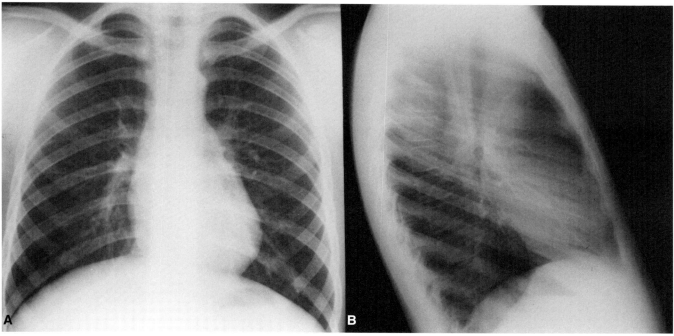

Fig. 46-1

Case 47

A 7-year-old boy has a heart murmur that was first heard when he was 2½ years old.

Pregnancy of mother was normal. He walked at 1 year.

Mother was 25 years old, father 32 years old when he was born; both were well. Maternal aunt, "hard of hearing," had heart surgery when she was a teenager. Paternal grandmother was born with cleft lip and palate. Paternal grandfather had throat cancer. Three siblings are well.

Weight at 7 years is 23 kg, height 116 cm, heart rate 110, respiratory rate 18, and blood pressure 90/78 mm Hg. A systolic murmur is present. The rest of the physical findings are normal.

ECG show left axis deviation.

In Figure 47-1, a curved shadow of water density is lateral to notched aortic arch, and barium is in stomach. Aortogram shows subclavian arteries, descending aorta, but not arch (Figure 47-2A). Right heart injection through saphenous vein shows left ventricle, carotid arteries, proximal subclavian arteries, and notch at junction of arch and descending aorta (Figure 47-2B).

He rides his bike "cross-town" and feels well at 17 years.

Weight at 17 years is 73 kg, height 157 cm, temperature 36.7°C, heart rate 80, respiratory rate 22, and blood pressure 102/72 mm Hg. Carotid pulses are strong. A systolic murmur is present. The rest of the physical findings are normal.

Hematocrit is 0.49. White cell count is 7.2×10^9/liter with 0.62 polymorphonuclear cells, 0.01 bands, 0.27 lymphocytes, 0.09 monocytes, and 0.01 eosinophils. Platelet count is 230×10^9/liter. Urine specific gravity is 1.014, pH 6. Urine has occasional white cells/HPF. Serum sodium is 140 mmol/liter, potassium 3.7, chloride 97, carbon dioxide 28, urea nitrogen 5.4, calcium 2.40, phosphorus 1.13, cholesterol 4.37, and glucose 5.1. Creatinine is 90 µmol/liter, uric acid 360, total bilirubin 5, and direct bilirubin 3. Total protein is 75 g/liter, albumin 47. Alkaline phosphatase is 85 U/liter, LDH 141, and SGOT 16.

Catheterization shows aortic systolic pressure 150 mm Hg above notch, 100 below notch.

At operation, diameter of aorta at notch is 8 mm, above and below notch diameter is 18. A woven polyester tube is used to bypass coarctation.

At 26 years, he feels well. Weight is 83 kg, blood pressure 122/106 in arm, 125/100 in leg. Scar and systolic murmur are present. Radial and femoral pulses are synchronous.

Diagnosis: Coarctation of aorta, subclavian arteries distal to coarctation.

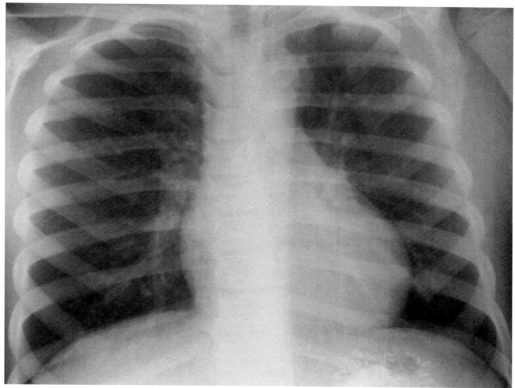

Fig. 47-1

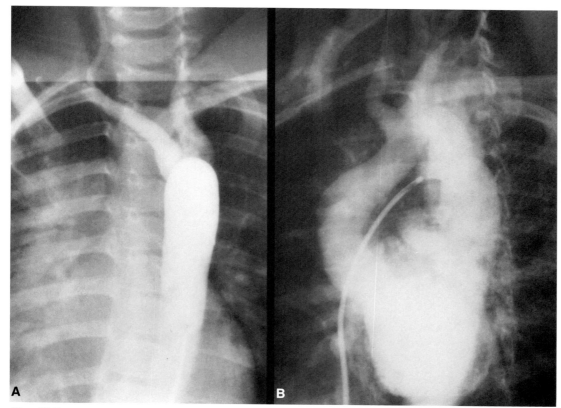

A   B

Fig. 47-2

Case 48

A 15-year-old girl is struck by a hit-and-run driver while trick-or-treating on Halloween. She is sitting up when paramedics arrive and then collapses, soon reviving enough to moan.

Heart rate is 140, respiratory rate 20–24. She is pale and cool. Dried blood is on face. Back of head and right elbow are scraped. She moans more when sternum, left side of chest, abdomen, and pelvis are palpated. Right shank is crooked. Radial pulses are impalpable, femoral pulses weak. Forty-five minutes later, heart rate is 130, blood pressure in left arm 106/78 mm Hg, and systolic pressure in right arm 108 mm Hg. Right calf is tense.

Hematocrit 45 minutes later is 0.32. White cell count is 15.6 × 10⁹/liter with 0.55 polymorphonuclear cells, 0.10 bands, 0.25 lymphocytes, 0.04 monocytes, 0.02 eosinophils, 0.01 basophils, 0.02 atypical lymphocytes, and 0.01 metamyelocytes. Platelet count is 334 × 10⁹/liter. Urine is turbid red, with specific gravity 1.020, pH 7.5. Urine has >0.30 g/liter protein, 13.9 mmol/liter glucose (after IV Ringer's lactate),

1.7 µmol/liter urobilinogen, nitrites, leukester, 0–1 white cell/HPF, occasional squamous epithelial cells/HPF, and >100 red cells/HPF. Serum sodium is 140 mmol/liter, potassium 3.6, chloride 108, carbon dioxide 20, urea nitrogen 5.0, and glucose 8.9. Creatinine is 90 µmol/liter. Amylase is 67 U/liter. Hematocrit is 0.15 after 5 hours.

Supracardiac shadow is widened in Figure 48-1A. Aortogram in Figure 48-1B shows widening of segment of aorta beyond left subclavian artery; widened segment is slightly more dense and its back wall slightly irregular.

At left posterolateral thoracotomy, a hematoma is around left subclavian artery. Aorta is transected at ligamentum arteriosum.

Diagnosis: Traumatic rupture of aorta with pseudo-aneurysm. (She also has fractured ribs, fifth lumbar vertebra, first sacral vertebra, right pubic bone, and right tibia and fibula with calf compartment syndrome.)

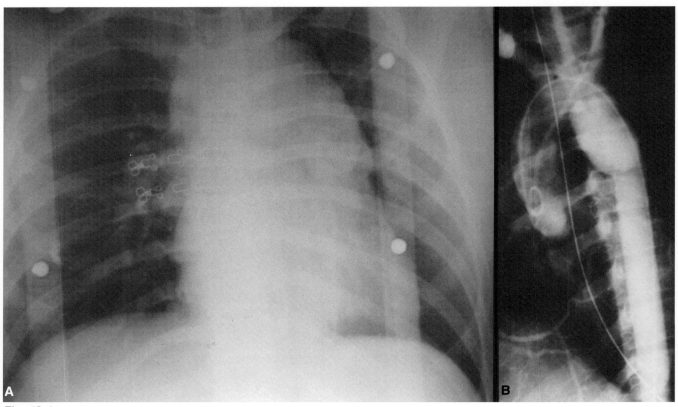

Fig. 48-1

Case 49

A 12-year-old boy has had epigastric and low chest pain since last night, despite narcotics.

Weight is 45 kg, height 152 cm, heart rate 80, and blood pressure 125/80 mm Hg. Physical findings are normal.

The next day he has spasms in which his expression becomes apprehensive and he writhes in pain. He is afebrile. Heart rate is 60–70, blood pressure 110/80 mm Hg. Hematocrit is 0.38. White cell count is 14.0×10^9/liter with 0.90 polymorphonuclear cells.

At 5:00 AM the second morning, 32 hours after first complaint, he sits up and screams, "There's a bone sticking through my back," and collapses. Pulse is weak and fast. He is pale and barely breathing. He revives briefly with IV fluids. Pulse is stronger, systolic blood pressure 110 mm Hg. Breath sounds are absent on right side. He dies a moment later.

Lateral aspect of descending aorta bulges slightly in examination soon after onset of pain (Figure 49-1A). Liquid is in right pleural space and around apex of left lung minutes before death (Figure 49-1B).

At necropsy, aorta is torn in two places, the upper tear between the fourth and fifth intercostal arteries, the lower near the tenth intercostal artery. A dissecting aneurysm extends from lower tear to ligamentum arteriosum. Blood is in retroperitoneum, mediastinum, and right pleural space. Heart, valves, and unaffected part of aorta are normal.

Diagnosis: Dissecting aneurysm and hemorrhage from aortic tears. (Later report is that the schoolboys were practicing the Heimlich maneuver the afternoon before the boy's pain began.)

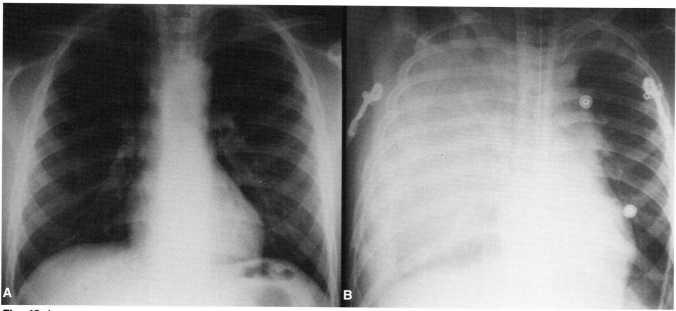

Fig. 49-1

Case 50

A 5-month-old boy has been vomiting for several days.

Mother (25 years old) was preeclamptic. Birth weight was 3.1 kg, length 53 cm, and Apgar score 8/10 at 1 and 5 minutes. Occasional afternoon fevers to 38.3–38.9°C began 6 weeks ago. He vomited several times and had a black stool 2½ weeks ago.

Weight at 5 months is 5.3 kg, temperature 36.4°C, heart rate 140, respiratory rate 40, and blood pressure 150/110 mm Hg to 190/130 mm Hg. He is limp. Mucous membranes are dry. A systolic murmur is present. Liver edge is 2 cm below costal margin. Fluids are infusing into a vein in the right foot. The rest of the physical findings are normal.

Hematocrit is 0.23 before transfusion, 0.35 after transfusion. White cell count is 19.2×10^9/liter with 0.40 polymorphonuclear cells, 0.28 bands, 0.24 lymphocytes, 0.06 monocytes, 0.01 eosinophils, and 0.01 basophils. Platelet count is 765×10^9/liter. Smear shows a few bizarre red blood cells. Urine specific gravity is 1.010, pH 7. Urine has protein, hemoglobin, 3–4 red cells/HPF, 10–12 white cells/HPF, few epithelial cells/HPF, hyaline and granular casts, mucus, and bacteria. Serum sodium is 132 mmol/liter, potassium 3.1, chloride 91, carbon dioxide 30, urea nitrogen 1.8, calcium 2.42, phosphorus 1.10, cholesterol 5.07, triglycerides 1.22, and glucose 6.2. Creatinine is 40 µmol/liter, uric acid 220, total bilirubin 9, and direct bilirubin 0. Total protein is 61 g/liter, albumin 27. Alkaline phosphatase is 360 U/liter, LDH 556, and SGOT 34. IgG is 20.6 g/liter (normal: 2.0–7.0), IgM 7.06 (normal: 0.25–1.00). Serum does not react in tests for antinuclear antibody, rheumatoid factor, ASO, syphilis, and toxoplasmosis. Anti-DNA antibody titers are 0.01 and 0.02 (normal: <0.10); rubella titer is <1:8. Urine epinephrine is 10 nmol/day (normal: 0–14), norepinephrine 70 (normal: 0–59).

ECG shows left ventricular hypertrophy.

He vomits bile a few days later.

Descending aorta is dilated in Figure 50-1A. In Figure 50-1B, stomach shows peristalsis, proximal small bowel is dilated, and gas is in distal gut.

At operation, jejunum is partly obstructed. Appendix is removed. Samples of kidney and liver are obtained.

Examination of resected jejunum shows ischemic mucosa, ulceration, subacute transmural inflammation, and thrombosis of submucosal vessels. Submucosal thrombosis is in appendix. Kidney wedge shows segmental mesangial sclerosis, IgM deposits, isolated tubular atrophy, and interstitial fibrosis. Electron microscopy of kidney shows increased mesangial matrix, irregularity of glomerular basement membrane, and collapse of epithelial foot processes. Fatty change is in liver.

In Figure 50-2, abdominal angiogram 12 days after operation shows occlusion of superior mesenteric artery approximately 4 cm from origin and stenosis at origin of inferior mesenteric artery (iM). Iliac arteries are in spasm (see Figure 50-2).

He is given antihypertensive and immunosuppressive treatment for approximately 1 year.

At 4½ years, he is well. Weight is 22 kg, height 107 cm, and blood pressure 98/60 mm Hg.

Diagnosis: Infantile arteritis, hypertensive dilation of descending aorta.

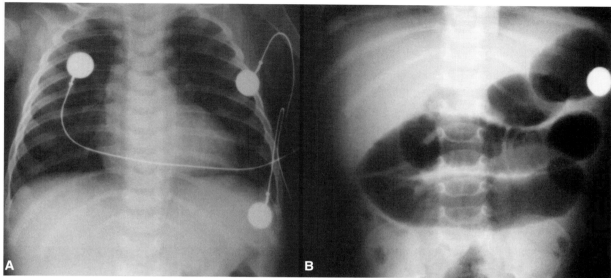

Fig. 50-1

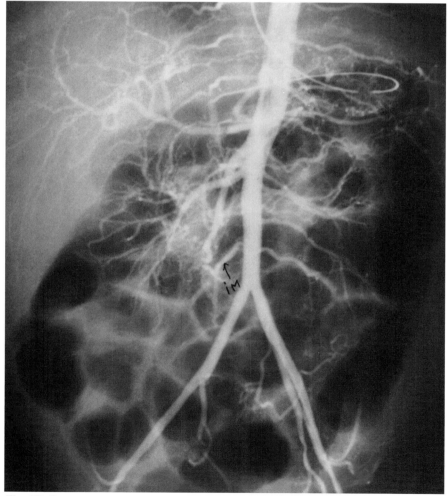

Fig. 50-2

Case 51

A 2½-month-old girl has an intracardiac mass that was discovered in prenatal ultrasound examination.

Pregnancy of mother was normal, birth weight 2.4 kg.

Mother (24 years old) is well. Maternal aunt has congenital heart disease. No one in family has seizures, mental retardation, or abnormal skin pigmentation.

Weight is 5.5 kg, length 55 cm, head circumference 38 cm, and heart rate 185. Short systolic murmur and diaper rash are present. The rest of the physical findings are normal.

ECG shows sinus rhythm and nonspecific anterolateral T-wave changes.

Roentgenographic findings in chest are normal. Echocardiogram in Figure 51-1 shows thickening of interventricular septum (2.6 × 1.3 cm) into right ventricle (and mild tricuspid regurgitation with flow velocity of approximately 2 m/sec).

At 3¼ years, growth and development are normal. Heart rate is 70, blood pressure 90/60 mm Hg. A soft systolic murmur is at lower left sternal border. The rest of the physical findings are normal.

Echocardiographic findings at 3½ years are like those of 3 years ago. The intracardiac mass is 2.5 × 1.3 cm.

Diagnosis: Rhabdomyoma of heart.

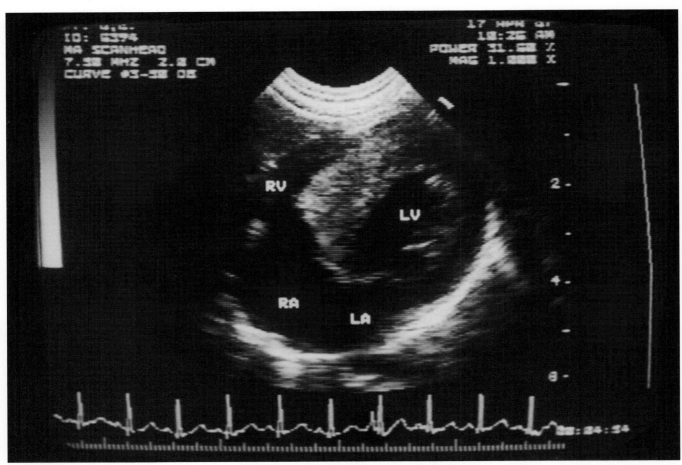

Fig. 51-1

Case 52

A 2-year-old boy has had 2- to 3-day periods with pain and 2- to 3-day periods without pain for 5 months when he urinates and for 3 weeks when he defecates.

Pregnancy of mother was normal, birth weight 3.0 kg. Skin tags were removed from a foot at 3 days. He walked at 1 year. Parents have been worried about his rapid heartbeat for 1 year. He had fever and ear infection 2 months ago.

Mother (20 years old) and father (22 years old) are well. He is their only child. Paternal uncle has asthma. Maternal grandmother had colon cancer.

Weight at 2 years is 11 kg, height 84 cm, temperature 38°C, heart rate 160, respiratory rate 28, and blood pressure 140/70 mm Hg. He is pale. Hair is blonde. A firm, irregular mass is in pelvis, palpable above and to left of rectum. The rest of the physical findings are normal.

Hematocrit is 0.32. White cell count is 10.6×10^9/liter with 0.40 polymorphonuclear cells, 0.02 bands, 0.48 lymphocytes, 0.07 monocytes, 0.02 eosinophils, and 0.02 basophils. Platelet estimate is adequate. Serum sodium is 130 mmol/liter, potassium 4.1, chloride 101, carbon dioxide 20, urea nitrogen 3.9, and glucose 4.4.

In Figure 52-1, interstitial markings in lungs are excessive. Excretory urogram in Figure 52-2 shows bladder pushed upward and forward and lower part of right ureter pushed laterally by a mass.

At operation, a tumor ($10 \times 7 \times 4$ cm) adherent to back of bladder is removed.

Outer surface of tumor is gray-tan, cut surface light tan and jellylike with hemorrhagic center. Microscopic examination shows (1) spindlelike cells with little eosinophilic cytoplasm; (2) round, ovoid, and oblong nuclei (most with fine reticular chromatin, some with clumped peripheral chromatin); and (3) stroma of delicate fibrous connective tissue infiltrated by lymphocytes and plasma cells.

One month later, he is coughing, short of breath, and "breathing funny." When he coughs, his lips are sometimes blue and he sweats and grunts. A systolic murmur is sometimes present. ECG shows sinus tachycardia and perhaps right ventricular hypertrophy. Chest roentgenogram shows larger heart and excess liquid in lungs. At cardiac catheterization, pulmonary artery pressure is 55/28 mm Hg, wedge pressure 38. Angiocardiogram shows left atrial mass that moves in and out of mitral valve with heartbeat. He dies before operation.

At necropsy, a translucent gray tumor ($4.5 \times 3.4 \times 2.0$ cm) is attached by a stalk to wall of left atrium. Microscopic examination shows (1) thin endothelial cover; (2) myxoid and fibrous connective tissue; (3) acellular, proteinaceous, eosinophilic ground substance; (4) aggregates of smooth muscle; and (5) many small, tortuous vascular channels. A microfocal Sertoli's cell adenoma in a dense fibrous sheath in a testicle consists of round aggregates of stellate cells with abundant, pale, eosinophilic cytoplasm; indefinable borders; and large round-to-oval vacuolated nuclei with fine reticular chromatin and occasional single or double central nucleoli. Lungs, liver, and kidney show passive congestion, and lungs show focal atelectasis.

Diagnosis: Liposarcoma in pelvis, left atrial myxoma, Sertoli's cell adenoma, skin tags (questionable myxoid neurofibromas) on foot; questionable syndrome myxoma.

(Continued)

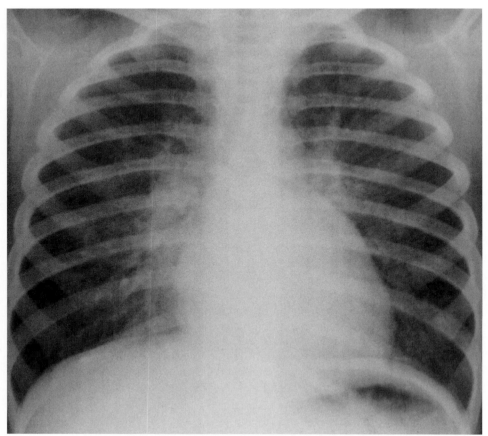

Fig. 52-1

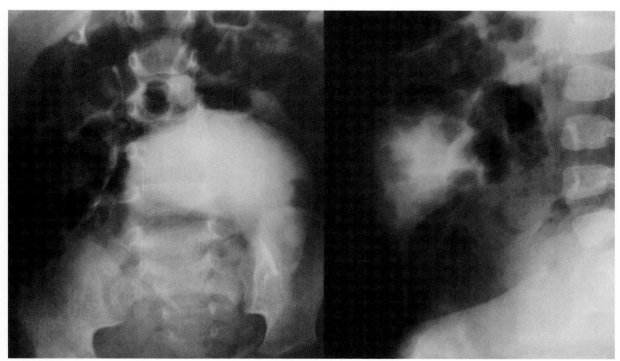

Fig. 52-2

Case 53

A 15-year-old boy has a "dull ache, a sore muscle feeling" in his chest.

He could not finish running laps in gym class 4 weeks ago because he was out of breath and his "heart was really pounding." He was tired and had a cough, sore throat, and fever 2 weeks ago. He has epigastric pain and sometimes vomits after he eats.

Mother (47 years old) is well. He has no siblings and knows nothing about his father.

Temperature is 36.1°C, heart rate 104, respiratory rate 18, blood pressure 110/66 mm Hg, and weight 58 kg. He is pale. Pimples and freckles are on face. Jugular veins are dilated. Heart beat is visible in left side of chest; point of maximal impulse is 11 cm from sternum. Heart sounds are loud with a gallop rhythm. A holosystolic murmur is loudest at apex and radiates to left axilla. Liver edge is 6 cm below costal margin. Ankles are swollen. The rest of the physical findings are normal.

Hematocrit is 0.38. White cell count is 11.8×10^9/liter with 0.79 polymorphonuclear cells, 0.14 lymphocytes, 0.03 monocytes, and 0.04 basophils. Platelet count is 377×10^9/liter. ESR is 1 mm/hr. MCV is 69 fl. MCH is 22 pg. MCHC is 320 g/liter. Fibrinogen is 2.6 µmol/liter (normal: 4.4–10.3). Smear shows poikilocytosis, anisocytosis, schistocytosis, and ovalocytosis. PT is 25.4 seconds, activated PTT 62.8. Serum ASO titer is 480 Todd units (normal: 0–250). Urine specific gravity is 1.026, pH 5. Urine has 0.30 g/liter protein, 1+ bilirubin, 0–1 red cell/HPF, 0–2 white cells/HPF, and 0–1 hyaline cast/LPF. Serum sodium is 130 mmol/liter, potassium 5.2, chloride 99, urea nitrogen 13.0, calcium 2.07, phosphorus 1.19, cholesterol 2.09, and glucose 6.6. Creatinine is 110

µmol/liter, uric acid 480, total bilirubin 67, and direct bilirubin 36. Total protein is 64 g/liter, albumin 28. Alkaline phosphatase is 234 U/liter, LDH 538, and SGOT 1128.

ECG shows sinus tachycardia, delayed right ventricular conduction, delayed interatrial conduction and/or enlargement of left atrium, and nonspecific ST-T wave abnormality.

In Figure 53-1, pericardiocardiac image is larger than normal, liquid is in right pleural space, and lung markings, which include Kerley's B lines near costophrenic angles, are prominent. Echocardiogram in Figure 53-2 shows a left atrial mass that goes into left ventricle during diastole.

At operation, right atrium and venae cavae are dilated. A mass in left atrium is attached to septum by a thin stalk. Mitral valve annulus fibrosus is dilated.

The glistening, gelatinous mass is yellow-green to brown-orange, its stalk firm and tan-white. Microscopic examination shows (1) organizing fibrin; (2) degenerating red cells; (3) small stellate cells with small hyperchromatic nuclei and eosinophilic cytoplasm; (4) larger cells with round-to-oval nuclei, some with two nuclei, and eosinophilic cytoplasm; (5) loose myxomatous stroma; and (6) many endothelium-lined channels, most occluded by red cells and clots.

Punch biopsy of a dark spot on the boy's back shows increased pigment along basal layer of epidermis and normal number of melanocytes.

Diagnosis: Left atrial myxoma, syndrome myxoma (cardiac myxoma, pigmented skin lesions, and peripheral and endocrine neoplasms).

(Continued)

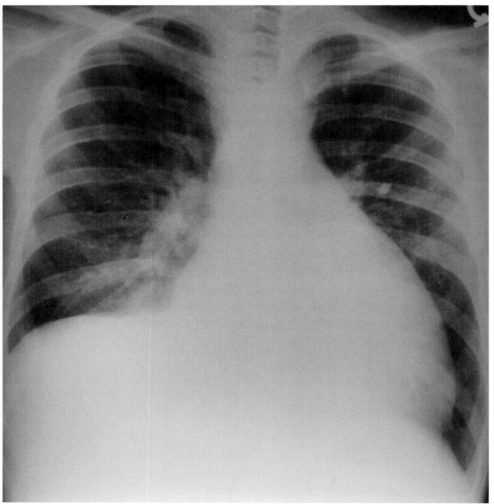

Fig. 53-1

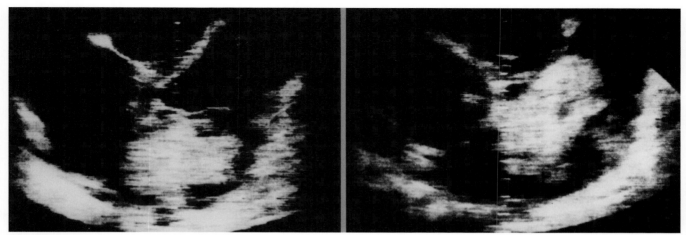

Fig. 53-2

Abdominal Wall

Case 1

A 2-month-old boy has a bleeding umbilicus and swelling and inflammation around it.

Pregnancy of mother (18 years old) was normal, birth weight 3.5 kg.

Weight is 4.8 kg, length 60 cm, temperature 37.2°C, heart rate 120, respiratory rate 46, and systolic blood pressure 90 mm Hg. The rest of the physical findings are normal.

Hematocrit is 0.29. White cell count is 10.6 × 10⁹/liter with 0.12 polymorphonuclear cells, 0.02 bands, 0.75 lymphocytes, 0.08 monocytes, and 0.03 eosinophils. Urine specific gravity is 1.005, pH 6.5. Urine has bacteria, occasional epithelial cells/HPF, red cells/HPF, and white cells/HPF. Serum sodium is 141 mmol/liter, potassium 5.0, chloride 106, carbon dioxide 22, urea nitrogen 2.1, calcium 2.57, phosphorus 1.97, cholesterol 2.66, and glucose 4.3. Creatinine is 40 μmol/liter,

uric acid 180, total bilirubin 3, and direct bilirubin 0. Total protein is 58 g/liter, albumin 38. Alkaline phosphatase is 232 U/liter, LDH 301, and SGOT 44.

In Figure 1-1, barium injected into opening in umbilicus goes into small bowel.

At operation, urachus and normal umbilical vessels are divided and ligated, omphalomesenteric duct and surrounding mesentery freed up by blunt dissection, and duct and segment of ileum excised.

The segment of ileum (2 cm long, 1 cm wide) is connected to a fistula (1.3 cm long, 0.9 cm wide) with cutaneous stoma surrounded by everted, ulcerated skin.

Diagnosis: Persistent omphalomesenteric (vitelline) duct.

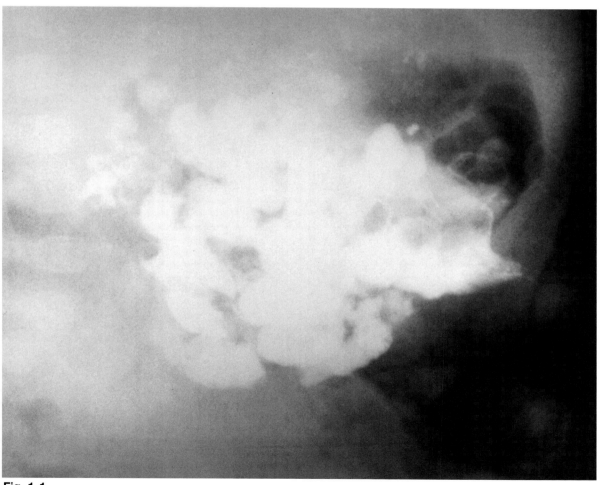

Fig. 1-1

Case 2

A 2-month-old girl has had a bulge in right groin and sometimes in left groin. Right bulge was occasionally present at 1–2 weeks, and is now always present.

Pregnancy of mother (28 years old) was marred by vaginal spotting. Birth weight was 2.4 kg. The girl had diarrhea and a bloody stool 3 days ago.

Weight at 2 months is 4.9 kg, temperature 36.3°C, heart rate 160, respiratory rate 40, and systolic blood pressure 85 mm Hg. The rest of the physical findings are normal.

Hematocrit is 0.29. White cell count is 11.7×10^9/liter with 0.05 polymorphonuclear cells, 0.01 bands, 0.76 lymphocytes, 0.15 monocytes, 0.01 eosinophils, and 0.02 atypical lymphocytes. Platelet count is 416×10^9/liter.

Both groins are swollen. In Figure 2-1, gas-containing gut is in right Nuck's diverticulum (peritoneal diverticulum that corresponds to male processus vaginalis).

At operation, sac in right inguinal canal contains ovary and fallopian tube; a smaller sac is in left inguinal canal.

Diagnosis: Bilateral inguinal hernias.

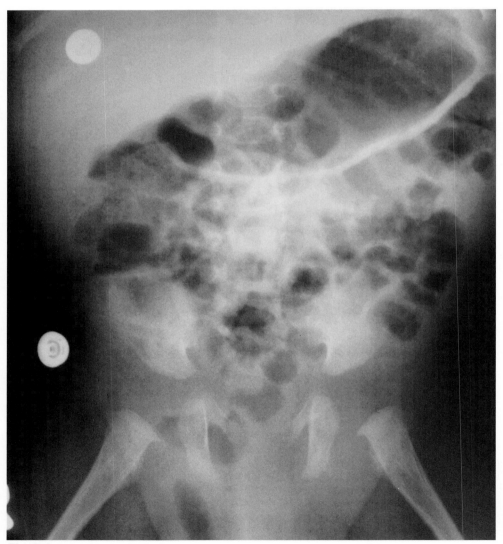

Fig. 2-1

Gastrointestinal Tract

Case 1

A newborn boy has Rh hemolytic disease.

Mother (24 years old), AB negative, had first trimester abortion 4 years ago. Intrauterine blood transfusion was performed 18 and 29 days ago after injection of contrast medium into baby's peritoneal cavity.

Weight is 2.5 kg, Apgar score 8/9 at 1 and 5 minutes, length 45 cm, head circumference 33 cm, temperature 35.6°C, heart rate 150, respiratory rate 80, and systolic blood pressure 62 mm Hg. Baby is jaundiced. Liver edge and spleen edge are 2 cm below costal margin. Left testicle is not in scrotum. The rest of the physical findings are normal.

Hematocrit is 0.44. Serum sodium is 136 mmol/liter, potassium 4.0, chloride 103, urea nitrogen 3.0, calcium 2.35, and glucose 3.1. Total bilirubin is 97 μmol/liter, direct bilirubin 38. Total protein is 55 g/liter.

Exchange transfusion is performed at 6½ hours. Abdomen is distended at 11 hours. A glycerine suppository is put in rectum at 11½ hours. Meconium is passed at 13 hours.

At 1¼ hours, gas is in stomach and undilated jejunum, and meconium opacified by contrast medium is in undilated rectum and sigmoid (Figure 1-1A). At 3¾ hours, gas is in stomach, undilated jejunum, and undilated ileum, and opacified meconium is in undilated rectum and sigmoid (Figure 1-1B). At 11 hours, gas is in stomach and rest of gut, including rectum. Contrast medium is in dilated rectum and sigmoid (Figure 1-2A). At 18 hours, pattern of intestinal gas is normal. Opacified meconium is gone (Figure 1-2B).

Diagnosis: Normal movement of gas through newborn gut and expulsion of meconium.

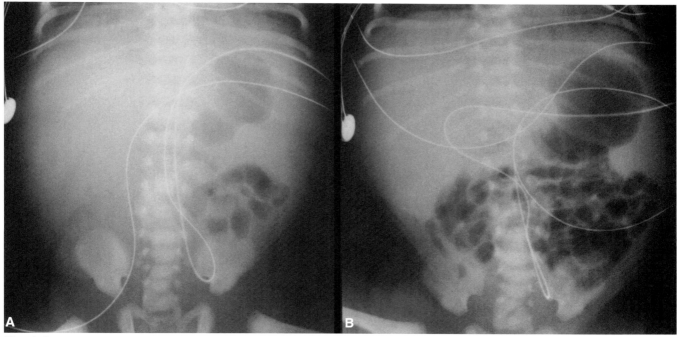

Fig. 1-1

(Continued)

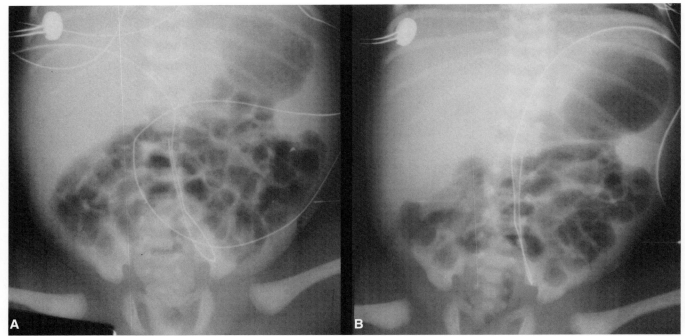

Fig. 1-2

Case 2

A premature girl has distended abdomen and has not passed meconium at 36 hours.

Birth weight is 1.6 kg, length 42 cm, head circumference 30 cm, and Apgar score 7/8 at 1 and 5 minutes. At 15 minutes, temperature is 36.8°C, heart rate 150, respiratory rate 65, blood pressure 61/32 mm Hg, and blood sugar 2.8 mmol/liter. At 36 hours, cry is loud. She is jaundiced. Distended abdomen is soft. Bowel sounds are normal. The rest of the physical findings are normal.

Serum sodium is 138 mmol/liter, potassium 5.1, chloride 105, and calcium 2.00. Total bilirubin is 113 μmol/liter.

In Figure 2-1, gut is uniformly dilated with gas at 36 hours.

She is not fed. She is given IV fluids.

In Figure 2-2A, barium enema at 4 days shows normal colon and medial displacement of ascending colon by dilated small bowel.

Most of barium is absent from colon at 5 days. She is given barium by mouth for GI series at 6 days. First feeding is at 10 days.

In Figure 2-2B at 11 days, barium is in distal colon and gut is not dilated.

Diagnosis: Normal premature gut in unfed baby.

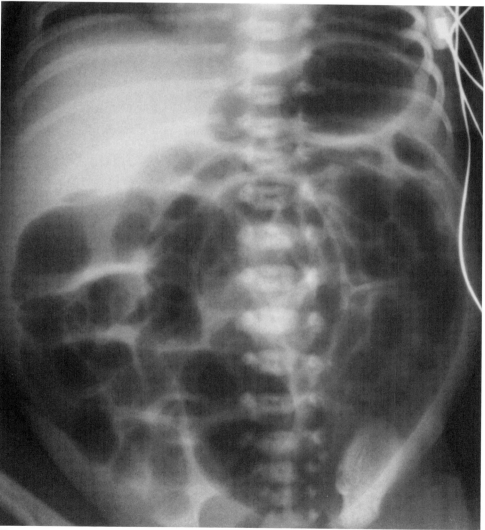

Fig. 2-1

(Continued)

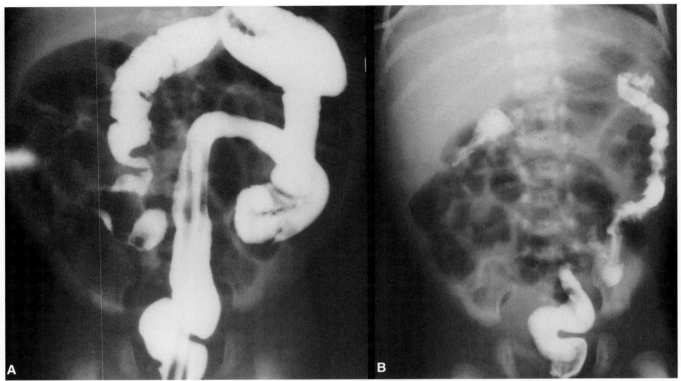

Fig. 2-2

Case 3

A 40-hour-old boy has a distended abdomen and has not passed meconium. He took glucose water followed by formula yesterday. Abdomen was distended at 31 hours. He vomited milk curds at 34 hours.

Birth weight is 2.5 kg, length 48 cm, and Apgar score 9/8 at 1 and 5 minutes. At 1 hour, temperature is 36.9°C, heart rate 140, respiratory rate 50, and blood pressure 62/23 mm Hg. At 40 hours, abdomen is distended, tense, and tympanitic. Bowel sounds are present. The rest of the physical findings are normal.

Hematocrit is 0.46. White cell count is 9.0×10^9/liter with 0.39 polymorphonuclear cells, 0.19 bands, 0.17 lymphocytes, 0.22 monocytes, 0.01 eosinophils, 0.01 basophils, and 0.01 metamyelocytes. Platelet count is 279×10^9/liter. Serum sodium is 135 mmol/liter, potassium 4.3, chloride 105, and calcium 2.15.

In Figure 3-1, gut is uniformly dilated with gas. Fluoroscopic spot films show meconium (Figure 3-2A) and then barium (Figure 3-2B) in gas-dilated rectum.

Meconium and barium are ejected a moment after the enema. He has large stools the next day. At 4 days, sweat chloride is 19 mmol/liter. Rectal suction biopsy shows submucosal ganglion cells.

Diagnosis: Meconium plug.

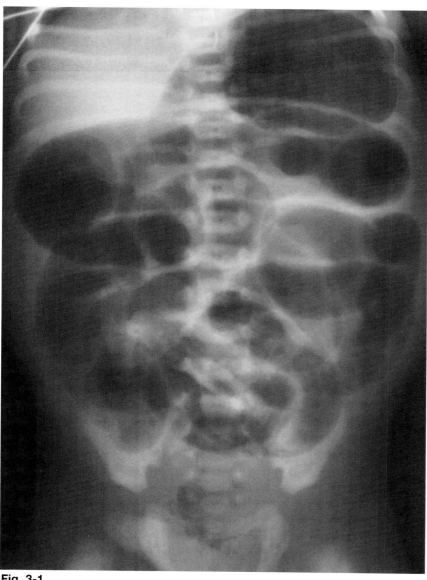

Fig. 3-1

(Continued)

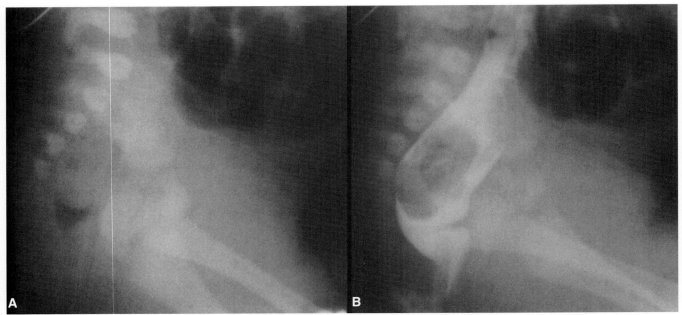

Fig. 3-2

Case 4

A 12-year-old boy has felt discomfort in midchest after swallowing food three times during the last 3 years. He swallowed a partly chewed piece of steak 2 weeks ago and felt uncomfortable for 2 hours until he vomited. Discomfort and sometimes panic usually last 10–15 minutes until food goes down or is spit out.

Birth weight was 3.8 kg. He was jaundiced until breast-feeding was stopped. He has had several ear infections. He broke a thumb.

Weight at 12 years is 44 kg, height 155 cm. Moles are on back. A systolic murmur is present. The rest of the physical findings are normal.

A constriction ring is in lower esophagus (Figure 4-1) only when boy exhales hard against closed glottis (Valsalva's maneuver) (Figure 4-2). GI series shows normal stomach and proximal small bowel.

Diagnosis: Schatzki's ring, normal esophagus.

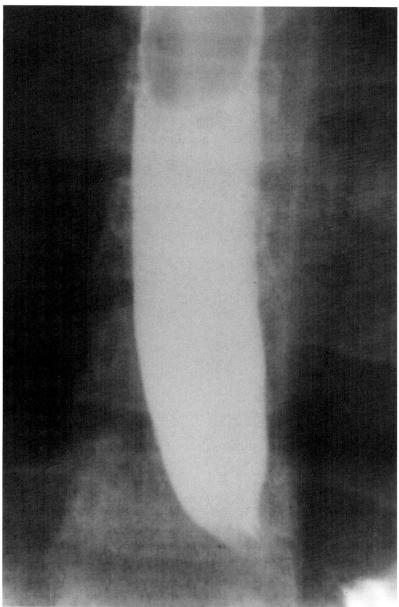

Fig. 4-1

(Continued)

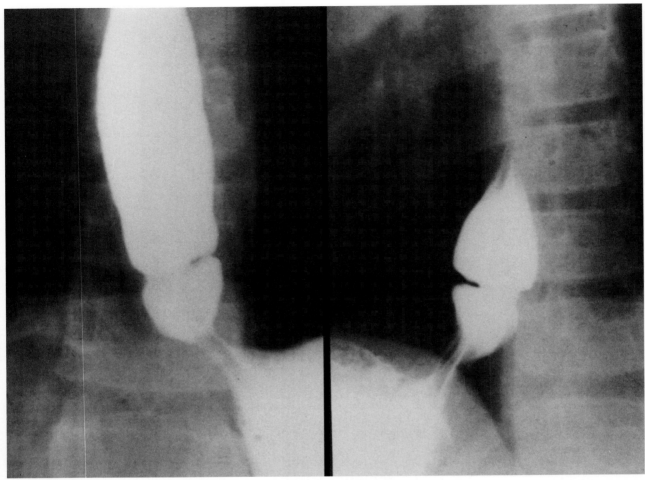

Fig. 4-2

Case 5

A 7-year-old girl has had blood-streaked stools for 1 week.

She has had watery stools several days per month for 1½ years. She has periumbilical pain in early morning and is sometimes awakened by it. She has frequent colds. She has had aphthae during the last 9 months. She had sore throat, fever, and a positive spot test for infectious mononucleosis 8 months ago. She has had swellings of knees and ankles during the last 5 months.

Older half brother has Crohn's disease.

Temperature at 7 years is 36.4°C, heart rate 76, respiratory rate 16, blood pressure 96/60 mm Hg, and weight 23.7 kg. Physical findings are normal.

Hematocrit is 0.37. White cell count is 6.9×10^9/liter with 0.62 polymorphonuclear cells, 0.03 bands, 0.26 lymphocytes, 0.06 monocytes, 0.02 eosinophils, and 0.01 atypical lymphocytes. Platelet count is 366×10^9/liter. ESR is 3 mm/hr.

One hour after girl drinks barium and water and eats breakfast, food is in dilated stomach, and barium is in ileum, colon, and appendix (Figure 5-1A). Barium is farther along in colon and almost out of appendix 5 minutes later (Figure 5-1B).

Diagnosis: Normal findings in GI tract, normal peristalsis of appendix.

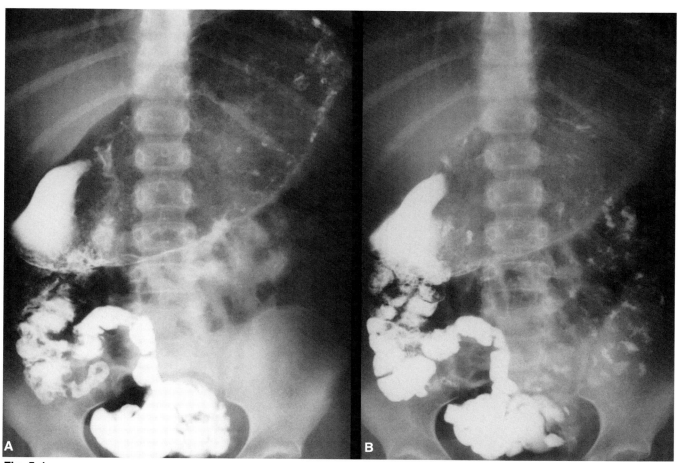

Fig. 5-1

Case 6

A 1-year-old girl has had two to three dark, loose stools per day for 2 weeks. Family lives on farm and drinks well water.

Physical findings are normal.

Stool is guaiac negative. It does not contain ova or parasites. Stool culture grows normal bowel flora.

Barium enema shows small, uniform filling defects throughout colon (Figure 6-1).

Diagnosis: Normal lymphoid follicles in colon.

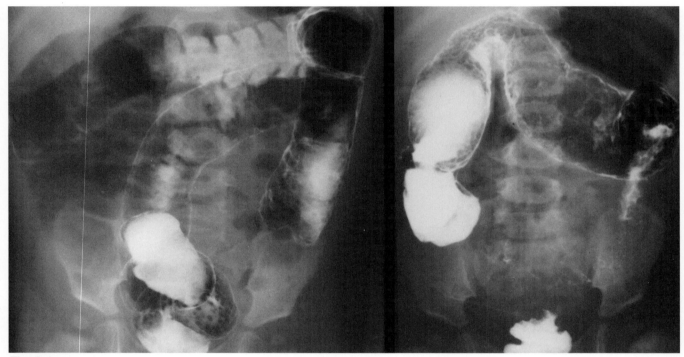

Fig. 6-1

Case 7

A newborn girl, whose Apgar score is 2 at 1 minute, cannot be intubated.

Mother (21 years old) had hypertension and edema during pregnancy. She was given magnesium sulfate during 3½-hour labor. Birth weight is 2.7 kg, length 52 cm, and head circumference 33 cm. At 2 minutes, she cries weakly. Mouth is full of mucus. Temperature is 36.3°C, heart rate 130, respiratory rate 30, and systolic blood pressure 70–90 mm Hg. She breathes easily in a few minutes. A membrane in back of mouth is fixed to soft palate, buccal mucosa, and back of tongue, and has a 2-mm hole through which uvula moves. Sucking and Moro's reflexes are depressed. The rest of the physical findings are normal.

Hematocrit is 0.54. White cell count is 9.9 × 10⁹/liter with 0.64 polymorphonuclear cells, 0.22 bands, 0.13 lymphocytes, and 0.01 eosinophils. Platelet estimate is adequate.

At 1 month, weight is 3.3 kg. At 2 months, she has cough, runny nose, and loose stools, and gains only 0.06 kg in the week before gastrostomy tube is placed.

At 9 months, barium fills mouth (Figure 7-1A) and trickles into throat before removal of membrane (Figure 7-1B).

At operation, soft palate is adherent to front of palatopharyngeal arch and base of tongue. Membrane is 1–2 mm thick in center and 5 mm thick at sides, and incorporates palatoglossus muscles. Lingual tonsil is large. Valleculae, epiglottis, and larynx are normal.

Diagnosis: Congenital stenosis of mouth.

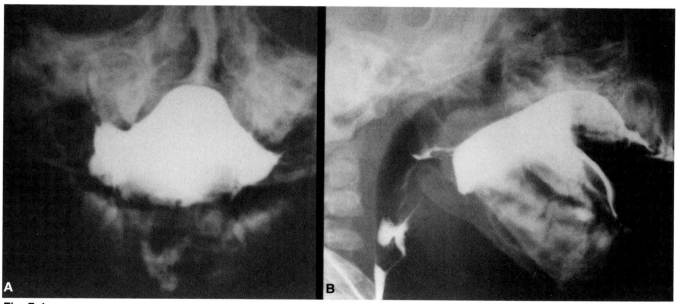

Fig. 7-1

Case 8

A 4-day-old boy has a "gurgly, hoarse" cry and yellow mucus in mouth.

Mother (31 years old) drank alcohol and smoked marijuana during pregnancy. Fetal heart rate slowed during labor. Forceps were used for delivery. Birth weight was 4 kg, Apgar score 3/6 at 1 and 5 minutes and 9 at 10 minutes. Meconium was in hypopharynx. Attempts to intubate failed. He is fed by gavage.

Weight is 3.7 kg, temperature 36.8°C, heart rate 124, respiratory rate 50, and blood pressure 79/56 mm Hg. Feet are clubbed. The rest of the physical findings are normal.

Hematocrit is 0.50. White cell count is 10.7×10^9/liter with 0.37 polymorphonuclear cells, 0.09 bands, 0.42 lymphocytes, and 0.12 monocytes. Platelet count is 274×10^9/liter. Serum sodium is 136 mmol/liter, potassium 4.2, chloride 107, carbon dioxide 16, urea nitrogen 15.7, calcium 2.15, phosphorus 2.81, cholesterol 4.27, and glucose 7.2. Creatinine is 90 µmol/liter, uric acid 370, total bilirubin 133, and direct bilirubin 9. Total protein is 57 g/liter, albumin 35. Alkaline phosphatase is 134 U/liter, LDH 496, and SGOT 25.

Swallowed barium goes into esophagus (Figure 8-1A) and a track to left of and behind esophagus (Figure 8-1B).

At laryngoscopy, epiglottis, aryepiglottic folds, and true vocal cords are slightly edematous.

Diagnosis: Traumatic pharyngeal pseudodiverticulum.

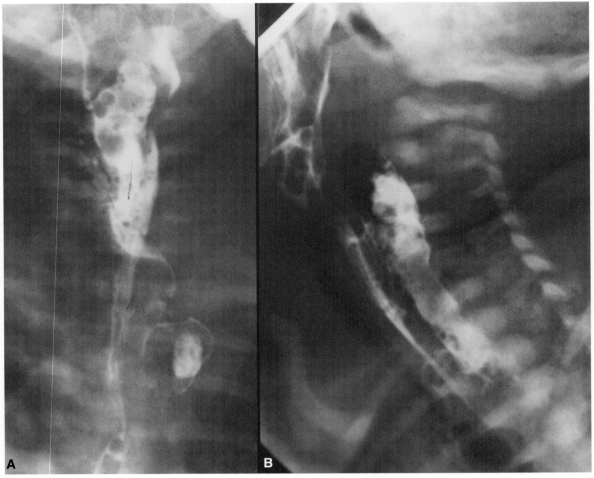

A   **B**

Fig. 8-1

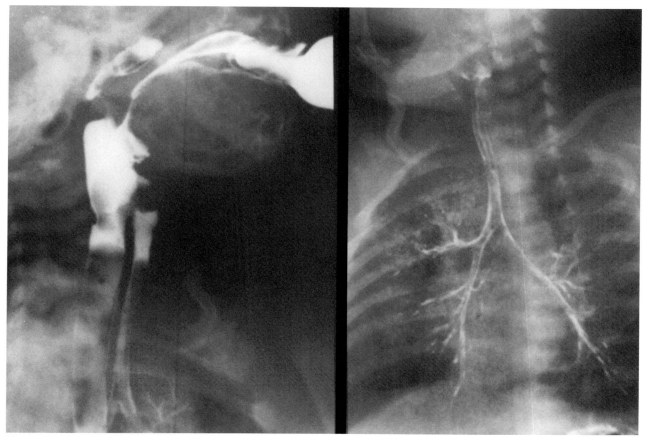

Fig. 10-1

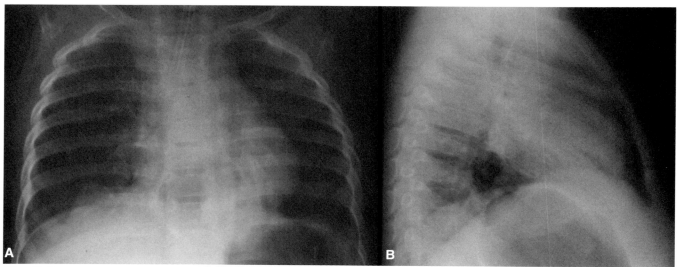

Fig. 10-2

Case 11

A 2-day-old boy vomits when feeding and has a distended abdomen.

Pregnancy of mother was normal, birth weight 3.7 kg. He coughs and chokes when he feeds and soon vomits. Recurrent cyanosis clears when thick mucus is aspirated from mouth and pharynx.

Mother (20 years old), father (28 years old), and sister (2 years old) are well.

Temperature is 37°C, heart rate 160, respiratory rate 60, systolic blood pressure 64 mm Hg, and weight 3.3 kg. Abdomen is distended and tympanitic. Skin veins are prominent. Bowel sounds are decreased. Rectal examination releases a lot of gas. The rest of the physical findings are normal.

Hematocrit is 0.47. Urine specific gravity is 1.005, pH 5. Urine has rare red cells/HPF and occasional epithelial cells/HPF. Serum sodium is 146 mmol/liter, potassium 4.6, chloride 114, urea nitrogen 5.6, and glucose 3.7.

Barium is in mouth, atretic esophagus, trachea, bronchi, distal tracheoesophageal fistula, and gas-distended stomach (Figure 11-1).

At operation, fistula is divided, two parts of esophagus are anastomosed, and gastrostomy is placed.

Diagnosis: Esophageal atresia with tracheoesophageal fistula.

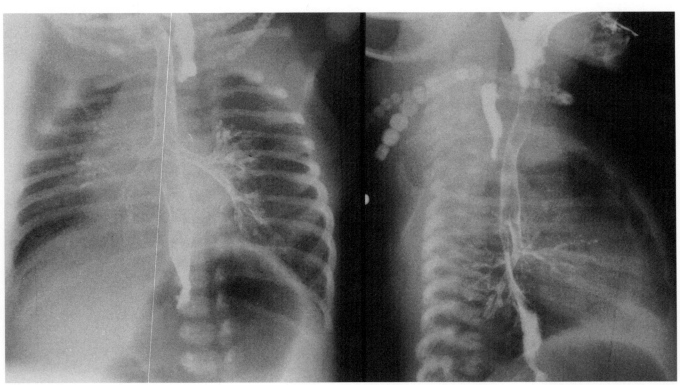

Fig. 11-1

Case 12

A 1-day-old girl chokes when fed.

Mother has been taking thyroid pills for 2 years. She bled from vagina during first trimester.

Weight is 2.1 kg, length 47 cm, temperature 37.2°C, heart rate 130, respiratory rate 40–50, and systolic blood pressure 64 mm Hg. She is jaundiced. The rest of the physical findings are normal.

Hematocrit is 0.63. Serum sodium is 145 mmol/liter, potassium 4.2, urea nitrogen 4.3, calcium 2.30, and glucose 2.5. Total bilirubin is 190 μmol/liter. Capillary blood pH is 7.40. P_{CO_2} is 31 mm Hg, P_{O_2} 49.

Air, liquid, and a coiled tube are in esophagus, and gas is in gut (Figure 12-1).

At operation, the coiled tube is in proximal atretic esophagus. Distal esophagus is connected to trachea.

Diagnosis: Esophageal atresia with tracheoesophageal fistula.

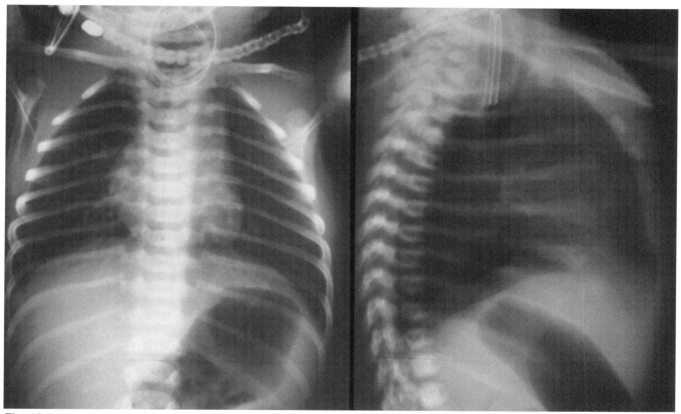

Fig. 12-1

Case 13

A newborn girl, who is retracting and dusky when handled, has a lot of thick white mucus in mouth.

Pregnancy of mother (22 years old) was normal. Birth weight is 2.2 kg, length 46 cm, head circumference 33 cm, and Apgar score 6/9 at 1 and 5 minutes. At 22 hours, temperature is 36.6°C, heart rate 110, respiratory rate 45, and systolic blood pressure 62 mm Hg. She is pink until handled. She retracts slightly and grunts occasionally. Abdomen is scaphoid. The rest of the physical findings are normal.

Hematocrit is 0.45. White cell count is 22.4×10^9/liter with 0.72 polymorphonuclear cells, 0.04 bands, 0.21 lymphocytes, 0.02 monocytes, and 0.01 eosinophils.

In Figure 13-1, a sac in upper mediastinum that contains air compresses and pushes trachea forward, and no gas is in gut.

At thoracotomy, an esophageal membrane is resected and the two parts of the esophagus are anastomosed.

Diagnosis: Esophageal atresia without tracheo-esophageal fistula.

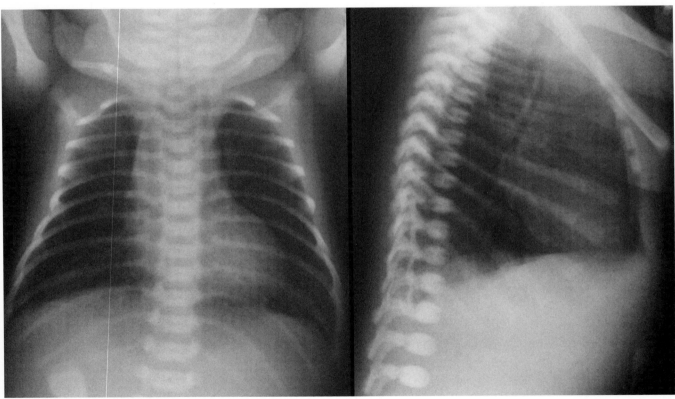

Fig. 13-1

Case 14

A newborn boy vomits 2–3 minutes after breast-feeding and sucks his fingers. He has stuffy nose, a lot of mucus in his mouth, and "seal bark" cough.

Mother (24 years old) and father (26 years old) are well. The boy is their only child.

Pregnancy of mother was normal. Birth weight is 3.2 kg, length 52 cm, head circumference 35 cm, Apgar score 9/10 at 1 and 5 minutes, temperature 36.8°C, heart rate 170, respiratory rate 40, and systolic blood pressure 70 mm Hg. The rest of the physical findings are normal.

Hematocrit is 0.52. White cell count is 10.1×10^9/liter with 0.34 polymorphonuclear cells, 0.06 bands, 0.52 lymphocytes, and 0.08 monocytes. Platelet count is 425×10^9/liter. Serum sodium is 148 mmol/liter, potassium 4.2, chloride 108, urea nitrogen 3.1, and glucose 4.8. At 68 hours, total bilirubin is 82 µmol/liter.

At right thoracotomy, esophageal atresia and tracheoesophageal fistula are found. Fistula is closed, esophagus anastomosed.

Barium swallow 5 days after esophageal anastomosis shows a stricture at anastomosis at level of T3 and another at T7 (Figure 14-1).

At 26 months, he says "stuck" and vomits an average of once per week. Weight is 13 kg, height 86 cm.

Diagnosis: Esophageal atresia with tracheoesophageal fistula and congenital stenosis. (Congenital stenosis at level of T7 is dilated to no. 24 French from above and, at 13 and 14 months, to no. 34 French from below through gastrostomy tube, which is then pulled. He can eat hamburger for the first time at 14 months.)

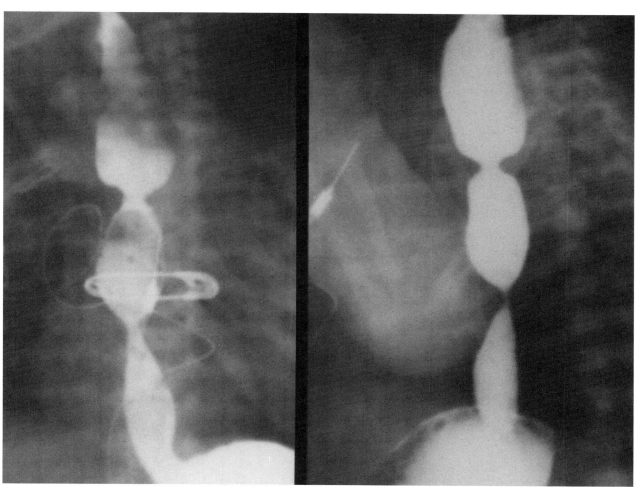

Fig. 14-1

Case 15

A newborn twin girl gags and spits up thick, frothy, pink mucus.

Mother (28 years old), father (31 years old), two brothers (2 and 9 years old), and sister (5 years old) are well. Twin sister, weight 2.4 kg, is normal.

Birth weight is 1.6 kg, length 44 cm, head circumference 31 cm, Apgar score 7/9 at 1 and 5 minutes. At 30 minutes, temperature is 35.8°C, heart rate 144, respiratory rate 52, and systolic blood pressure 74 mm Hg. At 5 hours, she gags on water. Water comes out of nose. Face is dusky. Attempt to pass a nasogastric tube fails. The rest of the physical findings are normal.

Hematocrit is 0.51. White cell count is 9.5×10^9/liter with 0.52 polymorphonuclear cells, 0.16 bands, 0.19 lymphocytes, 0.10 monocytes, 0.01 eosinophils, and 0.02 atypical lymphocytes. Platelet estimate is normal. Serum sodium is 137 mmol/liter, potassium 4.2, chloride 100, carbon dioxide 18, urea nitrogen 3.6, and glucose 7.5 (IV fluids).

In Figure 15-1 at 18½ hours, gas is in stomach and duodenal bulb but not beyond; a tube ends in neck.

At abdominal operation, stomach and proximal duodenum are dilated; rest of gut is collapsed. A small amount of meconium is in sigmoid colon. Gut is incompletely rotated. Small bowel is in front of transverse colon. Annular pancreas is present. A 0.5-cm mass is in antimesenteric subserosal tissue of jejunum, 6 cm beyond ligament of Treitz. Side-to-side duodenojejunostomy, gastrotomy, appendectomy, and resection of jejunal nodule are performed. Examination of the shiny smooth nodule (0.5 × 0.4 × 0.3 cm) shows dark black pancreas inside.

At thoracotomy at 6 days, esophageal anastomosis and division of tracheoesophageal fistula are performed. Gastrostomy tube is removed at 6 weeks. She chokes and vomits at 3 months. Esophageal anastomosis is dilated to no. 30 French. She is constipated at 5 months because of anal stenosis. At 23 months, she chokes on cereal and coughs when eating gelatin. Cry is hoarse. Temperature is 36.7°C, heart rate 100, respiratory rate 20, weight 9.3 kg, and height 77 cm. Chest and abdomen are scarred. The rest of the physical findings are normal.

In Figure 15-2, a mass of metal density is in esophagus.

Diagnosis: Esophageal atresia, tracheoesophageal fistula, annular pancreas, heterotopic pancreas (in jejunum), incomplete rotation of gut, anal stenosis, and mass at esophageal anastomosis. (Three pennies are removed at esophagoscopy.)

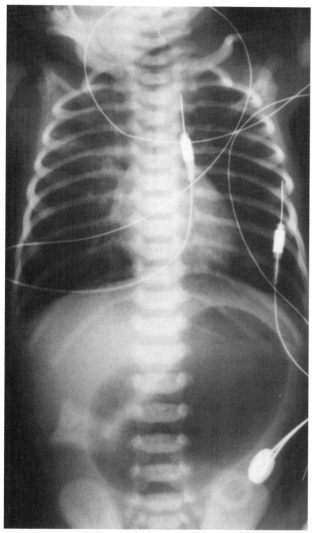

Fig. 15-1

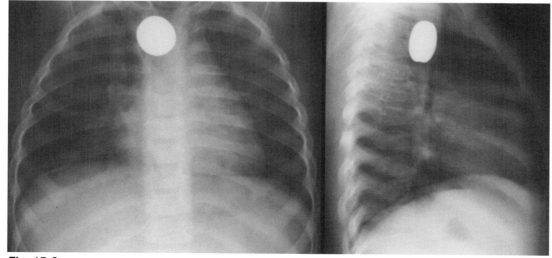

Fig. 15-2

Case 16

A newborn boy has imperforate anus discovered during attempt to take rectal temperature.

Pregnancy of mother (23 years old) was normal. Birth weight is 3.5 kg, Apgar score 8/9 at 1 and 5 minutes, length 52 cm, head circumference 35 cm, temperature 36°C, heart rate 130, respiratory rate 52, and systolic blood pressure 60 mm Hg. Umbilical cord has two vessels. A dimple is in place of anus. Perineal raphe is wide. The rest of the physical findings are normal.

In Figure 16-1 at 6 hours, gut is dilated with gas and liquid, and S5, partly hidden, looks dysplastic.

Right transverse colostomy is performed. Airway is full of secretions and breath sounds are coarse after operation. The baby coughs, gags, and turns blue when he tries to feed. Breathing is noisy.

Weight at 24 days is 3.5 kg, temperature 36.6°C, heart rate 144, respiratory rate 48, and systolic blood pressure 96 mm Hg. Rhonchi in chest clear when the baby cries. A colostomy is on right side.

Hematocrit is 0.29. White cell count is 11.3×10^9/liter with 0.25 polymorphonuclear cells, 0.10 bands, 0.60 lymphocytes, 0.02 monocytes, 0.02 eosinophils, and 0.01 basophils. Platelet count is 460×10^9/liter. Serum sodium is 136 mmol/liter, potassium 5.0, chloride 105, urea nitrogen 2.9. Creatinine is 40 µmol/liter.

Lateral examination of chest at 1 day shows (in retrospect) air in midesophagus (Figure 16-2A). Barium swallow at 24 days shows barium in hypopharynx, trachea, esophagus, fistula between trachea and esophagus, and gas-distended stomach (Figure 16-2B).

At bronchoscopy, a pit is in trachea several centimeters below vocal cords. Fistula (3-mm diameter) is divided at operation.

Diagnosis: Imperforate anus, tracheoesophageal fistula (H type).

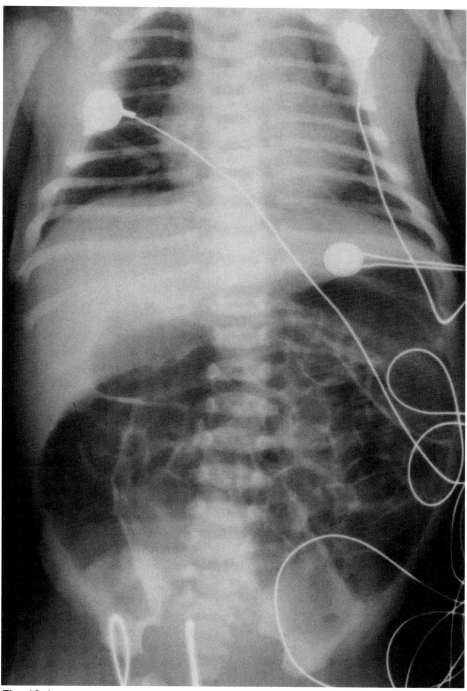

Fig. 16-1

(Continued)

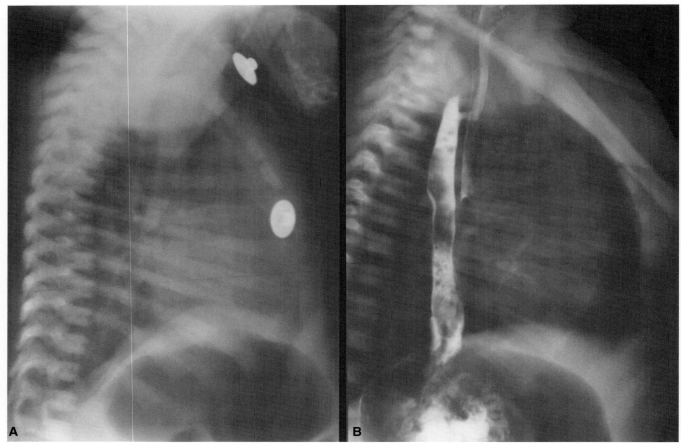

Fig. 16-2

Case 17

A 7-year-old girl has vomited mucus and undigested food "all her life." She eats, coughs, and then vomits.

Mother began taking levothyroxine for hypothyroidism 3 years before pregnancy. Birth weight was 2.8 kg, length 51 cm. Treatment was begun at 2 weeks for hypothyroidism found in neonatal screening examination. Bilateral inguinal herniorrhaphy was performed at 4 months.

Findings in physical examination are normal.

Chest roentgenogram at 7 years shows bilateral cervical ribs and narrowing of disc at T1–T2 and T3–T4. Esophagram in Figure 17-1 shows stenosis several centimeters above cardia.

At 11 years, weight is 44 kg, height 149 cm. Physical findings are normal. She is in the "Talented and Gifted" group of students and is active in sports.

Diagnosis: Congenital stenosis of esophagus, congenital hypothyroidism, rib and vertebral abnormality.

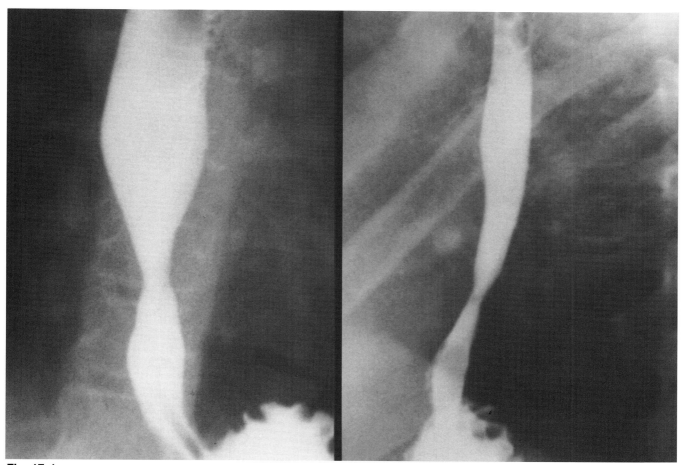

Fig. 17-1

Case 18

A 7-year-old girl eats mostly pureed food because coarse food often gets stuck in throat until she vomits.

Mother was aware of little fetal movement. Birth weight was 3.4 kg. The girl was floppy. She had a lot of mucus in her mouth. She vomited when she coughed or strained to move her bowels. She did not sit until after 1 year. She walked at 2 years. She recently learned to skip clumsily.

Mother (34 years old) wanted to be a ballet dancer but tired faster than other dancers, no matter how hard she tried to increase her stamina. She thinks husband screws bottle caps on too tight. Father (34 years old), who has had dislocating right knee since 16 years, has hyperextensible fingers and wrists and dry eyes. Brother (11 years old) has loose joints.

Weight at 7 years is 20.4 kg, height 121 cm, temperature 36.4°C, heart rate 96, respiratory rate 24, and blood pressure 90/60 mm Hg. Mouth droops when she laughs. She cannot whistle, sip through a straw, or touch chin to chest when supine. Proximal limb muscles are weak and thin. She cannot unclench her fist rapidly. Left first toe is bent toward second toe at interphalangeal joint. The rest of the physical findings are normal.

Hematocrit is 0.35. White cell count is 10.7×10^9/liter with 0.69 polymorphonuclear cells, 0.01 bands, 0.22 lymphocytes, 0.06 monocytes, 0.01 basophils, and 0.01 metamyelocytes. Platelet count is 530×10^9/liter. Urine specific gravity is 1.024, pH 7. Urine has occasional squamous epithelial cells/HPF, 3–6 white cells/HPF, and mucus. Serum sodium is 144 mmol/liter, potassium 5.1, chloride 106, carbon dioxide 24, urea nitrogen 3.6, calcium 2.57, phosphorus 1.52, cholesterol 4.27, and glucose 5.7. Creatinine is 40 µmol/liter, uric acid 140, total bilirubin 3, and direct bilirubin 0. Total protein is 73 g/liter, albumin 43. Alkaline phosphatase is 210 U/liter, LDH 254, and SGOT 32.

Barium suspension remains in pharynx, at junction of oropharynx and laryngopharynx (hypopharynx), after she swallows (Figure 18-1). Esophagus is irregularly narrow (see Figure 18-1).

She has myopia at 14 years, blepharitis at 16 years, and superficial corneal vascularization at 18 years. At 20 years, voice is nasal. She needs a deep breath to count to 6 or 7. Deep tendon reflexes are absent. ECG findings are normal.

Diagnosis: Myotonic dystrophy (Steinert's disease) in mother and daughter, worse in daughter, because of trinucleotide repeat instability* (genetic anticipation). Mother has 50–>200 cytosine thymine guanine repeat units, daughter >700.

---

*JF Gusella, ME McDonald. Trinucleotide repeat instability. Annu Rev Med 47;201, 1996.

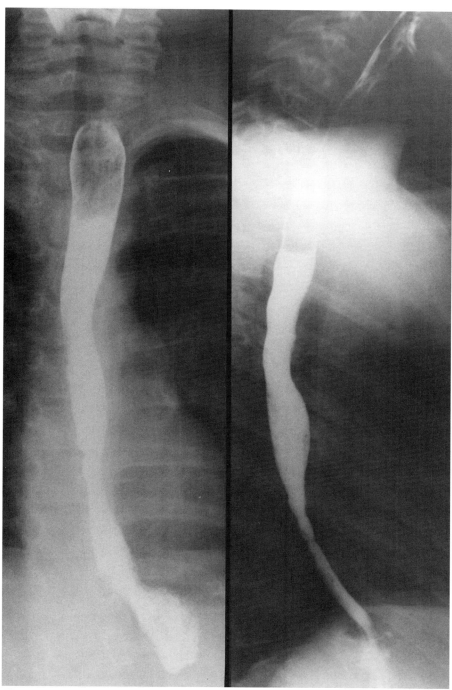

Fig. 18-1

Case 19

An 11-month-old girl vomits after feeding. She has one cold per month.

Pregnancy was normal, birth weight 3.6 kg. She stands and cruises.

Mother and father (both 16 years old) are well.

Weight is 7.4 kg, height 69 cm, head circumference 46 cm, temperature 37.3°C, heart rate 150, respiratory rate 22, and blood pressure 90/42 mm Hg. She has a diaper rash. The rest of the physical findings are normal.

A sliding esophageal hiatal hernia appears when she is supine and drinks barium suspension from a nipple (Figure 19-1).

Mother is advised about feeding. At 12 months, weight is 8.1 kg, height 70 cm.

Physical findings are normal when she returns the next time at 15 years with a sore throat.

Diagnosis: Sliding esophageal hiatal hernia.

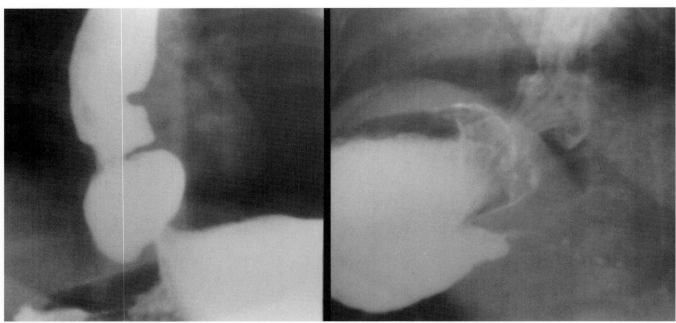

Fig. 19-1

Case 20

An 11-month-old boy is screaming and crawling in circles today. He has dry heaves.

Pregnancy of mother was normal. Birth weight was 3.2 kg, Apgar score 8/9 at 1 and 5 minutes. At 3 months, he spit up often and had a spell for less than 1 minute in which he was gray and did not breathe. Weight was 5.8 kg. GI series showed nonobstructive malrotation. Ladd operation, Nissen fundoplication, and appendectomy were performed at 3 months. He has been on Holter cardiorespiratory monitor since operation. Monitor sounds several times a night because heart rate goes below 70. He took 6–8 oz of feeding before operation, 3–4 oz after operation. He has had only 2 oz clear liquid today.

Mother (20 years old) and father (25 years old) are well. The boy is their only child.

Weight at 11 months is 8 kg, temperature 37.8°C, heart rate 136, respiratory rate 56, and systolic blood pressure 110 mm Hg. He is gagging but not belching. Abdomen is scarred, firm, and distended. Liver edge is 2–3 cm below costal margin. The rest of the physical findings are normal.

Hematocrit is 0.42. White cell count is 17.4×10^9/liter with 0.53 polymorphonuclear cells, 0.17 bands, 0.17 lymphocytes, 0.12 monocytes, and 0.01 metamyelocytes. Platelet count is 588×10^9/liter. Urine specific gravity is 1.016 (IV fluids), pH 8. Urine has trace protein and 6.5 mmol/liter glucose. Serum sodium is 133 mmol/liter, potassium 4.5, chloride 104, carbon dioxide 19, urea nitrogen 5.2, calcium 2.20, phosphorus 0.87, cholesterol 2.02, and glucose 10.5. Creatinine is 40 µmol/liter, uric acid 240, total bilirubin 5, and direct bilirubin 0. Total protein is 50 g/liter, albumin 36. Alkaline phosphatase is 152 U/liter, LDH 359, and SGOT 21.

Loops of gut, including pouch above diaphragm, are distended by gas; loops are separated by liquid or thickened wall (Figure 20-1).

At operation, a segment of gangrenous jejunum (29 cm long) that is twisted around an adhesive band is resected and an end-to-end anastomosis is performed.

Mucosa and submucosa of resected small bowel is ulcerated and necrotic.

GI series 4 days after second operation shows barium in esophagus, stomach, part of it herniated above diaphragm alongside esophagus, which ends below diaphragm, and proximal small bowel (Figure 20-2).

At third operation, esophageal hiatus (4-cm diameter) is reduced by crural sutures.

At 5 years, he chokes on food and turns blue every day. Weight is 16.8 kg. Esophagoscopy shows no stricture and no inflammation.

Diagnosis: Paraesophageal hiatal hernia.

(Continued)

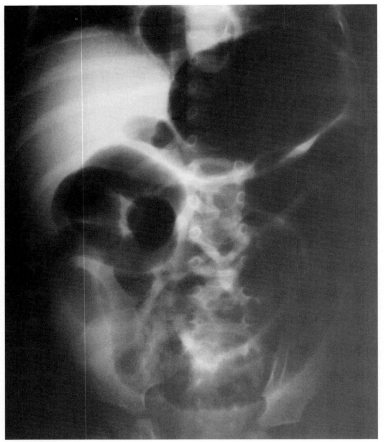

Fig. 20-1

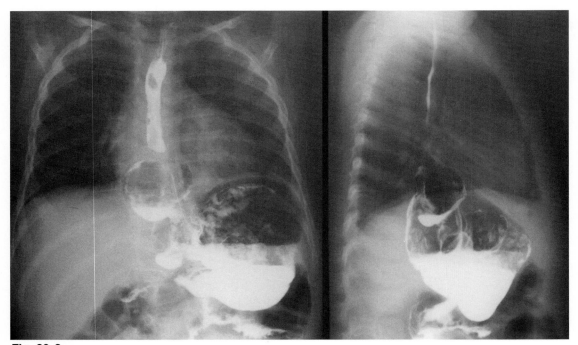

Fig. 20-2

Case 21

A 2½-year-old girl eats only soft and pureed foods and takes water in small sips. She has vomited mucus since birth and vomits digested or partially digested food soon after eating. Now she will not eat meat or bread crusts.

Pregnancy of mother was normal, birth weight 2.8 kg. She walked at 13 months. She has had several ear infections.

Mother had benign tumor of ovary. Father has hay fever.

Temperature is 36.6°C, heart rate 120, respiratory rate 24, blood pressure 110/74 mm Hg, weight 12.8 kg, and height 88 cm. Right eardrum is dull pink. A systolic murmur is present. The rest of the physical findings are normal.

Hematocrit is 0.35. White cell count is 9.8×10^9/liter with 0.58 polymorphonuclear cells, 0.03 bands, 0.26 lymphocytes, 0.09 monocytes, 0.02 eosinophils, and 0.02 basophils. Urine

specific gravity is 1.006, pH 6. Urine has occasional squamous epithelial cells/HPF.

When girl stands, swallowed barium suspension is held up in dilated esophagus that tapers to junction with cardiac opening of stomach (Figure 21-1).

At endoscopy, lower esophagus is dilated, gastroesophageal junction tight. Manometric findings are normal.

At operation, esophagus and stomach look normal. Heller's esophagomyotomy and Nissen fundoplication are performed.

Vomiting decreases to once every 10 days or so. At 3 years, weight is 13.8 kg, height 92 cm.

Diagnosis: Achalasia of esophagus.

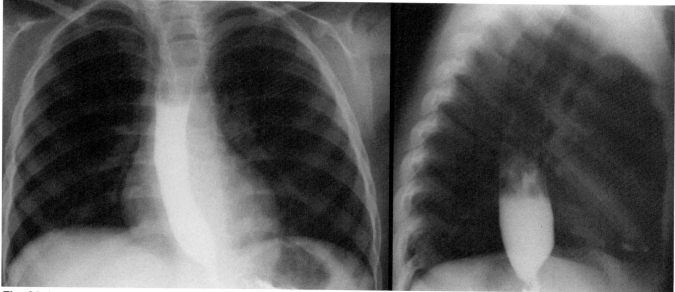

Fig. 21-1

Case 22

A newborn girl has petechiae.

Mother (17 years old) and father (22 years old) are well.

Mother took drugs during pregnancy and antibiotic in second trimester. Birth weight is 2.9 kg, length 49 cm, head circumference 33 cm, temperature 37.8°C, heart rate 140, respiratory rate 80, and systolic blood pressure 66 mm Hg. She is jaundiced. Abdomen is distended. Liver edge is 5 cm below costal margin, spleen edge 3 cm. The rest of the physical findings are normal.

Hematocrit is 0.54. White cell count is 19.3×10^9/liter with 0.33 polymorphonuclear cells, 0.13 bands, 0.51 lymphocytes, and 0.03 monocytes. Platelet count is 47×10^9/liter. Urine specific gravity is 1.006, pH 5. Urine has 0–1 white cell/HPF and 5–6 epithelial cells/HPF. Serum urea nitrogen is 6.8 mmol/liter, calcium 2.25, and glucose 15.2. Total bilirubin is 246 µmol/liter, direct bilirubin 178 (peak total at 5 days: 390, direct 277). IgA is trace (normal: 0.1–0.4 g/liter). IgG is 7.4 g/liter (normal: 6.5–16.0), IgM 0.08 (normal: <0.25), and complement component 3 1.5 (normal: 0.884 ± 0.117). SGOT is 142 U/liter.

Gut is displaced downward by large liver and spleen in Figure 22-1.

(Urine soon after birth has intranuclear inclusions. Culture of throat and urine grows cytomegalovirus. Later cultures do not.)

She has umbilical and bilateral inguinal hernias at 2 months and repair at 8 months. Spleen edge is 2 cm below costal margin, liver edge not palpable. Monthly nosebleeds begin at 1 year. At 16 months, she vomits blood. Spleen edge is 3 cm below costal margin. She is floppy. Babinski's sign is in feet. Ophthalmologic findings are normal.

Hemoglobin at 16 months is 55 g/liter. Serum total bilirubin is 3 µmol/liter, direct bilirubin 2. Total protein is 62 g/liter, albumin 35. Alkaline phosphatase is 56 U/liter, SGOT 31.

Barium swallow at 16 months shows varices in esophagus (Figure 22-2A) and gastric fundus (Figure 22-2B). Angiogram at 2½ years shows hepatofugal venous flow through gastric and esophageal collaterals (Figure 22-3A) and large spleen (Figure 22-3B).

At 2½ years, she walks unsteadily, feet wide apart and on toes. Reflexes in legs are brisk. GI bleeding is arrested with Sengstaken-Blakemore tube at 3¾ years. She dies of GI bleeding at 4 years.

At necropsy, spleen is firm, large, and weighs 450 g (normal: 39). Liver looks normal, is firm, and weighs 430 g (normal: 516). Dark blue, longitudinal ridges are in esophagus, longitudinal erosions in gastric mucosa; granulation tissue is at gastroesophageal junction. Microscopic examination shows (1) sclerosis of portal vein branches with concentric bands of collagen and elastic tissue under endothelium; (2) mild fibrosis around portal triads; (3) normal liver parenchyma; (4) thick fibrous trabeculae, diminished lymphoid tissue, and hyperemic red pulp in spleen; and (5) many thick-walled veins in distal esophagus and cardiac part of stomach.

Diagnosis: Portal hypertension, congenital cytomegalovirus infection.

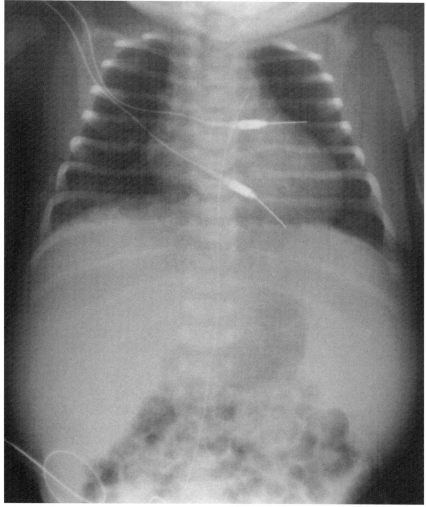

Fig. 22-1

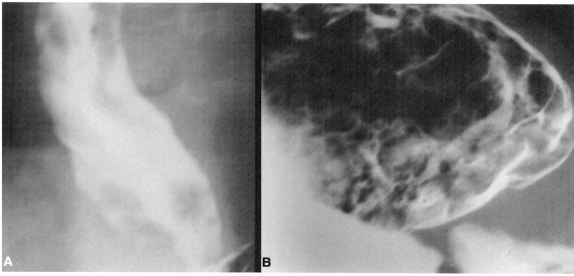

Fig. 22-2

(Continued)

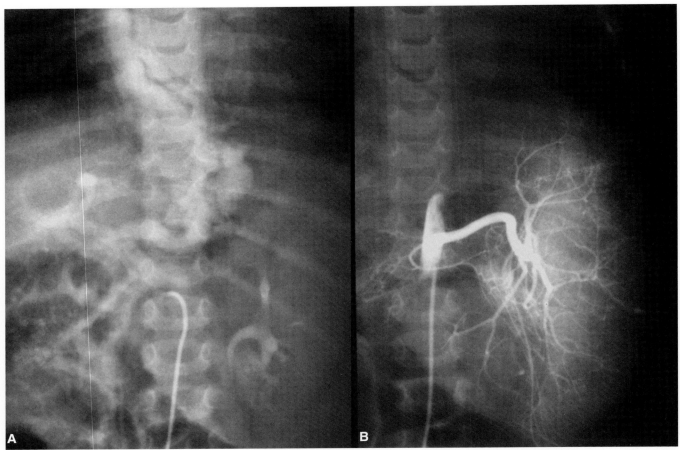

Fig. 22-3

Case 23

A 4-year-old boy swallowed an open safety pin 3 hours ago. He coughed for a while but now seems all right.

Liver lacerations sustained in a car crash 1 year ago healed without operation.

Temperature is 37.1°C, heart rate 108, respiratory rate 16, systolic blood pressure 90 mm Hg, and weight 17 kg. Physical findings are normal.

Hematocrit is 0.41. White cell count is 10.1×10^9/liter. Platelet count is 315×10^9/liter.

In Figure 23-1, an open safety pin is in midsagittal plane at level of aortic arch.

Pin goes into stomach during esophagoscopy and cannot be found at gastroscopy.

Pin is in stomach after esophagoscopy (Figure 23-2A) and in lower abdomen 2 days later (Figure 23-2B).

Open pin comes out anus, without pain or bleeding, hours after last roentgenogram.

Diagnosis: Passage of open safety pin through GI tract.

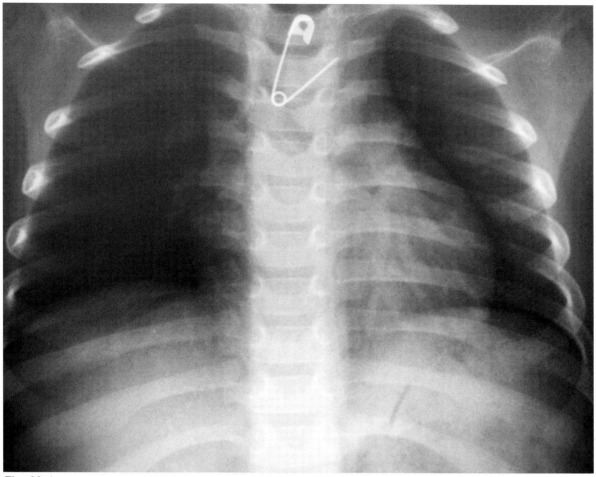

Fig. 23-1

(Continued)

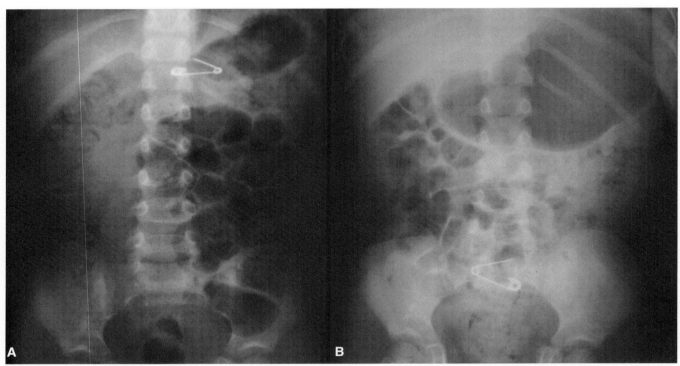

Fig. 23-2

Case 24

A 2-year-old girl swallows frequently. She has had a runny nose, occasional wheeze, and a wet cough for 2 weeks that got worse 2 days ago.

Temperature is 37.7°C, heart rate 124, respiratory rate 32, blood pressure 98/50 mm Hg, weight 11.9 kg, and height 92 cm. She has an expiratory wheeze. The rest of the physical findings are normal.

Hematocrit is 0.33. White cell count is 9.0×10^9/liter with 0.28 polymorphonuclear cells, 0.03 bands, 0.58 lymphocytes, 0.05 monocytes, 0.04 eosinophils, and 0.02 basophils.

In Figure 24-1, the metal clasp of a key chain is in midesophagus.

At endoscopy, esophageal mucosa is caught in slot of clasp. Granulation tissue is at site. A small amount of bleeding occurs when clasp is removed. Tan-brown matter is inside clasp.

Diagnosis: Metal clasp stuck in esophagus by mucosa inside clasp.

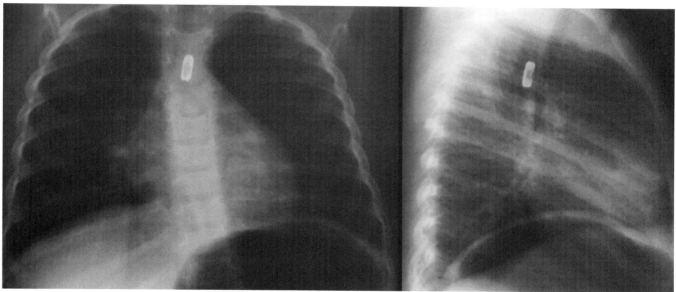

Fig. 24-1

Case 25

A 2½-year-old girl cannot swallow her spit.

She began to wheeze and cough 6 months ago. Four months ago, she began to vomit food as soon as she tried to swallow it. She later began to vomit liquids. Stools are infrequent. She has lost 2.7 kg in 3 weeks. She tilts head back to swallow. She has a brassy cough.

Pregnancy of mother was normal, birth weight 3.9 kg. At 14 months, she choked on a chicken bone that her father was able to remove with his finger.

Parents, two sisters, and one brother are well.

Temperature at 2½ years is 37.2°C, heart rate 128, respiratory rate 28, systolic blood pressure 96 mm Hg, weight 13.7 kg, and height 95 cm. She has a loud inspiratory wheeze. The rest of the physical findings are normal.

Hematocrit is 0.36. White cell count is 13.7 × 10⁹/liter. Serum sodium is 136 mmol/liter, potassium 4.2, chloride 100, carbon dioxide 20, urea nitrogen 2.5, calcium 2.47, phosphorus 1.13, cholesterol 5.17, and glucose 6.7. Creatinine is 40 µmol/liter, uric acid 120, total bilirubin 3, and direct bilirubin 0. Total protein is 74 g/liter, albumin 45. Alkaline phosphatase is 202 U/liter, LDH 113, and SGOT 37.

In Figure 25-1, barium trickles down from distended upper esophagus, barium is in colon from esophagram 1 day ago, and supracardiac shadow is widened.

Gastrostomy is placed and attempts at esophageal dilation are made. At right thoracotomy 3 months later, scar and perforation are at esophageal stricture and adhesions are around it. A piece of plastic doll (Figure 25-2) is removed from the esophagus. Partial esophagectomy, distal esophageal closure, and cervical esophagostomy are performed.

Diagnosis: Esophageal perforation, inflammation, and stricture from foreign body.

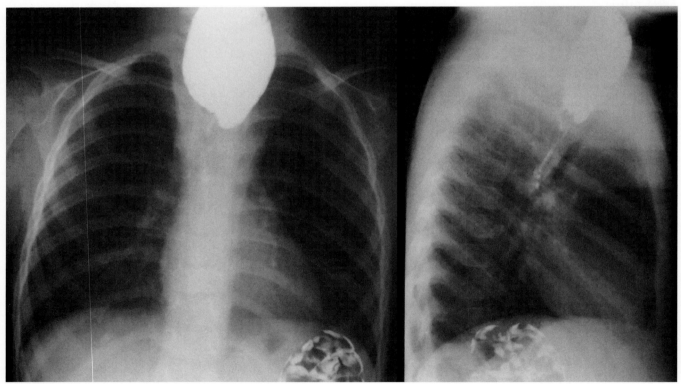

Fig. 25-1

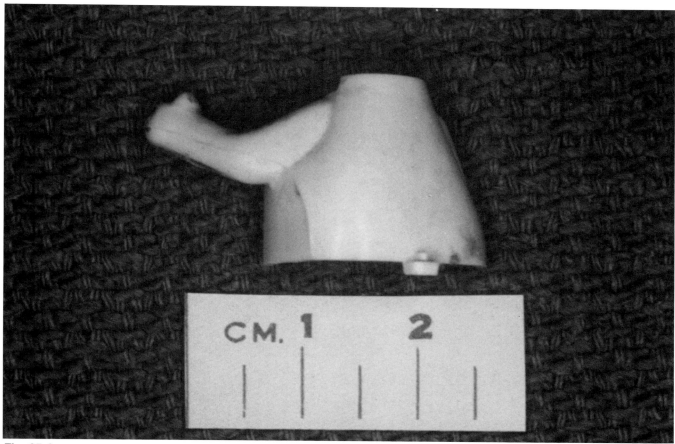

Fig. 25-2

Case 26

A 2-year-old boy swallowed Dynamite Pipe Cleaner, which contains lye, 4 hours ago. He has vomited brown liquid several times since then.

Temperature is 36.8°C, heart rate 152, respiratory rate 18, blood pressure 130/68 mm Hg, and weight 11.3 kg. Cheeks are red and shiny, lips red and blistered. Tongue and oropharynx are red. The rest of the physical findings are normal.

Hematocrit is 0.34. White cell count is 29.3×10^9/liter. Platelet count is 506×10^9/liter. Serum sodium is 140 mmol/liter, potassium 5.8, and chloride 111.

Vocal cords are edematous at laryngoscopy. Exudate lines whole esophagus at esophagoscopy the morning after lye ingestion.

Lateral examination of the chest 2 days (Figure 26-1A) and 2 weeks (Figure 26-1B) after lye ingestion shows air in trachea and in constricted esophagus behind trachea.

In esophagram 2 weeks after lye ingestion (Figure 26-2A), caliber of esophagus is normal. Barium is injected through a tube, which is looped in upper esophagus because boy will not swallow barium. Barium shows constriction of most of esophagus 6 weeks after lye ingestion (Figure 26-2B).

Diagnosis: Lye stricture of esophagus, apparent in plain film of chest 2 days after lye ingestion.

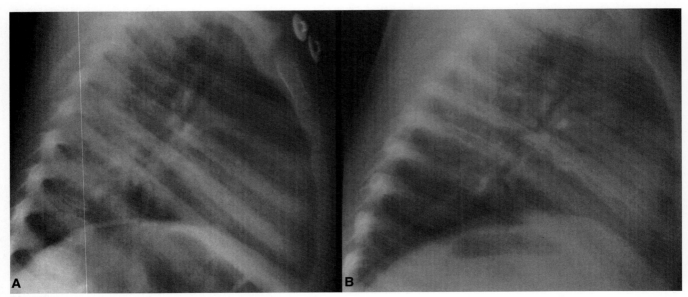

Fig. 26-1

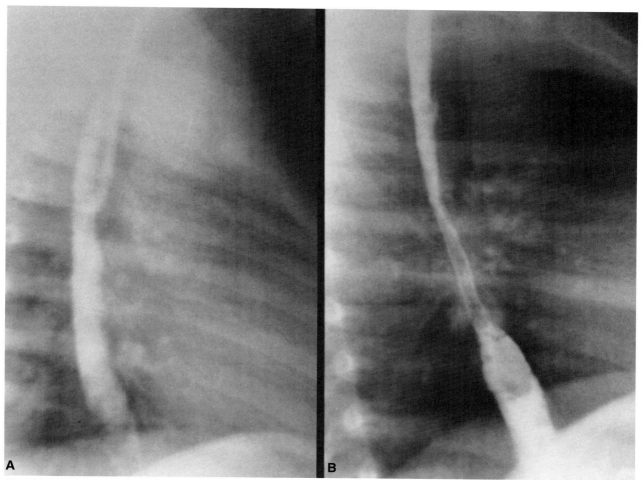

Fig. 26-2

Case 27

A newborn boy vomits bile and mucus at 7 hours.

Pregnancy of mother (29 years old) was normal. Birth weight is 2.6 kg, Apgar score 9/9 at 1 and 5 minutes, length 48 cm, and head circumference 35 cm. Temperature at 40 minutes is 36.3°C, heart rate 144, respiratory rate 44, and systolic blood pressure 58 mm Hg. Findings in physical examination are normal.

Hematocrit is 0.40. White cell count is 17.8×10^9/liter with 0.49 polymorphonuclear cells, 0.02 bands, 0.38 lymphocytes, 0.09 monocytes, 0.01 eosinophils, and 0.01 basophils. Platelet count is 318×10^9/liter. Serum sodium is 141 mmol/liter, potassium 5.2, chloride 106, urea nitrogen 8.2, and calcium 2. Total bilirubin is 116 µmol/liter.

Vomiting of bile and mucus persists. At operation on second day, nonrotation of intestine, Ladd's bands between gut and liver, duplication of ileum with segmental volvulus and distal atresia, and small stomach stuck to undersurface of liver are found. Duplication and atretic ileum are resected and end-to-end ileal anastomosis is performed.

He is hungry at 12 days. Bile is still coming out of naso-gastric tube. At operation, duodenal membrane obstructs just distal to major duodenal papilla. Duodenoduodenostomy is performed.

Examination after duodenoduodenostomy shows small, non-rotated stomach and intestine, and rib and thoracic vertebral abnormalities (Figure 27-1).

Diagnosis: Congenital microgastria, nonrotation of intestine, other intestinal abnormalities, and skeletal abnormalities.

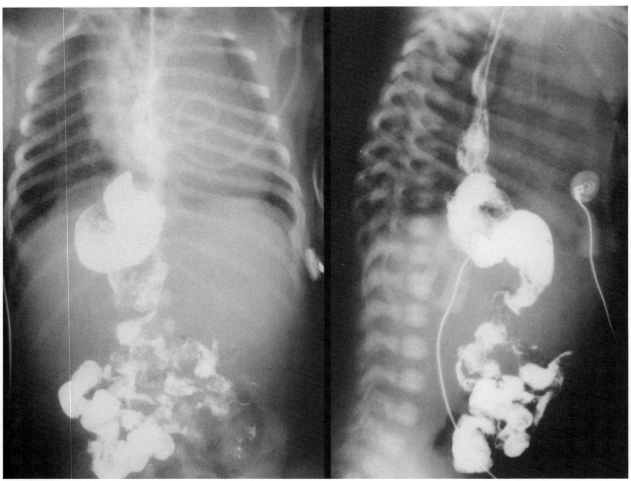

Fig. 27-1

Case 28

A newborn girl has a cyst behind stomach that was seen in prenatal ultrasound examination of her 19-year-old mother.

Birth weight is 2.8 kg, length 49 cm, head circumference 34 cm, Apgar score 8/9 at 1 and 5 minutes, temperature 36.7°C; heart rate 162, respiratory rate 52, and blood pressure 70/30 mm Hg. Physical findings are normal.

Hematocrit is 0.48. White cell count is 11.9×10^9/liter. Platelet count is 115×10^9/liter. Serum sodium is 140 mmol/liter, potassium 5.5, chloride 111, and urea nitrogen 3.0. Creatinine is 40 µmol/liter. Amylase is 25 U/liter.

Prenatal ultrasound examination in Figure 28-1 shows two collections of liquid in left upper quadrant of fetal abdomen.

Barium is in fundus and antrum but not body of stomach in GI series (Figure 28-2A). CT scan in Figure 28-2B shows a cyst between stomach and spine.

At operation, a cyst (2.0×1.5 cm) filled with mucus is stuck to back of stomach.

Inner wall of fibrous, tan-to-lavender cyst is smooth and glistening. Microscopic examination shows enteric epithelium.

Diagnosis: Gastric duplication.

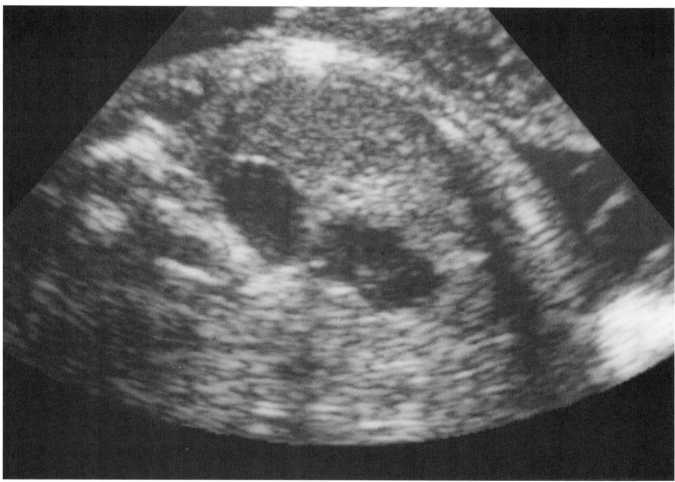

Fig. 28-1

(Continued)

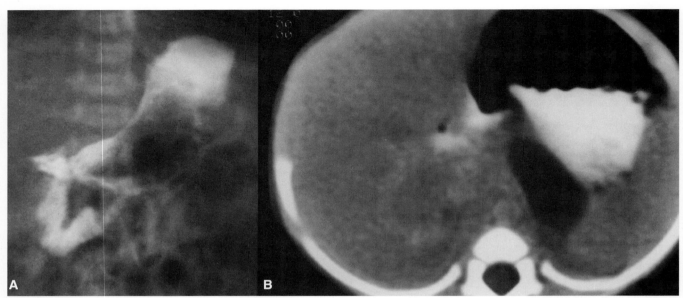

Fig. 28-2

Case 29

A 3-year-old boy cries a lot and is edematous and constipated.

He passed a worm 4 weeks ago and was given pyrvinium pamoate. He had a cough, fever, vomiting, and loose stools 3 weeks ago. He coughed and vomited off and on for the next 1–2 weeks. He began to eat less and drink more 1 week ago. Abdomen became distended. He has cried and not had a bowel movement for several days.

Pregnancy was normal, birth weight 3 kg. He sat at 6 months and walked at 1 year. He had otitis media at 2 years. He weighed 13.6 kg 1 month ago.

Mother (25 years old) and brother (5 years old) are well. Father (28 years old) had fever and pneumonia 3 weeks ago. Father is allergic to many things and sometimes swells with contact. Members of father's family have allergies.

Temperature at 3 years is 36.8°C, heart rate 98, respiratory rate 22, systolic blood pressure 100 mm Hg, weight 15 kg, and height 91 cm. Eyelids, scrotum, hands, and feet are edematous. Nasal turbinates are pale. Abdomen is distended and tender. The rest of the physical findings are normal.

Hematocrit is 0.38. White cell count is 9.8×10^9/liter with 0.26 polymorphonuclear cells, 0.14 bands, 0.31 lymphocytes, 0.08 monocytes, 0.03 eosinophils, and 0.18 atypical lymphocytes. Platelet count is 278×10^9/liter. PT is 9.2 seconds (control: 9.8), activated PTT 36.8 (control: 30.2). Urine specific gravity is 1.019, pH 6. Urine has rare epithelial cells/HPF. Serum sodium is 137 mmol/liter, potassium 3.6, chloride 112, carbon dioxide 23, urea nitrogen 1.0, calcium 1.92, phosphorus 1.32, cholesterol 3.65, and glucose 4.5. Creatinine is 40 μmol/liter, uric acid 180, total bilirubin 3, and direct bilirubin 0. Total protein is 33 g/liter, albumin 20. Alkaline phosphatase is 53 U/liter, LDH 287, and SGOT 32.

Subpulmonic pleural liquid is on both sides in erect roentgenogram (Figure 29-1). Defects are in fundus and body of stomach (Figure 29-2).

At endoscopy, folds in fundus and body of stomach are hypertrophied and hyperemic with scattered petechiae. Pyloric part of stomach is normal.

^{131}I-labeled serum albumin, 0.05, is in gastric aspirate 48 hours after IV injection, 0.01 in stool at 72 hours.

Microscopic examination of pieces of white, friable gastric mucosa removed at endoscopy shows long, tortuous glands with papillary infoldings near base and epithelium of tall, columnar, hypersecretory mucous cells.

Diagnosis: Ménétrier's disease (hypertrophic gastropathy).

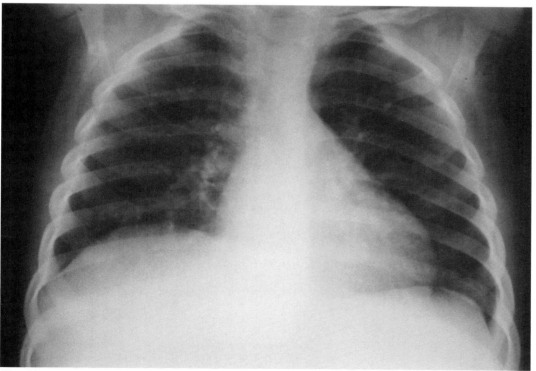

Fig. 29-1

(Continued)

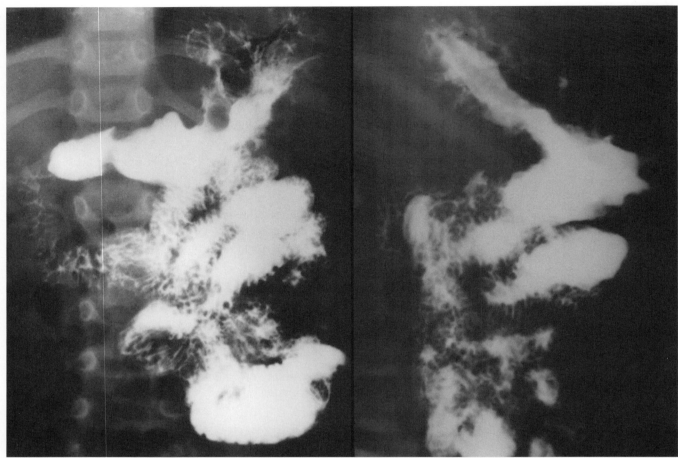

Fig. 29-2

Case 30

An 11-month-old girl has a swollen lip after falling down.

Birth weight was 2.2 kg. Weight at 5 months was 3.7 kg (when her face was bruised in a fall from a car seat).

She lives with parents and sister (2 years old) in one-bedroom apartment.

Temperature is 38.3°C, heart rate 100, respiratory rate 32, blood pressure not determined, weight 4.3 kg, length 61 cm, and head circumference 42 cm. She is skinny, pale, and apathetic. Round scabs are on forehead, nose, chin, and left arm; pustules on buttocks and perineum; and bruises on left thigh. Upper lip is swollen; a sore is inside lip. Eardrums are pink. Abdomen is protuberant. Lymph nodes are palpable in neck, axillas, and groins. She falls forward when placed sitting. The rest of the physical findings are normal.

Hematocrit is 0.32. White cell count is 20.0×10^9/liter with 0.68 polymorphonuclear cells, 0.13 bands, 0.17 lymphocytes, and 0.02 monocytes. Serum sodium is 148 mmol/liter, potas-sium 4.1, chloride 118, carbon dioxide 18, and urea nitrogen 6.4. The next morning, glucose is 3.9 mmol/liter.

A mottled mass of gas and water density is in distended stomach the morning after admission to hospital (Figure 30-1).

She sits and babbles after first feeding, which was taken eagerly. According to nurse, she "would not take eyes off the bottle" while being burped the next morning. She vomits after a feeding of cereal, fruit, and formula. She stands in crib on the third day. She is playful on the fifth day. She takes every feeding well, liquid and solid, until the seventh day when she is playing with the bottle during a feeding. She smiles and laughs aloud on the ninth day.

Weight is 4.3 kg the first day, 4.7 the second day, and 5.0 the thirteenth day.

Diagnosis: Starvation, acute repletion.

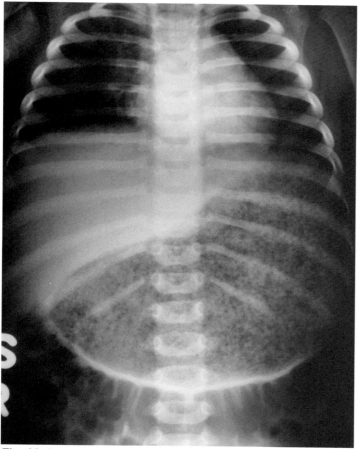

Fig. 30-1

Case 31

A 3-week-old girl is dusky and sleepy.

Mother used drugs during pregnancy and breast-feeding. She switched from breast milk to double-strength formula 1 week ago because baby was not gaining weight. Baby vomited yesterday and feeds slowly today. Birth weight was 3.3 kg.

Father uses drugs. Sister (5 years old) is well. Another sister (2 years old) is sick at home.

Temperature at 3 weeks is 36.7°C, heart rate 160, respiratory rate 52, systolic blood pressure 90 mm Hg, weight 3.0 kg, length 48 cm, and head circumference 35 cm. Skin is doughy. Mucous membranes are dry. Anterior fontanel and eyes are depressed. The rest of the physical findings are normal.

Hematocrit is 0.52. White cell count is 19.8 × 10⁹/liter with 0.38 polymorphonuclear cells, 0.52 lymphocytes, 0.06 mono-cytes, and 0.04 eosinophils. Platelet count is 475 × 10⁹/liter. Urine specific gravity is 1.005, pH 5. Urine has 0–1 white cell/HPF, bacteria, and amorphous urates. Serum sodium is 137 mmol/liter, potassium 5.1, chloride 105, carbon dioxide 24, urea nitrogen 1.4, calcium 2.50, phosphorus 2.32, cholesterol 1.94, and glucose 5.7. Creatinine is 30 μmol/liter, uric acid 110, total bilirubin 5, and direct bilirubin 0. Total protein is 52 g/liter, albumin 33. Alkaline phosphatase is 114 U/liter, LDH 337, and SGOT 44.

In Figure 31-1, a mass with convex top is in stomach.

Diagnosis: Milk bezoar.

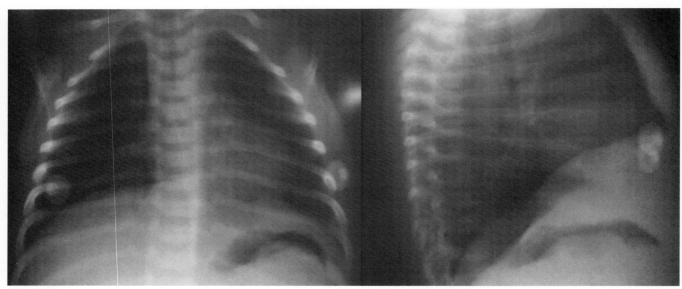

Fig. 31-1

Case 32

A 1-month-old boy stops breathing and turns blue during feeding.

Birth weight was 2.2 kg. He was switched from breast milk to formula at 1½ weeks. He had yellow discharge from nose 2 days ago and vomited once. He stopped breathing and turned blue tonight during feeding.

Mother (25 years old), father (22 years old), and brother (2 years old) are well.

Weight at 1 month is 2.2 kg, length 45 cm, head circumference 35 cm, temperature 37.2°C, heart rate 150, respiratory rate 52, and systolic blood pressure 96 mm Hg. Anterior fontanel is depressed. Yellow mucus is in nose. Lips are blue. Breathing is labored and wheezy. A systolic murmur is present. Liver edge is 1–2 cm below costal margin. The rest of the physical findings are normal.

Hematocrit is 0.25. White cell count is 19.4 × 10⁹/liter with 0.39 polymorphonuclear cells, 0.17 bands, 0.41 lymphocytes, 0.02 monocytes, and 0.01 eosinophils. Platelet estimate is adequate. Urine specific gravity is 1.010, pH 6. Urine is normal. Serum sodium is 141 mmol/liter, potassium 4.0, chloride 110, urea nitrogen 3.2, calcium 2.37, and glucose 3.8.

He has spells while sleeping and eating the next day. Eyes and mouth become dusky. Heart rate slows to 75–100. He has slight spells the second day and feeds slowly days 3 through 5.

Barium leaves coating around mass in stomach on the fifth day (Figure 32-1A). Mass is surrounded by gas from 7-Up in second fluoroscopic examination (Figure 32-1B) and gone 17 hours later, after he is given clear liquids to drink (Figure 32-2).

Diagnosis: Milk bezoar.

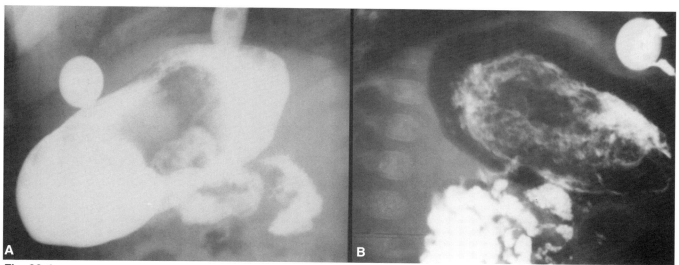

Fig. 32-1

(Continued)

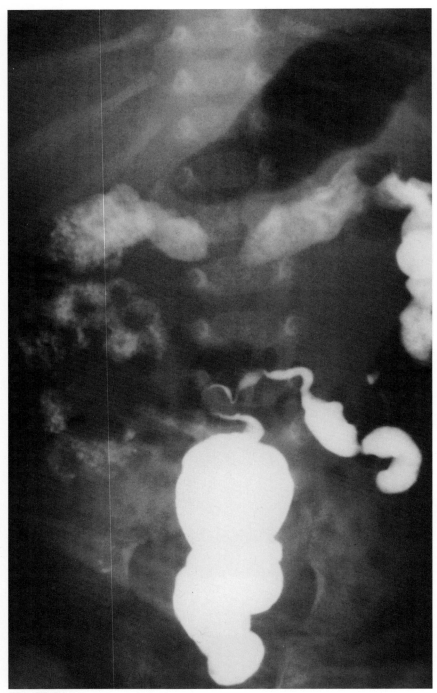

Fig. 32-2

Case 33

A 17-year-old girl is tired, dizzy, and has a bellyache.

She has lost 5–6 kg in the past year. She has been tired and had lower chest and epigastric pain for several months. For 2 weeks, she has been more tired with swollen ankles and worse pain that lasts for hours. She chewed on her hair and swallowed it from 5 to 12 years while living with father, mother, and two sisters. She has lived in another city with mother and two sisters for 1½ years. Menarche was at 12 years. Periods are normal. A sister (19 years old) had bowel infarction while taking birth control pills.

Temperature at 17 years is 37.4°C, heart rate 100, respiratory rate 24, blood pressure 110/65 mm Hg, weight 48 kg, and height 155 cm. She is pale. A systolic murmur is present. Epigastrium and left upper quadrant of abdomen are tender. The rest of the physical findings are normal.

Hematocrit is 0.22. Hemoglobin is 60 g/liter. Red blood cell count is 3.6×10^{12}/liter. Red-blood-cell distribution width is 20.3% (normal 11.5–15.0). MCV is 59 fl. MCH is 17 pg. MCHC is 280 g/liter. White cell count is 7.5×10^9/liter with 0.55 polymorphonuclear cells, 0.10 bands, 0.24 lymphocytes, 0.05 monocytes, 0.04 eosinophils, 0.01 basophils, and 0.01 atypical lymphocytes. Platelet count is 764×10^9/liter. Urine specific gravity is 1.022, pH 6. Urine has occasional squamous epithelial cells/HPF, 0–1 white cell/HPF, and mucus. Stool does not have occult blood. Serum sodium is 139 mmol/liter, potassium 4.1, chloride 109, carbon dioxide 23, urea nitrogen 5.0, calcium 2.05, phosphorus 1.61, cholesterol 4.50, and glucose 4.6. Creatinine is 50 μmol/liter, uric acid 120, total bilirubin 3, direct bilirubin 2, iron 2 (normal 9.0–30.4), and iron-binding capacity 48 (44.8–80.6). Total protein is 47 g/liter, albumin 29. Alkaline phosphatase is 62 U/liter, LDH 154, and SGOT 11.

Barium goes around a mass in stomach and duodenum, and into ulcer on lesser curvature of stomach (Figure 33-1).

At endoscopy, a trichobezoar is in stomach, a 1-cm ulcer on lesser curvature. Antral polyps go through pylorus. At operation, a hair cast of stomach, pylorus, and first part of duodenum is removed. Normal mucosa cover antral and pyloric polyps.

Hair cast weighs 260 g. The largest polyp ($2.5 \times 2.0 \times 2.0$ cm) is white-tan, soft, and multilobed. Microscopic examination shows inflammation and granulation tissue.

At endoscopy 1½ years later, polyps are small and few. Biopsy shows slight mucosal fibrosis.

Diagnosis: Trichobezoar.

(Continued)

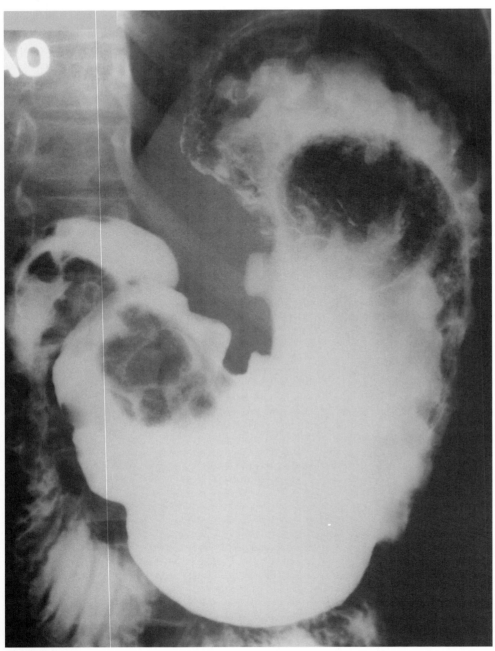

Fig. 33-1

Case 34

A 2-year-old boy is vomiting and has had two loose stools since he and his 4-year-old brother found a bottle of sustained-release ferrous sulfate capsules 3 hours ago. They have been treated with ipecac, gastric lavage, and magnesium sulfate. Vomit contains granules. Vomit and stool are guaiac positive.

Temperature is 37°C, heart rate 136, respiratory rate 24, systolic blood pressure 104 mm Hg, and weight 11 kg. He is sleepy. Eardrums are pink. The rest of the physical findings are normal.

Hematocrit is 0.37. White cell count is 14.6×10^9/liter with 0.66 polymorphonuclear cells, 0.16 bands, 0.12 lymphocytes, and 0.06 monocytes. Serum sodium is 141 mmol/liter, potassium 4.1, chloride 97, urea nitrogen 4.3, and glucose 7.6. Iron is 54 µmol/liter (normal: 9.0–21.5), iron-binding capacity 67 (normal: 17.9–71.6).

In Figure 34-1, particles of metal density are in gut.

Diagnosis: Iron ingestion, GI bleeding.

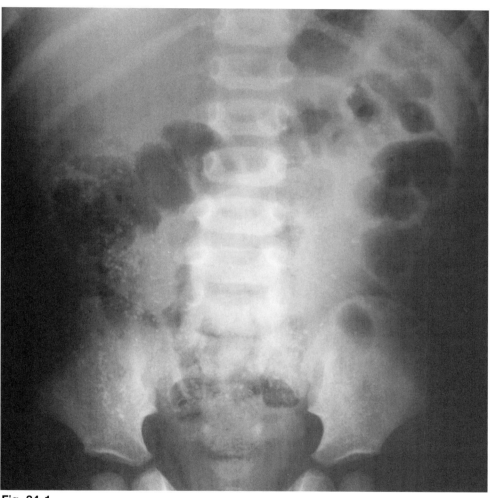

Fig. 34-1

Case 35

A 6-year-old boy has bellyaches, sometimes daily, sometimes months apart.

They began 3 years ago and come at various times during the day, last 5–10 minutes, and often cause him to lie on the floor and clutch at his belly. They do not wake him at night. Appetite is good. He does not vomit. Birth weight was 3.5 kg. He had tonsillitis and otitis media 1 year ago.

Mother (35 years old) has high blood pressure. Father (38 years old) is allergic to grasses. Brother (17 years old) has asthma, and brother (10 years old) has hay fever. Maternal grandmother has high blood pressure.

Temperature at 6 years is 36.6°C, heart rate 90, respiratory rate 20, blood pressure 100/60 mm Hg, weight 23.6 kg, and height 126 cm. Physical findings are normal.

Hematocrit is 0.38. White cell count is 9.7×10^9/liter with 0.59 polymorphonuclear cells, 0.02 bands, 0.32 lymphocytes, 0.02 monocytes, 0.04 eosinophils, and 0.01 basophils. Platelet count is 371×10^9/liter. ESR is 4 mm/hr. Urine specific gravity is 1.023, pH 8. Urine has occasional white cells/HPF and occasional epithelial cells/HPF. Serum sodium is 136 mmol/liter, potassium 4.2, chloride 103, carbon dioxide 25, urea nitrogen 4.6, calcium 2.40, phosphorus 1.65, and glucose 4.3. Total bilirubin is 5 μmol/liter, direct bilirubin 0. SGOT is 20 U/liter, amylase 152.

In Figure 35-1, a defect with central umbilication is in pyloric part of greater curvature of stomach.

At endoscopy, normal gastric mucosa covers a 1-cm mass and its central depression in pyloric part of stomach.

He has hay fever at 10 years. He does not complain of pain during visits between 6 and 13 years.

Diagnosis: Heterotopic pancreas.

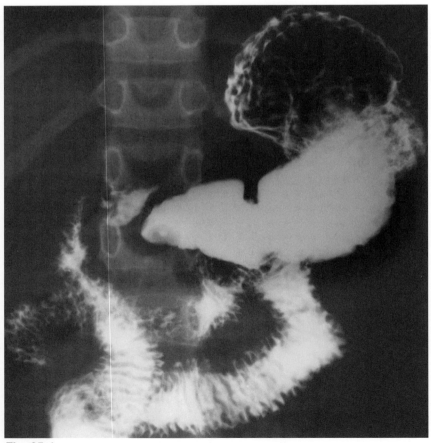

Fig. 35-1

Case 36

A 13-year-old girl is tired.

She has felt tired for 4 months, has sat around for 2 months, and has slept a lot for 2 weeks. She had pneumonia twice by 3 years and operation for cross-eyes at 5 years.

Mother (34 years old) has kidney disease; brother (15 years old) has hydrocephalus. Father (38 years old) is well. Paternal great-aunt had cancer of uterus.

Temperature at 13 years is 37.5°C, heart rate 103, respiratory rate 24, blood pressure 103/69 mm Hg, and weight 45.8 kg. She is pale. The rest of the physical findings are normal.

Hematocrit is 0.20. Hemoglobin is 58 g/liter. Red blood cell count is 2.7×10^{12}/liter. MCV is 73 fl. MCH is 22 pg. MCHC is 300 g/liter. Red-blood-cell distribution width is 32.3% (normal: 11.5–15.0). White cell count is 6.9×10^9/liter. Platelet count is 284×10^9/liter. Serum sodium is 140 mmol/liter, potassium 4.4, chloride 106, carbon dioxide 27, urea nitrogen 3.9, calcium 2.32, phosphorus 1.45, cholesterol 4.22, triglycerides 0.81, and glucose 4.7. Creatinine is 50 μmol/liter, uric acid 160, and total bilirubin 5. Total protein is 61 g/liter, albumin 41. Alkaline phosphatase is 75 U/liter, SGOT 19. Stool has occult blood. Bone marrow examination shows moderate erythroid hyperplasia with myeloid-to-erythroid ratio of 1.0 to 2.3.

Figure 36-1 shows a mass along greater curvature of stomach.

Partial gastrectomy is done. Tan-brown masses (0.5–2.5 cm) are in muscularis mucosae, submucosa, and subserosa along greater curvature.

Masses are tan in cut section. Microscopic examination shows tumors of epithelial cells with focal transition to spindle cells. Cells have (1) eosinophilic to clear cytoplasm; (2) oval to round nuclei with varying nuclear irregularity; (3) finely granular, evenly dispersed chromatin; and (4) prominent nucleoli. Cytoplasm is less well defined in spindle cells, and nuclei are more fusiform. Cells show 2–3 mitoses/HPF. Tumors are in muscularis mucosae and submucosa with focal hemorrhage and with focal serosal extensions covered by serosa one cell thick. Mucosa is spared except for ulcerated tips. Immunohistochemical analysis of tumor shows strong staining with antibodies to vimentin and neuron-specific enolase and occasional staining with antibody to smooth muscle actin.

Diagnosis: Gastric leiomyoblastoma.

(Continued)

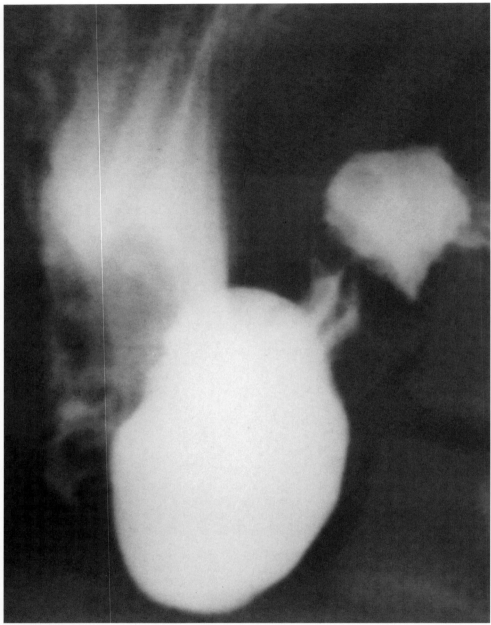

Fig. 36-1

Case 37

An 18-day-old boy is spitting up blood. He spit up after feedings several days ago. He is breast-fed and given supplemental formula. Mother's nipples were fissured 1 week ago.

Pregnancy of mother (18 years old) was normal. Birth weight was 3.3 kg, length 51 cm, and Apgar score 9/9 at 1 and 5 minutes.

Temperature at 18 days is 37.3°C, heart rate 128, respiratory rate 35, systolic blood pressure 85 mm Hg, and weight 3.6 kg. Umbilical cord is attached. The rest of the physical findings are normal.

Hematocrit is 0.32. White cell count is 13.4×10^9/liter with 0.22 polymorphonuclear cells, 0.02 bands, 0.70 lymphocytes, 0.02 monocytes, 0.03 eosinophils, and 0.01 basophils. Platelet count is 513×10^9/liter. Serum sodium is 138 mmol/liter, potassium 5.7, and chloride 105. Urine specific gravity is 1.010, pH 6.5. Urine has 3–5 white cells/HPF and 0–1 red cell/HPF.

In Figure 37-1, a thin defect is in pyloric canal <1 cm from sphincter.

At operation, external surface of stomach is normal. A circumferential band of fibrous tissue is in pyloric canal.

Diagnosis: Pyloric membrane.

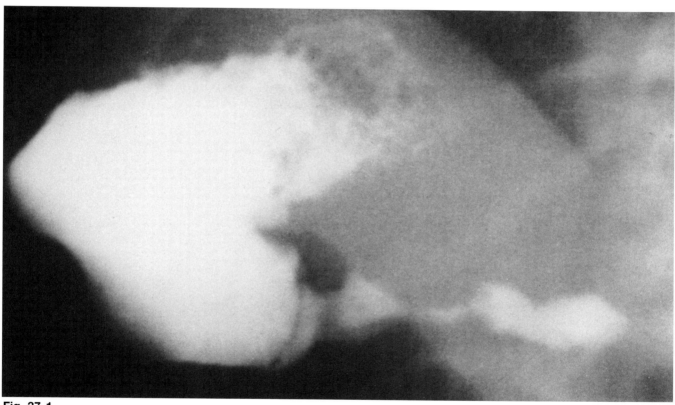

Fig. 37-1

Case 38

A 6-week-old boy is jaundiced and vomiting.

He is a "spitty" baby despite changes in formula. He has been vomiting curded milk for 9 days and has been jaundiced for 1 week. Stools are infrequent. He used to wet 10–12 diapers in 24 hours. He wet two yesterday.

Pregnancy of mother was normal. He weighed 2.9 kg at birth, 4.3 a week ago, and 4.0 yesterday. He lifts his head and smiles.

Mother (20 years old) has a "hole" in heart; father (21 years old) and brother (2 years old) are well.

Temperature at 6 weeks is 36.6°C, heart rate 108, respiratory rate 40, blood pressure 103/37 mm Hg, and weight 3.8 kg. Skin and sclerae are jaundiced. Mucous membranes are dry. The rest of the physical findings are normal.

Hematocrit is 0.44. White cell count is 15.5×10^9/liter with 0.19 polymorphonuclear cells, 0.74 lymphocytes, 0.03 monocytes, 0.03 eosinophils, and 0.01 atypical lymphocytes.

Platelet count is 361×10^9/liter. Serum sodium is 147 mmol/liter, potassium 5.5, chloride 96, carbon dioxide 25, urea nitrogen 3.9, calcium 2.67, phosphorus 1.68, cholesterol 2.77, and glucose 6.4. Creatinine is 40 μmol/liter, uric acid 290, total bilirubin 150, and direct bilirubin 15. Total protein is 51 g/liter, albumin 41. Alkaline phosphatase is 270 U/liter, LDH 327, and SGOT 34.

Between asterisks, ultrasound examination shows thick-walled (Figure 38-1A), long (Figure 38-1B) pyloric canal. Roentgenographic examination during fluoroscopy with baby obliquely prone, right side down, shows gastric peristalsis and long, curved, narrow pyloric canal between pyloric antrum and duodenal bulb (Figure 38-2).

At operation, circular muscle layer of pyloric canal is hypertrophied.

Diagnosis: Hypertrophic pyloric stenosis with jaundice.

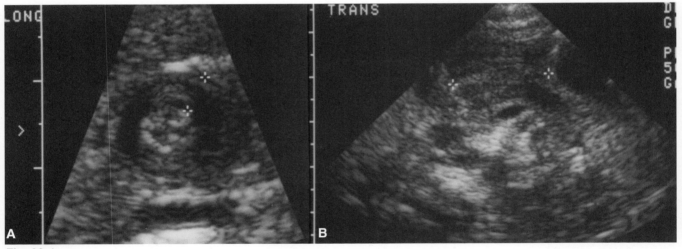

Fig. 38-1

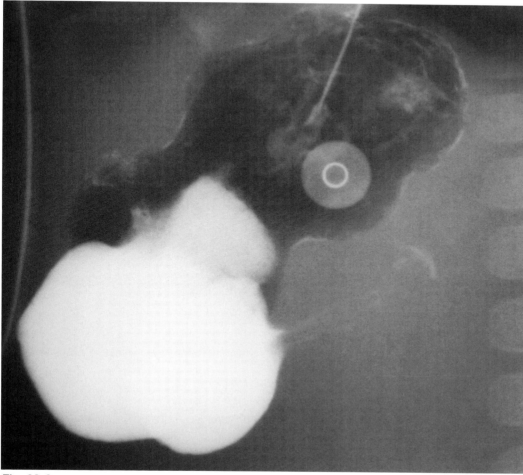

Fig. 38-2

Case 39

Twin brothers born prematurely 7½ weeks ago have been vomiting for 12 hours.

Each weighed 1.3 kg at birth and weighs 2.3 kg now.

Temperature of one twin is 35.6°C, heart rate 164, respiratory rate 20, and systolic blood pressure 60 mm Hg. Physical findings are normal.

Hematocrit is 0.34. White cell count is 9.3×10^9/liter with 0.13 polymorphonuclear cells, 0.26 bands, 0.50 lymphocytes, 0.09 monocytes, and 0.02 basophils. Platelet count is 500×10^9/liter. Serum sodium is 145 mmol/liter, potassium 4.1, chloride 97, urea nitrogen 6.8, and glucose 3.6.

Temperature of the other twin is 35.5°C, heart rate 168, respiratory rate 24, and systolic blood pressure 55 mm Hg. Physical findings are normal.

Hematocrit is 0.33. Urine specific gravity is 1.023, pH 6. Urine has 1+ protein and 1+ reducing substances. Serum sodium is 146 mmol/liter, potassium 4.4, and chloride 108. Vomit and stool are guaiac positive.

Roentgenograms with babies supine show gastric peristalsis in both twins (Figure 39-1). When they are lying obliquely prone, right side down, barium in stomach of first twin (Figure 39-2A) shows "shoulder" at angular notch on lesser curvature of stomach; barium in second twin shows narrow, curved, elongated pyloric canal (Figure 39-2B).

At operation, hypertrophied muscle around pyloric canal is divided and spread in an avascular plane down to mucosa and omentum sutured in gap.

Diagnosis: Hypertrophic pyloric stenosis in twin boys.

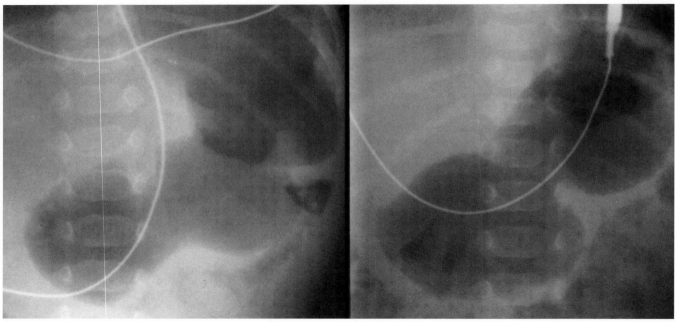

Fig. 39-1

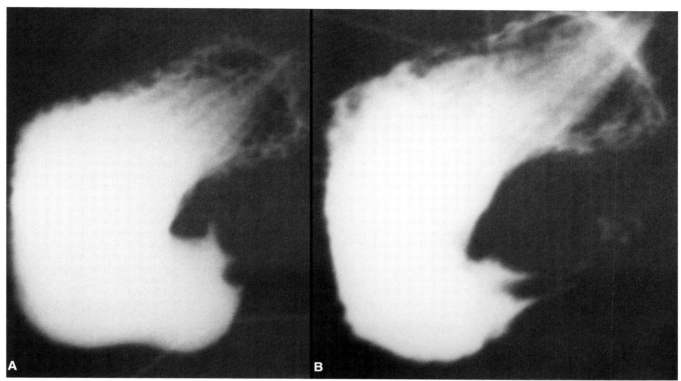

Fig. 39-2

Case 40

A 20-day-old boy, vomiting approximately 30 minutes after every feeding, is "shooting it out" today.

He began to vomit 5 days ago when changed from breast milk to formula. "He won't sleep at night, won't take a pacifier." Stools have been slimy for 2 days. Weight was 4.0 kg at birth and 4.0 kg 2 days ago.

Pregnancy of mother (20 years old) was normal. Membranes ruptured 15 hours before vaginal delivery. Mother was febrile. Baby smelled bad, cried quickly, and had acrocyanosis and caput succedaneum. Blood cultures showed no growth, gastric aspirate no β-hemolytic streptococci, and urine latex screen no group B streptococcal antigen. He was given six IM injections of ampicillin and gentamicin.

Temperature is 37.4°C, heart rate 140, respiratory rate 36, systolic blood pressure 82 mm Hg, and weight 3.9 kg. He is pale. Epigastric mass is questionably palpable. Bowel sounds are normal. The rest of the physical findings are normal.

Hematocrit is 0.40. White cell count is 15.5×10^9/liter with 0.10 polymorphonuclear cells, 0.26 bands, 0.54 lymphocytes, 0.09 monocytes, and 0.01 basophils. Platelet count is 655×10^9/liter. Serum sodium is 139 mmol/liter, potassium 5.4, chloride 95, carbon dioxide 29, urea nitrogen 2.1, and glucose 5.9. Creatinine is 60 μmol/liter. Blood culture shows no growth. Gram's stain of gastric aspirate shows 4+ gram positive cocci, 2+ gram positive bacilli, and 4+ white cells. Gastric aspirate grows 4+ α-hemolytic streptococci.

Gas is in wall of distended stomach. Gas and liquid are in stomach. Apparent asymmetry at hips results from pelvic tilt and abduction and external rotation of left femur (Figure 40-1).

At operation, stomach, boggy and friable, tears when a clamp is attached to it. Pyloric canal is long and thick.

Diagnosis: Hypertrophic pyloric stenosis, gastric emphysema.

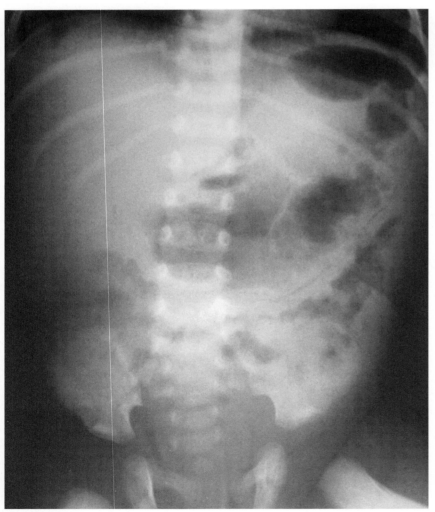

Fig. 40-1

Case 41

A 1-month-old boy is vomiting.

Pregnancy of mother was normal, birth weight 3.0 kg. He was slow to breathe. Supernumerary fifth fingers were tied off at birth. He slept a lot, fed slowly and poorly, and began to vomit milk curds 2 weeks ago. Weight was 2.6 kg.

Mother (22 years old), father (23 years old), and brother (3 years old) are well.

Temperature at 1 month is 36.7°C, heart rate 152, respiratory rate 44, systolic blood pressure 104 mm Hg, weight 2.5 kg, and head circumference 33 cm. He is floppy. Epicanthi are present. Ears are low. Nose is short and turned up. Chin is small, uvula cleft. A mass the size of an olive is in right hypochondrium. Penis is small. Urethra is near its base. Testes are not in scrotum. Second and third toes are partly fused on each foot. He vomits barium from an examination 12 hours ago.

Hematocrit is 0.46. White cell count is 16.4×10^9/liter. Serum sodium is 135 mmol/liter, potassium 6.0, chloride 97,

urea nitrogen 5.4, and glucose 6.7. Creatinine is 40 µmol/liter.

In roentgenogram with baby lying obliquely prone, right side down, barium is in stomach, pyloric canal, and small bowel 25 hours after GI series and soon after vomiting (Figure 41-1). Soft tissue partly fuses second and third toes of each foot (Figure 41-2).

Operation shows hypertrophic pyloric stenosis.

At 6 months, he coos and sometimes smiles. He does not follow with his eyes or reach for toys. Weight is 3.2 kg, length 57 cm, and head circumference 37 cm. Hands are closed, legs flexed and crossed. Neck and limbs are hypertonic. Testes are not palpable. He has right inguinal hernia.

Diagnosis: Pyloric stenosis, Smith-Lemli-Opitz syndrome.

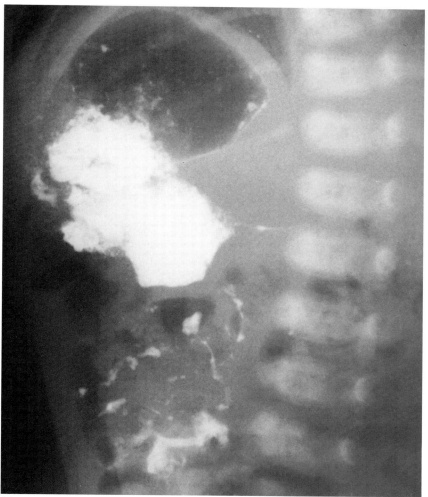

Fig. 41-1

(Continued)

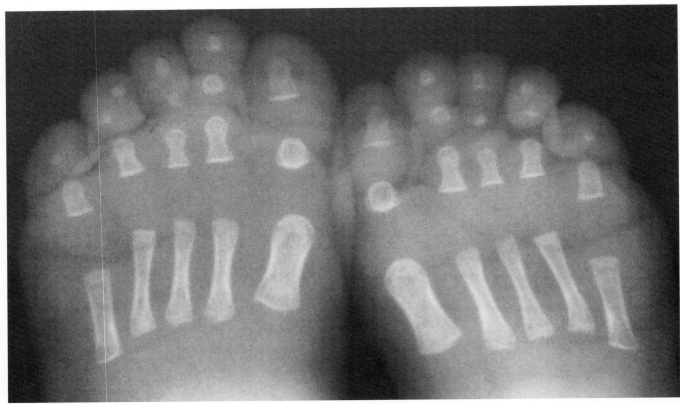

Fig. 41-2

Case 42

A 13-year-old girl has abdominal cramps 10–15 minutes after eating and epigastric and periumbilical tenderness.

One and one-half years ago, she had fever, rectal bleeding, and 5-kg weight loss. Weight was 35 kg, height 150 cm, and blood pressure 100/60 mm Hg. Right perianal tissues were swollen. The rest of the physical findings were normal.

Hematocrit 1½ years ago was 0.37. White cell count was 13.0 × 10⁹/liter with 0.45 polymorphonuclear cells, 0.31 bands, 0.15 lymphocytes, 0.05 monocytes, and 0.04 eosinophils. ESR was 45 mm/hr. Serum sodium was 138 mmol/liter, potassium 4.3, chloride 101, carbon dioxide 25, urea nitrogen 5.4, calcium 2.12, phosphorus 1.52, cholesterol 3.88, triglycerides 1.80, and glucose 5.0. Creatinine was 80 μmol/liter, uric acid 480, total bilirubin 3, and direct bilirubin 0. Total protein was 59 g/liter, albumin 26. Alkaline phosphatase was 124 U/liter, LDH 167, SGOT 19, and GGT 3. Sigmoidoscopy showed punctate ulcers.

She had three anal fissures 5 months ago. Colonoscopy showed edema distal to transverse colon. Two months ago, parents found 776 pills that she was supposed to have taken. She felt fine 1 month ago. Weight was 36 kg, height 150 cm, hematocrit 0.32. Cramps began 10 days ago.

Father has Crohn's disease; paternal grandfather had a fistula.

In Figure 42-1, her pyloric sphincter remains narrow and the base of the duodenal bulb is deformed. Loops of small bowel are narrow and separated in Figure 42-2.

Diagnosis: Pyloric stenosis, Crohn's disease.

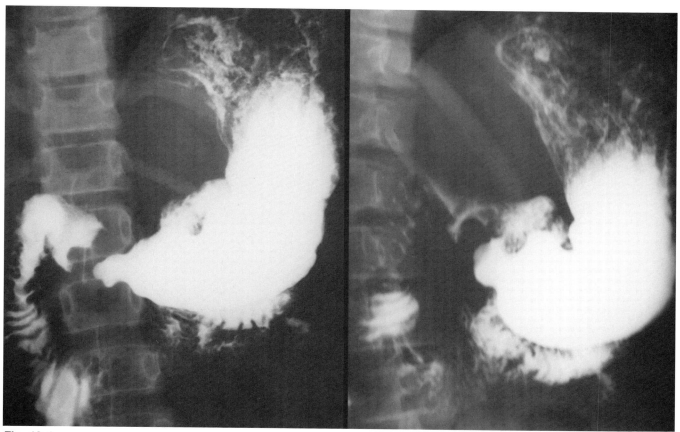

Fig. 42-1

(Continued)

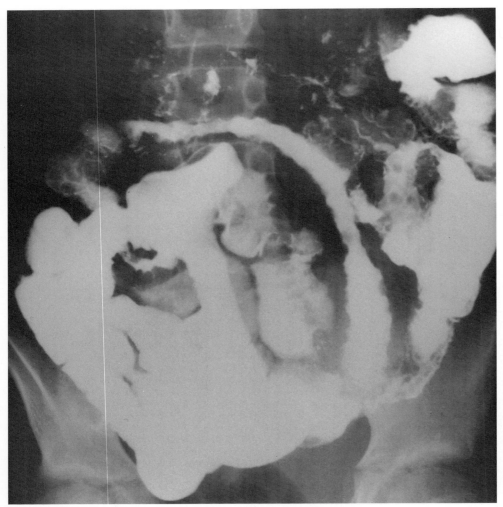

Fig. 42-2

Case 43

An 11-year-old boy feels "yucky."

He has had periumbilical pain for minutes to hours every few days for 1 month. Pain usually occurs during early morning or evening and is not relieved by food. He is nauseated. He goes to sleep when pain comes. It may or may not be gone when he wakes. He is sometimes barely able to get to the toilet in time for a loose stool. School grades are bad.

Parents and sibling (13 years old) are well.

Weight is 32.2 kg, height 139 cm. Physical findings are normal.

Hematocrit is 0.37. White cell count is 6.9×10^9/liter with 0.53 polymorphonuclear cells, 0.03 bands, 0.36 lymphocytes, and 0.08 monocytes. Platelet estimate is normal. Urine specific gravity is 1.011, pH 7. Urine is normal.

Barium goes into a defect in lower part of duodenal bulb (Figure 43-1) and remains there.

H_2-receptor antagonist alleviates his symptoms.

Diagnosis: Duodenal ulcer.

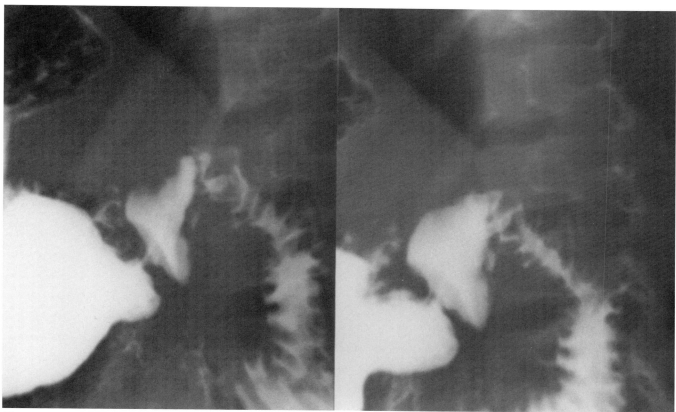

Fig. 43-1

Case 44

A 15-year-old girl has bloody vomit and black stools. She has had 25 blood transfusions since bleeding began 10 days ago.

She was cyanotic in infancy and operated on for Fallot's tetrad at 8 and 13 years. She has had epigastric pain when she eats for the past 3 months. She has been tired. Legs have felt so weak that she thinks she will collapse.

Mother died at 55 years with kidney disease; father died at 64 with leukemia. Maternal grandmother died with diabetes mellitus, maternal grandfather with cancer, and paternal grandmother with heart disease. Paternal grandfather died at 84.

Temperature at 15 years is 37°C, heart rate 120, respiratory rate 28, blood pressure 120/78, weight 34 kg, and height 137 cm. She is pale. Eyes bulge. Sclerae, lips, tongue, and nailbeds are blue; fingers and toes are clubbed. Neck veins are distended. Chest is scarred. Dullness to percussion and diminished breath sounds are on left side. Heart is large. Systolic murmur, diastolic murmur, and gallop rhythm are present. Palpation of abdomen is difficult because of guarding. Liver edge is at umbilicus. The rest of the physical findings are normal.

Hematocrit is 0.32. Platelet count is 10×10^9/liter. Serum sodium is 141 mmol/liter, potassium 4.7, chloride 103, urea nitrogen 9.6, and glucose 3.2.

The pylorus, duodenal bulb, and second part of duodenum are distorted and of fixed caliber (Figure 44-1A). A plaque of calcium density is above lesser curvature of stomach (Figure 44-1B).

At abdominal operation, a large, deep ulcer is at gastroduodenal junction. Tumor is in wall of duodenum, retroperitoneal lymph nodes, and liver. Spleen is three times larger than normal.

Surface of tumor is yellow-brown in cut section. Microscopic examination shows uniform cells (10–12-μm diameter) in regular branching trabeculae separated by fine, vascular septa and in lobules separated by broad bands of fibrous tissue. Tumor cytoplasm is eosinophilic and confluent; nuclei are round with a fine network of chromatin and 1 mitosis/HPF. At necropsy a week later, tumor is in liver, nodes, blood vessels, pancreatic bed, and behind stomach.

Diagnosis: Giant duodenal ulcer, gastrinoma (Zollinger-Ellison syndrome).

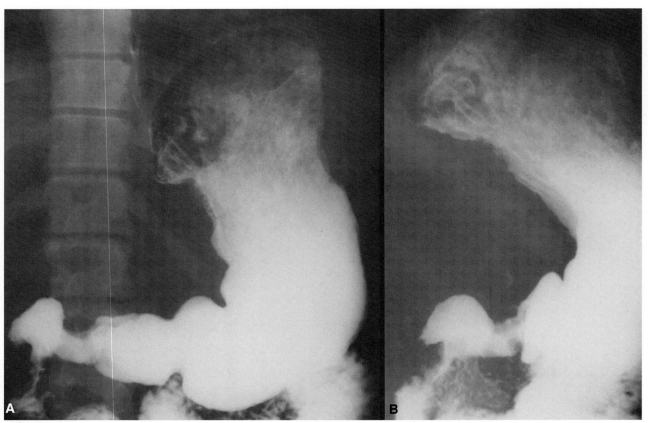

Fig. 44-1

Case 45

A premature newborn boy has a dilated, abnormally placed stomach in roentgenogram for catheter placement.

Mother (19 years old) had polyhydramnios. Labor began spontaneously 2 days ago. Birth weight is 1.1 kg, length 37 cm, head circumference 28 cm, temperature 36.8°C, heart rate 130, respiratory rate 50, and blood pressure 42/28 mm Hg. He breathes with expiratory grunt and alar flare. Skin is thin and gelatinous. Breast buds are not palpable. A single crease is on soles. A systolic murmur is present. Bile is aspirated from stomach. The rest of the physical findings are normal.

Hematocrit is 0.45. White cell count is 5.8×10^9/liter with 0.53 polymorphonuclear cells, 0.01 bands, 0.29 lymphocytes, 0.16 monocytes, and 0.01 eosinophils. Platelet count is 280×10^9/liter. Serum sodium is 135 mmol/liter, potassium 3.8, chloride 104, calcium 2.09, and glucose 5.5. Total bilirubin is 42 µmol/liter (peak bilirubin on third day: 193).

Air is in right pleural space, or a skinfold simulates right pneumothorax. Distended stomach is in right side of the abdomen, distended duodenal bulb in left side, and umbilical arterial catheter in aorta (Figure 45-1).

At operation, the whole gut is nonrotated. Liver is in right side, spleen left side, gall bladder midline. Small bowel adhesions are in left upper quadrant, cecum is in right lower quadrant, and transverse and descending parts of colon are fixed in mesentery in midline. Duodenum is distended to the crossing of portal vein in front of it. Caliber of small bowel beyond portal vein is 0.3 cm.

Diagnosis: Nonrotation of gut, obstruction at level of preduodenal portal vein.

(Continued)

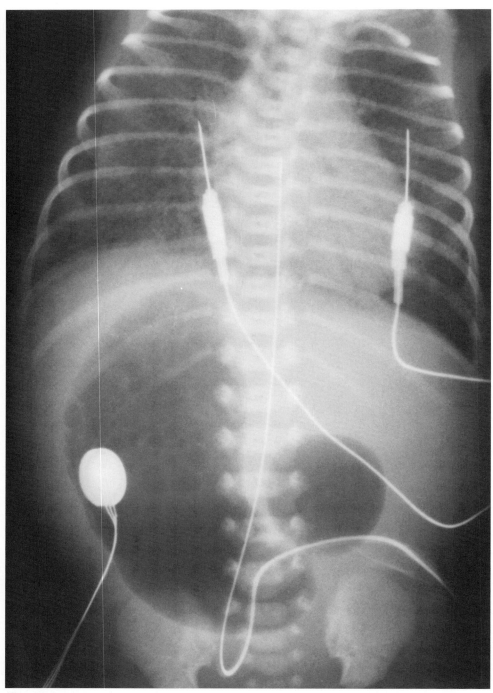

Fig. 45-1

Case 46

A 6-year-old boy has had abdominal cramps for a year. He goes to bed for the hour or so that they last and will not eat.

He is allergic to dairy products. Tonsils and adenoids were removed at 5 years, and tubes put in ears.

Mother (33 years old) has asthma. Father (31 years old) and two brothers (9 months and 7 years old) are well.

Temperature at 6 years is 36.5°C, heart rate 72, respiratory rate 16, blood pressure 100/60 mm Hg, weight 31 kg, and height 126 cm. Warts are on left hand and both knees. The rest of the physical findings are normal.

Hematocrit is 0.40. White cell count is 9.7×10^9/liter with 0.50 polymorphonuclear cells, 0.02 bands, 0.43 lymphocytes, 0.03 monocytes, 0.01 eosinophils, and 0.01 basophils. Urine specific gravity is 1.025, pH 5. Urine is normal. Serum sodium is 143 mmol/liter, potassium 4.2, chloride 106, carbon dioxide 28, urea nitrogen 4.3, calcium 2.59, phosphorus 1.71, cholesterol 2.61, and glucose 5.8. Creatinine is 40 μmol/liter, uric acid 260, total bilirubin 7, and direct bilirubin 0. Total protein is 66 g/liter, albumin 47. Alkaline phosphatase is 183 U/liter, LDH 288, and SGOT 25.

In Figure 46-1, a varying amount of barium and gas is in a pocket in second part of duodenum.

At operation, pancreas partly surrounds but does not obstruct duodenum. A blind pouch is in duodenum opposite major duodenal papilla (papilla of Vater). The resected pouch consists of mucosa without muscularis.

Diagnosis: Mucosal membrane in second part of duodenum.

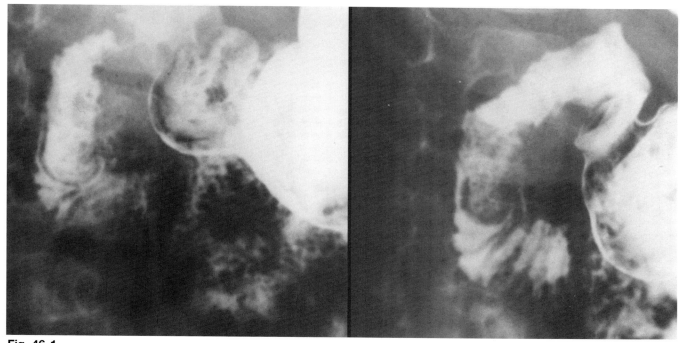

Fig. 46-1

Case 47

A 1-day-old boy is vomiting bright green liquid. He has had six meconium stools.

Mother (32 years old) had polyhydramnios and gestational diabetes. Two siblings are well.

Birth weight is 2.0 kg, Apgar score 8/9 at 1 and 5 minutes, temperature 37.2°C, heart rate 160, respiratory rate 52, and blood pressure 70/40 mm Hg. A systolic murmur is present. The rest of the physical findings are normal.

Hematocrit is 0.49. White cell count is 11.0×10^9/liter with 0.34 polymorphonuclear cells, 0.04 bands, 0.46 lymphocytes, 0.13 monocytes, 0.02 eosinophils, and 0.01 atypical lymphocytes. Platelet count is 319×10^9/liter. Serum sodium is 139 mmol/liter, potassium 6.7, chloride 106, urea nitrogen 6.1, calcium 2.17, phosphorus 1.74, cholesterol 1.94, and glucose 2.5. Creatinine is 100 µmol/liter, uric acid 440, and total bilirubin 33. Total protein is 57 g/liter, albumin 40. Alkaline phosphatase is 110 U/liter, LDH 973, and SGOT 68.

Ultrasound examination 3 weeks before birth shows excess amniotic fluid and double bubble—one with internal echoes, the other without—in baby's abdomen (Figure 47-1). GI series shows barium and gas in stomach and dilated first and second parts of duodenum, small amount of barium in normally placed jejunum, and gas and liquid in distal gut (Figure 47-2). Lower thoracic vertebral bodies are dysplastic in Figure 47-2.

At operation, a membrane is in third part of duodenum.

Diagnosis: Duodenal membrane.

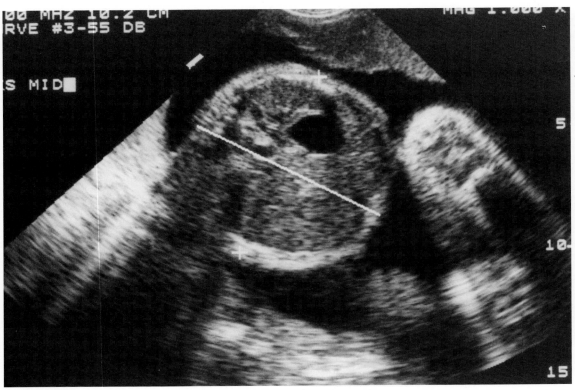

Fig. 47-1

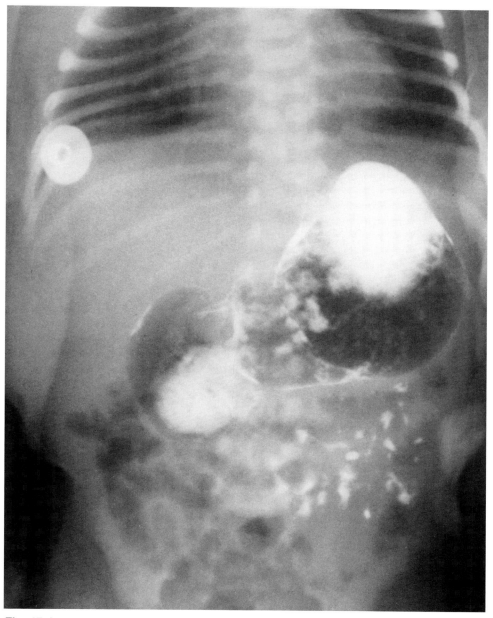

Fig. 47-2

Case 48

A 7-day-old boy who has Down syndrome is vomiting. He spit up first feedings, then vomited mucus, and now vomits green matter.

Pregnancy of mother was normal, birth weight 2.24 kg, and Apgar score 8/9 at 1 and 9 minutes.

Mother (27 years old) and father (31 years old) are well. The boy is their only child. Mother has normal older daughter by a different man. Mother's karyotype is 45,XXt(14/21); father's is 46,XY.

The boy's temperature is 38.3°C, heart rate 160, respiratory rate 60, systolic blood pressure 40 mm Hg, weight 2.15 kg, length 47 cm, and head circumference 30 cm. He is yellow. Breathing is noisy. Upper half of abdomen is more full than lower half. Liver edge is 3 cm below costal margin. Bowel sounds are absent. The rest of the physical findings are normal.

Hematocrit is 0.49. White cell count is 14.8×10^9/liter with 0.06 polymorphonuclear cells, 0.40 bands, 0.18 lymphocytes, 0.11 monocytes, 0.16 metamyelocytes, 0.08 myelocytes, and 0.01 promyelocytes. Platelet count is 150×10^9/liter. Urine specific gravity is 1.016, pH 5. Urine has 2+ protein and trace reducing substances. Serum sodium is 130 mmol/liter, potassium 5.1, chloride 94, carbon dioxide 24, urea nitrogen 8.9, calcium 1.95, phosphorus 1.68, cholesterol 3.08, and glucose 4.9. Creatinine is 150 μmol/liter, uric acid 570, total bilirubin 164, and direct bilirubin 75. Total protein is 42 g/liter, albumin 27. Alkaline phosphatase is 69 U/liter, LDH 972, and SGOT 84. Capillary blood pH is 7.27. P_{CO_2} is 52 mm Hg, P_{O_2} 44.

Figure 48-1A illustrates the following findings at 7 days: (1) gas is in stomach, first and second parts of duodenum, and not beyond; (2) air is in a few larger bronchi and not in rest of right lung; and (3) heart is positioned normally. Manubrium is bifid in lateral examination, and normal axial vascular grooves and coronal neurocentral synchondroses are prominent in some vertebral bodies (Figure 48-1B).

He dies at 11 days.

Diagnosis: Down syndrome, duodenal atresia (with possible annular pancreas).

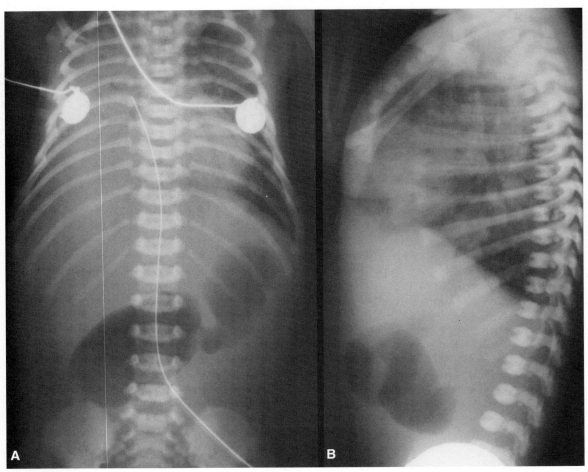

Fig. 48-1

Case 49

A newborn boy, who is breast- and bottle-fed, vomits milk curds at 10, 12, and 27 hours. He has not yet had a meconium stool at 36 hours.

Birth weight is 2.7 kg, Apgar score 8/9 at 1 and 5 minutes, length 48 cm, head circumference 32 cm, temperature 36.2°C, heart rate 146, respiratory rate 74, and systolic blood pressure 58 mm Hg. Physical findings are normal.

Hematocrit is 0.50. White cell count is 18.2×10^9/liter with 0.67 polymorphonuclear cells, 0.01 bands, 0.26 lymphocytes, and 0.06 monocytes. Platelet count is 307×10^9/liter. Serum sodium is 142 mmol/liter, potassium 5.5, chloride 105, calcium 2.17, and glucose 5.0.

Stomach and first and second parts of duodenum are dilated with gas and liquid; a small amount of gas is in distal gut (Figure 49-1).

At operation, annular pancreas and a membrane with a hole in it separating second from third part of duodenum are found.

Diagnosis: Duodenal membrane and annular pancreas.

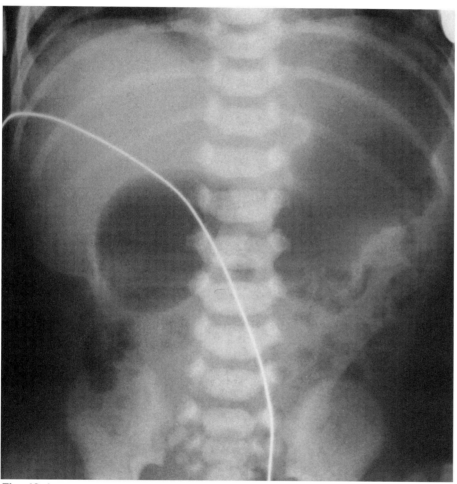

Fig. 49-1

Case 50

A newborn girl is breathing fast and chokes during first feeding.

Mother (29 years old) is well. She has two sons from an earlier marriage, both with defective vision. Father of the girl died 4 months ago in motorcycle crash.

Birth weight is 3.7 kg, length 51 cm, temperature 37.2°C, heart rate 154, respiratory rate 120, and blood pressure 79/49 mm Hg. Right upper eyelid droops. Diameter of right pupil is 2 mm, left 4. Right shoulder is smaller and more round than left. Proximal muscles of right arm are less full. A small hemangioma is over T1. The rest of the physical findings are normal.

Hematocrit is 0.61. Blood glucose is 2.3 mmol/liter.

Roentgenograms during GI series show barium going from proximal small bowel into cyst in back part of right side of chest, forward displacement of trachea (Figure 50-1), defects of cervical vertebrae and T1, and winged right scapula (Figure 50-2).

At operation, tubular upper part of cyst goes into spinal canal and dura. Clear yellow liquid drains from its transected end at C6–C7. Cyst goes through a 1-cm defect in right side of diaphragm and enters antimesenteric side of third part of duodenum. Ladd's bands cross duodenum. Cyst and third part of duodenum are removed, rest of duodenum is anastomosed end to end, appendix is removed, and ascending colon is placed in left lower quadrant of abdomen.

Diagnosis: Neurenteric cyst, malrotation of midgut.

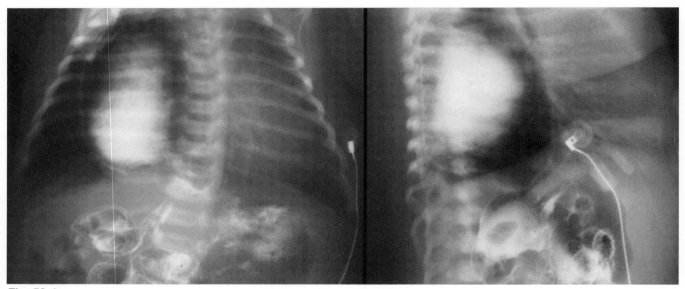

Fig. 50-1

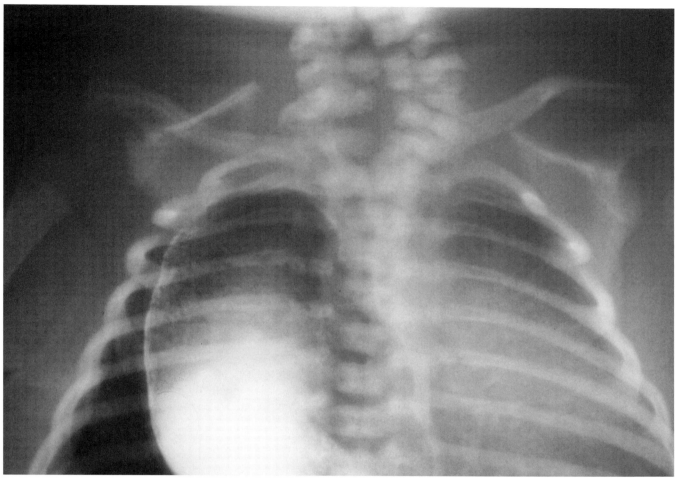

Fig. 50-2

Case 51

A 10½-year-old girl with diabetes mellitus, who "eats all day long" weighs less than she did at 7½ years.

Pregnancy of mother, who was diagnosed with diabetes at 17 years, was marred by toxemia and cesarean section. Birth weight was 3 kg. The girl walked at 13 months. She had mumps at 4 years, car door closed on left little finger at 6 years, and, from 7–9 years, she had four to six watery stools per day. At 7 years, weight was 24 kg, height 119 cm. Thyroid gland was rubbery, end of left little finger swollen. Blood glucose was 4.6 mmol/liter. Thyroid test results were normal. At 9 years, weight was 23 kg in school physical examination, height 126 cm. Thyroid gland was smooth and large. Urinalysis showed 4+ sugar and 3+ ketones. Serum thyroglobulin antibody titer was 80, thyroid antimicrosomal antibody titer 25,600 (normal: <100). Three months later, T_4 was 57 and 114 mmol/liter (normal: 51–142). Treatment with insulin was begun at 9 years, levothyroxine at 10 years, when TSH was 44 mU/liter (normal: 2–11).

Father has "thyroid growth" and takes thyroid pills. Four older half siblings are well. Paternal great-grandmother and maternal grandfather have diabetes mellitus. Maternal grandmother has goiter; maternal great-aunt has colitis.

Weight at 10½ years is 23.4 kg, height 128 cm, temperature 36.8°C, heart rate 100, respiratory rate 22, and blood pressure 90/70 mm Hg. Thyroid gland is not enlarged. Right eardrum is pink, abdomen protuberant. Liver edge and spleen edge are 5–6 cm below costal margin. Legs are thin. The rest of the physical findings are normal.

Hematocrit is 0.37. White cell count is 4.0×10^9/liter with 0.64 polymorphonuclear cells, 0.11 bands, 0.13 lymphocytes, 0.07 monocytes, 0.04 eosinophils, and 0.01 myelocytes. Platelet count is 274×10^9/liter. Urine specific gravity is 1.038, pH 6. Urine has >56 mmol/liter glucose and 3+ ketones. Serum sodium is 133 mmol/liter, potassium 4.2, chloride 103, carbon dioxide 6, urea nitrogen 6.1, calcium 2.42, phosphorus 2.13, cholesterol 6.39, and glucose 35.8. Creatinine is 115 µmol/liter, uric acid 190, total bilirubin 5, and direct bilirubin 3. Total protein is 71 g/liter, albumin 43. Alkaline phosphatase is 306 U/liter, LDH 378, and SGOT 32. T_3 resin uptake is 0.37 (normal: 0.25–0.35), T_4 95 nmol/liter (normal: 51–142), and TSH 16 mU/liter (normal: 2–11).

GI series shows jejunum in right side of abdomen at 15 minutes, ileum in left side at 2 hours (Figure 51-1). At 10½ years, bone age in left hand is about 8 years, 2–3 SDs below the mean. A cleft is in tuberosity of distal phalanx of little finger.

More insulin is given twice per day. Weight at 11 years is 27.5 kg, height 130 cm. Liver and spleen are not palpable.

Diagnosis: Diabetes mellitus, dwarfism, hepatosplenomegaly; hypothyroidism; nonrotation of midgut; traumatic acro-osteolysis.

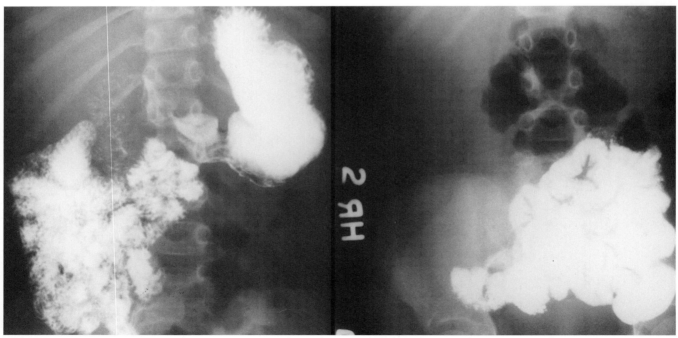

Fig. 51-1

Case 52

A 3-day-old boy is vomiting bile. He has been taking 1.5–2.0 oz of formula every few hours. He began to vomit bile 12 hours ago and has vomited many times since then. He takes formula eagerly but vomits 5–30 minutes afterward. He is not fussy.

Pregnancy of mother was normal, birth weight 4.0 kg, length 54 cm, head circumference 35 cm, and Apgar score 9/10 at 1 and 5 minutes.

Mother (22 years old), father (28 years old), and two sisters (1 and 3 years old) are well.

Temperature is 36.9°C, heart rate 164, respiratory rate 50, systolic blood pressure 64 mm Hg, and weight 3.7 kg. Light green vomit is around mouth and on blanket. Anterior fontanel is slightly depressed. Abdomen is distended until he vomits and then is soft without masses. Bowel sounds are normal. The rest of the physical findings are normal.

Hematocrit is 0.60. White cell count is 10.5×10^9/liter with 0.48 polymorphonuclear cells, 0.05 bands, 0.34 lymphocytes, 0.11 monocytes, and 0.02 eosinophils. Urine specific gravity is 1.019, pH 5. Urine has glucose (IV fluids). Serum sodium is 141 mmol/liter, potassium 5.6, and chloride 99.

Figure 52-1A shows gas in stomach; dilated superior, descending, and horizontal parts of duodenum; and a small amount in distal gut. Barium enema in Figure 52-1B shows a U-turn at hepatic flexure of colon.

At operation, chyle is in abdomen. Gut is dusky, mesentery engorged. Midgut is twisted clockwise four times on a short mesentery at Treitz's ligament. Peritoneal bands (Ladd's bands) from abdominal wall near liver cross duodenum to ectopic cecum.

Diagnosis: Nonrotation and volvulus of midgut.

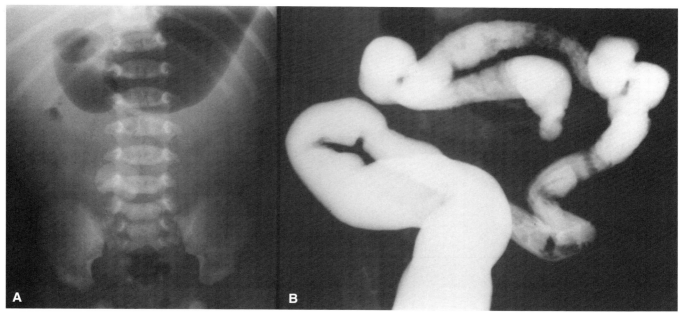

Fig. 52-1

Case 53

A 3-day-old boy is vomiting bile.

Birth weight was 3.1 kg. He had several meconium stools the first day. The next day he vomited mucus (clear at first, then green) and stopped having bowel movements. Later that day breathing was raspy. Eyes rolled back, and right arm and leg twitched.

Heart rate is 130, respiratory rate 36, and weight 2.8 kg. At start of operation, systolic blood pressure is 68 mm Hg. Abdomen is not distended. Liver edge is 4 cm below costal margin. Bowel sounds are absent. The rest of the physical findings are normal.

Hematocrit is 0.58. Serum sodium is 135 mmol/liter, potassium 4.4, chloride 95, calcium 2.54, and glucose 4.4.

Plain film of abdomen at 2 days shows normal findings.

At operation, volvulus of midgut is found. Gut is dusky. Color of gut becomes normal with reduction of volvulus and replacement of gut in abdomen.

At 11 days, he takes formula well. At 12 days, he has three seedy, green-yellow stools. He is irritable the evening of the eighteenth day, refuses to eat, and has a bloody stool. He vomits bile next morning. Temperature is 37.3°C, heart rate 120, respiratory rate 32, and systolic blood pressure 80 mm Hg. Abdomen is distended. Bowel sounds are absent.

Hematocrit at 19 days is 0.34. White cell count is 15.7 × 10⁹/liter with 0.03 polymorphonuclear cells, 0.45 bands, 0.37 lymphocytes, 0.05 monocytes, 0.02 eosinophils, 0.03 myelocytes, and 0.05 metamyelocytes.

Barium by mouth stops at junction of third and fourth parts of duodenum, by rectum at Cannon's ring in transverse colon (Figure 53-1).

At operation, midgut is gangrenous. Adhesions fix loops of gut. Cloudy liquid is in peritoneum.

Microscopic examination shows mesenteric venous thrombosis.

Diagnosis: Midgut volvulus, midgut gangrene.

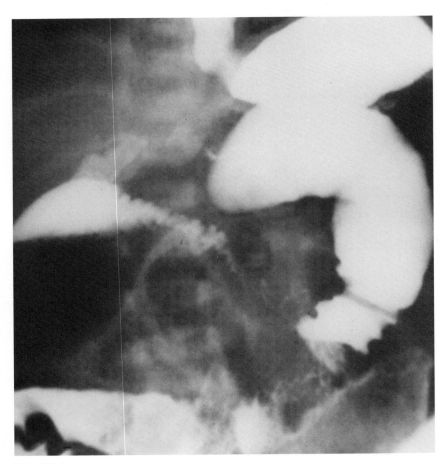

Fig. 53-1

Case 54

A 3-year-old girl vomits yellow liquid one day, green liquid the next day. She has had dark stools recently.

She lives with mother (24 years old), mother's boyfriend, and brother (1½ years old). Mother says that she got a new baby-sitter recently, that girl fell from bed onto toy cash register, and that daughter and son throw toys at each other. The girl is terrified when mother's boyfriend visits her in the hospital.

Weight is 16.8 kg, height 97 cm, temperature 37°C, heart rate 130, respiratory rate 28, and blood pressure 90/50 mm Hg. A dime-sized abrasion is on chin. Green and blue bruises of various age and size are on midback, right flank, lower part of right side of chest, right upper quadrant of abdomen, and left buttock. She cries when abdomen is palpated. Liver edge is 1 cm below costal margin. The rest of the physical findings are normal.

Hematocrit is 0.25. White cell count is 8.8×10^9/liter with 0.67 polymorphonuclear cells, 0.10 bands, 0.17 lymphocytes, and 0.06 monocytes. Platelet count is 174×10^9/liter. ESR is 37 mm/hr. Urine specific gravity is 1.017, pH 5. Urine has trace ketones, occasional white cells/HPF, and moderate urates. Serum sodium is 129 mmol/liter, potassium 4.7, chloride 74, urea nitrogen 3.3, and glucose 6.6.

Barium shows dilation of duodenum (Figure 54-1A) and partial obstruction beyond second part (Figure 54-1B). GI series 8 days later shows normal findings.

Diagnosis: Intramural duodenal hematoma.

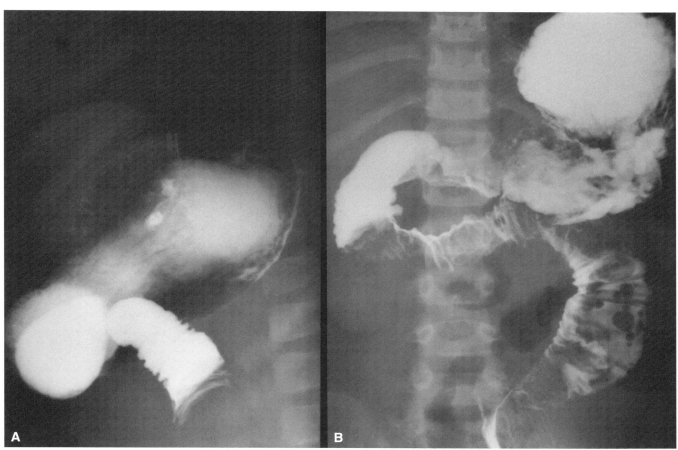

Fig. 54-1

Case 55

A newborn boy has meconium-stained amniotic fluid and 130 ml light green gastric aspirate.

Pregnancy of mother (16 years old) was normal. Birth weight is 2.5 kg, length 48 cm, head circumference 34 cm, Apgar score 8/9 at 1 and 5 minutes, temperature 36.4°C, heart rate 140, respiratory rate 70, and systolic blood pressure 42 mm Hg. Physical findings are normal.

Hematocrit is 0.48, blood glucose 2.8 mmol/liter.

Gas is in undistended stomach and proximal jejunum at 30 minutes (Figure 55-1A), no gas beyond distended stomach and distended proximal jejunum at 2 hours (Figure 55-1B). A clamp is on umbilical cord.

At operation, diameter of proximal jejunum is 4 cm and wall is thickened. A fibrous cord (2 cm long) connects proximal jejunum to distal small bowel. A gap is in mesentery. Superior mesenteric artery is absent. Blood flow to distal small bowel is from ileocolic artery.

Microscopic examination of the atretic cord shows complete muscular wall without identifiable mucosa. Dense fibrous tissue and a small amount of calcified matter are inside. Myenteric plexus is prominent and contains what appear to be immature ganglion cells.

Diagnosis: Jejunal atresia with fibrous obliteration of lumen.

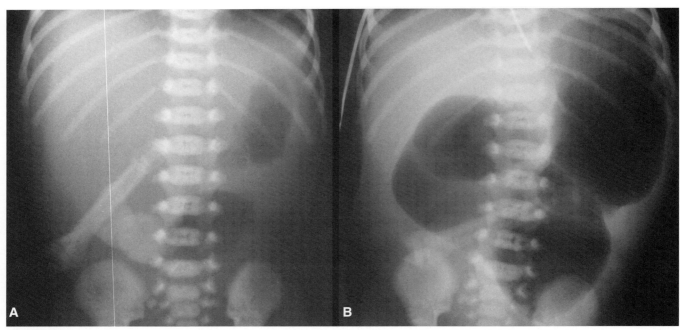

Fig. 55-1

Case 56

A newborn girl has 70 ml gastric aspirate.

Polyhydramnios, gestational diabetes, and meconium-stained amniotic fluid marred pregnancy.

Parents are well. She is their only child. Members of mother's family have diabetes mellitus.

Birth weight is 2.5 kg, Apgar score 10/10 at 1 and 5 minutes, length 47 cm, and head circumference 32 cm. Bowel sounds are absent. At 10 hours, temperature is 35.9°C, heart rate 120, respiratory rate 40, and systolic blood pressure 40 mm Hg. Abdomen is not distended. Liver edge is 1 cm below costal margin. Bowel sounds are absent. The rest of the physical findings are normal.

Hematocrit is 0.50. At 8½ hours, serum sodium is 141 mmol/liter, potassium 4.0, chloride 107, carbon dioxide 21, urea nitrogen 3.6, calcium 2.69, phosphorus 1.61, cholesterol 1.27, triglycerides 0.32, and glucose 8.3. Uric acid is 220 µmol/liter, total bilirubin 26, and direct bilirubin 3. Total protein is 49 g/liter, albumin 30. Alkaline phosphatase is 194 U/liter, LDH 328, SGOT 28, and CK 101. At 5 days, peak total bilirubin is 210 µmol/liter.

Gas is in moderately dilated proximal small bowel (Figure 56-1A). Barium shows meconium in colon and left displacement of colon (Figure 56-1B).

At operation, proximal small bowel is dilated with gas. Distal small bowel is coiled around a vascular pedicle. Two atretic segments are in distal small bowel. Appendix (3.5 × 0.3 cm) is normal.

At 1½ years, weight is 9.3 kg. Scar is on abdomen. The rest of the physical findings are normal.

Diagnosis: Jejunal atresia (apple peel or Christmas tree syndrome).

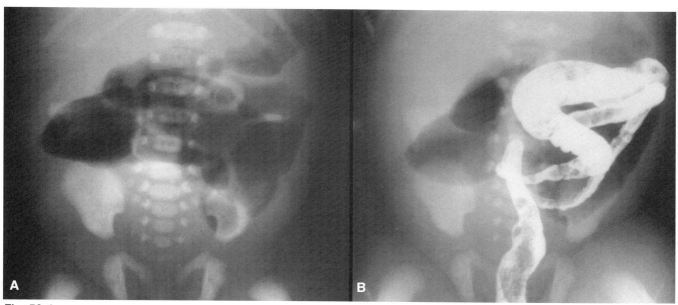

Fig. 56-1

Case 57

A newborn girl has a distended abdomen. Prenatal ultrasound examination 2 months ago showed polyhydramnios and, according to ultrasonographer, "cystlike structures, probably small bowel" in fetal abdomen.

Mother (26 years old), sister (9 years old), and brother (7 years old) are well.

Birth weight is 2.8 kg, Apgar score 8/9 at 1 and 5 minutes, temperature 36.5°C, heart rate 158, respiratory rate 50, and blood pressure 58/21 mm Hg. Abdomen is tense. Loops of bowel are palpable. The rest of the physical findings are normal.

Hematocrit is 0.54. White cell count is 16.6×10^9/liter. Platelet count is 224×10^9/liter. Serum sodium is 138 mmol/liter, potassium 5.2, chloride 111, urea nitrogen 2.9, and glucose 5.6. Creatinine is 90 µmol/liter. Capillary blood pH is 7.38 when $F_{IO_2} = 0.20$. P_{CO_2} is 41 mm Hg, P_{O_2} 31.

Dilated gut is in left side of abdomen, mass of water density is in right side, and thin band of calcium density is just under lateral end of right ninth rib (Figure 57-1).

At operation, 140 ml green meconium is in a cyst that is connected to dilated jejunum proximal to an atretic segment (5–6 cm long). Caliber of distal small bowel is 5–6 mm. Resection and end-to-end anastomosis are performed. Gastrostomy is placed.

Examination of resected jejunum shows dark, hemorrhagic mucosa; loss of mucosal folds; and gray-green exudate adherent to mucosa.

Diagnosis: Jejunal atresia, meconium peritonitis.

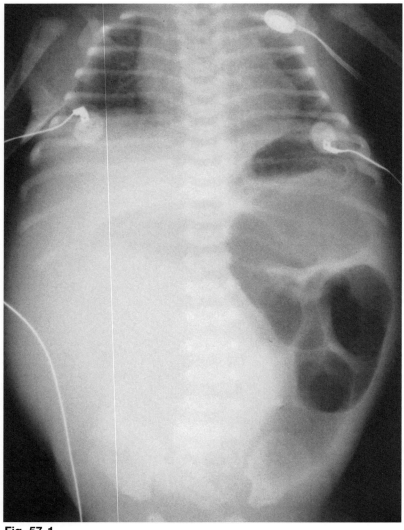

Fig. 57-1

Case 58

A 3-day-old girl vomits bile and has a small bloody stool.

Birth weight was 3.8 kg, Apgar score 8/10 at 1 and 5 minutes.

Weight is 3.6 kg, temperature 36.5°C, heart rate 130–150, respiratory rate 30–50, and systolic blood pressure 90 mm Hg. Bowel sounds are diminished. The rest of the physical findings are normal.

Hematocrit is 0.39. White cell count is 5.8 × 10⁹/liter with 0.42 polymorphonuclear cells, 0.53 lymphocytes, 0.04 monocytes, and 0.01 basophils. Serum sodium is 144 mmol/liter, potassium 5.1, chloride 104, carbon dioxide 26, urea nitrogen 1.0, calcium 2.54, phosphorus 1.65, cholesterol 4.40, and glucose 4.8. Creatinine is 50 μmol/liter, uric acid 170, and total bilirubin 135. Total protein is 57 g/liter, albumin 38. Alkaline phosphatase is 162 U/liter, LDH 612, and SGOT 37.

Barium enema in Figure 58-1 shows (1) defect in ascending colon, (2) barium in distal small bowel that remains from earlier GI series, and (3) dilated small intestine, its loops separated by excess liquid or thickened wall.

At operation, gelatinous, yellow liquid is in abdomen, and a firm mass is in ascending colon. Mass, cecum, appendix, and distal ileum are resected after mass is pushed back to cecum.

Examination of specimen shows an ischemic mass (2.4 × 1.8 cm) that contains yellow liquid in wall of ileum.

Diagnosis: Duplication of ileum, intussusception.

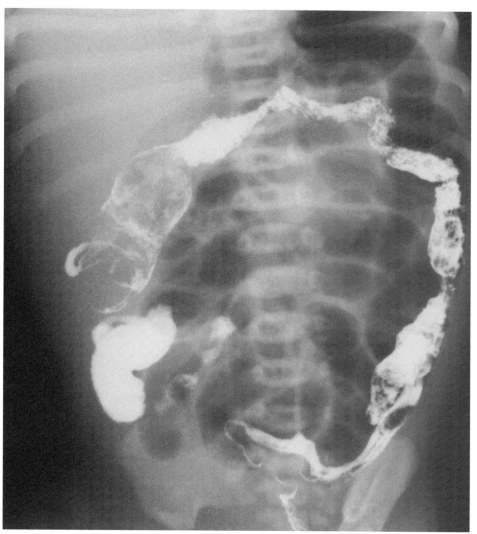

Fig. 58-1

Case 59

A 2-day-old girl, one of twins, has a distended abdomen.

Onset of labor was spontaneous, delivery by cesarean section because one twin was transverse in utero, the other oblique. Placenta was single with three membranes, two amnions and one chorion, between two umbilical cords.

Mother (31 years old), father (33 years old), three older siblings, and monozygotic twin are well.

Birth weight is 3.4 kg, length 50 cm, head circumference 34 cm, Apgar score 8/10 at 1 and 5 minutes, temperature 36.7°C, heart rate 150, and respiratory rate 38. Upper lids are bruised. The rest of the physical findings at birth are normal.

She feeds well at 1 day, poorly at 2 days. At 37 hours, she vomits and has first meconium stool. At 2 days, she is jaundiced. Systolic blood pressure is 60 mm Hg. Abdomen is tym-panitic. Bowel sounds are infrequent. Green liquid is aspirated from stomach.

Hematocrit is 0.61. White cell count is 10.0×10^9/liter with 0.42 polymorphonuclear cells, 0.05 bands, 0.45 lymphocytes, and 0.08 monocytes. Platelet count is 155×10^9/liter. Serum sodium is 146 mmol/liter, potassium 4.9, and chloride 107. Bilirubin is 169 μmol/liter.

Gut is distended with gas and liquid, especially in right upper quadrant (Figure 59-1).

At operation, diameter of midileum is 6–7 cm. A segment of distal ileum ends blindly and is resected. Ileoileostomy and gastrostomy are placed.

Diagnosis: Ileal atresia.

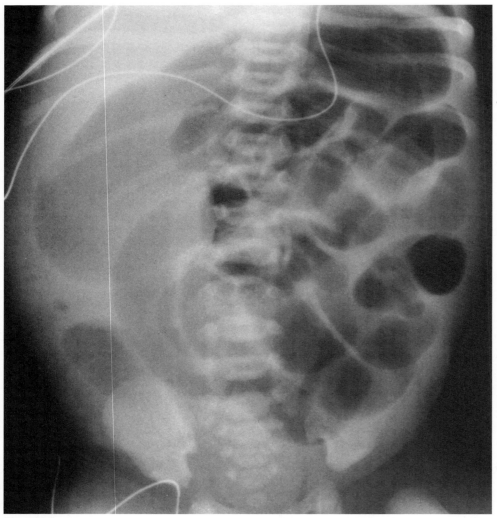

Fig. 59-1

Case 60

A newborn girl, one of twin sisters, has a distended abdomen.

Mother (26 years old) smoked one and a half packs of cigarettes per day during pregnancy. Labor and delivery of twins and two placentas were normal. Father (34 years old), two older siblings, and twin (birth weight 2.6 kg) are well.

Birth weight is 2.0 kg, length 44 cm, head circumference 31 cm, and Apgar score 6/8 at 1 and 5 minutes. At 25 minutes, temperature is 35.6°C, heart rate 128, and respiratory rate 56. She is lethargic and cries only when disturbed. Abdomen is distended at 12 hours. The rest of the physical findings are normal.

Umbilical venous blood hematocrit is 0.60. Green mucus is aspirated from stomach at 15 hours. She has not passed meconium at 22 hours.

Gut in right side of abdomen is moderately dilated at 22 hours, and a shadow of calcium density is in left upper quadrant of abdomen (Figure 60-1).

When operation is begun, systolic blood pressure is 70 mm Hg. Small bowel adhesions are in left upper quadrant. Distal ileum (2.5-cm diameter) is filled with meconium and ends blindly at a kinked, narrow segment of terminal ileum (3.5 cm long) that contains feces.

Diagnosis: Ileal atresia and meconium peritonitis.

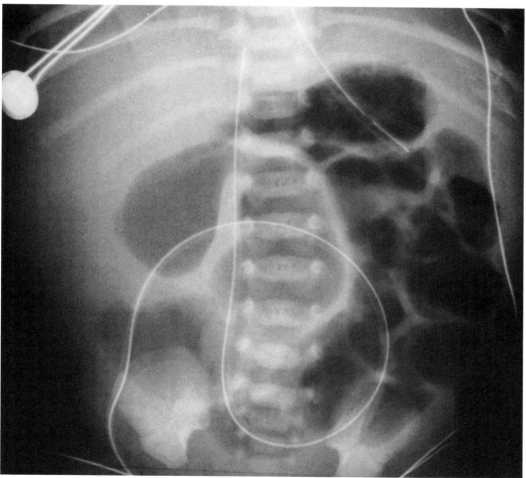

Fig. 60-1

Case 61

A newborn girl has a distended abdomen.

Mother (20 years old), father (28 years old), and sister (3 years old) are well. Sister (1½ years old) has cystic fibrosis and had meconium ileus.

Mother smoked half a pack of cigarettes per day during pregnancy. Amniotic fluid looks like thick pea soup and is at vocal cords. Birth weight is 3.0 kg, length 48 cm, head circumference 33 cm, Apgar score 8/9 at 1 and 5 minutes, and respiratory rate 68. At 6 hours, temperature is 36°C, heart rate 130, respiratory rate 62, and blood pressure 83/46 mm Hg. Blood glucose is 5.0 mmol/liter. Breath sounds are noisy. Abdomen is soft. The rest of the physical findings are normal.

Capillary blood pH is 7.41 while she breathes room air. P_{CO_2} is 38 mm Hg, P_{O_2} 49. Hematocrit is 0.44. White cell count is 11.3×10^9/liter. Platelet count is 268×10^9/liter. Serum sodium is 133 mmol/liter, potassium 5.6, chloride 107, carbon dioxide 21, urea nitrogen 2.9, calcium 2.40, phosphorus 1.52, and cholesterol 1.78. Creatinine is 70 μmol/liter, uric acid 310, and total bilirubin 72. Total protein is 59 g/liter, albumin 36. Alkaline phosphatase is 54 U/liter, LDH 821, and SGOT 60.

She passes a small amount of sticky, guaiac-negative meconium.

In Figure 61-1, little gas is in gut in right side of abdomen; barium enema shows that caliber and length of colon are normal and ascending colon is displaced to left.

At operation, distal ileum is beefy red and distended above a segment of axial volvulus and atresia.

Sweat chloride is 103 mmol/liter at 8 days.

Diagnosis: Cystic fibrosis, meconium ileus, axial ileal volvulus with atresia.

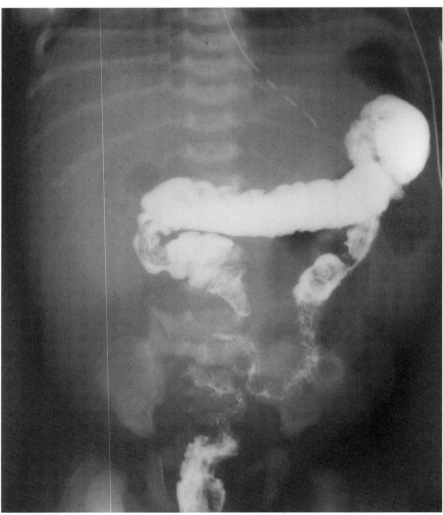

Fig. 61-1

Case 62

A 1-day-old boy has a distended abdomen and has not had a meconium stool. Birth weight was 3.5 kg, Apgar score 8/9 at 1 and 5 minutes.

Mother, father, and sister (4 years old) are well.

Temperature is 36.2°C, heart rate 160, respiratory rate 48, systolic blood pressure 60 mm Hg, and weight 3.4 kg. He has a systolic murmur. The rest of the physical findings are normal.

Hematocrit is 0.41. White cell count is 11.6×10^9/liter with 0.33 polymorphonuclear cells, 0.08 bands, 0.44 lymphocytes, 0.14 monocytes, and 0.01 myelocytes. Platelet estimate is normal. Urine specific gravity is 1.010, pH 6. Urine has 1+ protein, a few bacteria, occasional epithelial cells/HPF, and 0–2 white cells/HPF. Serum sodium is 141 mmol/liter, potassium 5.0, and chloride 106.

Gas and liquid are in unevenly dilated gut in left side and, to less degree, in right side of abdomen; bubbles of gas are in right side (Figure 62-1).

At operation, thick, sticky, dark green meconium is in small intestine from Treitz's ligament to ileocecal valve. A segment of jejunum that is damaged during removal of meconium is resected, end-to-end anastomosis performed, and gastrostomy placed.

He is obstructed at 5 months and treated successfully with saline enemas. He stops eating at 8 months, vomits, and has a distended abdomen.

At operation, kinks, adhesions, and inspissated stool in ileum are found.

He is lethargic, dusky, and 10% dehydrated on a summer day at 9 months when ambient temperature is 26.7°C.

Diagnosis: Cystic fibrosis (sweat chloride is 143 mmol/liter and 152 mmol/liter at 2 weeks); meconium ileus; intestinal obstruction by adhesions and/or meconium ileus equivalent at 8 months; questionable hyponatremia at 9 months.

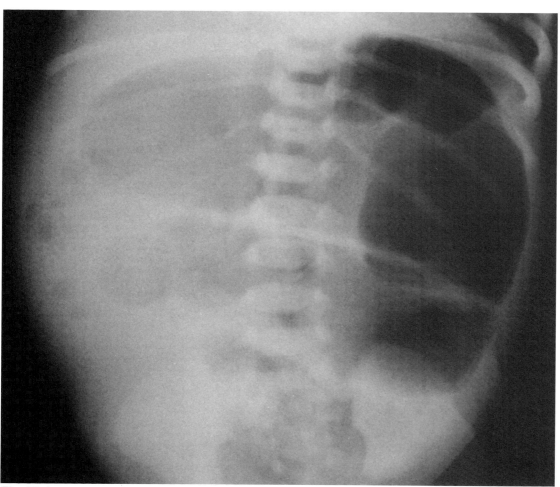

Fig. 62-1

Case 63

A 29-hour-old girl is vomiting green liquid and has not passed meconium. Pregnancy was normal.

Temperature is 37.2°C, heart rate 128, respiratory rate 40, blood pressure 71/30 mm Hg, and weight 3.7 kg. Abdomen is distended. Meconium is not in rectum. The rest of the physical findings are normal.

Hematocrit is 0.53. White cell count is 5.2×10^9/liter with 0.31 polymorphonuclear cells, 0.25 bands, 0.33 lymphocytes, 0.06 monocytes, 0.04 atypical lymphocytes, and 0.01 metamyelocytes. Platelet count is 211×10^9/liter. Serum sodium is 145 mmol/liter, potassium 4.8, chloride 102, carbon dioxide 21, urea nitrogen 6.8, calcium 2.17, phosphorus 2.26, cholesterol 1.94, and glucose 3.1. Creatinine is 70 µmol/liter, uric acid 430, total bilirubin 111, and direct bilirubin 7. Total protein is 53 g/liter, albumin 40. Alkaline phosphatase is 149 U/liter, LDH 449, and SGOT 34.

Gas-distended gut is in upper part of abdomen, constricted gut with gas is in pelvis and midabdomen, contrast medium is in constricted colon and around meconium pellets proximally, and an enteric tube ends in stomach (Figure 63-1).

At operation, small intestine is distended to a level 60 cm from Treitz's ligament and constricted beyond. Viscid pellets of meconium are in constricted segment.

Specimens of small bowel removed for frozen section show ganglion cells in dilated segment, none in distal constricted segment, and none in appendix.

Diagnosis: Hirschsprung's disease, long segment with transition zone in small intestine.

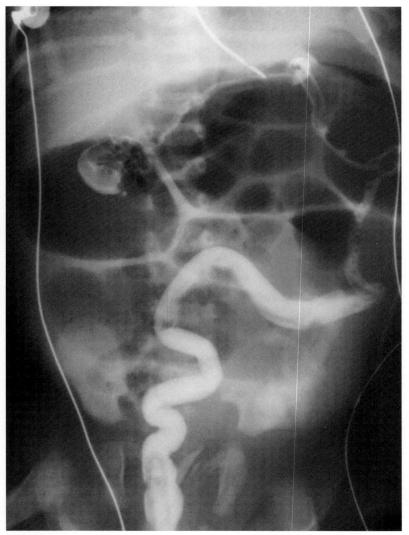

Fig. 63-1

Case 64

An 8-day-old girl has a distended, red-streaked abdomen.

Mother (40 years old) took phenelzine sulfate, propranolol hydrochloride, and levothyroxine during pregnancy and gained 24.5 kg. Membranes ruptured spontaneously 11 hours before baby was delivered by cesarean section.

Birth weight was 1.4 kg, Apgar score 7/8 at 1 and 5 minutes, temperature 35.6°C, heart rate 146, respiratory rate 66, and blood pressure 52/27 mm Hg. Physical findings were normal. Blood glucose was 6.7 mmol/liter. Grunting and retracting soon appeared. Umbilical arterial blood pH was 7.23. P_{CO_2} was 55 mm Hg, P_{O_2} 249. Bicarbonate was 22 mmol/liter. She was intubated, given oxygen for 12 hours, extubated, and then fed at 2 days. She had first stool after glycerine suppository at 4 days. She nippled weakly at 4 days and was fed by gavage. She had gastric residuals. She had apnea and bradycardia at 5 days. At 7 days, she vomited. Temperature was 36.8°C, heart rate 160, respiratory rate 60, and blood pressure 77/33 mm Hg. Girth of abdomen increased 3.5 cm and redness appeared around umbilicus. She had two small guaiac-negative stools after a rectal suppository was inserted. At 8 days, abdomen is softer, less red, and less distended.

Temperature is 35.5°C. Bowel sounds are normal. Two watery brown stools are guaiac negative.

Hematocrit is 0.39 at 8 days. White cell count is 8.6×10^9/liter with 0.35 polymorphonuclear cells, 0.05 bands, 0.38 lymphocytes, 0.10 monocytes, 0.10 eosinophils, and 0.02 metamyelocytes. Platelet count is 242×10^9/liter. Serum sodium is 137 mmol/liter, potassium 4.8, chloride 96, and calcium 2.07.

At 7 days, gut is dilated with gas and liquid. Figure 64-1A shows streaks of intramural gas in left upper quadrant and right lower quadrant, excess liquid in gut, and a tube ending in stomach. At 8 days, Figure 64-1B shows gas and excess liquid in dilated gut, as well as gas outside gut and on both sides of ligamentum teres.

At operation, stool is in peritoneum. A hole in cecum is surrounded by light green matter. Cecum, appendix, ascending colon, and terminal ileum are resected. Coagulase-negative staphylococci and *Eubacterium rectale* are cultured from peritoneum.

Diagnosis: Prematurity; necrotizing enterocolitis.

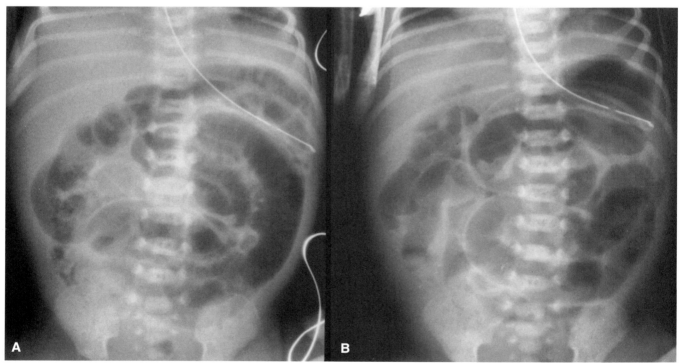

Fig. 64-1

Case 65

A premature girl is delivered by cesarean section because of prolapse of umbilical cord.

Pregnancy of mother (27 years old) was normal until spontaneous rupture of membranes 16 hours before delivery. Heart rate is under 100. She gasps several times in the minute it takes to intubate. Weight is 1.0 kg, Apgar score 3/6 at 1 and 5 minutes, temperature 35.6°C, systolic blood pressure 42 mm Hg, and respiratory rate 60 on ventilator. She is limp. She has a systolic murmur. Legs are bruised. The rest of the physical findings are normal.

Hematocrit is 0.66. White cell count is 10.1 × 10⁹/liter with 0.28 polymorphonuclear cells, 0.13 bands, 0.48 lymphocytes, 0.10 monocytes, and 0.01 eosinophils. Platelet count is 240 × 10⁹/liter. Blood glucose is between 3.8 and 5.6 mmol/liter in several determinations.

She is extubated at 4 days. Feeding is begun. Green liquid is aspirated from stomach at 7 days. Suck is weak, left lower quadrant of abdomen full at 8 days. Abdomen is distended from days 9 to 13. She has gastric residuals. Stools are runny from days 13 to 15. Heart rate increases from 140–160 to 190 at 15 days, then slows to 150 at 16 days. She is very pale at 16 days. She cries hard at 17 days. Abdomen is tense. Stool is bloody.

Hematocrit at 17 days is 0.35. White cell count is 13.0 × 10⁹/liter with 0.31 polymorphonuclear cells, 0.24 bands, 0.25 lymphocytes, 0.12 monocytes, 0.06 eosinophils, and 0.02 atypical lymphocytes. Platelet count is 453 × 10⁹/liter.

Roentgenogram at 17 days shows excess liquid in and around gut, gas in wall of gut in right side of abdomen, and gas in portal veins (Figure 65-1).

At operation, small bowel is necrotic. Subserosal blebs (1–2 cm) are in small and large intestine.

She dies soon after operation.

Diagnosis: Necrotizing enterocolitis.

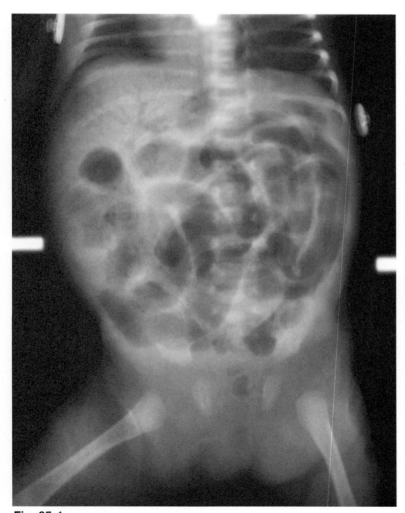

Fig. 65-1

Case 66

An 11-month-old boy has two black stools during the night.

Pregnancy of mother was normal, birth weight 3.1 kg. He had trouble breathing and was dusky during feedings until an operation at several weeks for overgrowth of nasal septal cartilage. He had an operation at 6 weeks for sagittal synostosis. He is now being given an antibiotic for ear infection.

Parents are well. He is their only child.

Temperature at 11 months is 36.8°C, heart rate 148, respiratory rate 44, systolic blood pressure 90 mm Hg, weight 8.1 kg, and head circumference 47 cm. Head is long. A midsagittal scar is on scalp. He has a systolic heart murmur and umbilical hernia. The rest of the physical findings are normal.

Hematocrit is 0.18. MCV is 83 fl. MCH is 27 pg. MCHC is 30 g/liter. White cell count is 13.1×10^9/liter with 0.30 polymorphonuclear cells, 0.03 bands, 0.66 lymphocytes, and 0.01 eosinophils. Platelet count is 285×10^9/liter. PT is 13.6 seconds, activated PTT 34.7. Fibrinogen is 1.8 g/liter (normal: 1.5–3.5). Serum sodium is 138 mmol/liter, potassium 4.1, and chloride 107. Total bilirubin is 5 μmol/liter. SGOT is 34 U/liter.

Technetium-99m pertechnetate scintiscan at 20 minutes shows accumulation of isotope in neck, heart, stomach, midabdomen, and urinary bladder (Figure 66-1).

At operation, a Meckel's diverticulum extends into umbilical hernia. Hernia is repaired. Diverticulum, a small segment of ileum, and appendix are removed.

Diverticulum (5 cm long, 1.5-cm diameter) has light purple serosa, smooth muscle, and gastric and small bowel mucosa. Appendix (5.5×0.5 cm) contains dark blood.

Abdomen is distended, and bowel sounds are absent 4 days after operation. Dark green liquid comes out of nasogastric tube. He passes a stool that looks like tarry clot.

In Figure 66-2, gas and excess liquid are in dilated gut.

He eats well and has normal stool 6 days after operation.

Diagnosis: Hemorrhage from Meckel's diverticulum that contains gastric mucosa, postoperative ileus.

(Continued)

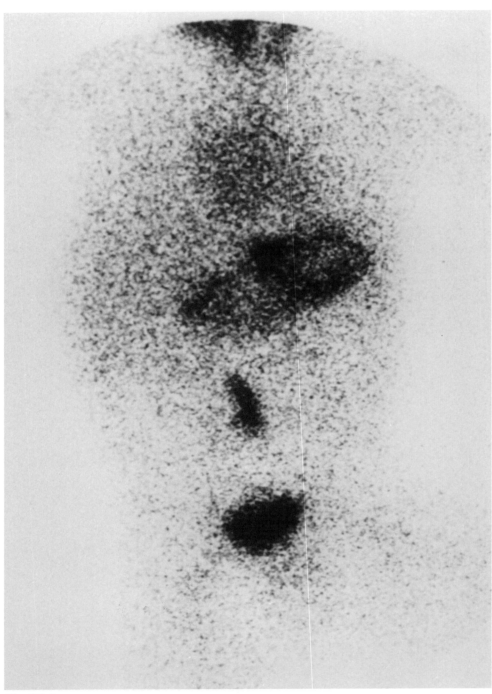

Fig. 66-1

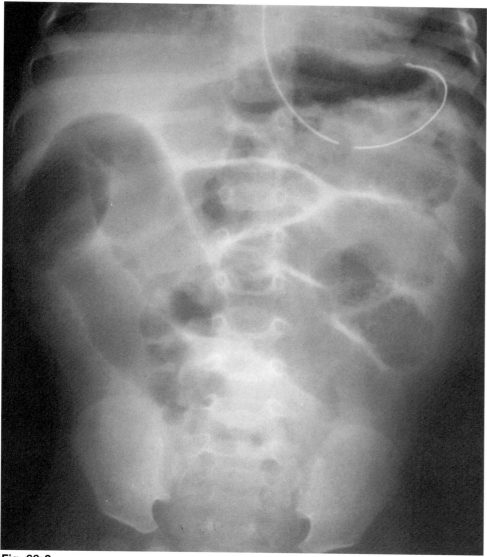

Fig. 66-2

Case 67

A 12-year-old girl vomits a lot of clear liquid several times per day.

Abdomen has always been bloated, more so in past year. Six months ago, she was sick for 1 week and vomited frequently. Since then she has had 5–7-day cycles of normal diet and activity, interrupted by spells of more bloating for several days and vomiting of up to 2 quarts of clear liquid several times per day. She has two to three soft stools per day. She was constipated from 13 months until 6 years. Colon biopsy at 18 months showed normal ganglion cells.

Temperature at 12 years is 36.9°C, heart rate 100, respiratory rate 20, blood pressure 110/65 mm Hg, weight 32.9 kg (5 months ago: 37.7), and height 153 cm. She is malnourished. Abdomen is distended, firm, and tympanitic. The rest of the physical findings are normal.

Hematocrit is 0.41. Urine specific gravity is 1.032, pH 7. Urine has 0.30 g/liter protein, 150 mg/liter ketones, and 4–6 white cells/HPF. Serum sodium is 137 mmol/liter, potassium 2.6, chloride 96, carbon dioxide 27, urea nitrogen 5.7, calcium 2.54, phosphorus 1.16, cholesterol 4.65, magnesium 0.86, and glucose 7.2. Creatinine is 80 μmol/liter, uric acid 330, total bilirubin 19, direct bilirubin 0, and zinc 11.3 (normal: 10.7–23.0). Total protein is 73 g/liter, albumin 46. Alkaline phosphatase is 109 U/liter, LDH 168, and SGOT 24.

In Figure 67-1, gut is dilated in varying degree with gas and liquid; barium shows change in caliber in descending colon.

Rectal biopsy shows ganglion cells.

Diagnosis: Intestinal pseudo-obstruction (questionable mitochondrial disease, questionable hypokalemia; repeat serum potassium is 3.1 mmol/liter).

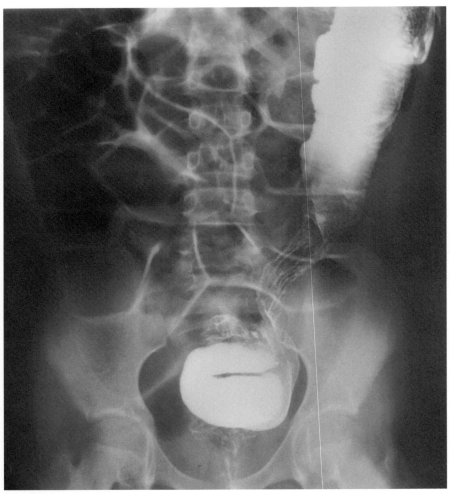

Fig. 67-1

Case 68

A 3-year-old girl is vomiting. She says her "belly button hurts." She has had a few freckles inside her lips since she was 1 year old.

Maternal grandmother had a section of bowel removed 4 years ago. Mother has buccal freckles and has been anemic.

Temperature is 37.2°C, heart rate 124, respiratory rate 32, blood pressure 98/62 mm Hg, and weight 13.8 kg. She is pale. Approximately 10 freckles are inside lips. Dilated gut is palpable. The rest of the physical findings are normal.

Hematocrit is 0.34. White cell count is 13.9×10^9/liter with 0.90 polymorphonuclear cells, 0.08 bands, and 0.02 lymphocytes. Platelet count is 481×10^9/liter. Serum sodium is 135 mmol/liter, potassium 4.7, chloride 104, carbon dioxide 15, urea nitrogen 4.6, calcium 2.37, phosphorus 1.61, cholesterol 4.65, and glucose 8.9 (IV fluids). Creatinine is 70 μmol/liter, uric acid 460, total bilirubin 5, and direct bilirubin 2. Total protein is 59 g/liter, albumin 41. Alkaline phosphatase is 238 U/liter, SGOT 32. Stool in rectum is guaiac negative.

Abdomen is tender next morning. Bowel sounds are diminished. Hematocrit is 0.26.

At operation, jejunojejunal intussusception, jejunal polyps, smaller ileal polyp, and many mesenteric lymph nodes are found. Sixty centimeters of necrotic jejunum is resected, end-to-end anastomosis performed, and appendix removed.

Dark red, firm resected gut contains a few pedunculated polyps (0.5–2.5 cm). Surface of appendix is beige to pink.

Microscopic examination shows hamartomatous polyps, normal appendix, and infarcted mesenteric lymph nodes.

She has occasional abdominal pain and black or blood-streaked stools. Pain is worse at 7 years. She vomits and will not eat. A mass is just to right of umbilicus. Hematocrit is 0.29 despite treatment with iron for 2 months.

GI series shows an intraluminal mass just beyond Treitz's ligament (Figure 68-1A) and small, round defects in stomach and small bowel (Figure 68-1B).

At operation, filmy adhesions are around gut. Two polyps (2.5 cm) on long stalks are removed from proximal jejunum.

She vomits and has abdominal pain and left lower quadrant fullness at 9 years. Hematocrit is 0.30. At operation, two polyps are in fourth part of duodenum, and duodenum is intussuscepted into jejunum. Distal duodenum, polyps, and proximal jejunum are removed, and end-to-end anastomosis is performed. She is jaundiced 10 days later. At endoscopy, small polyps are in stomach, a polyp is in third part of duodenum, and papilla of Vater is too ectopic to be cannulated. She is treated with sphincteroplasty and biliary stent, which is removed after 5 months.

Diagnosis: Peutz-Jeghers syndrome, intussusception.

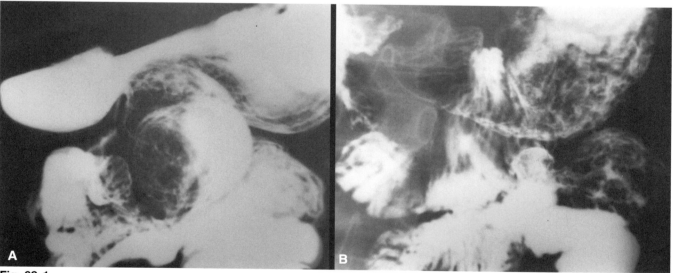

Fig. 68-1

Case 69

A 2½-month-old girl has puffy eyelids and feet.

Eyelids have been puffy since birth, feet for 1½ weeks. She has been fussy and gassy for 2 weeks. Eyes tear excessively.

Pregnancy of mother was normal, birth weight 3.5 kg, length 51 cm, head circumference 33 cm, and Apgar score 7/9 at 1 and 5 minutes. She is breast-fed. Weight at 3 weeks was 3.4 kg. Supplemental formula was added. Weight at 4 weeks was 3.1 kg. Rice and barley cereal were added.

Mother (25 years old) and father (29 years old) are well. She is their first child.

Weight at 2½ months is 5 kg, length 52 cm, head circumference 38 cm, temperature 36.7°C, heart rate 124, respiratory rate 60, and systolic blood pressure 78 mm Hg. Lids are edematous, corneas cloudy. Diameter of right cornea is 14–15 mm, left cornea 13 mm. Pressure in right eye is 45 mm Hg, left eye 44. Abdomen is protuberant and tense with taut skin, prominent veins, and umbilical hernia. Pitting edema is in feet and lower legs. The rest of the physical findings are normal.

Echocardiogram shows enlargement of left atrium and small pericardial effusion.

Hematocrit is 0.31. White cell count is 17.4 × 10⁹/liter with 0.41 polymorphonuclear cells, 0.02 bands, 0.50 lymphocytes, and 0.07 monocytes. Urine specific gravity is 1.005, pH 5. Urine has 15–20 white cells/HPF. Serum sodium is 141 mmol/liter, potassium 5.4, chloride 112, carbon dioxide 20, urea nitrogen 2.5, calcium 2.07, phosphorus 2.39, cholesterol 2.30, and glucose 6.8. Creatinine is 50 µmol/liter, uric acid 180, total bilirubin 5, and direct bilirubin 2. Total protein is 31 g/liter, albumin 21. Alkaline phosphatase is 255 U/liter,

LDH 265, and SGOT 32. Serum IgG is 0.49 g/liter (normal: 2.0–7.0), IgA 0.12 (normal: 0.04–0.80), and IgM 0.21 (normal: 0.25–1.00). T-lymphocyte number and function are normal. Serum VDRL test is nonreactive, rubella titer <1:8, toxoplasmosis IFA-IgM test negative, cytomegalovirus CF titer <1:8, and herpes CF titer <1:8. Stool fat on diet in which fat consists of medium chain triglycerides is 1.58 g/day (normal: <2). Duodenal trypsin activity is present at 1:320 dilution. Duodenal lipase is 122 units. A specimen of small bowel mucosa obtained by capsule is nondiagnostic.

Small bowel is featureless and contains excess liquid (Figure 69-1). A round shadow of water density in midabdomen (Figure 69-1A) is caused by an umbilical hernia. A bezoar, presumably inspissated milk and cereal, is in stomach (Figure 69-1B).

A brother is born 1 year later. He has episodes of puffy eyelids, distended abdomen, flatulence, and diarrhea. Left cornea is larger than right. Pressure in left eye is 49 mm Hg, right eye 17. He has epicanthi. Twenty-four–hour urine does not contain excess protein.

Serum vitamin E level in girl at 8 years is 5.6 µg/ml (normal: 5–20); in boy at 7 years, serum vitamin E level is 4 µg/ml. Her serum level of α_1-antitrypsin at 8 years is 1.8 g/liter (normal: 1.5–3.5), stool α_1-antitrypsin 1.1 mg/g stool, and clearance 152.0 ml/24 hr (normal: 0.0–12.5). His serum level of α_1-antitrypsin at 7 years is 1.9 g/liter, stool α_1-antitrypsin 0.9 mg/g stool, and clearance 246.0 ml/24 hr.

Diagnosis: Intestinal lymphangiectasia (without histologic proof), congenital glaucoma in sister and brother.

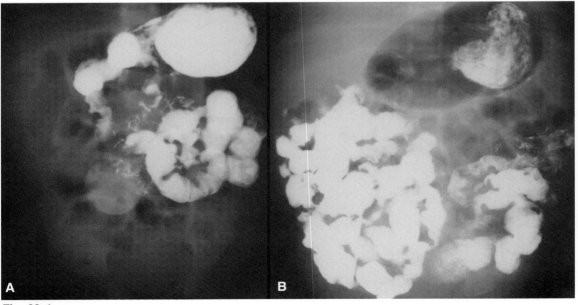

Fig. 69-1

Case 70

A 17-month-old girl vomits undigested food.

Two months ago, she vomited once per week, then several times per week, and now she vomits every day, usually after dinner. Abdomen has been protuberant for 2 months. She has gained 0.7 kg in 5 months. She is now crankier and less active. Stools are normal.

Pregnancy was normal, birth weight 4.2 kg. She was gray and breathed noisily at 6 hours and was given an antibiotic for 10 days. She walked at 10 months, used a few words at 1 year, and now climbs stairs. She was started on solid food and whole milk in place of formula at 1 year. She had chickenpox at 6 months.

Parents have hay fever. She is their only child. Maternal grandmother had colon cancer; paternal grandmother had hepatitis.

Temperature at 17 months is 37.2°C, heart rate 124, respiratory rate 36, systolic blood pressure 90 mm Hg, weight 9.3 kg, and height 80 cm. Limbs are thin. Abdomen protrudes and is tympanitic. Umbilicus protrudes. The rest of the physical findings are normal.

Hematocrit is 0.41. White cell count is 9.9×10^9/liter with 0.31 polymorphonuclear cells, 0.04 bands, 0.48 lymphocytes,

0.14 monocytes, 0.01 eosinophils, and 0.02 basophils. Serum sodium is 136 mmol/liter, potassium 5.2, chloride 99, carbon dioxide 20, urea nitrogen 5.0, calcium 2.44, phosphorus 1.29, cholesterol 3.13, and glucose 4.2. Creatinine is 50 µmol/liter, uric acid 330, total bilirubin 3, and direct bilirubin 0. Total protein is 66 g/liter, albumin 43. Alkaline phosphatase is 179 U/liter, LDH 443, and SGOT 59.

Barium puddles and flocculates in dilated gut, and contrast medium is in bladder from earlier excretory urogram (Figure 70-1).

D-xylose absorption is 0.7 mmol/liter (normal: >2.7). Serum carotenoids are 1.0 µmol/liter (normal: 1.5–7.4).

Microscopic examination of small bowel obtained with biopsy capsule at Treitz's ligament shows (1) loss of villi, (2) widely separated mucosal crypts, (3) mucosal epithelium consisting of a single layer of low columnar cells with atypical nuclei and poorly demarcated cytoplasmic boundaries, and (4) many plasma cells and normal lymphocytes in lamina propria.

Diagnosis: Celiac disease. (She is given a gluten-free diet. At 11 years, weight is 63 kg, height 163 cm. Physical findings are normal.)

(Continued)

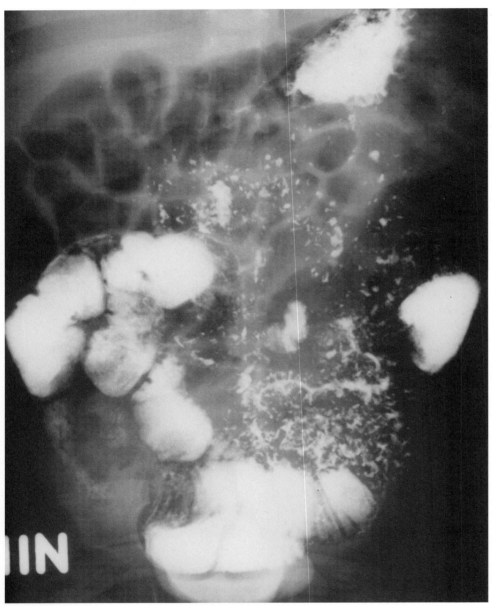

Fig. 70-1

Case 71

A 2-month-old girl will not eat and is lethargic. She was well until 2 days ago when she refused breast-feeding. She has not vomited. She has a stool every 3 days.

Parents are well. She is their only child.

Mother had vaginal discharge during third trimester. Birth weight was 3.5 kg. Breast-feedings were supplemented with 8 oz of formula per day at 5 weeks.

Weight is 5.1 kg, length 61 cm, temperature 37°C, heart rate 120, respiratory rate 30, and systolic blood pressure 140 mm Hg in arms and legs. Heart rate is suddenly 200 for several minutes, then 180, and then 130–140 during examination. Baby is alert. She lies with limbs flat on bed. She responds to pain with grimace and whimper. Cry is weak and gurgling. Eyes are glassy. Tongue protrudes. Gag reflex is absent. Abdomen is soft. Bowel sounds are normal. Muscle tone is decreased. Knee reflex is hyperactive. The rest of the physical findings are normal.

Hematocrit is 0.36. White cell count is 12.2×10^9/liter with 0.44 polymorphonuclear cells, 0.06 bands, 0.45 lymphocytes, and 0.05 monocytes. ESR is 6 mm/hr. Urine specific gravity is 1.025, pH 5. Urine has 1–3 epithelial cells/HPF. Serum sodium is 137 mmol/liter, potassium 3.6, chloride 101, and calcium 2.37. CSF has 5×10^6/liter white cells (all lymphocytes) and 2.3 mmol/liter glucose. Blood and spinal fluid are sterile.

Gas is in undilated gut throughout abdomen and displaced from pelvis by urinary bladder (Figure 71-1).

EMG shows normal conduction velocity and reduced amplitude of compound muscle potential.

Stool culture is positive for *Clostridium botulinum*, type A.

Diagnosis: Botulism.

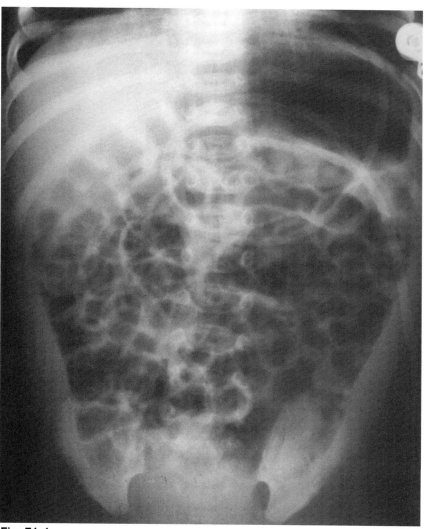

Fig. 71-1

Case 72

A 21-month-old girl has had occasional diarrhea for 5 months and vomiting and occasional fever for 1 month. Nose has been runny, and eyes have been watery for 3 days.

Temperature is 39.5°C, heart rate 140, respiratory rate 24, blood pressure 118/66 mm Hg, weight 8.7 kg, and head circumference 45 cm. A red papule is on soft palate. Small lymph nodes are in left side of neck. The rest of the physical findings are normal.

Hematocrit is 0.31. White cell count is 10.5×10^9/liter with 0.38 polymorphonuclear cells, 0.02 bands, 0.51 lymphocytes, 0.07 monocytes, and 0.02 eosinophils. Platelet count is 408×10^9/liter. Serum sodium is 136 mmol/liter, potassium 4.1, chloride 102, carbon dioxide 21, urea nitrogen 4.0, calcium 2.42, phosphorus 1.39, cholesterol 3.54, and glucose 4.3.

Creatinine is 30 μmol/liter, uric acid 250, total bilirubin 5, and direct bilirubin 2. Total protein is 75 g/liter, albumin 44. Alkaline phosphatase is 213 U/liter, LDH 236, and SGOT 25. Stool is pasty, light tan, and negative for blood and reducing substances.

In Figure 72-1, barium shows small, round defects in duodenum and jejunum.

Microscopic examination of stool shows (1) many *Giardia lamblia* cysts, (2) moderate *Endolimax* cysts, and (3) rare *Blastocystis hominis*.

Diagnosis: Lymphoid hyperplasia, small bowel; intestinal parasites.

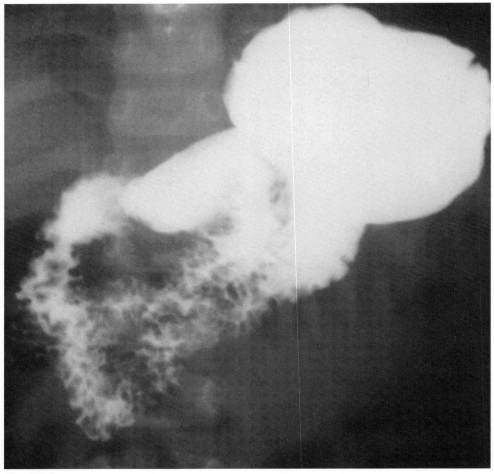

Fig. 72-1

Case 73

A 7-year-old girl has fever and diarrhea.

Pregnancy of mother was normal, birth weight 3.2 kg. At 5 years, she was occasionally constipated, sometimes had pain when she defecated, and sometimes soiled her pants. She had watery stools for a week 4 months ago, then firmer stools with mucus and streaks of blood. Two months ago, she had fever, aches in legs, abdominal cramps, and four to nine stools per day. One month ago, left knee was swollen and painful for 2 days. She had chickenpox 3 months ago.

Mother (33 years old), father (36 years old), and three younger sisters are well. Eleven months ago, she visited an uncle who was last week diagnosed with tuberculosis.

Temperature at 7 years is 38°C, heart rate 102, respiratory rate 20, weight 19 kg, and height 115 cm. She is pale. The rest of the physical findings are normal.

Hemoglobin is 90 g/liter. White cell count is 9.8×10^9/liter with 0.63 polymorphonuclear cells, 0.04 bands, 0.30 lym-phocytes, and 0.03 monocytes. ESR is 28 mm/hr. Urine specific gravity is 1.001, pH 6. Urine has 0–1 white cell/HPF and rare epithelial cells/HPF. Serum sodium is 140 mmol/liter, potassium 4.4, chloride 98, calcium 2.50, and phosphorus 1.39. Total protein is 75 g/liter, albumin 35. Iron is 4 µmol/liter (normal: 9.0–21.5), total iron-binding capacity 40 (normal: 44.8–80.6).

Skin test with intermediate strength PPD is negative.

Excretory urogram (Figure 73-1A) shows normal findings in urinary tract and constant, unusual collection of gas over right sacroiliac joint that is shown to be static terminal ileum by GI series at (7 years and) 11 years (Figure 73-1B). Both GI series show abnormal cecum and ascending colon.

Diagnosis: Crohn's disease.

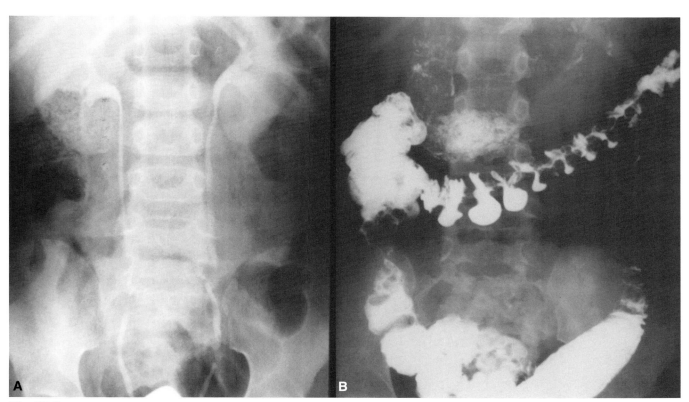

Fig. 73-1

Case 74

A 5-month-old girl is limp and barely responsive. She has vomited several times since yesterday. She has had a cough for 3 days.

Temperature is 38.4°C, heart rate 150, respiratory rate 50, blood pressure 84/60, and weight 7.0 kg. Mouth is dry. She has a systolic murmur. A mass is in right lower quadrant of abdomen. The rest of the physical findings are normal.

Hematocrit is 0.35. White cell count is 15.8×10^9/liter with 0.41 polymorphonuclear cells, 0.37 bands, 0.16 lymphocytes, and 0.06 monocytes. Platelet count is 411×10^9/liter. Urine specific gravity is 1.034, pH 6. Urine has 1+ ketones, amorphous urates, and uric acid crystals. Serum sodium is 143 mmol/liter, potassium 4.6, chloride 109, urea nitrogen 3.6, calcium 2.47, and glucose 6.1. Creatinine is 60 µmol/liter.

Barium enema (barium sulfate in equal amounts water and normal saline) shows normal colon and appendix and obstruction to retrograde flow of barium that is first encountered in distal ileum (Figure 74-1).

At operation, serous liquid is in peritoneum, and a dusky mass and intussuscepted Meckel's diverticulum are in ileum near ileocecal valve. Diverticulum, 12 cm of distal ileum, and appendix are resected. Ileoileal anastomosis is made.

Examination of resected ileum shows a fibrous loop 4 cm from one end and a Meckel's diverticulum 4 cm from other end, which slips through loop with diverticulum. Middle 4 cm of resected ileum is dusky purple. Microscopic examination of diverticulum (6.0 × 1.5 cm) shows blood clot and hemorrhagic, black, necrotic mucosa. Mucosa of middle 4 cm of ileum is hemorrhagic and necrotic. Lymphoid follicles are hyperplastic in rest of ileum. Appendix is normal.

Diagnosis: Ileoileal intussusception, Meckel's diverticulum in intussusceptum, lymphoid hyperplasia as lead point.

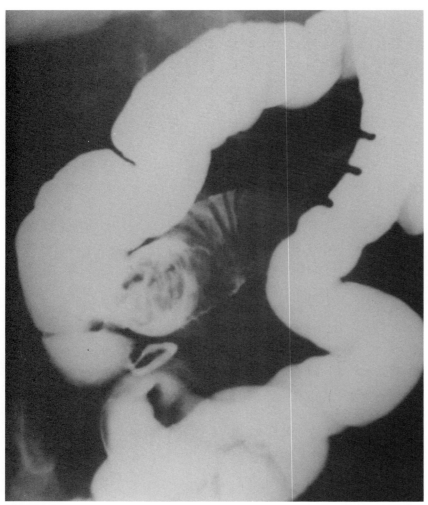

Fig. 74-1

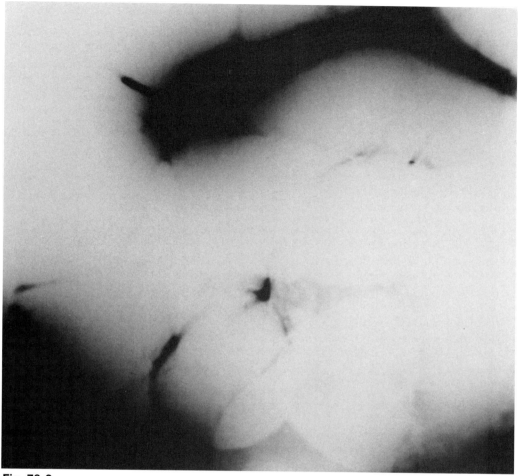

Fig. 76-2

Case 77

A 7-year-old girl is vomiting and has abdominal cramps during which she cries, holds her abdomen, and lies on side with knees drawn up.

Cramps began 1 week ago, vomiting yesterday. She is constipated and will not eat.

Birth weight was 3.7 kg. She had respiratory infections, wheezing, and ear infections during the first few years.

Weight is 23.8 kg, height 118 cm, temperature 36.9°C, heart rate 120, respiratory rate 26, and blood pressure 106/68 mm Hg. Abdomen is tender, especially in left lower quadrant, which feels full. Normal bowel sounds become louder and higher pitched during cramps. The rest of the physical findings are normal.

Hematocrit is 0.47. White cell count is 15.0×10^9/liter with 0.79 polymorphonuclear cells, 0.02 bands, 0.18 lymphocytes, and 0.01 monocytes. Platelet count is 507×10^9/liter. One hour after IV saline and glucose are begun, urine specific gravity is 1.033, pH 5. Urine has 5.6 mmol/liter glucose, >0.80 g/liter ketones, 0.30 g/liter protein, occasional squamous epithelial cells/HPF, and 5–10 white cells/HPF. Before IV fluids, serum sodium is 138 mmol/liter, potassium 4.5, chloride 97, carbon dioxide 23, urea nitrogen 3.6, and glucose 5.9. Creatinine is 70 μmol/liter.

Ultrasound examination in Figure 77-1 shows a hypoechoic mass in midabdomen (Figure 77-1). Barium outlines what seems to be a mass in transverse colon 5 hours after start of GI series (Figure 77-2A) and is around a mass after 18 hours (Figure 77-2B).

At operation, irreducible ileocolic intussusception and large mesenteric lymph nodes are found. Distal ileum, cecum, appendix, and three large mesenteric nodes are resected. Ileocolic anastomosis is made.

Examination of operative specimen (17 cm of ileum and cecum with appendix attached) shows intussusception (5-cm diameter) and three lymph nodes (≤3.5-cm diameter). Cut section of intussusception just distal to ileocecal valve is fish-flesh white with foci of hemorrhage and necrosis. Base of appendix is part of intussusceptum. Microscopic examination of intussusceptum shows uniform lymphoid cells and scattered histiocytes, like a starry sky. Cell margins of lymphocytes are indistinct. A thin rim of vacuolated cytoplasm is around nuclei, which have stippled chromatin and many nucleoli. Mitoses are many. Tumor cells are in all layers of wall of intussusceptum, in base of appendix, and not in intussuscipiens or mesenteric nodes. The monoclonal B cells are stained by antibodies to IgM, lambda, CALLA, and two pan B–cell antibodies.

Diagnosis: Ileocolic intussusception, Burkitt's lymphoma.

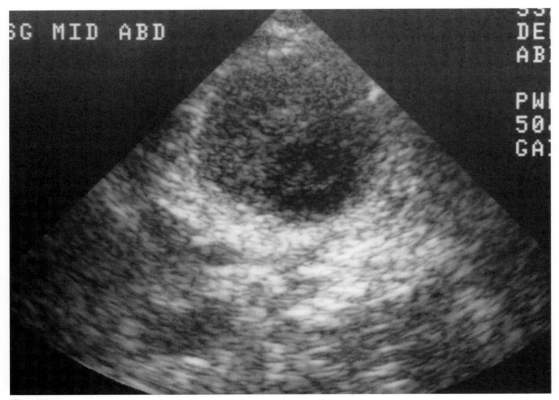

Fig. 77-1

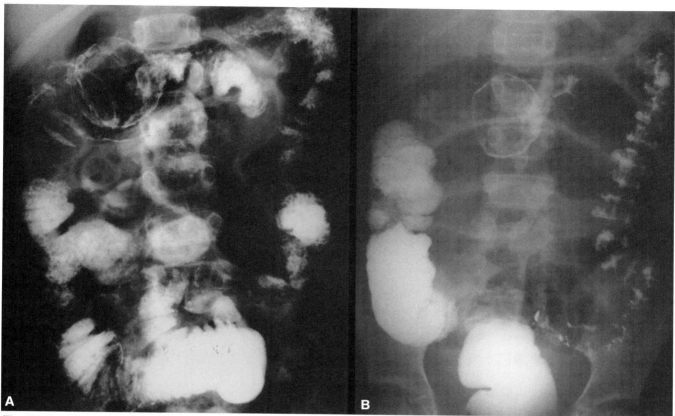

Fig. 77-2

Case 78

A 2-day-old boy has a distended abdomen.

Mother (27 years old) had poliomyelitis at 3 years and gestational diabetes. Members of her family have diabetes mellitus.

Birth weight is 3.3 kg, Apgar score 8/8 at 1 and 5 minutes, and temperature 35.6°C. At 2 days, heart rate is 150, respiratory rate 70, and systolic blood pressure 90 mm Hg. Abdomen is distended and tympanitic. Bowel sounds are few. The rest of the physical findings are normal.

Hematocrit is 0.42. White cell count is 13.5×10^9/liter with 0.74 polymorphonuclear cells, 0.05 bands, 0.08 lymphocytes, 0.11 monocytes, 0.01 metamyelocytes, and 0.01 myelocytes. Platelet count is 338×10^9/liter. Serum sodium is 122 mmol/liter, potassium 5.4, chloride 96, calcium 1.57, and glucose 5.0. Total bilirubin is 97 μmol/liter.

Sigmoid and part of descending colon are constricted (Figure 78-1).

He has first stool 3 hours after barium enema, next small one at 78 hours when green liquid comes out of nasogastric tube. He has two large stools at 6 days, no abdominal distension, and no drainage from nasogastric tube.

Diagnosis: Small left colon syndrome in newborn of mother with gestational diabetes.

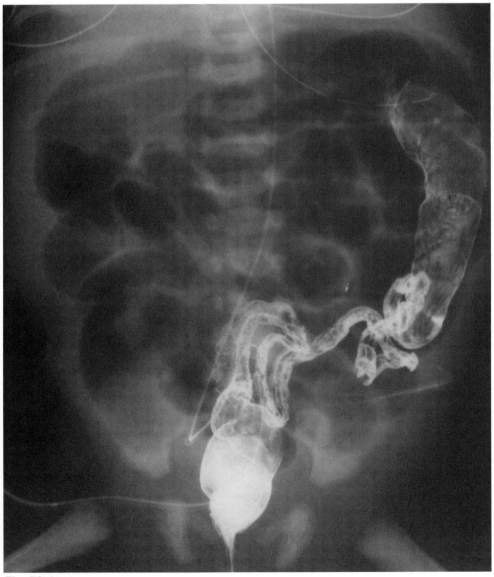

Fig. 78-1

Case 79

A 6-day-old boy is vomiting. He is hard to feed and cries a lot.

Pregnancy of mother was normal, birth weight 2.9 kg, and Apgar score 9/9 at 1 and 5 minutes. At 4 days, he refused a feeding and vomited twice. He was cranky yesterday while feeding. Temperature at 5 days was 36.6°C, heart rate 160, and respiratory rate 60.

Temperature is 38.3°C, systolic blood pressure 70 mm Hg, and head circumference 33 cm. Abdomen is slightly distended. A reducible hydrocele is in right side of scrotum. Mucousy, guaiac-positive stool is in rectum. The rest of the physical findings are normal.

Hematocrit at 5 days was 0.39. White count was 14.8×10^9/liter with 0.61 polymorphonuclear cells, 0.12 bands, 0.14 lymphocytes, 0.09 monocytes, and 0.04 eosinophils. Serum sodium at 6 days is 142 mmol/liter, potassium 4.8, and urea nitrogen 4.0. Total bilirubin is 115 µmol/liter, direct bilirubin 39.

In Figure 79-1, barium enema shows mass at hepatic flexure.

Abdomen is more distended after barium enema. Bowel sounds are diminished.

At operation, 50 ml cloudy yellow liquid is in abdomen. Gut is matted and edematous. Mesentery is short. A mass is in cecum, a perforation is 3 cm distal to mass, and white matter is on serosa. Distal ileum and ascending colon are resected.

Outer surface of spherical mass (2-cm diameter) is brown-tan, inner surface is white.

Culture of abdominal liquid grows *Escherichia coli* and *Bacteroides fragilis*.

Barium is in peritoneum and right scrotal hydrocele 2 weeks after operation (Figure 79-2A) and 8 years later in roentgenogram made before cystogram for urinary frequency (Figure 79-2B).

Diagnosis: Duplication of colon, perforation during barium enema.

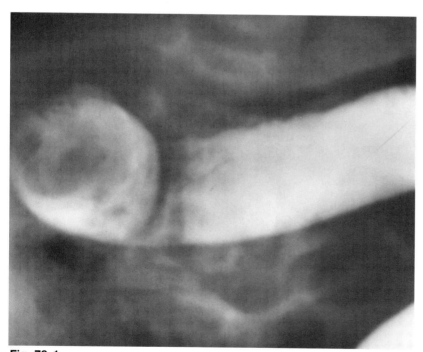

Fig. 79-1

(Continued)

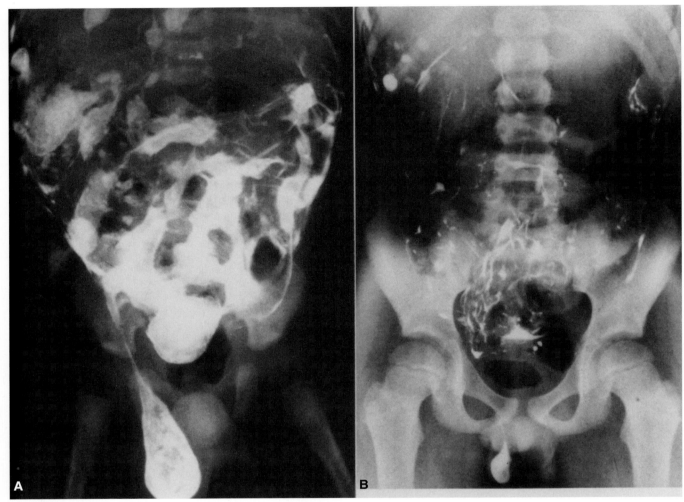

Fig. 79-2

Case 80

A 1-day-old girl has a distended abdomen.

Mother (27 years old) is well. Maternal grandmother has diabetes mellitus; maternal grandfather has lung cancer.

Pregnancy of mother was normal, amount of amniotic fluid normal. Birth weight was 3 kg, Apgar score 7/8 at 1 and 5 minutes. At 1 hour, heart rate was 120, respiratory rate 64, and systolic blood pressure 64 mm Hg. Abdomen is flaccid, doughy, and distended at 1 day. The rest of the physical findings are normal.

Hematocrit at 1 day is 0.50. White cell count is 19.1 × 10⁹/liter with 0.64 polymorphonuclear cells, 0.30 lymphocytes, 0.03 monocytes, 0.01 eosinophils, and 0.02 basophils. Serum calcium is 2.64 mmol/liter, glucose 4.2. Total bilirubin is 67 µmol/liter.

She urinates the first day but does not pass meconium.

Moderately dilated gut is displaced up and left by mass of water density, which cystogram shows to be bladder. Barium shows hypoperistalsis and narrow distal colon at 30 hours (Figure 80-1A) and 54 hours (Figure 80-1B).

At 3 days, serum sodium is 143 mmol/liter, potassium 3.7, chloride 106, carbon dioxide 25, urea nitrogen 2.8, calcium 2.32, phosphorus 2.10, cholesterol 4.22, and glucose 7.8. Creatinine is 70 µmol/liter, uric acid 210, total bilirubin 195, and direct bilirubin 12. Total protein is 56 g/liter, albumin 35. Alkaline phosphatase is 156 U/liter, LDH 526, and SGOT 29.

She still has not passed meconium at 85 hours. Abdomen is distended and soft. She has runny stools at 4 days. She is hypotonic at 5 days. Abdomen is still lax at 13 days, when she goes home.

Diagnosis: Intestinal hypoperistalsis, megacystis-microcolon type.

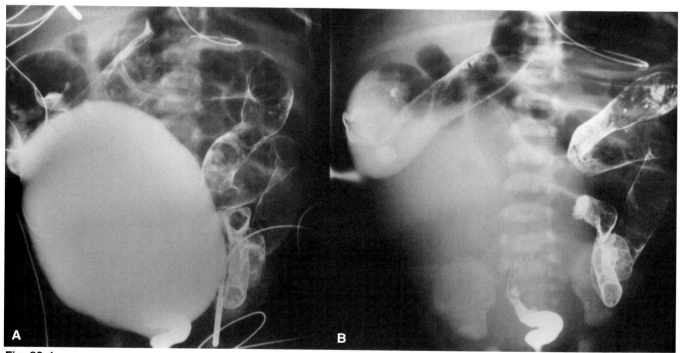

Fig. 80-1

Case 81

A 2-day-old boy is vomiting bile and has not passed meconium.

Pregnancy of mother was normal. Birth weight was 3.8 kg, Apgar score 7/9 at 1 and 15 minutes, temperature 36.1°C, heart rate 150, and respiratory rate 60. At 2 days, systolic blood pressure is 60 mm Hg. Thick yellow liquid, 15 ml, is aspirated from stomach. Abdomen is distended and tympanitic. The rest of the physical findings are normal.

Hematocrit is 0.44. Serum sodium is 136 mmol/liter, potassium 5.1, and chloride 96. Urine specific gravity is 1.016, pH 5.5. Urine has 2+ protein, 2+ glucose, 1–3 white cells/HPF, occasional epithelial cells/HPF, uric acid crystals, and amorphous sediment.

In Figure 81-1, a large sac of gas and liquid is in right side of abdomen, gas is in stomach and undilated small bowel in left side and in pelvis.

At operation, cecum and ascending colon are distended proximal to atresia at hepatic flexure.

Diagnosis: Colon atresia, competent ileocecal valve.

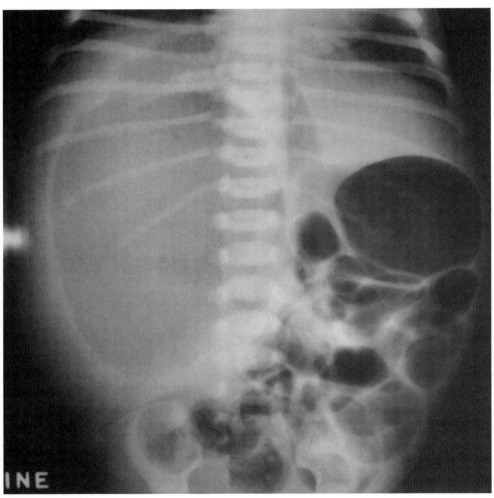

Fig. 81-1

Case 82

A 7-month-old boy is vomiting and constipated.

He was weaned at 5 months. He has been vomiting for 2 months, constipated 1 month.

Pregnancy of mother was normal.

Parents and sister, who is thought to have food allergy, are well.

Weight at 7 months is 7.1 kg, temperature 37°C, heart rate 140, respiratory rate 24, and blood pressure 104/68 mm Hg. He is pale, irritable, and lethargic. Back is arched. Abdomen is distended and tympanitic. Liver edge is 1 cm below costal margin. The rest of the physical findings are normal.

Hematocrit is 0.20. White cell count is 18.2 × 10⁹/liter with 0.32 polymorphonuclear cells, 0.19 bands, 0.40 lymphocytes, 0.08 monocytes, and 0.01 metamyelocytes. ESR is 30 mm/hr. Urine specific gravity is 1.009, pH 6. Urine has trace glucose, 1–2 red cells/HPF, 40–50 white cells/HPF, and 6–8 casts/LPF. Serum sodium is 139 mmol/liter, potassium 3.7, chloride 101, calcium 1.92, and glucose 2.7. Total bilirubin is 3 μmol/liter, direct bilirubin 2. Total protein is 41 g/liter, albumin 19.

Preliminary roentgenogram shows a mass of water density in right side of abdomen (Figure 82-1A). Caliber and length of colon are normal in barium enema with barium sulfate and equal amounts of water and normal saline (Figure 82-1B). Small diverticula protrude from ascending colon, which is displaced medially (see Figure 82-1B).

At operation, small bowel is dilated, especially distal ileum.

Biopsy at various levels of colon and terminal ileum shows isolated nerve trunks and no ganglion cells.

Diagnosis: Hirschsprung's disease, total colonic aganglionosis.

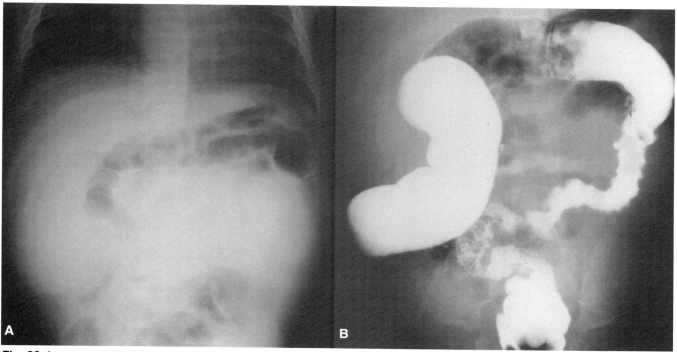

Fig. 82-1

Case 83

A 4-day-old boy is vomiting.

Mother (28 years old), father (30 years old), and two sisters (2 and 6 years old) are well. Paternal grandmother had cancer; maternal great-grandmother had diabetes mellitus.

Pregnancy of mother was normal, birth weight 3.1 kg, length 51 cm, head circumference 35 cm, Apgar score 8/10 at 1 and 5 minutes, and blood glucose 3.3 mmol/liter. He fed poorly or not at all, vomited yellow mucus, vomited feedings, and did not have a meconium stool until glycerine rectal suppository at 4 days.

Weight is 2.7 kg, temperature 37.1°C, heart rate 156, respiratory rate 48, and systolic blood pressure 78 mm Hg. He is jaundiced. Skin turgor is poor. Abdomen is distended, firm, and tympanitic. Bowel sounds are decreased. The rest of the physical findings are normal.

Hematocrit is 0.47. White cell count is 3.9×10^9/liter with 0.18 polymorphonuclear cells, 0.11 bands, 0.40 lymphocytes, 0.26 monocytes, 0.02 eosinophils, and 0.03 basophils. Serum sodium is 147 mmol/liter, potassium 4.8, and chloride 103. Total bilirubin is 200 μmol/liter, direct bilirubin 36 (peak total bilirubin: 280 at 8 days).

Throughout abdomen, gut is uniformly dilated with gas and liquid (Figure 83-1A). Barium enema with barium sulfate and equal amounts water and normal saline suggests change in colonic caliber at splenic flexure; barium has been put into stomach through a tube because of uncertainty about change in colonic caliber (Figure 83-1B).

He is treated by colostomy at 7 days and by colorectal anastomosis at 8 months. He vomits and has watery stools at 10 months. Vomiting is worse at 1 year, abdomen is distended, and he has no bowel movement for 3 days.

Temperature at 1 year is 37.4°C, heart rate 136, respiratory rate 36, systolic blood pressure 90 mm Hg, weight 10.2 kg, and height 76 cm. Abdomen is distended and scarred. Bowel sounds are increased.

Barium put into rectum at 1 year flows back through small anastomosis into colon, which has filling defects (Figure 83-2).

Colorectal anastomosis (1.5 cm) is enlarged at proctoscopy. A new colorectal anastomosis is made at 3½ years.

Diagnosis: Hirschsprung's disease with aganglionosis to splenic flexure, obstruction at Duhamel's anastomosis, questionable secondary mural irregularity.

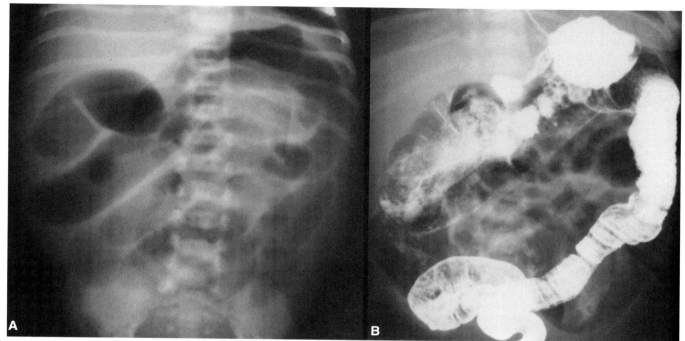

Fig. 83-1

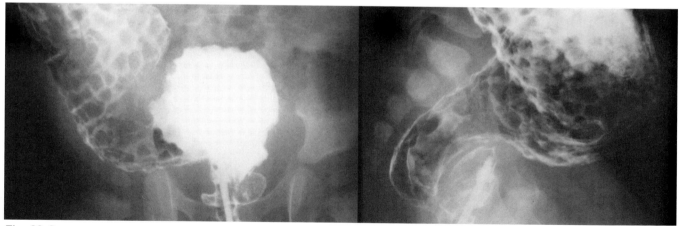

Fig. 83-2

Case 84

A 40-hour-old boy is vomiting bile and has had no stool.

Pregnancy of mother was normal, Apgar score 9/10 at 1 and 5 minutes, birth weight 4.5 kg, length 56 cm, and head circumference 38 cm. He breast-fed well until he vomited mucus at 18 and 20 hours. He refused to feed and went to sleep. He began to vomit bile at 24 hours. Abdomen was tight and shiny at 37 hours. He was uncomfortable when moved.

Mother, sister (3 years old), and brother (1½ years old) are well. Father has macular degeneration. Grandfathers have diabetes mellitus.

Temperature at 40 hours is 36.5°C, heart rate 145, respiratory rate 50, systolic blood pressure 75 mm Hg, and weight 4.1 kg. Abdomen is distended. Bowel sounds are absent. The rest of the physical findings are normal.

Hematocrit is 0.60. White cell count is 13.7 × 10⁹/liter with 0.78 polymorphonuclear cells, 0.15 lymphocytes, 0.05 mono-cytes, and 0.02 eosinophils. Platelet estimate is normal. Serum sodium is 143 mmol/liter, potassium 4.0, chloride 105, and carbon dioxide 21. Total bilirubin is 149 µmol/liter.

Gut is uniformly dilated with gas and liquid in frontal examination (Figure 84-1A). Rectum and part of sigmoid are constricted in lateral examination (Figure 84-1B). Barium enema with barium sulfate and equal amounts water and normal saline shows distal rectosigmoid constriction and proximal sigmoid dilation.

At colostomy, ganglion cells are in dilated proximal sigmoid and not in constricted distal sigmoid.

Diagnosis: Hirschsprung's disease with transition zone in sigmoid colon.

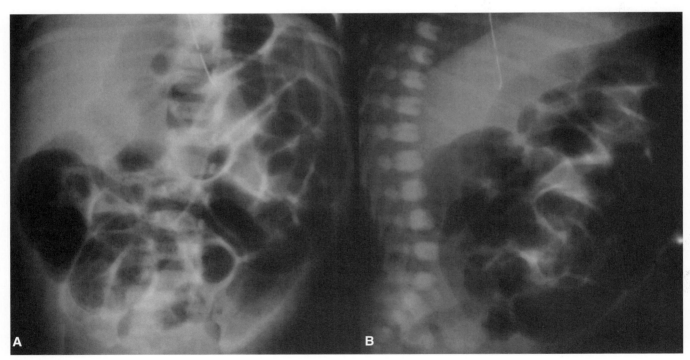

Fig. 84-1

Case 85

An 8½-month-old boy is constipated. Stools are infrequent, usually small, and sometimes blood streaked. Birth weight was 3.3 kg.

Weight is 7.5 kg, length 70 cm, head circumference 45 cm, temperature 36.5°C, heart rate 135, respiratory rate 40, and systolic blood pressure 90 mm Hg. Stool is palpable in lower part of distended abdomen. Hard stool is in rectum. The rest of the physical findings are normal.

Hematocrit is 0.36. White cell count is 12.6×10^9/liter with 0.29 polymorphonuclear cells, 0.01 bands, 0.63 lymphocytes, and 0.07 monocytes. Platelet count is 590×10^9/liter. Urine specific gravity is 1.016, pH 7. Urine is normal.

Plain film shows stool in distended, elongated, ectopic sigmoid colon (Figure 85-1). Barium enema with barium sulfate and equal amounts water and normal saline shows abnormal sigmoid (Figure 85-2A) and change in caliber and transition zone at rectosigmoid junction in lateral examination (Figure 85-2B).

Biopsy of rectal mucosa shows no ganglion cells in frozen section. At operation for diverting colostomy, wall of sigmoid is 0.2 cm thick. Ganglion cells are in sigmoid myenteric plexus. Soave anastomosis is performed at 1 year.

Diagnosis: Hirschsprung's disease, rectosigmoid transition zone.

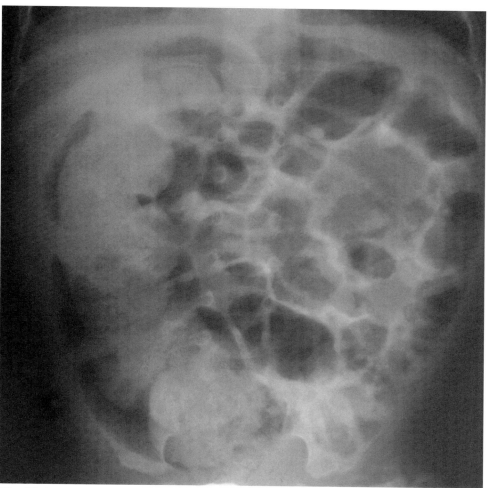

Fig. 85-1

(Continued)

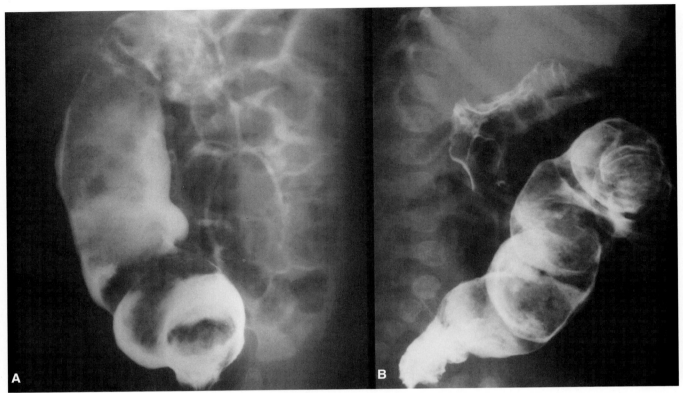

Fig. 85-2

Case 86

A newborn girl vomits green mucus.

Father had Hirschsprung's disease. The girl is his first child.

Pregnancy of mother (22 years old) was normal. Birth weight is 3.4 kg, length 53 cm, head circumference 34 cm, and Apgar score 8/9 at 1 and 5 minutes. Green bile is on blanket near baby's head at 18 hours. Temperature is 37°C, heart rate 140, respiratory rate 20, and blood pressure 79/64 mm Hg. Abdomen is round. The rest of the physical findings are normal. She has had a meconium stool.

Hematocrit is 0.54. White cell count is 28.6 × 10^9/liter with 0.67 polymorphonuclear cells, 0.06 bands, 0.21 lymphocytes, 0.05 monocytes, and 0.01 eosinophils. Platelet count is 466 × 10^9/liter.

Her brother, born 20 months later, vomits water at 2 days.

His temperature is 37.6°C, heart rate 142, respiratory rate 42, blood pressure 82/63 mm Hg, weight 3.4 kg, length 54 cm, and head circumference 36 cm. Anterior fontanel is slightly depressed, mouth dry. The rest of the physical findings are normal.

He has first meconium stool just before roentgenographic examination.

His hematocrit is 0.47. White cell count is 15.5 × 10^9/liter. Platelet count is 311 × 10^9/liter.

Throughout girl's abdomen, gut is uniformly dilated with gas and liquid at 20 hours (Figure 86-1A). Boy's abdomen looks normal at 3 days (Figure 86-1B).

At operation, distal ileum is constricted in both infants.

Microscopic examination shows myenteric ganglion cells to 20 cm proximal to ileocecal valve in girl, and to 5 cm proximal to ileocecal valve in boy, and none in distal ileum, appendix, or colon in either.

Diagnosis: Familial Hirschsprung's disease.

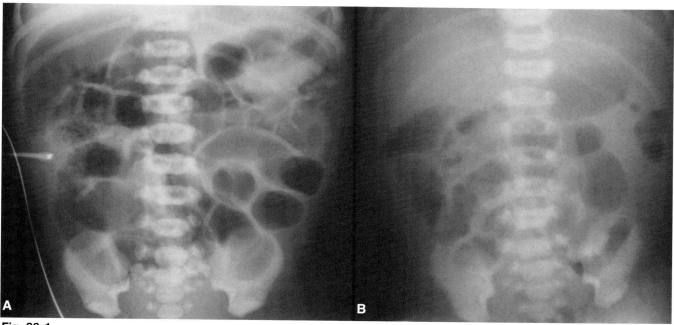

Fig. 86-1

Case 87

A 29-month-old girl is constipated. She has a bowel movement at 7- to 10-day intervals after an enema and does not soil herself between bowel movements. Stools were normal until breast-feeding was stopped at 3 months.

Weight is 11 kg, temperature 36.6°C, heart rate 132, respiratory rate 20, and blood pressure not recorded. A mass is in left lower quadrant of abdomen. The rest of the physical findings are normal.

Hematocrit is 0.37. White cell count is 9.0×10^9/liter. Urine specific gravity is 1.003, pH 7. Urine has 0–1 white cell/HPF.

Barium enema with barium sulfate and equal amounts of water and normal saline shows rectum distended with stool to anatomic anal canal (Figure 87-1).

At posterior rectal myomectomy, a strip of light tan muscle (7–8 cm long) from just above anus to coccyx is removed. Ganglion cells are infrequent in proximal half and many nerve bundle fibers are between layers of muscularis externa and interna. Distal half has no ganglion cells and increased number of nerve bundle fibers.

Diagnosis: Hirschsprung's disease, ultrashort segment.

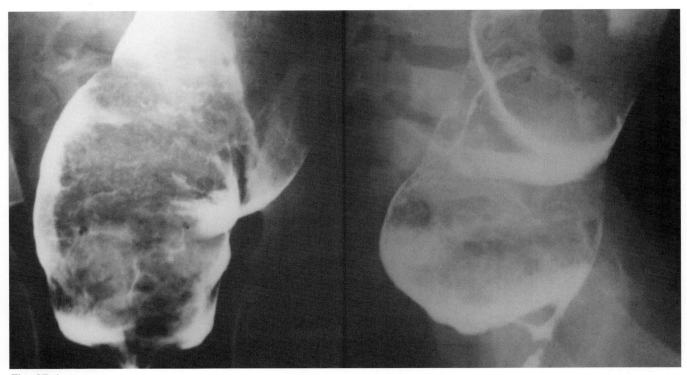

Fig. 87-1

Case 88

A newborn boy has dimple instead of anus. Passage of naso-gastric tube is blocked at 10 cm.

Pregnancy, mother's third, was normal. First pregnancy produced an abortus with anatomic abnormalities, the second a normal infant.

Mother (20 years old), father (21 years old), and brother (1 year old) are well.

Birth weight is 3.0 kg, Apgar score 9/9 at 1 and 5 minutes, length 51 cm, and head circumference 35 cm. At 1½ hours, temperature is 39°C, heart rate 154, respiratory rate 54, and blood pressure 69/48 mm Hg. Penis with hypospadias is bound to scrotum. Right testis is in scrotum, left is not. At 12 hours, he drools. Abdomen is distended. Right foot is slightly rocker-bottom. The rest of the physical findings are normal.

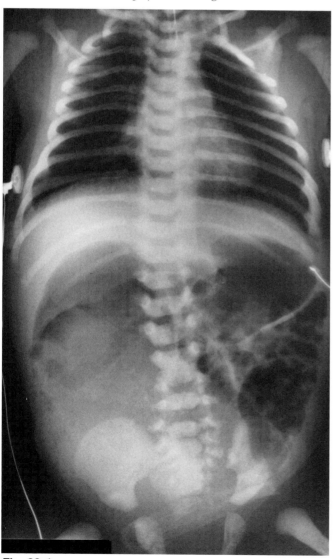

Fig. 88-1

Hematocrit is 0.65. White cell count is 19.2 × 10⁹/liter with 0.66 polymorphonuclear cells, 0.08 bands, 0.20 lymphocytes, 0.05 monocytes, and 0.01 basophils. Platelet count is 199 × 10⁹/liter. Serum sodium is 133 mmol/liter, potassium 4.8, chloride 107, urea nitrogen 2.5, and calcium 2.47. Creatinine is 100 µmol/liter, highest total bilirubin 229 at 4 days. Chromosomes are 46,XY.

Roentgenogram in Figure 88-1 shows (1) distended gut and small shadows of calcium density in right side of abdomen; (2) dysplastic and fused left first and second ribs; (3) ossified ischia and ilia, without pubic ossification; (4) 13 ribs on left side; (5) two fused midlumbar vertebrae; and (6) an enteric tube that ends at the level of T2.

At operation at 2 days, distal tracheoesophageal fistula is divided, two ends of esophagus are anastomosed, and right transverse colostomy with mucous fistula is made.

Cystogram shows urethra, bladder, urogenital sinus, and rectum (Figure 88-2). Ultrasound examination and later excretory urogram show right pyelocaliectasis and do not show left kidney.

Nissen fundoplication is performed at 3 months; posterior sagittal anorectoplasty at 19 months; closure of colostomy at 23 months; and removal of fibrotic, atrophic testicle from left inguinal canal at 2½ years.

At 3½ years, weight is 12 kg. Left femur is 3 cm shorter than right.

Diagnosis: Esophageal atresia with tracheo-esophageal fistula, cloaca, skeletal abnormalities.

(Continued)

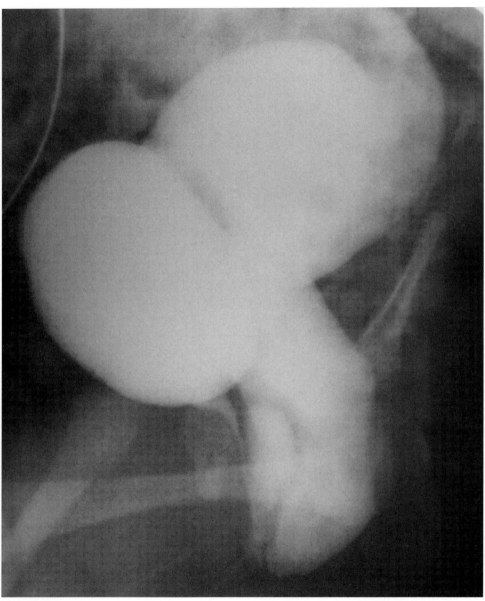

Fig. 88-2

Case 89

A 25-year-old man has had lumps in right side of neck for 3 weeks. He is tired, has frontal headache, feels full after eating little, needs laxatives, and has lost 9 kg in 3 weeks. He has "never been to a doctor before."

Mother (60 years old), three brothers, and one sister are well.

Temperature is 37.5°C, heart rate 72, respiratory rate 16, blood pressure 102/76 mm Hg, weight 54.5 kg, and height 175 cm. Conjunctivae are reddened. Lower halves of eyeballs are prominent. Lips are thick. Edge of tongue is uneven. Several firm masses are in right side of neck. The largest mass (3 cm diameter) moves with swallowing and seems to be in right lobe of thyroid gland. An ill-defined mass is in left upper quadrant of abdomen. Abdomen is tympanitic. Bowel sounds are normal. The rest of the physical findings are normal.

Hematocrit is 0.49. White cell count is 9.4×10^9/liter with 0.65 polymorphonuclear cells, 0.07 bands, 0.20 lymphocytes, and 0.08 monocytes. Platelet count is 351×10^9/liter. ESR is 22 mm/hr. Urine specific gravity is 1.024, pH 6. Urine has 2+ ketones. Serum sodium is 143 mmol/liter, potassium 4.5, chloride 104, carbon dioxide 23, urea nitrogen 6.8, calcium 2.72, phosphorus 1.32, cholesterol 5.28, and glucose 6.7.

Creatinine is 70 µmol/liter, uric acid 290, total bilirubin 10, and direct bilirubin 3. Total protein is 83 g/liter, albumin 53. Alkaline phosphatase is 114 U/liter, LDH 184, and SGOT 6. T_3 resin uptake is 0.34 (normal: 0.28–0.38), T_4 total 124 nmol/liter (normal: 52–154). Isotope scan shows cold nodules in the right lobe of the thyroid.

Colon is unevenly dilated in Figure 89-1.

At total thyroidectomy, a firm mass in right lobe of thyroid surrounds recurrent laryngeal nerve. Firm nodes (1.5–3-cm diameter) are in right internal jugular chain. A right paratracheal node is large and firm. Nodes are yellow to brown, gritty on section. Microscopic examination of mass in thyroid gland shows (1) collections of round to polygonal cells and (2) nests and cords of round and spindle-shaped cells with few mitoses in eosinophilic stroma, which stains for amyloid with Congo red. Similar cells and stroma are in lymph nodes.

Diagnosis: Metastatic medullary carcinoma of the thyroid gland, multiple endocrine neoplasia type III, ganglioneuromatosis of alimentary tract.

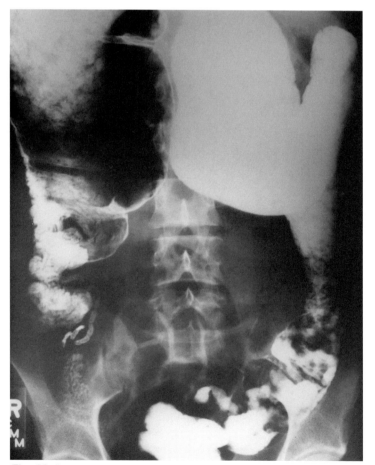

Fig. 89-1

Case 90

A 4-year-old girl has had runny stools for 2–3 days. Then, after mother, who was constipated herself, puts a glycerine suppository into the girl's rectum, the girl has a large, hard stool.

Barium enema with barium sulfate and equal amounts water and normal saline shows stool-distended rectum and normal colon (Figure 90-1A). One hour later, barium has leaked from rectum into anal canal (Figure 90-1B) and onto underwear.

She comes back at 7 years, after seeing one psychiatrist and two psychologists. She is unaware, still soiling herself, and fighting attempts to get her to go to the toilet. Rectum is full of hard stool.

She soils herself occasionally at 7⅔ years if she does not get enough daily stool softener. Weight is 28.3 kg, height 128 cm. Physical findings are normal.

Diagnosis: Chronic constipation.

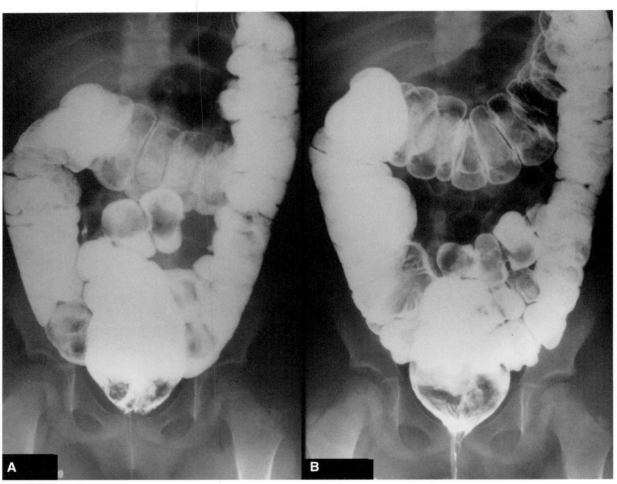

A   B

Fig. 90-1

Case 91

A 3-year-old girl who is examined for suspected urinary tract infection has a pin in abdomen.

Temperature is 37.8°C, heart rate 104, respiratory rate 28, blood pressure 90/60 mm Hg, weight 16.6 kg, and height 95 cm. Physical findings are normal.

Hematocrit is 0.35. White cell count is 8.5×10^9/liter with 0.48 polymorphonuclear cells, 0.03 bands, 0.39 lymphocytes, 0.05 monocytes, 0.04 eosinophils, and 0.01 basophils. Urine specific gravity is 1.017, pH 5. Urine has few epithelial cells/HPF, occasional red cells/HPF, and 0–2 white cells/HPF. Serum urea nitrogen is 6 mmol/liter, creatinine 30 μmol/liter.

Roentgenograms of abdomen over a 3-week period, including those in Figure 91-1 (21 days apart), show a pin swinging full circle in right lower quadrant of abdomen.

At operation, appendix is thickened and contains a pin.

Examination of appendix shows smooth, shiny serosa and thickened, corrugated mucosa.

Diagnosis: Pin in appendix.

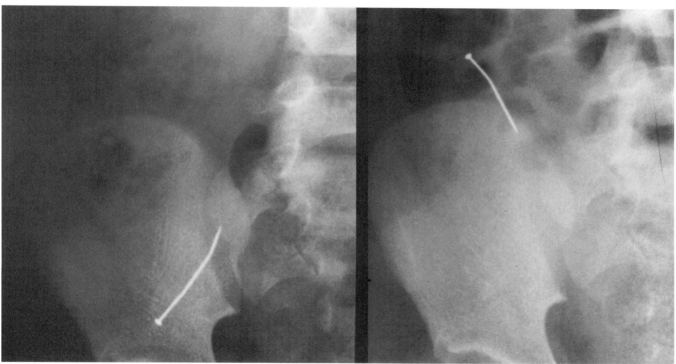

Fig. 91-1

Case 92

A 3-year-old boy has bellyaches that began 4 days ago, last about 5 minutes, and interrupt play and sleep. He grabs his abdomen and occasionally vomits. Appetite is normal.

Parents and two siblings are well.

Temperature is 36.8°C, heart rate 100, respiratory rate 24, blood pressure 122/78 mm Hg, weight 15 kg, and height 91 cm. Bowel sounds are increased. The rest of the physical findings are normal.

Hematocrit is 0.38. White cell count is 16.0×10^9/liter with 0.40 polymorphonuclear cells, 0.30 lymphocytes, 0.04 monocytes, and 0.26 eosinophils. Urine pH is 6. Urine has 3+ ketones, 3–5 epithelial cells/HPF, and rare white cells/HPF. Serum sodium is 135 mmol/liter, potassium 4.2, and chloride 103. Stool is guaiac positive.

Barium enema with barium sulfate and equal amounts water and normal saline shows an intussusceptum at hepatic flexure (Figure 92-1A) and flow into ileum before cecum (Figure 92-1B). Pain recurs. Three attempts to reduce intussusception are made, but boy suffers three recurrences in 2 days with same sequence of flow of barium into ileum before cecum (Figure 92-2A). Barium is in ileum, and a defect is in cecum after partial evacuation (Figure 92-2B).

At operation, appendix is intussuscepted into cecum and cannot be pushed out until appendiceal ring is enlarged with a hemostat. Appendix is edematous (6 cm long, 1.3 cm wide).

Examination of resected appendix shows smooth, pale tan–gray serosal surface and no fecalith. Microscopic examination shows chronic inflammation.

Diagnosis: Appendicocolic intussusception.

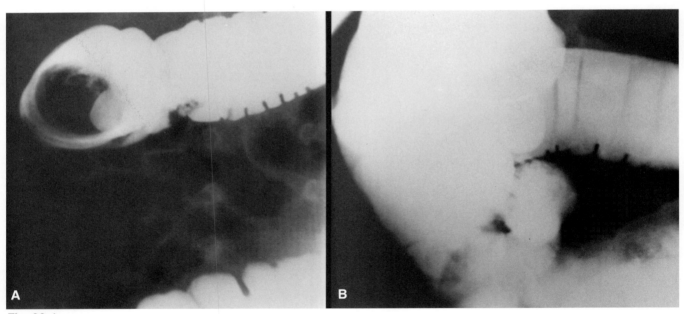

Fig. 92-1

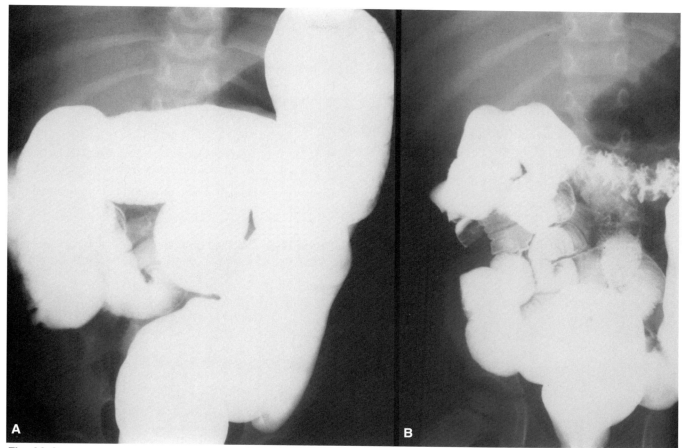

Fig. 92-2

Case 93

A 2½-week-old boy has an abdominal mass.

Birth weight was 2.1 kg, length 45 cm, head circumference 32 cm, and Apgar score 1/8 at 1 and 5 minutes. Testes were not in scrotum. Scrotum had few rugae.

Mother (29 years old) has been taking dapsone for 8 months for leprosy. Mother and father are tuberculin positive.

Weight is 2.3 kg, temperature 37.9°C, heart rate 140, and respiratory rate 48. A mass (1–2 cm) is in right lower quadrant of abdomen. Right testis is not palpable. Left testis is in inguinal canal. The rest of the physical findings are normal.

Hematocrit is 0.36. White cell count is 9.3 × 10⁹/liter. Platelet count is 560 × 10⁹/liter. Urine specific gravity is 1.060, pH 8. Urine has few epithelial cells/HPF and 2–3 white cells/HPF. Serum sodium is 139 mmol/liter, potassium 4.7, and chloride 102. Total protein is 56 g/liter, albumin 35.

Excretory urogram in Figure 93-1A shows normal urinary tract. In Figure 93-1B, a calcified mass is forward in right lower quadrant.

At beginning of operation, systolic blood pressure is 82 mm Hg. Appendix is stuck to cecum and ileum by a calcified mass at its tip. Appendix and mass are removed.

Examination shows light-tan to pink appendix (1.8 × 0.5 cm) and an irregular gray to green-black mass (1.5 × 0.8 cm) at one end. The firm, gritty mass contains necrotic, granular, yellow to green-black matter. Culture grows *Klebsiella pneumoniae*.

Right testis is brought down into scrotum from inguinal ring at 5 years.

Diagnosis: Calcified granulomatous inflammation of fibroareolar tissue at tip of appendix.

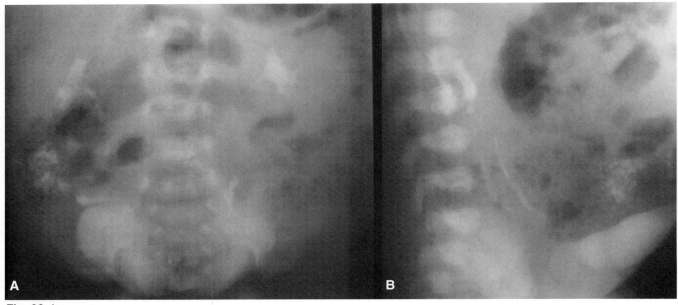

Fig. 93-1

Case 94

A 1-year-old boy is vomiting and febrile.

Parents (both 19 years old) are well. He is their only child.

Pregnancy was normal, birth weight 3.4 kg, and Apgar score 8/9 at 1 and 5 minutes. Left side of scrotum was blue, left testis enlarged without inguinal hernia. The rest of the physical findings were normal. At operation the day after birth, swelling and torsion of left testis were found, and lower half of left testis was removed. Right tunica vaginalis was thickened and adherent to tunica albuginea, and right testis was pale with a few blue spots. Microscopic examination of black, gelatinous lower half of left testis showed hemorrhagic infarction. Biopsy of right testis showed (1) coagulation necrosis, (2) hemorrhage around necrotic zones, (3) hemosiderin and calcification, and (4) connective tissue. He takes 1.0–1.5 qt milk and little table food each day. He began to vomit 2 days ago. Temperature was 38.9°C yesterday.

Weight at 1 year is 8.8 kg, length 77 cm, head circumference 46 cm, temperature 39°C, heart rate 168, respiratory rate 36, and systolic blood pressure 88 mm Hg. He is pale. A systolic heart murmur is present. Abdomen is soft and nontender. The rest of the physical findings are normal.

Hemoglobin is 39 g/liter. Hematocrit is 0.14. Red blood cell count is 3.2×10^{12}/liter. MCV is 43 fl. MCH is 12 pg. MCHC is 290 g/liter. Reticulocyte fraction is 11×10^{-3}. White cell count is 8.2×10^9/liter with 0.24 polymorphonuclear cells, 0.49 bands, 0.21 lymphocytes, and 0.06 monocytes. Platelet count is 740×10^9/liter. Blood smear shows hypochromia, microcytosis, anisocytosis, poikilocytosis, and Döhle inclusion bodies. Urine specific gravity is 1.019, pH 5. Urine has trace protein, trace ketones, and many uric acid crystals. Serum sodium is 138 mmol/liter, potassium 4.0, chloride 104, urea nitrogen 3.9, and glucose 9.3.

Vomit is green the next day. He cries when diapered the third day and resists being turned onto right side. He pulls legs up. Abdomen is distended, tense, and tympanitic. Bowel sounds are absent.

Gas and excess liquid are in gut, some of gut dilated, some constricted; small shadows of calcium density are on right side near iliac crest (Figure 94-1).

At operation, pus is in right lower quadrant of abdomen, and fibrinous exudate is around appendix, behind cecum. A perforation is approximately 1 cm from base of appendix.

Appendix is $5.0 \times 1.1 \times 0.7$ cm. Its surface is white to tan, and dark brown where covered with thin exudate. Tan granules (<0.1 cm) are in lumen.

Diagnosis: Acute suppurative appendicitis with calcified fecaliths, intrauterine torsion of left testis (questionable torsion and detorsion of right testis), iron-deficiency anemia.

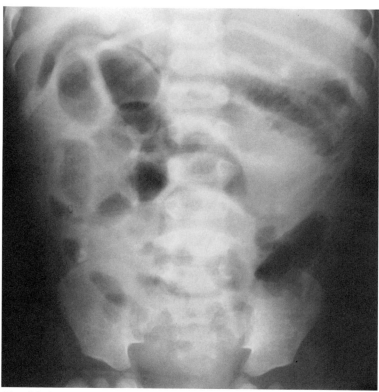

Fig. 94-1

Case 95

A 2-year-old girl vomits dark brown matter and is limp and pale. She opens her eyes occasionally and moves slightly with venipuncture. She was fussy and febrile 4 days ago, less active last night, and hard to wake this morning. She has had almost no food or drink since yesterday.

Temperature is 39.7°C, heart rate 160, respiratory rate 40, systolic blood pressure 116 mm Hg, weight 10.1 kg, and height 82 cm. Abdomen is firm. Bowel sounds are absent. Left arm stiffens 1 hour later, and legs extend and cross at ankles. The rest of the physical findings are normal.

Hematocrit is 0.39. White cell count is 34.3×10^9/liter with 0.64 polymorphonuclear cells, 0.18 bands, 0.12 lymphocytes, and 0.06 monocytes. Platelet count is 532×10^9/liter. Serum sodium is 141 mmol/liter, potassium 4.5, chloride 102, carbon dioxide 9, urea nitrogen 3.9, no calcium measurement due to machine error, phosphorus 1.74, cholesterol 3.15, and glu-

cose 7.4 (IV fluids). Creatinine is 50 μmol/liter, uric acid 570, total bilirubin 5, and direct bilirubin 0. Total protein is 66 g/liter, albumin 44. Alkaline phosphatase is 222 U/liter, LDH 477, SGOT 32, and amylase 26.

In Figure 95-1, gas and liquid are in dilated gut; a loop of gut, presumably ascending colon, is concave along lower, medial aspect ("cecal cut-off" sign).

At operation, tan-gray liquid is in right lower quadrant of abdomen. A perforation is at base of swollen, friable appendix. Culture of peritoneal liquid grows *Escherichia coli*, *Streptococcus viridans*, and *Bacteroides*.

The appendix (6.0 × 0.5 cm) is soft, tan to red, and contains a fecalith.

Diagnosis: Acute appendicitis.

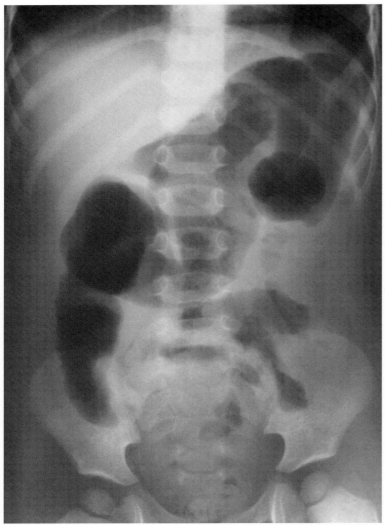

Fig. 95-1

Case 96

A 15-year-old boy has a cough and abdominal "tightness." He coughed up sputum 2 days ago, woke up yesterday with pain in right lower quadrant of abdomen that is worse with deep inspiration, and vomited four times. His head hurts when he sits up. His left leg feels weak and his left thigh and calf hurt.

Temperature is 40.1°C, heart rate 120, respiratory rate 40, blood pressure 118/62 mm Hg, and weight 54 kg. One examiner thinks breath sounds are diminished on right side. Two other examiners think breath sounds are normal. A systolic murmur is present. Abdomen is tender, most marked in right lower quadrant, where there is guarding and rebound tenderness. Rectal examination causes pain on right side. The rest of the physical findings are normal.

Hematocrit is 0.35. White cell count is 21.8×10^9/liter with 0.48 polymorphonuclear cells, 0.42 bands, and 0.10 lymphocytes. ESR is 18 mm/hr. Serum sodium is 129 mmol/liter, potassium 3.4, chloride 93, carbon dioxide 18, urea nitrogen 6.4, and glucose 7.8. Amylase is 25 U/liter.

Erect and supine roentgenograms of abdomen show slight dilation of gut with gas and liquid throughout abdomen (Figure 96-1). A shadow of water density is behind heart along right side of spine in the erect roentgenogram (Figure 96-1B).

Appendix is removed at operation.

Appendix is smooth and translucent, its wall 2 mm thick. Pinworms are in appendix.

Diagnosis: Pneumonia, right lower lobe (medial basal segment in chest roentgenogram), pinworms in appendix.

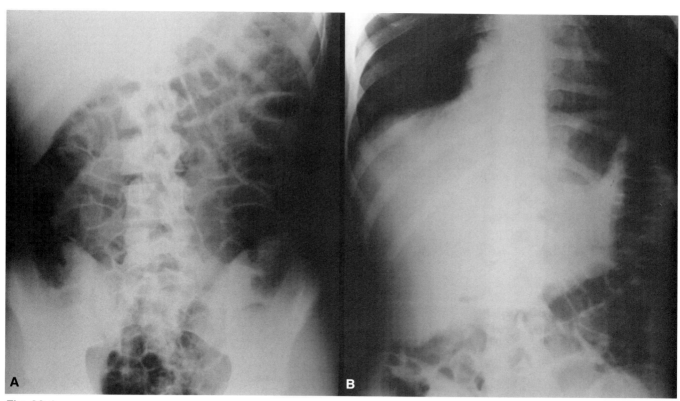

Fig. 96-1

Case 97

A 7-year-old girl woke up early today retching and leaking urine. She vomited and had suprapubic pain 4 days ago.

She had chickenpox at 3 years; headache, bellyache, and fever for a week at 3½ years while her mother was hospitalized for a miscarriage; right pink eye and abrasions of shoulder and flank at 4 years; and scarlet fever 3 months ago.

Temperature at 7 years is 37.6°C, heart rate 90, respiratory rate 20, blood pressure 124/90 mm Hg, height 119 cm, and weight 23.2 kg (down 0.4 kg from 2 days ago). She is shivering. She tenses abdomen and is diffusely tender. The rest of the physical findings are normal.

Hematocrit is 0.36. White cell count is 8.6×10^9/liter with 0.87 polymorphonuclear cells, 0.05 bands, 0.07 lymphocytes, and 0.01 atypical lymphocytes. Two days ago, urine had pH 6, 5–7 white cells/HPF, 1–3 red cells/HPF, trace protein, and bacteria. Culture is sterile. Serum sodium is 135 mmol/liter, potassium 3.7, chloride 105, carbon dioxide 20, urea nitrogen 2.5, calcium 2.50, phosphorus 1.23, cholesterol 4.40, and glucose 6.6. Creatinine is 50 µmol/liter, uric acid 140, total bilirubin 3, and direct bilirubin 2. Total protein is 76 g/liter, albumin 50. Alkaline phosphatase is 269 U/liter, LDH 205, and SGOT 102.

Roentgenographic findings are normal in Figure 97-1.

She is nauseated the second day. Abdominal pain is greater on right side of umbilicus. Operative findings in abdomen are normal. Normal appendix is removed. She goes home 2 days after operation and eats well for 5 days. She returns on the sixth day vomiting yellow liquid, doubled over with pain, and nervous.

Red blotches are on body. She tenses abdomen during examination and says, "Don't do that or I'll cry harder." She complains of pain, then watches TV, or walks around. The medical psychologist finds her cheerful until "bad touches" and sexual encounters are brought up. She then cries and refuses to talk. The psychologist learns that the mother married the stepfather 4 years ago. He hits the mother in the girl's presence. He spanks the girl hard and often. He confesses to sexually abusing the girl three times.

Diagnosis: Normal appendix, sexual abuse.

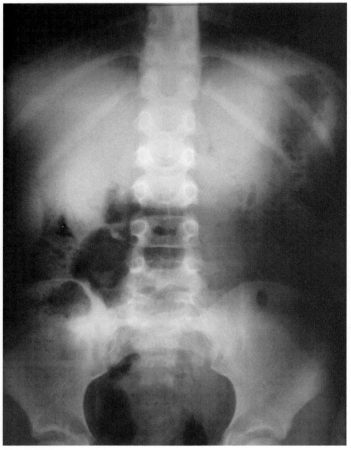

Fig. 97-1

Case 98

A 6-month-old boy has a mass at anus three times in 2 weeks and blood at anus the last time.

Weight is 8 kg, height 66 cm. A stalked mass (1 × 1 cm) is on back wall of rectum. The rest of the physical findings are normal.

Laboratory data are not obtained.

In Figure 98-1, barium enema with barium sulfate and equal amounts water and normal saline shows a mobile mass in rectum.

Examination of pedunculated mass removed at proctoscopy shows spherical, soft, tan cyst (1.2-cm diameter) made up of (1) colonic mucosa, (2) smooth muscle, (3) connective tissue, (4) lymphoid aggregates, (5) pseudostratified columnar epithelium, (6) lamina propria, and (7) crypts lined by epithelium and mucus-producing cells.

Diagnosis: Benign epithelial polyp (juvenile polyp, retention cyst).

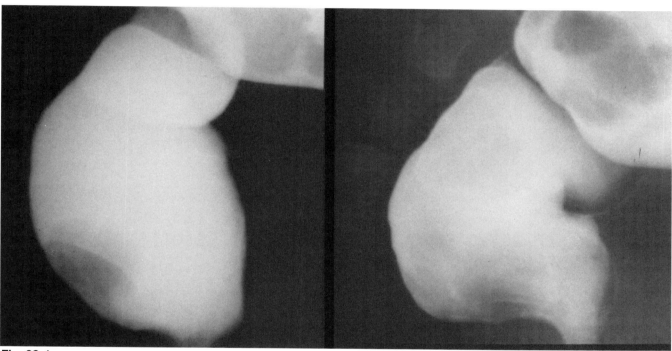

Fig. 98-1

Case 99

A 15-year-old boy has cramps before bowel movements. He used to have one bowel movement per day but has had two or three movements per day, some with blood, for 1 month. A sebaceous cyst behind left ear was removed recently.

Mother had colectomy and ileostomy for colonic polyps. Maternal uncles have colonic polyps. Some maternal relatives have died of cancer, including bowel cancer, in middle age. Father had rheumatic heart disease.

Temperature is 37.6°C, heart rate 86, respiratory rate 18, blood pressure 110/60 mm Hg, weight 40 kg, and height 146 cm. Sebaceous cysts are on neck and back. A scar is behind left ear. A streak of dark retinal pigment is lateral to right optic disc. Small polyps are palpable in rectum. The rest of the physical findings are normal.

Hematocrit is 0.48. White cell count is 11.7×10^9/liter with 0.57 polymorphonuclear cells, 0.01 bands, 0.36 lymphocytes, 0.03 monocytes, 0.02 eosinophils, and 0.01 basophils. Urine specific gravity is 1.023, pH 5. Urine has occasional epithelial cells/HPF, 0–1 white cell/HPF, and mucus. Serum sodium is 144 mmol/liter, potassium 4.4, chloride 105, carbon dioxide 23, urea nitrogen 3.6, calcium 2.59, phosphorus 1.94, cholesterol 4.19, and glucose 5.3. Creatinine is 80 µmol/liter, uric acid 410, total bilirubin 7, and direct bilirubin 2. Total protein is 75 g/liter, albumin 46. Alkaline phosphatase is 279 U/liter, LDH 226, and SGOT 20. Carcinoembryonic antigen is 1.1 µg/liter (normal: <3).

Small, round defects are in large bowel from appendix to anus in Figure 99-1.

Colonoscopy shows small, smooth, pink polyps.

Microscopic examination of a rectal polyp shows (1) normal rectal glands, (2) surface crowding of epithelial cells, (3) decreased goblet cells, and (4) tubular glands and crowded goblet cells on a stalk of connective tissue.

Colon is removed, and ileostomy with normal ileal mucosa is placed.

Diagnosis: Familial adenomatous polyposis coli, sebaceous cysts, hypertrophy of retinal pigment epithelium; Gardner's syndrome.

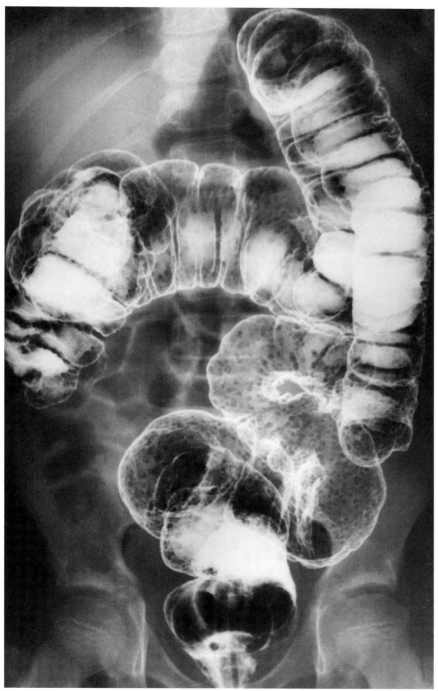

Fig. 99-1

Case 100

A 52-year-old man has bloody vomit, black stools, and no appetite. He has had abdominal pain for several years that has worsened the last 2 weeks. He says that he came in to die.

Temperature is 36.7°C, heart rate 100, respiratory rate 18, and blood pressure 128/82 mm Hg. He is thin. Abdomen is tender, especially in epigastrium and left lower quadrant. Left inguinal hernia is present. Testes are atrophied. The rest of the physical findings are normal.

Hematocrit is 0.47. White cell count is 7.8 × 10⁹/liter with 0.29 polymorphonuclear cells, 0.48 bands, 0.02 lymphocytes, 0.12 monocytes, 0.01 eosinophils, and 0.08 metamyelocytes. Platelet count is 179 × 10⁹/liter. Serum sodium is 130 mmol/liter, potassium 2.6, chloride 86, carbon dioxide 24, urea nitrogen 15.0, calcium 1.85, phosphorus 1.16, cholesterol 3.10, and glucose 8.2. Creatinine is 120 µmol/liter, uric acid 600, total bilirubin 24, and direct bilirubin 10. Total protein is 57 g/liter, albumin 23. Alkaline phosphatase is 101

U/liter, LDH 324, SGOT 21, and amylase 72. Stool shows many amoeba/HPF, some of them containing red cells. Stool contains 4+ *Entamoeba histolytica* trophozoites.

Figure 100-1 shows gut dilated with gas and liquid, and ulcers (broader at bottom than at surface) in what appears to be transverse colon.

Sigmoidoscopy is limited to 14 cm by pain. Blood is in colon. An ulcer is near dentate (anorectal) line. Smaller white plaques are scattered across normal-looking mucosa.

Rectal biopsy shows (1) patches bare of mucosa; (2) slightly thickened connective tissue in lamina propria; and (3) infiltrates of plasma cells, eosinophils, lymphocytes, but no polymorphonuclear cells.

Diagnosis: Amebic colitis.

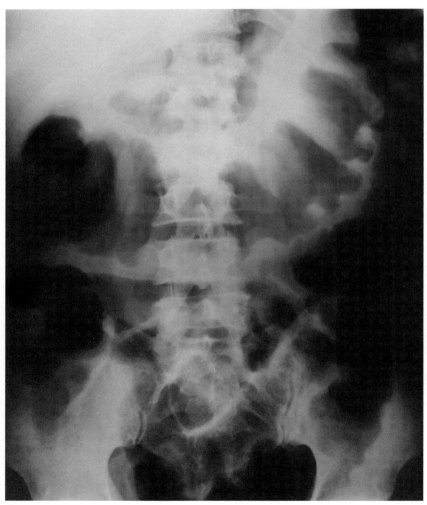

Fig. 100-1

Case 101

A 33-month-old girl is vomiting round, white worms and excreting round, white worms in her stools.

Activity diminished 2 months ago. She cries intermittently with pain. She began to vomit yellow liquid and worms as long as 10 cm 1 month ago. Stools are liquid and contain worms.

Siblings are excreting worms.

Temperature is 37.9°C, heart rate 124, respiratory rate 24, weight 8.8 kg, and height 84 cm. A systolic murmur is present. Liver edge is 2 cm below costal margin. Bowel sounds are hyperactive. The rest of the physical findings are normal.

Hematocrit is 0.38. White cell count is 22.4 × 10⁹/liter with 0.50 polymorphonuclear cells, 0.16 bands, 0.01 eosinophils, 0.27 lymphocytes, and 0.06 monocytes. Urine specific gravity is 1.015, pH 7. Urine has 1+ acetone. Serum sodium is 130 mmol/liter, potassium 4.4, and chloride 92. SGOT is 38 U/liter.

Figure 101-1 shows coiled tubular shadows in left upper quadrant of abdomen below nasogastric tube.

Stool contains ova and adult *Ascaris lumbricoides*. One stool contains a cyst of *Giardia lamblia* and a cyst of *Endolimax nana*.

Diagnosis: Ascariasis and other intestinal parasites.

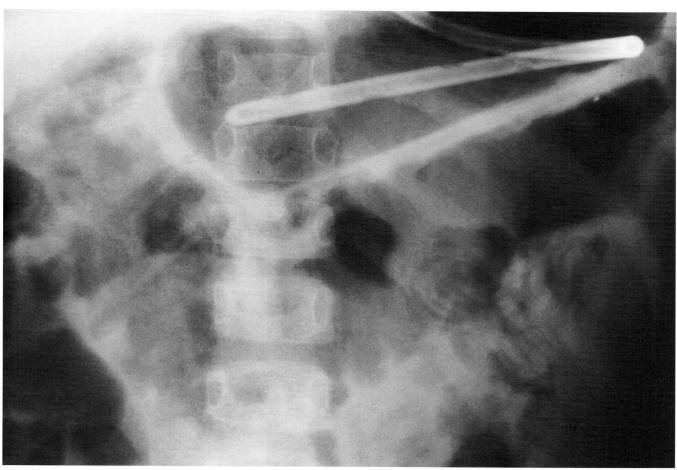

Fig. 101-1

Case 102

A 10-month-old boy has had fever, vomiting, and diarrhea for 3 days. Stools are green, slimy, and frequent. He cries when he is moved and trembles when his diapers are changed. He was given an antibiotic for an ear infection 3 weeks ago.

Parents are well. He is their only child.

Temperature is 38.2°C, heart rate 120, respiratory rate 24, and blood pressure 100/60 mm Hg. He has a faint, blotchy rash. Lids are half closed, eyes sunken. Abdomen is scaphoid and silent. Muscle tone is poor. The rest of the physical findings are normal.

Hematocrit is 0.32. White cell count is 22.9 × 10⁹/liter with 0.52 polymorphonuclear cells, 0.31 bands, 0.02 lymphocytes, 0.12 monocytes, 0.02 metamyelocytes, and 0.01 myelocytes. Platelet count is 132 × 10⁹/liter. Urine specific gravity is 1.012, pH 6.5. Urine is normal. Serum sodium is 134 mmol/liter, potassium 2.0, chloride 100, and urea nitrogen 1.1. Total protein is 41 g/liter, albumin 25. Stool has blood in it. Stool culture grows *Yersinia enterocolitica*.

Figure 102-1 shows barium mixed with liquid in colon and thumbprinting in descending colon.

Sigmoidoscopy shows edematous mucosa, decreased vascular pattern, raised yellow plaques, and small patches of exudate.

Diagnosis: Enterocolitis, *Y. enterocolitica.*

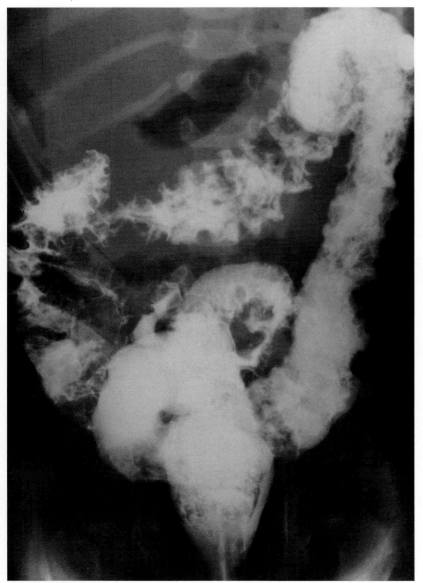

Fig. 102-1

Case 103

A 13-year-old girl has several loose, bloody stools a day. Diarrhea began 3 months ago. Blood appeared 2 weeks later.

Pregnancy of mother was normal, birth weight 3.1 kg. She was breast-fed for 9 months. She began to wheeze at 1 year, to have eczema at 2 years, and to have a runny nose and sneezing in early summer at 3 years. She had bellyaches until she stopped drinking milk at 6 years. Eczema gets better, wheezing worse in summer.

Mother and one brother (10 years old) are well. Father had asthma and died at 40 years. Two sisters (16 and 18 years old) and another brother (17 years old) have allergies. Maternal grandmother had diabetes mellitus; maternal grandparents had strokes. Maternal uncle has colitis. Paternal grandmother had duodenal ulcer.

Temperature at 13 years is 37.0°C, heart rate 66, respiratory rate 17, blood pressure 100/65 mm Hg, weight 29 kg (3 months ago: 34 kg), and height 149 cm. Lower abdomen is tender. The rest of the physical findings are normal.

Hematocrit is 0.36. White cell count is 10.3×10^9/liter with 0.13 polymorphonuclear cells, 0.48 bands, 0.29 lymphocytes, 0.05 monocytes, and 0.05 eosinophils. Platelet count is 400×10^9/liter. ESR is 20 mm/hr.

She is treated with salicylazosulfapyridine and then prednisone. Loose, bloody stools continue. Sigmoidoscopy 4 months later shows "cobblestones" and red mucosa that bleeds easily. Prednisone is increased. Stools become normal. Sigmoidoscopy shows pale mucosa at 14⅓ years. Prednisone is stopped at 15½ years. Loose, bloody stools recur. She has chills, fever, and abdominal pain at 15¾ years. Weight is 38.6 kg, height 158 cm, temperature 36.7°C, heart rate 80, respiratory rate 18, and blood pressure 100/70. She has eczema on hands and neck. Lower abdomen is tender.

Hematocrit at 15¾ years is 0.33. White cell count is 7.6×10^9/liter with 0.36 polymorphonuclear cells, 0.45 bands, 0.12 lymphocytes, 0.04 monocytes, 0.02 eosinophils, and 0.01 basophils. Total protein is 88 g/liter, albumin 25.

Barium enema shows colonic haustrations only in ascending part at 14 years (Figure 103-1A) and 15¾ years (Figure 103-1B) and reflux into ileum both times. Transverse and descending parts of colon are featureless and a pill is in stomach, partly hidden by splenic flexure, in Figure 103-1A.

Sigmoidoscopy at 15¾ years shows pale, friable, granular mucosa and rectal ulcers.

At operation, colon, rectum, and appendix are removed, and ileostomy is placed.

Length of colon and rectum is 76.5 cm; length of resected ileum is 3.5 cm. Colonic serosa is dark and smooth. Blood is in lumen. A thin white film covers rough mucosa of distal third of colon. Mucosa of middle third is smooth. Petechiae that stop at ileocecal valve are in mucosa of haustrated proximal third of colon. Microscopic examination shows (1) absence of colonic glands; (2) vascular congestion; (3) necrosis; (4) extravasated red cells; (5) fibrin thrombi; (6) a cover of inflammatory cells and thick fibrin; (6) mucosal and submucosal neutrophils; (7) submucosal plasma cells and lymphocytes, the changes less marked in ascending colon and appendix than in rest of colon. Granulomas are not present. Muscularis externa, serosa, and ileum are normal. Lymph nodes show follicular hyperplasia.

Diagnosis: Ulcerative colitis.

(Continued)

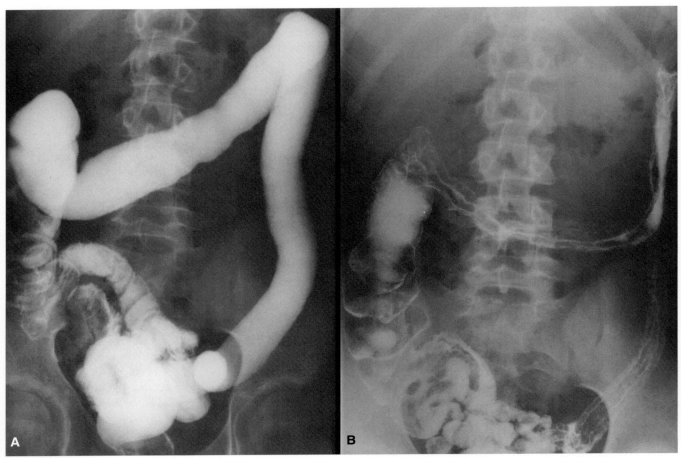

Fig. 103-1

Case 104

A 2-year-old girl has melena today.

Tantrums began 6 weeks ago, urinary frequency 5 weeks ago, and night restlessness 3 weeks ago. She had an earache and runny ear 2 weeks ago and red, swollen, painful knees, ankles, and toes 3 days ago. She vomited dark matter 2 days ago and then would not eat.

Pregnancy was normal, birth weight 2.4 kg. She sat at 6 months, began to walk at 9 months. She has had colds and urinary tract infection.

Parents, brother (4 years old), and sister (8 months old) are well.

Temperature at 2 years is 40°C, heart rate 160, respiratory rate 30, and systolic blood pressure 30 mm Hg. She is pale. Lips and nailbeds are blue. Pulse is weak. Right external acoustic meatus is crusted. Dry mucus is in nose. Tonsils are large. A systolic murmur is present. Abdomen is distended and tender. Bowel sounds are diminished. Blood is at anus. Old bruises are on shins. Purpuric nodules (2–3-mm diameter) are on feet. The rest of the physical findings are normal.

Hemoglobin is 127 g/liter. Hematocrit is 0.37. Reticulocyte fraction is 11×10^{-3}. White cell count is 7.6×10^9/liter with 0.20 polymorphonuclear cells, 0.40 bands, 0.21 lymphocytes, 0.11 monocytes, 0.01 basophils, 0.03 atypical lymphocytes, 0.01 myelocytes, and 0.03 metamyelocytes. Platelet count is 657×10^9/liter. ESR is 13 mm/hr. Urine specific gravity is 1.023, pH 5.5. Urine has trace albumin, 3–4 red cells/HPF, and many hyaline casts/LPF. Serum sodium is 134 mmol/liter, potassium 4.1, chloride 92, and urea nitrogen 6.8. Creatinine is 60 µmol/liter. Total protein is 50 g/liter, albumin 23. SGOT is 103 U/liter.

Adenoids are small or absent (Figure 104-1A). Barium enema shows defects (thumbprinting) near splenic and hepatic flexures and constriction of distal ileum (Figure 104-1B).

Diagnosis: Henoch-Schönlein purpura, intramural hematomas in colon.

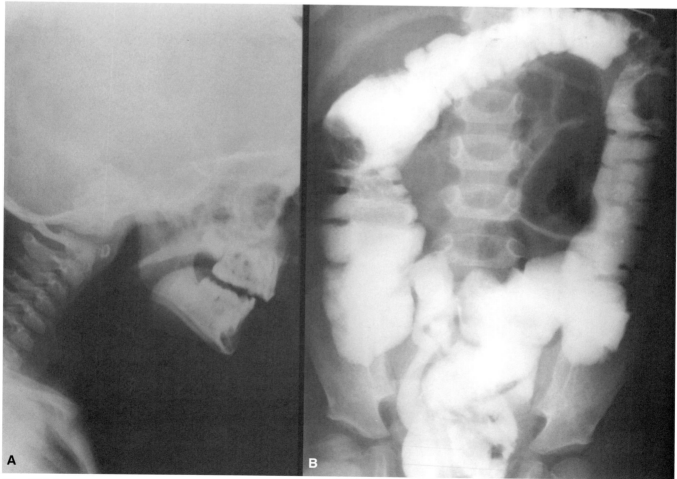

A   B

Fig. 104-1

Case 105

A 12-year-old girl has stopped growing. She has had abdominal pain during meals for 5–6 weeks, has vomited occasionally, and has had one to two loose stools per week. A stool specimen contained *Giardia lamblia* cysts, for which she was treated.

Birth weight was 3.6 kg. At 10 years, weight was 29.5 kg, height 137 cm.

Parents and two brothers (10 and 20 years old) are well.

Weight at 12 years is 29 kg, height 137 cm, temperature 36.5°C, heart rate 72, respiratory rate 14, and blood pressure 100/54 mm Hg. No secondary sexual characteristics are present. The rest of the physical findings are normal.

Hematocrit is 0.42. White cell count is 10.3×10^9/liter with 0.77 polymorphonuclear cells, 0.19 lymphocytes, 0.03 monocytes, and 0.01 eosinophils. ESR is 22 mm/hr. Serum sodium is 142 mmol/liter, potassium 3.8, chloride 107, carbon dioxide 30, urea nitrogen 5.4, calcium 2.25, phosphorus 1.23, cholesterol 4.32, and glucose 3.8. Creatinine is 50 μmol/liter, uric acid 330, total bilirubin 5, and direct bilirubin 2. Total protein is 58 g/liter, albumin 35. Alkaline phosphatase is 168 U/liter, LDH 181, and SGOT 18. T_4 is 99 nmol/liter (normal: 51–142). T_3 resin uptake is 0.35 (normal: 0.25–0.35). TSH is 5 mU/liter (normal: 2–11). FSH is <2 IU/liter (normal: <10), LH <3 (normal: <12). Growth hormone at 60 minutes after L-dopamine injection is 8.0 μg/liter (normal: >5), at 90 minutes 7.1, and mean 24-hour growth hormone 0.9.

Appetite is worse for the next 3 months. She has left lower quadrant pain during meals and dull periumbilical pain all day long. She has aphthae. Two stools are blood streaked.

In Figure 105-1, barium enema shows a defect in ascending colon around ileocecal valve. Bone age in left hand is 10 years.

Symptoms and vomiting persist during the next 3 months despite daily prednisone, and she has fever. At colonoscopy, colon is normal; distal ileum is erythematous and ulcerated. At operation, fat is in mesentery of distal ileum, and wall of distal ileum is thickened.

Examination of resected piece of ileum and ascending colon shows dark red–brown ulcerated mucosa in distal ileum, at ileocecal valve, and in cecum.

Diagnosis: Crohn's disease, growth retardation.

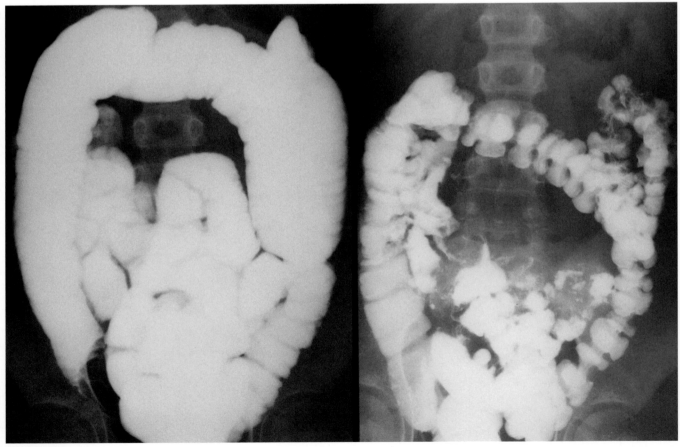

Fig. 105-1

Case 106

A 1-month-old boy is cranky and will not eat today. He grunts and draws knees up to chest. He is belching and passing gas. He was switched from breast milk to formula 5 days ago.

Birth weight was 3.4 kg. Mother had gestational diabetes. She and brother (2½ years old) are well.

Temperature is 38.6°C, heart rate 140, respiratory rate 40, systolic blood pressure 92 mm Hg, weight 4 kg, and length 55 cm. He is jaundiced. Abdomen is distended, firm, and tender. The rest of the physical findings are normal.

Hematocrit is 0.41. White cell count is 9.1×10^9/liter with 0.40 polymorphonuclear cells, 0.17 bands, 0.26 lymphocytes, and 0.17 monocytes. Platelet count is 387×10^9/liter. Urine specific gravity is 1.018, pH 6. Urine has 0.30 g/liter protein and 1–2 white cells/HPF. Serum sodium is 144 mmol/liter, potassium 5.6, chloride 107, carbon dioxide 20, urea nitrogen 4.0, calcium 2.45, phosphorus 1.97, cholesterol 2.28, and glucose 5.1. Creatinine is 40 μmol/liter, uric acid 240, total bilirubin 168, and direct bilirubin 9. Total protein is 57 g/liter, albumin 41. Alkaline phosphatase is 249 U/liter, LDH 343, and SGOT 23.

In Figure 106-1, undistended, gas-containing gut is displaced by a midabdominal mass. Ultrasound examination in Figure 106-2 shows that the mass is a septate cyst.

At operation, a cyst (6 × 4 cm) is in mesentery of ileum. Surface of cyst is bright yellow; contents are milky yellow liquid. Resected cyst is multilocated with thin outer wall and focal acute inflammation.

Diagnosis: Mesenteric (chylous) cyst.

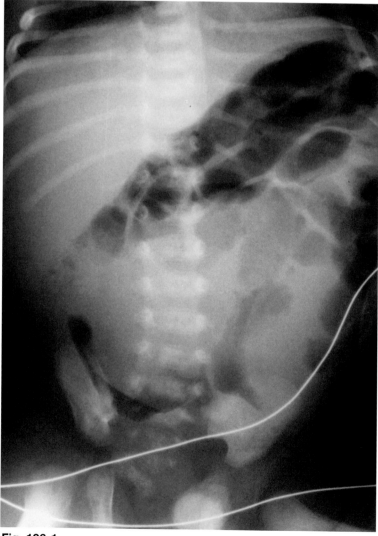

Fig. 106-1

(Continued)

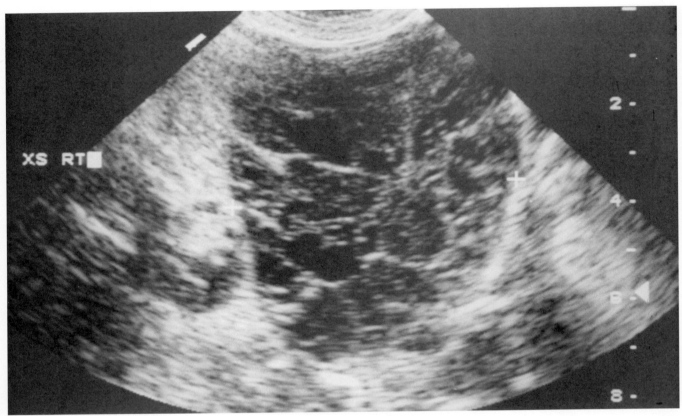

Fig. 106-2

Case 107

A 3-year-old boy has a "bloated stomach" and has not eaten much for 2 weeks. He began to complain of bellyache 1 week ago. He will not walk or play, but just watches his 5-year-old brother.

His face was bruised at 1 year, chest scalded at 1½ years. Buttocks and thighs were bruised 6 months ago.

Mother (25 years old) and father (28 years old) are separated. They have used illegal drugs. Mother's boyfriend lives with her.

Temperature at 3 years is 37.4°C, heart rate 120, respiratory rate 20, blood pressure 98/50 mm Hg, weight 13.6 kg, height 98 cm, and head circumference 50 cm. Arms are bruised. Abdomen is distended and dull to percussion. Bowel sounds are diminished. The rest of the physical findings are normal.

Hematocrit is 0.29. White cell count is 9.0×10^9/liter with 0.43 polymorphonuclear cells, 0.43 lymphocytes, 0.09 monocytes, and 0.05 eosinophils. Platelet count is 677×10^9/liter. Urine is clear yellow with pH 6, specific gravity 1.018, and 2–4 white cells/HPF. Serum sodium is 136 mmol/liter, potassium 3.8, chloride 102, carbon dioxide 27, urea nitrogen 3.6, calcium 1.92, phosphorus 1.36, cholesterol 3.93, triglycerides 1.48, and glucose 5.6. Creatinine is 40 µmol/liter, uric acid

70, total bilirubin 5, and direct bilirubin 2. Total protein is 51 g/liter, albumin 34. Amylase is 36 U/liter, alkaline phosphatase 106, LDH 28, and SGOT 24.

CT scan in Figure 107-1 shows ascites and enlarged left adrenal gland.

Two liters of peritoneal liquid are suctioned from abdomen at operation. A mass is in base of mesentery of small bowel. Mesentery is torn near base. Hard lumps are in omentum and along antimesenteric border of transverse colon. Duodenum is scarred.

Cytologic examination of peritoneal liquid shows many lymphocytes. Microscopic examination of left adrenal gland shows blood and necrotic tissue inside a rim of adrenal tissue. Lumps in omentum consist of fat; dilated blood vessels; and fibrotic, necrotic granulation tissue. A lump along transverse colon consists of fat, fibrous tissue, and hemorrhage. Lymph nodes have fibrous tissue, hemorrhage, granulation tissue, and benign lymphoid aggregates; one node shows sinus histiocytosis.

Diagnosis: Chylous ascites and left adrenal hemorrhage, child abuse.

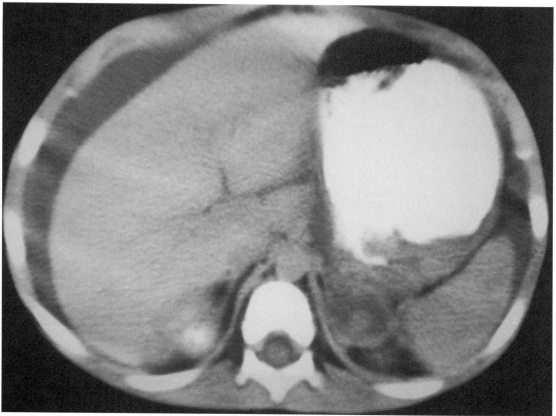

Fig. 107-1

Case 108

A 2½-year-old girl has been vomiting bile for 1½ days.

Temperature is 38.4°C, heart rate 160, respiratory rate 32, systolic blood pressure 85 mm Hg, and weight 11.7 kg. She lies quietly. Skin turgor is poor. Abdomen is firm, tender, and quiet. The rest of the physical findings are normal.

Hematocrit is 0.38. White cell count is 17.6 × 10⁹/liter with 0.88 polymorphonuclear cells, 0.06 bands, and 0.06 lymphocytes. Serum sodium is 138 mmol/liter, potassium 3.9, and chloride 98.

In Figure 108-1, excess liquid is in dilated gut throughout abdomen, and an enteric tube ends near pylorus.

At operation, cloudy yellow liquid is in peritoneum. Spots of erythema and small deposits of fibrin are on appendix and small bowel.

Peritoneal liquid contains white cells and gram-negative bacilli. Appendix is normal. Culture of peritoneal liquid grows *Salmonella infantis* (group C1).

She vomits and has abdominal pain occasionally over the next 4½ months. She then has cramps that last several minutes several times per hour for 12 hours. She vomits several times.

Temperature at 2 years, 10½ months, is 36.7°C, heart rate 100, respiratory rate 20, blood pressure 108/60 mm Hg, and weight 12.7 kg. Abdomen is flat and soft. Bowel sounds are increased.

Hematocrit is 0.38. White cell count is 7.0 × 10⁹/liter with 0.68 polymorphonuclear cells, 0.07 bands, 0.18 lymphocytes, 0.06 monocytes, and 0.01 atypical lymphocytes.

Proximal gut is distended with gas and liquid in Figure 108-2.

At operation, an internal hernia is in a band across mid–small bowel. Gut is normal after release.

She wakes at midnight 7 weeks later, cries, vomits nonbilious liquid several hours later, and then has dry heaves.

Temperature at 3 years is 36.6°C, heart rate 137, respiratory rate 24, blood pressure 100/60 mm Hg, and weight 12.4 kg.

Eyes are sunken. Mouth is dry. Abdomen is soft, distended, tympanitic, and tender in left upper quadrant. Bowel sounds are diminished.

Hematocrit is 0.46. White cell count is 28.8 × 10⁹/liter with 0.88 polymorphonuclear cells, 0.01 bands, 0.07 lymphocytes, and 0.04 monocytes.

In Figure 108-3, excess liquid is in gut; a cluster of dilated loops is in left upper quadrant.

At operation, 5 cm of gangrenous mid–small bowel in left lower quadrant is twisted around a band.

Resected gut is purple-brown and has small serosal adhesions, patches of red-brown mucosa on granular, red-brown base, and intraluminal blood.

She has abdominal cramps for a week at 5½ years. She vomits several times and has small, hard stools.

Temperature at 5½ years is 37°C, heart rate 104, respiratory rate 20, blood pressure 100/57 mm Hg, weight 16.5 kg, and height 110 cm. Abdomen is soft. A nontender, mobile mass is just to right of umbilicus.

Hematocrit is 0.37. White cell count is 10.0 × 10⁹/liter with 0.66 polymorphonuclear cells, 0.02 bands, 0.20 lymphocytes, 0.08 monocytes, and 0.04 eosinophils. Platelet count is 314 × 10⁹/liter.

Ultrasound examination in Figure 108-4 shows cyst in abdomen.

At operation, a cyst (9 × 9 × 8 cm) is in mesentery of transverse colon.

Cyst is tan to light brown, surface smooth. Two lumens are inside, each lined by intestinal mucosa and containing gray-tan serofibrinous liquid.

Diagnosis: Peritonitis at 2½ years; small bowel obstruction by adhesions at 2 years, 10½ months; segmental volvulus, transmural hemorrhagic infarction at 3 years; colonic duplication at 5½ years.

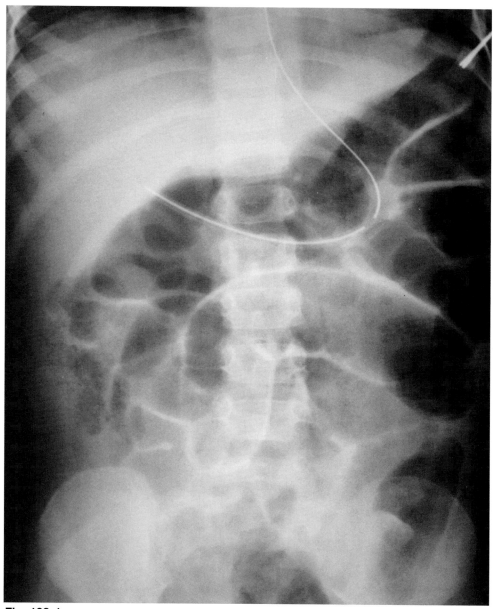

Fig. 108-1

(Continued)

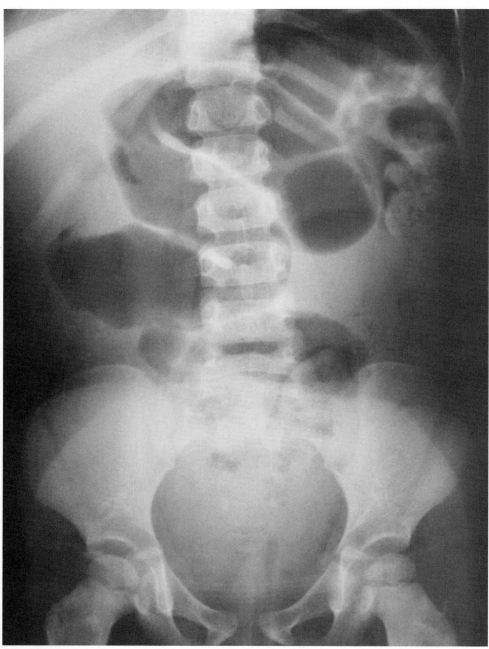

Fig. 108-2

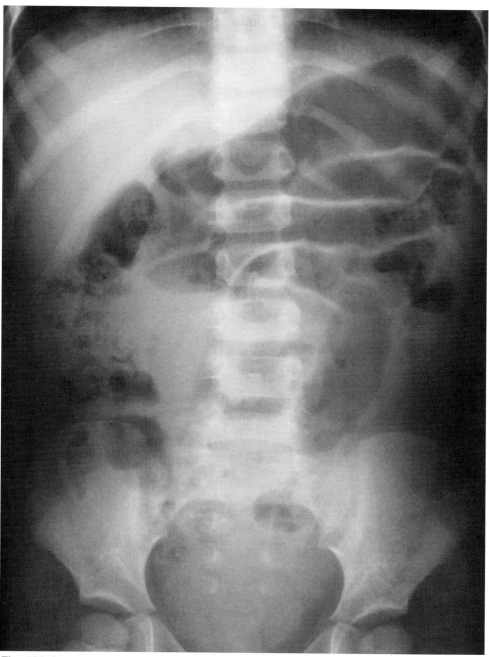

Fig. 108-3

(Continued)

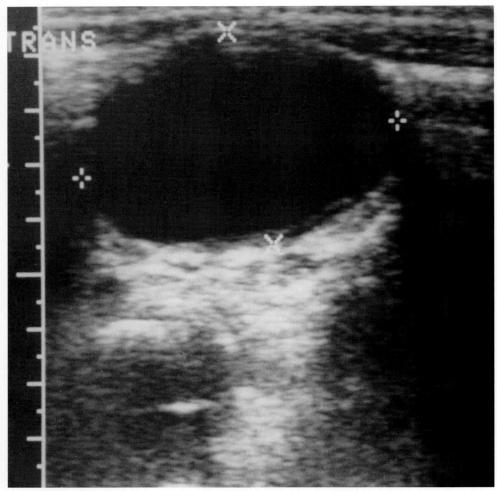

Fig. 108-4

Peritoneum and Abdominal Viscera

Case 1

A 1-month-old girl coughs, fusses, and will not eat.

Pregnancy of mother was normal, birth weight 3.4 kg.

Weight is 2.8 kg, temperature 37.6°C, heart rate 140, respiratory rate 40, and systolic blood pressure 60 mm Hg. She is pale and breathing hard. Lips are blue, neck veins distended. Hemangiomas are on left side of face and neck, left buttock, and right thigh. Precordium heaves. A holosystolic murmur is present. Abdominal veins are prominent. Liver is firm, edge below umbilicus. A thrill and bruit are in epigastrium. Peripheral pulses are full. The rest of the physical findings are normal.

Hematocrit is 0.33. White cell count is 10.5×10^9/liter with 0.51 polymorphonuclear cells, 0.04 bands, 0.31 lymphocytes, 0.06 monocytes, and 0.08 eosinophils. Platelet count is 449×10^9/liter. Serum sodium is 130 mmol/liter, potassium 5.5, chloride 89, carbon dioxide 31, urea nitrogen 18.0, calcium 2.50, phosphorus 2.13, cholesterol 3.08, and glucose 3.9. Creatinine is 70 µmol/liter, uric acid 780, total bilirubin 31, and direct bilirubin 10. Total protein is 64 g/liter, albumin 46. Alkaline phosphatase is 144 U/liter, LDH 297, and SGOT 35. PT is 11.9 seconds, activated PTT 30.2.

Heart and liver are large (Figure 1-1). Contrast medium is in right kidney 2 days after its injection for the CT scan. CT scan (Figure 1-2A) shows defects in liver as does ultrasound examination (Figure 1-2B). Contrast medium puddles in liver and flows into large veins in angiogram (Figure 1-3A). Intrahepatic blood flow is decreased after injection of metal coils (Figure 1-3B).

Diagnosis: Hemangiomas in liver; heart failure, high-output state.

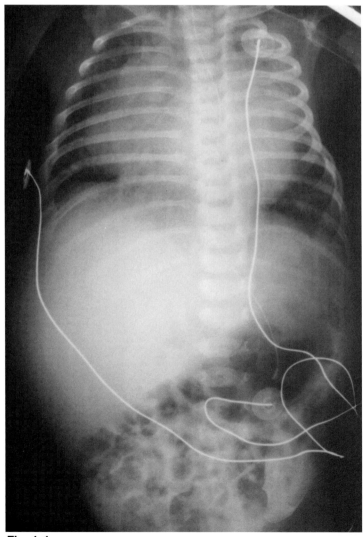

Fig. 1-1

(Continued)

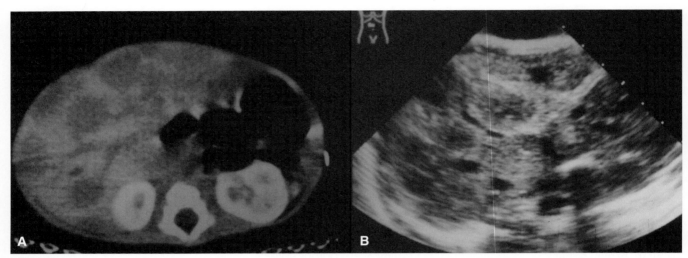

Fig. 1-2

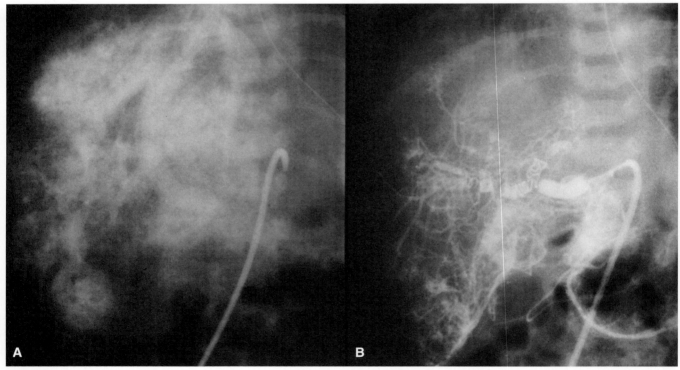

Fig. 1-3

Case 2

An 8-day-old girl has a big liver.

Mother had proteinuria in last week of pregnancy. Birth weight was 2.5 kg. The infant had right parietal cephalohematoma, petechiae, and purpura. Infant's platelet count was 49×10^9/liter, mother's was 125×10^9/liter. Baby is breast-fed. Liver was big yesterday.

Parents and brother (3 years old) are well. Two maternal aunts had breast cancer.

Weight is 2.4 kg, length 47 cm, head circumference 32 cm, temperature 36.8°C, heart rate 152, respiratory rate 60, and systolic blood pressure 80 mm Hg. A right parietal cephalohematoma is present. She is jaundiced. Abdomen is distended. Liver edge is near right iliac crest and umbilicus. The rest of the physical findings are normal.

Hematocrit is 0.51. White cell count is 12.2×10^9/liter with 0.23 polymorphonuclear cells, 0.01 bands, 0.60 lymphocytes, 0.11 monocytes, and 0.05 eosinophils. Platelet count is 598×10^9/liter. PT is 13.3 seconds. At 9 days, serum sodium is 137 mmol/liter, potassium 3.8, chloride 108, carbon dioxide 21, urea nitrogen 1.8, calcium 2.50, phosphorus 1.87, cholesterol 2.69, and glucose 5.7. Creatinine is 60 µmol/liter, uric acid 140, total bilirubin 265, and direct bilirubin 10. Total protein is 47 g/liter, albumin 33. Alkaline phosphatase is 262 U/liter, LDH 416, and SGOT 53.

Ultrasound examination in Figure 2-1A shows cysts in liver. CT scan after IV injection of contrast medium shows that cysts are not vascular (Figure 2-1B).

At operation, large cysts with fine gelatinous septa and clear yellow liquid are in right lobe of liver, one or two small cysts in left lobe. One surface of excised pink-yellow cyst is glistening and has a network of small vessels, other surface mucoid and semitranslucent. Cross section is green-yellow. Microscopic examination shows (1) edematous connective tissue of fine strands of collagen, (2) occasional fibroblasts, (3) small blood vessels, and (4) thin rim of hepatocytes and proliferating bile ducts. Cyst liquid has 1×10^6/liter white cells, 0.12 polymorphonuclear cells, 0.60 lymphocytes, 0.24 monocytes, 0.04 histiocytes, 850×10^6/liter red cells, 1.1 mmol/liter glucose, 36 g/liter protein, and 162 µmol/liter total bilirubin. Cyst liquid is sterile.

Diagnosis: Mesenchymal hamartoma of liver.

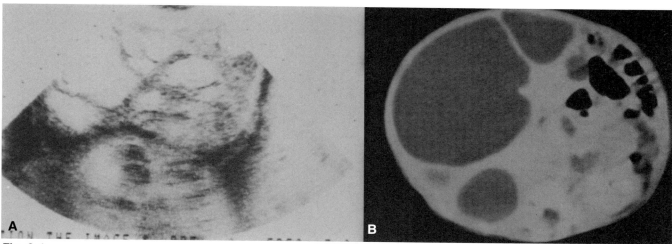

Fig. 2-1

Case 3

A 16-year-old girl is jaundiced and itchy.

She had periumbilical cramps and vomiting 3 weeks ago, followed by jaundice, itching, dark urine, and light stools. She has lost 1.4 kg in the past week and has had headache, dizziness, and nausea for 2 days.

Birth weight was 3.5 kg.

Mother, father, and eight siblings were well when she was born. Maternal grandfather had died with cirrhosis of liver and cancer; paternal grandfather had died with diabetes mellitus.

She was jaundiced at 2 months. At 3 months, liver edge was 3 cm below costal margin. Total bilirubin was 200 µmol/liter, direct bilirubin 164. Alkaline phosphatase was 402 U/liter, SGOT 520. At 3 years, liver edge was 7–8 cm below costal margin, spleen edge 7 cm below costal margin. Serum total bilirubin was 12 µmol/liter, direct bilirubin 5. Alkaline phosphatase was 151 U/liter, SGOT 96. Liver biopsy showed (1) thick capsule from which broad bands of fibrous tissue went into liver and encased bile ductules, (2) collections of lymphocytes and plasma cells, (3) proliferating bile ductules, (4) dilated interlobular veins, and (5) normal lobules. She vomited blood from age 6 to 10 years. Tonsils were removed at 10 years. Menarche was at 13 years. At 15 years, she had epigastric and left upper quadrant pain. Liver edge was not palpable, spleen edge 8 cm below costal margin. Spleen (852 g) was removed and splenorenal shunt made. Examination of spleen showed thick capsule; dense fibrous, hyalinized bands; and sinusoidal congestion.

Weight at 16 years is 72 kg, height 152 cm, temperature 36.9°C, heart rate 80, respiratory rate 20, and blood pressure 108/70 mm Hg. Scar is on upper abdomen. The rest of the physical findings are normal.

Hematocrit is 0.37. White cell count is 12.1×10^9/liter with 0.57 polymorphonuclear cells, 0.03 bands, 0.24 lymphocytes, 0.11 monocytes, 0.03 eosinophils, and 0.02 basophils. Platelet count is 457×10^9/liter. Smear shows Howell-Jolly bodies. PT is 9.9 seconds, activated PTT 34. Serum sodium is 142 mmol/liter, potassium 4.7, chloride 104, carbon dioxide 24, urea nitrogen 3.6, calcium 2.50, phosphorus 1.00, cholesterol 7.53, and glucose 5.0. Creatinine is 70 µmol/liter, uric acid 230, total bilirubin 282, and direct bilirubin 215. Total protein is 61 g/liter, albumin 34. Alkaline phosphatase is 600 U/liter, LDH 402, and SGOT 162.

At operation, liver is small, green, and fibrotic. Wall of gallbladder is thick and edematous. A cyst (6 × 4 cm) is in common hepatic duct just above entrance of adherent cystic duct. Cholecystectomy, cystectomy, and Roux-en-Y anastomosis are performed.

Angiogram before splenectomy at 15 years shows normal renal calyces and pelvises. Operative cholangiogram at 16 years (Figure 3-1) shows (1) intrahepatic ducts, some of them slightly dilated; (2) dilated right and left hepatic ducts; (3) distended common hepatic duct; and (4) gallbladder and cystic duct.

Microscopic examination of gallbladder shows serosal edema and fibrosis and submucosal chronic inflammation. Cyst has fibrous wall and columnar epithelium. Liver biopsy shows (1) stellate fibrosis in portal triads, (2) bile ductule proliferation, (3) increased bile pigment, (4) dilated bile canaliculi, (5) decreased number of portal venous radicles, and (6) foamy hepatocytes.

She is pregnant at 21 years.

Diagnosis: Congenital hepatic fibrosis, dilation of bile ducts.

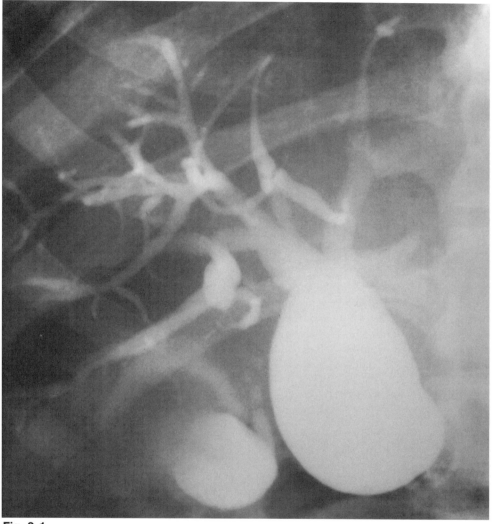

Fig. 3-1

Case 4

A 6-week-old boy has been slightly jaundiced for 3 weeks and is more so today. Stools are green.

Mother had herpetic blisters on lower abdomen during thirty-fourth week of pregnancy and perineal blister at time of vaginal delivery. Birth weight was 3.2 kg.

Parents and sister (2 years old) are well.

Weight is 3.5 kg, length 52 cm, head circumference 37 cm, temperature 37.2°C, heart rate 140, respiratory rate 60, and systolic blood pressure 100 mm Hg. He is pale yellow, tinged green. Liver edge is 1–2 cm below costal margin. The rest of the physical findings are normal.

Hematocrit is 0.41. White cell count is 9.3×10^9/liter with 0.20 polymorphonuclear cells, 0.01 bands, 0.63 lymphocytes, 0.13 monocytes, and 0.03 eosinophils. Platelet count is 611×10^9/liter. Urine specific gravity is 1.006, pH 5. Urine has trace glucose, 1+ bilirubin, and occasional squamous epithelial cells/HPF. Serum sodium is 138 mmol/liter, potassium 5.6, chloride 106, carbon dioxide 20, urea nitrogen 2.9, calcium 2.52, phosphorus 1.94, cholesterol 5.17, and glucose 4.3. Creatinine is 40 µmol/liter, uric acid 130, total bilirubin 152, and direct bilirubin 124. Total protein is 56 g/liter, albumin 39. Alkaline phosphatase is 461 U/liter, LDH 365, and SGOT 191. Serum does not contain HBsAg, HBsAb, or HBcAb. Urine culture does not grow cytomegalovirus. Throat culture does not grow herpesvirus.

Duodenal aspirate is bile tinged. At operation, liver is large.

Operative cholangiogram in Figure 4-1 shows contrast medium in gallbladder, extrahepatic bile ducts, pancreatic duct (Wirsung's duct), duodenum, and faintly in intrahepatic bile ducts.

Liver biopsy shows (1) enlarged portal triads; (2) increased bile in canaliculi; (3) increased biliary epithelium; (4) few swollen, bile-containing hepatocytes; (5) bile in scattered lymphocytes and macrophages; (6) collagen around central veins; and (7) no globules of α_1-antitrypsin with PAS stain after diastase digestion in periportal cells. Electron microscopy shows increased bile in canaliculi and segmental dilation of endoplasmic reticulum with electron dense material.

α_1-Antitrypsin level is 0.57 g/liter (normal: 1.5–3.5), phenotype ZZ. Mother's phenotype is MZ, father's is MZ.

He vomits blood and has tarry stools at 10 months. Hematocrit is 0.23. Serum cholesterol is 6.23 mmol/liter. Ammonia is 68 µmol/liter (normal: 5–50), total bilirubin 24, and direct bilirubin 12. Esophageal varices are injected with sclerosant three times between 12 and 14 months. At 3⅔ years, he has black stools. Weight is 10.9 kg. He has prominent abdominal veins and ascites. Liver transplantation is performed at 4 years.

Diagnosis: α_1-Antitrypsin deficiency.

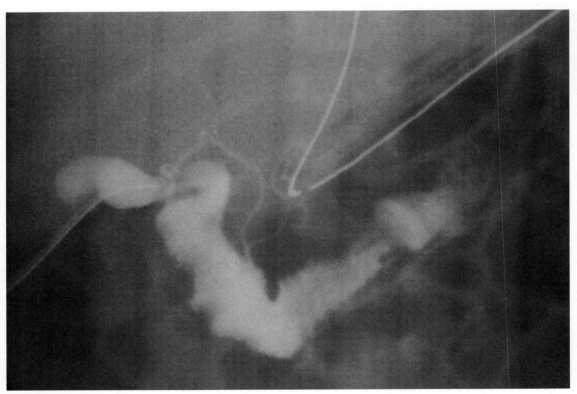

Fig. 4-1

Case 5

A 10-month-old boy has had 10–12 watery stools today.

Pregnancy of mother was normal, birth weight 3.6 kg, length 52 cm, head circumference 37 cm, and Apgar score 9/9 at 1 and 5 minutes. At 36 hours, he refused breast-feeding. Respirations were grunty. He looked distressed. At 39 hours, neck was stiff. Capillary blood glucose was <2.2 mmol/liter, CSF glucose 0.2. He was fed frequently and given glucose by nasogastric tube. At 4 months, he was lethargic and breathing fast. Liver edge was at iliac crest. Venous blood pH was 7.23. Blood was lipemic with cholesterol 6.67 mmol/liter, triglycerides 29.35 (normal: <1.80), lactic acid 6.7 (normal: 0.5–2.0), and uric acid 680 μmol/liter. Fasting blood glucose at start of glucose tolerance test was 0.7 mmol/liter, lactate 11.9. At 2 hours, glucose was 10.8 mmol/liter, lactate 6.1. At 4 hours, glucose was 1.1 mmol/liter, lactate 4.2. He was alert and happy. He had seven seizures at start of feedings from 5 to 7 months.

Temperature at 10 months is 37.7°C, heart rate 140, respiratory rate 36, systolic blood pressure 80 mm Hg, weight 10.2 kg, and length 70 cm. He is pale. Cry is weak. Eyes are glazed and sunken. Skin turgor is poor. Liver edge is 6 cm below costal margin. He is receiving electrolyte and glucose solution by nasogastric tube. The rest of the physical findings are normal.

Hematocrit is 0.33. White cell count is 11.6×10^9/liter with 0.36 polymorphonuclear cells, 0.02 bands, 0.49 lymphocytes, 0.10 monocytes, 0.01 atypical lymphocytes, 0.01 metamyelocytes, and 0.01 myelocytes. Venous blood pH is 7.25. Stool contains blood. Serum sodium is 164 mmol/liter, potassium 4.6, chloride 138, carbon dioxide 8, urea nitrogen 10.0, and glucose 4.7.

Roentgenogram in Figure 5-1 shows that (1) dilated gut, which contains gas and liquid, is displaced to left by enlarged liver; (2) an enteric tube ends in stomach; (3) heart is small; and (4) lungs are normal.

Glycogen in piece of liver obtained at operation is 7.3% by wet weight (normal: 2.5–6.0%), in right rectus 0.02% by wet weight (normal: 0.1–5.4). Liver glucose-6-phosphatase activity is 0 (normal: 4.7 ± 1.9 μmol/Pi/g/min).

Diagnosis: Glycogenosis, type IA (von Gierke's disease).

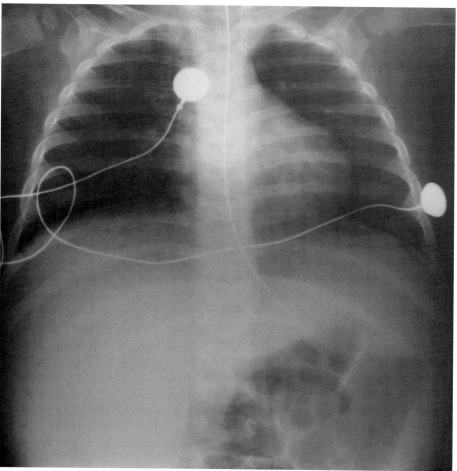

Fig. 5-1

Case 6

A 4½-month-old girl feeds erratically several times per week. She will breast-feed for 1–2 minutes, turn away, become bloated, and then refuse to feed for as long as 18 hours. She has four to five bowel movements per day and then none for 5 days. Mother thinks girl's abdomen has been large for several months.

Mother and sister (1 year old) are well. Father (38 years old) had a coronary bypass operation 1 year ago.

Pregnancy of mother was normal, birth weight 3.9 kg, length 48 cm, and head circumference 37 cm. Guthrie spot tests of blood obtained at 3 days and 1 month showed 550 µmol/liter tyrosine (normal: 20–90). Weight was 5.3 kg at 2 months. She reaches for toys and holds them.

Temperature at 4½ months is 37.7°C, heart rate 132, respiratory rate 32, systolic blood pressure 98 mm Hg, weight 5.8 kg, length 61 cm, and head circumference 41 cm. Left pupil is larger than right. Liver edge is 6 cm below costal margin, spleen edge 5 cm. A capillary hemangioma is on right buttock. The rest of the physical findings are normal.

Hematocrit is 0.39. White cell count is 12.6×10^9/liter with 0.15 polymorphonuclear cells, 0.03 bands, 0.79 lymphocytes, 0.01 monocytes, and 0.02 eosinophils. Platelet count is 155×10^9/liter. Urine specific gravity is 1.005, pH 7. Urine has rare red and white cells/HPF, bacteria, and mucus. Serum sodium is 140 mmol/liter, potassium 4.7, chloride 112, carbon dioxide 17, urea nitrogen 1.8, calcium 2.52, phosphorus 0.81, cholesterol 5.61, triglycerides 2.17, and glucose 3.4. Creatinine is 40 µmol/liter, uric acid 200, total bilirubin 26, direct bilirubin 15, and ammonia 43 (normal: 5–50). Total protein is 65 g/liter, albumin 45, and α_1-antitrypsin 2.8 (normal: 1.5–3.5). Alkaline phosphatase is 1,854 U/liter, LDH 276, and SGOT 75. Ceruloplasmin is 400 mg/liter (normal: 200–350). PT is 15.1 seconds, activated PTT 54.6 with no response to vitamin K. Urine has succinylacetone and 1,068 µmol/liter ∂-aminolevulinic acid (normal: 0–42). Plasma tyrosine is 230 µmol/liter (normal: 72–216).

Excretory urogram shows normal renal pelves and calyces and displacement of gut by enlarged liver (Figure 6-1). Metaphyses at knees (Figure 6-2A) are not rachitic at 4½ months; those at ankles are, and, at 1 year, those at knees are (Figure 6-2B).

At 1 year, she sits and pulls to stand. Weight is 7.5 kg, length 72 cm. Serum calcium is 2.37 mmol/liter, phosphorus 0.58, and magnesium 0.66 (normal: 0.8–1.2). α-Fetoprotein is 213 µg/liter (normal: 0–20).

She vomits frequently and has abdominal pain. She is unresponsive at 4 years because of hepatic encephalopathy. She undergoes liver transplantation at 4 years, 2 months, and dies with metastatic hepatocellular carcinoma at 5 years, 4 months.

Diagnosis: Tyrosinemia, rickets.

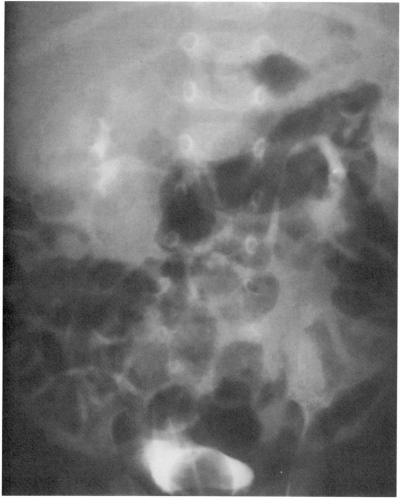

Fig. 6-1

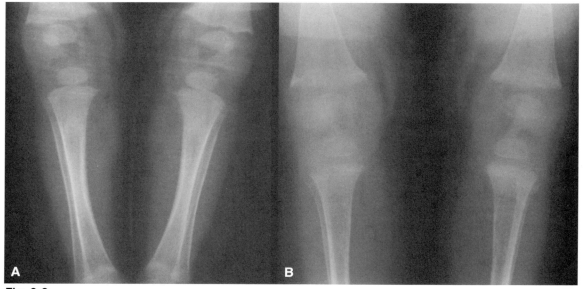

Fig. 6-2

Case 7

A 14-year-old girl with cystic fibrosis has lower abdominal cramps.

She has had many ear infections and myringotomies and a tonsillectomy. She has been coughing more for 2 months, bringing up green, blood-streaked sputum and vomiting after some coughing spells. Cramps began 2 days ago; they start in early morning, last all day, are worse approximately 20 minutes after she eats, and do not wake her at night. Appetite is good. She has several bowel movements per day.

Temperature is 37.8°C, heart rate 100, respiratory rate 24, blood pressure 115/76 mm Hg, and weight 34 kg. Eardrums are opaque. Nasal mucosa is injected. Rales are in right upper lobe. Nailbeds are blue. Lower abdomen is tender. The rest of the physical findings are normal.

Hematocrit is 0.37. White cell count is 7.4×10^9/liter with 0.68 polymorphonuclear cells, 0.23 lymphocytes, and 0.09 monocytes. Platelet count is 416×10^9/liter. Urine specific gravity is 1.025, pH 7. Urine has trace ketones, 3–6 white cells/HPF, occasional squamous epithelial cells/HPF, and 1–3 hyaline casts/LPF. Serum sodium is 142 mmol/liter, potassium 3.4, chloride 103, carbon dioxide 20, urea nitrogen 2.9, calcium 2.32, phosphorus 1.19, cholesterol 2.33, and glucose 10.3. Creatinine is 70 µmol/liter, uric acid 210, total bilirubin 5, and direct bilirubin 2. Total protein is 79 g/liter, albumin 44. Alkaline phosphatase is 230 U/liter, LDH 188, and SGOT 24. Venous blood pH is 7.46. P_{CO_2} is 24 mm Hg, P_{O_2} 53. HCO_3 is 16 mmol/liter.

Pulmonary function tests show moderate obstruction.

Front part of liver is hyperechoic with a sharp edge between it and less echogenic back part (Figure 7-1).

Diagnosis: Fatty liver in a girl with cystic fibrosis and hyperglycemia.

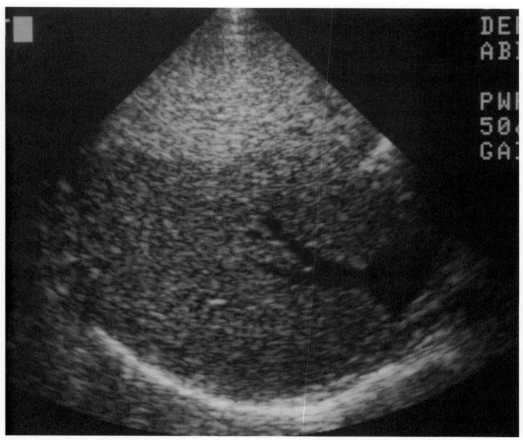

Fig. 7-1

Case 8

A 9-year-old girl who was knocked out in a car crash complains of pain in right side of chest, right flank, and left leg 15 minutes later.

Temperature is 37.6°C, heart rate 140, respiratory rate 24, blood pressure 116/70 mm Hg, and weight 22 kg. She is drowsy at times and does not remember the crash. She is pale. A bruise is on left side of forehead. Teeth marks are on tongue. Neck is tender at C4 and C5. Left clavicle is tender. Abdomen is tender. Bowel sounds are diminished. Blood is at urethral meatus. A bruise is on left thigh. The rest of the physical findings are normal.

Hematocrit is 0.37. White cell count is 11.6×10^9/liter with 0.23 polymorphonuclear cells, 0.18 bands, 0.41 lymphocytes, 0.04 monocytes, 0.06 atypical lymphocytes, 0.05 metamyelocytes, and 0.03 myelocytes. Platelet count is 603×10^9/liter. Serum sodium is 139 mmol/liter, potassium 3.3, chloride 110, carbon dioxide 21, urea nitrogen 6.4, and glucose 10.0. Bloody urine comes out of bladder catheter.

Cystogram in Figure 8-1A shows extravasation of contrast medium from bladder into right side of pelvis, contrast medium in both ureters, and medial displacement of right ureter. CT scan after IV and oral contrast media shows jagged strips of diminished density in liver (Figure 8-1B). Roentgenogram of chest shows fracture of left clavicle.

At operation, blood is in space of Retzius between pubic bone and bladder. A 2-mm hole is in right side of bladder. A laceration is in dome of right lobe of liver, a smaller one in left lobe near falciform ligament, a small one in top of spleen, and a small serosal tear in cecum.

She is well 3 weeks later. Urine has a few epithelial cells/HPF and 1–2 white cells/HPF.

Diagnosis: Laceration of liver and perforation of urinary bladder.

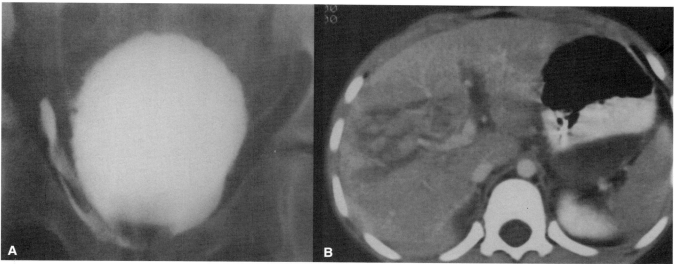

Fig. 8-1

Case 9

A 10-year-old girl, who was injured 13 days ago while horse-back riding, had a bellyache this morning and is vomiting blood clots. She vomits unclotted blood 12 hours later.

Liver laceration was closed at operation 11 days ago. She has been taking aspirin for 13 days.

Weight is 29.2 kg, temperature 38°C, heart rate 100, respiratory rate 20, and blood pressure 120/80 mm Hg. Breath sounds are diminished at right base. An incision is in abdomen, a drain site incision in right flank. Right side of abdomen is tender. Liver edge is 1–2 cm below costal margin. The rest of the physical findings are normal.

Hematocrit is 0.36. White cell count is 18.1×10^9/liter with 0.57 polymorphonuclear cells, 0.11 bands, 0.21 lymphocytes, 0.10 monocytes, and 0.01 eosinophils. Platelet count is 604×10^9/liter. Urine specific gravity is 1.018, pH 8. Urine has occasional white cells/HPF and amorphous phosphates.

Straw-colored liquid, 250 ml, is aspirated from right side of chest. GI series and endoscopic findings in esophagus, stomach, and duodenum are normal. Ultrasound examination of gallbladder shows small, dense echoes without shielding that are gone several days later.

She has black stools 23 days after injury. She vomits blood 28 days after injury. Fifty-eight days after injury, she vomits again and has epigastric pain.

Metal clips are in liver; injection of contrast medium into celiac arterial trunk shows pseudoaneurysm in branch of right hepatic artery, stretching of branches of right and left hepatic arteries, and tortuosity of upper right branches (Figure 9-1).

She has no more GI bleeding after selective embolization with gelfoam of artery that has pseudoaneurysm.

Diagnosis: Hematobilia.

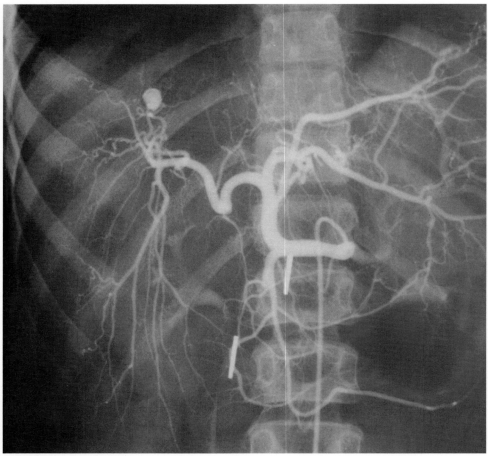

Fig. 9-1

Case 10

A 22-year-old woman has bruised easily for 1 month. She bruised a thigh when she got into a car too fast. Nose and gums bleed.

Weight is 57 kg, temperature 36.9°C, heart rate 80, respiratory rate 20, and blood pressure 118/70 mm Hg. A systolic murmur is present. Old and new bruises are on legs. The rest of the physical findings are normal.

Hematocrit is 0.32. White cell count is 11.0×10^9/liter with 0.13 polymorphonuclear cells, 0.04 bands, 0.66 lymphocytes, 0.01 monocytes, 0.01 eosinophils, 0.02 atypical lymphocytes, 0.01 metamyelocytes, and 0.12 blasts. Platelet count is 116×10^9/liter. PT is 16.9 seconds, activated PTT 39.4. Fibrinogen level is 0.5 g/liter (normal: 1.5–3.5). D-Dimer level is 8–16 mg/liter (normal: <0.5).

Bone marrow biopsy shows 90–100% immature cells, smear of marrow aspirate blasts with abundant vacuolated cytoplasm and large nuclei with prominent nucleoli and dispersed chromatin. Peroxidase stain is negative; butyrate esterase stain is positive.

Treatment is begun for acute monocytic leukemia. She begins to have temperature of 38.3–40.0°C on the fourteenth day. Hematocrit is 0.24 on the fifteenth day. White cell count is 0.4×10^9/liter with 1.0 lymphocytes. Platelet count is 26×10^9/liter. Chemotherapy for infection is begun on the six-teenth day. Hematocrit is 0.28 on the thirty-seventh day. White cell count is 8.6×10^9/liter (3 days earlier: 8.7×10^9/liter with 0.78 polymorphonuclear cells, 0.01 bands, 0.06 lymphocytes, 0.14 monocytes, and 0.01 basophils). Platelet count is 291×10^9/liter.

Ultrasound examination of spleen on the thirty-seventh day (Figure 10-1A) and CT scan on the thirty-eighth day (Figure 10-1B) show uniform round defects, fewer in liver, more in spleen.

Six months after diagnosis and first treatment for leukemia, CT scan shows larger defects in liver, fewer and smaller defects in spleen. At operation, adhesions and firm, yellow implants are on capsules of liver and spleen. Spleen is removed. It is $20.0 \times 10.0 \times 3.5$ cm, weighs 350 g, and is covered by gray, glistening fibrous capsule and white-yellow firm nodules (0.1–0.9 cm). Cut section shows well-circumscribed, yellow-white cheesy nodules. Biopsy of liver shows similar surface nodule. Microscopic examination shows fungus inside necrotizing granulomas.

Blood and urine cultures on sixteenth day grow *Candida paratropicalis*.

She dies 9 months after diagnosis of leukemia.

Diagnosis: Acute monocytic leukemia, disseminated candidiasis.

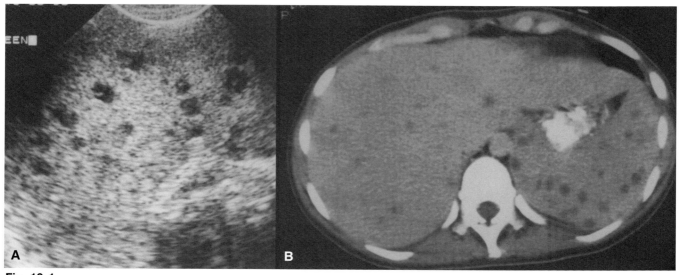

Fig. 10-1

Case 11

A 7-month-old boy has cried whenever left arm or left leg is moved during past 3 days. He has been cranky and belching for a week. Abdomen is swollen today.

Pregnancy of mother was normal, birth weight 5 kg. Left humerus was fractured 2 months ago when he rolled from sister's lap onto a soft couch.

Mother (36 years old), father, and sister (12 years old) are well. Paternal grandmother had colon cancer; paternal great-grandmother had lung cancer.

Temperature is 37.2°C, heart rate 140, respiratory rate 40, systolic blood pressure 100 mm Hg, and weight 8.6 kg. Cheeks are flushed, sclerae jaundiced. Left arm is flexed and resists movement. Abdominal veins are prominent. A hemangioma is below umbilicus. A mass fills right side of abdomen and crosses midline. The rest of the physical findings are normal.

Hematocrit is 0.36. White cell count is 13.7×10^9/liter with 0.35 polymorphonuclear cells, 0.08 bands, 0.45 lymphocytes, and 0.12 monocytes. Platelet count is 1.2×10^{12}/liter. Urine specific gravity is 1.013, pH 5. Urine has 2+ protein, 5–6 red cells/HPF, 40–50 white cells/HPF, and 1–2 hyaline casts/LPF. Serum sodium is 126 mmol/liter, potassium 8.7, chloride 89, carbon dioxide 13, urea nitrogen 16.8, calcium 3.02, phosphorus 2.39, cholesterol 16.30, and glucose 2.3. Creatinine is 110 µmol/liter, uric acid 640, total bilirubin 87, and direct bilirubin 67. Total protein is 75 g/liter, albumin 44. Alkaline phosphatase is 149 U/liter, LDH 484, and SGOT 132. PT is 11.9 seconds (control: 9.9), activated PTT

37.4 (normal: 30.6). Urinary calcium/creatinine is 1.8 to 2.7 (normal: <0.4), urinary phosphorus/creatinine is 0.5 to 1.2 (normal: <0.4). Serum calcitonin is 430 ng/liter (normal: <400). α-Fetoprotein is 509,000 µg/liter. Urine vanillylmandelic acid is 15.5 mmol/mol$_{creatinine}$ (normal: 0–12.7).

Roentgenogram in Figure 11-1 shows (1) rarefied bones; (2) fractures in left humerus; and (3) newer fracture near proximal metaphysis of left radius, in right femur, and in distal part of left fibula. Angiogram in Figure 11-2 shows tumor vessels in large liver.

At operation, tumor is solid and partly necrotic. Bleeding at operative wound persists. He dies later the same day.

Necropsy shows (1) tumor cells in sheets, nests, trabeculae, and acini, and (2) thick fibrous septa that contain benign, intense proliferation of bile ductules in branching network. Parenchymal tumor cells are of fetal cell type, smaller than normal hepatocytes. The tumor cells have increased nucleus-to-cytoplasm ratio, amphophilic cytoplasm, clumped and peripherally marginated chromatin, eccentric prominent nucleoli, and 1–3 mitoses/HPF. Proliferating bile ductules are lined by cuboidal and columnar epithelium with round, oval, or polygonal nuclei and evenly dispersed chromatin. Large clusters of islet cells are in pancreas. Rib metaphysis is fibrotic. Osteoclasts line thin spicules of bone. Cortex is thin, absent in places. Bone is normally mature and has normal amount of calcification. Parathyroid glands are normal.

Diagnosis: Hepatoblastoma, osteoporosis.

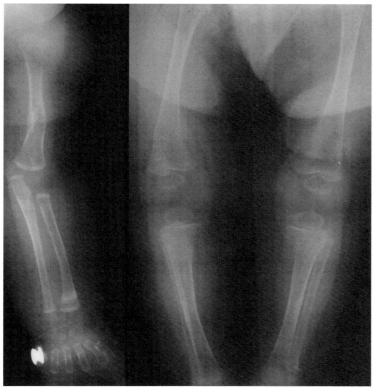

Fig. 11-1

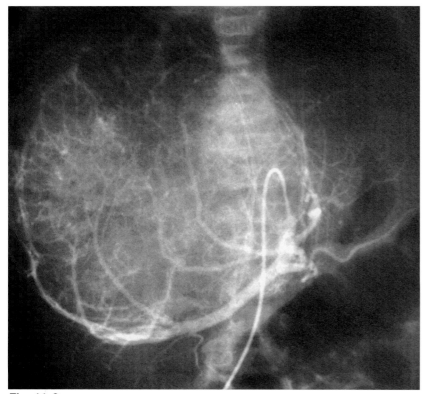

Fig. 11-2

Case 12

A 1-month-old boy has a mass in abdomen.

Pregnancy of mother was normal, birth weight 4.4 kg, and Apgar score 7/9 at 1 and 5 minutes. He is breast-fed. A dense central cataract was in right lens at 2 weeks. At operation, lens, dense plaque in its back part, part of a hyaloid vessel, and surrounding vitreous were removed. He has had several episodes of flushing and crying loudly, and sleeps more than his two older siblings did at that age. A mass was felt yesterday.

Parents and two siblings are well.

Weight at 1 month is 5.4 kg, length 55 cm, head circumference 40 cm, temperature 36.7°C, heart rate 175, respiratory rate 40, and blood pressure 110/35 mm Hg. Red papules are on face. Liver edge is below umbilicus and crosses midline. Three subcutaneous nodules (1.0–1.5 cm), two on chest, one on back of right thigh, are present. The rest of the physical findings are normal.

Hematocrit is 0.44. White cell count is 20.5×10^9/liter with 0.16 polymorphonuclear cells, 0.02 bands, 0.70 lymphocytes, 0.09 monocytes, and 0.03 eosinophils. Platelet count is 357×10^9/liter. Serum sodium is 143 mmol/liter, potassium 5.4, chloride 107, carbon dioxide 23, urea nitrogen 2.5, calcium 2.74, phosphorus 1.81, cholesterol 3.34, and glucose 4.6. Creatinine is 40 µmol/liter, uric acid 170, total bilirubin 15, and direct bilirubin 0. Total protein is 61 g/liter, albumin 40. Alkaline phosphatase is 549 U/liter, LDH 447, and SGOT 79.

CT scan after IV injection of contrast medium shows mottled liver and round mass in front of upper part of left kidney, and smaller mass in front of spine between aorta and inferior vena cava (Figure 12-1).

Urine vanillylmandelic acid is 128 $mmol/mol_{creatinine}$ (normal: 0–32.4), homovanillic acid 79.5 (normal: 0–28.6). Bone marrow is normal.

At operation, liver is hard and nodular. Left adrenal tumor, nodule on back of right thigh, and two cores of liver are removed.

Adrenal tumor ($2.5 \times 1.9 \times 0.8$ cm) is encapsulated, its cut surface hemorrhagic, subcutaneous nodule gray-tan. Microscopic examination of all specimens shows neuroblastoma.

More subcutaneous nodules are present at 3 months, original ones smaller. At 16 months, he is well. Liver edge is 3 cm below costal margin. No subcutaneous nodules are present. Urine vanillylmandelic acid is 25 µmol/day (normal: <10).

Diagnosis: Neuroblastoma, stage IV S, congenital cataract, and persistent hyperplastic primary vitreous.

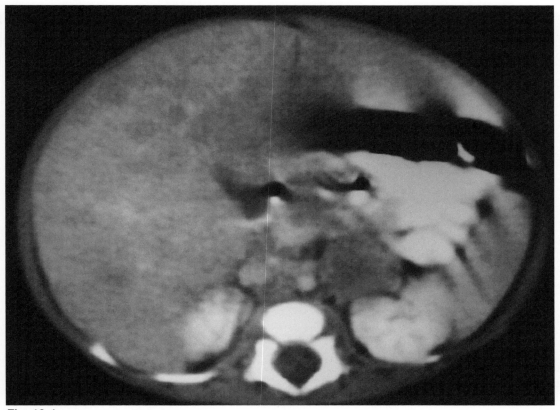

Fig. 12-1

Case 13

A newborn girl has a gallstone found in prenatal ultrasound examination.

Mother (19 years old) is well. Pregnancy was normal. Birth weight is 2.7 kg, Apgar score 9/9 at 1 and 5 minutes, length 47 cm, head circumference 31 cm, temperature 36.7°C, heart rate 132, and respiratory rate 48. Physical findings are normal.

Serum total bilirubin is 67 μmol/liter at 18 hours.

Ultrasound examinations a month before birth (Figure 13-1A) and 1 day after birth (Figure 13-1B) show echogenic focus in region of gallbladder with shadowing.

At 14 days, hematocrit is 0.44, serum sodium 141 mmol/liter, potassium 4.9, chloride 108, carbon dioxide 21, urea nitrogen 1.8, calcium 2.62, phosphorus 2.10, cholesterol 3.49, and glucose 5.1. Creatinine is 40 μmol/liter, uric acid 180, total bilirubin 60, and direct bilirubin 7 (she is breast-fed). Total protein is 51 g/liter, albumin 34. Alkaline phosphatase is 252 U/liter, LDH 282, and SGOT 29.

At 6 weeks, weight is 4 kg. Physical findings are normal.

Diagnosis: Prenatal and neonatal cholelithiasis.

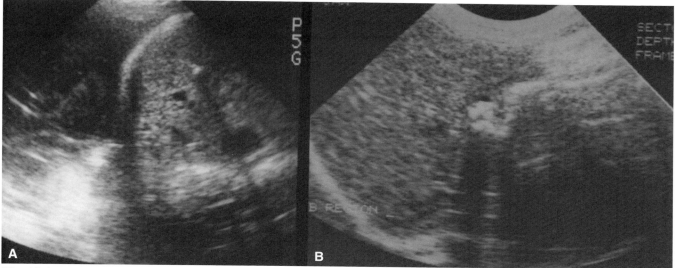

Fig. 13-1

Case 14

A 10-day-old girl has a mass in right upper quadrant of abdomen.

Labor began prematurely, was stopped with ritodrine, and resumed when ritodrine was stopped 2 weeks later. Delivery was by cesarean section because of previous cesarean section.

Mother (22 years old) is well. Sister (2 years old) has ear infections and cold sores.

Birth weight was 2.8 kg, Apgar score 8/8 at 1 and 5 minutes, temperature 36.7°C, heart rate 145, respiratory rate 80, and blood pressure 60/40 mm Hg. Liver edge was 4 cm below costal margin. The rest of the physical findings were normal. She was soon dusky and retracting, then pale and flaccid.

Hematocrit was 0.40. White cell count was 18.4×10^9/liter. Platelet count was 309×10^9/liter. Serum sodium was 141 mmol/liter, potassium 4.2, chloride 100, calcium 1.95, and glucose 5.6. Arterial blood pH was 7.21. P_{CO_2} was 58 mm Hg, P_{O_2} 72. At 8 days, serum bilirubin was 85 µmol/liter.

At 8 days, feeding was begun and stopped because she vomited and had bile in gastric aspirate. A mobile mass is in right upper quadrant of abdomen at 10 days.

In Figure 14-1 at 10 days, nonshadowing echogenic matter is in dilated gallbladder.

At 11 days, serum total bilirubin is 44 µmol/liter, direct bilirubin 7. Liver edge is 2–3 cm below costal margin at 12 days.

Diagnosis: Biliary sludge.

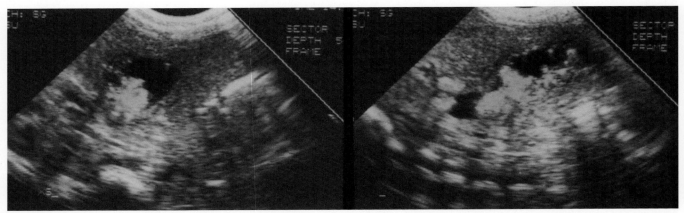

Fig. 14-1

Case 15

A 3½-year-old girl has had abdominal cramps for 3 days and vomiting for 2 days.

Parents and sister (5 years old) are well.

Temperature is 37.6°C, heart rate 92, respiratory rate 20, blood pressure 92/48 mm Hg, weight 13 kg, and height 98 cm. Physical findings are normal.

Hematocrit is 0.34. White cell count is 12.7 × 10⁹/liter with 0.67 polymorphonuclear cells, 0.15 bands, 0.15 lymphocytes, 0.02 monocytes, and 0.01 basophils. Platelet count is 488 × 10⁹/liter. Urine specific gravity is 1.012, pH 6. Urine has >56 mmol/liter glucose, 0.40 g/liter ketones, and occasional squamous epithelial cells/HPF. Serum sodium is 138 mmol/liter, potassium 3.9, chloride 104, carbon dioxide 24, urea nitrogen 3.6, calcium 2.47, phosphorus 1.03, cholesterol 4.71, and glucose 6.7. Creatinine is 50 μmol/liter, uric acid 330, total bilirubin 21, and direct bilirubin 15. Total protein is 62 g/liter, albumin 43. Alkaline phosphatase is 440 U/liter, LDH 232, SGOT 116, and amylase 17.

A shadow of calcium density is in right side of abdomen at level L3–L4; smaller shadows of calcium density are closer to right side of spine at level L2–L3 (Figure 15-1). Ultrasound examination shows echogenic object in gallbladder with shadowing (Figure 15-2A), another in common bile duct with shadowing (Figure 15-2B).

At operation 4 days later, gallbladder is slightly edematous and contains a stone. Cholangiogram shows normal bile ducts without stone.

Microscopic examination of gallbladder shows chronic cholecystitis.

Diagnosis: Cholecystitis, cholelithiasis, choledocholithiasis, and spontaneous passage of ductal stone.

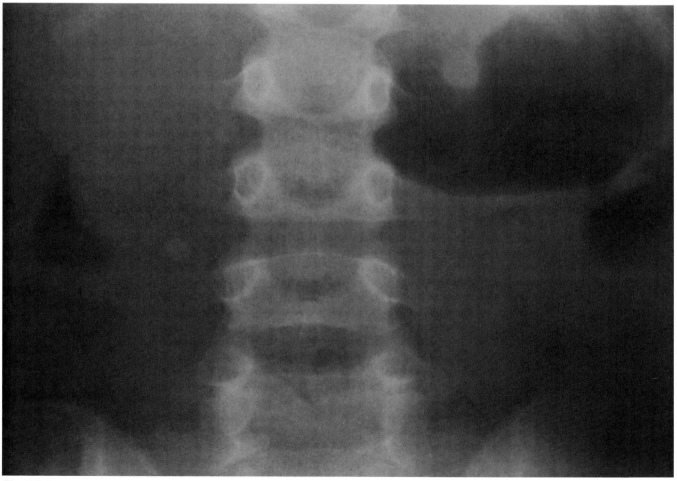

Fig. 15-1

(Continued)

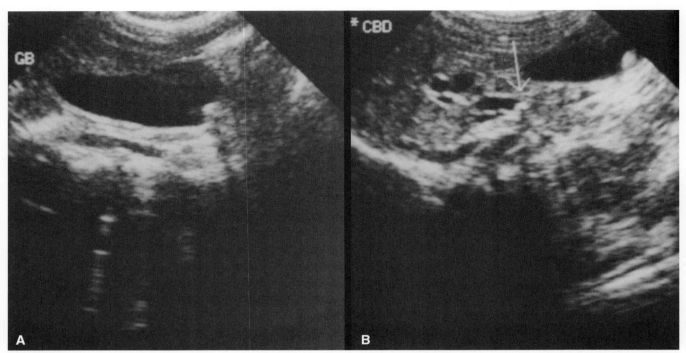

Fig. 15-2

Case 16

A 5-year-old girl has abdominal pain.

Pregnancy of mother was normal, birth weight 3 kg. She has had epigastric pains radiating to back for a year. She is pale and lies on side with legs flexed when she has pain and feels better after she vomits. Pain used to last from a few hours to all day. Three times in the last month, she has had pain and fever lasting 4–5 days.

Parents are well. Father has similar pain.

Weight is 15 kg, height 105 cm, temperature 37.4°C, heart rate 100, respiratory rate 24, and blood pressure 86/60 mm Hg. Epigastrium and right upper quadrant of abdomen are tender. The rest of the physical findings are normal.

Hematocrit is 0.40. White cell count is 9.2×10^9/liter with 0.72 polymorphonuclear cells, 0.03 bands, 0.21 lymphocytes, and 0.04 monocytes. Platelet count is 284×10^9/liter. Serum sodium is 137 mmol/liter, potassium 4.3, chloride 102, carbon dioxide 28, urea nitrogen 2.5, calcium 2.27, phosphorus 1.49, cholesterol 3.15, and glucose 4.7. Creatinine is 50 µmol/liter, uric acid 100, total bilirubin 3, and direct bilirubin 0. Total protein is 75 g/liter, albumin 32. Alkaline phosphatase is 111

U/liter, LDH 260, SGOT 22, and amylase 1,132 (normal: 0–130). Urine amylase is 486 U/liter. PT is 12 seconds, activated PTT 29.6.

Ultrasound examination shows normal kidneys and dilated extrahepatic bile ducts (Figure 16-1A). Paraisopropyliminodiacetic acid isotope scan shows dilated common hepatic duct (Figure 16-1B). Endoscopic retrograde cholangiopancreatogram shows dilated common hepatic duct, dilated gallbladder, and long, dilated cystic duct; common bile duct is undilated, short and joined by undilated pancreatic duct (Figure 16-2).

At operation, gallbladder, choledochal cyst, and normal appendix are removed. Roux-en-Y anastomosis is created.

Gross and microscopic examinations show mucosal hyperplasia and slight chronic inflammation in gallbladder, and dilation and focal mucosal ulceration of cystic duct and common bile duct.

Diagnosis: Recurrent pancreatitis, choledochal cyst.

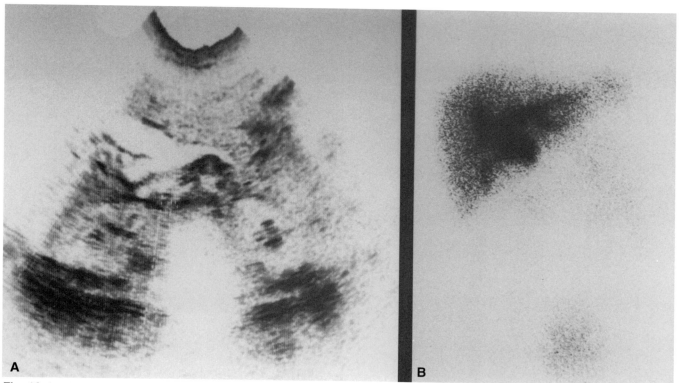

Fig. 16-1

(Continued)

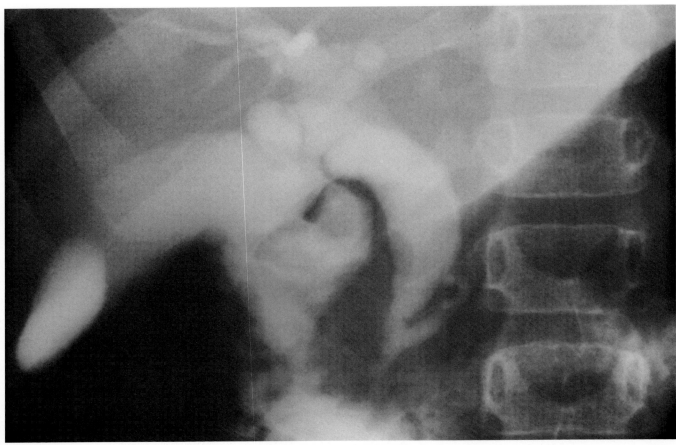

Fig. 16-2

Case 17

A 75-year-old woman has an unusual finding in CT scan of abdomen.

She had cervical cancer that was treated by irradiation at 44 years. Diabetes mellitus was diagnosed at 54 years. Cholecystectomy was performed at 64 years. She has been taking insulin for 3 years. She had rectal bleeding at 74 years, ascribed to colonic diverticula found at barium enema and colonoscopy. GI series showed sliding hiatal hernia.

Temperature at 75 years is 36.2°C, heart rate 72, respiratory rate 16, blood pressure 148/70 mm Hg, weight 73 kg, and height 163 cm. A scar is on abdomen. The rest of the physical findings are normal.

CT scan in Figure 17-1 shows a round mass in right side of abdomen, superior mesenteric vein medial to it, inferior vena cava behind and medial, and descending second part of duodenum with contrast medium between it and right kidney, and cysts in left kidney. Endoscopic retrograde cholangiopancreatography in Figure 17-2 shows (1) contrast medium that has been injected into major papilla in common bile duct, main hepatic ducts, and pancreatic duct; (2) contrast medium that has been injected into dorsal minor papilla in second pancreatic duct; (3) contrast medium in gallbladder or duodenum; and (4) barium in colonic diverticula.

Diagnosis: Pancreas divisum.

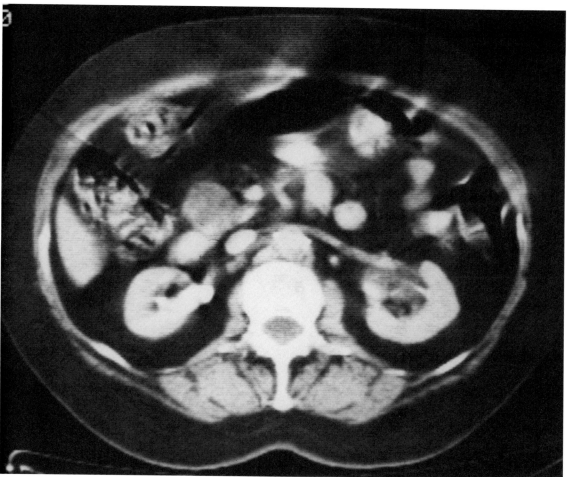

Fig. 17-1

(Continued)

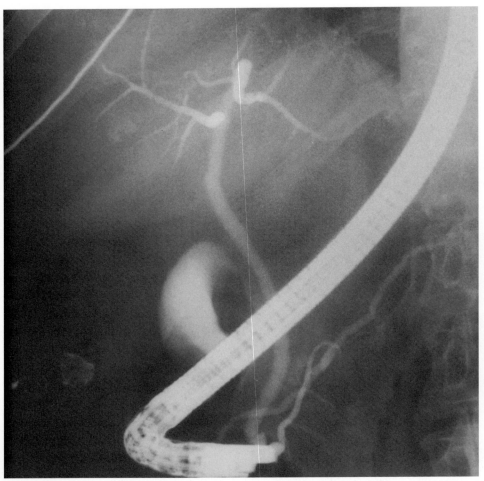

Fig. 17-2

Case 18

An 8-year-old boy has abdominal pain that goes through to back, gets worse for 1–2 days, and then subsides during next 2–3 days. He has been hospitalized four times for pain since age 4 years.

Mother has similar pain once per year; maternal grandfather, who died with pancreatic cancer, and maternal great-grand-mother had similar pain. Maternal great-great-grandmother, maternal great-grandmother, two maternal great-aunts, and maternal aunt had pancreatitis.

Temperature is 37.3°C, heart rate 66, respiratory rate 14, blood pressure 90/60 mm Hg, and weight 32.5 kg. Ten months ago, height was 127 cm. Epigastrium is tender. The rest of the physical findings are normal.

Hemoglobin is 145 g/liter. White cell count is 6.9×10^9/liter with 0.58 polymorphonuclear cells, 0.04 bands, 0.29 lymphocytes, 0.07 monocytes, and 0.01 eosinophils. Serum sodium is 140 mmol/liter, potassium 4.4, chloride 106, carbon dioxide 24, urea nitrogen 6.4, calcium 2.37, phosphorus 1.81, cholesterol 4.24, and glucose 4.8. Creatinine is 50 µmol/liter, uric acid 320, total bilirubin 9, and direct bilirubin 3. Total protein is 72 g/liter, albumin 48. Alkaline phosphatase is 321 U/liter, LDH 245, SGOT 32, and amylase 50 (242 and 840 during last two attacks; normal: 0–130). α_1-Antitrypsin is 2.5 g/liter.

His 16-year-old cousin, son of healthy maternal uncle, had constant abdominal pain once at 5 years and twice at 15 years, at 5-month intervals with serum amylase 385 U/liter in last episode. He was treated by cholecystectomy, followed by transduodenal sphincteroplasty, Roux-en-Y anastomosis, and, for a while, feeding jejunostomy.

Endoscopic retrograde pancreatography shows slight, uneven dilation of pancreatic duct in tail of pancreas in 8-year-old boy (Figure 18-1A) and aneurysms and tortuosity of pancreatic duct in 16-year-old boy (Figure 18-1B). Contrast medium is also in bile ducts of younger boy (see Figure 18-1A) and in small bowel of both boys (see Figure 18-1); two metal clips are in upper abdomen of older boy (see Figure 18-1B).

Diagnosis: Hereditary pancreatitis.

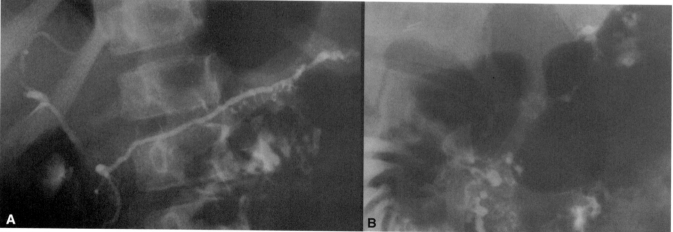

Fig. 18-1

Case 19

A 6-year-old girl has had epigastric pain for 3 days. She began to vomit 2 days ago. Pain and vomiting are worse today.

She told her parents this morning that she had the wind knocked out of her a week and a half ago when she fell off a picnic table and hit her abdomen on a corner of the table. She broke an arm 2 years ago.

Temperature is 37°C, heart rate 100, respiratory rate 20, blood pressure 110/70 mm Hg, and weight 18.2 kg. Tongue is dry. Eyes are sunken. Epigastrium is tender. Bowel sounds are increased. The rest of the physical findings are normal.

Hematocrit is 0.35. White cell count is 11.3×10^9/liter with 0.65 polymorphonuclear cells, 0.13 bands, 0.09 lymphocytes, and 0.13 monocytes. Platelet count is 409×10^9/liter. Urine specific gravity is 1.016, pH 7. Urine has 0–1 white cell/HPF,

0–1 red cell/HPF, and mucus. Serum sodium is 140 mmol/liter, potassium 4.3, chloride 103, carbon dioxide 24, urea nitrogen 2.1, calcium 2.37, phosphorus 1.19, cholesterol 3.49, triglycerides 0.71, and glucose 6.1. Creatinine is 40 μmol/liter, uric acid 170, total bilirubin 15, and direct bilirubin 5. Total protein is 61 g/liter, albumin 42. Alkaline phosphatase is 176 U/liter, LDH 197, SGOT 30, and amylase 2,075 (on sixteenth day: 150; normal: 0–130).

Ultrasound examination on the thirteenth day (Figure 19-1A) shows echolucent defect in head of pancreas (medial to right kidney). Defect is gone a month later (Figure 19-1B).

Diagnosis: Questionable traumatic pancreatitis; pseudocyst.

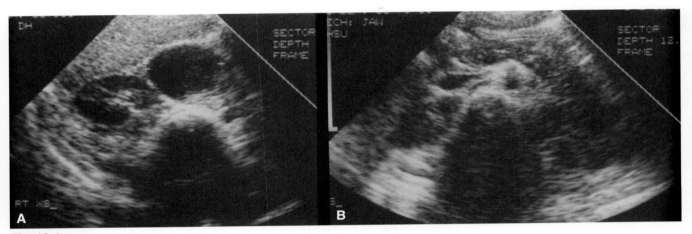

Fig. 19-1

Case 20

A newborn boy has petechiae and purpura.

Mother (27 years old) and sister (4 years old) are well.

Pregnancy was normal, presentation breech, and delivery by cesarean section. Birth weight is 4.3 kg, length 53 cm, head circumference 38 cm, and Apgar score 8/8 at 1 and 5 minutes. At 5 hours, he is blue around lips and pale. Respiratory rate is 85. The rest of the physical findings are normal. At 3 days, temperature is 36.8°C, heart rate 140, respiratory rate 78, and systolic blood pressure 70 mm Hg. He has petechiae, purpura, and papules and pustules with 1-cm red rim. A continuous heart murmur is present. Liver edge and spleen edge are 6 cm below costal margin. The rest of the physical findings are normal.

At 19 hours, hematocrit is 0.41. White cell count is 60.0 × 10⁹/liter with 0.12 polymorphonuclear cells, 0.07 bands, 0.80 lymphocytes, and 0.01 monocytes. Platelet count is 330 × 10⁹/liter. Urine specific gravity is 1.009, pH 6. Urine has trace protein, 0–2 epithelial cells/HPF, 0–2 white cells/HPF, 0–2 granular casts/LPF, and mucus. Serum sodium is 141 mmol/liter, potassium 4.5, chloride 107, carbon dioxide 20, urea nitrogen 3.6, calcium 2.40, phosphorus 2.00, cholesterol 1.60, and glucose 4.6. Creatinine is 110 μmol/liter, uric acid 310, total bilirubin 68, and direct bilirubin 2. Total protein is 56 g/liter, albu-

min 36. Alkaline phosphatase is 134 U/liter, LDH 774, and SGOT 51. Smear of peripheral blood at 3 days shows that approximately half the white cells are large and immature with little cytoplasm and one to four distinct nucleoli.

Roentgenogram at 3 days shows umbilical arterial catheter kinked at umbilicus and displacement of gas-containing gut by large liver and spleen (Figure 20-1).

At 3 days, nearly two-thirds of bone marrow cells are immature myeloid cells, some blastic, many promyelocytic with dark staining granules, 0.63 blasts, 0.20 myeloid cells, 0.10 erythrocytes, and 0.07 lymphocytes. Karyotype of bone marrow cells obtained at 8 days shows 18 of 20, 47,XY,+21; two of 20, 46,XY. Of peripheral cells, eight of 21 are 47,XY,+21, and 13 of 21 are 46,XY. Liver and spleen are not palpable on day 10. At 12 days, hematocrit is 0.45. White cell count is 21.5 × 10⁹/liter with 0.26 polymorphonuclear cells, 0.02 bands, 0.42 lymphocytes, 0.02 monocytes, 0.26 blasts, 0.01 myelocytes, and 0.01 metamyelocytes. Rash is gone at 1 month. All 40 marrow cells karyotyped at 2 months are 46,XY. Weight is 23.6 kg at 4½ years, height 114 cm. Physical findings are normal.

Diagnosis: Neonatal erythema toxicum and blastic bone marrow with leukemoid reaction.

(Continued)

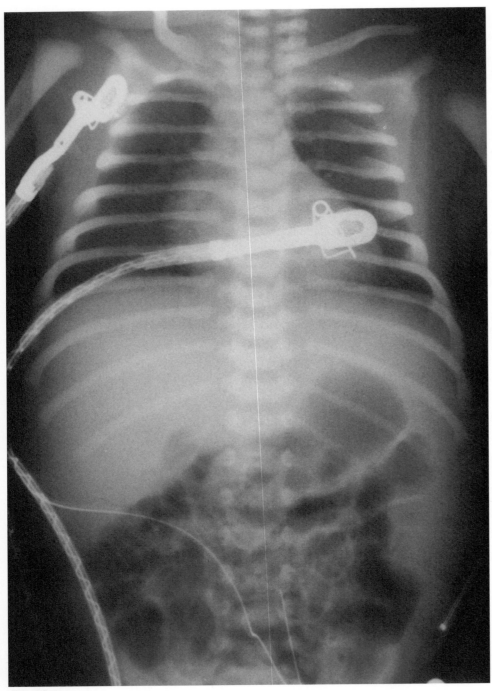

Fig. 20-1

Case 21

An 8-year-old girl who feels well has a lump in abdomen that was noticed by her mother 5 months ago.

Temperature is 37.9°C, heart rate 117, respiratory rate 28, blood pressure 112/76 mm Hg, weight 23 kg, and height 123 cm. A nontender mass is in left upper quadrant of abdomen. The rest of the physical findings are normal.

Hematocrit is 0.39. White cell count is 6.7×10^9/liter with 0.63 polymorphonuclear cells, 0.30 lymphocytes, 0.05 monocytes, 0.01 eosinophils, and 0.01 basophils. Platelet count is 254×10^9/liter. Urine specific gravity is 1.020, pH 7.5. Urine has trace protein, trace urobilinogen, 0–1 white cell/HPF, and occasional squamous and nonsquamous epithelial cells/HPF. Serum sodium is 137 mmol/liter, potassium 4.4, chloride 104, carbon dioxide 26, urea nitrogen 2.5, calcium 2.35, phosphorus 1.36, cholesterol 4.24, and glucose 6.8. Creatinine is 60 μmol/liter, uric acid 180, total bilirubin 20, and direct biliru-

bin 5. Total protein is 79 g/liter, albumin 47. Alkaline phosphatase is 206 U/liter, LDH 229, and SGOT 32.

A large cyst with uniform internal echoes occupies most of spleen in sonogram (Figure 21-1A) and contains liquid in CT scan (Figure 21-1B).

At operation, spleen is large, its top infarcted and fixed by adhesions.

Resected spleen ($13 \times 11 \times 5$ cm) is round, soft, deep brown to red and pale white in one part. Inside is a cyst (10-cm diameter) that contains brown liquid and has an inner wall crossed by white fibrous bands.

Diagnosis: Epidermoid or traumatic cyst of spleen (pseudocyst).

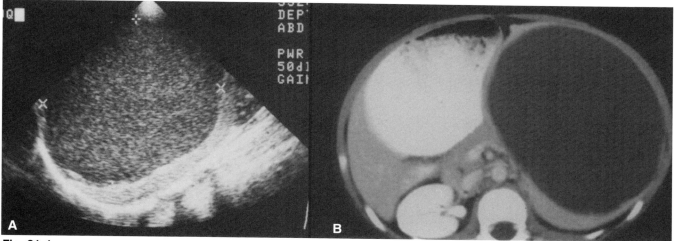

Fig. 21-1

Abdominal Vessels

Case 1

A 6½-year-old boy riding his bike was hit by a car and knocked 10 ft into a hedge. He opens his eyes when spoken to and complains of abdominal pain.

Heart rate is 126, blood pressure 79/32 mm Hg. He is pale. An 8-cm laceration is on forehead. Abdomen is distended and tender. Bowel sounds are absent. Left forearm is swollen near elbow. Bloody urine drains from bladder catheter. The rest of the physical findings are normal. One hour later, weight is 20 kg, heart rate 120, respiratory rate 24, and blood pressure 102/60 mm Hg.

Thirty minutes after injury, hematocrit is 0.36. White cell count is 9.3 × 10⁹/liter with 0.53 polymorphonuclear cells, 0.46 lymphocytes, and 0.01 monocytes. Platelet count is 297 × 10⁹/liter. Urine has protein, glucose, ketones, and blood.

CT scan 1 hour after injury (Figure 1-1A) shows uneven radiodensity in spleen and in enlarged left kidney, where it does not change after IV injection of contrast medium (Figure 1-1B). Left transverse process of L1 is fractured.

At operation 2 hours after injury, 300 ml blood is in abdomen. Spleen, fractured into four pieces, is removed. Retroperitoneal blood covers left kidney. Laceration of forehead is sutured.

Aortogram performed on evening after operation shows no flow beyond left renal artery (Figure 1-2). Left tenth rib is fractured.

Parents oppose blood transfusion. Lowest hematocrit is 0.19, 4 days after injury. Urine is clear 5 days after injury. Twelve days after injury, hematocrit is 0.24. Seven weeks after injury, he is well. Weight is 21 kg, height 122 cm, temperature 37.8°C, and blood pressure 90/60 mm Hg. Midline abdominal scar is thick. Roentgenographic examination shows good alignment and thickened cortex at fracture of left ulna and fracture of left radius. Urine does not have blood.

Diagnosis: Fracture of spleen and left kidney, occlusion of left renal artery.

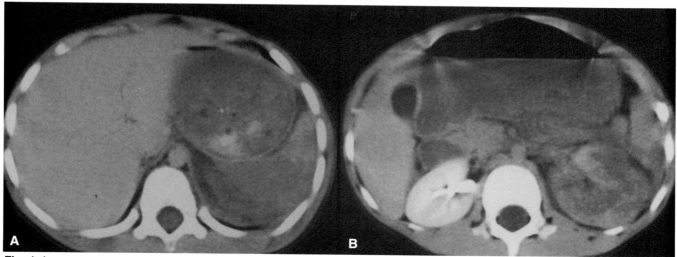

Fig. 1-1

(Continued)

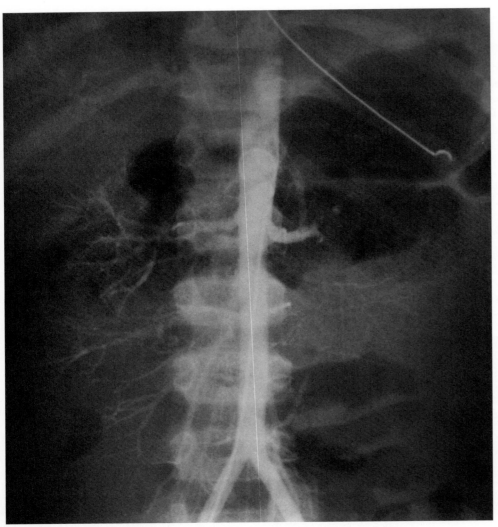

Fig. 1-2

Case 2

An 8-year-old girl "sees double" in right eye. Legs hurt. Fingers fall asleep.

Pregnancy of mother was normal, birth weight 3 kg. She had measles at 6 years. She was treated for amoebas and pin-worms. Ten months ago, she had a rash on her shins that faded after several months and left hypopigmented spots. Daily fever, 38–39°C, began 6 months ago. Three and a half months ago, she and two sisters, all given BCG in infancy, started treatment with isoniazid and ethambutol. Her vision was blurred 2½ months ago, then back to normal until 1½ months ago when right eye turned upward and outward, and right upper lid drooped. For the past 1½ months, she has sometimes slept all day. Calves hurt. Gait was stiff.

Mother (30 years old), father (33 years old), and two sisters (4 and 6 years old) are well.

Temperature at 8 years is 37.7°C, heart rate 96, respiratory rate 20, blood pressure 110/70 mm Hg, weight 23 kg, and height 124 cm. Right eye turns outward and cannot be adducted fully or raised above midline. She has "jelly" nystagmus when she tries to look up. Hypopigmented spots are on shins. Calves are tender and hurt when ankles are dorsi-flexed. Hands twitch. Tandem gait is clumsy. The rest of the physical findings are normal.

Hematocrit is 0.32. Hemoglobin is 102 g/liter. Red blood cell count is 5.0×10^{12}/liter. MCV is 64 fl. MCH is 20 pg. MCHC is 320 g/liter. Red-blood-cell distribution width is 11.2% (normal: 11.5–15.0). Reticulocyte fraction is 8×10^{-3}. White cell count is 8.5×10^9/liter with 0.62 polymorphonuclear cells, 0.01 bands, 0.28 lymphocytes, 0.08 monocytes, and 0.01 basophils. Eosinophils are 299×10^6/liter. ESR is 83 mm/hr. Urine specific gravity is 1.016, pH 7. Urine has occa-sional squamous epithelial cells/HPF. Serum sodium is 137 mmol/liter, potassium 4.4, chloride 104, carbon dioxide 23, urea nitrogen 3.2, calcium 2.27, phosphorus 1.42, cholesterol 3.44, and glucose 5.4. Creatinine is 60 µmol/liter, uric acid 110, total bilirubin 14, direct bilirubin 2, iron 3.0 (normal: 9.0–21.5), and iron-binding capacity 31.0 (normal: 44.8–80.6). Ferritin is 170 µg/liter (normal: 70–140). Total protein is 78 g/liter, albumin 36. Alkaline phosphatase is 108 U/liter, LDH 244, and SGOT 29. CSF has 0.15 g/liter protein, 2.2 mmol/liter glucose (blood glucose: 4.7), 3×10^6/liter red cells, 1×10^6/liter white cells, and 14 µg/liter myelin basic protein (normal: <40). Serum complement component 3 is 1.8 g/liter (normal: 0.7–1.6), complement component 4 0.6 (normal: 0.2–0.4). Functional hemolytic complement is 174 U/liter (normal: 75–160). Serum does not have rheumatoid factor, antinuclear antibodies, HBsAg, or HBsAb. Cultures of blood, urine, CSF, and bone marrow are sterile.

Vision is better for 4 months and then worse. She sleeps a lot, vomits, and acts silly. Speech slurs. Eyes turn left when she wants to look straight. Hands tremble so that she knocks over her milk and cannot feed herself. Blood pressure is 130–140/110 mm Hg. Hematocrit is 0.29. Platelet count is 731×10^9/liter. ESR is 58 and 95 mm/hr.

Angiography shows aneurysms in branches of celiac trunk (Figure 2-1A) and in superior mesenteric (Figure 2-1B) and renal arteries (Figure 2-2).

She can run, ride her bike, and write legibly 2 years later. She is cushingoid from treatment. Blood pressure is 102/68 mm Hg.

Diagnosis: Polyarteritis nodosa.

(Continued)

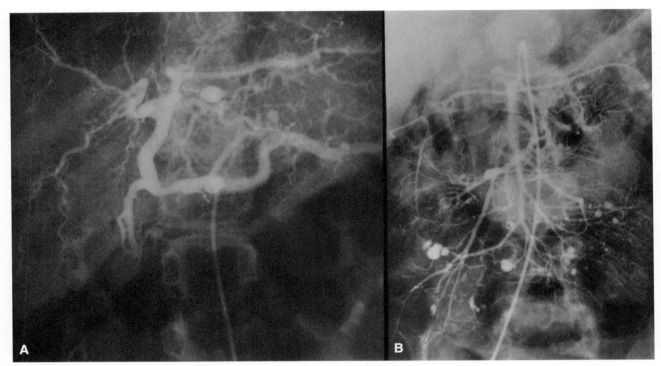

Fig. 2-1

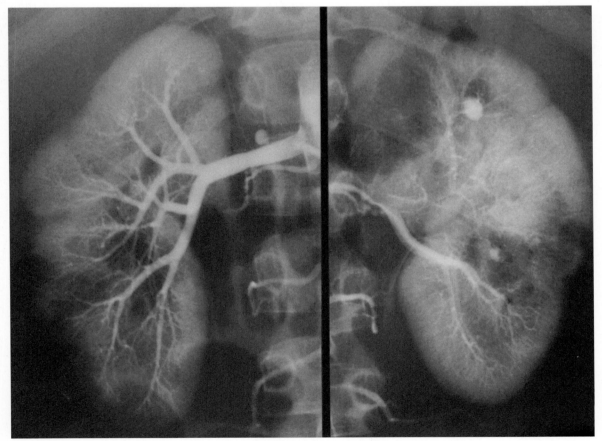

Fig. 2-2

Case 3

A 7-month-old boy who is breast-fed is vomiting blood.

Pregnancy was normal, birth weight 3.3 kg. He vomited right after feeding 3 weeks ago and then vomited small amounts of thin, yellow-green liquid. Vomit resembled coffee grounds 2 days later. Stool was guaiac positive. He was treated with metoclopramide hydrochloride and mixture of breast milk and solid food. He has sucked poorly since then and is now fed by syringe. He began to vomit again 4 days ago.

Mother (17 years old) and father (23 years old) are well. He is their only child.

Weight is 5.9 kg, temperature 37°C, heart rate 140, respiratory rate 56, and blood pressure 115/50 mm Hg. He is weak and has wet cough, occasional basal rales, and skinny limbs. The rest of the physical findings are normal.

Hematocrit is 0.27. White cell count is 15.4×10^9/liter with 0.17 polymorphonuclear cells, 0.05 bands, 0.69 lymphocytes, and 0.09 monocytes. Platelet count is 474×10^9/liter. Serum sodium is 141 mmol/liter, potassium 3.8, chloride 93, carbon dioxide 28, urea nitrogen 3.6, calcium 2.22, phosphorus 1.78, cholesterol 3.65, and glucose 4.6. Creatinine is 40 μmol/liter,

uric acid 290, total bilirubin 5, and direct bilirubin 2. Total protein is 57 g/liter, albumin 34. Alkaline phosphatase is 150 U/liter, LDH 254, and SGOT 39. Five days later, hematocrit is 0.22, hemoglobin is 74 g/liter, red blood cell count is 2.9×10^{12}/liter, MCV is 78 fl, MCH is 26 pg, and MCHC is 330 g/liter.

A shadow of calcium density is in right side of abdomen at level of L1 in plain film examination (Figure 3-1A). Barium shows gastric mucosal folds above diaphragm and shadow of calcium density in front of spine in lateral examination (Figure 3-1B). Ultrasound examination shows echogenic mass in inferior vena cava and shadowing (Figure 3-2).

A no. 22, but not no. 24, French dilator can be passed through esophagus. Esophagoscopy shows friable mucosa and white fibrinous exudate at gastroesophageal junction.

Microscopic examination of dark red tissue resected at esophagoscopy shows fragments of ulcer bed.

Diagnosis: Esophageal hiatal hernia, esophagitis, calcified thrombus in inferior vena cava.

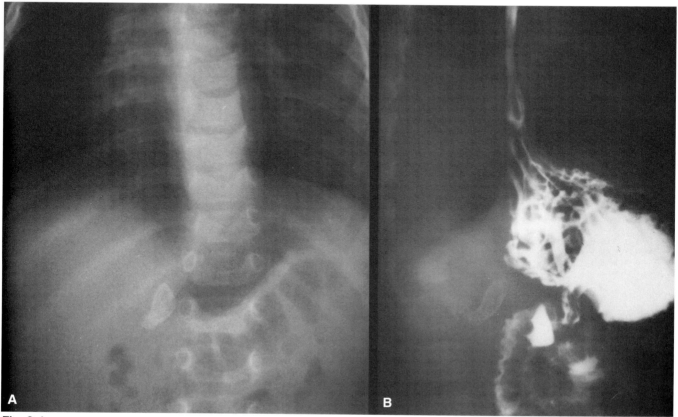

Fig. 3-1

(Continued)

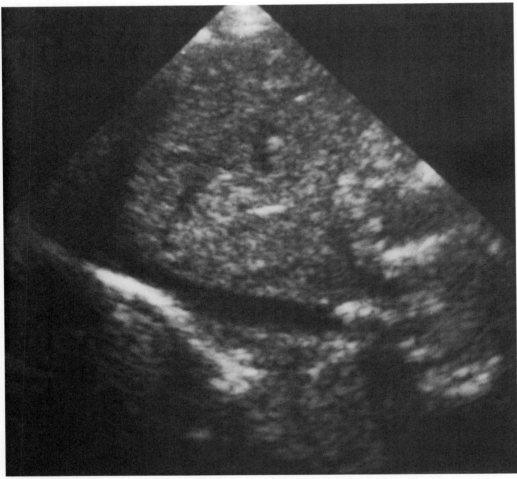

Fig. 3-2

Abdominal Tumors

Case 1

A 20-month-old girl is ataxic and has "strange eye movements."

Birth weight was 4.5 kg. She began to walk at 1 year. She fell from a step and bloodied her nose at 18 months. Arms and legs began to shake 7 weeks ago. She stopped walking and began to crawl 6 weeks ago. She began to walk holding onto furniture 3 weeks ago. Now she gurgles and vomits once per day, wakes up at night, and seems scared. Mother has just noticed strange eye movements.

Parents are well. She is their only child. Maternal grandmother died with heart attack at 49 years. Paternal grandfather has arthritis.

Temperature at 20 months is 36°C, heart rate 120, respiratory rate 24, blood pressure 120/50 mm Hg, weight 12.8 kg, and height 87 cm. She fixes her gaze momentarily until eyeballs begin to jerk from side to side. Arms sway when she reaches out. A few small lymph nodes are in neck. A pink rash is on chin and right thigh. The rest of the physical findings are normal.

Hematocrit is 0.38. White cell count is 12.0×10^9/liter with 0.23 polymorphonuclear cells, 0.01 bands, 0.66 lymphocytes, 0.07 monocytes, 0.01 eosinophils, and 0.02 basophils.

Platelet count is 512×10^9/liter. Blood glucose is 4.1 mmol/liter. CSF has 2.4 mmol/liter glucose, 0.30 g/liter protein, 2×10^9/liter red cells, 12×10^6/liter white cells, 1.00 lymphocytes, and is sterile. Urinary homovanillic acid is 27 μmol/day (normal: <45), vanillylmandelic acid 21 (normal: <10). Vanillylmandelic acid/creatinine is 13.3 mmol/mol (normal: 0–7.8).

CT scan after IV injection of contrast medium shows a mass between right kidney and inferior vena cava and inside back layer of renal fascia (Figure 1-1).

At operation, a tumor in medial part of right adrenal gland and right adrenal gland are removed.

Gland is $3.0 \times 3.0 \times 1.6$ cm; tumor is $1.4 \times 1.0 \times 0.8$ cm, encapsulated, tan, and glistening.

She is treated with methylprednisolone. A month later she walks with help, feeds herself with a spoon, puts objects into containers, talks more, and has less opsoclonus and ataxia.

Diagnosis: Ganglioneuroblastoma with marked lymphohistiocytic infiltrate.

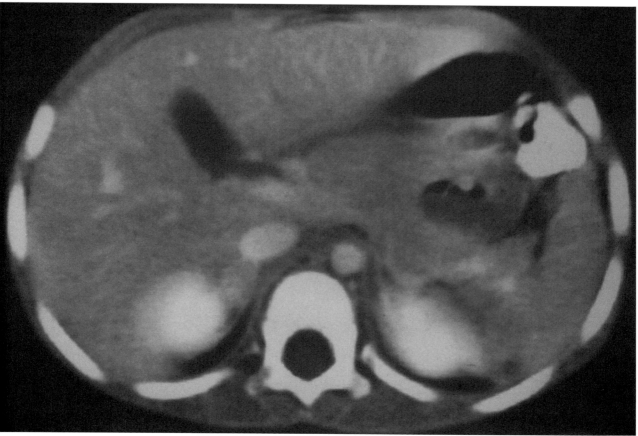

Fig. 1-1

Case 2

A 3-year, 10-month-old girl is pale and has had a swollen abdomen for 2 weeks. She has been eating and playing less and napping more for 2 months.

Pregnancy was normal. She has had ear infections and placement of tubes.

Mother (31 years old), father (35 years old), brother (8 years old), and sister (2 years old) are well. Paternal grandfather died with prostate cancer; maternal grandfather died with a heart attack.

Temperature is 38.8°C, heart rate 160, respiratory rate 40, blood pressure 84/50 mm Hg, weight 13.8 kg, and height 92 cm. She is pale. A systolic murmur is present. A mass is in left side of abdomen. The rest of the physical findings are normal.

Hematocrit is 0.20. Hemoglobin is 66 g/liter. Red blood cell count is 3.2×10^{12}/liter. MCV is 64 fl. MCH is 21 pg. MCHC is 330 g/liter. Red-blood-cell distribution width is 17.1% (normal: 11.5–15.0). White cell count is 6.5×10^9/liter with 0.58 polymorphonuclear cells, 0.03 bands, 0.35 lymphocytes, 0.02 monocytes, 0.01 eosinophils, and 0.01 basophils. Platelet count is 539×10^9/liter. ESR is 120 mm/hr. Serum sodium is 136 mmol/liter, potassium 3.8, chloride 100, carbon dioxide 24, urea nitrogen 1.8, calcium 2.37, phosphorus 1.07, cholesterol 4.01, and glucose 7.2. Creatinine is 40 µmol/liter, uric acid 230, total bilirubin 3, direct bilirubin 0, and iron 1.3 (normal: 9.0–21.5). Alkaline phosphatase is 123 U/liter, LDH >2,000, SGOT 49, and SGPT 9. Urinary homovanillic acid is 10 µmol/day (normal: 8–24).

Excretory urogram in Figure 2-1 shows displacement of left collecting system and stomach by a mass. CT scan shows a hypovascular mass that contains calcium (Figure 2-2A) and seems to be separate from left kidney, and retroperitoneal tumor along left side of aorta (Figure 2-2B).

At operation, soft, friable material is under capsule of retroperitoneal tumor, and tail of pancreas is stuck to front of tumor. Enlarged lymph nodes are along left side of aorta. Left ovarian vein is dilated. Part of tumor is removed.

Microscopic examination shows (1) necrosis and cells with little eosinophilic cytoplasm; (2) large pleomorphic, basophilic nuclei with smudged chromatin and rare nucleoli; and (3) abnormal mitoses. Electron microscopy shows (1) cells without core granules, (2) a cluster of cells with dense core granules (70–140-nm diameter), and (3) thick, long neuritic processes that contain microtubules. Immunoperoxidase stain of touch preparation with pan-leukocyte antibody, T-cell antibody, and B-cell antibody is negative and with neuron-specific enolase probably negative. Bone marrow is normal.

She has a lump above left eye, a lump in mouth, and pain and swelling in right thigh 5 months later. She dies at 4 years, 3 months.

Diagnosis: Neuroblastoma.

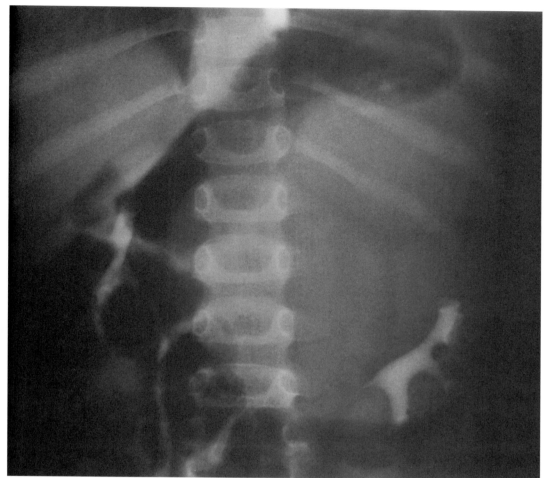

Fig. 2-1

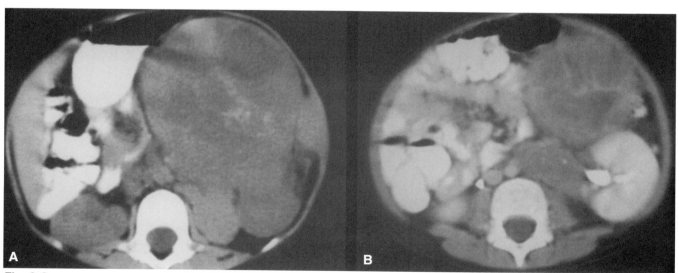

Fig. 2-2

Case 3

A 4-year, 8-month-old boy has had a large left breast for 11 months and has grown 6 cm in the last 9 months. Bone age in left hand is between 9 and 10 years.

Birth weight was 3.2 kg, length 52 cm. First tooth came in at 6 months. He walked at 17 months. He has had ear infections, placement of tubes, and, 7 months ago, adenoidectomy.

Weight is 20 kg, head circumference 54 cm, and height 109 cm. At 4 years, 11 months, height is 112 cm, temperature 37.4°C, heart rate 92, and blood pressure 84/48 mm Hg. Diameter of left breast is 5–6 cm, right breast 1 cm, and testes 1.5 cm. Length of penis is 5 cm. The rest of the physical findings are normal.

Hematocrit is 0.38. White cell count is 9.3×10^9/liter. Platelet count is 333×10^9/liter. Serum sodium is 143 mmol/liter, potassium 5.4, and chloride 106. Estrone is three to four times normal level and unresponsive to adrenocorticotropic hormone or HCG. Levels of other hormones are juvenile or prepubertal.

MRI shows a mass with bright T2 signal in right adrenal gland in axial (Figure 3-1A) and coronal (Figure 3-1B) views.

At operation, a mass ($2.0 \times 1.5 \times 1.0$ cm) in right adrenal gland has a white fibrous capsule and contains red and beige nodules of soft tissue.

Microscopic examination shows (1) nodules of abnormal cells, variable in size, with round nuclei and prominent nucleoli, and (2) broad fibrous bands.

Diagnosis: Adrenal cortical adenoma.

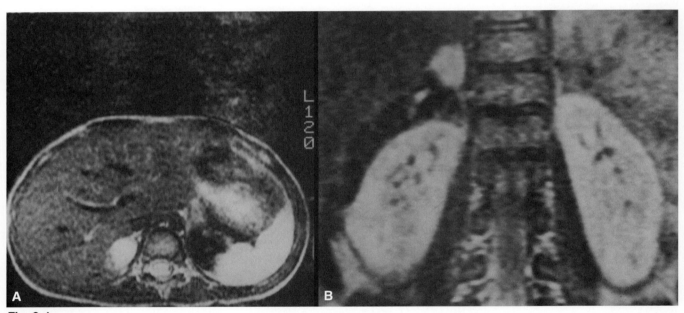

Fig. 3-1

Case 4

A 9-year-old boy has fever and anorexia. He has not felt well for 1 month.

He has had acute glomerulonephritis and is allergic to some foods.

Temperature is 38.2°C, heart rate 128, respiratory rate 28, blood pressure 88/48 mm Hg, weight 34 kg, and height 139 cm. He wants to stay in bed. He is pale. Cervical and axillary lymph nodes are large. Liver edge is 8 cm below costal margin, spleen edge 12 cm. A fluid wave is in abdomen. The rest of the physical findings are normal.

Hematocrit is 0.24. Hemoglobin is 82 g/liter. Red blood cell count is 3.1×10^{12}/liter. MCV is 76 fl. MCH is 26 pg. MCHC is 350 g/liter. White cell count is 0.7×10^9/liter with 0.56 polymorphonuclear cells, 0.08 bands, 0.32 lymphocytes, and 0.04 monocytes. Platelet count is 75×10^9/liter. Urine specific gravity is 1.014, pH 6. Urine has few epithelial cells/HPF, 1–2 red cells/HPF, 2–3 white cells/HPF, and bacteria. Serum sodium is 126 mmol/liter, potassium 3.6, chloride 91, carbon dioxide 23, urea nitrogen 2.5, calcium 1.82, phosphorus 0.87, cholesterol 3.98, and glucose 5.7. Creatinine is 60 μmol/liter, uric acid 70, total bilirubin 14, direct bilirubin 9, iron 33.0

(normal: 9.0–21.5), and iron-binding capacity 35.0 (normal: 44.8–80.6). Total protein is 46 g/liter, albumin 29. Alkaline phosphatase is 348 U/liter, LDH 1,782, and SGOT 312. CSF has 1.4 mmol/liter glucose, 0.11 g/liter protein, $<1 \times 10^6$/liter red cells, 1×10^6/liter white cells, 0.60 lymphocytes, 0.07 plasmacytoid lymphocytes, and 0.33 polymorphonuclear cells.

Excretory urogram 1 minute after IV injection of contrast medium shows enlarged kidneys (Figure 4-1).

Smear of bone marrow aspirate shows increased histiocytes, biopsy fibrosis. Microscopic examination of axillary lymph node shows (1) sheets of pleomorphic cells in medulla with primary follicles and paracortical tissue at periphery, (2) a few small lymphocytes, (3) rare plasma cells, (4) 3–8 mitoses/HPF, and (5) necrosis. The abnormal cells are large with ill-defined cytoplasm and large nuclei that have coarsely reticular or clumped, marginated chromatin and one or two prominent chromocenters. Many of the cells are lymphoblastic or plasmacytoid.

Diagnosis: Malignant lymphoreticular disease (questionable malignant histiocytosis), visceromegaly.

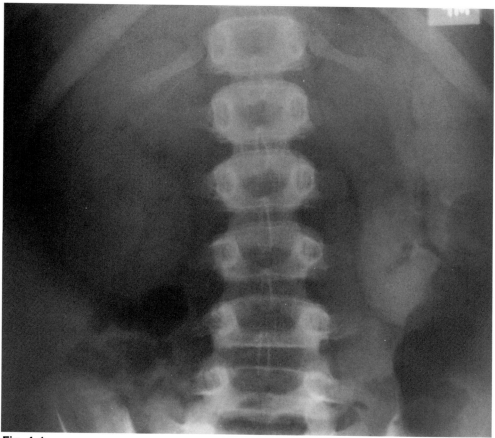

Fig. 4-1

Case 5

A 9-year-old boy has a distended abdomen. He has not felt well for 1 month.

Birth weight was 4.7 kg. He walked at 11 months. He had an ear infection at 15 months. He had pneumonia at 21 months. He limped for 2 months and then had pain and tenderness in left hand at 4 years and said his "stomach feels like it is going to break." Temperature was 39.3°C. Red macules and papules that blanched with pressure and bruises were on skin. Sternum was tender. Systolic murmur was present. Liver edge was 5 cm below costal margin, spleen edge 2 cm. Hematocrit was 0.28. White cell count was 1.5×10^9/liter with 0.09 polymorphonuclear cells, 0.01 bands, 0.83 lymphocytes, and 0.07 monocytes. Platelet count was 50×10^9/liter. He was treated for T-cell ALL.

Left testis was large, firm, and irregular at 5½ years; right testis was normal. He was given more treatment.

Temperature at 9 years is 36.8°C, heart rate 100, respiratory rate 20, and blood pressure 118/80 mm Hg. A mass is palpable in pelvis. The rest of the physical findings are normal.

Hematocrit is 0.27. White cell count is 6.7×10^9/liter with 0.65 polymorphonuclear cells, 0.07 bands, 0.14 lymphocytes, 0.04 monocytes, 0.09 eosinophils, and 0.01 basophils. Platelet estimate is normal. Urine specific gravity is 1.008, pH 5. Urine has occasional squamous epithelial cells/HPF and 4–6 white cells/HPF. Serum sodium is 140 mmol/liter, potassium 4.6, chloride 103, carbon dioxide 18, urea nitrogen 21.0, calcium 2.50, phosphorus 1.65, cholesterol 5.33, and glucose 4.9. Creatinine is 200 μmol/liter, uric acid 480, total bilirubin 7, and direct bilirubin 2. Total protein is 81 g/liter, albumin 48. Alkaline phosphatase is 137 U/liter, LDH 406, and SGOT 24. CSF has 3×10^6/liter white cells, 0.59 lymphocytes, 0.38 blasts, 0.03 pia-arachnoid cells, $<1 \times 10^6$/liter red cells, 4.2 mmol/liter glucose, and 0.17 g/liter protein. Bone marrow is normal.

Ultrasound examination at 9 years shows a mass of mixed echoes behind compressed bladder (Figure 5-1), left pyelocaliectasis, and right caliectasis.

Bone marrow at 4 years had small lymphoblasts which were TdT and sheep erythrocyte rosette receptor–positive in immunologic analyses. Biopsy of both testes at 5½ years showed (1) groups of round to polygonal cells with little cytoplasm and indistinct borders, (2) irregular nuclei with granular chromatin, (3) prominent nucleoli, (4) atypical mitoses, (5) dense connective tissue, and (6) obliteration of seminiferous tubules. Retrovesical tumor at 9 years has sheets and strands of abnormal lymphoid cells with little cytoplasm, irregular nuclei, dustlike chromatin, mitoses, and necrosis. Lymphoid cells are of mixed lineage T-cell phenotype.

Diagnosis: T-cell ALL, at 4 years with testicular and CNS relapse; T-cell malignant lymphoblastic lymphoma, at 9 years.

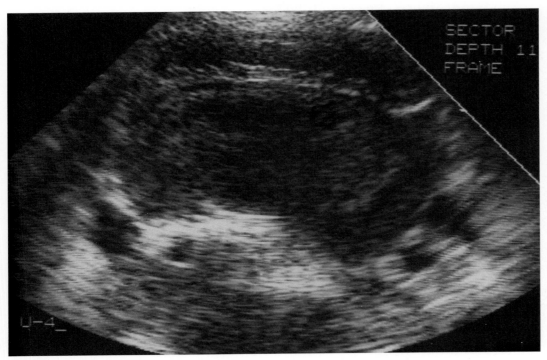

Fig. 5-1

Case 6

A 6-week-old girl has a mass between sacrum and anus.

Pregnancy of mother was normal, birth weight 3.9 kg. A soft perineal swelling (2–3 cm) appeared at 2 weeks. The girl has been straining with bowel movements for several days.

Mother (19 years old), father (22 years old), and sibling (18 months old) are well.

Weight is 4.3 kg, temperature 37.2°C, heart rate 142, respiratory rate 38, and systolic blood pressure 85 mm Hg. A red rash is in diaper area, a fluctuant swelling (3–4-cm diameter) between anus and sacrum. The rest of the physical findings are normal.

Hematocrit is 0.36. White cell count is 11.6×10^9/liter. Urine specific gravity is 1.004, pH 5.5. Urine has few squamous epithelial cells. Serum sodium is 135 mmol/liter, potassium 6.0, chloride 105, and urea nitrogen 2.9.

Buttocks are large. Rectum, anus, bladder, and urethra are pushed forward in Figure 6-1.

At operation, a cystic tumor (6 × 4 × 2 cm) deep to gluteus maximus muscles extends from sacral promontory to ischial tuberosities. Encapsulated tumor, its attachment to tip of coccyx, and coccyx are removed.

Cross section of tumor shows a cyst with white mucinous material and several solid white foci.

Diagnosis: Benign sacrococcygeal teratoma.

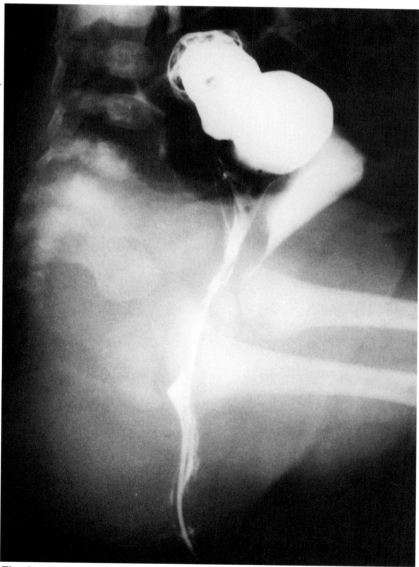

Fig. 6-1

Urinary Tract

Case 1

An 8-year-old girl, who became occasionally incontinent of urine at 6 years, has had several episodes of low backache since then.

Birth weight was 2.7 kg. Health is good.

Temperature is 36.7°C, heart rate 100, respiratory rate 30, blood pressure 98/60 mm Hg, weight 21.8 kg, and height 122 cm. Physical findings are normal.

Hematocrit is 0.41. White cell count is 12.4×10^9/liter with 0.32 polymorphonuclear cells, 0.16 bands, 0.47 lymphocytes, and 0.06 monocytes. Urine specific gravity is 1.023, pH 7.

Urine has few epithelial cells/HPF, several nonsquamous epithelial cells/HPF, 4–5 red cells/HPF, and 15–20 white cells/HPF and is sterile. Serum sodium is 140 mmol/liter, potassium 4.2, chloride 99, carbon dioxide 21, urea nitrogen 3.9, and glucose 5.9. Creatinine 40 is μmol/liter.

Excretory urogram in Figure 1-1 shows cortical groove in right kidney.

She is well and pregnant at 24.

Diagnosis: Normal kidneys; fetal lobation, right kidney.

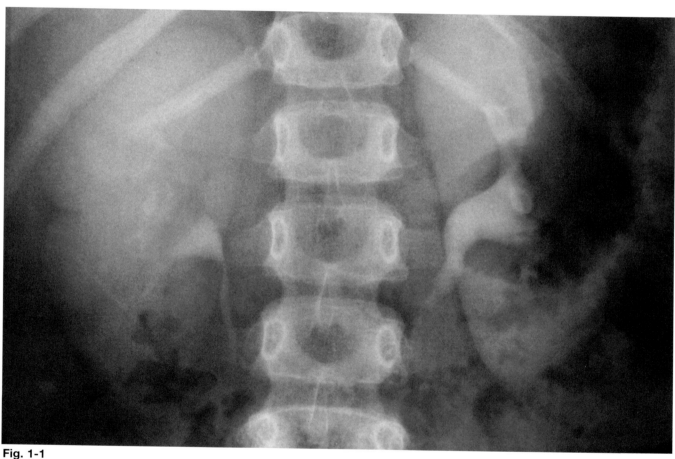

Fig. 1-1

Case 2

A 13-year-old girl wakes up with frontal headaches that last all day.

Tonsils and adenoids were removed at 11½ years because of ear infections. She was pale and had puffy eyelids and bloody urine at 12 years. Blood pressure was 220/160 mm Hg. Excretory urogram and arteriogram showed small left kidney and normal right kidney, 10.5 cm long. Cystogram showed no vesicoureteral reflux. At nephroureterectomy, left kidney (4 cm long and 2.3 cm from ureteropelvic junction to lateral edge) was free of adhesions. Capsule stripped easily from smooth surface. Cortex was thin. Calyces were dilated. Lymphocytic infiltrates with germinal centers were in parenchyma around calyces; around sclerotic, hyalinized glomeruli; and around collapsed and dilated tubules. Walls of arterioles of all sizes were thickened by intimal fibrosis and medial hypertrophy. Foci of medullary deposits of calcium and of normal glomeruli and tubules were present.

Father and older sister have headaches.

In last examination 6 months ago, weight was 27 kg, height 141 cm, temperature 37.2°C, and blood pressure 112/88 mm Hg. A scar was on left flank. The rest of the physical findings were normal.

Culture of urine was sterile 4 months ago.

Supine voiding cystogram at 13 years shows normal bladder (Figure 2-1A) and reflux of contrast medium into stump of left ureter. Erect voiding cystogram at 18 years, when she has headache, blood pressure 120/90 mm Hg, >10⁵ colonies *Escherichia coli*/ml urine, and normal right kidney in excretory urogram, shows normal bladder with bladder ears (Figure 2-1B).

Diagnosis: Normal bladder with and without bladder ears.

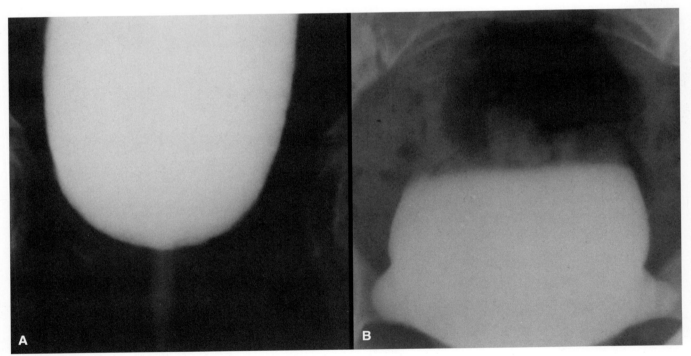

Fig. 2-1

Case 3

A 3-day-old girl is tachypneic. Pregnancy was normal, birth weight 5.2 kg, and Apgar score 8/10 at 1 and 5 minutes.

Mother (25 years old), father (24 years old), and two sisters (2 and 4 years old) are well.

Temperature is 37.7°C, heart rate 140, respiratory rate 80, and head circumference 35 cm. A firm, smooth mass is in each flank. The rest of the physical findings are normal.

Hematocrit is 0.57. White cell count is 15.7×10^9/liter with 0.49 polymorphonuclear cells, 0.19 bands, 0.23 lymphocytes, and 0.09 monocytes. Urine specific gravity is 1.020, pH 5.5. Urine has 1+ protein, 4–6 epithelial cells/HPF, 4–6 white cells/HPF, 2–5 red cells/HPF, uric acid crystals, and amorphous urates. Serum sodium is 142 mmol/liter, potassium 6.6, chloride 103, urea nitrogen 25.0, and glucose 4.9. Urea nitrogen is 17.9 at 4 days, 8.9 at 5 days.

In excretory urogram at 4 days, contrast medium is in large kidneys and bladder 7 hours after IV injection (Figure 3-1A). In excretory urogram at 19 days, contrast medium is in normal calyces, pelves, and bladder 20 minutes after IV injection (Figure 3-1B).

Diagnosis: Nephromegaly in infant of prediabetic mother. (Results of mother's glucose tolerance test 6 weeks after delivery are "abnormal.")

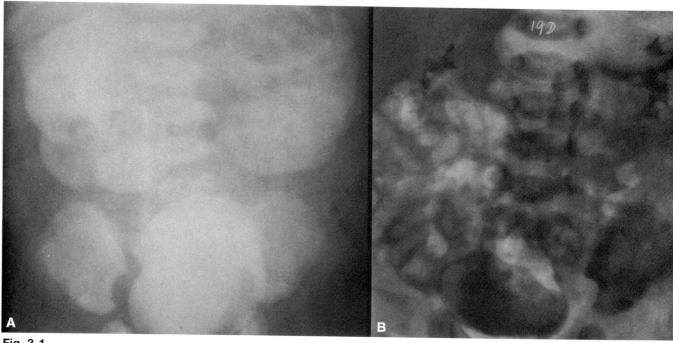

Fig. 3-1

Case 4

An 8-day-old boy has dilated left renal pelvis and calyces that were found in prenatal ultrasound examination.

Birth weight was 3.3 kg, length 52 cm, head circumference 35 cm, and Apgar score 9/9 at 1 and 5 minutes.

Temperature at 8 days is 36.4°C, heart rate 160, respiratory rate 50, systolic blood pressure 88 mm Hg, and weight 3.3 kg. Physical findings are normal.

Hematocrit is 0.49. White cell count is 11.6×10^9/liter with 0.35 polymorphonuclear cells, 0.05 bands, 0.40 lymphocytes, 0.16 monocytes, and 0.04 eosinophils. Platelet count is 337×10^9/liter. Serum sodium is 140 mmol/liter, potassium 5.1, chloride 104, carbon dioxide 17, urea nitrogen 3.2, calcium 2.45, phosphorus 2.39, cholesterol 3.08, and glucose 4.6. Creatinine is 50 μmol/liter, uric acid 170, total bilirubin 100, and direct bilirubin 10. Total protein is 65 g/liter, albumin 36. Alkaline phosphatase is 198 U/liter, LDH 393, and SGOT 23.

Ultrasound examination at 9 days shows dilation of left renal pelvis and calyces (Figure 4-1A) and normal right kidney. Excretory urograms at 9 days (Figure 4-1B), 7 months (Figure 4-2A), and 2½ years (Figure 4-2B) show quick appearance of contrast medium in both kidneys and dilation of left renal pelvis and calyces.

Diagnosis: Normal kidneys.

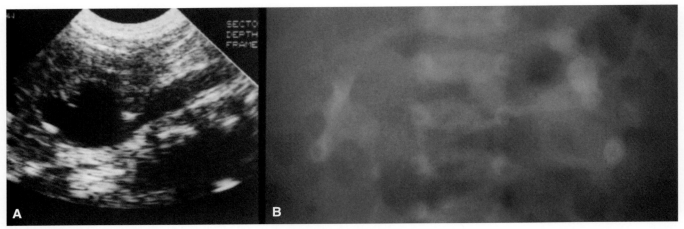

Fig. 4-1

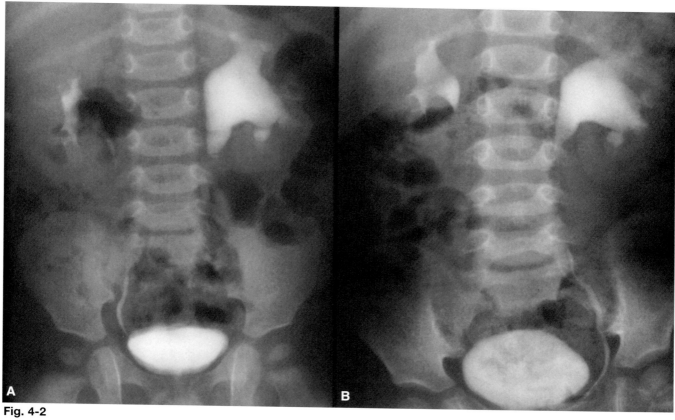

Fig. 4-2

Case 5

A 7½-year-old boy, who had excretory urogram and urethral meatotomy at 3 years after red blood cells were found in urinalysis for fever, comes in for follow-up examination.

Weight is 25 kg, height 124 cm, temperature 36.7°C, and blood pressure 80/30 mm Hg. Physical findings are normal.

Hematocrit is 0.39. White cell count is 4.3×10^9/liter with 0.42 polymorphonuclear cells, 0.44 lymphocytes, 0.11 monocytes, and 0.03 basophils. Platelet count is 358×10^9/liter. Urine specific gravity is 1.021. Urine is normal with 6.2 mmol creatinine/liter and no protein. Serum sodium is 141 mmol/liter, potassium 4.7, chloride 109, carbon dioxide 21, urea nitrogen 6.8, calcium 2.62, phosphorus 1.52, cholesterol 3.39, and glucose 5.2. Creatinine is 60 μmol/liter, uric acid 210, total bilirubin 7, and direct bilirubin 0. Total protein is 70 g/liter, albumin 46. Alkaline phosphatase is 268 U/liter, LDH 274, and SGOT 33.

Renal calyces and pelves are dilated in excretory urogram at 7½ (Figure 5-1A) and 8½ years (Figure 5-1B).

Diagnosis: Normal kidneys, megacalycosis.

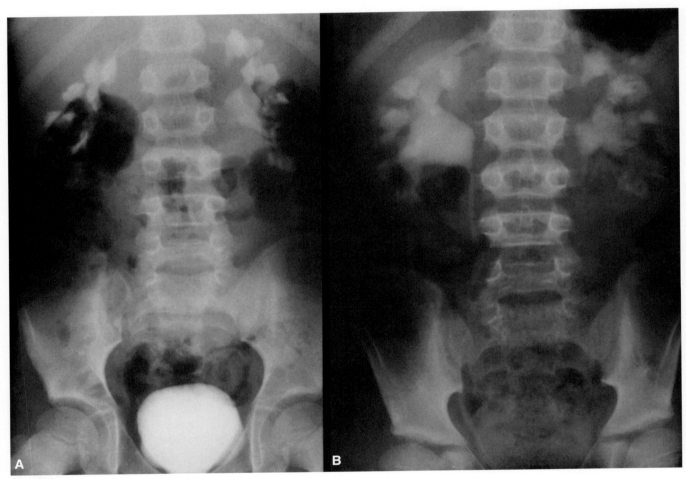

Fig. 5-1

Case 6

A 6-year-old girl has bacteriuria.

Parents and three sisters are well.

Temperature is 37°C, heart rate 114, respiratory rate 24, blood pressure 112/76 mm Hg, weight 19 kg, and height 112 cm. Heart sounds are in right side of chest. The rest of the physical findings are normal.

Hematocrit is 0.43. White cell count is 7.4×10^9/liter with 0.61 polymorphonuclear cells, 0.08 bands, 0.27 lymphocytes, and 0.04 monocytes. Platelet estimate is adequate. Urine specific gravity is 1.021, pH 6. Urine has occasional epithelial cells/HPF, occasional red cells/HPF, 2–3 white cells/HPF, and bacteria. Serum urea nitrogen is 6.1 mmol/liter. Creatinine is 50 µmol/liter. Chromosomes in peripheral white cells are 46,XX.

Excretory urogram in Figure 6-1 shows two renal pelves on left side, none on right side, a ureter on each side of bladder, and stomach on right side. Urogram also shows apex of heart in right side. Cervical and upper thoracic vertebrae and upper ribs are dysplastic in Figure 6-2.

A lump (3 × 2 cm) is in right inguinal canal 3 months later. At operation, right and left uterus, neither communicating with shallow vagina (0.5–1.0 cm long), hypoplastic uterine tubes, and right and left ovary are found. Right ovary, uterus, and tube are in right inguinal canal; left ovary, uterus, and tube are in pelvis.

Biopsy of both ovaries shows normal findings.

Diagnosis: Crossed ectopy of kidneys, situs inversus, and skeletal and genital abnormalities (questionable Rokitansy-Küster-Hauser syndrome).

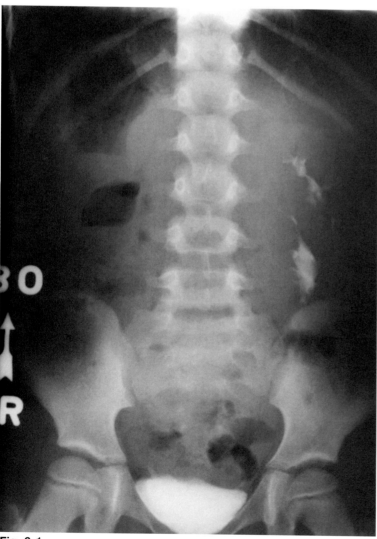

Fig. 6-1

(Continued)

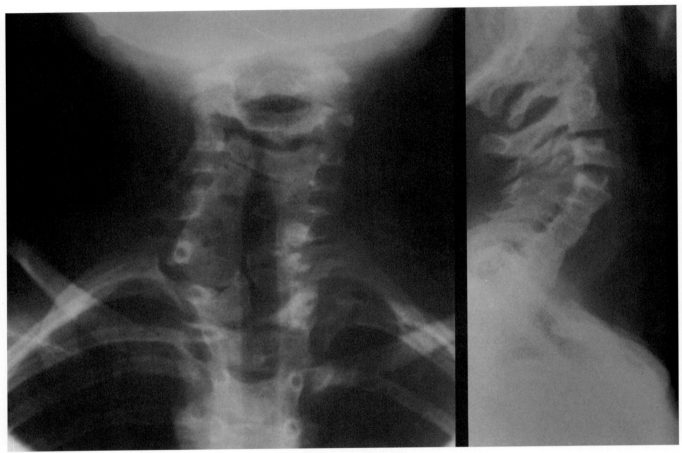

Fig. 6-2

Case 7

A newborn boy is dusky. His mouth is full of mucus.

Mother (18 years old) smoked during pregnancy. Birth weight is 2.0 kg, length 44 cm, head circumference 32 cm, Apgar score 3/8 at 1 and 5 minutes, temperature 36.2°C at 5 minutes, heart rate 146, respiratory rate 56, systolic blood pressure 50 mm Hg, and blood glucose 4.4 mmol/liter. Thumbs are fingerlike. A supernumerary digit is lateral to right second finger. Second and third toes of both feet are partly fused. The rest of the physical findings are normal. Hematocrit is 0.50.

Roentgenogram at 45 minutes shows endotracheal tube and a kinked tube in neck, gas in gut, umbilical cord clamp, and slight dysplasia of sacrum. Excretory urogram at 3 weeks shows ectopy of right kidney (Figure 7-1).

Esophagoesophagostomy, division of tracheoesophageal fistula, gastrotomy, and excision of supernumerary finger, which contains bone, cartilage, and soft tissue, are performed at 1 day. Gastrostomy is placed.

Gastrostomy tube is removed at 3 months. He has choking apneic spells during feedings. Systolic murmur and diastolic murmur are present at 6 months. Audiogram shows normal hearing. Gastrostomy is placed. Nissen fundoplication is performed at 6 months. Ductus arteriosus is ligated 2 weeks later.

Treatment with mitomycin-C of peripheral lymphocyte culture obtained at 5 months causes multiple breaks, rearrangements, rings, and triradials in 75 of 100 cells and gaps or breaks in seven of 100 control cells. At 10 months, hematocrit is 0.42. Platelet count is 246×10^9/liter. At 21 months, hematocrit is 0.46. Platelet count is 159×10^9/liter. At 33 months, bruises are on legs. Hematocrit is 0.36. Platelet count is 61×10^9/liter. At 3½ years, gastrostomy tube is removed. Bone marrow is hypocellular. At 4 years, weight is 10.4 kg, height 93 cm. Bruises are on arms and legs. Hematocrit is 0.31. Hemoglobin is 103 g/liter. Red blood cell count is 2.8×10^{12}/liter. MCV is 110 fl. MCH is 37 pg. MCHC is 340 g/liter. Red-blood-cell distribution width is 16.4% (normal: 11.5–15.0). White cell count is 5.1×10^9/liter with 0.29 polymorphonuclear cells, 0.02 bands, 0.51 lymphocytes, 0.12 monocytes, 0.04 eosinophils, and 0.02 basophils. Platelet count is 23×10^9/liter. At 4½ years, hematocrit is 0.14. Platelet count is 14×10^9/liter.

Diagnosis: Skeletal abnormalities, esophageal atresia and tracheoesophageal fistula, ductus arteriosus, pelvic kidney, Fanconi's hypoplastic anemia.

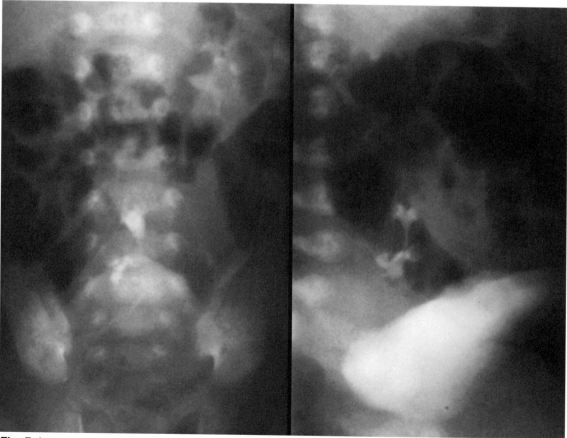

Fig. 7-1

Case 8

A 13-year-old girl has not grown for 1 year. Schoolmates and brothers make fun of her. She is irritable and inattentive in school. She has had headaches, cramps, and backaches for 2 months.

Birth weight was 2.4 kg. She vomited and did not gain weight. Weight at 9 months was 4 kg. She was put on soybean milk. Weight at 14 months was 10 kg. She walked at 1 year. She had headaches at 7 and 8 years, pneumonia at 8 years, and scarlet fever at 9 years. She has had measles, mumps, and chickenpox. Tonsils and adenoids were removed at 8 years. She has not begun to menstruate.

Mother (33 years old), father (33 years old), and two brothers (8 and 15 years old) are well. Another brother (9 years old) has asthma. Paternal grandmother and maternal grandfather have diabetes mellitus.

Temperature at 13 years is 37.2°C, heart rate 76, respiratory rate 18, blood pressure 82/56 mm Hg, weight 31.7 kg, and height 124 cm. Breasts are underdeveloped. Pubic hair is absent. The rest of the physical findings are normal.

Hematocrit is 0.41. White cell count is 6.5×10^9/liter with 0.68 polymorphonuclear cells, 0.04 bands, 0.22 lymphocytes, 0.04 monocytes, 0.01 eosinophils, and 0.01 basophils. Platelet estimate is adequate. Urine specific gravity is 1.018, pH 6.5. Urine has occasional white cells/HPF. Serum sodium is 144 mmol/liter, potassium 4.1, chloride 98, carbon dioxide 24, urea nitrogen 6.1, and glucose 4.9. Creatinine is 60 µmol/liter. Her buccal smear is Barr-body negative. Chromosomes in her peripheral blood lymphocytes are 45,XO.

Excretory urogram shows that renal pelves do not have normal lower lateral divergence from spine (Figure 8-1) and that proximal part of ureters curves forward (Figure 8-2).

Diagnosis: Horseshoe kidney in girl who has Turner's syndrome.

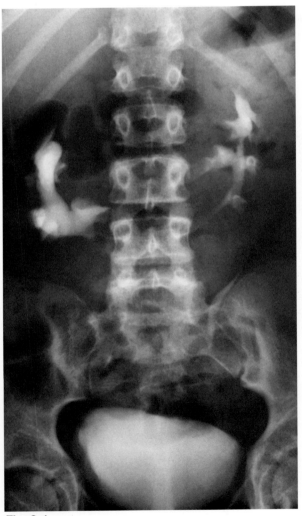

Fig. 8-1

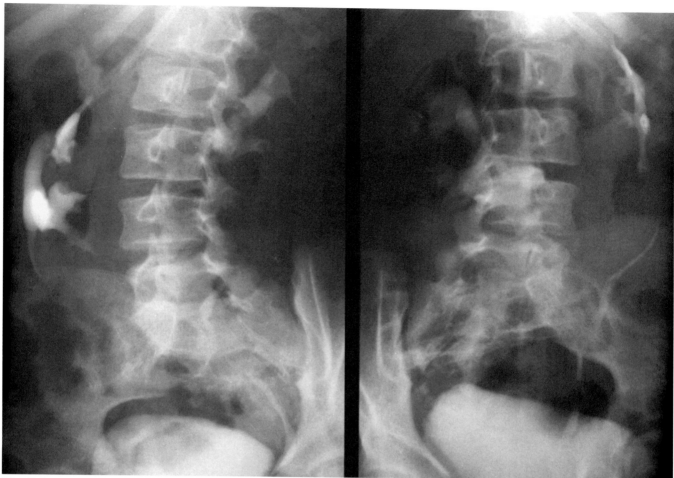

Fig. 8-2

Case 9

A 2-month-old boy who has been breathing fast for 2 weeks has tachycardia and high blood pressure. Pregnancy was normal, birth weight 3.5 kg.

Mother (22 years old) and father (27 years old) are well. The boy is their only child.

Temperature is 37°C, heart rate 150, respiratory rate 40, systolic blood pressure 130 mm Hg in right arm, 150 mm Hg in right leg, weight 5.9 kg, length 63 cm, and head circumference 41 cm. Pulses are strong in arms and legs. Liver edge is 2 cm below costal margin. The rest of the physical findings are normal.

ECG findings are normal.

Hematocrit is 0.32. White cell count is 7.6×10^9/liter with 0.21 polymorphonuclear cells, 0.11 bands, 0.63 lymphocytes, 0.04 monocytes, and 0.01 eosinophils. Urine specific gravity is 1.008, pH 7. Urine has rare squamous epithelial cells/HPF. Serum sodium is 136 mmol/liter, potassium 5.5, chloride 104, and urea nitrogen 7.5. Creatinine is 40 μmol/liter. Peripheral plasma renin is 1.40 mmol/liter/hr (normal: 0.30–0.59) on a diet restricted to 10 mmol sodium/kg.

Excretory urogram shows (1) quick appearance of contrast medium in both renal pelves, (2) a defect in left side of bladder (Figure 9-1A), and (3) later accumulation of contrast medium in dilated left renal pelvis, dilated left ureter (which did not show peristalsis during fluoroscopic examination), and bladder, where defect is now obscured (Figure 9-1B).

At cystoscopy, a left ureterocele is resected.

Peripheral renin on salt-restricted diet is 1.42 mmol/liter/hr the next day, 0.83 on normal diet 3 days after resection, and 0.21 on normal diet 7 days after resection.

Blood pressure is 95/55 mm Hg 3 weeks after resection, 110/70 mm Hg 5 years later, and 120/60 mm Hg 11 years later, when physical findings are normal and excretory urogram shows normal left ureter and slight dilation of left calyces.

Diagnosis: Hyperreninemic hypertension, simple ureterocele.

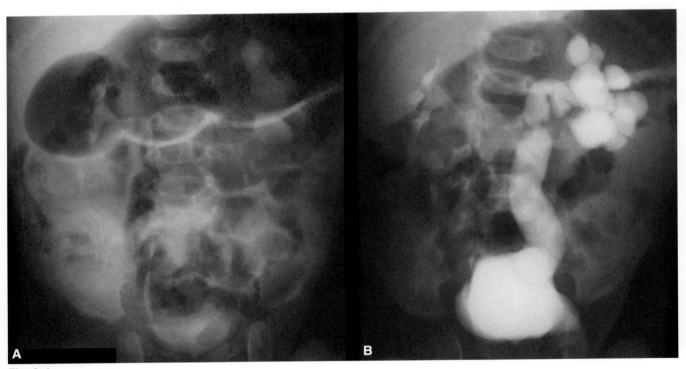

Fig. 9-1

Case 10

A 3-month-old girl has had loose stools and fevers to 40°C for 3 weeks, since she began formula.

Pregnancy was normal, birth weight 4.4 kg.

Temperature is 36.8°C, heart rate 160, respiratory rate 44, systolic blood pressure 80 mm Hg, weight 5.5 kg, length 62 cm, and head circumference 41 cm. A systolic murmur is present. The rest of the physical findings are normal.

Hematocrit is 0.29. White cell count is 16.1 × 10⁹/liter with 0.43 polymorphonuclear cells, 0.02 bands, 0.46 lymphocytes, and 0.09 monocytes. Platelet count is 918 × 10⁹/liter. Urine specific gravity is 1.012, pH 7. Urine has trace protein, 1+ hemoglobin/myoglobin, few nonsquamous epithelial cells/HPF, few squamous epithelial cells/HPF, >100 white cells/HPF, and amorphous sediment. Serum sodium is 137 mmol/liter, potassium 5.8, chloride 107, carbon dioxide 19, urea nitrogen 1.8, calcium 2.52, phosphorus 2.55, cholesterol 3.78, and glucose 4.6. Creatinine is 40 μmol/liter, uric acid 100, total bilirubin 7, and direct bilirubin 0. Total protein is

56 g/liter, albumin 37. Alkaline phosphatase is 186 U/liter, LDH 312, and SGOT 42.

Ultrasound examination shows cyst in upper part of left kidney, dilated left upper pelvis and ureter (Figure 10-1A), and cyst in bladder (Figure 10-1B). Excretory urogram in Figure 10-2 shows duplication of right renal pelvis, lateral and downward displacement of left pelvis, and spherical defect in bladder.

At cystoscopy, right and left ureteral openings are normally placed in trigone; a mucosal blister is below and medial to left opening.

At left upper nephroureterectomy and ureterocelectomy, two left ureters are in common sheath (continuation of renal fascia).

Diagnosis: Duplication of pelvis of left kidney and ureter and left ectopic ureterocele.

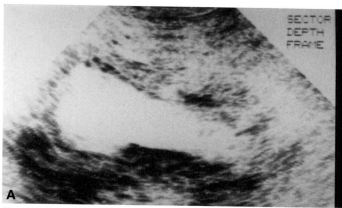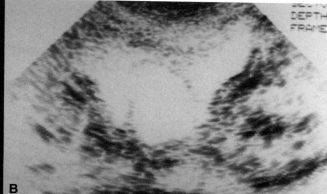

Fig. 10-1

(Continued)

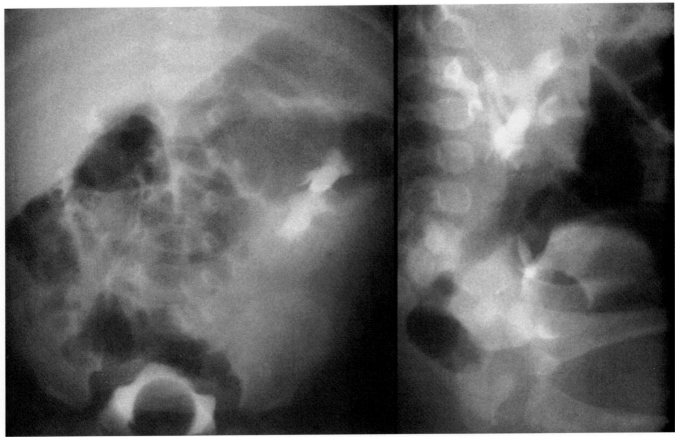

Fig. 10-2

Case 11

A 7-month-old boy has right pyelocaliectasis that was found in prenatal ultrasound examination.

Weight is 10 kg, temperature 38.2°C, heart rate 144, respiratory rate 42, and blood pressure 99/63 mm Hg. Physical findings are normal.

Excretory urogram in Figure 11-1 shows dilated right calyces and ureter, undilated left calyces of duplicated pelvis, undilated left ureter, and defect in lower part of large bladder. Contrast medium injected during cystoscopy is in upper right ureter and lower left pelvis and ureter (Figure 11-2).

Right ureterocelectomy is performed at 8 months, right upper nephroureterectomy at 3½ years. Culture of bladder swab obtained during ureterocelectomy is sterile. Weight at 3½ years is 18.5 kg, blood pressure 109/61 mm Hg, serum urea nitrogen 6.1 mmol/liter, and creatinine 40 μmol/liter. Physical findings are normal.

Ureterocele is of transitional epithelium and has submucosal edema and chronic inflammation. Upper part of right kidney has focal dysplasia and crystalline matter in tubules.

Diagnosis: Duplication of pelves of kidneys, right ectopic ureterocele that obstructs both right ureters and not left ureters.

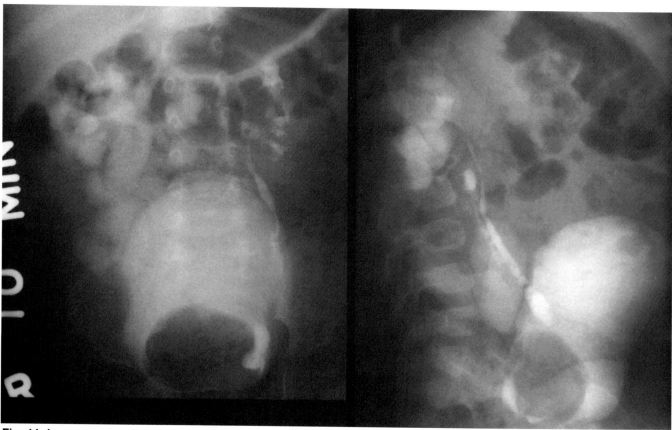

Fig. 11-1

(Continued)

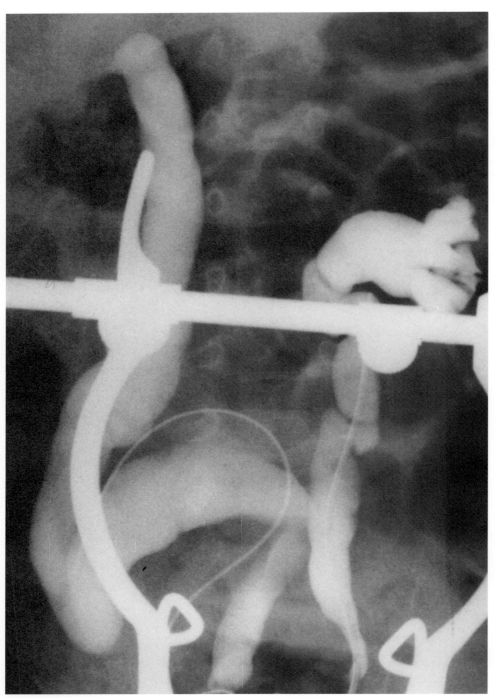

Fig. 11-2

Case 12

A 7-year-old boy's underpants and pajama bottoms are always damp.

Pregnancy was normal. He has had pneumonia, viral meningitis at 5 years, and a fractured nose at 6 years.

Mother (25 years old), father (27 years old), and brother (10 months old) are well.

Weight at 7 years is 22 kg, height 117 cm, temperature 36.8°C, heart rate 72, respiratory rate 12, and blood pressure 100/60 mm Hg. Physical findings are normal.

Hematocrit is 0.40. White cell count is 5.9×10^9/liter with 0.40 polymorphonuclear cells, 0.07 bands, 0.41 lymphocytes, 0.07 monocytes, and 0.04 eosinophils. Platelet count is 340×10^9/liter. Urine specific gravity is 1.011, pH 5. Urine is normal. Serum sodium is 134 mmol/liter, potassium 3.6, chloride 97, carbon dioxide 20, urea nitrogen 3.6, calcium 2.27, phosphorus 1.13, cholesterol 4.89, and glucose 8.0. Creatinine is 60 µmol/liter, uric acid 200, total bilirubin 7, and direct bilirubin 2. Total protein is 77 g/liter, albumin 43. Alkaline phosphatase is 200 U/liter, LDH 252, and SGOT 59.

Figure 12-1 shows duplicated right renal pelvis and ureters. One right ureter enters bladder at same level as single left ureter. Second right ureter goes lower than left ureter and first right ureter.

At operation, both right ureters are in same sheath of renal fascia. Right upper pole ureter continues to opening just to right of seminal colliculus (verumontanum). The transected right upper pole ureter is put into bladder through a tunnel below and medial to normal opening in trigone of right lower pole ureter.

Diagnosis: Urinary incontinence, ectopic ureteral opening in urethra.

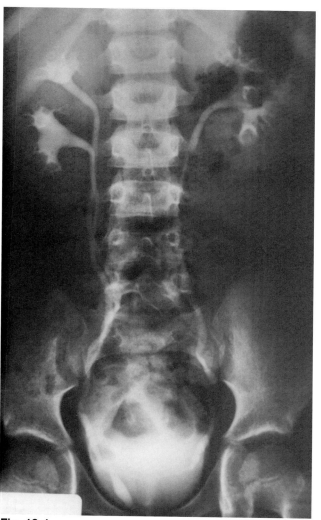

Fig. 12-1

Case 13

A newborn boy is retracting, grunting, and blue.

Pregnancy was normal, delivery by cesarean section for breech presentation. No amniotic fluid is present. Thick vernix covers baby. Apgar score is 9/8 at 1 and 5 minutes, birth weight 3.3 kg, length 50 cm, head circumference 35 cm, heart rate 180, systolic blood pressure 67 mm Hg, and respiratory rate soon 80–100. Respirations are shallow, breath sounds decreased. A nodular mass is in left flank. Testes are not in scrotum. Feet are clubbed. The rest of the physical findings are normal.

When FIO_2 = 0.40, arterial blood pH is 7.04, PCO_2 94 mm Hg, and PO_2 35 mm Hg. When FIO_2 = 1.0, arterial blood pH is 7.37, PCO_2 38 mm Hg, and PO_2 44 mm Hg.

Roentgenogram at 17 minutes and before intubation (Figure 13-1) shows mediastinal air, indicated by thymus dissected from pericardium and extending obliquely across upper part of chest and air below heart between parietal pleura and left side of diaphragm. Right pleural air is above thymus in Figure 13-1. Ultrasound examination shows small, partly cystic right kidney (Figure 13-2A) and large multicystic left kidney (Figure 13-2B).

He dies at 32 hours, 30 minutes after extubation.

At necropsy, left kidney weighs 30 g. Many cysts (0.2–1.0 cm) on its surface contain clear yellow liquid and are separated by bands of tough, pale fibrous tissue without normal parenchyma. Right kidney (weight: 6 g) has purple-brown nodular upper part with thin, dark cortical tissue around randomly arranged, pale pyramids and multicystic lower part. A probe cannot pass down either ureter. Microscopic examination shows (1) no normal parenchyma in left kidney; (2) well-developed glomeruli, primitive glomeruli, normal looking tubules grouped in unusual, circumscribed medullary zones, and primitive tubules lined by columnar epithelium in upper part of right kidney; and (3) cysts lined by cuboidal and flattened epithelial cells in lower part of right kidney. Lungs contain mixture of small alveoli in immature interstitium, hyperaerated alveoli, cartilaginous bronchi almost to pleural surface, thin eosinophilic hyaline membranes, and interstitial hemorrhage.

Diagnosis: Dysplasia of kidneys, hypoplasia of lungs.

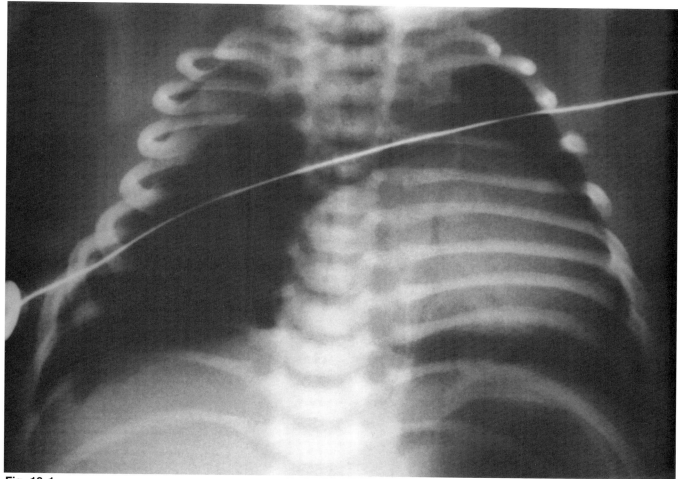

Fig. 13-1

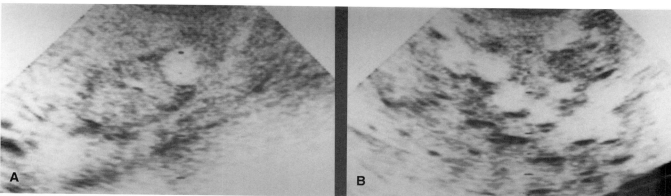

Fig. 13-2

Case 14

A 10-year-old boy will not walk because legs ache. He stopped running 1½ years ago, then walked knock-kneed, with feet turned out, and now will take a few short steps only when he has to. He stopped growing 2 years ago. Appetite is bad. He drinks a lot, especially soda, and gets up twice per night to urinate.

Birth weight was 4.5 kg, length 55 cm. Flank masses were found during 6-week checkup. Systolic blood pressure was 200 mm Hg. Urine specific gravity was 1.005, pH 6. Urine had occasional epithelial cells/HPF and 3–4 white cells/HPF. Creatinine clearance was 26 ml/min/1.73 m² (SI: 0.25 ml/sec/m²). Serum urea nitrogen at 4 years was 28.9 mmol/liter. Creatinine was 240 µmol/liter. Calcium was 2.40 mmol/liter, phosphorus 1.55. C-terminal parathyroid hormone was 329 mlEq/liter (normal: <50).

Mother and sister (16 years old) are well. Father (39 years old) has had insulin-dependent diabetes mellitus for 13 years.

Temperature at 10 years is 36.9°C, heart rate 108, respiratory rate 16, blood pressure 120/72 mm Hg, weight 24 kg, and height 115 cm. Complexion is pasty. Large freckles are on face. Head is large. Biting surfaces of teeth are gray. Sternum protrudes. A systolic murmur is present. A mass (10-cm diameter) is in each flank. Legs move mostly at knees when he walks. The rest of the physical findings are normal.

Hematocrit is 0.19. Hemoglobin is 64 g/liter. Red blood cell count is 2.4 × 10¹²/liter. MCV is 79 fl. MCH is 26 pg. MCHC is 330 g/liter. White cell count is 3.6 × 10⁹/liter with 0.50 polymorphonuclear cells, 0.04 bands, 0.39 lymphocytes, 0.03 monocytes, 0.03 eosinophils, and 0.01 basophils. Platelet count is 113 × 10⁹/liter. Urine specific gravity is 1.008, pH 7. Urine has 0.03 g/liter protein, trace glucose, and 1–2 white cells/HPF. Serum sodium is 139 mmol/liter, potassium 4.1, chloride 107, carbon dioxide 21, urea nitrogen 38.0, calcium 2.15, phosphorus 2.62, magnesium 0.82, cholesterol 4.71, and glucose 4.2. Creatinine is 430 µmol/liter, uric acid 390, total bilirubin 3, and direct bilirubin 0. Total protein is 62 g/liter, albumin 36. Alkaline phosphatase is 948 U/liter, LDH 192, SGOT 17, and amylase 87. N-terminal parathyroid hormone is 397 ng/liter (normal: 8–24).

At 6 weeks, streaks of contrast medium are in much of both flanks 24 hours after IV injection (Figure 14-1). CT scan in Figure 14-2 at 10 years shows large, knobby kidneys. Proximal metaphyses of femurs have little bone at 10 years and abnormal relation to epiphyses (Figure 14-3).

Diagnosis: Infantile polycystic kidneys (Potter-Osathanondh type 1), secondary hyperparathyroidism.

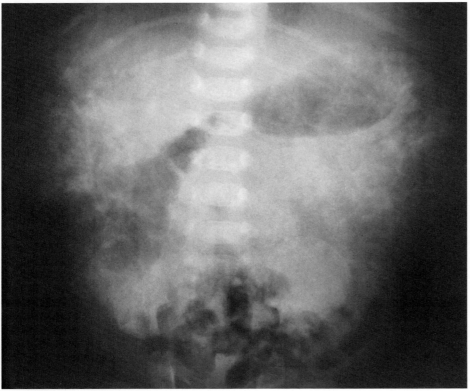

Fig. 14-1

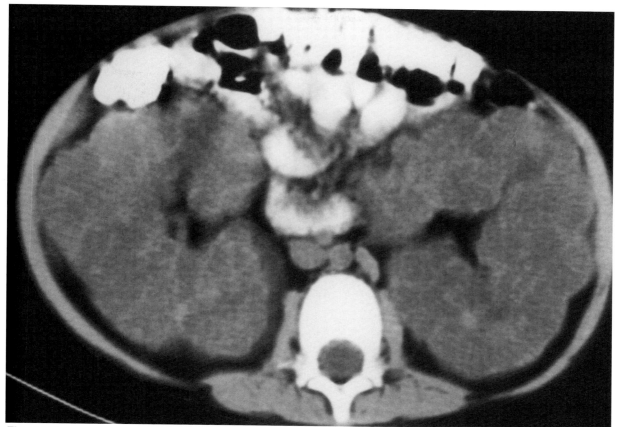

Fig. 14-2

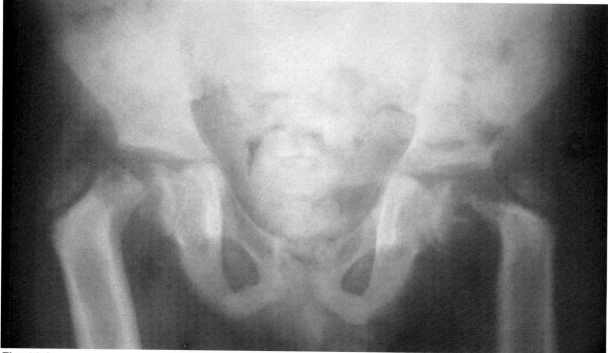

Fig. 14-3

Case 15

A 3-week-old boy has a mass in right flank. The rest of the physical findings are normal.

Pregnancy was normal, birth weight 3.5 kg.

Parents and one sibling are well.

Serum sodium is 138 mmol/liter, potassium 5.3, chloride 105, carbon dioxide 22, urea nitrogen 5.7, calcium 2.54, phosphorus 2.29, cholesterol 2.87, and glucose 4.3. Creatinine is 40 μmol/liter, uric acid 140, total bilirubin 3, and direct bilirubin 0. Total protein is 59 g/liter, albumin 41. Alkaline phosphatase is 341 U/liter, LDH 308, and SGOT 40.

Excretory urogram shows contrast medium in normal left renal pelvis and calyces and in bladder, but not in right pelvis (Figure 15-1A). Contrast medium injected percutaneously into mass in right flank shows cysts, irregular tubes, and part of stenotic ureter (Figure 15-1B).

Weight at 3 months is 5.4 kg, length 62 cm, head circumference 41 cm, and systolic blood pressure 122 mm Hg. The rest of the physical findings are normal.

Diagnosis: Multicystic right kidney (Potter-Osathanondh type 2).

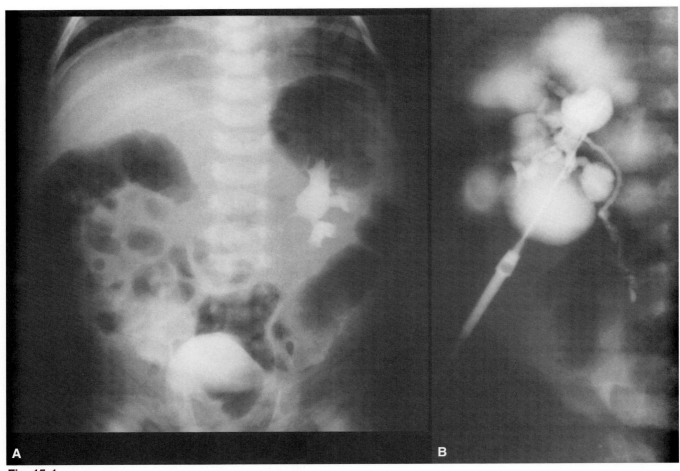

Fig. 15-1

Case 16

A 32-year-old woman has pain in left upper quadrant of abdomen that sometimes makes it hard to breathe.

She has had pain that is brief, unpredictable, and varying in intensity for several years. Liquid was aspirated from left side of chest or left upper quadrant of abdomen when she was 14. She has smoked half a pack of cigarettes per day for 15 years.

Parents died of old age. Two brothers, three sisters, and her two children are well.

Weight is 48 kg, height 155 cm, heart rate 55, respiratory rate 14, and blood pressure 140/90 mm Hg. A burn scar is on right forearm. Left upper quadrant of abdomen is tender. The rest of the physical findings are normal.

Hematocrit is 0.37. White cell count is 4.9×10^9/liter with 0.53 polymorphonuclear cells, 0.01 bands, 0.36 lymphocytes, 0.09 monocytes, and 0.01 basophils. Platelet estimate is normal. ESR is 4 mm/hr. Urine specific gravity is 1.023, pH 8. Urine has many squamous epithelial cells/HPF and 1–2 red cells/HPF. Serum sodium is 141 mmol/liter, potassium 4.1, chloride 108, carbon dioxide 27, urea nitrogen 7.1, calcium 2.37, phosphorus 1.13, cholesterol 4.42, and glucose 5.3. Creatinine is 80 μmol/liter, uric acid 290, total bilirubin 10, and direct bilirubin 2. Total protein is 71 g/liter, albumin 43. Alkaline phosphatase is 33 U/liter, LDH 111, and SGOT 20. Urine creatinine is 5.0 and 9.0 mmol/day (normal: 7.0–15.8).

Curved shadows of calcium density are in right side of abdomen; L5 is transitional (Figure 16-1).

At cystoscopy, left ureteral orifice is normal, right is absent.

Diagnosis: Congenital multicystic right kidney.

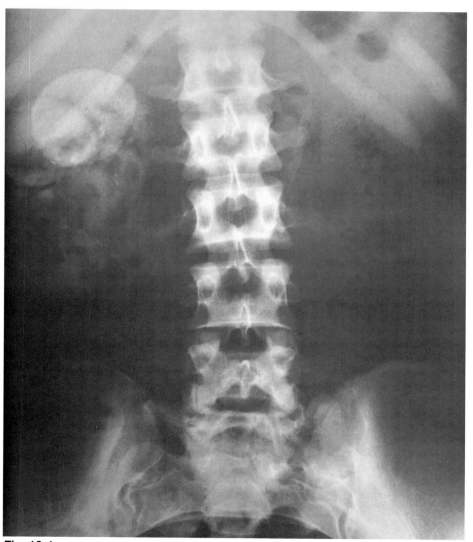

Fig. 16-1

Case 17

A 5-year-old girl examined for respiratory infection has hepatosplenomegaly.

She was delivered prematurely by cesarean section for abruptio placentae. Birth weight was 870 g, Apgar score 5/6 at 1 and 5 minutes. Physical findings were normal. She was intubated and given oxygen for 2 days. Total bilirubin peak was 108 μmol/liter at 7 days. Weight at 2½ months was 2.1 kg, length 44 cm. She has had many colds and often has bellyaches.

Mother (25 years old), father, and sister (3 years old) are well. Maternal grandmother had leukemia.

Temperature at 5 years is 36.5°C, blood pressure 110/70 mm Hg, weight 14 kg, and height 95 cm. Skin under eyes is loose. Right eardrum is red. Tonsils are large. Small lymph nodes are in neck. Liver edge is 4 cm below costal margin, spleen edge 3 cm. Fingers are slightly clubbed. The rest of the physical findings are normal.

Hematocrit is 0.34. White cell count is 7.0×10^9/liter with 0.64 polymorphonuclear cells, 0.05 bands, 0.25 lymphocytes, 0.01 monocytes, 0.02 eosinophils, 0.01 basophils, and 0.02 atypical lymphocytes. Platelet count is 249×10^9/liter. Urine specific gravity is 1.014, pH 7. Urine has 1+ hemoglobin/myoglobin, few bacteria, 10–15 red cells/HPF, and 3–5 white cells/HPF. Serum sodium is 137 mmol/liter, potassium 4.2, chloride 101, carbon dioxide 25, urea nitrogen 7.0, calcium 2.37, phosphorus 1.07, cholesterol 3.47, and glucose 9.1. Creatinine is 50 μmol/liter, uric acid 180, total bilirubin 3, direct bilirubin 2, and ceruloplasmin 3.3 (normal: 1.8–2.5). Total protein is 74 g/liter, albumin 47. Alkaline phosphatase is 157 U/liter, LDH 187, and SGOT 27. α_1-Antitrypsin is 2.0 g/liter (normal: 1.5–3.5). Free T_4 is 141 nmol/liter (normal: 77–155), total T_3 2.0 (normal: 1.2–3.4). TSH is 3.5 mU/liter (normal: 0.4–5.4). Sweat chloride is 21 mmol/liter. Serum is negative for hepatitis A antigen, HBsAg, HBcAg, and HBsAb. Chromosomes are 46,XX.

Cysts are in kidneys and liver (Figure 17-1).

She vomits blood at 9 years. Esophagoscopy shows esophageal and small gastric varices. Sclerosant is injected. She has ascites despite diuretics. Weight is 23.5 kg, heart rate 96, respiratory rate 20, and blood pressure 98/63 mm Hg. Liver edge is 2 cm below costal margin, spleen edge at umbilicus. Hematocrit is 0.29. Urine specific gravity is 1.010, pH 7. Urine has bacteria, trace blood, 0.2 AU urobilinogen, and 0–3 white cells/HPF. Serum urea nitrogen is 5.4 mmol/liter. Creatinine is 60 μmol/liter, total bilirubin 7, and direct bilirubin 0. Total protein is 67 g/liter, albumin 41. Alkaline phosphatase is 183 U/liter, LDH 238, SGOT 28, and amylase 81. Prothrombin ratio is 1 to 1. Activated PTT is 30.4 seconds. At operation at 10 years to make portocaval shunt, liver is scarred and has small cysts; coronary and left gastric veins are dilated. Wedge biopsy of liver shows white fibrous patches on capsule and homogeneous tan parenchyma that contains many small cysts that look like vessels filled with blood.

Diagnosis: Autosomal dominant polycystic kidney disease with liver cysts and hepatic fibrosis (Potter-Osathanondh type 3 cystic kidneys).

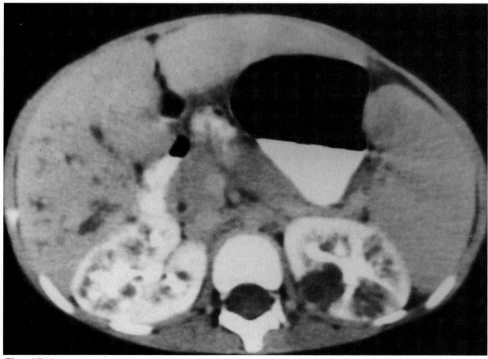

Fig. 17-1

Case 18

A 2-week-old boy has a mass in each flank.

Pregnancy of mother was normal, birth weight 3.5 kg. Lungs were mucousy at 1 hour. He was jaundiced. Flank masses were felt at 4 days. He urinates small amounts with 15- to 30-cm stream. He has been cranky and lethargic for 2 days. He is breast-fed.

Weight is 3.8 kg, temperature 36.8°C, heart rate 120, and respiratory rate 40. Two weeks later, systolic blood pressure is 78 mm Hg. He is jaundiced. The rest of the physical findings are normal.

Hematocrit is 0.30. Hemoglobin is 101 g/liter. MCV is 99 fl. MCH is 34 pg. MCHC is 340 g/liter. White cell count is 14.9 × 10^9/liter with 0.41 polymorphonuclear cells, 0.04 bands, 0.29 lymphocytes, 0.14 monocytes, 0.07 eosinophils, and 0.05 atypical lymphocytes. Platelet estimate is normal. Urine specific gravity is 1.010, pH 5. Urine has occasional squamous epithelial and nonsquamous epithelial cells/HPF, 4–5 red cells/HPF, and 0–1 white cell/HPF. Capillary blood pH is 7.27. P_{CO_2} is 29 mm Hg, P_{O_2} 34. Total carbon dioxide is 14 mmol/liter. Serum sodium is 136 mmol/liter, potassium 5.6, chloride 105, carbon dioxide 14, urea nitrogen 28.6, calcium 2.42, phosphorus 1.71, cholesterol 5.22, triglycerides 1.82, and glucose 5.3. Creatinine is 470 μmol/liter, uric acid 690, total bilirubin 205, and direct bilirubin 31. Total protein is 69 g/liter, albumin 43. Alkaline phosphatase is 273 U/liter, LDH 420, and SGOT 36. Creatinine clearance is 0.0037 ml/sec/m^2 (normal: >0.02).

Cystogram in Figure 18-1 shows (1) reflux into ureters as he expels contrast medium from bladder; (2) dilation of prostatic urethra, grooved along floor by seminal colliculus (verumontanum); and (3) membranous and bulbous urethra.

Renal biopsy shows (1) increased interstitial matrix, (2) foci of spindle-shaped cells with eosinophilic cytoplasm, (3) fascicles of cells that look like smooth muscle cells, (4) atrophic tubules, (5) microcysts lined by cuboidal epithelium, and (6) immature glomeruli.

At cystoscopy, valves are at seminal colliculus.

Diagnosis: Posterior urethral valves (Potter-Osathanondh type 4 subcapsular cystic kidneys).

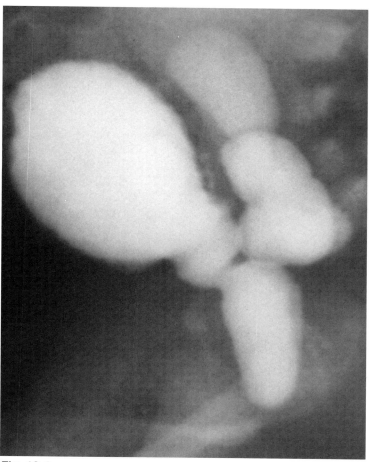

Fig. 18-1

Case 19

A 7-year-old boy has had aches in back and right thigh for 3 days. His teacher says he has recently been tired and inattentive in the afternoon.

He was born 1 month prematurely and spent 1 week in neonatal intensive care unit. He has had ear infections.

Parents and brother (12 years old) are well.

Temperature is 38°C, heart rate 126, respiratory rate 28, blood pressure 116/84 mm Hg, weight 25 kg, and height 120 cm. Flanks and right thigh are tender. A mass (7-cm diameter) is in left side of abdomen. The rest of the physical findings are normal.

Hematocrit is 0.24. White cell count is 24.8×10^9/liter with 0.03 polymorphonuclear cells, 0.27 lymphocytes, 0.01 atypical lymphocytes, and 0.69 blasts. Platelet count is 42×10^9/liter. Urine specific gravity is 1.025, pH 5. Urine has 0.2 AU urobilinogen, mucus, calcium oxalate crystals, and occasional squamous epithelial cells/HPF. Serum sodium is 140 mmol/liter, potassium 4.3, chloride 101, carbon dioxide 27, urea nitrogen 3.6, calcium 2.35, phosphorus 1.36, cholesterol 3.75, and glucose 5.9. Creatinine is 60 µmol/liter, uric acid 200, total bilirubin 9, and direct bilirubin 2. Total protein is 67 g/liter, albumin 44. Alkaline phosphatase is 161 U/liter, LDH 550, and SGOT 58. CSF has 3.8 mmol/liter glucose, 0.17 g/liter protein, $<1 \times 10^6$/liter red cells, $<1 \times 10^6$/liter white cells, 0.47 lymphocytes, and 0.53 monocytes of 17 cells counted.

CT scan after oral and IV contrast media shows cyst with contrast medium in it in left kidney, ureters, and compressed kidney parenchyma medial to and in front of cyst, all confined by renal fascia (Figure 19-1).

Examination of bone marrow aspirate shows (1) 19 of 20 homogeneous lymphoblasts with 47,XXY karyotype in Wright's stain of cytocentrifuge preparation and (2) staining with antibodies to TdT, CALLA, B4, and CD34 in immunologic analysis of Ficoll-Paque suspension (Pharmacia Biotech, Piscataway, NJ).

Clear liquid is aspirated from cyst. Treatment is begun for precursor B-cell ALL. Weight at 10 years is 43.6 kg, height 141 cm. Left side of abdomen is slightly full. Bone marrow is normal. At operation at 10 years, a cyst that contains 500 ml clear liquid is removed from left kidney.

Cyst membrane (0.2-cm thick) is smooth tan. A piece of attached tissue consists of compressed atrophic renal parenchyma and connective tissue.

Diagnosis: Simple renal cyst.

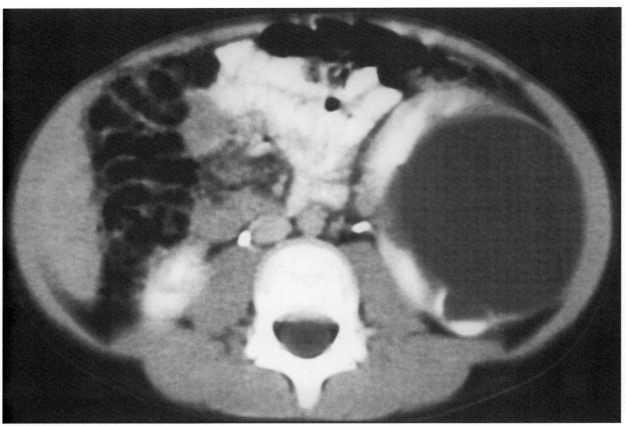

Fig. 19-1

Case 20

An 11-year-old girl drinks and urinates a lot, has not grown much recently, is less active, eats less than she used to, and bruises easily. The quality of her school work has decreased. Right knee "locks" and aches.

She had a mouth infection at 3 years, nasal fracture at 4 years, removal of tonsils and adenoids at 5 years, pustules on right hand 6 months ago, and otitis externa 5 months ago, when blood pressure was 120/70 mm Hg.

Father (45 years old) and two brothers (13 and 16 years old) are well. Mother (41 years old) has headaches and high blood pressure and has had several operations. Maternal grandfather has high blood pressure.

Weight at 11 years is 38 kg, height 144 cm, temperature 36.3°C, heart rate 80, respiratory rate 20, and blood pressure 106/66 mm Hg. Complexion is muddy. Conjunctivae are pale, retinal vessels tortuous. Breasts are beginning to develop. She has a systolic murmur and knock-knees. The rest of the physical findings are normal.

Urine specific gravity 5 months ago was 1.007, pH 6. Urine had no sugar, protein, casts, or cells.

Hematocrit at 11 years is 0.20. White cell count is 4.1×10^9/liter with 0.60 polymorphonuclear cells, 0.03 bands, 0.32 lymphocytes, 0.04 monocytes, and 0.01 eosinophils. Platelet count is 148×10^9/liter. Serum sodium is 143 mmol/liter, potassium 3.2, chloride 105, carbon dioxide 18, urea nitrogen 22.0, calcium 2.32, phosphorus 1.65, cholesterol 5.51, and glucose 5.9. Creatinine is 330 μmol/liter, uric acid 410, total bilirubin 5, and direct bilirubin 0. Total protein is 72 g/liter, albumin 45. Alkaline phosphatase is 1,197 U/liter, LDH 146, and SGOT 27.

Because of findings in girl, her two brothers are examined. Blood urea nitrogen and creatinine of the 13-year-old brother are normal. Blood urea nitrogen of the 16-year-old brother is 15.4 mmol/liter, creatinine 340 μmol/liter.

The 16-year-old brother feels well. Appetite is good. He gets up once per night to urinate. Five months later, he says that he tires quickly, that his back tingles after exercise, and that

he has lost 4.5 kg in 1 month despite having grown 8 cm in the past year.

Tonsils of 16-year-old brother were removed at 9 years.

His weight is 58 kg, height 170 cm, temperature 36.9°C, heart rate 80, respiratory rate 20, and blood pressure 120/68 mm Hg. A systolic murmur is present. The rest of the physical findings are normal.

His hematocrit is 0.32. White cell count is 7.1×10^9/liter with 0.57 polymorphonuclear cells, 0.01 bands, 0.31 lymphocytes, 0.06 monocytes, 0.03 eosinophils, and 0.02 basophils. Serum sodium is 141 mmol/liter, potassium 3.4, chloride 108, carbon dioxide 24, urea nitrogen 10.4, calcium 2.50, phosphorus 1.78, cholesterol 4.63, and glucose 5.4. Creatinine is 320 μmol/liter, uric acid 390, total bilirubin 5, and direct bilirubin 5. Total protein is 69 g/liter, albumin 43. Alkaline phosphatase is 230 U/liter, LDH 69, and SGOT 12. Twelve-hour urine collection of 3,170 ml has no protein. In 6 hours after start of water deprivation test, he loses 2 kg and passes 2,220 ml urine with specific gravity 1.004 and osmolality 138 mmol/kg. Four months later, plasma C-terminal parathormone is 536 mlEq/liter (normal: <50). Serum calcium is 2.74 mmol/liter.

Roentgenographic examination of girl's abdomen shows small kidneys (Figure 20-1A). Figure 20-1B shows a radiolucent defect in expanded superior ramus of right pubic bone and deep and poorly mineralized growth plates of femurs. Mineralization of calvaria is speckled like salt and pepper (Figure 20-2). Laminae dura in mandible are not mineralized. Cystogram in 16-year-old boy shows large bladder (Figure 20-3A) and retrograde pyelogram normal pelves and calyces (Figure 20-3B). Normal urethra in cystogram is not shown. Selective renal angiograms show excessive tapering of interlobar arteries and thin cortices (Figure 20-4).

Diagnosis: Familial juvenile nephronophthisis (nephronophthisis–medullary cystic disease complex). Renal rickets, secondary hyperparathyroidism, and brown tumor of right pubic bone, in girl.

(Continued)

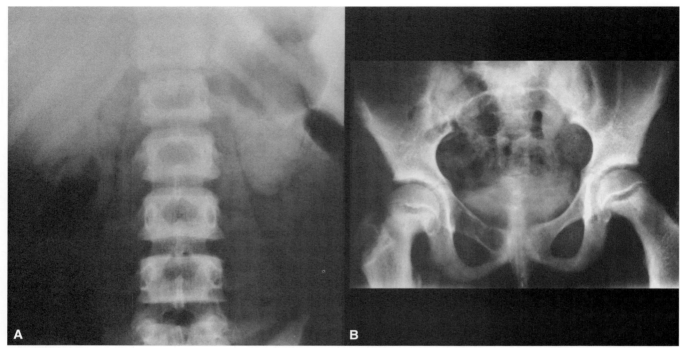

Fig. 20-1

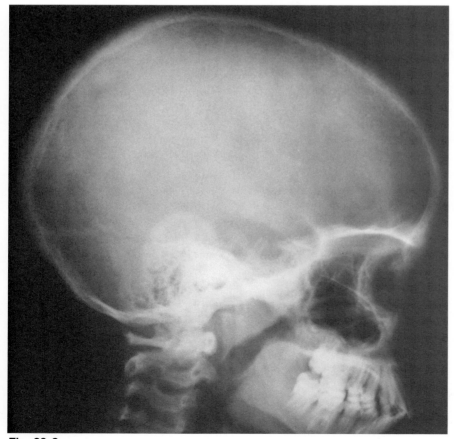

Fig. 20-2

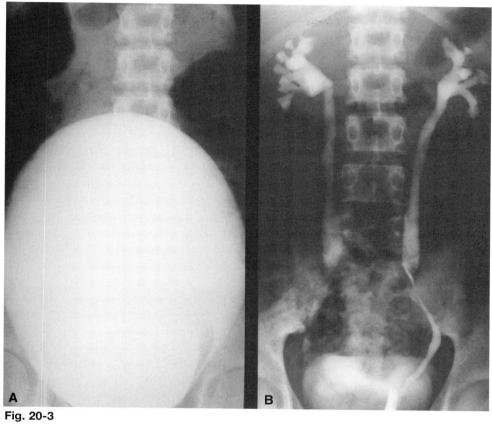

Fig. 20-3

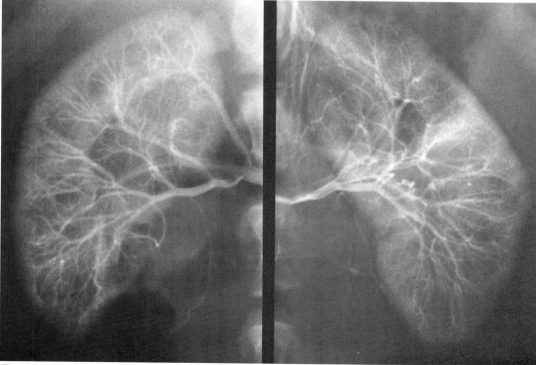

Fig. 20-4

Case 21

A newborn girl is large and edematous.

Mother (23 years old), father (28 years old), and brother (2 years old) are well. Mother had a stillborn son by a different father at 17 years. The stillborn baby had hypoplastic lungs, subendocardial fibrosis, no kidneys, and no urinary bladder. Maternal grandfather had tuberculosis; paternal grandfather had emphysema.

Pregnancy was normal. Birth weight is 4.7 kg, length 52 cm, head circumference 34 cm, temperature 36.6°C, heart rate 128, respiratory rate 24, and blood glucose >2.5 mmol/liter. A bruise is on forehead. Tongue is large. A systolic murmur is present. A gap is between rectus abdominis muscles. The rest of the physical findings are normal.

Right leg is larger than left at 2½ months. Tongue is large at 2 years. She wears size 9½ right shoe, size 8½ left shoe at 32 months. She has diastasis recti at 5 years. Right arm is 53 cm long at 6½ years, left arm 51. Right leg is thicker and 4 cm longer than left. A café au lait spot is on abdomen. Liver edge is 2–3 cm below costal margin. Right leg is 6 cm longer than left at 11½ years. Distal right femoral and proximal right tibial and fibular epiphysiodeses are performed.

Urine specific gravity at 2 years is 1.015, pH 6. Urine has 3–5 epithelial cells/HPF, 10–15 white cells/HPF, and mucus.

Excretory urograms at 2½ (Figure 21-1A) and 6½ years (Figure 21-1B) show a haze of contrast medium in medullas (pyramids) of kidneys.

Diagnosis: Beckwith-Wiedemann syndrome, medullary sponge kidneys.

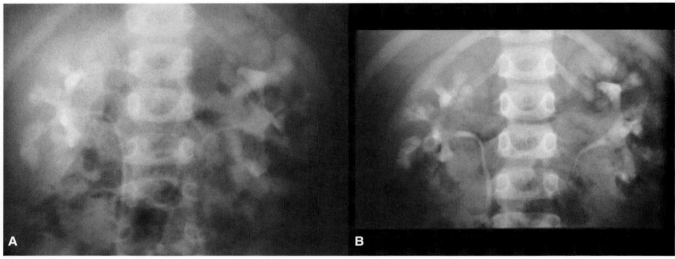

Fig. 21-1

Case 22

An 8-day-old boy is jaundiced and hypertensive.

Pregnancy of mother was normal, membranes ruptured spontaneously, labor lasted 3 hours, presentation was vertex, and forceps were used during delivery. Birth weight was 4.3 kg, length 52 cm, head circumference 36 cm, Apgar score 8/8 at 1 and 5 minutes, heart rate 160, respiratory rate 50, systolic blood pressure 56 mm Hg, and blood glucose 3.9 mmol/liter. Lips were blue at 12 hours. Baby was yellow at 24 hours. At 54 hours, hematocrit was 0.62. Hemoglobin was 200 g/liter. White cell count was 11.6 × 10⁹/liter with 0.35 polymorphonuclear cells, 0.04 bands, 0.41 lymphocytes, 0.13 monocytes, 0.05 eosinophils, and 0.02 basophils. Serum total bilirubin was 371 mmol/liter, direct bilirubin 24. Total bilirubin was 402 mmol/liter, direct bilirubin 58 just before exchange transfusion at 94 hours.

Systolic blood pressure at 8 days is 110 and 112 mm Hg in arms, 102 and 104 mm Hg in legs. Testes are in inguinal canals. The rest of the physical findings are normal.

Serum sodium is 140 mmol/liter, potassium 5.5, chloride 108, carbon dioxide 18, urea nitrogen 4.3, calcium 2.50, phosphorus 2.07, cholesterol 5.30, and glucose 4.0. Creatinine is 90 µmol/liter, uric acid 230, total bilirubin 137, and direct bilirubin 10. Total protein is 61 g/liter, albumin 45. Alkaline phosphatase is 197 U/liter, LDH >600, and SGOT 30.

Excretory urogram at 8 days (Figure 22-1A) shows downward displacement of pelvis of right kidney and a round, relatively radiolucent shadow above it 10 minutes after injection of contrast medium. Findings in excretory urogram at 3 months are normal (Figure 22-1B). A shadow of calcium density that is on right side at level of T12 at 14 months (Figure 22-2A) is smaller, better defined, and slightly higher at 4 years (Figure 22-2B).

Diagnosis: Right adrenal hematoma in newborn boy, later calcification.

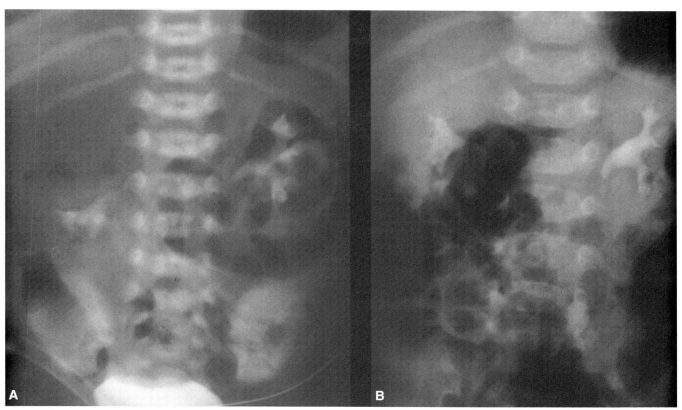

Fig. 22-1

(Continued)

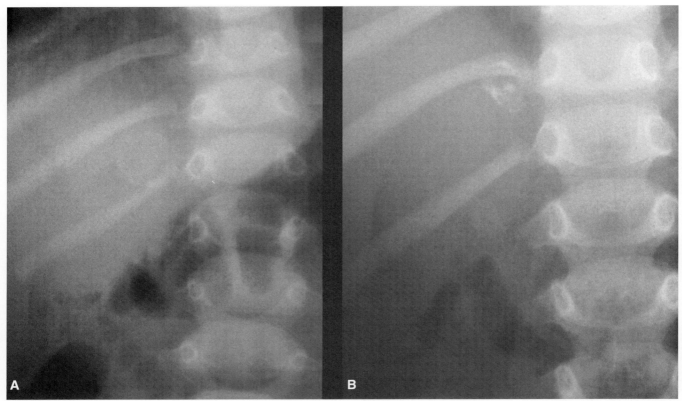

Fig. 22-2

Case 23

A 10-year-old boy is shivering and vomiting.

He hit left side of abdomen on the edge of a board 2 hours ago when he fell 4 ft.

Temperature is 36.1°C, heart rate 88, respiratory rate 20, blood pressure 128/80 mm Hg, and weight 36 kg. He is pale and cool. A bruise is under left ribs front and back 2 hours after the fall; left upper quadrant is tender and full 8 hours after fall. The rest of the physical findings are normal.

Hematocrit is 0.32. White cell count is 10.4 × 10⁹/liter with 0.69 polymorphonuclear cells, 0.08 bands, 0.14 lymphocytes, 0.06 monocytes, and 0.03 eosinophils. Platelet count is 276 × 10⁹/liter. Urine is red and cloudy; specific gravity is 1.023, pH 6. Urine has 4+ protein, 1+ glucose, <1.7 µmol/liter urobilinogen (normal: 0.5–3.6 µmol/2 hours), bacteria, 0–1 white cell/HPF, and many red cells/HPF. Eight hours after the fall, serum sodium is 135 mmol/liter, potassium 4.3, chloride 105, carbon dioxide 22, urea nitrogen 2.9, calcium 2.27, phosphorus 0.97, cholesterol 3.59, and glucose 11.4 (IV fluids). Creatinine is 70 µmol/liter, uric acid 160, total bilirubin 7, and direct bilirubin 2. Total protein is 56 g/liter, albumin 40. Alkaline phosphatase is 221 U/liter, LDH 308, and SGOT 50.

CT scan after IV and oral contrast media shows varying densities in and around large left kidney; contrast medium leaks back from left pelvis to renal fascia (Figure 23-1).

Abdomen hurts more and is more distended 3 days later. Blood pressure is 160/100 mm Hg. At operation, blood is in peritoneum and retroperitoneum behind descending colon. A contusion is in small bowel. Blood is around left kidney. A transverse tear bisects left kidney from hilum to cortex. Left kidney is removed.

Microscopic examination of pale tan tissue around tear shows hemorrhagic infarction and necrosis.

After operation, he occasionally cannot eat and other times "he eats everything in sight." He wakes up one morning 3 months after operation vomiting and in pain. Abdomen is tender. Bowel sounds are infrequent. At operation, adhesions are around gut. A distended loop is herniated under a hemorrhagic band of fibroadipose tissue between abdominal scar and bed of left kidney.

Diagnosis: Traumatic rupture and infarction of left kidney, intestinal obstruction by postoperative or posthemorrhagic adhesion.

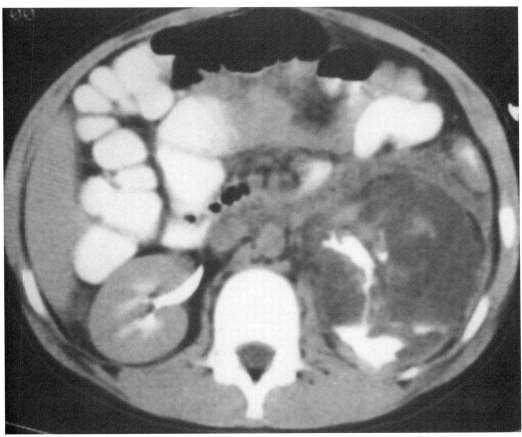

Fig. 23-1

Case 24

A 10-year-old girl has left flank pain and urinary frequency.

Pregnancy was normal. She had a seizure at 14 months.

Mother (29 years old), maternal grandfather, and maternal great-grandfather have had blood in urine. Father (30 years old), brother (8 years old), and sister (6 years old) are well.

Temperature is 37°C, heart rate 68, respiratory rate 22, blood pressure 112/60 mm Hg, weight 47 kg, and height 137 cm. A systolic heart murmur is present. The rest of the physical findings are normal.

Hematocrit is 0.36. White cell count is 7.1×10^9/liter. Platelet count is 307×10^9/liter. Urine specific gravity is 1.005, pH 5. Urine has packed white cells, occult blood, and $>10^5$ colonies *Escherichia coli*/ml. Two weeks later, urine specific gravity is 1.007, pH 7. Urine has 20–25 red cells/HPF, few epithelial cells/HPF, and bacteria. Serum sodium is 139 mmol/liter, potassium 5.7, chloride 103, carbon dioxide 22, urea nitrogen 5.4, calcium 2.52, phosphorus 1.39, cholesterol 5.51, and glucose 5.1. Creatinine is 60 µmol/liter, uric acid 290, total bilirubin 9, and direct bilirubin 2. Total protein is 81 g/liter, albumin 47. Alkaline phosphatase is 293 U/liter, LDH 439. Two months later, SGOT is 16 U/liter.

Figure 24-1 shows a staghorn calculus in pelvis and some of major calyces of left kidney, and small stones of calcium density in minor calyces.

Bladder and ureteral orificia are normal at cystoscopy.

Urine has 1,272 mmol lysine/mol$_{creatinine}$ (normal: 6.2 ± 1.5), 684 mmol arginine/mol$_{creatinine}$ (normal: 1.3 ± 0.7), 369 mmol ornithine/mol$_{creatinine}$ (normal: 1.1 ± 0.3), and 437 and 723 mmol cystine/mol$_{creatinine}$ (normal: 7–28).

She has occasional ureteral colic despite medical treatment and irrigations through nephrostomy tubes and ureteral catheters. Stones are removed at ureteroscopy and fragmented by extracorporeal shock wave lithotripsy. Blood pressure at 21 years is 140/102 mm Hg. Serum urea nitrogen is 3.9 mmol/liter, carbon dioxide 33, calcium 2.27, and phosphorus 0.97. Creatinine is 90 µmol/liter.

Diagnosis: Cystinuria. (Parents have trace cystine in urine. Sister has cystinuria; brother does not.)

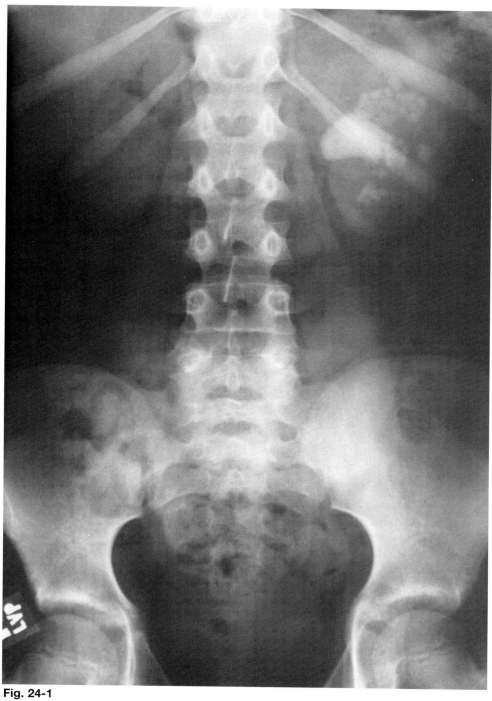

Fig. 24-1

Case 25

A 13-year-old boy has right flank pain down to right testicle. He has vomited three times.

He cried and had pink urine at 2 years. He had right flank pain, fever, and gravel in urine at 7 years. Since then he has had stones in his urine without pain about once per month.

Mother (47 years old) had first attack of renal colic at 17 years and kidney transplant at 40 years. Two maternal aunts, two maternal uncles, and two of mother's first cousins have had kidney stones. Maternal grandfather (85 years old) has calcifications in both kidneys. Sister (15 years old) has had renal colic and hematuria. Father (42 years old) is well.

Weight is 32 kg, height 130 cm, temperature 36.7°C, heart rate 88, respiratory rate 20, and blood pressure 104/50 mm Hg. Right flank is tender despite treatment with meperidine. The rest of the physical findings are normal. Pain subsides after he passes several brown stones, the largest 5 × 4 mm.

Hematocrit is 0.40. White cell count is 14.9×10^9/liter with 0.92 polymorphonuclear cells, 0.04 bands, 0.02 lymphocytes, 0.01 monocytes, and 0.01 eosinophils. Platelet estimate is adequate. Urine specific gravity is 1.007, pH 7. Urine contains hemoglobin, 15–20 white cells/HPF, and 60–80 red cells/HPF. Serum sodium is 141 mmol/liter, potassium 3.8, chloride 110, carbon dioxide 12, urea nitrogen 5.0, calcium 2.37, phosphorus 1.29, cholesterol 4.37, triglycerides 0.45, and glucose 6.7. Creatinine is 70 µmol/liter, uric acid 260, total bilirubin 5, and direct bilirubin 0. Total protein is 77 g/liter, albumin 44. Alkaline phosphatase is 223 U/liter, LDH 308, SGOT 23, and CK 62. Venous blood pH is 7.30. P_{CO_2} is 33 mm Hg, P_{O_2} 48. Bicarbonate is 16 mmol/liter, total carbon dioxide 17.

Calcium deposits are in medullas of kidneys (Figure 25-1A). Excretory urogram the next day shows contrast medium in renal cortices 1 minute after IV injection and a calcified stone in right side of bony pelvis (Figure 25-1B). Contrast medium is in bladder at 30 minutes.

Diagnosis: Nephrocalcinosis, distal renal tubular acidosis. (A sister, born 2 years after mother had renal transplant, is now 23 and, when asked about symptoms of her brother's says, "I never had any of that." She enjoys mountain biking and volleyball and wants to play tennis again with her brother [now 33 years old] who has not played for years and has been undergoing peritoneal dialysis 9 hours a day for the last 8 months. She is well and wants to donate a kidney to her brother. The human leukocyte antigenic match between them is favorable.)

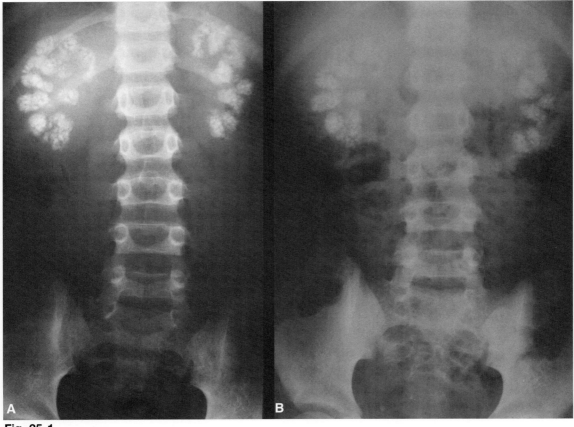

Fig. 25-1

Case 26

A 10-year-old boy drinks and urinates a lot. In the last few months he has not played as much football and soccer as he used to.

Blood was in urine for 1 month at 4 years. His teeth worried his parents at 7 years. Stones were found in kidney biopsy at 7 years.

Mother took phenytoin during pregnancy for seizures that started at 28 years. Birth weight was 4 kg. He has had chickenpox.

Mother (39 years old), father (41 years old), and brother (7 years old) are well.

Weight at 10 years is 39 kg, height 147 cm, temperature 36.4°C, heart rate 80, respiratory rate 20, and blood pressure 120/70 mm Hg. A small dark nevus is on forehead, a larger, hairier one on left upper arm. Teeth are chalky, chipped, and mottled. A scar is in right flank. The rest of the physical findings are normal. Ophthalmologic findings are normal.

Hematocrit is 0.24. Hemoglobin is 81 g/liter. Red blood cell count is 2.9×10^{12}/liter. MCV is 81 fl. MCH is 28 pg. MCHC is 340 g/liter. White cell count is 8.0×10^9/liter with 0.50 polymorphonuclear cells, 0.02 bands, 0.40 lymphocytes, 0.02 monocytes, 0.04 eosinophils, and 0.02 basophils. Platelet count is 346×10^9/liter. Urine specific gravity is 1.008, pH 6. Urine has trace protein, 0–1 red cell/HPF, 15–20 white cells/HPF, and bacteria. Culture shows no growth. Serum sodium is 142 mmol/liter, potassium 5.6, chloride 107, carbon dioxide 14, urea nitrogen 26.4, calcium 2.40, phosphorus 2.00, magnesium 0.91, cholesterol 3.47, and glucose 5.4. Creatinine is 450 µmol/liter, uric acid 330, total bilirubin 15, and direct bilirubin 0. Total protein is 77 g/liter, albumin 47. Alkaline phosphatase is 474 U/liter, LDH 111, SGOT 28, and amylase 200. Intact parathormone is 43 pmol/liter (normal: 1.0–6.0) when calcium is 2.37 mmol/liter.

Deposits of calcium are in kidneys and cortex looks thin (Figure 26-1).

Urine volume is 2,225 ml/day. Urine protein is 0.32 g/day (normal: <0.15). Urine creatinine is 5.9 mmol/day (normal: 7.1–15.9). Creatinine clearance is 0.12 ml/sec/m² (mean: 0.86). Urine oxalate is 1,444 µmol/day (normal: 110–440). Urine glycolic acid is 0.77 mmol/day (normal: 0.20–0.79).

Diagnosis: Oxalosis type I.

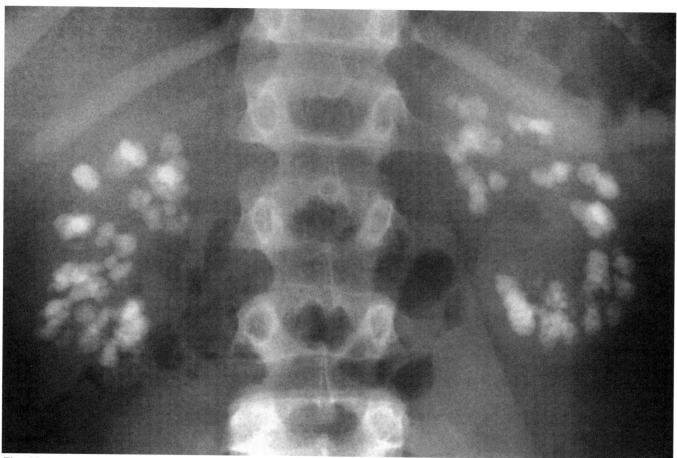

Fig. 26-1

Case 27

A 13-year-old boy has right flank pain.

Pain in flank and right side of abdomen began yesterday morning. He vomited and had a headache last night. He feels better when prone. He is in too much pain to sit or walk.

Tonsils and adenoids were removed "long ago." He broke his right forearm at 5 years.

Temperature is 40°C, heart rate 96, respiratory rate 28, blood pressure 114/64 mm Hg, weight 28 kg, and height 138 cm. He is thin and pale. Right flank is tender. Slight rebound tenderness is in right side of abdomen. The rest of the physical findings are normal.

Hematocrit is 0.43. White cell count is 15.9×10^9/liter with 0.83 polymorphonuclear cells, 0.10 bands, 0.05 lymphocytes, and 0.02 monocytes. Platelet count is 247×10^9/liter. Urine specific gravity is 1.020, pH 7. Urine has 0.40 g/liter ketones, 0.30 g/liter protein, trace blood, 0.34 μmol/liter urobilinogen (normal: 0.5–3.6 μmol/2 hrs), amorphous phosphates, 5–10 white cells/HPF, and many gram-positive cocci. Serum sodium is 134 mmol/liter, potassium 4.5, chloride 96, carbon dioxide 22, urea nitrogen 3.9, calcium 2.35, phosphorus 0.65, cholesterol 4.16, and glucose 10.3 (IV fluids). Creatinine is 70 μmol/liter, uric acid 160, total bilirubin 7, and direct bilirubin 2. Total protein is 67 g/liter, albumin 41. Alkaline phosphatase is 206 U/liter, LDH 215, and SGOT 15.

Ultrasound examination in Figure 27-1 shows increase in central echoes in right kidney around a cyst that contains sediment.

Culture of urine grows >10^5 colonies coagulase-negative staphylococci/ml.

He feels well 5 days later.

Diagnosis: Abscess, right kidney.

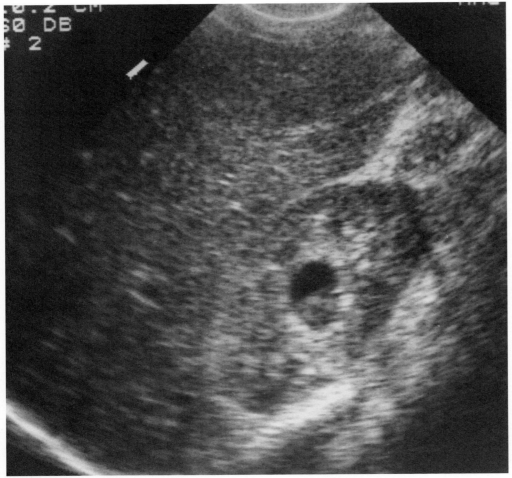

Fig. 27-1

Case 28

A 2-year-old boy has white sludge in his urine. He has "felt warm" and been sick for several days.

Weight is 10.4 kg, height 84 cm, temperature 37.4°C, heart rate 104, respiratory rate 32, and blood pressure 108/74 mm Hg. Right flank feels full. The rest of the physical findings are normal.

Hematocrit is 0.27. Hemoglobin is 89 g/liter. Red blood cell count is 4.4×10^{12}/liter. MCV is 61 fl. MCH is 20 pg. MCHC is 340 g/liter. Red-blood-cell distribution width is 13.5% (normal: 11.5–15.0). White cell count is 11.2×10^9/liter with 0.44 polymorphonuclear cells, 0.06 bands, 0.35 lymphocytes, 0.12 monocytes, 0.02 eosinophils, and 0.01 basophils. Platelet count is 458×10^9/liter. After blood transfusion 4 days later, ESR is 34 mm/hr. Urine is cloudy with specific gravity 1.029, pH 6, 1.0 g/liter protein, 2+ hemoglobin/myoglobin, few squamous epithelial cells/HPF, 10–20 red cells/HPF, and >100 white cells/HPF. Serum sodium is 136 mmol/liter, potassium 4.1, chloride 98, carbon dioxide 19, and urea nitrogen 5.7. Creatinine is 40 µmol/liter. SGOT is 30 U/liter.

Excretory urogram 5 minutes after IV injection (Figure 28-1A) shows contrast medium in bladder and in normal left calyces and pelvis but not in right calyces and pelvis.

At cystoscopy, sludge is in bladder and right ureter. Right ureteral orifice is large and red.

Retrograde pyelogram (Figure 28-1B) shows contrast medium around matter in dilated pelvis and calyces of right kidney.

Culture of urine grows 9,000 colonies *Proteus mirabilis*/ml.

At right nephroureterectomy, adhesions surround kidney. A focus of calcification is in kidney. A lymph node (1.5 cm) is in hilum.

Right kidney (6.5 × 3.5 × 3.0 cm, 51 g) has mottled purple capsule, liquefied necrotic medulla, and 1–2 cm lumps of soft, yellow-white matter. Similar matter is in right ureter, which has 1.5-cm circumference. Microscopic examination shows (1) pelvic urothelial granulomas with polymorphonuclear cells in necrotic center, (2) other granulomas encroaching on medulla with multinucleated giant cells in center, (3) peripheral histiocytes, (4) cortical histiocytes and lymphocytes, (5) lymphoid follicles with active germinal centers, (6) necrotic matter in pelvis, and (7) intact transitional cell epithelium in ureter with submucosal lymphoid aggregates, dilated vessels, and small collections of foam cells.

Diagnosis: Xanthogranulomatous pyelonephritis.

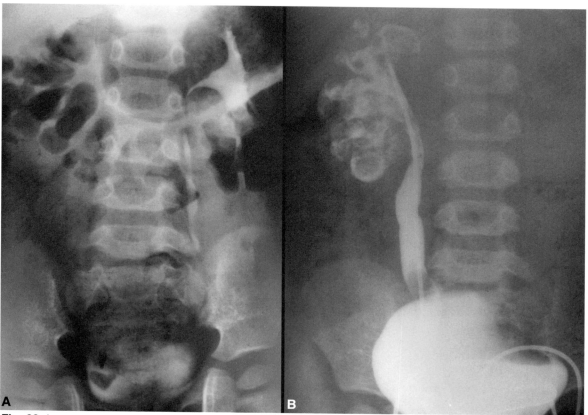

A   **B**

Fig. 28-1

Case 29

A 15-year-old boy, whose blood pressure was normal 4 months ago, has high blood pressure in school examination. He is on school wrestling and football teams and runs 60 track laps per day.

Appendix was removed several years ago.

Parents and sister are well.

Temperature is 36.8°C, heart rate 72, respiratory rate 16, blood pressure in arms 150–152/102–104 mm Hg, in legs 154–164/110–114 mm Hg, weight 69 kg, and height 175 cm. A scar is in right lower quadrant of abdomen. The rest of the physical findings are normal.

Hematocrit is 0.42. White cell count is 5.5×10^9/liter with 0.43 polymorphonuclear cells, 0.44 lymphocytes, 0.10 monocytes, and 0.03 eosinophils. Urine specific gravity is 1.013, pH 7. Urine has occasional epithelial cells/HPF and 0–1 white cell/HPF. Three earlier specimens of urine have 4+, 2+, and 0 protein. Six of 25 random specimens of urine, three of them first-morning specimens, now have no protein; seven of 25 have trace protein; five of 25 have 1+ protein; four of 25 have 2+ protein; and three of 25 have 3+ protein. Three 24-hour collections of urine have 0.40, 1.80, and 0 g protein/day. Serum sodium is 140 mmol/liter, potassium 3.5, chloride 96, carbon dioxide 26, urea nitrogen 4.6, calcium 2.27, phosphorus 1.16, and cholesterol 3.67. Creatinine is 100 μmol/liter,

uric acid 280, total bilirubin 9, and direct bilirubin 0. Total protein is 69 g/liter, albumin 44. Alkaline phosphatase is 163 U/liter, LDH 217, and SGOT 28. Urine epinephrine is 16 nmol/day (normal: <55), norepinephrine 260 (normal: <590).

Plasma renin* on normal diet is 1.58 ng/(L · s) (normal: 0.30–1.14) before he gets out of bed and 4.17 ng/(L · s) after he walks. Right renal vein renin is 5.00 ng/(L · s), left renal vein renin 1.25 ng/(L · s).

Renal arteriogram shows normal left renal artery, three branch right renal arteries, and occlusion of lowest right renal branch 1.5 cm distal to its origin. In nephrogram, right kidney is smaller than left and has a lateral defect (Figure 29-1A). Excretory urogram shows normal renal pelves and calyces that descend the height of two vertebral bodies and change in axis of right kidney when he stands up (Figure 29-1B).

He is treated medically for hypertension. Cortical defect in right kidney is smaller, lowest right renal artery uneven but patent in angiogram 2½ years later.

Diagnosis: Renal artery occlusion, renovascular hypertension, orthostatic proteinuria.

---

*2.778 ng/(L · s) renin = 1 μg angiotensin I × h^{-1} × liter^{-1}.

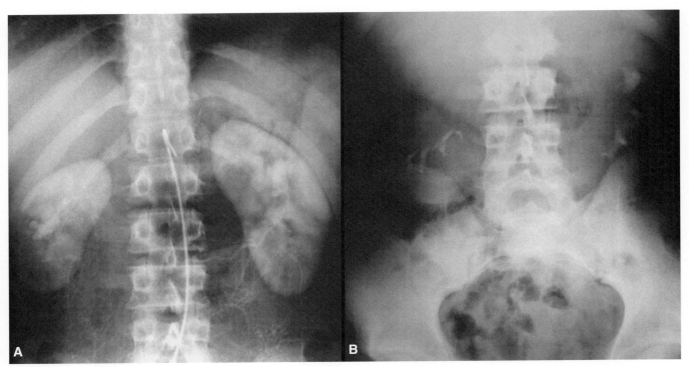

Fig. 29-1

Case 30

A 15-year-old girl has had headaches and nosebleeds for 2 months.

Birth weight was 3.6 kg. At 4 years, she had urinary tract infection with >10^5 colonies *Escherichia coli*/ml in two urine specimens. Cystography showed normal findings and no vesico-ureteral reflux. Cystoscopy showed bullous cystitis. Urethral dilation was performed. She had vomiting and abdominal pain at 8 years. Blood pressure was 110/60 mm Hg. Physical findings were normal. Urine specific gravity varied from 1.012 to 1.020, pH from 5 to 7. Urine had few white cells/HPF and many red cells/HPF. Three urine cultures were sterile. Serum urea nitrogen was 7.5 mmol/liter. Creatinine was 70 μmol/liter. Cystography showed normal findings and no vesicoureteral reflux. Cystoscopy showed cystitis. Menarche was at 13 years.

Parents and two half brothers are well.

Temperature at 15 years is 37.5°C, heart rate 80, respiratory rate 24, blood pressure 132/96 mm Hg, weight 54 kg, and height 161 cm. The rest of the physical findings are normal.

Hematocrit is 0.39. White cell count is 5.9 × 10^9/liter with 0.49 polymorphonuclear cells, 0.02 bands, 0.36 lymphocytes, 0.12 monocytes, and 0.01 eosinophils. Platelet count is 265 × 10^9/liter. Serum urea nitrogen is 5.7 mmol/liter, calcium 2.30, and phosphorus 1.09. Creatinine is 80 μmol/liter.

Excretory urogram shows normal findings at 4 years (Figure 30-1A), small left kidney at 8 years (Figure 30-1B).

Angiography at 15 years shows (1) normal right renal artery and right kidney, (2) small left renal artery that tapers slightly several millimeters beyond origin, and (3) small left kidney, similar to appearance of kidney at 8 years.

At left nephrectomy, kidney is 5 × 3 × 1 cm. Gross and microscopic examinations show parenchymal atrophy.

Diagnosis: Atrophy of left kidney between 4 and 8 years.

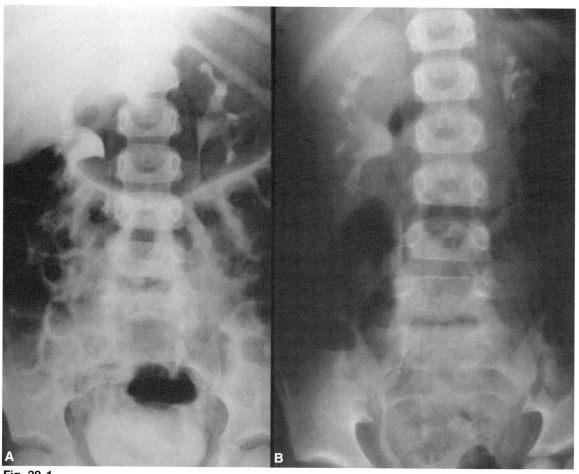

Fig. 30-1

Case 31

A 12-year-old girl has had frontal headaches for 2 weeks. Today, headache is accompanied by fever.

Pregnancy of mother was normal, birth weight 3.7 kg. She had a systolic murmur at 3 months. Hemoglobin was 89 g/liter at 3 months, 55 at 5 months when she had cough, fever, wheezing, umbilical hernia, and hepatosplenomegaly. Reticulocyte fraction was 208×10^{-3}. Blood smear showed target and sickle cells. Red cells sickled in sodium bisulfide. Hemoglobin electrophoresis showed Hb SS, parents' hemoglobin Hb SA. She had a rash and fever at 9 months. Liver and spleen were not palpable. She walked at 11 months. She had pneumonia at 2, 3, and 4 years. Tracheal aspirate grew *Klebsiella aerogenes*, *Neisseria catarrhalis*, and staphylococcus at 4 years. She had fever, abdominal pain, headache, limb pain, and jaundice five times at 9 years. She was enuretic. Liver was tender, its edge 3 cm below costal margin. Left forearm was swollen and tender for 1½ weeks during the fifth episode.

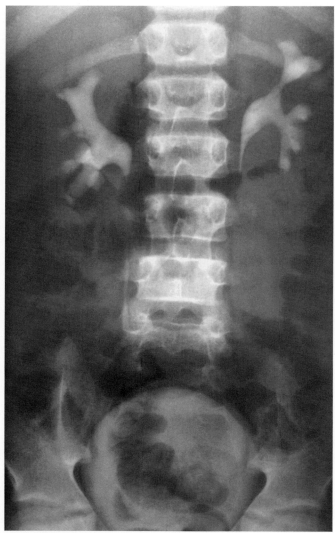

Fig. 31-1

Urine specific gravities were between 1.003 and 1.010, pH between 5.5 and 8. Urine was sterile. Gallbladder, which contained nonopaque stones, was removed.

Temperature at 12 years is 38.4°C, heart rate 110, respiratory rate 24, blood pressure 112/40 mm Hg, weight 33 kg, and height 144 cm. She has yellow sclerae; small, tender anterior cervical nodes; systolic murmur; and abdominal scar. Liver is not palpable in one examination, its edge is 4 cm below costal margin 4 days later. Spleen edge is 2 cm below costal margin in one examination, only tip palpable in another examination 3 days later. The rest of the physical findings are normal.

Hematocrit is 0.18. Hemoglobin is 67 g/liter. Red blood cell count is 2.2×10^{12}/liter. MCV is 84 fl. MCH is 31 pg. MCHC is 370 g/liter. Reticulocyte fraction is 110×10^{-3}. White cell count is 14.7×10^{9}/liter with 0.41 polymorphonuclear cells, 0.18 bands, 0.26 lymphocytes, 0.11 monocytes, and 0.04 eosinophils. Blood smear shows sickle cells. Urine specific gravity is 1.004, pH 5.5. Urine has occasional epithelial cells/HPF, occasional red cells/HPF, 1–2 white cells/HPF, and 70,000 colonies *Escherichia coli*/ml. Serum sodium is 132 mmol/liter, potassium 4.8, chloride 98, and urea nitrogen 3.0. Total bilirubin is 74 µmol/liter, direct bilirubin 2. Throat culture grows normal flora. Cultures of blood and CSF are sterile. Bone marrow is hypercellular with increase in erythrocyte series, especially normoblasts. Sinusoidal red cells are sickled.

Excretory urogram at 12 years (Figure 31-1) shows blunt calyces and contrast medium collected in papilla of lowest pyramid of right kidney. Roentgenogram of skull at 2 years shows thickening of frontal diploë. At 4 years, heart is large and shadows of water density are in lungs. At 9 years, nonopaque stones are in gallbladder in oral cholecystogram.

Diagnosis: Sickle cell anemia with pneumonia at 4 years; cholelithiasis at 9 years; isosthenuria and renal papillary necrosis at 12 years.

Case 32

A 3-year-old boy has painful, bloody bowel movements. He began to grimace, cry, and double up before bowel movements 3 days ago. Stools were loose and frequent. They were streaked with blood 2 days ago and became grossly bloody 1 day ago. He has slept a lot the last 3 days. His mother vomited and had abdominal pain 3 days ago. The family drinks well water.

He had tonsillectomy, adenoidectomy, and placement of tubes in ears 3 months ago.

Temperature is 38.3°C, heart rate 137, respiratory rate 28, blood pressure 128/88 mm Hg, and weight 12 kg. He is pale. Skin turgor is poor. Lips are dry. Mucus and blood clots are at anus. The rest of the physical findings are normal.

Two days ago, hematocrit was 0.41. White cell count was 14.9 × 10⁹/liter with 0.80 polymorphonuclear cells, 0.06 bands, 0.11 lymphocytes, and 0.03 monocytes. Platelet count was 207 × 10⁹/liter. Today, hematocrit is 0.33. White cell count is 24.7 × 10⁹/liter with 0.09 polymorphonuclear cells, 0.39 bands, 0.35 lymphocytes, 0.11 monocytes, 0.04 atypical lymphocytes, and 0.02 metamyelocytes. Platelet count is 36 × 10⁹/liter. Schistocytes are in blood smear. Urine is bloody with specific gravity 1.015, pH 5.5, 3 g/liter protein, 15–20 white cells/HPF, 3–5 hyaline casts/LPF, and 20–30 granular casts/LPF. PT is 13.9 seconds, activated PTT 36.1. Serum sodium is 127 mmol/liter, potassium 4.3, chloride 96, and urea nitrogen 23.6. Creatinine is 140 μmol/liter.

Figure 32-1 shows narrow sigmoid and lower descending colon, and thumbprints in transverse and ascending colon.

Diagnosis: Hemolytic-uremic syndrome.

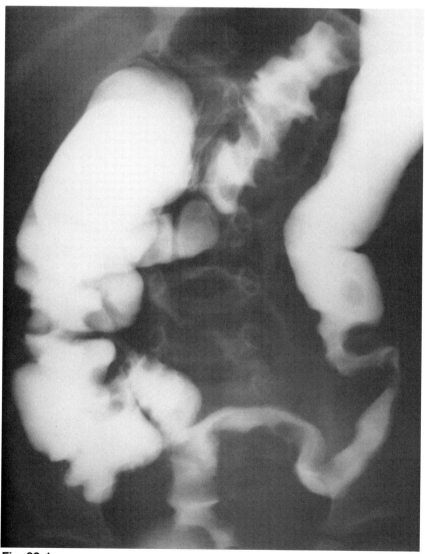

Fig. 32-1

Case 33

A newborn boy, born prematurely after spontaneous onset of labor and delivered by cesarean section for breech presentation, begins to grunt and breathe hard at 30 minutes.

A peripheral infarct is in placenta. Birth weight is 1.12 kg, Apgar score 8/10 at 1 and 5 minutes, heart rate 150, and respiratory rate 50. Auricles are soft. Liver edge is 1 cm below costal margin. The rest of the physical findings are normal.

Hematocrit is 0.45. White cell count is 21.0×10^9/liter with 0.73 polymorphonuclear cells, 0.07 bands, 0.10 lymphocytes, 0.08 monocytes, 0.01 eosinophils, and 0.01 metamyelocytes. Platelet count is 88×10^9/liter. Serum calcium is 2.47 mmol/liter. At 20 minutes, umbilical arterial blood pH while he breathes room air is 7.21. P_{CO_2} is 65 mm Hg, P_{O_2} 53.

At 1 hour, he is intubated and put on respirator. Umbilical arterial catheter is removed because left leg is pale. At 7 days, respiratory rate is 60, systolic blood pressure 60 mm Hg. Physical findings are normal. At 9 days, stools are guaiac positive. At 12 days, he is pale. Systolic blood pressure is 85 mm Hg. A mass is in left flank. Hematocrit is 0.32. White cell count is 24.3×10^9/liter with 0.71 polymorphonuclear cells, 0.01 bands, 0.08 lymphocytes, 0.18 monocytes, and 0.02 eosinophils. Platelet estimate is low. Smear shows few schistocytes and many burr cells. Urine has occasional squamous and nonsquamous epithelial cells/HPF, 0–2 white cells/HPF, and >100 red cells/HPF. Serum sodium is 139 mmol/liter,

potassium 6.0, chloride 104, carbon dioxide 19, urea nitrogen 4.6, calcium 2.54, phosphorus 2.32, cholesterol 3.57, and glucose 4.7. Creatinine is 110 μmol/liter, uric acid 210, total bilirubin 10, and direct bilirubin 3. Total protein is 56 g/liter, albumin 35. Alkaline phosphatase is 350 U/liter, LDH 1,152, and SGOT 88. Capillary blood pH is 7.37 while he breathes room air. P_{CO_2} is 38 mm Hg, P_{O_2} 36. He has three spells of apnea and bradycardia late in the day at 12 days, many at 13 days. Mass is larger. Isotope scan shows no excretion by left kidney.

At 14 days, aortogram through left umbilical artery shows corkscrew pattern of poor perfusion in liver, diminished right nephrogram, and absent left nephrogram with retention of contrast medium in left renal arteries during venous phase.

Mass is gone at 23 days. Abdomen is distended at 2 months. Weight is 2.3 kg, systolic blood pressure 78–88 mm Hg.

At 2 months, stringy shadows of water density are in lungs, excess liquid is in gut, and a strip of calcium density is in upper left quadrant of abdomen at about level of T12 (Figure 33-1).

He is alert, smiling, and tracking objects at 6 months. Weight is 6.3 kg, length 63 cm, and head circumference 41 cm. Physical findings are normal.

Diagnosis: Thrombosis, left renal vein.

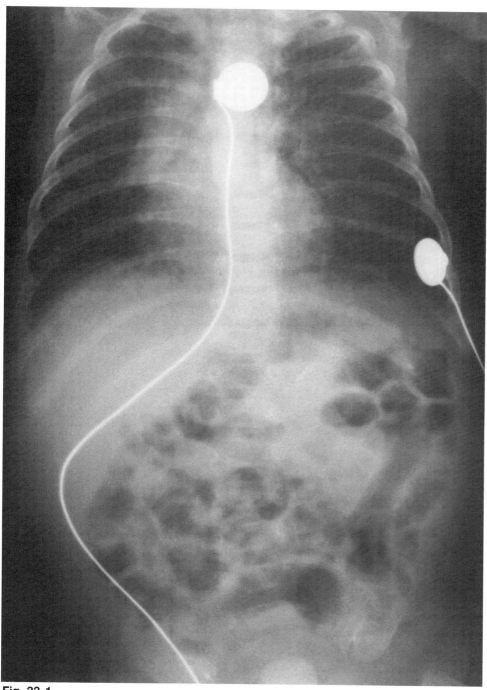

Fig. 33-1

Case 34

An 8-week-old girl has a mass in right side of abdomen, found during examination for stuffy nose.

Weight is 4.9 kg, length 51 cm, head circumference 39 cm, temperature 36.6°C, heart rate 140, respiratory rate 56, and systolic blood pressure 80 mm Hg. The rest of the physical findings are normal.

Hematocrit is 0.32. White cell count is 11.6×10^9/liter. Platelet count is 436×10^9/liter. Serum sodium is 138 mmol/liter, potassium 6.6, and chloride 103.

Ultrasound examination in Figure 34-1 shows mass in hilum of right kidney and dilated calyces. Findings are similar in excretory urogram.

At right nephrectomy, a firm white mass ($5.8 \times 4.5 \times 4.3$ cm) with thin transparent membrane is in central and lower part of light gray–purple kidney. Microscopic examination shows (1) packed fibromyomatous cells with large vesiculated nuclei, clumped chromatin, and little foamy eosinophilic cytoplasm; (2) as many as 5 mitoses/HPF; (3) dysplastic tubules, some with smooth muscle around them; (4) cysts, some with red blood cells in them; (5) focal hemorrhage; and (6) normal kidney.

Diagnosis: Mesoblastic nephroma.

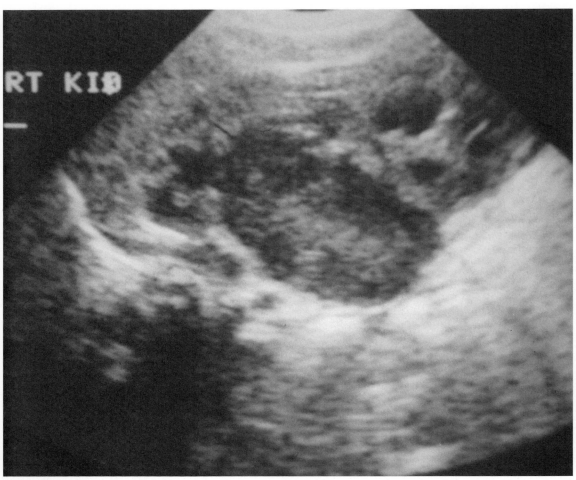

Fig. 34-1

Case 35

A 9-month-old boy has a large abdomen. It was firm 1 month ago, enlarged 2 weeks ago.

Pregnancy was normal, birth weight 4.3 kg.

Parents, two brothers, and one sister are well. A paternal great-aunt died at 6 years with a large abdomen. Three maternal great-aunts had cancer.

Temperature is 36.8°C, heart rate 148, respiratory rate 30–40, blood pressure 126/81 mm Hg, and weight 11 kg. A mass is in left flank, a mass or large liver in right flank. The rest of the physical findings are normal.

Hematocrit is 0.37. White cell count is 9.0×10^9/liter with 0.09 polymorphonuclear cells, 0.84 lymphocytes, and 0.07 monocytes. Platelet count is 391×10^9/liter. Urine specific gravity is 1.005, pH 6. Urine has 1–5 red cells/HPF. Serum sodium is 141 mmol/liter, potassium 3.9, chloride 105, carbon dioxide 24, urea nitrogen 3.0, calcium 2.45, phosphorus 1.55,

cholesterol 2.35, and glucose 7.4. Creatinine is 40 µmol/liter, uric acid 290, total bilirubin 7, and direct bilirubin 2. Total protein is 52 g/liter, albumin 35. Alkaline phosphatase is 115 U/liter, LDH 251, and SGOT 24. α-Fetoprotein is 10 µg/liter (normal: 0–20).

Figure 35-1 shows large kidneys and a round mass near each hilum.

At operation, a mass is in lower part of each kidney. Focal hemorrhages are in left kidney. Left hilar node and wedge sections from masses and from kidneys are removed.

A pink-purple capsule is over beige or white fishlike flesh. Microscopic examination shows (1) Wilms' tumor and nephroblastomatosis in masses, (2) nephroblastomatosis in kidneys, and (3) lymphoid hyperplasia in lymph node.

Diagnosis: Nephroblastomatosis and Wilms' tumor.

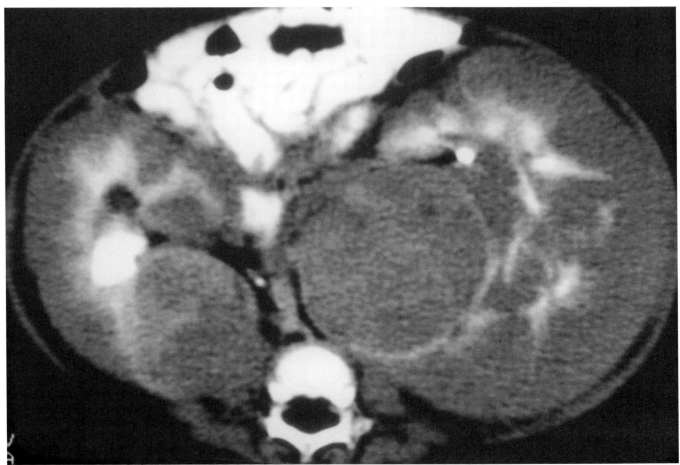

Fig. 35-1

Case 36

A 4½-year-old girl has abdominal pain.

Pain in left upper quadrant began suddenly yesterday, followed by vomiting. Pain is worse today, especially in a bumpy car ride. She walks bent over. She has vomited four times today.

Temperature is 38.7°C, heart rate 144, respiratory rate 36, blood pressure 150/100 mm Hg, weight 20 kg, and height 112 cm. Left upper quadrant is guarded, full, and tender with diminished bowel sounds. The rest of the physical findings are normal.

Three days after pain begins, hematocrit is 0.32. White cell count is 24.0 × 10⁹/liter with 0.89 polymorphonuclear cells, 0.03 lymphocytes, and 0.08 monocytes. Platelet count is 304 × 10⁹/liter. Urine specific gravity is 1.025, pH 6. Urine has 2+ ketones, 1.00 g/liter protein, 1+ bacteria, 2+ amorphous sediment, 20–30 white cells/HPF, and 75–100 red cells/HPF. Five days after pain begins, serum sodium is 137 mmol/liter, potassium 3.7, chloride 103, carbon dioxide 22, urea nitrogen 4.5, calcium 2.35, phosphorus 1.26, cholesterol 4.29, and glucose 3.7. Creatinine is 50 μmol/liter, uric acid 220, total bilirubin 32, and direct bilirubin 5. Total protein is 64 g/liter,

albumin 39. Alkaline phosphatase is 188 U/liter, LDH 844, and SGOT 22.

Ultrasound examination shows a mass in left renal fossa. CT scan after IV injection of contrast medium shows left perirenal mass confined by renal fascia (Figure 36-1). Density of mass is the same in CT scan without IV contrast medium.

At operation, blood is around left kidney, yellow tumor in kidney. Tumor (3.3-cm diameter) extends from hilum to within 0.2 cm of lateral cortex.

Microscopic examination shows sheets and cords of neoplastic blastemic cells mixed with stromal and epithelial neoplastic cells. The blastemic cells are packed oval cells that have little cytoplasm and large hyperchromatic oval to polygonal nuclei. Epithelial cells form tubules with lumens. Stroma has dense oval to spindle fibroblasts with large hyperchromatic nuclei. Mitoses are many.

She is well at 13 years. Weight is 48 kg, height 166 cm.

Diagnosis: Wilms' tumor.

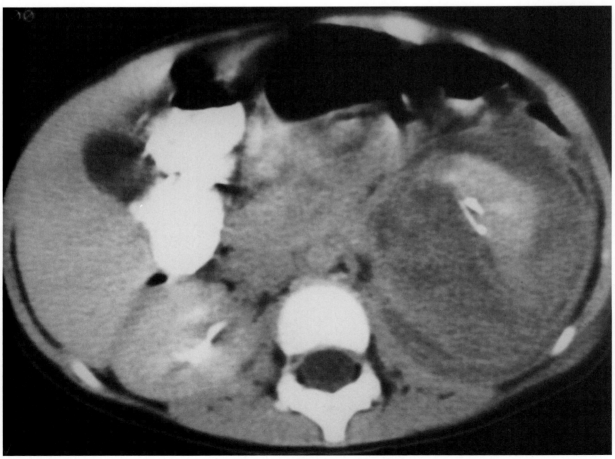

Fig. 36-1

Case 37

A 3-year-old boy says, "My body hurts." He complained 2 weeks ago and put his hand on right side of abdomen. He felt warm 1–2 days later. Weight has decreased from 16.3 to 12.3 kg in 2 weeks. He "just lies around." He drinks a lot of apple juice. Two days ago, abdominal pain was worse, he could not sleep, and temperature was 39.4°C.

Parents are well. Maternal grandmother and maternal great-aunt have diabetes mellitus. Two great-grandparents had tuberculosis.

Temperature is 37.1°C, heart rate 140, respiratory rate 30, blood pressure 120/86 mm Hg, and height 92 cm. He is thin, pale, and lethargic. A loud systolic heart murmur is at left sternal border. A smooth, firm mass extends approximately 12 cm below right costal margin. The rest of the physical findings are normal.

Hematocrit is 0.32. White cell count is 23.9×10^9/liter with 0.52 polymorphonuclear cells, 0.01 bands, 0.31 lymphocytes, 0.15 monocytes, and 0.01 basophils. Platelet count is 665×10^9/liter. Urine specific gravity is 1.015, pH 6. Urine has trace protein. Serum sodium is 136 mmol/liter, potassium 4.6, chloride 100, carbon dioxide not determined, urea nitrogen 2.7, cholesterol 2.43, triglycerides 0.95, calcium 2.17, phosphorus 1.13, and glucose 5.4. Creatinine is 40 µmol/liter, uric acid 290, total bilirubin 10, and direct bilirubin 3. Total protein is 54 g/liter, albumin 32. Alkaline phosphatase is 130 U/liter, LDH 657, SGOT 121, and GGT 36.

Echocardiogram shows dilated hepatic veins and a mass in right atrium that goes through tricuspid valve.

Selective renal arteriogram shows tumor in right kidney, in streaks of tumor vessels along right side of spine (Figure 37-1), and in left kidney, in addition to contrast medium in cortices and distorted calyces and pelves of both kidneys.

At operation, a mass (4 × 4 cm) is removed from right atrium. The mass obstructs tricuspid valve and extends into inferior vena cava. Liver is congested. Right kidney, large right hilar lymph nodes, and caval mass are removed. Left kidney is biopsied.

Capsule of right kidney is intact. Nodules of white tumor are visible through capsule. Microscopic examination of kidneys shows (1) aggregates of small uniform cells with little cytoplasm, (2) scattered tubular structures, and (3) loose stroma. Similar nests of cells and scattered tubules are in caval tumor.

Diagnosis: Bilateral Wilms' tumor, tumor in right renal vein, inferior vena cava, and right atrium.

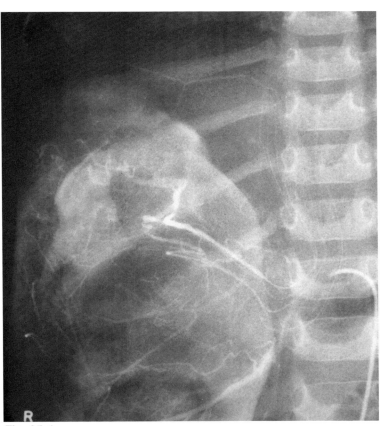

Fig. 37-1

Case 38

An 8-year-old girl with a lump on right shoulder screams in pain. She was found to have a kidney tumor at laminectomy for new paraplegia 3 years ago.

Roentgenogram 3 years ago (Figure 38-1), minutes after L4 laminectomy and IV injection of contrast medium with girl 20 degrees upright, shows (1) intraspinal block at L3–L4 in myelogram performed earlier, (2) collapse of body of L4, (3) contrast medium in normal pelvis and calyces of left kidney and in widely separated calyces of right kidney, and (4) crescents of calcium density that are also in plain roentgenogram before laminectomy just above and in line of top of right ilium.

Laminectomy, excision of extradural tumor, and right nephrectomy were performed and chemotherapy and radiation therapy begun.

Tumor that appeared in lung 14 months after operation was resected. She had pain in right leg 2 years after operation and a lytic lesion in right femur that was biopsied and treated with irradiation and additional chemotherapy. She used crutches at 7½ years because of pain in right thigh until treatment with local irradiation, after which she was able to "skip down the hall." A lump appeared on right shoulder 3 weeks ago.

Temperature at 8 years is 40.1°C, heart rate 144, respiratory rate 28, blood pressure 108/50 mm Hg, weight 15.6 kg, and height 110 cm. Hair is thick except for bald spots on back of head. Optic fundi and lips are pale. Scars are on chest, abdomen, lower back, and inner right knee. S_3 is intermittent. The rest of the physical findings are normal.

Hematocrit is 0.11. White cell count is 1.0×10^9/liter with 0.36 polymorphonuclear cells, 0.52 bands, and 0.12 monocytes. Platelet count is 22×10^9/liter. Serum sodium is 137 mmol/liter, potassium 4.0, chloride 104, carbon dioxide 24, urea nitrogen 8.6, calcium 2.57, phosphorus 1.03, cholesterol 3.47, and glucose 7.5. Creatinine is not determined. Uric acid is 420 µmol/liter, total bilirubin 14, and direct bilirubin 3. Total protein is 74 g/liter, albumin 37. Alkaline phosphatase is 87 U/liter, LDH 195, and SGOT 9.

She dies 2 days later. Necropsy shows tumor in skull, thoracic right paraspinal soft tissues, right iliac fossa, humeri, femurs, body of T10, left lung, and liver. Microscopic examination shows (1) necrotic tumor cells in lung; (2) pale cells with little eosinophilic cytoplasm and pale, oval to spindle nuclei in liver; (3) bizarre mitoses; (4) similar but more spindle cells in tumor of right shoulder; (5) ulcers in esophagus; and (6) lymphocyte depletion and no follicles in lymph node.

Diagnosis: Clear cell sarcoma of kidney (bone metastasizing renal tumor of childhood).

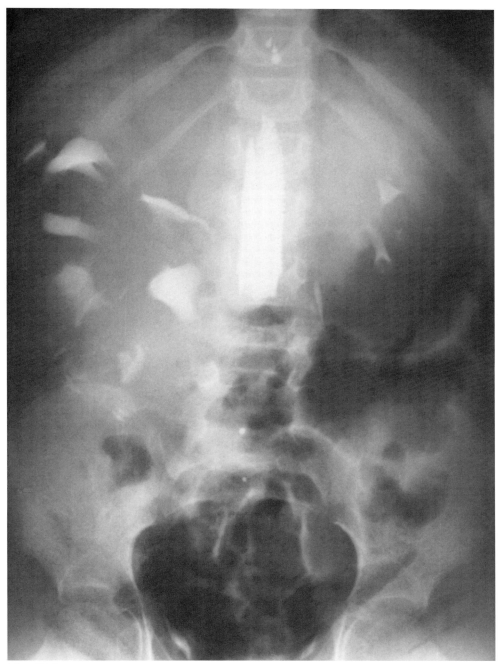

Fig. 38-1

Case 39

A 2-year-old boy, who comes in for routine examination, has a mass in left side of abdomen. Physical findings in abdomen were normal when he was examined for rash 6 weeks ago.

Birth weight was 4 kg. He has had some colds. He had roseola at 1 year.

Parents and brother (6 weeks old) are well. Father's right arm and right foot are larger than left. A paternal aunt has hypoglobulinemia. Members of father's family are hypertensive. A maternal aunt died with lymphatic cancer.

Weight is 14 kg, height 89 cm, temperature 36.7°C, heart rate 140, respiratory rate 25, and blood pressure 90/60 mm Hg. A firm, rough mass is in left side of abdomen. The rest of the physical findings are normal.

Hematocrit is 0.38. White cell count is 10.9×10^9/liter with 0.53 polymorphonuclear cells, 0.15 bands, 0.29 lymphocytes, 0.02 monocytes, and 0.01 basophils. Platelet count is 332×10^9/liter. Urine specific gravity is 1.050, pH 5. Urine has many uric acid crystals. Serum sodium is 138 mmol/liter, potassium 4.0, chloride 103, carbon dioxide 15, urea nitrogen 5.4, calcium 2.79, phosphorus 1.29, cholesterol 4.24, and glucose 11.7. Creatinine is 70 μmol/liter, uric acid 350, total bilirubin 7, and direct bilirubin 2. Total protein is 68 g/liter, albumin 48. Alkaline phosphatase is 185 U/liter, LDH 495, and SGOT 39.

Pelvis of left kidney is dilated, distorted, and displaced upward in excretory urogram (Figure 39-1).

At operation, a pale-gray to blue-gray mass (10-cm diameter) is in left kidney. Microscopic examination of tumor shows (1) islands of small, round deeply basophilic cells with large round nuclei; (2) irregular tubules in some islands; and (3) less cellular eosinophilic bands.

The boy has abnormal crossbite and jaw asymmetry at 4 years. Panoramic roentgenogram of mouth shows that lower left first molar is larger than right.

Diagnosis: Nephroblastoma (Wilms' tumor) in boy whose father has hemihypertrophy.

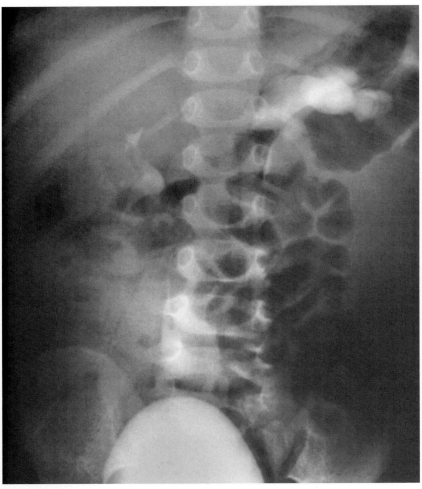

Fig. 39-1

Case 40

A 2½-year-old girl has been wakeful at night for several weeks, screams frequently, and does not urinate as often as she used to.

Mother, a dental x-ray technician, performed 50 examinations per day during middle trimester and had cough and rash at about the twentieth week. Birth weight was 2.4 kg, Apgar score 9/10 at 1 and 5 minutes. Weight was 5.3 kg at 7 months. Head was small, occiput flat, anterior fontanel larger on left than right, right auricle larger than left. Eyes were deep and small and had epicanthi, only a thin stub of iris, hypoplastic maculae, and hypoplastic, doubly margined discs. She squinted and moved her head until she could locate objects. Nose was small, bridge flat, tip turned up. Anus was slightly forward. The rest of the physical findings were normal. Short arm of one chromosome 11 was missing. She has had ear infections. She stands with help. She bites fingers and bangs head on floor.

Mother (28 years old), father (29 years old), brother (10 years old), and sister (6 months old) are well. Parents' chromosomes are normal.

Temperature at 2½ years is 37.9°C, heart rate 120, respiratory rate 28, blood pressure 98/60 mm Hg, weight 9.8 kg, height 78 cm, and head circumference 43 cm. A firm mass (6 × 5 cm) is in right side of abdomen.

Hematocrit is 0.41. White cell count is 11.8×10^9/liter with 0.83 polymorphonuclear cells, 0.04 bands, 0.03 lymphocytes, and 0.10 monocytes. Platelet estimate is normal. Urine specific gravity is 1.012, pH 7. Urine has 1+ ketones, few squamous epithelial cells/HPF, and rare nonsquamous epithelial cells/HPF. Serum sodium is 141 mmol/liter, potassium 4.8, chloride 104, carbon dioxide 24, urea nitrogen 2.1, calcium 2.62, phosphorus 1.55, cholesterol 8.07, and glucose 4.5. Creatinine is 40 μmol/liter, uric acid 360, total bilirubin 12, and direct bilirubin 2. Total protein is 70 g/liter, albumin 44. Alkaline phosphatase is 189 U/liter, LDH 1420, and SGOT 54.

Excretory urogram shows normal findings at 2 years (Figure 40-1A), displacement and distortion of right renal pelvis and displacement of gut at 2½ years (Figure 40-1B).

At operation, right kidney and encapsulated tumor, part of right ureter, and a lymph node are removed. Cecum in right upper quadrant is placed in left lower quadrant, and Ladd's bands are lysed.

Tumor (12.0 × 8.5 × 7.0 cm) is tan to dark blue on outside, tan and solid on inside. Microscopic examination shows Wilms' tumor without spread or lymph node involvement.

She dies with small bowel perforation and peritonitis at 3½ years.

Diagnosis: Aniridia, malrotation of midgut, chromosome 11p−, Wilms' tumor.

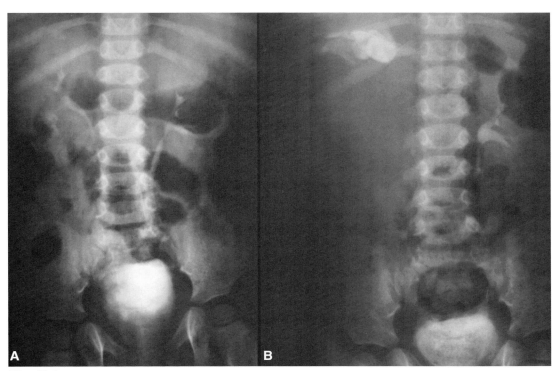

Fig. 40-1

Case 41

A 2-year-old boy has pain when he urinates. He vomited and had a fever 6 days ago and has had dysuria since then. Urine has occasionally been bloody and once had a clot.

Pregnancy was normal. Mother (25 years old) took no medicine during pregnancy. Birth weight was 3.5 kg, length 53 cm, head circumference 35 cm, and Apgar score 9/9 at 1 and 5 minutes. External genitalia were ambiguous with chordee, hypospadias, and impalpable testes.

Weight is 12.5 kg, temperature 37.3°C, heart rate 162, respiratory rate 36, and blood pressure 145/73 mm Hg. He has hypospadias. Testes are not in scrotum. The rest of the physical findings are normal.

Hematocrit is 0.40. White cell count is 16.0×10^9/liter with 0.43 polymorphonuclear cells, 0.45 lymphocytes, 0.01 monocytes, and 0.11 eosinophils. Platelet count is 667×10^9/liter. Urine specific gravity is 1.016, pH 5. Urine has 0.3 g/liter protein and 20–30 white cells/HPF. Serum sodium is 136 mmol/liter, potassium 5.0, chloride 112, carbon dioxide 15, and urea nitrogen 7.0. Creatinine is 50 µmol/liter. Chromosomes are 46,XY.

He passes a brown fibrin clot through urethra 2 days later.

Cystogram at 2 days shows contrast medium in bladder, urethra, and vagina (Figure 41-1). Ultrasound examination at 2 years shows mass in pelvis of right kidney and in right ureter. CT scan at 2 years (Figure 41-2) shows mass in pelvis of right kidney and in right ureter; contrast medium is around mass in right kidney and in normal left pelvis.

At operation, right kidney is purple-gray and firm. Soft hemorrhagic tumor is in right renal parenchyma and pelvis. Blood clot and tumor are in right ureter. Fragments of tumor are in bladder.

Microscopic examination of tumor shows sheets of blastema and aggregates of tubules on background of spindle cells. Tumor is in lymph node. Tumor, blood, and fibrous tissue are in ureter and bladder.

Diagnosis: Wilms' tumor in a boy with abnormal gonadal differentiation (Denys-Drash syndrome).

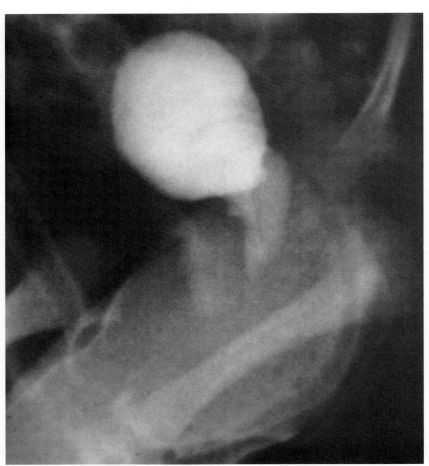

Fig. 41-1

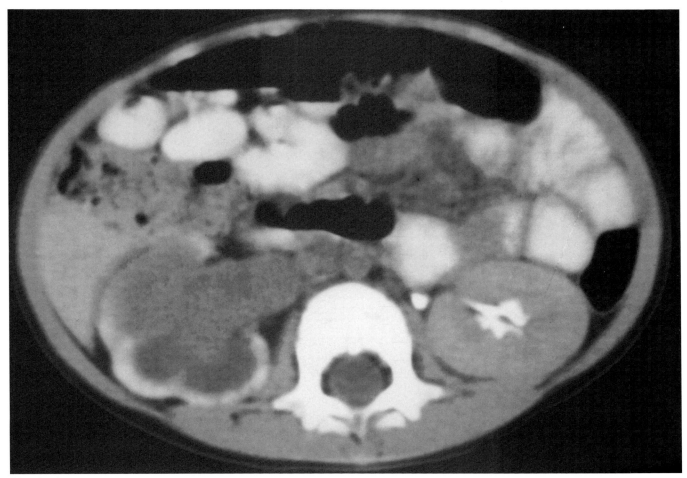

Fig. 41-2

Case 42

A 15-year-old boy has been incontinent of urine for 8 years, worse recently. He drips constantly without urgency. He had bladder infections until 2 years ago.

Birth weight was 3 kg. He had pneumonia two or three times during first year. He began to walk at 13 months. He was slow to speak. Tonsils and adenoids were removed at 11 years. A bladder operation was performed at 13 years. He tires faster than his friends. He drinks about 10 glasses of water a day.

Mother (55 years old) had Hodgkin's disease. Father, three older sisters, and an older brother are well. Maternal aunt has kidney disease. Two grandparents, an aunt, and an uncle have diabetes mellitus.

Temperature is 37°C, heart rate 88, respiratory rate 16, blood pressure 140/80 mm Hg, weight 50 kg, and height 161 cm. He is frail and immature. Fundus of bladder is 7 cm above symphysis pubis. Right testicle is not palpable. The rest of the physical findings are normal.

At cystoscopy, bladder is trabeculated, verumontanum prominent, and prostatic urethra short.

Self-catheterization ameliorates incontinence.

Excretory urogram 8 months later shows bilateral ureteropyelocaliectasis and suggests a mass in lower part of right kidney. Ultrasound examination shows an echogenic mass in right kidney. Skeletal examination shows Schmorl-Scheuermann herniation of disc into several thoracic vertebral bodies (Figure 42-1) and focal cortical thickening along lateral aspect of right humerus and medial aspect of left ulna. Renal angiogram in Figure 42-2 shows a vascular tumor in lower part of right kidney; tumor is supplied by a peripheral artery and contains a network of uniform vessels.

Blood pressure at 16 years is 130/70 mm Hg, weight 55 kg. A systolic murmur is present.

Hematocrit is 0.40. White cell count is 8.1×10^9/liter with 0.51 polymorphonuclear cells, 0.12 bands, 0.29 lymphocytes, and 0.08 monocytes. Platelet estimate is adequate. Urine specific gravity is 1.017, pH 6. Urine contains few squamous and nonsquamous epithelial cells/HPF, 15–20 white cells/HPF, mucus, and >10^5 colonies *Escherichia coli*/ml. Serum sodium is 145 mmol/liter, potassium 4.2, chloride 105, carbon dioxide 29, urea nitrogen 6.4, calcium 2.72, phosphorus 1.32, cholesterol 4.68, and glucose 5.8. Creatinine is 90 μmol/liter, uric acid 410, total bilirubin 19, and direct bilirubin 0. Total protein is 84 g/liter, albumin 52. Alkaline phosphatase is 229 U/liter, LDH 225, SGOT 26, and CK 169. Chromosomes are 46,XY.

At operation, a smooth, round tumor is removed. Upper part of right kidney (not removed) has thin, soft cortex and dilated pelvis. Tumor ($7 \times 6 \times 5$ cm, 145 g) is covered by clear glistening capsule except for a bit of kidney at the upper margin.

Cut section shows brown to gray vascular tissue with small hemorrhages. Microscopic examination shows (1) tightly arranged tubules, most of them like normal proximal tubules; (2) scattered isolated tubules like distal convoluted tubules and cortical collecting tubules; (3) many tubules dilated, some with blood, some separated by edema; (4) bland cells with focal moderate pleomorphism; (5) little hyaline stroma; and (6) no mitoses. Capsule is intact. Attached kidney shows patchy tubular interstitial fibrosis and inflammation.

Right inguinal herniorrhaphy and orchiectomy are performed at 22 years. An atrophic testicle is at internal inguinal ring in hernia sac. Seminiferous tubules have thick basement membrane, Sertoli's cells, and no germ cells.

Diagnosis: Renal oncocytoma, Scheuermann's thoracic kyphosis.

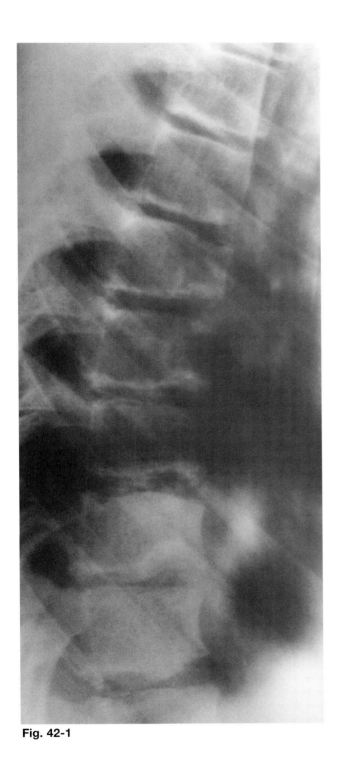

Fig. 42-1

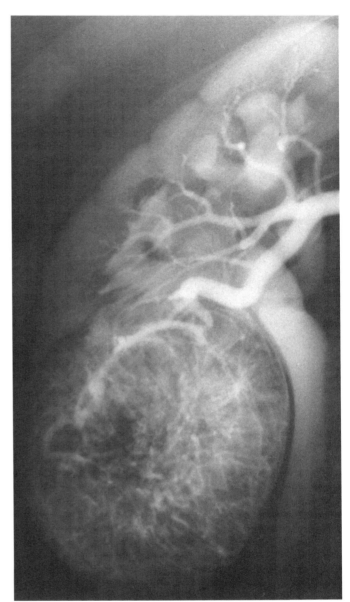

Fig. 42-2

Case 43

A 19-year-old man has urinated more easily sitting than standing for 1 year and has had vague discomfort in left lower quadrant of abdomen during meals. Appendix was removed 1 year ago. Urination burned 1 month ago.

Parents and two sisters are well.

Weight is 100 kg, temperature 36.7°C, heart rate 76, respiratory rate 24, and blood pressure 130/78 mm Hg. Liver edge is 4 cm below costal margin. Right kidney is palpable. A fixed, nontender mass (6 × 5 cm) in region of prostate is palpable through rectum. The rest of the physical findings are normal.

Hematocrit is 0.45. White cell count is 4.8×10^9/liter with 0.49 polymorphonuclear cells, 0.33 lymphocytes, 0.14 monocytes, and 0.04 eosinophils. Urine specific gravity is 1.021, pH 6. Urine has occasional squamous epithelial cells/HPF. Serum sodium is 139 mmol/liter, potassium 4.0, chloride 103, carbon dioxide 26, urea nitrogen 4.6, calcium 2.30, phosphorus 1.25, cholesterol 3.70, and glucose 4.6. Creatinine is 100 µmol/liter, uric acid 430, total bilirubin 18, and direct bilirubin 2. Total protein is 66 g/liter, albumin 42. Alkaline phosphatase is 59 U/liter, LDH 164, and SGOT 21.

Ultrasound examination in longitudinal plane shows compressed bladder above and in front, cyst behind (Figure 43-1). Excretory urogram in Figure 43-2 shows pelvis of right kidney, right ureter, and bladder, where most of contrast medium is squeezed into fundus. Metal clips are from appendectomy.

At cystoscopy, right ureteral orifice is normal, left not seen.

At operation, a retroperitoneal cyst that contains 350 ml of cloudy, whitish liquid extends from left pelvic wall across midline behind bladder, elevates trigone, and stretches prostatic urethra. A tube that looks like a ureter at upper left aspect of cyst has focal narrowing and dilation and seems to end blindly several centimeters higher up.

Cyst wall is rubbery; 0.5–1.2 cm thick; white, tan, and dark brown in places; slightly wrinkled and focally edematous on outside; and tan, brown, gray-purple, and ragged on inside.

Diagnosis: Seminal vesicle cyst, absence of left kidney.

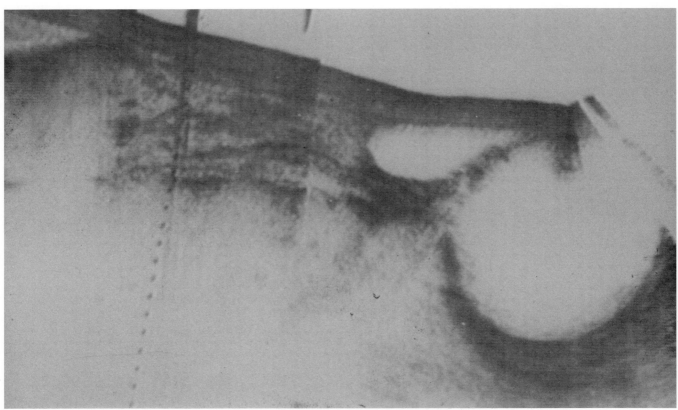

Fig. 43-1

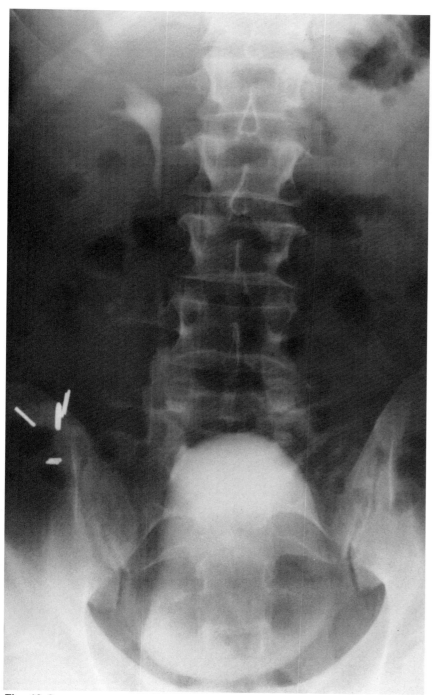

Fig. 43-2

Case 44

A newborn boy has only a dimple where anus should be.

Pregnancy of mother (21 years old) was normal. Birth weight is 3.3 kg, length 50 cm, head circumference 35 cm, Apgar score 9/9 at 1 and 5 minutes, temperature 36.4°C, heart rate 164, respiratory rate 60, and systolic blood pressure 56 mm Hg. Head is molded. Right testis is not in scrotum. Testis and hydrocele are in left side of scrotum. The rest of the physical findings are normal.

Hematocrit is 0.60. White cell count is 27.1×10^9/liter, and blood glucose 5.0 mmol/liter. Serum sodium is 147 mmol/liter at 3 days, potassium 4.8, chloride 105, carbon dioxide 25, urea nitrogen 5.0, calcium 2.52, phosphorus 2.26, cholesterol 4.22, and glucose 4.8. Creatinine is 80 µmol/liter, uric acid 170, total bilirubin 200, and direct bilirubin 14. Total protein is 59 g/liter, albumin 35. Alkaline phosphatase is 104 U/liter, LDH 597, and SGOT 36. Urine specific gravity is 1.003 at 3 days, pH 5. Urine is clear and has rare squamous epithelial cells/HPF. Urine has 3×10^4 colonies *Escherichia coli*/ml at 11 days.

Right transverse colostomy is performed at 1 day.

Roentgenogram at 2 days (Figure 44-1A) shows (1) a gas-dilated viscus in pelvis and lower abdomen, (2) dysplastic sacrum, and (3) butterfly T8. Faint shadows of calcified meconium are in right side of abdomen at 2 days (left side at 3 days). Excretory urogram at 7 days (Figure 44-1B) shows contrast medium in left renal calyces and pelvis, left ureter, bladder, and not in right kidney or right ureter. Colostomy bag is on right side.

At sacroabdominal pull-through operation at 13 months, rectum ends at level of iliococcygeus muscle. A fistula between rectum and lower back part of bladder is excised and closed. Right testis is in abdomen, right inguinal canal absent.

Microscopic findings in resected right testis are normal.

Diagnosis: Imperforate anus, fistula between rectum and bladder, nonvisualization of right kidney.

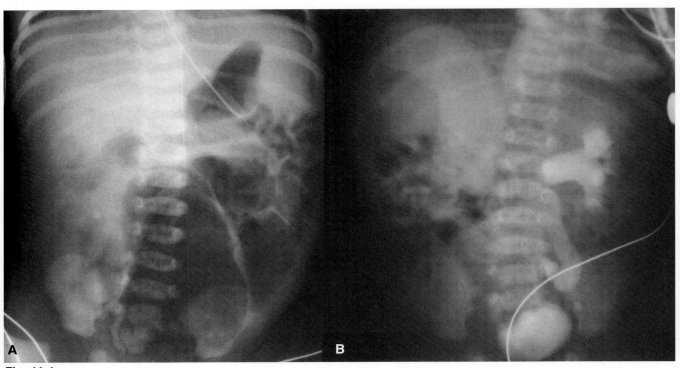

A   B

Fig. 44-1

Case 45

A newborn boy has a large, lax abdomen.

Pregnancy of mother (19 years old) was normal. The boy is her first child. A son born 2 years later also has a large, lax abdomen.

Birth weight is 4.1 kg, length 53 cm, head circumference 36 cm, temperature 36.2°C, heart rate 130, and respiratory rate 60. Abdominal skin is loose and dry. Flanks bulge. Kidneys are easily felt. Penis is small. Testes are not in scrotum. Feet are edematous, clubbed, and mobile. The rest of the physical findings are normal.

He urinates 150 ml soon after birth. Hematocrit is 0.67. Serum urea nitrogen is 7.1 mmol/liter. Urine specific gravity is 1.003 at 2 days, pH 6. Urine has trace albumin, bacteria, 2–3 white cells/HPF, 4–5 red cells/HPF, and 1–2 epithelial cells/HPF. Urine stream, seen twice at 4 days, is strong. Chromosomes are 46,XY.

Cystogram at 12 days shows irregular bladder (Figure 45-1A) with urachal extension; dilated, redundant ureters; and dilated prostatic urethra in lateral view (Figure 45-1B).

Loop ureterostomies are performed at 17 days. Feet are normal at 2 months. At cystoscopy at 5½ years, urethra is normal, left ureteral opening at trigone large, and right ureteral opening not seen. Urine specific gravity is 1.002, pH 6. Urine has rare white cells/HPF. Serum sodium is 135 mmol/liter, potassium 4.9, chloride 97, and urea nitrogen 8.6. Creatinine is 90 μmol/liter. Ureters are reimplanted, ureterostomies closed. Serum urea nitrogen is 8.9 mmol/liter at 9 years, creatinine 110 μmol/liter. Testes are found in abdomen at operation at 11 years. Microscopic examination of right testis, which is resected with ductus deferens and epididymis, and biopsy of left testis, which is placed in scrotum, shows atrophy and no germ cells in testes. Epididymis and ductus deferens are normal. At 13 years, weight is 46 kg, height 152 cm, and blood pressure 112/68 mm Hg. He has axillary and pubic hair. Volume of left testis is 6 ml.

Diagnosis: Prune-belly syndrome in two brothers.

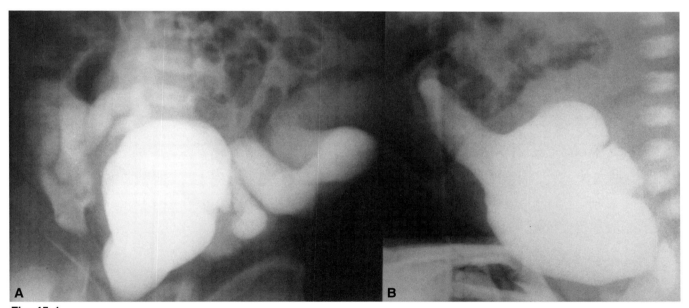

Fig. 45-1

Case 46

A 16-year-old boy wets bed and sometimes pants.

Birth weight was 3.4 kg. He was given oxygen for the first 2 days. Herniorrhaphy was performed at 1 year. He fractured a clavicle at 7 years, left femur at 9 years. Intelligence is low normal.

Parents, brother (19 years old), and sister (15 years old) are well. Grandmother and cousin have diabetes mellitus.

Weight is 58 kg, blood pressure 120/80 mm Hg. Eyes are wide set. Nasal bridge is flat. The rest of the physical findings are normal.

Cystogram shows bladder diverticula, left vesicoureteral reflux (Figure 46-1), and normal urethra.

Diagnosis: Hutch bladder diverticula.

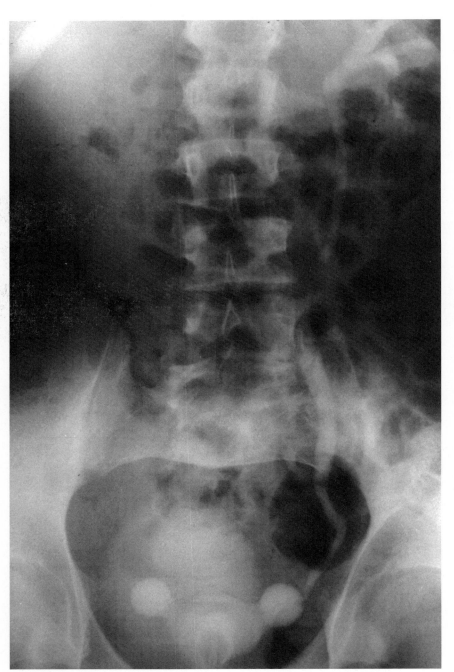

Fig. 46-1

Case 47

A 7-year-old boy, who has had occasional left flank pain for 1 year, has hematuria today.

Birth weight was 1.4 kg, Apgar score 8/8 at 1 and 5 minutes. He had hypospadias, which was repaired at 5 years.

Weight at 7 years is 23 kg, temperature 36.4°C, heart rate 96, respiratory rate 20, and blood pressure 96/62 mm Hg. Left flank is tender. The rest of the physical findings are normal.

Hematocrit is 0.44. White cell count is 10.0×10^9/liter. Platelet count is 305×10^9/liter. Serum sodium is 139 mmol/liter, potassium 4.9, chloride 109, and urea nitrogen 6.4. Creatinine is 60 µmol/liter.

Excretory urogram in Figure 47-1 shows dilated renal pelves and calyces and narrow ureters with filling defects from ureteropelvic junction down.

At operation, soft, glistening, white and tan polyps are removed from both ureters.

Diagnosis: Fibroepithelial polyps.

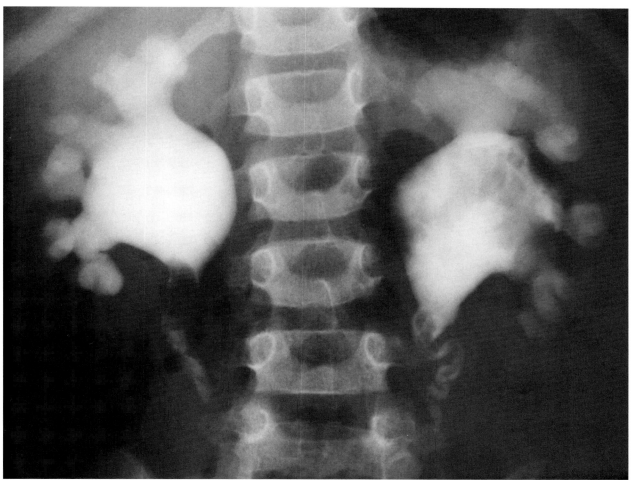

Fig. 47-1

Case 48

An 8-month-old girl has recurrent urinary tract infections with *Escherichia coli*, treated with amoxicillin, which was thought to have caused diarrhea 3 weeks ago. Infections are now suppressed with nightly trimethoprim-sulfamethoxazole.

Pregnancy of mother was normal.

Weight is 8.6 kg, length 71 cm, and head circumference 44 cm. Abdomen, external genitalia, and urethral meatus are normal. Urine, 20 ml, that is microscopically and biochemically normal is obtained through a no. 8 French catheter.

Excretory urogram in Figure 48-1 shows normal urinary tract. Contrast medium is in vagina when she is supine (Figure 48-1A), in bladder a moment later when she is prone (Figure 48-1B).

She returns at 2 years because she has swallowed a penny, at 7 years because she is vomiting. Weight at 7 years is 21.6 kg, height 121 cm. Physical findings are normal.

Diagnosis: Escherichia coliuria.

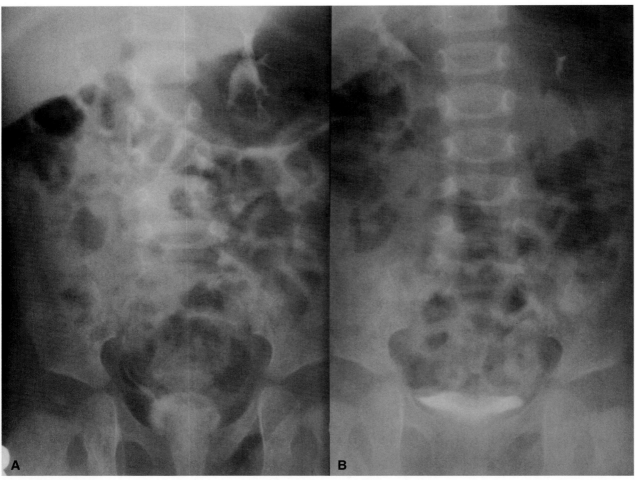

Fig. 48-1

Case 49

A 5-year-old boy cannot urinate.

Pregnancy was normal, birth weight 3.9 kg. He was pale "like a china doll." Hair looked like it would be curly. He was alert and smiling at 5½ months, turning toward noise and following objects with his eyes, but unable to lift his head or grasp objects. He cried "uncontrollably" at 6 months and had jack-knife seizures. He was plump and smiling at 1 year. Hair was coarse, light brown, and almost gone from occiput. He could barely lift his head from prone. He did not kick or lift his legs when supine and barely moved his arms. Deep tendon reflexes were normal. The rest of the physical findings were normal. EEG was normal. Tube feedings were begun when he was hospitalized for dehydration at 1½ years. A leg was broken during diaper change at 3 years. Gastrostomy was placed at 3 years.

He is constipated and cannot urinate on his own at 5 years. He needs regular bladder catheterization and frequent upper airway suctioning.

Parents, sister (7 years old), and brother (2 years old) are well.

Serum copper at 8 months was 5.5 µmol/liter (normal: 11–22), ceruloplasmin 0.8 (normal: 1.8–2.5). Urine copper was 0.5 µmol/day (normal: <0.6). Serum copper at 1 year was 9.1 and 14.3 µmol/liter, ceruloplasmin 0.9, 1.3, and 1.5. Urine copper was 1.1 µmol/day.

Hematocrit at 5 years is 0.31. White cell count is 6.4 × 10⁹/liter. Platelet count is 352 × 10⁹/liter. Serum sodium is 137 mmol/liter, potassium 3.8, chloride 100, carbon dioxide 27, urea nitrogen 5.0, calcium 2.47, phosphorus 1.16, cholesterol 4.34, and glucose 4.2. Creatinine is 40 µmol/liter, uric acid 120, total bilirubin 3, direct bilirubin 0, and ceruloplasmin 2.5. Total protein is 67 g/liter, albumin 41. Alkaline phosphatase is 137 U/liter, LDH 295, and SGOT 73.

Much subcutaneous fat and little muscle are in legs at 1 year; metaphyses are normal (Figure 49-1). Diverticula are in bladder at 5 years (Figure 49-2).

Diagnosis: Menkes' kinky hair syndrome.

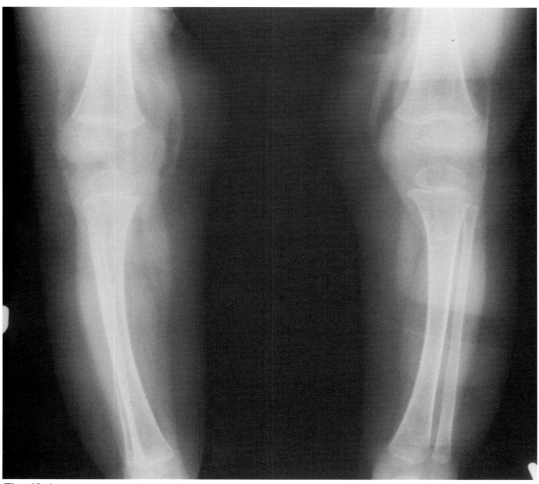

Fig. 49-1

(Continued)

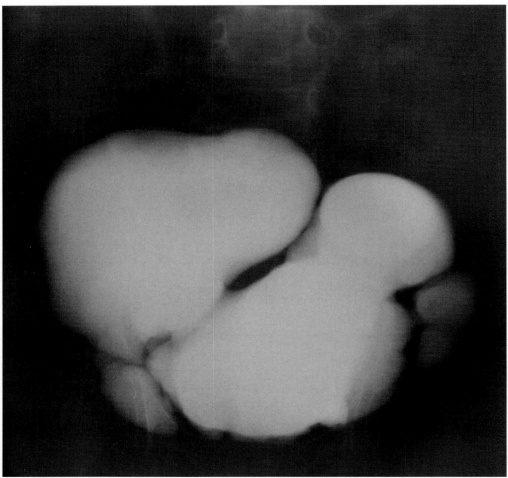

Fig. 49-2

Case 50

A 3⅚-year-old boy has strained to urinate for the past 7 days.

He urinated small amounts every 5–10 minutes 7 days ago; said, "It tickles"; and wet his bed that night. Six days ago, he had a runny nose, had temperature 38.7°C, and could not urinate. He was catheterized the next day. He drank 1,320 ml liquid 3 days ago, urinated 270 ml, and wet his bed that night.

Weight is 19 kg, height 105 cm. Physical findings are normal.

Cystogram in Figure 50-1 shows normal bladder and urethra.

He empties his bladder during cystography. Straining with urination is about the same as before for the next 6 days. He strains and sometimes fails. He has a cough and temperature of 39.4°C 6 days after cystography. Mother says that he is "a lot better" and almost well 22 days after he first began to strain.

Impression: Viral infection, acute neurogenic bladder.

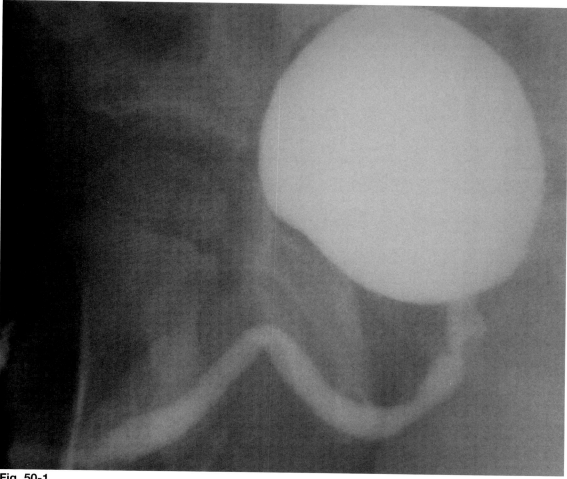

Fig. 50-1

Case 51

A 12-year-old boy has been drinking and urinating a lot by day for several years. Six months ago, he had early morning nausea and vomiting every 2 weeks. Now, he has nausea and vomiting almost daily. He also gets up at night and sometimes wets bed.

Pregnancy was normal, birth weight 3.2 kg.

Mother, who had ectopic ureter to urethra; father; two brothers; and one sister are well. Paternal uncle died at 14 years with kidney disease. Maternal great-grandfather and maternal grandfather had kidney stones.

Temperature is 36.9°C, heart rate 80, respiratory rate 20, blood pressure 115/70 mm Hg, weight 45.4 kg, and height 145 cm. Physical and ophthalmologic findings are normal.

Hematocrit is 0.42. White cell count is 7.1×10^9/liter. Urine specific gravity is 1.002, pH 5. Urine has occasional white cells/HPF. Serum sodium is 146 mmol/liter, potassium 4.4, chloride 109, carbon dioxide 27, urea nitrogen 5.0, calcium 2.42, phosphorus 1.49, and glucose 5.1. Creatinine is 80 μmol/liter, uric acid 400, total bilirubin 5, and direct bilirubin 3. Total protein is 78 g/liter, albumin 48. Alkaline phosphatase is 159 U/liter, LDH 260, SGOT 34, and CK 72. Eight months later, cholesterol is 5.74 mmol/liter, triglycerides 1.83.

Figure 51-1 shows dilated renal pelves and left ureter, and distended bladder.

Results of test with deprivation of water and injection of aqueous pitressin are (1) at start, urine osmolality is 145 mOsm/kg, serum 289, and serum sodium 140 mmol/liter; (2) at 7 hours, urine osmolality is 150 mOsm/kg, serum 301, and serum sodium 152 mmol/liter; and (3) at 11 hours, urine osmolality is 528 mOsm/kg, serum 304, and urine specific gravity 1.014.

Treatment for diabetes insipidus is begun. He is operated on for left slipped capital femoral epiphysis at 14½ years. He is prepubertal at 14¾ years. Treatment for hypothyroidism is begun. Growth hormone is added at 15 years. He fails vision test for driver's license at 16 years and again, with glasses, at 18 years, when he is found to lack medial vision in right eye and central vision in left. At craniotomy, optic nerves and chiasm are large. Tumor bulges toward right internal carotid artery and into sella turcica.

Biopsy shows (1) slightly atypical astrocytes, (2) many perivascular lymphocytes, and (3) scattered histiocytes and plasma cells. He has non–insulin dependent diabetes mellitus at 19 years. Weight at 22 years is 114.6 kg, blood glucose 24.8 mmol/liter. He dies suddenly at 23 years, 10 months. Necropsy shows (1) hypothalamic ganglioglioma that extends to floor of third ventricle and to optic chiasm, (2) demyelination and calcification of pons, and (3) atrophy and demyelination of medulla.

Diagnosis: Central diabetes insipidus.

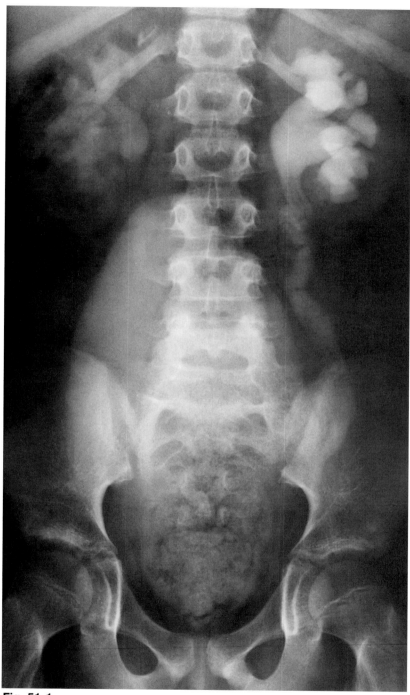

Fig. 51-1

Case 52

A 27-year-old man has a deep ulcer behind sacrum.

Pregnancy of mother was normal, birth weight 3.4 kg, and head circumference 38 cm. He was born with ruptured lumbosacral meningomyelocele and absent sensation below T7–T8. Rectal sphincter was lax. Legs were flaccid. Meningomyelocele was operated on, and ventriculoatrial shunt was placed. Urine came out in drips when he cried or grunted and occasionally in a stream 12–13 cm long. Right inguinal hernia was repaired at 2½ months. A plaster cast was applied at 1 year for hip contracture. He was always wet at 2½ years despite Credé's pressure. He was usually wet at 4 years. He started self-catheterization of bladder at 11 years. Spine was operated on at 12 years. *Citrobacter diversus*, *Escherichia coli*, and *Klebsiella pneumoniae* were cultured from urine at 13 years. Buttocks were ulcerated at 21 years and covered with skin flaps at 23 years.

A sibling of his father died soon after birth with meningomyelocele and hydrocephalus.

Temperature at 27 years is 37.5°C, heart rate 74, respiratory rate 18, and blood pressure 90/60 mm Hg. He is alert and oriented. A cleft is in left side of tongue. Rales are at lung bases. Surgical scars are on body. Back of sacrum is visible at bottom of ulcer. Legs are flaccid and child size. The rest of the physical findings are normal.

Hematocrit is 0.26. White cell count is 10.7×10^9/liter with 0.71 polymorphonuclear cells, 0.17 lymphocytes, 0.08 monocytes, 0.03 eosinophils, and 0.01 basophils. Platelet count is 605×10^9/liter. Urine specific gravity is 1.015, pH 7. Urine has 0.2 AU urobilinogen, small amount leukocyte esterase, 4–7 white cells/HPF, occasional squamous and nonsquamous epithelial cells/HPF, and 0–3 granular casts/LPF, and is sterile. Serum sodium is 138 mmol/liter, potassium 4.1, chloride 107, carbon dioxide 26, urea nitrogen 1.4, calcium 2.05, phosphorus 1.39, cholesterol 3.47, and glucose 5.3. Creatinine is 60 μmol/liter, uric acid 200, total bilirubin 7, direct bilirubin 3, iron 5 (normal: 14–32), and iron-binding capacity 29 (normal: 45–82). Ferritin is 500 μg/liter (normal: 18–300). Total protein is 65 g/liter, albumin 24. Alkaline phosphatase is 273 U/liter, LDH 112, and SGOT 17.

Lumbar and sacral neural arches are defective. Cystograms at 1 year (Figure 52-1A), 2¾ years, 7 years, and 13 years (Figure 52-1B) show gradual evolution of changes in bladder. Contrast medium is in dilated prostatic urethra and in urethral sinus in each lateral lobe of prostate at 13 years. Spine is braced with orthopedic apparatus (see Figure 52-1B).

Diagnosis: Neurogenic bladder.

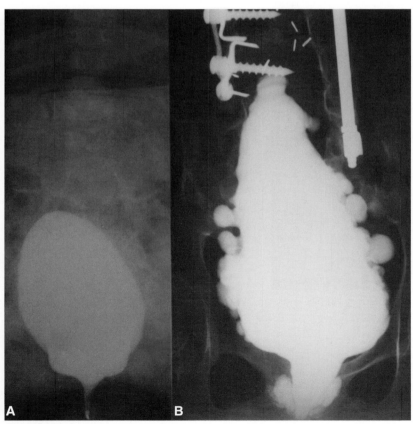

Fig. 52-1

Case 53

A newborn boy, the smaller of twins, has esophageal atresia that was diagnosed after two attempts to aspirate stomach.

Mother (19 years old), father (22 years old), and sister (16 months old) are well.

Birth weight is 2.2 kg, length 46 cm, Apgar score 9/9 at 1 and 5 minutes, and blood glucose 2.7 mmol/liter at 30 minutes. Temperature is 36.6°C at 9 hours, heart rate 130, respiratory rate 60, and systolic blood pressure 58 mm Hg. Umbilical cord is odd looking. The rest of the physical findings are normal.

Hematocrit is 0.63. White cell count is 13.6 × 10^9/liter. Serum sodium is 135 mmol/liter, potassium 5.9, chloride 101, and calcium 2.30.

Liquid drips from umbilicus the day after division of tracheoesophageal fistula and esophageal anastomosis. He urinates through urethra and umbilicus simultaneously later in the day and then soaks umbilical dressings.

Cystogram in Figure 53-1 shows contrast medium in bladder, urethra, and urachus, and end of catheter in urachus. Chest roentgenogram shows dysplasia of bodies of T2, T3, and T5.

At operation, urachus between bladder and lower end of umbilicus is excised.

Diagnosis: Skeletal abnormalities, esophageal atresia with tracheoesophageal fistula, and patent urachus.

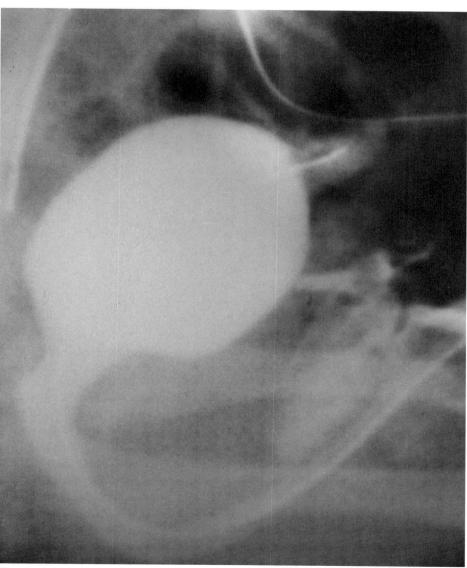

Fig. 53-1

Case 54

A 3-year-old girl has been urinating less often for 2 weeks because of lower abdominal pain while she urinates. She has played and eaten less for 1 week. A tender, midline mass below the umbilicus appeared 2 days ago. She has had several ear infections.

Temperature is 38.1°C, heart rate 120, respiratory rate 24, systolic blood pressure 78 mm Hg, and weight 13 kg. A mobile, tender mass is between umbilicus and pelvis. The rest of the physical findings are normal.

Hematocrit is 0.33. White cell count is 22.0×10^9/liter with 0.61 polymorphonuclear cells, 0.11 bands, 0.23 lymphocytes, 0.03 monocytes, and 0.02 eosinophils. Platelet estimate is high.

Longitudinal ultrasound examination in Figure 54-1 shows a variably echogenic mass indenting fundus of dilated bladder.

At operation, phlegmon and wall (1–2 cm thick) surround a cyst that is attached to umbilicus and fundus of urinary bladder. Cyst has 10–15 ml pus.

Excised mass (7.5 × 4.5 × 2.4 cm) has a white-tan wall with gray, glistening fibrous membrane around it; rough, ridged lining in it; and a firm lump (2.8-cm diameter) at one pole. Microscopic examination shows fibrous tissue, muscle, adipose tissue, granulation tissue, and acute and chronic inflammation.

Culture of pus grows coagulase-positive *Staphylococcus aureus*.

Diagnosis: Infected urachal cyst.

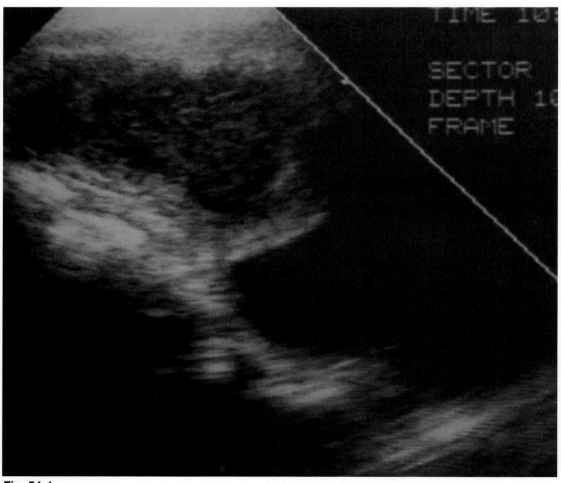

Fig. 54-1

Case 55

A 4-year-old boy, who was recently operated on for first-degree hypospadias, is thought to have a pelvic mass.

He was delivered by cesarean section for abruptio placentae. Birth weight was 2.4 kg, Apgar score 5/8 at 1 and 5 minutes. Mouth was full of mucus. Anus was ectopic. Meconium was at junction of perineum and scrotum. Esophageal anastomosis, division of tracheoesophageal fistula, sigmoid colostomy, and gastrostomy were performed at 2 days. Nissen gastric fun-doplication was performed at 3 months, and, later, colon reanastomosis and anoplasty.

Cystogram in Figure 55-1 shows (1) contrast medium in bladder, in prostatic and membranous urethra, and between urethra and rectum; (2) residual barium in rectum; and (3) dysplastic sacrum.

Diagnosis: Reflux into elongated prostatic utricle.

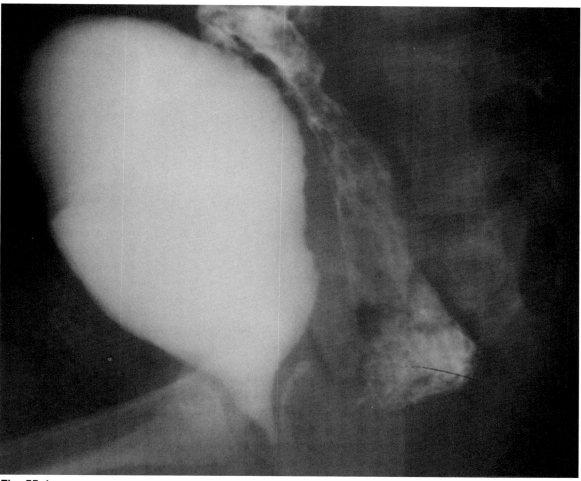

Fig. 55-1

Case 56

A newborn baby has dimple in place of anus and penoscrotal hypospadias.

Pregnancy of mother (24 years old) was normal until cesarean section was performed because of earlier cesarean section. Birth weight is 2.5 kg, length 48 cm, head circumference 33 cm, Apgar score 8/9 at 1 and 5 minutes, temperature 35.6°C, heart rate 156, and respiratory rate 42. At 2 days, systolic blood pressure is 80 mm Hg. The rest of the physical findings are normal.

Blood glucose is 2.8 mmol/liter. At 2 days, hematocrit is 0.60. White cell count is 13.8×10^9/liter with 0.57 polymorphonuclear cells, 0.12 bands, 0.29 lymphocytes, and 0.02 monocytes. Platelet count is 174×10^9/liter. Serum sodium is 144 mmol/liter, potassium 4.9, chloride 109, urea nitrogen 3.6, and calcium 2.47. Creatinine is 80 µmol/liter. Peak total bilirubin at 5 days is 251 µmol/liter.

Transverse colostomy is performed at 2 days.

Plain film at 5 days shows dysplastic sacrum. Cystogram at 6 weeks (Figure 56-1) shows normal bladder and, when he voids, two small collections of contrast medium behind the urethra, one at level of urogenital diaphragm, the other below it at the level of bulbous urethra.

At posterior sagittal anorectoplasty at 9 months, end of rectum without fistula is adherent to prostate.

He weighs 31.3 kg at 8 years, has loose anal sphincter and "daily accidents."

Diagnosis Imperforate anus, hypospadias, reflux of contrast medium from urethra into bulbourethral duct and gland (Cowper's gland).

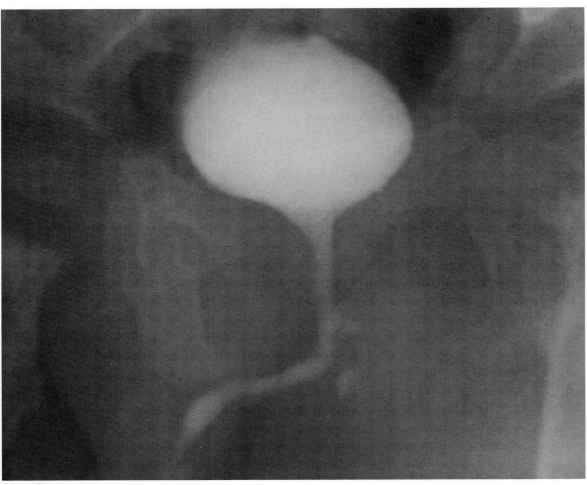

Fig. 56-1

Case 57

A 5½-year-old girl cannot start school because she wears diapers. She is continent of stool but not of urine.

Birth weight was 2.3 kg. She was born with a small cervical meningocele that has been removed. She sat at 6 months, walked at 1 year. She had a febrile convulsion. Right eye turns in less than it used to.

Mother (28 years old), father, and brother (7 years old) are well.

Temperature is 37.4°C, heart rate 100, respiratory rate 20, blood pressure 84/50 mm Hg, height 107 cm, and weight 22 kg. Epicanthi are in eyes. Nasal bridge is broad. A dimple is in front of each ear. A scar is on back of neck. Systolic murmur and click are along left sternal border. Labia majora are not fused in front. Clitoris is bifid. Little fingers curve in. First toes are broad and have two nails. The rest of the physical findings are normal.

Hematocrit is 0.42. White cell count is 14.4×10^9/liter with 0.38 polymorphonuclear cells, 0.50 lymphocytes, 0.04 monocytes, and 0.08 eosinophils. Platelet estimate is adequate. Urine specific gravity is 1.028, pH 6.5. Urine has 1–2 white cells/HPF and 10–12 epithelial cells/HPF. Chromosomes are 46,XX.

Excretory urogram (Figure 57-1) 10 minutes after injection of contrast medium shows (1) contrast medium in renal substance, in duplicated renal pelves and ureters, and on perineum; and (2) wide pubic symphysis.

At cystoscopy, diameter and length of urethra are 1 cm. Vagina and cervix are normal.

Diagnosis: Diastasis of symphysis pubis, short urethra, female suprasymphyseal epispadias. Clinical diagnosis of heart abnormality is aortic stenosis and bicuspid aortic valve.

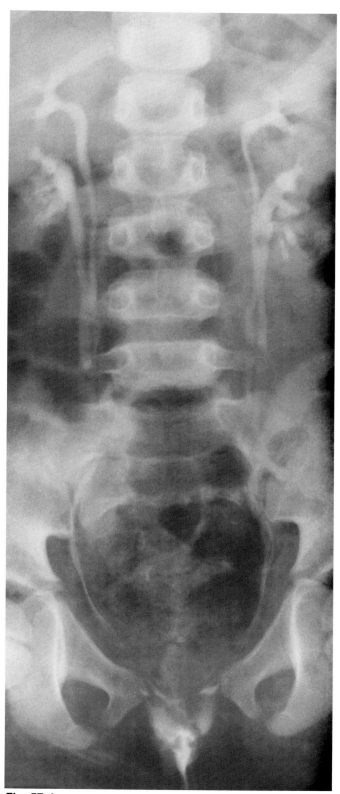

Fig. 57-1

Case 58

A newborn baby has a lower abdominal defect that discharges stool and urine.

Pregnancy of mother (37 years old) was normal. Amniocentesis at 16 weeks showed fetal chromosomes 46,XX, and amniotic fluid α-fetoprotein 24.0 mg/liter (median 12.3, SD 3).

Mother, father, and two sisters (10 and 14 years old) are well.

Birth weight is 2.6 kg, length 46 cm, temperature 36°C, heart rate 150, and respiratory rate 50. Stool is in defect; ureteral openings are at sides of defect. An omphalocele merges with top of defect. Labia majora gape around defect and fuse behind it. Perineum lacks vaginal and anal openings. The rest of the physical findings are normal.

Hematocrit is 0.55. White cell count is 22.4×10^9/liter with 0.21 polymorphonuclear cells, 0.07 bands, 0.62 lymphocytes, 0.09 monocytes, and 0.01 eosinophils. Platelet estimate is low. Serum sodium is 138 mmol/liter, potassium 9.3, urea nitrogen 6.8, calcium 2.35, and glucose 5.9. Total bilirubin is 32 μmol/liter.

A mass of soft tissue is between widely separated pubic bones and sacrum is dysplastic (Figure 58-1A). Barium goes into small bowel and not colon when injected into the opening from which stool comes (Figure 58-1B).

She dies at 6 days.

At necropsy, cecum merges into abdominal wall. Colon is 1 cm long and has two appendixes. Ureters open to abdominal wall. Right kidney is in pelvis, along with two uteri, each uterus with one tube and one ovary. Vagina is atretic. A gap separates rectus muscles. Subarachnoid blood is in posterior cranial fossa.

Diagnosis: Exstrophy of cloaca.

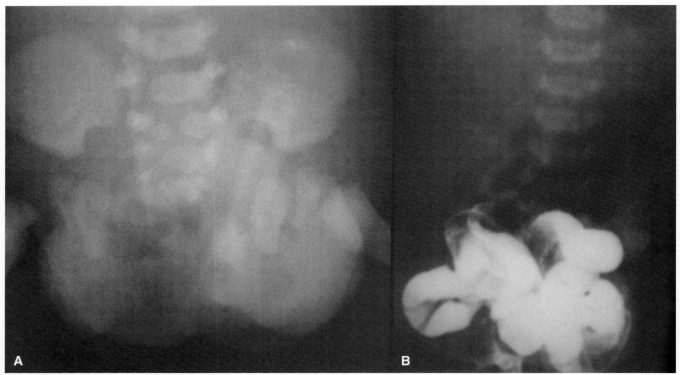

Fig. 58-1

Case 59

A 10½-year-old boy wets his pants after he thinks he is done urinating. Urine came from end of penis and an opening near junction of penis and abdominal wall until upper opening was surgically closed at 3 years.

Weight is 38.8 kg, height 149 cm, and blood pressure 110/80 mm Hg. Stream of urine is normal but is resumed by stripping penis and followed by drips.

Cystogram in Figure 59-1 shows two penile urethras, the lower one beginning in bulbous urethra at level of opening of bulbourethral ducts, and a blind-ending stub midway along upper penile urethra. Width of symphysis pubis is normal.

Diagnosis: Duplication (questionable original triplication) of urethra.

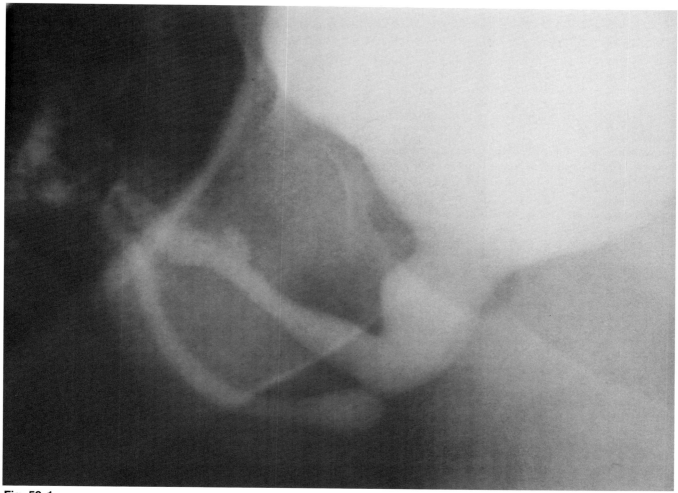

Fig. 59-1

Case 60

A 14-month-old boy urinated blood 5 days ago.

Birth weight was 3.3 kg. He walked at 9 months and can say a few words.

Parents are well. Maternal grandmother and both great-grandmothers have diabetes mellitus.

Temperature is 38.0°C, heart rate 120, respiratory rate 22, systolic blood pressure 88 mm Hg, weight 11.1 kg, and height 83 cm. A hard, mobile mass is in front of rectum in rectal examination. The rest of the physical findings are normal.

Hematocrit is 0.36. White cell count is 12.9×10^9/liter with 0.27 polymorphonuclear cells, 0.07 bands, 0.50 lymphocytes, 0.11 monocytes, 0.03 eosinophils, 0.01 basophils, and 0.01 atypical lymphocytes. Platelet count is 328×10^9/liter. Urine specific gravity is 1.021, pH 5.5. Urine has trace protein, hemoglobin, 2–3 red cells/HPF, 5–10 white cells/HPF, bacteria, and amorphous urates. Serum sodium is 138 mmol/liter, potassium 5.1, chloride 108, carbon dioxide not determined, urea nitrogen 8.2, calcium 2.52, phosphorus 1.61, cholesterol 3.62, and glucose 4.6. Creatinine is 40 μmol/liter, uric acid 260, total bilirubin 3, and direct bilirubin 0. Total protein is 59 g/liter, albumin 40. Alkaline phosphatase is 363 U/liter, LDH 297, and SGOT 42.

Excretory urogram in Figure 60-1 shows mass at base of bladder.

At cystoscopy, bladder and urethra are normal. A hard mass (2-cm diameter) is in prostate.

Two cores of tissue from mass are obtained transperineally.

Biopsy of white mucinous tumor shows (1) round to oval cells with eosinophilic granular cytoplasm and eccentric flattened nuclei with granular chromatin; (2) spindle-shaped cells with eosinophilic, vacuolated cytoplasm, and elongated nuclei; (3) stellate cells with eosinophilic cytoplasm and central round to oval nuclei; and (4) myxoid stroma infiltrated by eosinophils, rare mitoses, and occasional strap cells with cross striations. Bone marrow is normal.

Tumor is smaller after 3 months of chemotherapy.

At operation, bladder, prostate, prostatic and membranous parts of urethra, seminal vesicles, part of spermatic cords, and appendix are removed. Ureters are anastomosed to an ileal-abdominal conduit.

Shiny gray mucus membrane in bladder covers mucoid, grapelike tumor in prostate. Wall of bladder is thickened. Microscopic examination shows sheets of tumor cells, crowded together or separated by loose, eosinophilic myxoid stroma in prostate, bladder, spermatic cords, and seminal vesicles. Tumor does not have a cambium layer and does not cross epithelial surfaces.

Bile continuously comes out of nasogastric tube 1 day after operation. Bowel sounds are absent, rare, or high pitched; abdomen is distended and tympanitic. He vomits bile and then feculent liquid.

Gut is distended by gas and liquid 12 days after operation (Figure 60-2A). Barium enema shows displacement of ascending colon by distended ileum (Figure 60-2B).

Diagnosis: Rhabdomyosarcoma of prostate (sarcoma botryoides), postoperative intussusception. (At operation, ileoileal intussusception is easily reduced.)

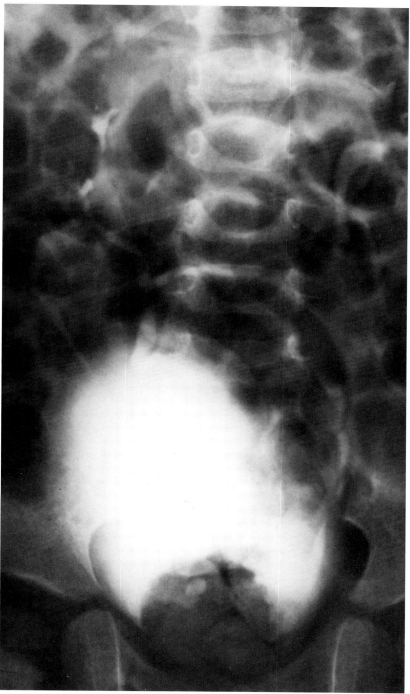

Fig. 60-1

(Continued)

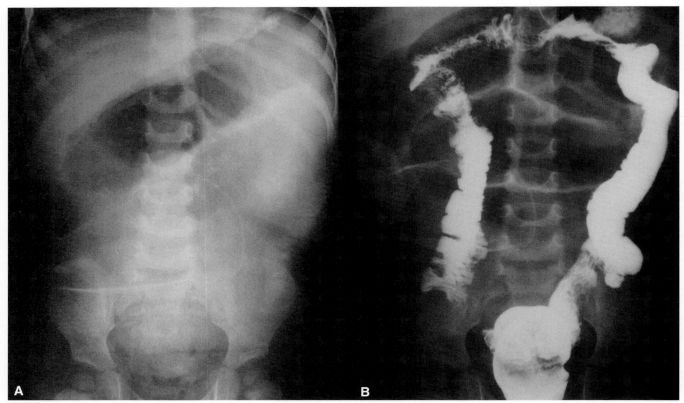

Fig. 60-2

Urogenital System

Case 1

A 15-month-old girl has a lump in left labium majus.

Pregnancy was normal, birth weight 3.8 kg, and length 53 cm. Labia majora were swollen. Mother felt a lump in left labium. Girl was jaundiced at 5 days. A gonad was mobile in larger left labium majus; a smaller gonad was higher on right side. Serum FSH at 2 weeks and 2½ months was <10 U/liter (normal: 1–4), LH 7 and 4 (normal: 1–18). Testosterone at 2 weeks was <10 nmol/liter (normal: 2.6–13.9). Chromosomes in peripheral blood cells were 46,XY.

Mother (32 years old), father (38 years old), and brother (5 years old) are well. Father has first degree hypospadias. Brother had an undescended testis during first year.

Weight at 15 months is 10.5 kg, height 83 cm, head circumference 49 cm, temperature 36.8°C, heart rate 108, respiratory rate 24, and blood pressure 80/50 mm Hg. A gonad (volume: 1 cm) is in left labium majus, a smaller gonad is in right groin. Clitoris is normal. Labia minora are thinly fused in back. The rest of the physical findings are normal.

Hematocrit is 0.33. Before and after three daily IM injections of 3,333 U HCG, serum progesterone is <0.3 nmol/liter (normal: 0.2–1.7), 17α-hydroxyprogesterone 0.5 and 1.7 (normal: 0.1–2.7), dehydroepiandrosterone 2.0 and 3.1 (normal: 0.7–4.5), androstenedione 0.6 and 1.2 (normal: 0.3–1.7), testosterone 1.04 and 3.47 (normal: 0.10–0.35), and dihydrotestosterone 0.31 and 1.14 (normal <0.10). Chromosomes are again 46,XY.

Cystogram while bladder is emptying shows bladder, urethra, and vagina without cervical impression (Figure 1-1). Ultrasound examination does not show uterus or ovaries behind bladder.

At cystoscopy, vagina, urethra, and bladder are normal.

At operation, tunica vaginalis, testis, epididymis, and part of ductus deferens are removed from each inguinal canal.

Left testis (3.0 × 2.5 × 1.0 cm) and right testis (2.5 × 2.0 × 0.8 cm) are light blue, smooth, and contain immature testicular tissue in microscopic examination.

Diagnosis: Androgen insensitivity syndrome.

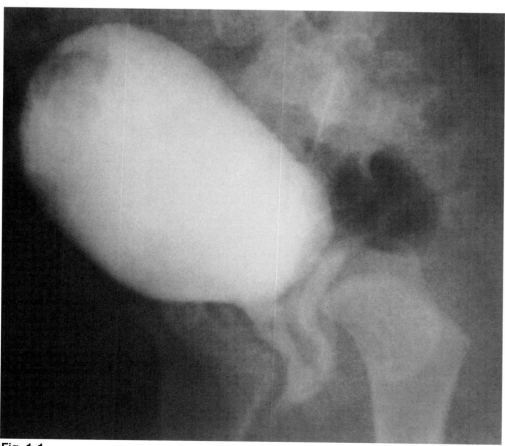

Fig. 1-1

Case 2

A 1-month-old girl has been vomiting for 3 days. Abdomen has been distended for 2 days.

Temperature is 36.6°C, heart rate 140, respiratory rate 40, blood pressure 120/67 mm Hg, weight 5 kg, length 54 cm, and head circumference 38 cm. Left thigh is swollen and purplish. Hymen bulges. The rest of the physical findings are normal.

Hematocrit is 0.40. White cell count is 15.9×10^9/liter with 0.43 polymorphonuclear cells, 0.03 bands, 0.45 lymphocytes, 0.07 monocytes, 0.01 eosinophils, and 0.01 atypical lympho-cytes. Platelet count is 396×10^9/liter. Serum sodium is 136 mmol/liter, potassium 5.7, chloride 106, and carbon dioxide 16.

Longitudinal ultrasound examination shows mass with sedimented matter behind thick-walled bladder (Figure 2-1) and bilateral pyelocaliectasis.

At operation, 175 ml of turbid, white liquid is released when hymen is nicked.

Diagnosis: Imperforate hymen, hydrocolpos.

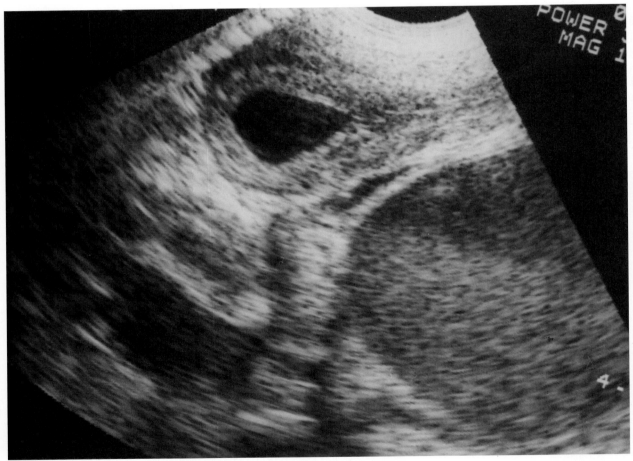

Fig. 2-1

Case 3

An 8-year-old girl has been bleeding from vagina for 1 week.

She bled from vagina for several days 4 months ago. Breasts were "puffy."

Mother and father are well. Mother's menarche was at 12–13 years. A maternal aunt had ovarian cancer; another maternal aunt had ovarian cysts.

Weight is 31.6 kg, height 134 cm, temperature 37.9°C, heart rate 104, respiratory rate 28, and blood pressure 98/56 mm Hg. Breast development is Tanner stage II. Fine hair is on labia majora. The rest of the physical findings are normal.

Hematocrit is 0.37. White cell count is 12.7×10^9/liter with 0.70 polymorphonuclear cells, 0.27 lymphocytes, and 0.03 monocytes. Platelet count is 321×10^9/liter. Urine specific gravity is 1.022, pH 6. Urine has 1–3 white cells/HPF. Serum sodium is 145 mmol/liter, potassium 3.8, chloride 113, carbon dioxide 24, urea nitrogen 3.6, calcium 2.25, phosphorus 1.74, cholesterol 3.83, and glucose 4.6. Creatinine is 50 μmol/liter, uric acid 230, total bilirubin 9, and direct bilirubin 2. Total protein is 62 g/liter, albumin 42. Alkaline phosphatase is 972 U/liter, LDH 198, and SGOT 24. Thyroid function tests are normal. Serum estradiol is 170 pmol/liter (normal: 18–184). 17α-hydroxyprogesterone is 3.3 nmol/liter (normal: 0.5–4.5).

HCG is <2 U/liter. α_1-Fetoprotein is <10 μg/liter, carcinoembryonic antigen <2. Serum FSH is <2 IU/liter, LH <3 during 2 hours after IV injection of 85 μg gonadotropin-releasing hormone.

Transverse ultrasound examination in Figure 3-1 shows ovaries and uterus behind bladder; right ovary is larger than left. Bone age in left hand is normal.

At operation, serous liquid is aspirated from a cyst (2 × 1 cm) in left ovary. A cyst (2.5-cm diameter) that makes up half of right ovary is removed.

Outer surface of right ovarian cyst is smooth and gray-white; wall is 1–4 mm thick. Several cysts (2–5 mm) are on inner surface.

Breasts resume growth at 8½ years. A café au lait spot is on abdomen at 9 years. Menarche is at 12 years. Periods are regular.

Diagnosis: Follicular cyst, right ovary; gonadotropin-independent precocious puberty; questionable McCune-Albright syndrome.

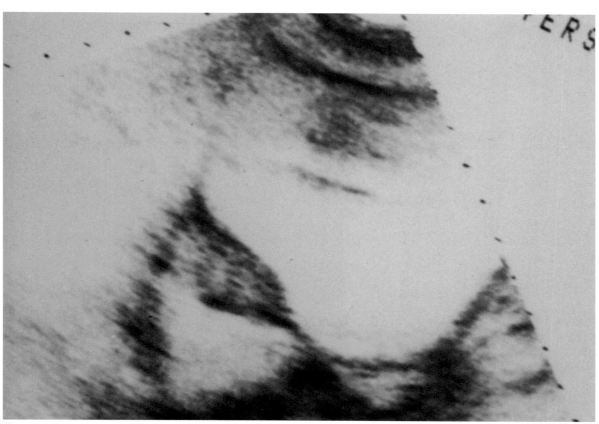

Fig. 3-1

Case 4

A 22-month-old girl is bleeding from the vagina. Mother saw blood 1 week ago and 3 days ago. She found a blood stain (4–5 cm) on diaper today. She then saw tissue at vaginal opening while she was drying her daughter after a bath.

Temperature is 36.3°C, respiratory rate 24, weight 11.8 kg, and length 83 cm. A small spot of blood is at vagina. A bloody, cystic mass protrudes from vagina when the girl cries. The rest of the physical findings are normal.

Hematocrit is 0.36. White cell count is 6.2×10^9/liter with 0.18 polymorphonuclear cells, 0.78 lymphocytes, 0.02 monocytes, 0.01 eosinophils, and 0.01 atypical lymphocytes. Platelet count is 290×10^9/liter. Serum sodium is 141 mmol/liter, potassium 3.9, chloride 104, carbon dioxide 25, urea nitrogen 2.1, calcium 2.62, phosphorus 1.49, cholesterol 3.00, and glucose 4.8. Creatinine is 40 µmol/liter, uric acid 280, total bilirubin 5, and direct bilirubin 2. Total protein is 62 g/liter, albumin 44. Alkaline phosphatase is 181 U/liter, LDH 274, and SGOT 45.

Ultrasound examination in Figure 4-1A shows a mass with mixed echoes behind bladder. CT scan in Figure 4-1B shows a mass between bladder and rectum.

Vaginoscopy shows a mass attached to upper back part of vagina. Edematous translucent white and blood-stained tissue is removed for microscopic examination.

She is incontinent of stool at 6 years, soiling underpants and passing small stools when she urinates. Weight is 16.7 kg, temperature 36.9°C, heart rate 70, respiratory rate 16, and blood pressure 86/42 mm Hg. Blood vessels are prominent around anus that barely admits fingertip. Sigmoidoscopy shows increased vascular pattern.

Diagnosis: Rhabdomyosarcoma (sarcoma botryoides), radiation proctitis.

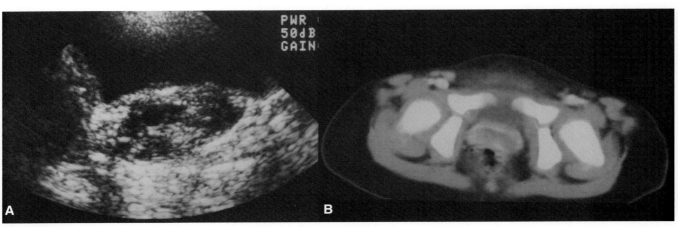

Fig. 4-1

Case 5

A 15-year-old girl has a distended, painful abdomen.

Last menstrual period was 3½ months ago. She bled from vagina 13 days ago. Ultrasound examination showed a molar pregnancy. Urine βHCG level was >10⁶ U/liter. Uterine contents were removed by dilation and curettage 10 days ago. Abdominal pain and distention began 7 days ago. She has gained 8 kg in the last week.

Menarche was at 13 years.

Temperature is 37.7°C, heart rate 128, respiratory rate 32, and blood pressure 100/70 mm Hg. Breathing is labored and shallow. Alae nasi flare. Breath sounds are diminished at bases. Abdomen is tense and tender. Bowel sounds are diminished. Vulva is swollen. The rest of the physical findings are normal.

Hematocrit is 0.29. She received a transfusion of packed red cells 5 days ago. White cell count is 15.8 × 10⁹/liter with 0.69 polymorphonuclear cells, 0.07 bands, 0.21 lymphocytes, 0.02 monocytes, and 0.01 basophils. Platelet count is 621 × 10⁹/liter. Serum sodium is 133 mmol/liter, potassium 3.5, chloride 102, carbon dioxide 22, urea nitrogen 5.0, calcium 1.95, phosphorus 1.19, cholesterol 3.23, and glucose 6.5.

Total bilirubin is 10 μmol/liter, direct bilirubin 2. Total protein is 43 g/liter, albumin 22. Amylase is 30 U/liter, alkaline phosphatase 93, LDH 182, and SGOT 14. First specimen of urine on second day is amber and turbid with specific gravity 1.030 and pH 5. It has trace ketones, 1–2 white cells/HPF, many amorphous crystals/HPF, and 4–6 granular casts/LPF. Peritoneal liquid obtained at paracentesis is sterile.

Ultrasound examination shows uterus, large cystic ovaries, and peritoneal liquid. CT scan in Figure 5-1 shows large cystic ovaries, uterus, and uterine (fallopian) tubes and peritoneal liquid behind them.

Microscopic examination of material obtained at dilation and curettage of uterus shows (1) a few small villi and large edematous villi with trophoblastic proliferation; (2) central cisternae; (3) irregular scalloped borders with inclusions lined with syncytial trophoblasts that show mild to moderate atypia; and (4) syncytial, intermediate, and cytotrophoblastic cells.

Diagnosis: Ovarian hyperstimulation syndrome in molar pregnancy.

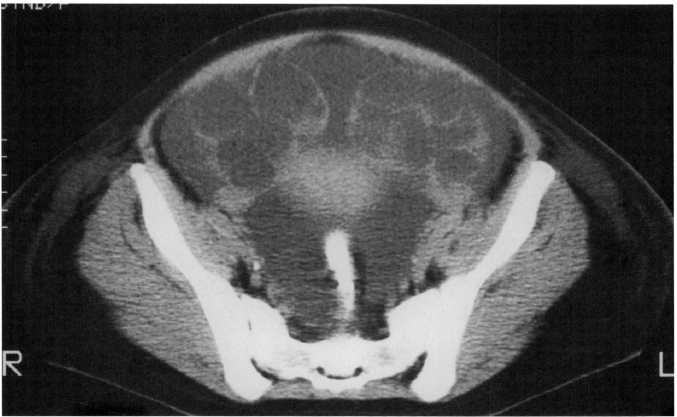

Fig. 5-1

Case 6

A 7-year-old girl has slight abdominal pain.

She vomited and had abdominal cramps and temperature 38.3°C for several hours 1 month ago and then did not feel right for several days. She broke her left arm 3 years ago. She has had chickenpox.

Mother (29 years old), father (31 years old), and sister (9 years old) are well.

Weight is 21.5 kg, height 115 cm, temperature 37.2°C, heart rate 100, respiratory rate 20, and blood pressure 108/60 mm Hg. Physical findings are normal.

Hematocrit is 0.37. White cell count is 4.9×10^9/liter with 0.57 polymorphonuclear cells, 0.37 lymphocytes, 0.03 monocytes, 0.02 eosinophils, and 0.01 basophils. Urine specific gravity is 1.007, pH 5. Urine has occasional squamous and nonsquamous epithelial cells/HPF and 2–4 white cells/HPF.

In Figure 6-1A, an object of calcium density is in pelvis. Excretory urogram in Figure 6-1B shows the object outside urinary tract and in different part of pelvis.

At operation, a rubbery white mass is loose behind uterus. Left ovary and uterine tube are missing. Right ovary, right uterine tube, and uterus are normal. Mass and normal appendix are removed.

Mass (2.0 × 1.0 × 0.8 cm) is gritty when cut. Microscopic examination shows necrotic, calcified tissue.

Diagnosis: Necrosis of left ovary and uterine tube.

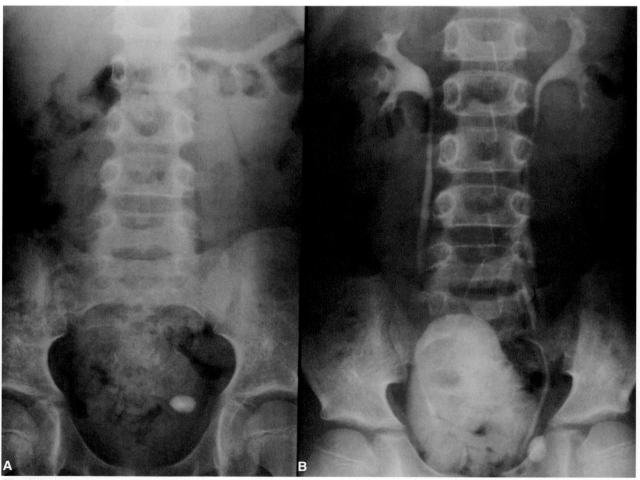

Fig. 6-1

Case 7

A 16-year-old girl with scoliosis that has remained slight and unchanged in roentgenographic examinations since discovery by a school nurse 2 years ago has another roentgenographic finding. Menarche was at 13 years.

Parents, five sisters, and three brothers are well. Maternal grandmother has breast cancer.

Temperature is 37°C, heart rate 76, respiratory rate 16, blood pressure 100/60 mm Hg, weight 63 kg, and height 180 cm. A right adnexal mass (10 × 10 cm) and a smaller left adnexal mass are in pelvis. The rest of the physical findings are normal.

Hematocrit is 0.40. White cell count is 7.3×10^9/liter with 0.60 polymorphonuclear cells, 0.02 bands, 0.26 lymphocytes, 0.09 monocytes, and 0.03 eosinophils. Platelet count is 191×10^9/liter. Serum sodium is 139 mmol/liter, potassium 4.0, and chloride 108. HCG is 16 U/liter (normal: <5). α_1-Fetoprotein is <15 µg/liter (normal: <25).

Figure 7-1 shows a round shadow of fat density in each side of pelvis, both of which contain a shadow of calcium density, the one on left like a tooth.

At operation, a smooth, reddish bilobed cyst is removed from right ovary; a smooth, smaller single-lobed cyst and two other small cysts are removed from left ovary.

Right ovarian cyst (10.8 × 6.5 × 4 cm) is multiloculated; contains hair and yellow, cheesy, greasy matter; and feels as if it contains calcium deposits when cut across. The largest left ovarian cyst contains similar matter and three rudimentary teeth. Another left ovarian cyst (2.0 × 0.7 × 0.3 cm) is glistening purple with a rim of soft orange tissue and a purple rough inner surface. The smallest is a 1-cm white nodule that has a 0.2-cm cyst within.

Diagnosis: Mature teratoma in each ovary; old corpus luteum cyst and 1-cm nodule that contains cyst lined by benign squamous epithelium in left ovary.

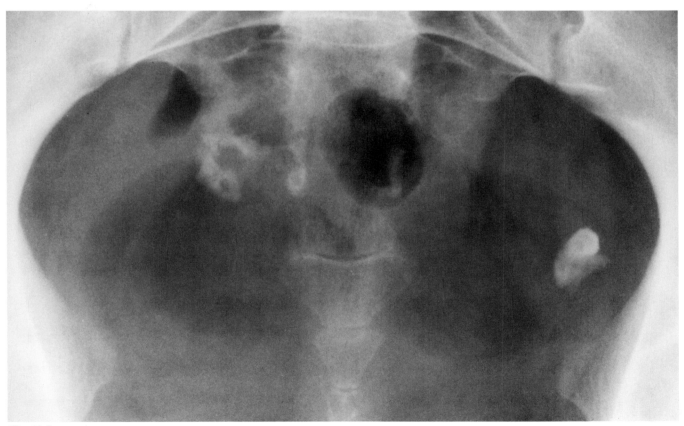

Fig. 7-1

Case 8

A 2½-year-old girl is vomiting bile.

Parents noticed abdominal distention 2 weeks ago when she had a bellyache. Appetite is decreased. She has lost 2 kg. She urinates frequently. She has loose stools some days, none other days.

Temperature is 37.6°C, heart rate 100, respiratory rate 24, blood pressure 102/60 mm Hg, and weight 28.3 kg. Abdomen is large. A firm, tender mass is palpable from epigastrium to rectum. The rest of the physical findings are normal.

Hematocrit is 0.31. White cell count is 12.8×10^9/liter with 0.85 polymorphonuclear cells, 0.03 bands, 0.07 lymphocytes, and 0.05 monocytes. Platelet count is 534×10^9/liter. Serum sodium is 137 mmol/liter, potassium 4.5, chloride 101, carbon dioxide 20, urea nitrogen 6.4, calcium 2.05, phosphorus 1.49, cholesterol 4.45, and glucose 4.8. Creatinine is 90 μmol/liter, uric acid 310, total bilirubin 9, and direct bilirubin 0. Total

protein is 60 g/liter, albumin 32. Alkaline phosphatase is 150 U/liter, LDH 984, and SGOT 37.

CT scan in Figure 8-1 shows a mass of varying density that almost fills pelvis.

At operation, a red-to-yellow, friable, gelatinous mass, much of it necrotic, seems to come from left ovary and is stuck to uterus and bladder in front, rectum and retroperitoneum behind, and left side of the colon. Mass, uterus, tubes, left ovary, and some omentum are removed.

Microscopic examination shows (1) malignant germ cell tumor with yolk sac component, (2) dysgerminoma, (3) chronic inflammation, and (4) mesothelial hyperplasia. Parts of tumor react with antibody to α_1-fetoprotein.

Diagnosis: Teratoma of left ovary.

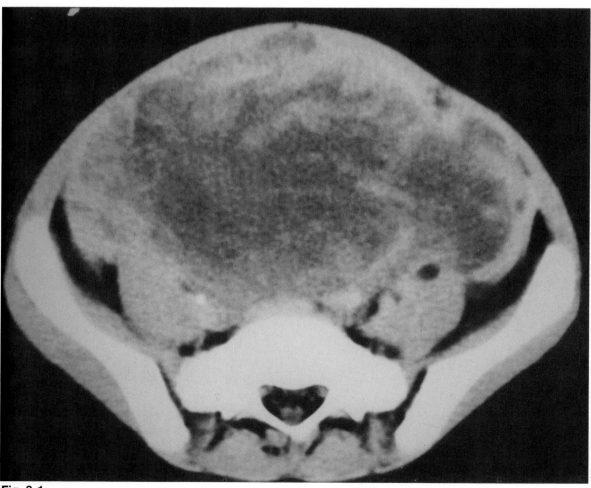

Fig. 8-1

Case 9

A 3-month-old boy is vomiting and febrile.

Pregnancy was normal, birth weight 3.7 kg.

Temperature is 38°C, heart rate 158, respiratory rate 56, systolic blood pressure 110 mm Hg, and weight 6.5 kg. Mouth is dry. A mass (3 × 3 cm) is in lower abdomen. Left testis is not in scrotum. The rest of the physical findings are normal.

Hematocrit is 0.23. White cell count is 15.0×10^9/liter with 0.56 polymorphonuclear cells, 0.05 bands, 0.33 lymphocytes, and 0.06 monocytes. Platelet count is 457×10^9/liter. Urine specific gravity is 1.027, pH 5. Urine has trace protein, trace ketones, amorphous sediment, bacteria, 0–3 white cells/HPF, and occasional epithelial cells/HPF.

Figure 9-1 shows a mass of water density with calcium in it in abdomen and normal colon and bladder. Ultrasound exami-nation of mass shows part with mixed echoes, part with shad-owing, and part without echoes.

At operation, a smooth, round mass (5 × 5 × 4 cm) is attached to spermatic cord at left deep inguinal ring.

Mass, covered by glistening gray membrane, contains blood clot and pale tan lobular tissue that is covered by tunica vaginalis. Microscopic examination of mass shows skin, hair, neural tis-sue, mature adipose tissue, cartilage, bone, and hemorrhage. Ductus deferens is in attached twisted spermatic cord.

Diagnosis: Mature teratoma, left testis.

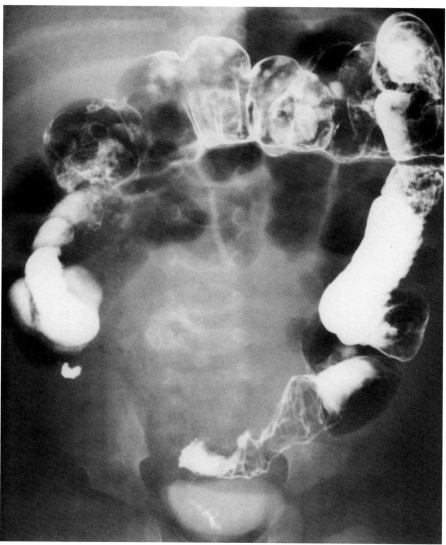

Fig. 9-1

Normal
Skeleton

Case 1

A 14-year-old girl has had pain in left shoulder for 1 month. She recently had spinal fusion for scoliosis. Left arm has always been weak.

A skin tag is in front of left ear. Left thumb is small; left first metacarpal bone is short. Left thenar muscles are hypoplastic. Thoracic spine is convex left. A scar is over it. The rest of the physical findings are normal.

Hematocrit is 0.33. White cell count is 11.5×10^9/liter. Platelet count is 312×10^9/liter.

Figure 1-1 shows bone between left acromion and head of left humerus.

Diagnosis: Os acromiale.

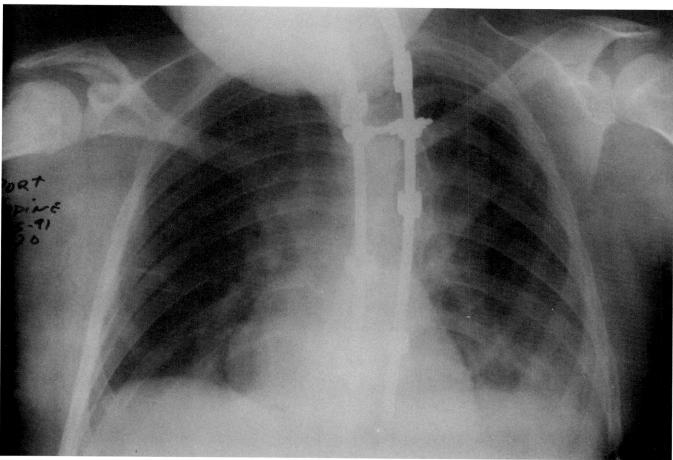

Fig. 1-1

Case 2

An 8-year-old girl has a lump on right side of chest that has been getting larger for 6 months.

Temperature is 37°C, weight 25.4 kg, and height 128 cm. A bony lump (5 cm) is just to right of sternum. The rest of the physical findings are normal.

Figure 2-1 shows bifid right fifth rib.

Diagnosis: Bifid rib (Luschka's forked rib), normal variant.

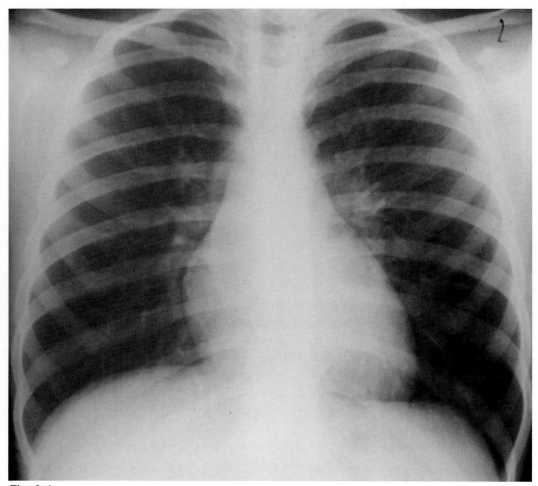

Fig. 2-1

Case 3

A 2-month-old girl, who suffered a left parietal skull fracture in a car crash 3 weeks ago, has roentgenographic examination for other fractures.

Pregnancy of mother (17 years old) was normal, delivery by cesarean section for slow labor. Birth weight was 3.2 kg, length 49 cm, head circumference 34 cm, and Apgar score 5/8 at 1 and 5 minutes. Physical findings were normal.

Weight at 2 months is 5.2 kg, length 56 cm, and head circumference 39 cm. A bony gap is palpable in left parietal bone. The rest of the physical findings are normal.

Lateral roentgenogram of spine in Figure 3-1 shows clefts in lumbar and lower thoracic vertebrae. A fracture is in left parietal bone. Roentgenographic findings in rest of skeleton are normal.

Diagnosis: Normal coronal clefts in vertebrae.

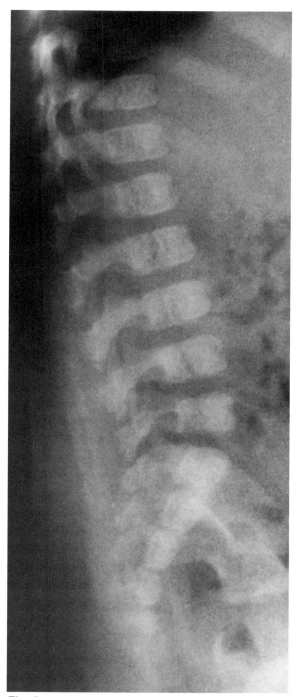

Fig. 3-1

Case 4

An 11-year-old girl has leg cramps when she gets up in the morning.

For the past 2 years, she has frequently walked on tiptoes for 5–15 minutes in the morning, until cramps subside.

She walked at 1 year. She has had otitis media. She wets bed about once per month. She occasionally takes pills for allergies to dust and pollen. She is active in ball games and gymnastics.

Weight at 11 years is 39 kg, height 142 cm. Physical findings are normal.

Hematocrit is 0.38. White cell count is 4.4×10^9/liter.

Figure 4-1 shows fragments of bone in grooves at top and bottom of front edge of some of the vertebral bodies.

Diagnosis: Normal ossification of ring cartilage of vertebral bodies.

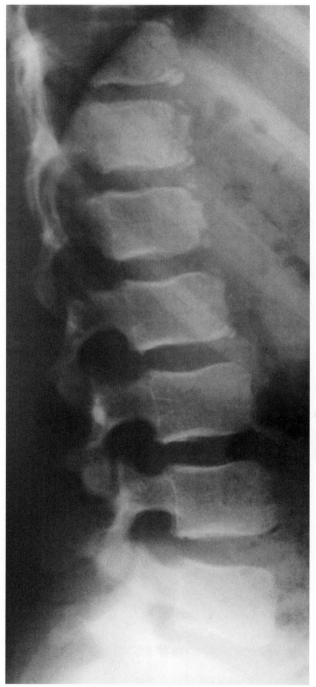

Fig. 4-1

Case 5

A 26-month-old girl had left pyeloplasty 2 months ago.

Pregnancy was normal. Bacteriuria was found in well-baby examination and persisted despite various antibiotics.

Weight at 24 months was 11.7 kg, height 95 cm, temperature 37.3°C, heart rate 85, respiratory rate 20, and blood pressure 100/60 mm Hg. Physical findings were normal.

Hematocrit was 0.37. White cell count was 6.2×10^9/liter with 0.45 polymorphonuclear cells, 0.06 bands, 0.39 lymphocytes, and 0.10 monocytes. Platelet estimate was adequate. Urine specific gravity was 1.012, pH 5.5. Urine had occasional squamous epithelial cells/HPF and occasional white cells/HPF. Culture of urine grew >10^5 colonies *Streptococcus fecalis*/ml. Excretory urogram showed left pyelectasis. Left pyeloplasty was performed.

Excretory urogram in lateral view at 26 months shows dilated left renal pelvis, forward displacement of L5 on S1, and thinning and perhaps interruption of pars interarticularis of vertebral (neural) arch of L5 (Figure 5-1A). Excretory urogram in lateral view at 32 months shows discontinuity of vertebral arch of L5 (Figure 5-1B).

Diagnosis: Spondylolisthesis, L5–S1; spondylolysis, L5.

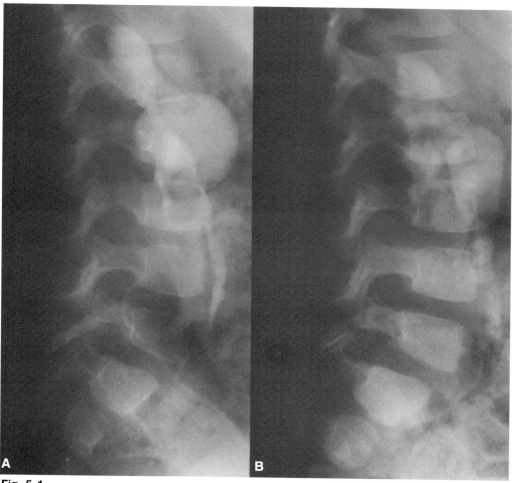

Fig. 5-1

Case 6

A 15-year-old boy has a sore, tender left elbow after being hit in a basketball game.

Movement at elbow and rest of physical findings in left arm are normal.

Medial one-third of palm and palmar side of left little finger are numb 16 months later, after a blow to medial side of left arm. Soft tissues along medial side of left elbow are swollen and tender. Volar aspect of left forearm is bruised. Touch sen-sation is impaired in numb part of left hand. The rest of the findings in the arms are normal.

Roentgenograms at 15 years show a spur of bone on antero-medial aspect of left humerus (Figure 6-1).

Diagnosis: Supracondylar spur of humerus, a normal variant; questionable association with numbness of left hand (median nerve and superficial branch of ulnar nerve).

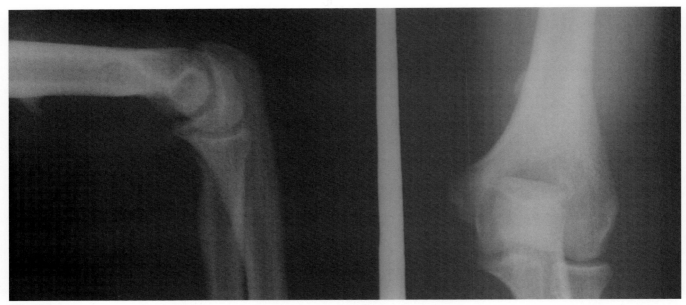

Fig. 6-1

Case 7

A 15-year-old boy fell today and hurt his right elbow.

He has had ear infections. A lump that appeared on his tongue at 9 years was removed at 11 years and diagnosed as benign fibroepithelial papilloma.

Right elbow is swollen, tender, and abraded along medial side.

An elliptical bone is in right olecranon fossa (Figure 7-1A) and not in left olecranon fossa (Figure 7-1B) in comparison view.

Diagnosis: Supratrochlear foraminal bone, right humerus.

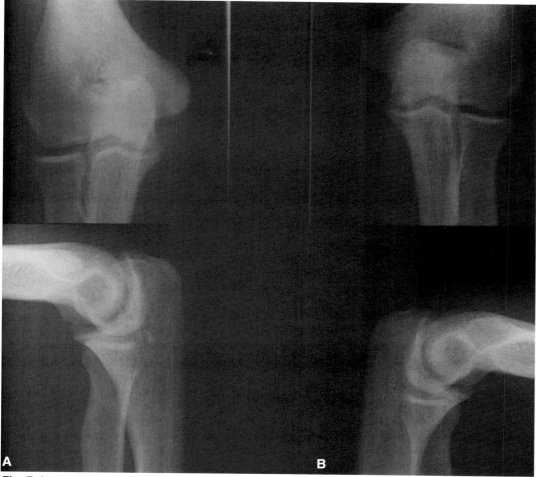

Fig. 7-1

Case 8

A 9-year-old boy fell today and hit flexed left elbow.

Elbow is bruised and scratched. Initially, he cannot straighten it, later he can.

Roentgenographic findings are normal. A sesamoid bone is in each triceps brachii tendon below olecranon fossa of humerus, visible in lateral (Figure 8-1) but not frontal view.

Diagnosis: Bilateral patella cubiti.

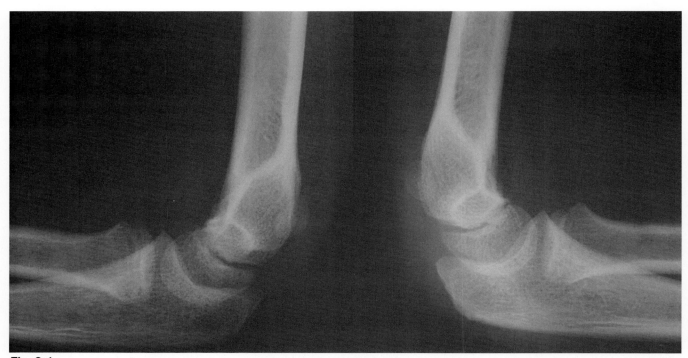

Fig. 8-1

Case 9

A 7-year-old boy, who hurt his right arm in a fall 2 months ago and had a cast on it for 1 month, cannot fully flex or extend right arm.

Weight is 23.8 kg, height 122 cm. Flexion at right elbow is 45 degrees, extension 120 degrees. The rest of the physical findings in arms are normal.

Ossification center of right capitulum (Figure 9-1A) is smaller than that of left (Figure 9-1B) and slightly sclerotic. Right elbow is not fully extended but is flexed almost 90 degrees (Figure 9-2).

Three months later, flexion at right elbow is normal, extension 160 degrees. He has full motion at right elbow at 14 years and cannot remember when it returned. He is right-handed and plays defensive tackle on high school football team.

Diagnosis: Normal ossification of right capitulum or Panner's abnormality.

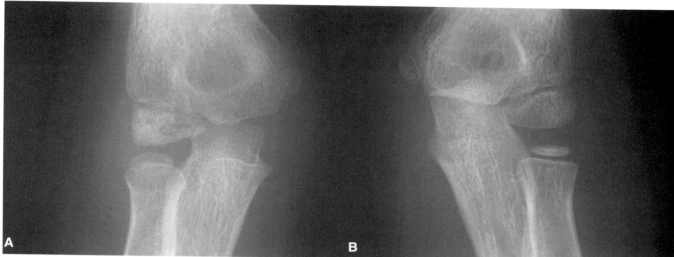

Fig. 9-1

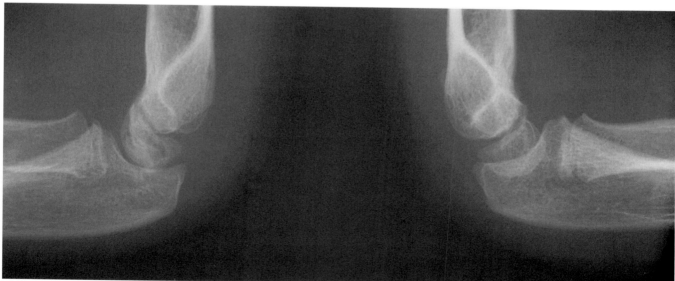

Fig. 9-2

Case 10

A 3½-year-old boy, who fell from a slide, has a swollen left thigh.

Parents (both 31 years old) and brother (7 years old) are well.

Heart rate is 80, respiratory rate 12, and blood pressure 120/70 mm Hg. The rest of the physical findings are normal.

Hematocrit is 0.33. Urine specific gravity is 1.029, pH 6.5. Urine has a few epithelial cells/HPF, occasional white cells/HPF, and bacteria.

Figure 10-1 shows (1) an oblique fracture and ossified callus in left femur 16 days after fall from sliding board, and (2) small, fragmented proximal epiphyseal ossification center. When fracture is healing 2 months later, proximal epiphyseal ossification center of right femur is small and scooped out in upper part (Figure 10-2A). At 6 years, proximal epiphyseal ossification center of right femur is still not smoothly ossified (Figure 10-2B) and bone age in left hand is 4 years, 2–3 SDs below the mean. Findings are normal at 10 years (Figure 10-3).

At 18 years, he has played for his high school football team for 4 years and is given an award for being the Outstanding Defensive Player.

Diagnosis: Meyer's dysplasia of capital femoral epiphyses.

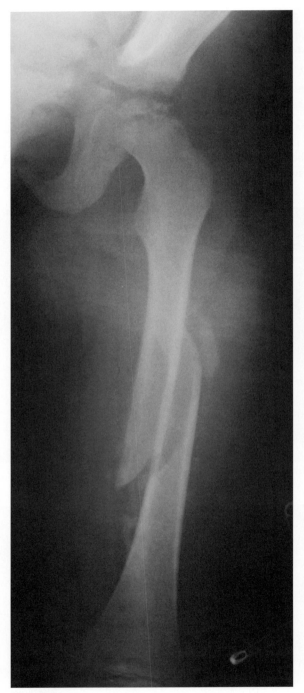

Fig. 10-1

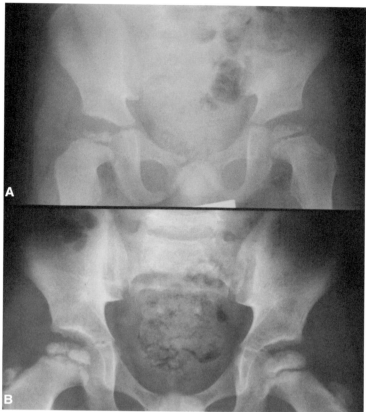

Fig. 10-2

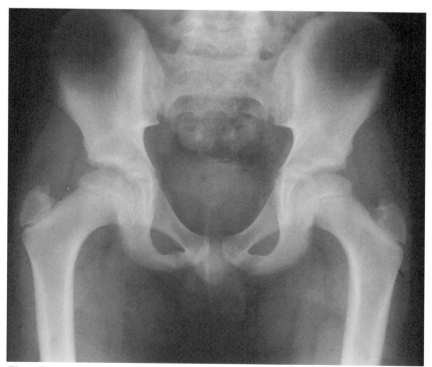

Fig. 10-3

Case 11

A 3⅚-year-old boy sometimes limps and has complained of pain in left groin for 2 months.

Pregnancy was normal, birth weight 3.5 kg. He has had otitis media.

Mother (30 years old), father (33 years old), and two brothers (7 and 12 years old) are well.

Weight is 17 kg, height 101 cm. He moves around the examining room with enthusiasm. Motion at right hip is normal with 70-degree abduction, 45-degree internal and external rotation, and full flexion. Motion at left hip is restricted with 20-degree abduction, no internal rotation, and 20-degree external rotation. He has no pain at 4⅙ years. Abduction at left hip is 40 degrees, internal rotation 20 degrees, and external rotation 45 degrees. "He never slows down" at 5¾ years. Left leg is slightly shorter than right at 8⅓ years. Flexion and rotation at left hip are normal; abduction is slightly limited.

Bone age in left hand is normal. At 4⅙ years, Figure 11-1 shows (1) small and sclerotic left femoral epiphyseal ossification center, (2) small and slightly sclerotic right femoral epiphyseal ossification center, (3) cystic defects in left metaphysis, (4) slightly unevenly mineralized right metaphysis, (5) neck of left femur shorter and broader than right, and (6) left neck-shaft angle less than that of right. At 6¼ years, Figure 11-2A shows (1) right femur not displaced from acetabulum, (2) left femur displaced from acetabulum, (3) most of head of left femur not ossified, and (4) edge of left epiphysis shown by gas in hip in abduction view, the antivacuum phenomenon. Right hip is normal at 8⅓ years, gas shows edge of right epiphysis, and more bone is in left epiphysis (Figure 11-2B).

Diagnosis: Perthes' disease, left hip; normal right hip with slow epiphyseal ossification (Meyer's dysplasia epiphysealis capitis femoris).

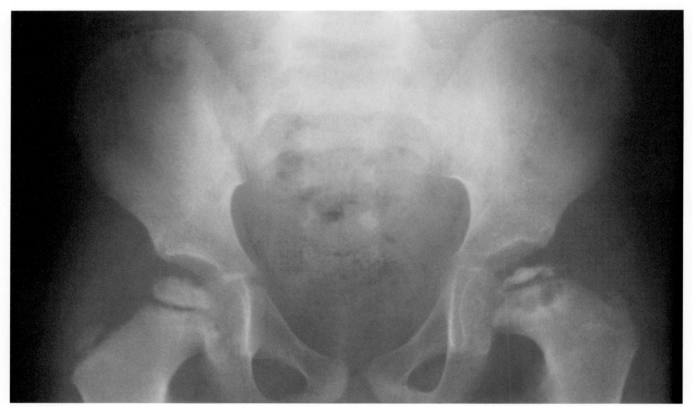

Fig. 11-1

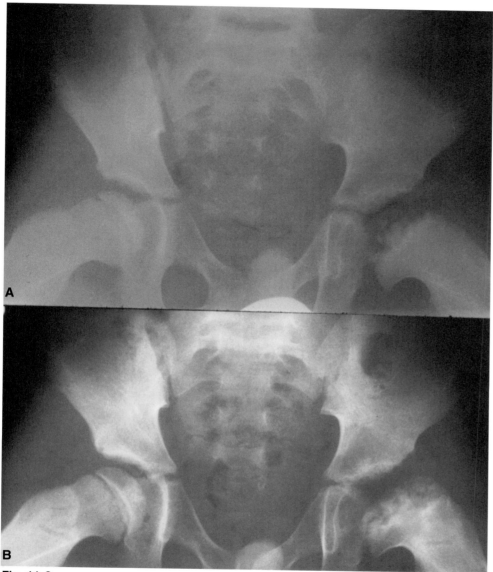

Fig. 11-2

Case 12

A 6-year-old boy, who was just hit by a truck, says he is sleepy.

Heart rate is 112, respiratory rate 24, and systolic blood pressure 55 mm Hg by palpation. He revives quickly and complains of pain in head and left leg. Systolic blood pressure is 124 mm Hg, temperature 37.8°C, heart rate 130, respiratory rate 28, and weight 20 kg. A stellate laceration (5 cm) is on left side of forehead. A small laceration and hematoma are on left side of occiput. Upper central incisors are broken at gumline. Bruises are on abdomen. Left leg is several centimeters shorter than right. Left thigh is swollen. An abrasion is in front of right knee. Back of right thigh is bruised. The rest of the physical findings are normal.

Hematocrit is 0.36. White cell count is 14.6×10^9/liter with 0.66 polymorphonuclear cells, 0.04 bands, 0.25 lymphocytes, 0.02 monocytes, and 0.03 eosinophils. Platelet count is 543×10^9/liter. Urine specific gravity is 1.045, pH 6. Urine has 0.4 g/liter ketones, 1+ hemoglobin/myoglobin, 7–8 red cells/HPF, 0–1 white cell/HPF, and few calcium oxalate crystals. Serum sodium is 136 mmol/liter, potassium 3.5, chloride 105, carbon dioxide 21, urea nitrogen 5.7, and glucose 9.5.

Figure 12-1 shows cystlike defects in medial part of distal metaphysis of right femur. A comminuted fracture is in left femur.

Diagnosis: Normal cystlike defects in femur at site of origin of medial head of gastrocnemius muscle.

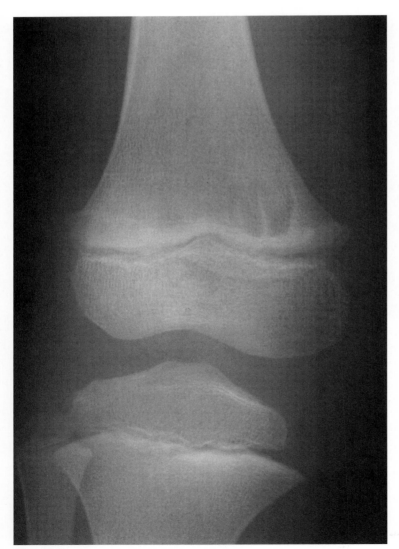

Fig. 12-1

Case 13

A 15-year-old high-school wrestler has had deep, throbbing, and diffuse pain at right knee for 1 month. Pain is slight at rest and worse with exercise such as wrestling and bowling. He has lost 11 kg in the last 3 weeks because of "dieting for a wrestling match." He has had a cough for a week.

Parents and three sisters are well.

Temperature is 37.3°C, heart rate 96, respiratory rate 20, blood pressure 120/80 mm Hg, weight 53 kg, and height 166 cm. Throat is injected. Deep, diffuse tenderness is behind right knee. The rest of the physical findings are normal.

Hemoglobin is 161 g/liter. White cell count is 6.8 × 10⁹/liter with 0.56 polymorphonuclear cells, 0.30 lymphocytes, 0.13 monocytes, and 0.01 eosinophils. ESR is 2 mm/hr. Urine specific gravity is 1.017, pH 7. Urine has occasional squamous epithelial cells/HPF and occasional white cells/HPF.

Medial part of metaphysis of right femur is irregular in frontal and lateral views (Figure 13-1). An exostosis protrudes back from right tibia (Figure 13-1B). Fluoroscopy shows similar irregularity behind left femur when left femur is turned into similar position.

Diagnosis: Normal cortical irregularity near adductor tubercle at site of insertion of adductor magnus muscle.

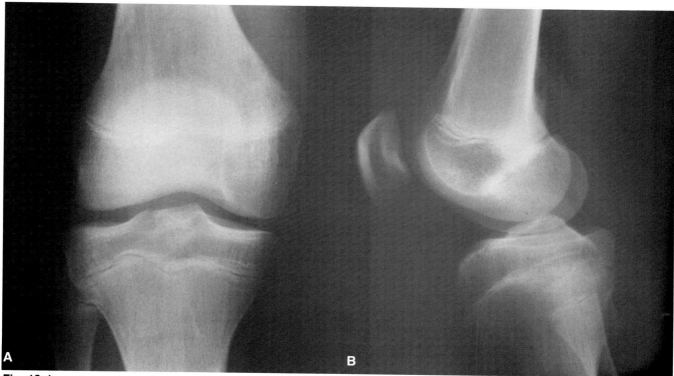

Fig. 13-1

Case 14

A 23-month-old boy is bowlegged and cross-eyed.

Birth weight was 3.0 kg. He rolled over at 2 months and walked at 13 months. He runs and jumps normally. Left eye has occasionally turned out since he was 6 months old.

Mother (19 years old), father (21 years old), and sister (2 years old) are well.

Weight at 23 months is 12.9 kg, height 84 cm, and head circumference 47 cm. Left eye turns out briefly. A systolic murmur is present. External rotation is limited at hips. Legs are bowed. The rest of the physical findings are normal.

Roentgenograms show bowlegs at 2 years (Figure 14-1A), knock-knees at 3 years (Figure 14-1B).

No mention of eye or leg abnormality is made in examinations at 5, 7, and 9 years.

Diagnosis: Normal juvenile bowlegs, normal juvenile knock-knees.

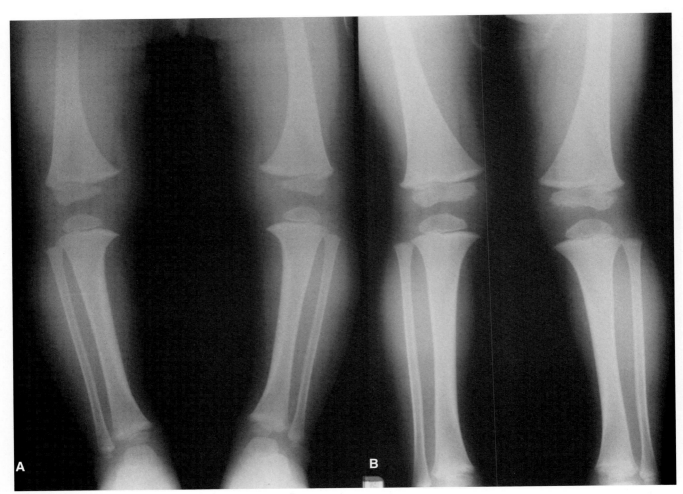

Fig. 14-1

Case 15

A 13-year-old boy has a "sore right knee and a lump." Right knee hurt for the first time 2 years ago. Since then, he has hurt it several times while running, playing ball, or riding his bicycle.

Parents and three brothers are well.

Temperature is 37°C, heart rate 80, respiratory rate 18, blood pressure 106/66 mm Hg, weight 48 kg, and height 160 cm. A hard, nontender lump is on medial aspect of upper part of right tibia. The rest of the physical findings are normal.

Hematocrit is 0.38. White cell count is 6.4×10^9/liter with 0.58 polymorphonuclear cells, 0.05 bands, 0.29 lymphocytes, 0.05 monocytes, and 0.03 eosinophils. Urine specific gravity is 1.015, pH 6. Urine is normal. Serum sodium is 141 mmol/liter, potassium 4.0, chloride 108, carbon dioxide 25, urea nitrogen 3.9, calcium 2.30, phosphorus 1.39, cholesterol 3.20, and glucose 5.3. Creatinine is 70 μmol/liter, uric acid 220, total bilirubin 17, and direct bilirubin 3. Total protein is 64 g/liter, albumin 46. Alkaline phosphatase is 312 U/liter, LDH 284, and SGOT 39.

A defect in back of proximal part of right tibia protrudes medially (Figure 15-1). Sclerotic rim of defect is thicker at diaphyseal than at metaphyseal edge in Figure 15-1.

At operation, yellow-brown cheesy material in defects under cortex of tibia tracks into cancellous bone.

Microscopic examination shows (1) whorls of spindle-shaped fibroblasts infiltrating cortical bone; (2) blood vessels; (3) large deposits of hemosiderin in phagocytes; (4) clumps of multinucleated giant cells; (5) clumps of histiocytes with foamy, vacuolated cytoplasm; (6) new bone surrounded by osteoblasts; (7) foci of capillary bleeding; and (8) an incomplete rim of thick collagen.

Impression: Benign cortical defect.

Surgical and Microscopic Diagnosis: Nonossifying fibroma.

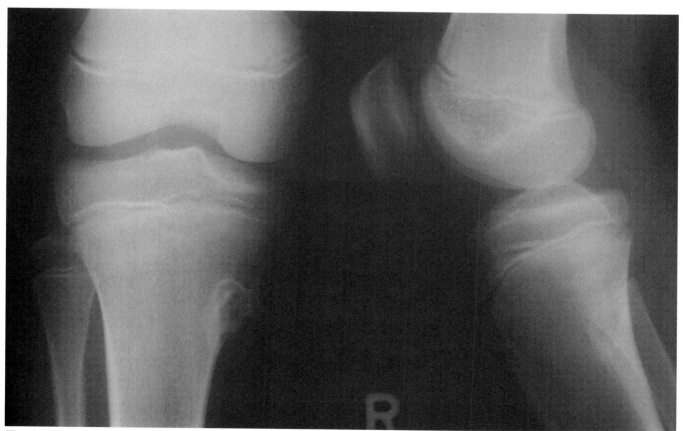

Fig. 15-1

Case 16

An 11⅚-year-old boy, who complains of fatigue, headache, and runny nose but is "otherwise well," also says that after a hard session of soccer his knees hurt until he rests for several hours.

Weight is 45 kg, height 155 cm, and temperature 35.7°C. Medial femoral condyles are tender when knees are flexed. The rest of the physical findings are normal.

Figures 16-1, with knees extended, and 16-2, with knees partly flexed, show medial femoral condyles that are unevenly mineralized along posteromedial aspect.

He continues to play soccer "all the time." He also plays football and skateboards. He has no knee pain. At 13⅓ years, physical and roentgenographic findings are normal.

Diagnosis: Normal knees, normal uneven mineralization of medial femoral condyles.

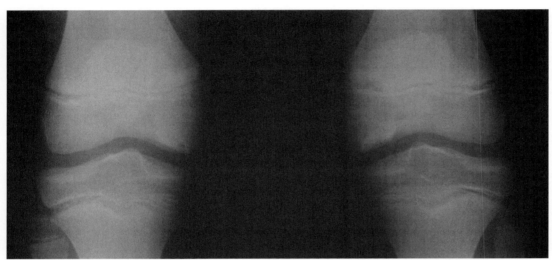

Fig. 16-1

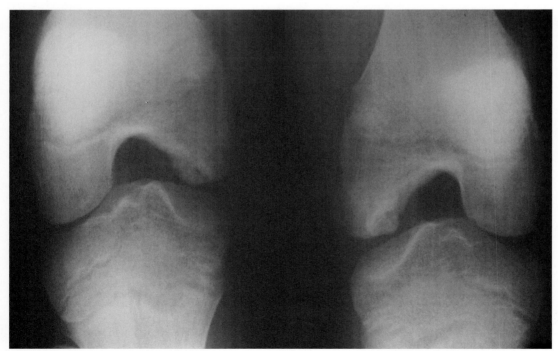

Fig. 16-2

Case 17

A 14-year-old boy's right knee has given way, sometimes painfully, while he is running or walking, one to three times per year for the last 2 years.

Medial condyle of right femur is tender. The rest of the physical findings at knees are normal.

Figure 17-1 shows a curved radiolucent defect with central radiodensity in front part of medial condyle of right femur.

Diagnosis: Osteochondrosis dissecans, right femur.

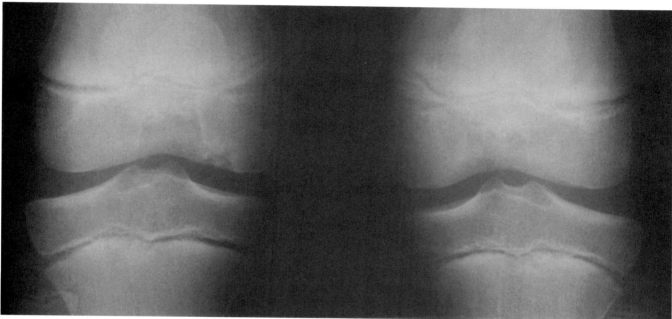

Fig. 17-1

Case 18

An 11-year-old boy has had pain in knees and, less often, in elbows, wrists, and ankles for 1 year. Running and jumping, such as when playing tennis, bring on knee pain that lasts several minutes.

He has 1+ left patellofemoral crepitus. The rest of the findings in examination of arms, legs, and pelvis are normal.

Figure 18-1 shows patellas ossifying from more than one center.

Orthopedic Diagnosis: Chondromalacia patellae.

Roentgenographic Diagnosis: Normal ossification of patellas.

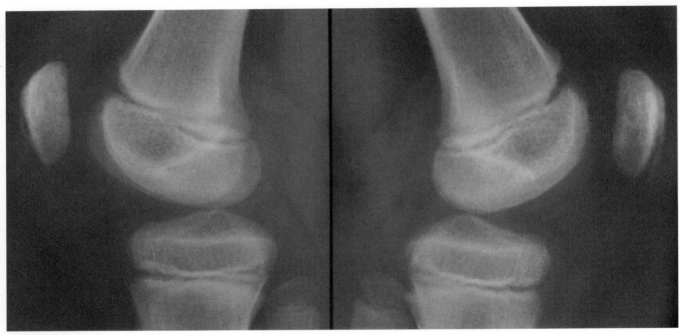

Fig. 18-1

Case 19

A 1-month-old boy has bowlegs.

Mother (19 years old) had bloody vaginal discharge at 6 months and painful contractions during last trimester. She says boy was active but did not change position during last trimester. Birth weight was 2.3 kg, length 43 cm, and head circumference 30 cm.

Parents are well. The boy is their first child. Mother's teeth were yellow and wore down quickly. She now has false teeth. Two first cousins, who are siblings, have Lowe oculocerebrorenal syndrome.

Temperature is 37°C, heart rate 160, respiratory rate 34, length 48 cm, weight 3.1 kg, and head circumference 34 cm. He turns his head toward sounds and follows objects with his eyes. Neck and limbs are stubby, shanks bowed. Movement at hips is limited. The rest of the physical findings are normal.

Hematocrit is 0.38. White cell count is 10.0×10^9/liter with 0.31 polymorphonuclear cells, 0.05 bands, 0.50 lymphocytes, 0.09 monocytes, and 0.03 eosinophils. Urine specific gravity is 1.003, pH 5. Urine is normal. Serum sodium is 143 mmol/liter, potassium 6.9, chloride 99, urea nitrogen 6.0, calcium 2.30, and phosphorus 2.26. Alkaline phosphatase is 236 U/liter.

Humeri, femurs, tibias, and fibulas are laterally convex at 1 month (Figure 19-1).

At 9 months, sclerae are blue. At 6 years, bowing of legs is gone. He has knock-knees. At 9½ years, weight is 25 kg, height 123 cm. At 10 years, he is one of the two best players on his baseball team. Sclerae are blue; teeth are yellow and translucent. The rest of the physical findings are normal.

Ankles are separated when he stands with knees together at 10 years and tibias are slightly laterally convex (Figure 19-2).

His brother, 3 years younger, has similar sclerae and teeth. Brother's legs, bowed at birth, are straight at 8 years.

Diagnosis: Prenatal bowing of limbs; dentinogenesis imperfecta.

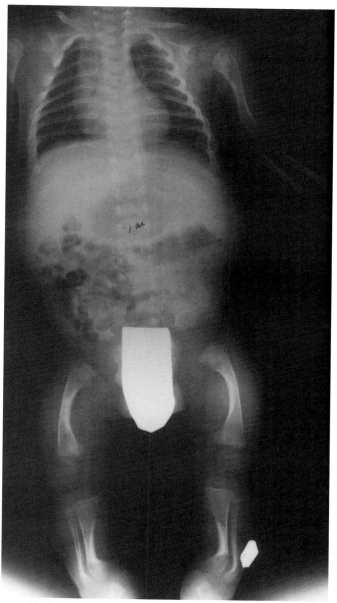

Fig. 19-1

(Continued)

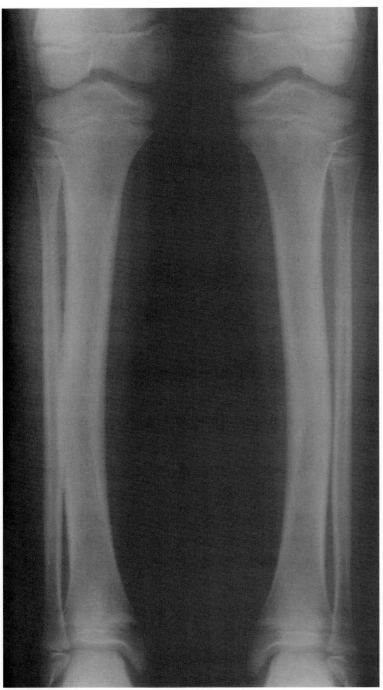

Fig. 19-2

Case 20

An 11-year-old girl had swelling and pain at right ankle after she ran in 400-m race yesterday. She has had recurrent swelling and tenderness at right ankle since she hurt it when she fell from a tree at 6 years.

Circumduction at right ankle is slightly limited. Lateral soft tissues at right ankle are puffy and tender. The rest of the physical findings at the ankles are normal.

Figure 20-1A shows uneven and sclerotic trochlea of right talus and a bone fragment in right ankle above and lateral to

talus. Findings at left ankle are normal (Figure 20-1B). A bone is below (see Figure 20-1) and in front of (Figure 20-2) right medial malleolus.

Diagnosis: Old fracture and aseptic necrosis of right talus; os subtibiale, right.

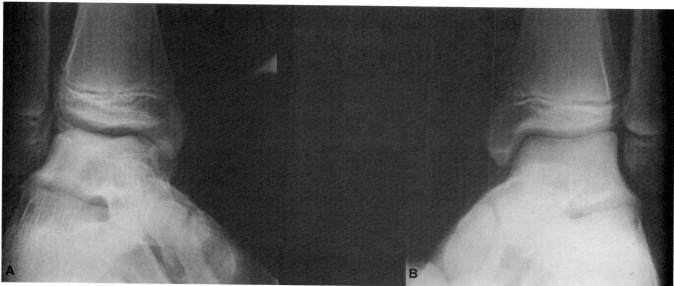

Fig. 20-1

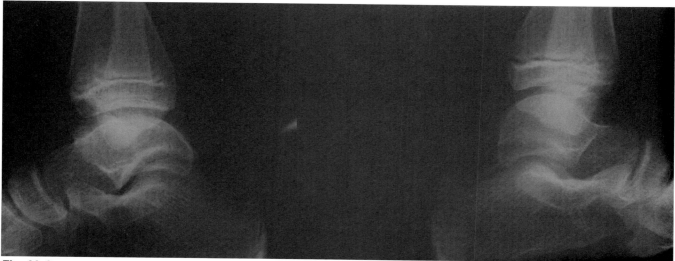

Fig. 20-2

Case 21

A 13-year-old girl has pain across front of left ankle. She twisted it 1½ hours ago when she slid into second base.

Temperature is 37°C, heart rate 68, respiratory rate 14, and blood pressure 100/70 mm Hg. Soft tissues along left lateral malleolus are swollen. The rest of the physical findings are normal.

Roentgenogram shows a small bone beneath epiphysis of right fibula (Figure 21-1A) and swelling along left lateral malleolus (Figure 21-1B).

Diagnosis: Sprain, left ankle; os subfibulare, right ankle.

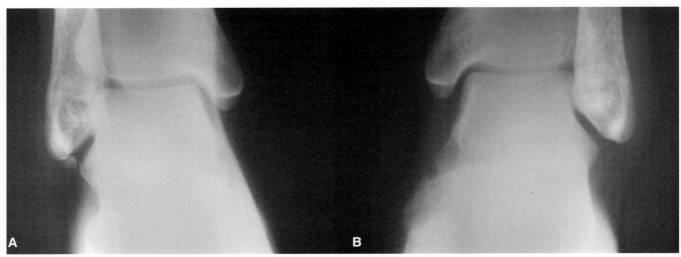

Fig. 21-1

Case 22

A 5⅔-year-old boy has pain in right foot "because of shoes" that were prescribed for him, his mother says.

He limped after jumping from bed 4 months ago. Roentgenographic examination was performed and left foot was in a cast for 6 weeks. He has worn the prescribed shoes since then.

Weight is 28.6 kg, height 125 cm. Midtarsal part of left foot is tender. The rest of the physical findings are normal.

Mother is worried by his limp at 9 years. He is very active and has no pain. Gait is normal. Examination of feet shows normal findings.

Left navicular bone is sclerotic at 5⅔ years (Figure 22-1) and normal at 9 years (Figure 22-2), when calcaneal apophyses are sclerotic.

Diagnosis: Normal feet at 5⅔ years and not Köhler's bone disease; normal feet at 9 years and not Sever's disease.

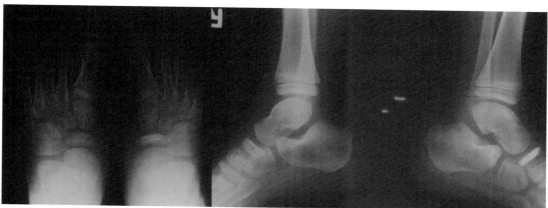

Fig. 22-1

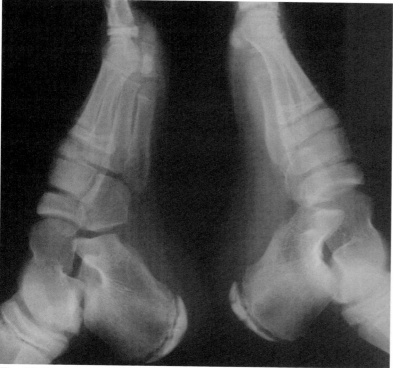

Fig. 22-2

Case 23

A 10-year-old girl has a fever, and pain in right heel that began yesterday while she was playing. She felt hot last night and did not eat much. Temperature was 38.3°C this morning, then 40°C despite taking aspirin. She complains of "sharp" pain and will not bear weight on right heel.

She had otitis media twice in infancy, chickenpox at 3 years, and left leg infection treated with oral antibiotics at 6 years.

Parents and brother (7 years old) are well. Maternal grandmother had breast cancer, maternal grandfather had heart disease, and paternal grandfather had diabetes mellitus.

Temperature is 38.9°C, heart rate 120, respiratory rate 20, blood pressure 104/70 mm Hg, weight 36 kg, and height 142 cm. Pus is on left tonsil. Small lymph nodes are in neck. A soft systolic murmur is present. Right heel is tender along lateral side. The rest of the physical findings are normal. Temperature is 39.5°C the next day. Right heel does not hurt.

Hematocrit is 0.42. White cell count is 2.5×10^9/liter with 0.49 polymorphonuclear cells, 0.02 bands, 0.28 lymphocytes, 0.20 monocytes, and 0.01 basophils. Platelet count is 161×10^9/liter. ESR is 13 mm/hr. Urine specific gravity is 1.007, pH 5. Urine has 3–5 white cells/HPF. Two days later, white cell count is 2.0×10^9/liter with 0.38 polymorphonuclear cells, 0.03 bands, 0.47 lymphocytes, 0.10 monocytes, and 0.02 atypical lymphocytes.

Figure 23-1A shows a cystlike defect in right calcaneum and a bone island in right talus. Roentgenographic findings in left foot are normal (Figure 23-1B).

Throat culture grows normal flora. Monospot test is positive. Serum contains heterophile antibodies.

Diagnosis: Infectious mononucleosis; calcaneal pseudocyst (normal).

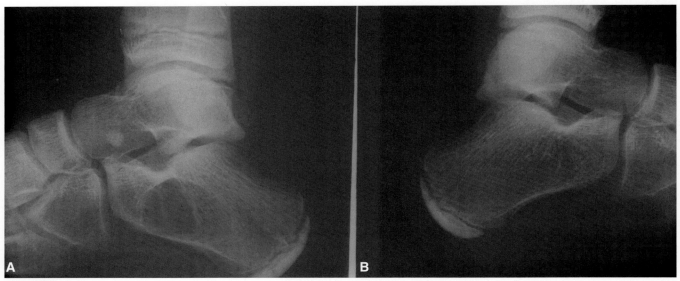

Fig. 23-1

Case 24

A 12¾-year-old boy has pain in right ankle but can bear weight on right foot. Right foot turned in while he was playing basketball today.

Soft tissues are swollen over right lateral malleolus. Inversion of right foot hurts. The rest of the physical findings in right ankle and foot are normal.

A 26-year-old woman cannot bear weight on left foot. She fell while dancing last night and turned left ankle.

Soft tissues are swollen over left lateral malleolus. Left ankle is tender at tibiofibular ligaments and tibiocalcaneal ligament.

Separate fragments of bone are under lateral part of right calcaneum of boy (Figure 24-1A). A knob of bone is under lateral part of left calcaneum of woman (Figure 24-1B).

Diagnosis: Sprained ankle; normal peroneal trochlea, ossifying in boy, ossified in woman.

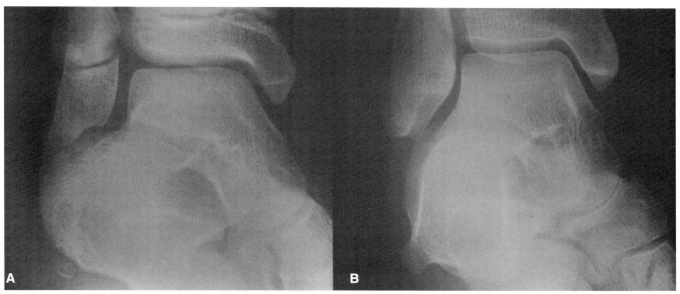

Fig. 24-1

Case 25

A 15-year-old girl, who had cadaver renal transplant 2 years ago, has had pain in feet, right foot more than left, for 2 years. Pain is worse when she walks and has been so for the last several months.

Pregnancy of mother (then 16 years old) was normal, birth weight 3 kg. Proteinuria was found at 2 years. She tired quickly at 8 years, vomited, and had headaches and muscle cramps. Weight was 26.3 kg, height 128 cm, temperature 36.7°C, heart rate 100, respiratory rate 20, and blood pressure 164/108 mm Hg. She was thin and sallow and had periorbital edema, basal rales in lungs, systolic murmur, and large liver.

Hematocrit was 0.24. White cell count was 7.6×10^9/liter with 0.59 polymorphonuclear cells, 0.03 bands, 0.31 lymphocytes, 0.04 monocytes, and 0.03 basophils. Platelet count was 268×10^9/liter. Urine specific gravity was 1.015, pH 6. Urine had >3.0 g/liter protein, occasional squamous epithelial cells/HPF, 4–6 red cells/HPF, and 10–15 white cells/HPF, and was sterile. Serum sodium was 140 mmol/liter, potassium 5.1, chloride 103, urea nitrogen 32.8, calcium 2.02, phosphorus 0.84, glucose 8.8, carbon dioxide 16, and cholesterol 7.71. Creatinine was 950 μmol/liter (2 days later: 940), uric acid 580, total bilirubin 3, and direct bilirubin 2. Total protein was 57 g/liter, albumin 27. Alkaline phosphatase was 166 U/liter, LDH 372, and SGOT 27.

Biopsy of left kidney showed (1) diffuse glomerulosclerosis and hyalinosis, (2) extensive subacute interstitial nephritis,
(3) diffuse segmental deposits of IgM and complement component 3, and (4) moderately severe arteriosclerosis. Continuous ambulatory peritoneal dialysis was begun at 8 years, cadaver renal transplant performed at 13 years.

Examination of feet at 15 years shows (1) redness and tenderness along medial aspect of head of first right metatarsal bone, (2) right hallux valgus 30 degrees, and (3) left hallux valgus 16 degrees.

An ossicle separate from calcaneal anterior articular surface for talus is in transverse tarsal joint of left foot (Figure 25-1A). Another separate ossicle is at proximal dorsal edge of navicular bone in left transverse tarsal joint (Figure 25-1B), and a third separate ossicle is behind posterior process of talus in left foot (Figure 25-2), where all three ossicles are apparent. Right foot lacks separate ossicle at calcaneal anterior articular surface for talus but has the other two.

At 21 years, renal function is stable, weight 77 kg, and blood pressure 140/98 mm Hg. She has headache, papilledema, CSF pressure 250 mm H_2O, glucose 4.0 mmol/liter, protein 0.24 g/liter, and diagnosis of pseudotumor cerebri.

Diagnosis: Bunion at 15 years; os trigonum and os supranaviculare in both feet, calcaneum secondarium in left foot.

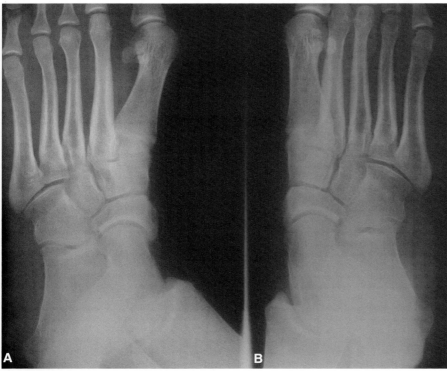

Fig. 25-1

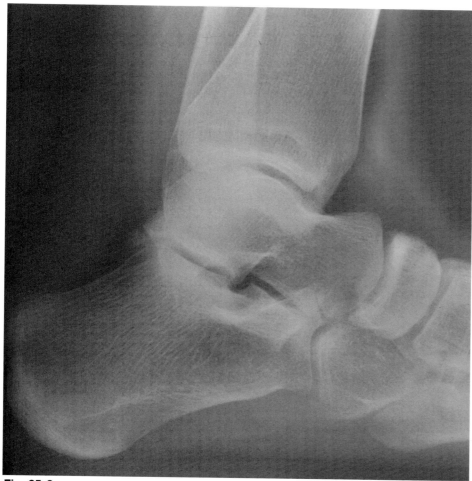

Fig. 25-2

Case 26

A 15-year-old girl has swollen joints.

Grip weakened 7 months ago. Wrists and hands swelled 2 months ago. Knees, ankles, and feet swelled 3 weeks ago. She aches behind eyes when she wakes up. She tires quickly. She has lost 2 kg in the last 1½ weeks.

She had many sore throats in childhood. Myringotomies and removal of tonsils and adenoids were performed at 5 years. She fractured right humerus at 8 years. She hurt left knee and had left knee effusion at 11 years. Menarche was at 12 years. She was found to have slight scoliosis with thoracic right convexity at 13 years. She is allergic to dust and dander.

Parents and twin siblings (girl and boy, 12 years old) are well. Maternal grandmother had cancer; paternal grandfather had asthma.

Temperature at 15 years is 36.6°C, heart rate 64, respiratory rate 18, blood pressure 114/80 mm Hg, weight 57 kg, and height 173 cm. A right rib hump appears when she bends forward. Right elbow is deformed. Left second and fourth fingers are swollen, tender, and not fully extensible. Right Achilles tendon and right first toe are tender. The rest of the physical findings are normal.

Hematocrit is 0.38. White cell count is 4.1×10^9/liter with 0.51 polymorphonuclear cells, 0.10 bands, 0.29 lymphocytes, 0.06 monocytes, and 0.04 eosinophils. Platelet count is 250×10^9/liter. ESR is 50 mm/hr. Urine specific gravity is 1.012, pH 5. Urine has moderate squamous epithelial cells/HPF and occasional white cells/HPF. Serum sodium is 139 mmol/liter, potassium 5.1, chloride 102, carbon dioxide 25, urea nitrogen 3.6, calcium 2.45, phosphorus 1.52, cholesterol 3.15, and glucose 5.1. Creatinine is 50 μmol/liter, uric acid 260, total bilirubin 21, and direct bilirubin 3. Total protein is 87 g/liter, albumin 41. Alkaline phosphatase is 80 U/liter, LDH 214, and SGOT 14. Complement component 3 is 1.0 g/liter (normal: 1.412 ± 0.149), complement component 4 0.10 (normal: 0.12–0.36). Serum is positive for antinuclear antibody and anti-DNA.

A separate ossicle is medial to each navicular bone (Figure 26-1), another under each cuboid bone (Figure 26-2).

She is treated with corticosteroids and able to do farm chores until 25 years, when she has cough, shortness of breath, and "burning" in her chest. She can walk only 10 steps before she feels light-headed during a trip to the mountains. She faints occasionally. Weight is 79 kg at 26 years, height 173 cm, temperature 36.7°C, heart rate 74, respiratory rate 22, and blood pressure 114/82 mm Hg. She has large heart, sternal heave, and gallop rhythm. Scintiscan shows patchy lung perfusion. At catheterization, pulmonary artery pressure is 106/57 mm Hg, mean 74, and wedge 8. She dies at 27 years.

Diagnosis: Normal bilateral os tibiale externum (insertion of posterior tibial tendon) and os peroneum (peroneus longus tendon under cuboid) in 15-year-old girl with lupus erythematosus who dies at 27 years with pulmonary hypertension.

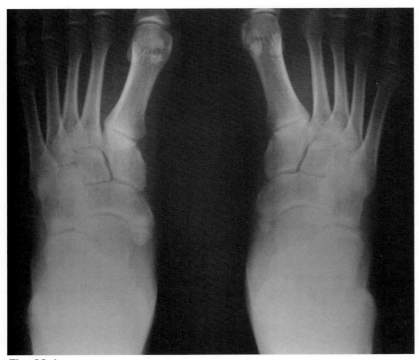

Fig. 26-1

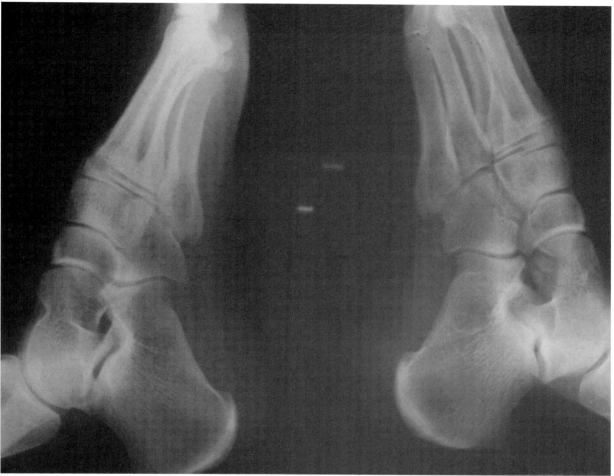

Fig. 26-2

Case 27

A 12-year-old boy has pain in left elbow.

Swelling and redness of left thumb 6 weeks ago were followed several days later (despite antibiotic treatment) by a red streak along front of left arm, discharge of pus from thumb, and redness and swelling of tip of left third finger. He also had right lower quadrant pain and findings of normal appendix and mesentery at appendectomy 1 month ago, swelling and redness of left first toe 3 weeks ago, fever and headache during last week, and pain in left elbow yesterday.

Pregnancy was normal, birth weight 3.6 kg. A dermoid cyst (1 cm), unchanged since birth, was removed from left brow at 6 months. He walked at 10 months. He likes to play football.

Mother (32 years old), father (35 years old), and sister (9 years old) are well.

Temperature is 38.8°C, heart rate 104, respiratory rate 16, blood pressure 120/80 mm Hg, weight 32.8 kg, and height 142 cm. Left elbow is tender and hurts when flexed more than 90 degrees. Left thumb and left first toe are purplish along medial side. Suprasternal thrill, ejection click, systolic murmur, and diastolic murmur are present. The rest of the physical findings are normal.

Hematocrit is 0.36. White cell count is 9.0×10^9/liter with 0.48 polymorphonuclear cells, 0.03 bands, 0.36 lymphocytes, 0.11 monocytes, and 0.02 eosinophils. Platelet count is 305×10^9/liter. ESR is 50 mm/hr. Urine specific gravity is 1.028, pH 5.5. Urine is normal. Serum sodium is 137 mmol/liter, potassium 5.1, chloride 101, carbon dioxide 23, urea nitrogen 4.6, calcium 2.40, phosphorus 1.42, cholesterol 4.50, and glucose 4.7. Creatinine is 70 μmol/liter, uric acid 140, total bilirubin 5, and direct bilirubin 0. Total protein is 69 g/liter, albumin 39. Alkaline phosphatase is 165 U/liter, LDH 187, and SGOT 17.

Figure 27-1 shows metatarsal bones with distal epiphyseal ossification centers and some, besides first, with what look like proximal epiphyseal ossification centers.

Streptococcus mutans grows in blood culture.

He dies 1 month later of transtentorial herniation of brain. Necropsy also shows bicuspid aortic valve with vegetations on ventricular surface that show focal necrosis in microscopic examination.

Diagnosis: Bicuspid aortic valve, bacterial endocarditis, normal metatarsal pseudoepiphyses.

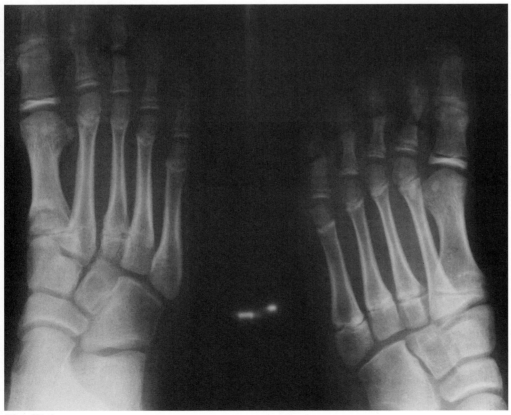

Fig. 27-1

Case 28

A 15-year-old girl, who tripped going upstairs 2 hours ago, cannot walk on right foot.

Temperature is 36.2°C, heart rate 96, respiratory rate 16, and blood pressure 120/80 mm Hg. Dorsum of right foot is tender, bruised, and swollen. Passive movement of right toes hurts. The rest of the physical findings in feet are normal.

Figure 28-1 shows a small piece of bone between proximal part of first and second metatarsal bones in each foot.

Diagnosis: Intermetatarsal bones.

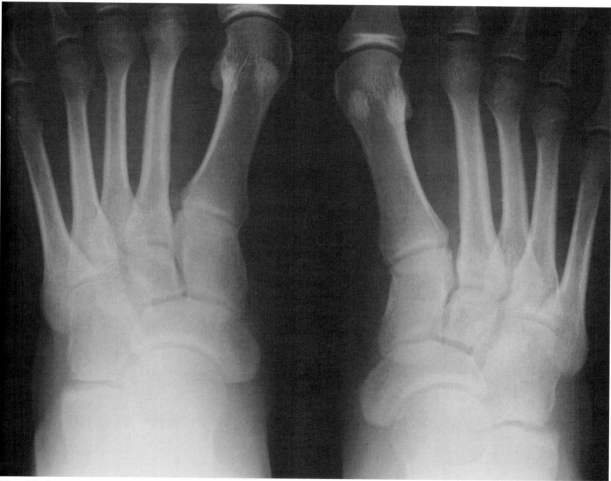

Fig. 28-1

Skeletal Dysplasia

Case 1

A newborn girl is blue and apneic. She was delivered by cesarean section for slow heart rate.

Mother (36 years old), father (41 years old), and 10 siblings are well. One sibling died in infancy.

Birth weight is 1.6 kg, Apgar score 2/3 at 1 and 5 minutes. Treatment with endotracheal tube and oxygen is begun immediately. Head is soft, without palpable fontanels or sutures, and large relative to trunk and limbs. Respirations are irregular at 10 minutes; breath sounds are diminished and rattly. Limbs are short and misshapen. Moro's reflex is absent. The rest of the physical findings are normal.

Figure 1-1A shows small, irregular plaques of bone in calvaria. Figure 1-1B shows knobby and corrugated clavicles, ribs, and bones of limbs, and possibly left scapula; and flat vertebrae, especially T7.

She dies soon after birth.

Diagnosis: Mosaic rarefaction in calvaria, fractures in skeleton; osteogenesis imperfecta.

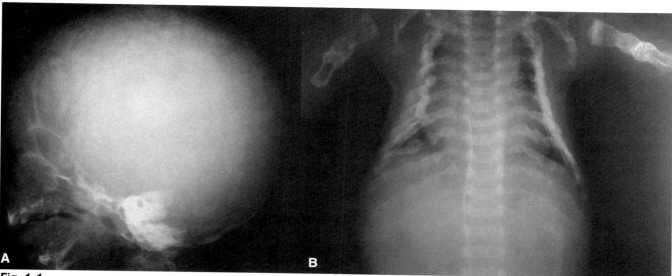

Fig. 1-1

Case 2

A 10-month-old boy breathes noisily. "His eyes roll up most of the time he's awake, and he won't turn his head" to loud sounds.

Mother (21 years old) used illegal drugs and alcohol during pregnancy and had needle marks on legs at labor. Birth weight was 3.2 kg. Blood cysts were on gums, petechiae on body. Platelet count was 38×10^9/liter. Serologic tests for prenatal infection were negative. Blood cysts were on gums at 1 month. Weight was 5 kg at 4½ months. Head was large. Eardrums were dull. Nose was stuffy. Eyes wandered. Pupils (4 mm) barely contracted in bright light. Discs were white, their size normal. His only movement when prone at 8 months was turning of head. Muscle tone was increased. Reflexes were those of a newborn infant.

Weight at 10 months is 6.2 kg, length 68 cm, head circumference 46 cm, temperature 37.8°C, heart rate 156, respiratory rate 48, and systolic blood pressure 96 mm Hg. Face is without expression. He rolls from front to back but cannot sit. Scabs and dry pustules are on body. Anterior fontanel bulges. Eyes wander. Discs are small and pale. Nose is stuffy. Left eardrum is dull red; right eardrum cannot be seen. He retracts during inspiration. Liver edge is 2 cm below costal margin. Knees are large. Back is stiff. Muscle tone is increased. The rest of the physical findings are normal.

Hematocrit is 0.28. Hemoglobin is 92 g/liter. Red blood cell count is 3.3×10^{12}/liter. MCV is 83 fl. MCH is 28 pg. MCHC is 330 g/liter. Red-blood-cell distribution width is 24.0 (normal: 11.5–15.0). White cell count is 7.9×10^9/liter with 0.27 polymorphonuclear cells, 0.11 bands, 0.27 lymphocytes, 0.16 monocytes, 0.16 eosinophils, and 0.03 myelocytes. Platelet estimate is normal. Serum sodium is 142 mmol/liter, potassium 4.2, chloride 104, carbon dioxide 29, urea nitrogen 3.6, calcium 2.17, phosphorus 1.16, cholesterol 3.96, and glucose 5.6. Creatinine is 30 µmol/liter, uric acid 330, total bilirubin 3, and direct bilirubin 0. Total protein is 62 g/liter, albumin 41. Alkaline phosphatase is 153 U/liter, LDH 295, and SGOT 24.

Roentgenogram shows sclerotic bones, including base of skull (Figure 2-1), and expanded metaphyses (Figure 2-2) that contain lucent and sclerotic bands. Tarsal bones have sclerotic center and less sclerotic rim (see Figure 2-2), as do some vertebral bodies. Vertebral nutrient canals are tall, deep wedges. CT scan in Figure 2-3 shows dilated ventricles, deep sulci, and excess subdural liquid.

Biopsy of cores of bone from iliac crest shows (1) translucent white tissue made up of thick spicules of interlacing bone with nucleated cells in the bone, (2) small islands of hematopoiesis, (3) a focus of enchondral ossification with a zone of proliferating cartilage, and (4) no osteoclasts.

Diagnosis: Osteopetrosis, hydrocephalus, scabies.

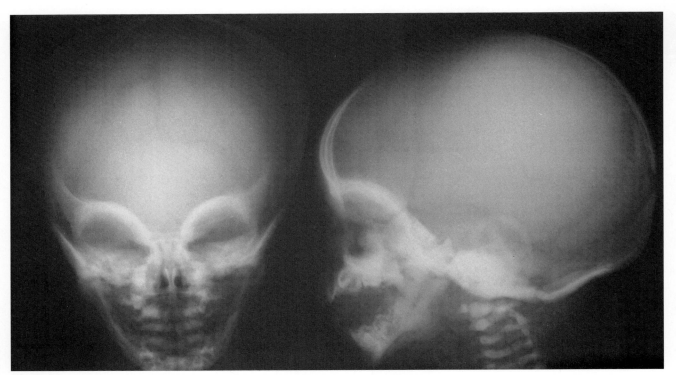

Fig. 2-1

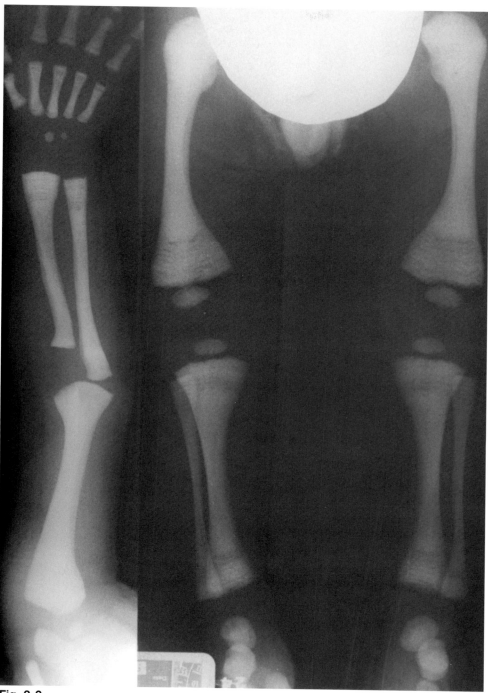

Fig. 2-2

(Continued)

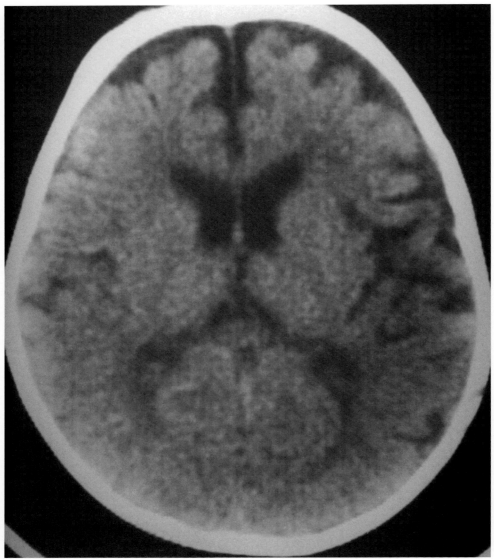

Fig. 2-3

Case 3

A 14-year-old dwarf girl, who has felt tired for 1 month, has had a cough and stabbing pain in right side of chest for 2 weeks.

Birth weight was 3.6 kg, length 53 cm. She was weak at 1 year. Growth slowed. Appetite was bad. Hair fell out at 2 years. She was cross-eyed; eyes were operated on at 4 years. Postoperative infection caused blindness in right eye. She has had measles and chickenpox. She broke tibia and fibula 2 years ago when she fell from a bicycle. She bruises easily. She wears a wig. She is an A student who keeps up with 3 normal teenage sisters and resents being treated like a child.

Mother (38 years old), father (36 years old), and three sisters are well. Paternal aunt and maternal aunt have cancer; two maternal great-aunts died with cancer. Paternal great-uncle died with a stroke.

Weight at 14 years is 13 kg, height 112 cm, temperature 37.6°C, heart rate 144, respiratory rate 28, and blood pressure 110/64 mm Hg. Skin is thin, wrinkled, and spotted brown. Scalp veins are prominent. Anterior fontanel is open. Right eye is small and opaque. Face looks too small for head. Nose is thin. Earlobes are absent. Lips are thin. Chin is small. Teeth are crooked. Small lymph nodes are in neck. She has no breast tissue. A 10-cm bulge is below right scapula. Spine is convex left. Breath sounds are tubular and diminished and inspiratory rales are on right side. Liver edge is 4–5 cm below costal margin. Limbs are bony and weak. Fingers, toes, and nails are short. Genitalia are prepubertal. The rest of the physical findings are normal.

Hematocrit is 0.39. White cell count is 6.2×10^9/liter with 0.20 polymorphonuclear cells, 0.14 bands, 0.53 lymphocytes, 0.07 monocytes, 0.05 eosinophils, and 0.01 basophils. Platelet estimate is adequate. Reticulocyte fraction is 11×10^{-3}. ESR is 33 mm/hr. Urine specific gravity is 1.020, pH 6. Urine has few epithelial cells/HPF, calcium oxalate crystals, and mucus. Serum carbon dioxide is 21 mmol/liter, cholesterol 3.54, triglycerides 1.52, and phosphorus 1.78. Uric acid is 160 μmol/liter, total bilirubin 3, and direct bilirubin 0. Total protein is 76 g/liter, albumin 44. Alkaline phosphatase is 68 U/liter, LDH 234, and SGOT 14. PT is 11.8 seconds, PTT 31.1.

Figure 3-1A shows open cranial sutures. Figure 3-1B shows calcified pineal gland. Figure 3-2 shows a mass of calcium and water density in right side of chest, spine concave right, thin clavicles and ribs, and fractured right seventh rib. Vertebral ring apophyses are ossifying; anterior edge of L1 and L2 is concave. A wedge of calcium density is in aorta at level of T12. Neck-shaft angle of femurs is almost 180 degrees. Fingers, especially distal phalanges, are short; body, tuberosity, and head of distal phalanges of first and second digits are absent; and growth plates are closed in hands, open in radius and ulna (Figure 3-3).

At right thoracotomy, a posterolateral mass that involves 5 ribs is stuck to lung and diaphragm. Mass and part of right upper lobe are removed.

Surface of mass is white to ivory to tan. Cut section shows yellow bone, gray-red cartilage, and yellow-gray fibrous tissue flecked with calcification. Microscopic examination shows (1) cartilage cells in lacunae; (2) packed spindle cells separated by amorphous eosinophilic matter; (3) endothelium-lined spaces of different sizes; (4) foci of calcification; and (5) pleomorphic, hyperchromatic cells of different sizes with vacuolated eosinophilic cytoplasm and different sized hyperchromatic nuclei that contain clumped chromatin and occasionally prominent nucleolus. Electron microscopy shows spindle-shaped cells that contain (1) distended cisternae of endoplasmic reticulum, (2) lipid droplets, (3) well-developed Golgi apparatus, (4) round or irregular nuclei, and (5) prominent nucleoli in a matrix of fine collagen fibrils and amorphous ground substance.

She dies at 15 years, 2 months. Necropsy shows (1) almost no subcutaneous or mesenteric fat; (2) atherosclerotic narrowing of first 2 cm of left coronary artery; and (3) atheromatous plaques on a mitral cusp, in sinuses of Valsalva, in aorta at ligamentum arteriosum, at superior mesenteric artery, and at bifurcation. Atelectasis and changes of irradiation are in right lung; viral and bacterial inflammatory changes are in left lung. An increased number of corpora amylacea are in some brain sections.

Diagnosis: Progeria, chondrosarcoma or osteosarcoma, acro-osteolysis.

(Continued)

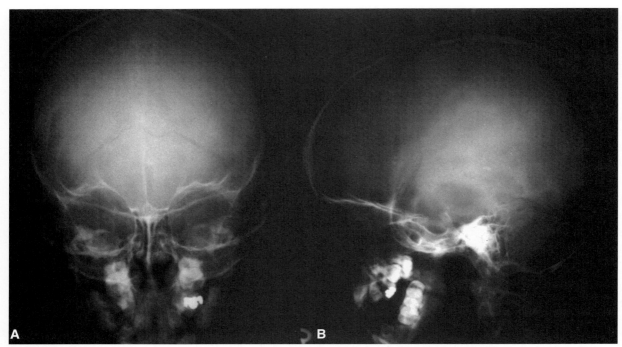

Fig. 3-1

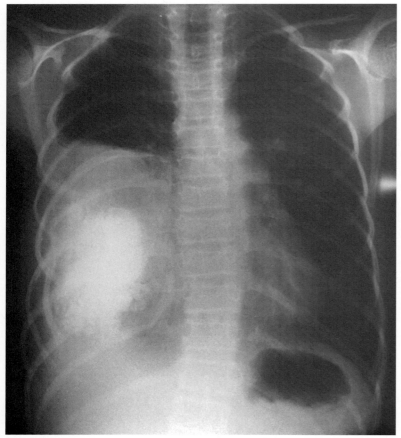

Fig. 3-2

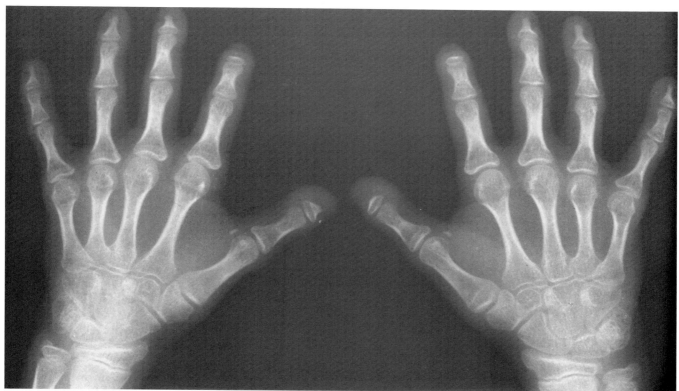

Fig. 3-3

Case 4

Roentgenograms of an adult for whom no clinical information can be had show acro-osteolysis in hands and feet and short metatarsal bones, especially fourth (Figure 4-1), and open calvarial sutures and absent angles of mandible (Figure 4-2).

Diagnosis: Pyknodysostosis.

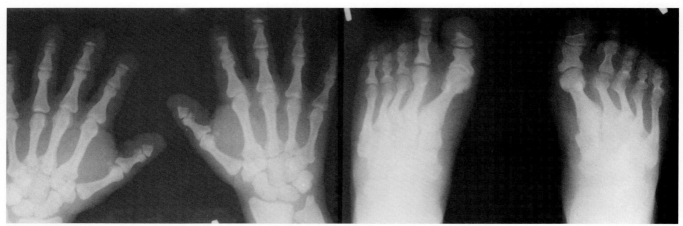

Fig. 4-1

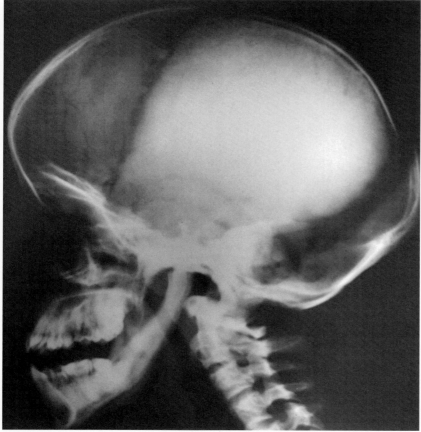

Fig. 4-2

Case 5

A 16-year-old girl and her 13-year-old brother look older than their ages and are dwarfed, mentally retarded, and clumsy. They also "sunburn earlier in spring than anyone else."

Pregnancies were normal. The girl weighed 2.8 kg at birth, sat at 6 months, walked at 1 year, and talked at 2 years. She walked with stiff legs, head and body bent forward as if "trying to catch up with herself." Her forehead and backs of hands and feet were burned at 27 months in a house fire in which a 5-year-old sister died. Growth slowed. She did not run; she did not squat. She fell a lot. She failed first grade. Arms were too stiff for her to wash her back at 6 years. Hands trembled. Ophthalmologic findings were normal. Menarche was at 10 years. Feet were operated on several times for cavus and equinovarus deformity between 10 and 16 years. Ability to learn leveled at 14 years when she was in the fourth grade.

The boy weighed 3.3 kg at birth, sat at 8 months, crawled at 11 months, and walked at 15 months. He bent forward and feet slapped the ground when he walked. He did not run; he did not squat. He fell a lot. Clumsiness increased until he was 7 years old. At 7 years, right heel cord lengthening was performed. Weight was 9.5 kg at 2½ years, 12 kg at 9½ years. Height was 102 cm at 9½ years.

Mother, father, and two sisters (1 and 9 years old) are well. Father has mild to moderate sensorineural hearing loss. He and 16-year-old daughter, but none of the other members of the family, have type IV hyperlipoproteinemia.

The girl's height at 16 years is 114 cm, weight 22 kg, temperature 37.1°C, heart rate 84, respiratory rate 22, blood pressure 115/80 mm Hg, head circumference 45 cm, and IQ 56. Skin is mottled. Forehead and backs of hands and feet are scarred from burns. Thumbs and left third digit are the only fingernails that have regrown since the fire. Face is birdlike. Eyes are deep. Visual acuity is 20/80 OU. Punctate opacities are in lenses, clumped pigment is in maculae and retinal periphery, and discs are pale and cupped. Voice is high, speech halting. Teeth are crowded. Muscles are small, deep tendon reflexes weak. Babinski's sign is in feet. Operative scars and little movement are at ankles and feet. The rest of the physical findings are normal.

The boy's height at 13 years is 105 cm, weight 13.6 kg, temperature 37.4°C, heart rate 82, respiratory rate 20, blood pressure 90/56 mm Hg, and IQ 58. He is ataxic with hand tremor and Romberg's sign. Skin is mottled. Face is thin, skin tight and scaly. Vision is 20/200 OU. Opacities are in lenses. Anterior chambers are shallow, maculae are degenerated, and discs are cupped and pale. He is nearly deaf. Right testis (2

cm) is in scrotum; left is not. Thin limbs look too long for trunk. Feet are cavus. An operative scar is at right ankle. Deep tendon reflexes are brisk. Babinski's sign is in feet. The rest of the physical findings are normal. Head circumference is 45 cm at 18 years.

The girl's hematocrit is 0.44. White cell count is 6 × 10⁹/liter. Urine specific gravity is 1.024, pH 6.5. Urine has 1+ white cells/HPF, 2+ epithelial cells/HPF, and few bacteria. Serum sodium is 137 mmol/liter, potassium 4.0, chloride 103, carbon dioxide 30, urea nitrogen 4.6, calcium 2.94, phosphorus 1.10, and cholesterol 5.77. Total protein is 76 g/liter, albumin 49. The boy's hematocrit is 0.49. White cell count is 7.9 × 10⁹/liter. Urine specific gravity is 1.022, pH 6. Urine has 1+ white cells/HPF, occasional epithelial cells/HPF, and few bacteria. Serum sodium is 137 mmol/liter, potassium 4.4, chloride 101, carbon dioxide 28, urea nitrogen 7.5, calcium 2.79, and phosphorus 1.26. Total protein is 76 g/liter, albumin 53.

Boy's skull is small. Symmetric deposits of calcium density are in basal ganglia of boy at 13 years (Figure 5-1), in those of girl at 16 years. Deposits are more dense in boy's brain at 24 years (Figure 5-2). Boy's iliac wings lack normal flare at 13 years (Figure 5-3A). At 24 years, his vertebral bodies are slightly flat, and T12–L1 and L1–L2 intervertebral discs are partly calcified (Figure 5-3B).

Biopsy of forearm skin of both children shows normal histologic findings. The boy's chromosomes show increased aneuploidy, increased polyploidy, and increased breakage in fibroblast culture, consistent with premature senescence at 19 years. At 27 years, he uses a walker, is deaf, is almost blind, cannot feed himself, and wears a coat even on hot days. Blood pressure is 130/110 mm Hg. Peripheral pulses are not palpable. Deep tendon reflexes are absent. Serum cholesterol is 6.05 mmol/liter, triglycerides 3.27. He dies at 30 years.

The girl is wrinkled and deaf at 25 years and dies at 28 years. Her necropsy shows (1) few but not excessive plaques in aorta, (2) infantile internal genitalia, (3) patchy bronchopneumonia, (4) a few bloody spots in dura, (5) thickened pia-arachnoid, (6) thin cerebral gyri, (7) wide sulci, and (8) dilated ventricles. Lentiform and dentate nuclei are gritty. White matter looks like cottage cheese. Microscopic examination with hematoxylin-and-eosin stain shows dark blue granules that do not stain for iron with Prussian blue in basal ganglia, granular layer, and subcortical folia of cerebellum.

Diagnosis: Cockayne's syndrome.

(Continued)

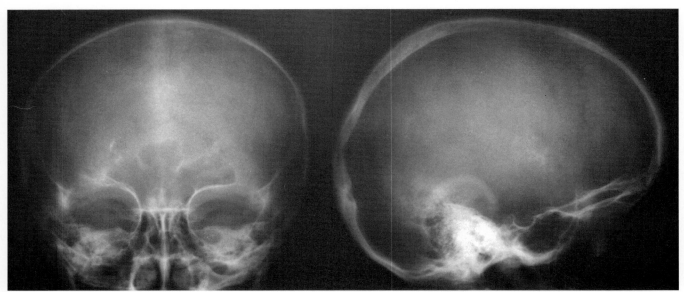

Fig. 5-1

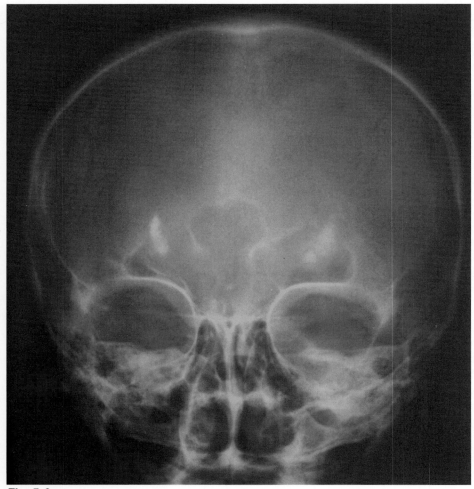

Fig. 5-2

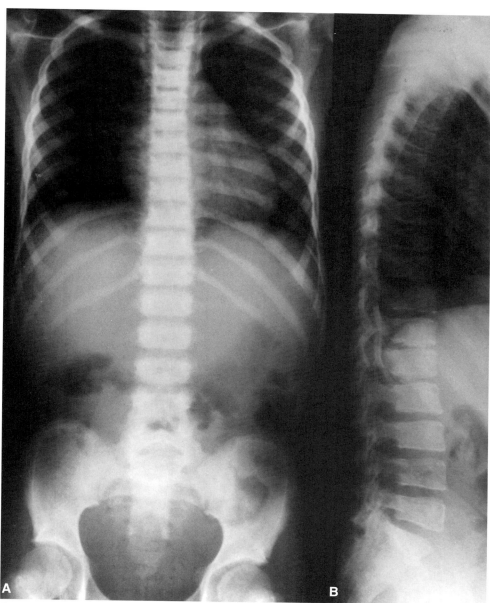

Fig. 5-3

Case 6

A 26-month-old boy (one of twins) has a short, flail left thumb.

Pregnancy was normal, his birth weight 2.2 kg, length 44 cm, and twin brother's weight 3.0 kg. He sat at 6 months, walked at 21 months. He has had ear infections. Ear tubes were placed at 21 months.

Mother (34 years old), father (32 years old), brother (3 years old), and twin brother are well.

Weight at 26 months is 8.2 kg, height 76 cm, head circumference 47 cm, temperature 36°C, heart rate 128, respiratory rate 32, and blood pressure 74/41 mm Hg. His skin, originally fair, is now more tan than twin's. Hair is blond and sparse. Eyes are widely spaced, auricles small and folded. Nasal bridge is wide, tip up. Mandible is small. Teeth are crowded. Supination and extension of right elbow are limited. Left thumb is fleshy, right thumb short, little finger of both hands curved inward. He walks bowlegged. The rest of the physical findings are normal.

Hematocrit is 0.39. White cell count is 8.4×10^9/liter with 0.43 polymorphonuclear cells, 0.47 lymphocytes, 0.08 monocytes, 0.01 eosinophils, and 0.01 basophils. Platelet count is 463×10^9/liter. Serum sodium is 139 mmol/liter, potassium 4.6, chloride 108, carbon dioxide 22, urea nitrogen 6.8, calcium 2.52, phosphorus 1.91, cholesterol 4.24, and glucose 5.4. Creatinine is 50 µmol/liter, uric acid 150, total bilirubin 3, and direct bilirubin 0. Total protein is 69 g/liter, albumin 48. Alkaline phosphatase is 279 U/liter, LDH 308, and SGOT 42. Chromosomes are 46,XY.

Left second digit is pollicized at operation. Hair does not grow as fast as twin's. Brows and lashes are thin at 3½ years, medial lower lashes absent. Skin of face is blotchy, forehead high, philtrum flat, and mandible small. Lids are puffy, auricles folded, and patellas absent. Cheeks, auricles, hands, and buttocks are mottled with telangiectases at 5 years. Height at 8 years is 116 cm, twin's height 124 cm. Hair is blond and thin. Brows and lashes are almost absent.

Figure 6-1A shows corner defects in metaphyses at right knee and distal metaphysis of left femur at 26 months. Distal metaphysis of right ulna shows similar defects. Bones of forearms are too short at 8 years. At 8 years, Figure 6-1B shows (1) hypoplastic middle phalanges of right second and fifth fingers, (2) right ulna that is longer than radius at wrist, (3) delayed and abnormal carpal ossification, (4) fused capitate and trapezoid bones, and (5) trapezium bone, which normally appears before trapezoid, absent or fused to trapezoid. Left middle second and fifth phalanges and patellas are not ossified at 8 years.

Diagnosis: Rothmund-Thomson syndrome.

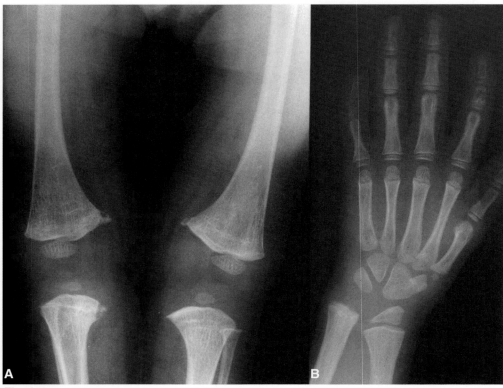

Fig. 6-1

Case 7

A 2-day-old girl has limited extension of limbs and long fingers and toes that are flexed and hard to straighten.

Mother (32 years old), father (33 years old), sister (6 years old), and brother (4 years old) are well.

Pregnancy was normal, birth weight 3.1 kg, length 53 cm, head circumference 34 cm, and Apgar score 8/9 at 1 and 5 minutes.

Temperature at 2 days is 36.6°C, heart rate 130, respiratory rate 50, and blood pressure 79/62 mm Hg. Nose is pushed to the right. Limbs are flexed. Extension is limited. The rest of the physical findings are normal.

Hematocrit is 0.53. White cell count is 17.7×10^9/liter with 0.44 polymorphonuclear cells, 0.02 bands, 0.39 lymphocytes, 0.14 monocytes, and 0.01 eosinophils. Platelet count is 315×10^9/liter. Urine specific gravity is 1.025, pH 5. Urine has 0.30 g/liter protein, 0.2 AU urobilinogen, moderate bacteria, few nonsquamous epithelial cells/HPF, and moderate squamous cells/HPF. Serum sodium is 141 mmol/liter, potassium 4.7, chloride 102, carbon dioxide 20, urea nitrogen 5.7, calcium 2.62, phosphorus 2.45, cholesterol 1.76, and glucose 5.7. Creatinine is 50 μmol/liter, uric acid 320, total bilirubin 113, and direct bilirubin 5. Total protein is 57 g/liter, albumin 39. Alkaline phosphatase is 126 U/liter, LDH 410, and SGOT 50.

Figure 7-1 shows long metacarpals and phalanges. Metatarsals are also long.

At 4 days, a systolic heart murmur is present. Echocardiography shows redundant atrioventricular valves and mitral and aortic regurgitation. At 5 days, lenses are displaced upward. At 45 days, a holosystolic heart murmur is present. Heart rate is 90. Liver edge is 2 cm below costal margin. At 5 months, she is fussy and breathing hard. She does not have enough energy to nipple. Heart rate is 180, respiratory rate 40, and blood pressure 131/95 mm Hg. A holosystolic murmur is present. Liver edge is 4–5 cm below costal margin.

At operation at 5 months, right atrium and annulus fibrosis of atrioventricular valves are dilated. Left ventricular papillary muscles and chordae are long. Posterior cusp of mitral valve is herniated and flail. Mitral valve is replaced with a prosthetic valve, and tricuspid annuloplasty is performed. She is treated with warfarin. At 17 months, she vomits for 2 days. Right arm and right leg twitch. She is unresponsive. Heart rate is 170, pulse thready. Hematocrit is 0.20. PT is 20 seconds, PTT 32.

At 17 months, parenchymal and old and new subdural blood are on left side (Figure 7-2A). Patency of temporal horn of right lateral ventricle, compression of left, and indentation in left side of interpeduncular cistern (Figure 7-2B) result from herniation of uncus of left temporal lobe into incisura of tentorium cerebelli.

Diagnosis: Neonatal Marfan syndrome; uncal herniation.

(Continued)

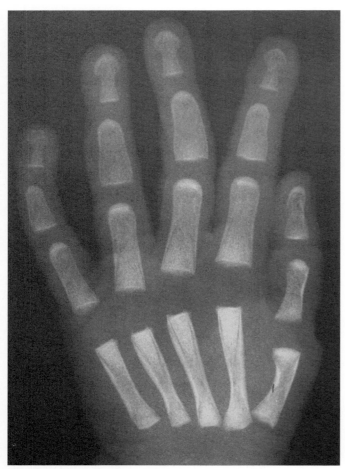

Fig. 7-1

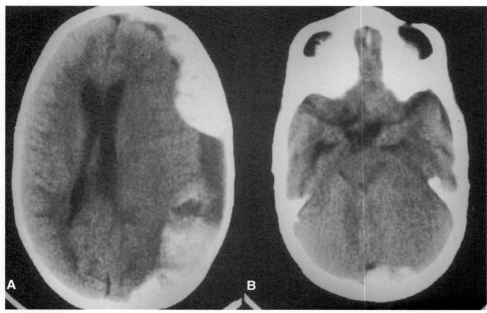

Fig. 7-2

Case 8

A newborn boy has short upper arms and flexed arms and legs.

Mother (16 years old) and father (19 years old) are well. Two siblings of mother died in infancy, one with meningitis, the other with heart disease. Maternal grandmother has had six miscarriages.

Birth weight is 2.6 kg, length 46 cm, head circumference 32 cm, Apgar score 7/7 at 1 and 5 minutes, temperature 37.1°C, heart rate 148, respiratory rate 52, and systolic blood pressure 80 mm Hg. Cry is high pitched. Ends of fingers and toes are blue. Movement at shoulders is limited. Elbows extend 30 degrees. Hands are pronated. Hips are flexed. Femurs abduct 60 degrees. Knees are flexed 90 degrees. Feet are supinated. Testes are not palpable. The rest of the physical findings are normal.

Hematocrit is 0.62. White cell count is 11.3×10^9/liter with 0.17 polymorphonuclear cells, 0.20 bands, 0.53 lymphocytes, 0.07 monocytes, and 0.03 eosinophils. Platelet estimate is adequate. Urine specific gravity is 1.007, pH 5. Urine has 4+ hemoglobin, 60–70 red blood cells/HPF, and rare squamous epithelial cells/HPF. Serum sodium is 129 mmol/liter, potassium 6.5, chloride 98, carbon dioxide 15, calcium 2.50, phosphorus 1.94, urea nitrogen 5.0, and glucose 4.2.

Figure 8-1 shows short humeri, deposits of calcium in and near shoulders, elbows, hips, and knees and in soft tissue of wrist and heel at 2 days. Figure 8-2 shows coronal clefts in thoracic vertebrae. Similar deposits of calcium are in arms and legs at 1 year. Femurs are displaced laterally from acetabulums. Figure 8-3 shows (1) flat and pointed vertebral bodies in neck at 20 months, (2) calcium in corniculate and arytenoid cartilage and in C5–C6 intervertebral disc, and (3) flecks of calcium and little bone in manubrium.

At 2 weeks, corneas are cloudy. A systolic heart murmur is present. Cataracts are present at 4 months, removed at 8 months. He has ear infections. Neck is stiff. At 1 year, he has right optic atrophy. At 20 months, he does not sit or crawl. At 23 months, length is 58 cm, head circumference 39 cm, and weight 5 kg. He has poor head control. He can roll front to back. Left eardrum cannot be seen because external acoustic meatus is too narrow. Nasal bridge is flat. Systolic murmur and diastolic murmur are present, as are inguinal hernias. Testes are not in scrotum. Arms and legs are flexed, forefeet adducted.

Diagnosis: Chondrodysplasia punctata, rhizomelic type.

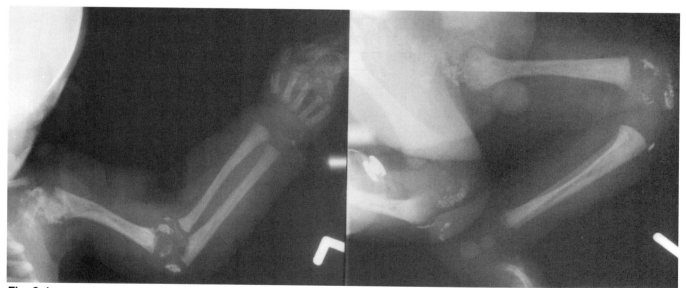

Fig. 8-1

(Continued)

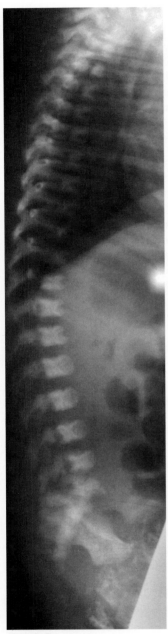

Fig. 8-2

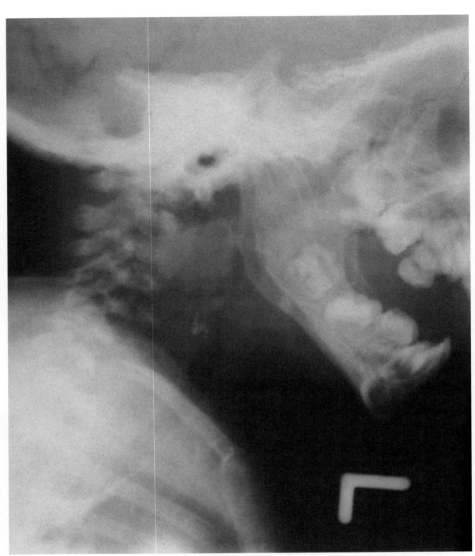

Fig. 8-3

Case 9

A 2-month-old boy has lumps on back of hands and right instep that were discovered by his mother at 2 weeks.

Mother (26 years old) and father (30 years old) are well. The boy is their only child. Parents have same great-great-grandfather.

Weight is 4.9 kg, length 61 cm, and head circumference 39 cm. He has epicanthi, depressed nasal bridge, and right scrotal hydrocele. Movement at wrists is limited. He cries when wrists are flexed. The rest of the physical findings are normal.

Lumps are gone at 4 months. He holds hands flexed and cries when movement is forced. Ophthalmologic findings are normal.

Para-articular calcifications are at shoulders (Figure 9-1), knees (Figure 9-2A), and hips. Carpus (see Figure 9-1) and tarsus (Figure 9-2B) are shallow and spotted with calcifications at 4 months.

He is crawling and pulling to stand at 7 months. Weight at 13 years is 44.5 kg, height 164 cm. He compensates for lack of wrist extension beyond 20 degrees by bending fingers backward when he shoots a basketball in games at 13 years. A younger sister is normal.

Diagnosis: Chondrodysplasia punctata, Conradi-Hünermann type.

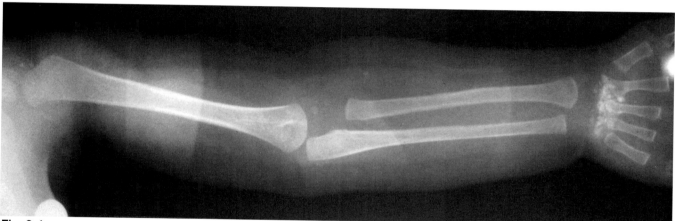

Fig. 9-1

(Continued)

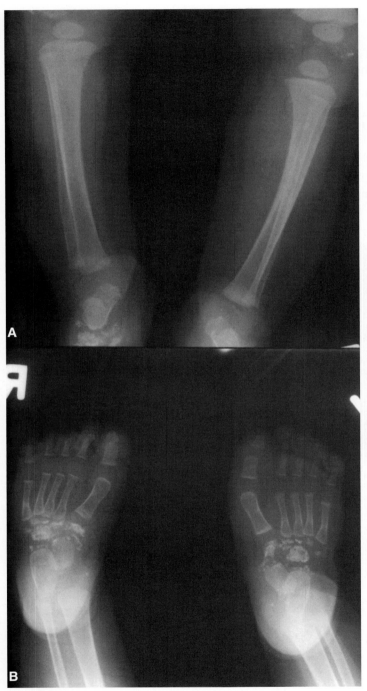

Fig. 9-2

Case 10

A 15-day-old girl is too weak to suck. She was limp at birth, convulsed for 1–2 minutes with jerking limbs and rolling eyes at 2 days, and was jaundiced at 1 week.

Pregnancy of mother was normal.

Parents have been treated for tuberculosis.

Weight is 3.6 kg, length 56 cm, temperature 37.2°C, heart rate 150, respiratory rate 60, and systolic blood pressure 100 mm Hg. Face is expressionless. Skull is narrow. Calvarial sutures are wide. Eyes are prominent with lateral nystagmus and opaque lenses. Respirations are shallow. Liver edge is 1 cm below costal margin. A mass (6 × 3 cm) is in left side of abdomen. Gag reflex is weak. Deep tendon reflexes are absent. The rest of the physical findings are normal. Ophthalmologic examination shows zonular cataracts.

Hematocrit is 0.49. Urine specific gravity is 1.018, pH 6. Urine is normal. Serum sodium is 143 mmol/liter, potassium 4.8, chloride 102, urea nitrogen 3.6, calcium 2.50, phosphorus 1.50, and glucose 4.9. Creatinine is 30 μmol/liter, uric acid 130, and iron 55.7 (normal: 17.9–44.8). CSF glucose is 2.8 mmol/liter, protein 1.01 g/liter. CSF has 11 × 10⁶

small lymphocytes/liter. Total bilirubin at 22 days is 113 μmol/liter, direct bilirubin 110. Total bilirubin at 29 days is 287 μmol/liter, direct bilirubin 149. LDH at 22 days is 1,150 U/liter, CK 29. GGT is 51 U/liter at 22 days and 39 at 29 days. IgA at 22 days is <0.2 g/liter (normal: 0.20–0.50), IgM 0.25 (normal: 0.20–0.80), and IgG 11.80 (normal: 2.5–9.0). CSF glucose at 15 days is 2.8 mmol/liter, protein 1.01 g/liter. CSF at 15 days has 11 × 10⁶ small lymphocytes/liter. At 15 days, serologic complement fixation titer is herpes simplex virus 1:128, cytomegalovirus 1:32, rubeola 1:8, rubella hemagglutination titer negative, and toxoplasmosis test negative.

EEG shows generalized paroxysmal discharge beginning in the left central region.

At 15 days, spotty calcifications are in front of cervical vertebrae and in arytenoid cartilage (Figure 10-1A) and at hips and near knees (Figure 10-1B). Spotty calcifications are also in shoulders.

Diagnosis: Cerebrohepatorenal syndrome (Zellweger syndrome).

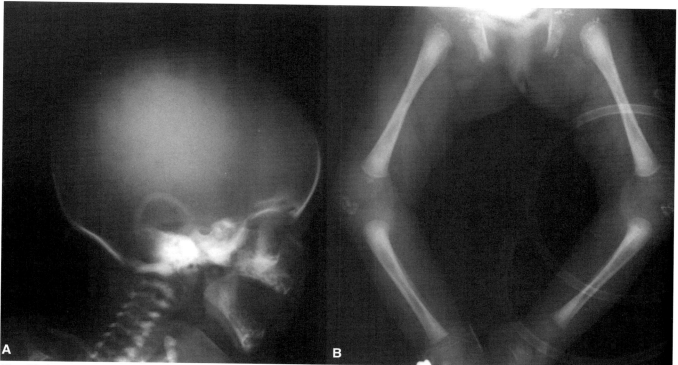

Fig. 10-1

Case 11

A newborn dwarf boy does not breathe.

Pregnancy was marred by polyhydramnios and premature onset of labor.

Mother (35 years old), father (37 years old), and brother (10 years old) are well.

Birth weight is 940 g. He is hydropic. Calvaria is soft. Face is flat. Eyeballs are bulging, auricles small and low. Arms are flipperlike, legs stubby. Chest is small. Ribs end at midaxilla. Sternum is not palpable. Bowel sounds are absent. Testes are not in scrotum. The rest of the physical findings are normal. Chromosomes are 46,XY.

Figure 11-1 shows (1) vertebrae that are not mineralized; (2) faintly mineralized calvaria, clavicles, and ilia; (3) short,

thin ribs; (4) bones of arms and legs that are curved stubs; and (5) five metatarsal bones in left foot. In Figure 11-2, facial bones are slightly mineralized.

Necropsy shows (1) airless lungs that are uniformly pink in cross section, (2) normal heart, and (3) normal abdominal viscera. Testes are in inguinal canals. Microscopic examination shows (1) cartilaginous vertebral bodies, (2) calcification of vertebral laminas, and (3) immature alveolar ducts and no alveoli in lungs.

Diagnosis: Achondrogenesis, type I.

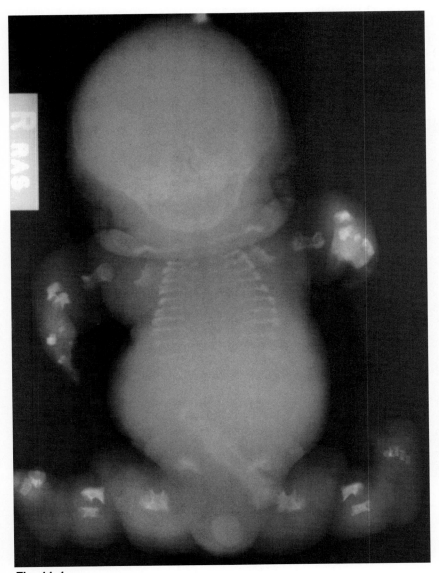

Fig. 11-1

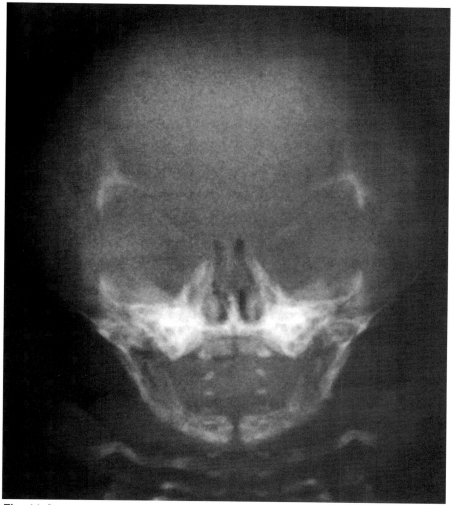

Fig. 11-2

Case 12

A newborn dwarf boy is not breathing. Heart rate is 60.

Mother (23 years old) smoked 15 cigarettes per day during pregnancy and had polyhydramnios. She had vaginal discharge of "green slime" 2 days ago.

Birth weight is 2.2 kg, Apgar score 1/4 at 1 and 10 minutes, heart rate 110 after intubation, temperature 36.3°C, and systolic blood pressure 42 mm Hg. He is hydropic. Head is large and edematous. Nasal bridge is depressed. Eyes are widely set and without lashes. Mouth is small. Limbs are short. Moro's reflex is present. The rest of the physical findings are normal.

Hematocrit is 0.54. White cell count is 21.6×10^9/liter with 0.53 polymorphonuclear cells, 0.13 bands, 0.08 lymphocytes, 0.07 monocytes, 0.01 eosinophils, 0.06 metamyelocytes, and 0.12 myelocytes. Platelet count is 234×10^9/liter. Venous blood pH is 6.81 when $FIO_2 = 1.0$. PCO_2 is 132 mm Hg, PO_2 34. Chromosomes are 46,XY.

He dies at 9 hours.

Roentgenogram after death shows small vertebral ossification centers, short bones with metaphyseal flare in arms and legs, bent tibias and fibulas, thin ribs, and unmineralized ischia and pubic bones (Figure 12-1) and large calvaria (Figure 12-2).

At necropsy, clear yellow liquid is in body cavities. Combined weight of lungs is 10 g (normal: 44 g); cut surface is dense and soggy. Palate is cleft. Olfactory tracts are absent. Microscopic examination shows small alveoli in lungs and hyaline membranes. Cartilage cells are not in normal columns at ends of bones, and penetration by blood vessels is irregular and incomplete. Vertebrae are almost all cartilage and loose fibrillar connective tissue.

Diagnosis: Achondrogenesis, type II.

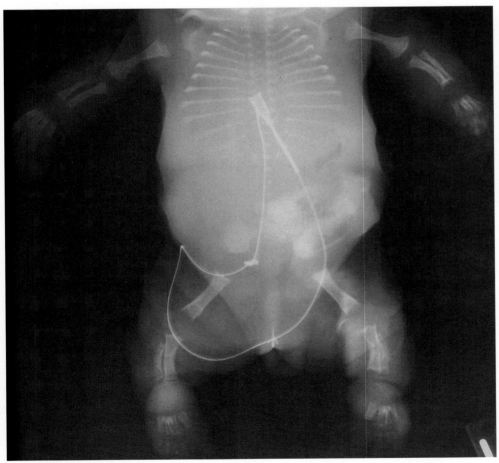

Fig. 12-1

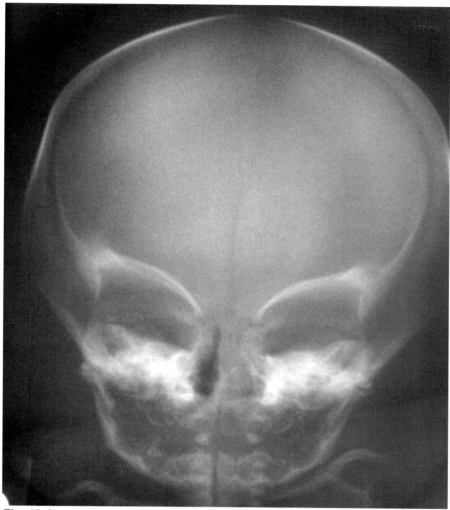

Fig. 12-2

Case 13

A newborn dwarf girl can breathe only with neck extended.

Pregnancy of mother (18 years old) was normal. Birth weight is 3.2 kg, Apgar score 6 at 5 minutes, heart rate 140, and head circumference 34 cm. Limbs are short. Nasal bridge is depressed, tip of nose anteverted. Eyes are widely set. Soft palate is cleft. Neck is short. Hands are broad and simian creased. Fingers flex only at metacarpophalangeal joints. Legs are abducted at hips and flexed at knees. Skin in front of right knee is dimpled. Second and third toes are fused. The rest of the physical findings are normal.

Hematocrit is 0.42. White cell count is 38.1×10^9/liter with 0.75 polymorphonuclear cells, 0.05 bands, 0.18 lymphocytes, 0.01 monocytes, and 0.01 eosinophils. Urine specific gravity is 1.019, pH 6. Urine has 0.10 g/liter protein, 3+ hemoglobin/myoglobin, 2+ reducing substances, and 5–6 red cells/HPF. Serum sodium is 141 mmol/liter, potassium 6.0, chloride 105, calcium 105, calcium 2.61, and urea nitrogen 3.6. Creatinine is 110 µmol/liter, total bilirubin 43. Chromosomes are 46,XX.

Figure 13-1A shows (1) short bones in arms and legs, (2) peg-like humeri, (3) fibulas not ossified, (4) flat vertebrae (especially cervical), (5) hypoplastic sacrum, and (6) pubis that is only a fragment of bone. Bone fragments are in only some metacarpals and phalanges (Figure 13-1B).

At necropsy, lungs are hemorrhagic, other viscera normal. Microscopic examination shows (1) disarray of proliferating and hypertrophied chondrocytes at costochondral junctions; (2) sparsity and disarray in vertebral growth plate with only two or three chondrocytes (nonproliferating) in column; and (3) disorganization at humeral, femoral, and tibial growth plates with fibrovascular tissue, degenerating chondrocytes, and empty lacunae. Fibulas are all cartilage. Tracheal cartilage contains enlarged chondrocytes; dark, unevenly staining matrix; empty lacunae; and focal necrosis.

Diagnosis: Atelosteogenesis.

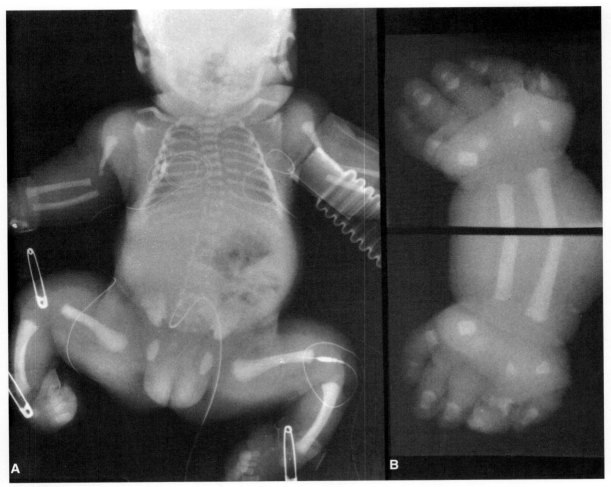

Fig. 13-1

Case 14

A newborn dwarf boy does not breathe.

Pregnancy of mother (22 years old) was marred by polyhydramnios and delivery by cesarean section because of genital herpes. Birth weight is 2.7 kg, length 40 cm, head circumference 35 cm, and heart rate 60. Upper lip has right cleft. Thorax is small. Abdomen and scrotum are distended. Limbs are short. Supernumerary fifth digits are on hands, seven toes on right foot, and six on left foot. The rest of the physical findings are normal.

Complement fixation titer for cytomegalovirus is 1:32, herpes simplex virus 1:16. Chromosomes are 46,XY.

Roentgenogram in Figure 14-1 shows airless lungs, gasless abdomen, short ribs, vertebra plana, and dysplastic T6. Figure 14-2 shows short bones in arms and legs, especially tibias; proximal humeral and femoral epiphyseal ossification centers; and polydactyly. Skull is normal.

At necropsy, microscopic examination shows (1) lung alveoli lined by cuboidal-to-columnar epithelium, (2) eosinophilic cytoplasm in tracheal and bronchial chondrocytes, (3) diminution of proliferating zone of chondrocytes at costochondral junction, and (4) irregularity in alignment at provisional zone of calcification. Abdominal viscera are normal except for high cecum.

Diagnosis: Short rib-polydactyly syndrome (Majewski type).

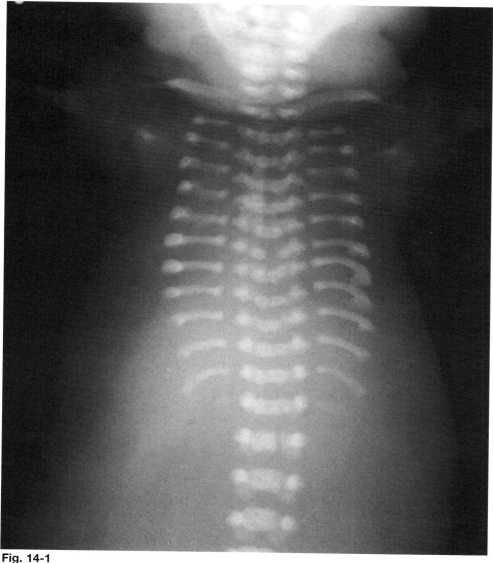

Fig. 14-1

(Continued)

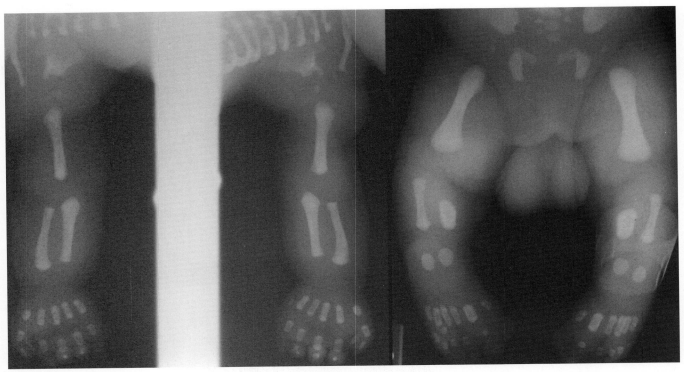

Fig. 14-2

Case 15

A newborn dwarf boy has a protruding tongue and is cyanotic.

Mother (21 years old) and father (24 years old) are well. The boy is their only child.

Pregnancy was normal. Birth weight is 2.8 kg, Apgar score 5/7 at 1 and 5 minutes, and temperature 35.9°C. Nasal bridge is depressed. Tongue is too large for small mouth. Thorax is small. Limbs are short. The rest of the physical findings are normal.

Hematocrit is 0.35. White cell count is 11.1 × 10⁹/liter.

Figure 15-1 shows (1) humeri that are shorter than radii and ulnae, (2) flaring metaphyses of ribs and bones of limbs, (3) interpediculate distance of lumbar vertebrae that does not increase at L4 and L5, (4) square ilia, and (5) small sciatic notches. Calvaria is normal.

Diagnosis: Achondroplasia.

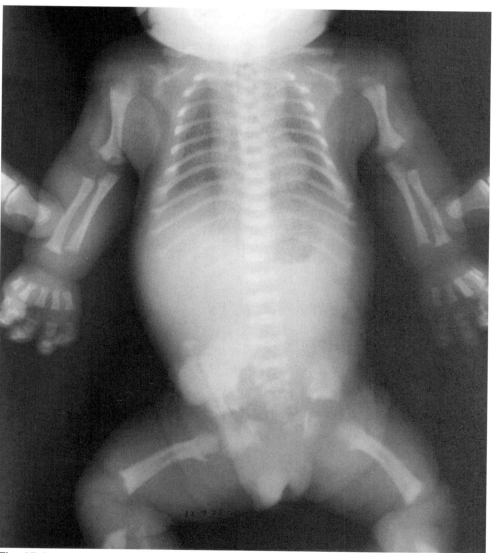

Fig. 15-1

Case 16

An 11½-year-old dwarf girl walks on outside edge of left foot.

Parents and six older siblings are well.

Pregnancy of mother (then 31 years old) was normal. Birth weight was 3.6 kg, length 46 cm. At 7 months, she could sit, spine humped, for short periods. At 9 months, head circumference was 50 cm, anterior fontanel large and flat. She had one tooth. At 22 months, she began to walk. At 5 years, height was 82 cm, weight 14.5 kg. Elbow extension was limited to 45 degrees. Lumbar spine was deeply lordotic. Legs were bowed and curved backward at knees. At 6 years, short arms made it difficult for her to dress and undress. Her father put a step in front of the toilet so she could get on and off. At 8 years, left shank was bowed. At 10 years, she had headaches for a while.

Height at 11½ years is 107 cm, weight 28 kg, head circumference 60 cm, temperature 36.7°C, heart rate 88, respiratory rate 20, and blood pressure 100/80 mm Hg. Teeth are crowded. Breasts are developing. Knees are lax. Lower part of left tibia is bowed. The rest of the physical findings are normal.

Hematocrit is 0.43. White cell count is 7.3×10^9/liter with 0.43 polymorphonuclear cells, 0.08 bands, 0.45 lymphocytes, and 0.04 basophils. Platelet estimate is adequate. Urine specific gravity is 1.027, pH 7. Urine has 25–30 white cells/HPF, occasional epithelial cells/HPF, and moderate amorphous crystals. Serum sodium is 140 mmol/liter, potassium 4.4, chloride 107, urea nitrogen 4.3, and glucose 5.5.

Forehead (membranous bone) protrudes beyond face. Basal view of skull shows small bones and smaller than normal foramen magnum. Clavicles are too long for short ribs (Figure 16-1A). Spinal canal is narrow, especially between pedicles of L4 and L5 (Figure 16-1B). Bones of arms and hands are short, broad, and knobby (Figure 16-2A). Fibulas are longer than tibias and left foot is turned in (Figure 16-2B).

At operation to straighten left shank, a wedge of tibia and proximal part of fibula are resected.

Microscopic examination of fibular growth plate shows random array of chondrocytes and no normal columns.

Diagnosis: Achondroplasia.

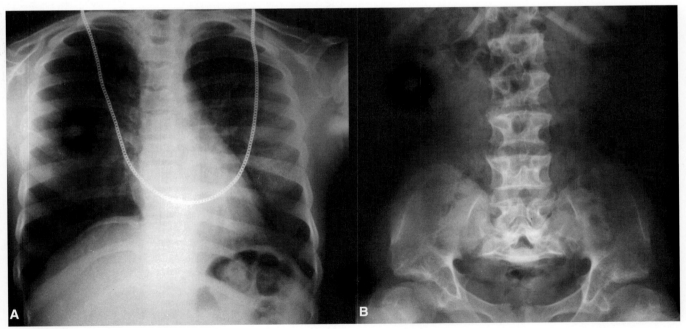

Fig. 16-1

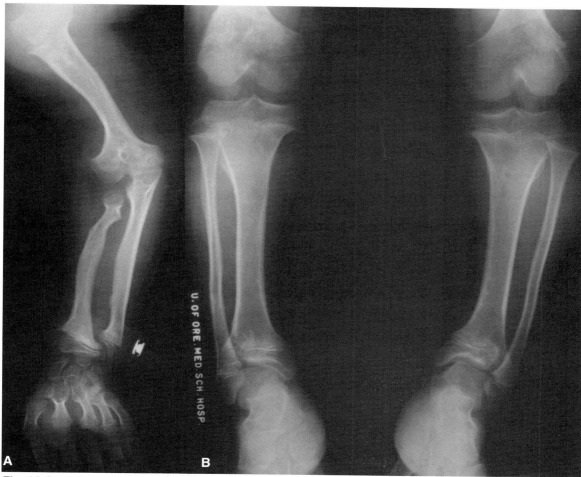

Fig. 16-2

Case 17

A 9-year-old boy is a dwarf.

Birth weight was 3.4 kg, length 50 cm. He walked at 14 months. He limped at 2 years. Height was 81 cm at 2 years. He often has nose bleeds. He is weak and stumbles a lot.

Mother (27 years old) is well. Father (28 years old), 114 cm tall, a professional musician, is well.

Height is 96 cm, weight 21 kg. Head and face are normal. He has knobby joints, pectus carinatum, protuberant abdomen, and moderate thoracic kyphosis and lumbar lordosis. Extension and supination are limited at elbows. Hands are floppy, fingers spread apart. Hip abduction is 45 degrees. Knees are unstable and lack a few degrees of full extension. He walks with toes pointed inward. The rest of the physical findings are normal.

Roentgenogram in Figure 17-1A shows flat vertebrae, normal lumbar interpediculate distance, small greater sciatic notches, and thickening and irregular edges of the three parts of the innominate bones. Figure 17-1B shows short bones in legs; broad, irregular metaphyses; small epiphyses with spotty ossification; and bowed legs.

Height at 15 years is 101 cm, weight 29 kg. He cannot stand for long at 22 years because left hip hurts.

Diagnosis: Pseudoachondroplastic dysplasia (formerly hyperplastic achondroplasia).

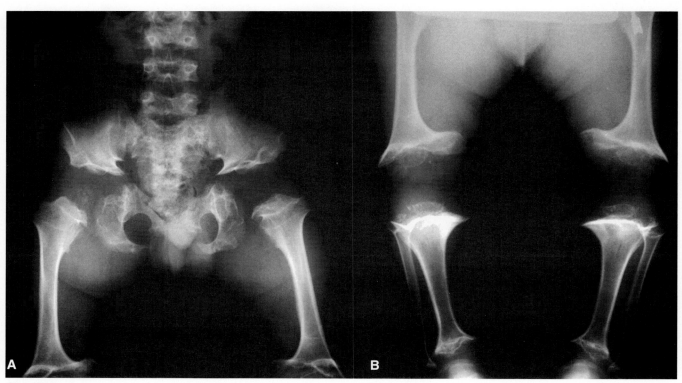

Fig. 17-1

Case 18

A 10-year-old girl is short. Classmates make fun of her.

Pregnancy was normal, birth weight 4.1 kg, and length 51 cm. Growth slowed at 1–2 years. Height was below third percentile at 5 years. She wears glasses and has nosebleeds and several carious teeth.

Mother (42 years old), 165 cm tall; father (57 years old), 170 cm tall; and four older siblings, whose heights are normal, are well.

Height is 114 cm, weight 28 kg, and head circumference 57 cm. Chest is shallow. Rib ends flare. Limbs, fingers, and toes are short. The rest of the physical findings are normal.

Interpediculate distance in Figure 18-1A is 21 mm at L4, 25 mm at L5. Spinal canal is shallow front to back in Figure 18-1B. Necks of femurs are short in Figure 18-1A; fibulas are elongated at ankles, and legs bow when she stands (Figure 18-2).

Diagnosis: Hypochondroplasia.

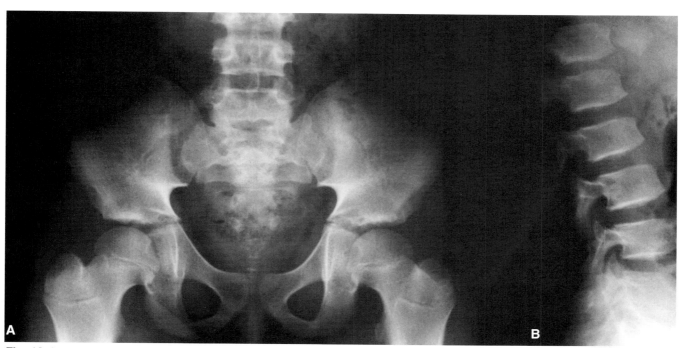

Fig. 18-1

(Continued)

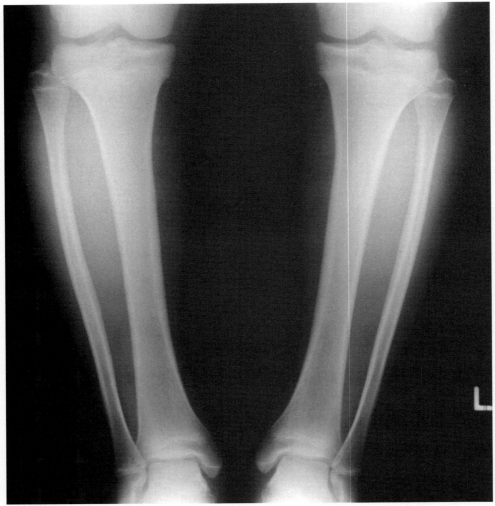

Fig. 18-2

Case 19

A 2½-month-old boy has "lumps at all joints" and has wheezed since birth.

Pregnancy was normal, birth weight 2.6 kg.

Mother (23 years old) had rheumatic fever. Father (28 years old) and sister (19 months old) are well. A grandfather died with Addison's disease.

Weight is 3.6 kg, heart rate 130, and respiratory rate 60. He is pale. Left side of head is flat. Neck is short and stiff, spine kyphotic and stiff. Chest is narrow side to side and deep front to back. Abdomen is tense. Testes are not in scrotum. Ilia are broad. Coccyx sticks out 5 cm from sacrum like a tail. Joints are stiff, fingers and toes immobile. A hemangioma is at right ankle. The rest of the physical findings are normal.

Hemoglobin is 98 g/liter. White cell count is 11.8×10^9/liter with 0.60 polymorphonuclear cells, 0.37 lymphocytes, 0.01 monocytes, and 0.02 eosinophils. Urine has 1+ albumin, 3+ white cells/HPF, and a few red cells/HPF. Serum calcium is 2.22 mmol/liter.

Figure 19-1 shows that (1) bones of limbs are short and flare at metaphyses; (2) carpal and tarsal ossification is advanced although epiphyses are not ossified; (3) deposits of calcium density are in para-articular soft tissues, especially at knees; and (4) ilia are broad and square.

Diagnosis: Metatropic dysplasia.

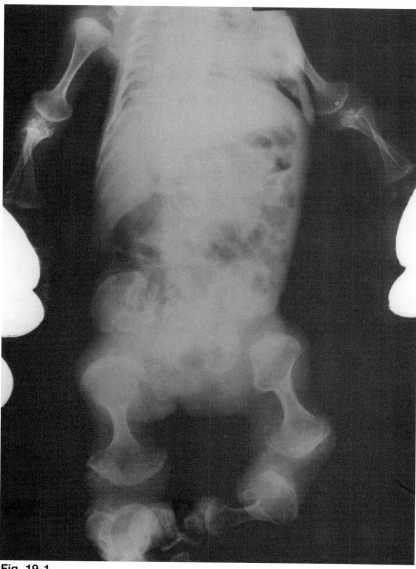

Fig. 19-1

Case 20

A 17-year-old boy, who is in his third year of high school, is short.

Pregnancy was normal, birth weight 3.2 kg. Limbs were short at 5 months. Bridge of nose was depressed. Arms were pudgy and pronated; extension was limited. Fingers were short, nails broad. Lower sternum was depressed. Limbs were lax at 2 years, hands floppy. At 6½ years, he was shorter than his 3-year-old sister. At 10 years, writing hurt his hand. Grip was weak. He could not flex metacarpophalangeal joints.

Parents (both 42 years old) and sister (14 years old) are well.

Height at 17 years is 130 cm, weight 37 kg.

Bones of arms, especially forearms, are short at 4½ years (Figure 20-1A). Bones of hands are short at 9 years (Figure 20-1B). Similar findings are in feet. First toes are larger than other toes. Roentgenograms of spine at 2, 5, and 9 years show vertebra plana.

Diagnosis: Acromesomelic dysplasia.

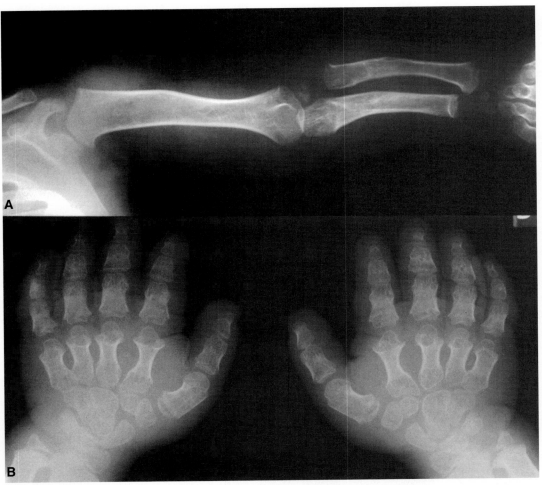

Fig. 20-1

Case 21

A 9-year-old boy needs to rest when he walks 100 yd. He goes down steps one at a time, on his rear end. He cannot put on socks or button his shirt and has trouble with zippers. Joints are stiff. Knees, left wrist, and right ankle sometimes ache. Feet sometimes tingle.

Mother had vaginal discharge and labor pains 2½ months before he was born. Birth weight was 3.5 kg, length 46 cm, and head circumference 37 cm. He was blue at birth and given oxygen. Limbs were short, joints large. Motion was limited at hips. He held his head up at 2 months, rolled over at 3–4 months, sat at 6 months, talked at 8–10 months, and walked at 19 months. He had right inguinal herniorrhaphy at 6 months and right ear infection and perforation of eardrum at 26 months. At 2½ years, he used the top of his head to shift his weight toward his feet when he moved from supine to erect. He walked heel to toe, with shoulders back, chest forward, and lordosis. He had ear infections from 2–4 years. At 4 years, hearing was bad. He was nearsighted. Face was flat, bridge of nose depressed, and neck short. He had diastasis recti, right inguinal scar, and limited movement at all joints. He could not make a fist or touch his feet. He grasped small objects, such as pellets and string, between second and third fingers; he grasped larger objects, such as pencils, between thumb and side of hand or second finger.

Mother (43 years old) and two sisters (21 and 23 years old) are well. Father (46 years old) has allergies. Another sister, born 6 weeks early, died at 24 hours with respiratory distress. Paternal grandfather died with high blood pressure and stroke.

Height is 108 cm, weight 29 kg. Spine has 40-degree thoracic kyphosis and 90-degree lumbar lordosis when he stands, less kyphosis and lordosis when prone. He stands leaning forward with flexed elbows, flexed hips, flexed and knock-knees, and pronated feet.

He begins to use a wheelchair at 9 years. He is sometimes incontinent of urine at 10 years. He swims regularly at 13 years and finds it helpful and enjoyable. Height is 142 cm at 13 years, 9 months.

Roentgenogram in Figure 21-1, at 5 years, shows short, deformed bones of limbs; large joints; and epiphyseal and metaphyseal irregularity. Pelvis and hips are dysplastic at 5 years in Figure 21-2. Examination also shows stubby bones of hands and feet, knobby joints in hands, Freiburg-like change in right second metatarsal bone, flat vertebral bodies that are long front to back, and shallow neural canals.

Diagnosis: Kniest dysplasia.

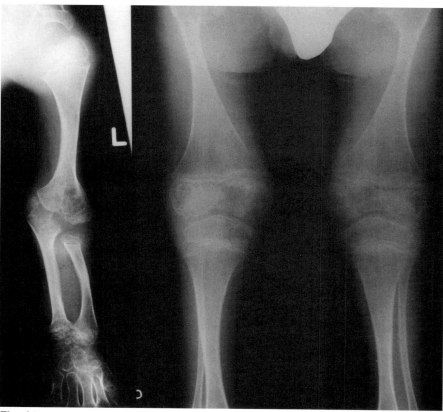

Fig. 21-1

(Continued)

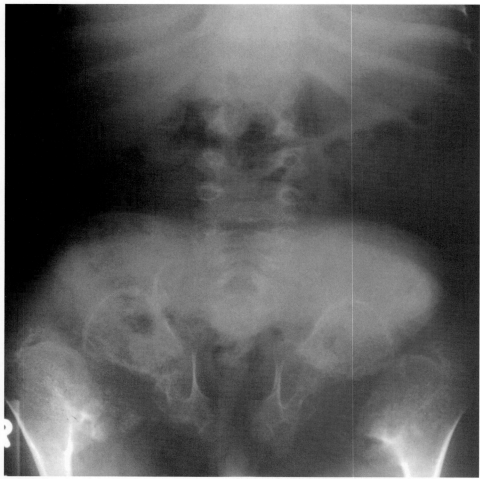

Fig. 21-2

Case 22

A newborn boy has short limbs, thick gums, left central maxillary incisor, and flail extra little finger on each hand.

Pregnancy of mother (25 years old) was normal. Birth weight is 3.0 kg, Apgar score 8/9 at 1 and 5 minutes, length 43 cm, head circumference 34 cm, temperature 37.1°C, heart rate 140, respiratory rate 50, and blood pressure 76/28 mm Hg. Tooth is 8 mm wide, 2 mm high. Fingers are short and tapered, fingernails hypoplastic. The rest of the physical findings are normal.

Hematocrit is 0.44. White cell count is 17.7×10^9/liter with 0.48 polymorphonuclear cells, 0.01 bands, 0.23 lymphocytes, 0.12 monocytes, 0.14 eosinophils, 0.01 metamyelocytes, and 0.01 myelocytes. Platelet count is 190×10^9/liter. Serum sodium is 134 mmol/liter, potassium 4.6, chloride 101, carbon dioxide not determined, calcium 2.47, phosphorus 1.61, magnesium 0.70, cholesterol 1.47, bicarbonate 26 mmol/liter, and glucose 2.4. Creatinine is 70 µmol/liter, uric acid 240, total bilirubin 58, and direct bilirubin 3. Total protein is 56 g/liter, albumin 38. Alkaline phosphatase is 89 U/liter, LDH 680, SGOT 132, and SGPT 26. Capillary blood pH is 7.37 when $F_{IO_2} = 0.20$. P_{CO_2} is 44 mm Hg, P_{O_2} 40. Oxygen saturation is 0.74.

Figure 22-1 shows bell-shaped chest, short arms with relatively long humeri, serrated iliac bases, and shallow sciatic notches. A flail extra stub of finger is on ulnar side of each hand, a small piece of bone in right stub.

Echocardiogram shows common atrium, atrioventricular canal, and mitral and tricuspid regurgitation. Ultrasound examination shows normal kidneys.

Diagnosis: Chondroectodermal dysplasia (Ellis–van Creveld syndrome).

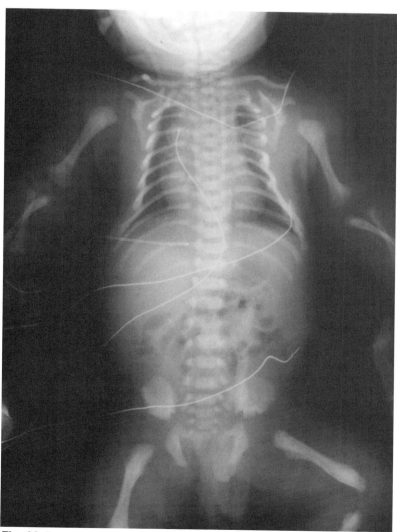

Fig. 22-1

Case 23

A 6-month-old girl has had an intermittent heart murmur since she was 2 days old. She tires during feedings. She wheezes, gets short of breath, and turns blue around mouth when she cries.

Pregnancy was normal, birth weight 4.1 kg. She rolls over, reaches for toys, and is beginning to sit up.

Mother (24 years old) and father (23 years old) are well. The girl is their only child.

Temperature is 36.8°C, heart rate 140, respiratory rate 40, systolic blood pressure 90 mm Hg, weight 6.3 kg, length 64 cm, and head circumference 47 cm. Chest is small. Expiration is prolonged. A systolic heart murmur is present. Liver edge and spleen edge are 1 cm below costal margin. Limbs are short. Six fingers are on each hand. Right third and fourth toes are fused. The rest of the physical findings are normal.

Hematocrit is 0.44. White cell count is 15.2×10^9/liter with 0.13 polymorphonuclear cells, 0.82 lymphocytes, 0.04 monocytes, and 0.01 eosinophils. Platelet estimate is normal. Urine specific gravity is 1.018, pH 5. Urine has rare red cells/HPF and rare white cells/HPF.

Ribs are short. Heart is large, diaphragm depressed. Lumbar and lower thoracic vertebrae are square in lateral view. Ilia flare, with bases that are irregularly ossified and greater sciatic notches that are small (Figure 23-1). Tibial plateau is triangular, proximal tibial epiphysis is medial (see Figure 23-1). Extra digits are at broad ends of fifth metacarpal bones; metacarpals, metatarsals, and phalanges, especially distal phalanges, are short (Figure 23-2). Distal phalanges in toes are unossified.

At cardiac catheterization, right ventricular pressure is 76/9 mm Hg, mean pulmonary artery pressure 56, and left ventricular systolic pressure 82. Oxygen saturation is 0.48 in superior vena cava and right atrium, 0.79 in right upper pulmonary vein, 0.69 in right ventricle, and 0.76 in ascending aorta. Angiocardiogram shows membranous ventricular septal defect.

Teeth are small and deformed at 4 years, nails dysplastic.

Diagnosis: Chondroectodermal dysplasia (Ellis–van Creveld syndrome), pulmonary hypertension, ventricular septal defect with bidirectional shunt.

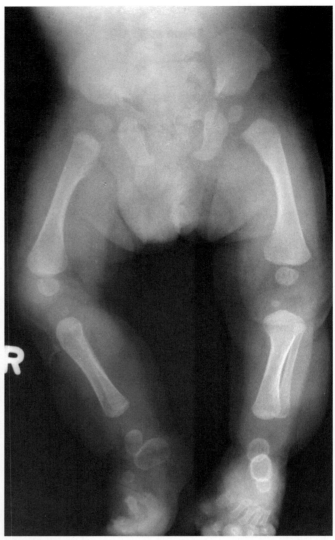

Fig. 23-1

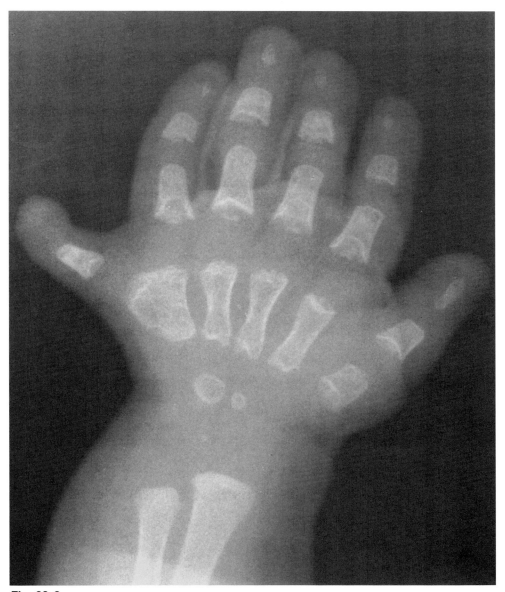

Fig. 23-2

Case 24

A newborn girl has large head; short limbs; bent, dimpled shins; and respiratory distress.

Mother (28 years old), father, and older sibling are well.

Pregnancy was normal, presentation brow. Birth weight is 2.4 kg, length 45 cm, head circumference 36 cm, Apgar score 5/8 at 1 and 5 minutes. Heart rate at 4 hours is 170, respiratory rate 70, systolic blood pressure 48 mm Hg, and blood glucose 2.5 mmol/liter. Head is large, occiput prominent, forehead high and bruised, hair abundant, and anterior fontanel large. Face and nasal bridge are flat. Nose is grooved at junction of alar cartilage and alar fibrofatty tissue. Neck is short and stiff. Chest is small. Femurs are bent. Shins are dimpled over forward convexity of tibias. Hands and feet are small. Fingers, especially thumbs, are small. Nails are small. Knees are deformed. All joints in limbs are hypermobile except ankles, which are equinus. The rest of the physical findings are normal.

Hematocrit is 0.43. White cell count is 25.3×10^9/liter with 0.78 polymorphonuclear cells, 0.08 bands, 0.04 lymphocytes, 0.09 monocytes, and 0.01 metamyelocytes. Platelet count is 305×10^9/liter. Capillary blood pH is 7.15 when FIO_2 = 0.35. PCO_2 is 83 mm Hg, PO_2 48. Serum sodium is 132 mmol/liter, potassium 3.1, chloride 103, and calcium 2.30. Creatinine is 120 µmol/liter, total bilirubin 55.

Pubic cartilage is not ossified, right femur is displaced laterally at hip, femurs are convex forward, and left tibia and hypoplastic left fibula are displaced forward at knee and convex forward (Figure 24-1A). First metacarpals and all phalanges are hypoplastic (Figure 24-1B). Vertebrae are flat (Figure 24-2). Roentgenogram of chest at 3 days (see Figure 24-2) shows 11 pairs of thin ribs, ossified spines but little else of scapulas, high diaphragm, and partial atelectasis of left lower lobe.

She dies at 3 days.

Diagnosis: Camptomelic dysplasia.

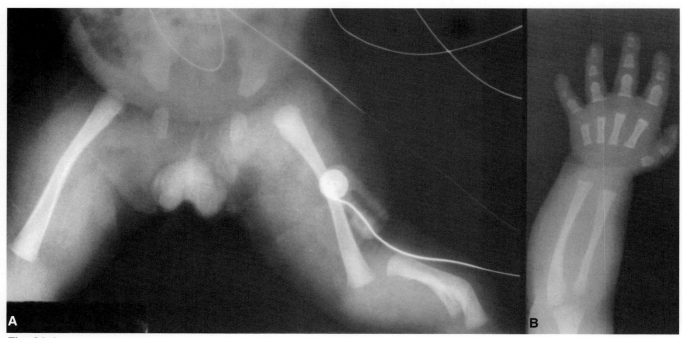

Fig. 24-1

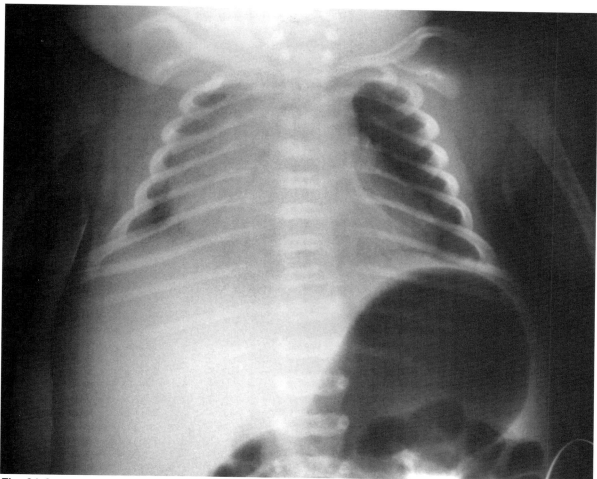

Fig. 24-2

Case 25

A short, 19-year-old man has a first-grade intellect.

Pregnancy was marred by little fetal movement, birth weight 2.0 kg. Cry was weak. He had many colds. At 9 months, hairline was low. Eyebrows met. No teeth had erupted. Neck was short. A systolic heart murmur was present. Elbow extension was limited. Thumbs were short. Lower back was hairy. The rest of the physical findings were normal. He sat at 15 months and walked at 2 years. His thick tongue made spoon-feeding difficult. At 3 years, right inguinal herniorrhaphy and lacrimal duct probing were performed. Nose was stubby. Lips were thin, angles of mouth down turned. At 14 years, feet were so short and broad that he could not find shoes that were comfortable. At 17 years, hands trembled when he was agitated. He had nystagmus with lateral gaze. Eyelashes were long. Deep tendon reflexes were weak; relaxation was slow.

Serum sodium at 17 years was 141 mmol/liter, potassium 5.2, chloride 103, carbon dioxide 24, urea nitrogen 5.0, calcium 2.72, phosphorus 1.10, cholesterol 4.50, and glucose 5.5. Creatinine was 90 µg/liter, uric acid 450, total bilirubin 14, and direct bilirubin 2. Total protein was 86 g/liter, albumin 51. Alkaline phosphatase was 251 U/liter, LDH 232, and SGOT 18. T_3 uptake was 0.29 (normal: 0.25–0.35), T_4 117 nmol/liter (normal: 51–142).

Parents, sister (20 years old), and brother (15 years old) are well.

Height at 19 years is 159 cm, weight 74 kg, and head circumference 51 cm. Serum FSH is 9 IU/liter (normal: 1–10), LH 13 (normal: 3–25). Testosterone is 21.7 nmol/liter (normal: 10.4–34.7). Chromosomes are 46,XY.

Radii are dislocated dorsad at elbows at 17 years (Figure 25-1A); first metacarpals and middle phalanges of fifth digits are too small (Figure 25-1B).

Diagnosis: Cornelia de Lange syndrome.

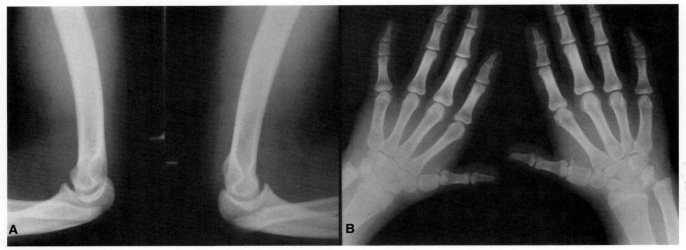

Fig. 25-1

Case 26

A 12-year-old girl has clubfeet.

Mother took levothyroxine during pregnancy. Birth weight was 3.7 kg, length 38 cm, and Apgar score 7/8 at 1 and 5 minutes. Breathing was noisy. Fingers were blue. Weight was 3.5 kg at 5 weeks, length 46 cm, head circumference 37 cm, heart rate 150, and respiratory rate 40. A flame nevus was on forehead. Nose was small and tipped upward. Mandible was small, soft palate cleft. A systolic heart murmur was present. Limbs were stubby, thumbs short, and feet clubbed. The rest of the physical findings were normal. Cardiac catheterization showed pulmonary artery mean pressure of 68 mm Hg. Glossopexy was performed at 2 months, soft palate repair at 6 months, and lengthening of calcaneal tendons at 11 months. Spine was straight at 3½ years. Flexion contractures were at hips and knees. Knees were operated on at 4½ years.

Mother (34 years old), father (38 years old), and two brothers (11 and 12 years old) were well when the girl was 2 years old.

Weight at 12 years is 30 kg, heart rate 80, respiratory rate 12, and blood pressure 104/68 mm Hg. Spine is straight. Flexion contractures are at hips and knees.

Radius is dislocated dorsad at elbow, and left thumb is short at 2 months (Figure 26-1). Right thumb is also short. Interpediculate distances of sacrum and lower lumbar vertebrae are shortened at 4 years, hips and knees dysplastic (Figure 26-2). Feet are dysplastic at 12 years (Figure 26-3). Vertebrae are bulky, and pedicles are large at 12 years.

Diagnosis: Diastrophic dwarfism.

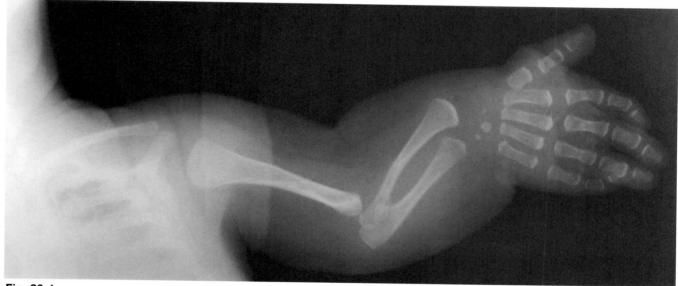

Fig. 26-1

(Continued)

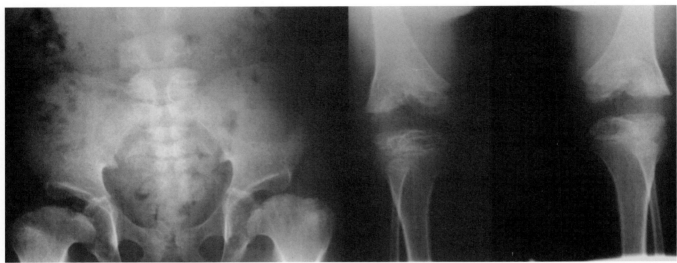

Fig. 26-2

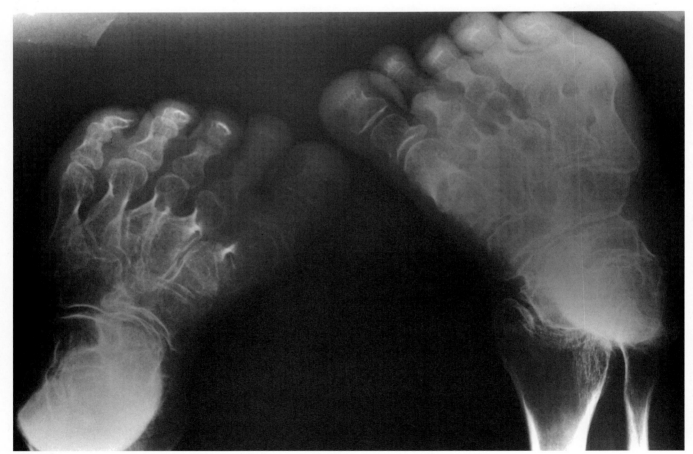

Fig. 26-3

Case 27

A newborn girl has broad thumbs and broad first toes.

Pregnancy was normal, amniotic fluid muddy. Birth weight is 3.2 kg, length 50 cm, head circumference 35 cm, temperature at 10 minutes 36.6°C, heart rate 172, and respiratory rate 64. Third and fourth fingers of hands and right second and third toes are fused. The rest of the physical findings are normal.

Phalanges of fingers, especially distal phalanges of thumbs (Figure 27-1), and phalanges of first toes (Figure 27-2) are short and broad. Proximal phalanges of first toes are displaced medially in Figure 27-2. Skull is bathrocephalic; prognathism suggests that brain growth is slow compared to somatic growth in Figure 27-3. Sternal segments are ossified and fused early. Ilia flare.

She falls asleep during feedings. She has esotropia at 7 months. She does not babble at 1 year. Development is estimated to be at least 3 months behind normal.

Diagnosis: Rubinstein-Taybi syndrome.

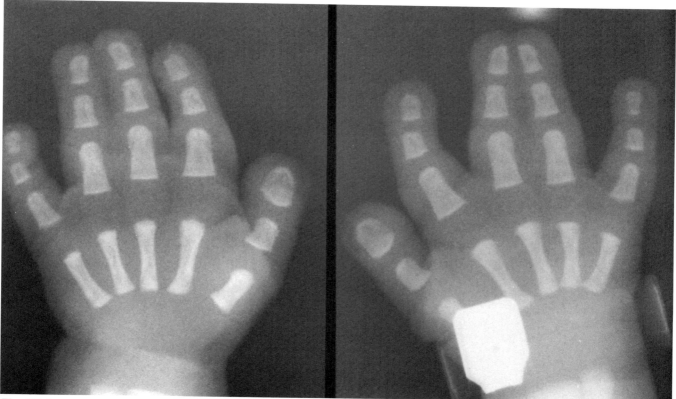

Fig. 27-1

(Continued)

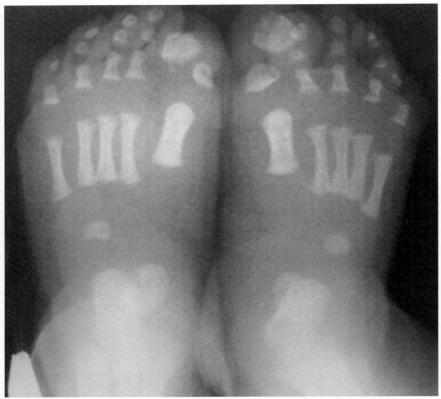

Fig. 27-2

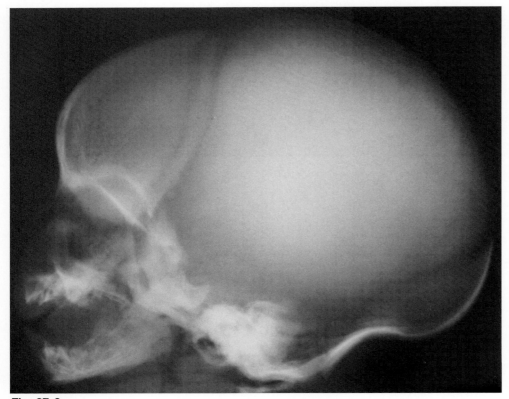

Fig. 27-3

Case 28

A 5-year-old girl limps and has had hip pain for 4 months.

Pregnancy was normal, birth weight 3.5 kg, and length 53 cm. Hair on head and in eyebrows and lashes has always been sparse. She sat at 8 months, walked at 19 months. She has had many ear infections. Tonsils and adenoids were removed, and myringotomy tubes placed at 3 years. Intelligence is above average.

Mother (28 years old), father (39 years old), and brother (4 years old) are well. Paternal grandfather had a stroke; paternal grandmother had tuberculosis.

Heart rate is 72, respiratory rate 16, blood pressure 102/72 mm Hg, weight 26.5 kg, height 106 cm, and head circumference 52 cm. Hair is blonde, sparse, and fine; hairline is high. Nose is pear shaped, columella broad. The rest of the physical findings are normal.

She has pain in lower back, right leg, and occasionally in hands at 17 years. She can walk two blocks. Weight is 91 kg, height 145 cm. Rotation hurts at right hip, and abduction and flexion are limited. Movement at other joints is normal.

Middle phalanges are short with cone-shaped epiphyses that are partly fused at 5 years. Middle phalanges are short with wedged bases at 17 years (Figure 28-1). Femoral epiphyseal ossification centers are small at 5 years (Figure 28-2A). Epiphyses and metaphyses at hips are deformed at 17 years (Figure 28-2B).

Diagnosis: Trichorhinophalangeal dysplasia, dysplasia and osteoarthropathy at hips.

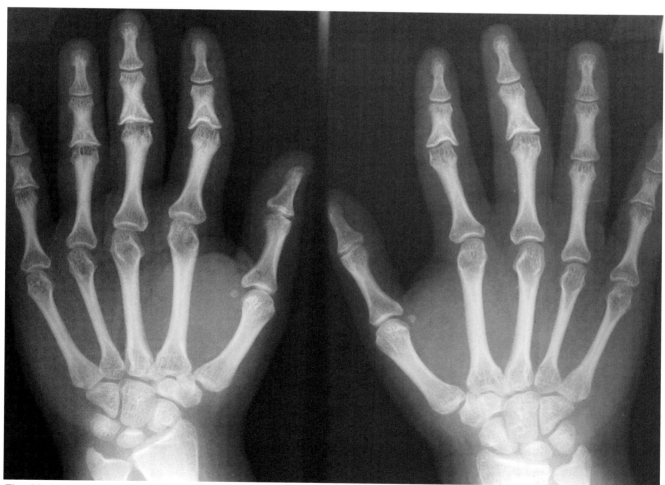

Fig. 28-1

(Continued)

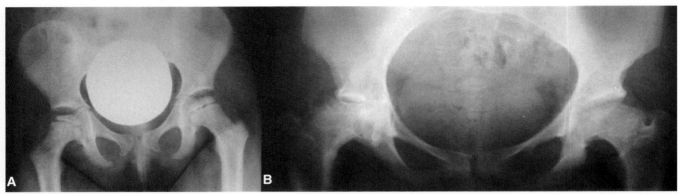

Fig. 28-2

Case 29

A 15-year-old boy has seizures. Head turns right or left, arms jerk, then sometimes legs, and then he sleeps, sometimes wetting himself. He had similar seizures during the first year and has had these during the last year.

He sat at 9 months, walked at 19 months, and spent 2 years in first grade.

Mother and two sisters are well.

He is "cheerful but doesn't understand very much." He is short. Weight is 49 kg, heart rate 92, respiratory rate 16, and blood pressure 152/108 mm Hg. He has pimples on forehead and a small, pug nose. Hands and feet are short and broad. Palms are thick. Fingers and toes, except for relatively large first toes, are stubby. The rest of the physical findings are normal.

Hemoglobin is 150 g/liter. White cell count is 7.0×10^9/liter with 0.57 polymorphonuclear cells, 0.09 bands, 0.29 lymphocytes, and 0.05 monocytes. Urine pH is 1.019, reaction acid. Urine has occasional white cells/HPF and occasional epithelial cells/HPF. Serum calcium is 3.12 mmol/liter in only determination.

In Figure 29-1, metacarpals two through five are short, broad, and without growth plates, and all phalanges except proximal phalanx of thumbs are stubby with flared metaphyses, cupped epiphyses, and most without growth plates. Figure 29-2 shows small nasal bone and absent anterior nasal spine.

Diagnosis: Acrodysostosis.

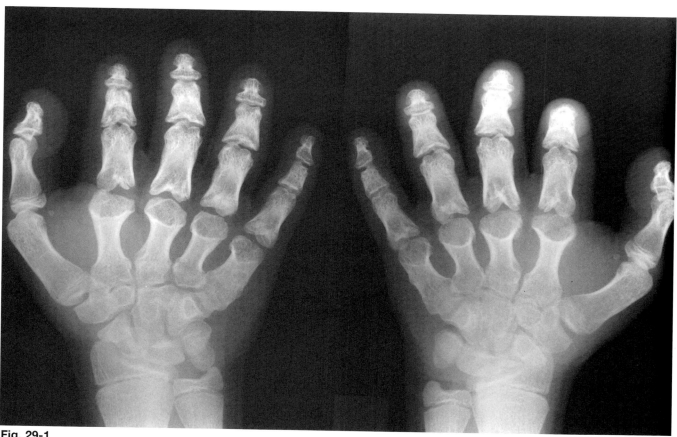

Fig. 29-1

(Continued)

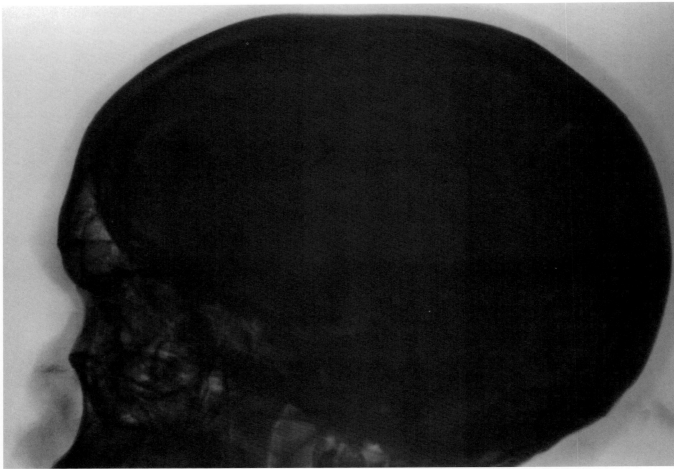

Fig. 29-2

Case 30

A 2½-year-old boy will not walk and cries "like it hurts to stand." He clutched his belly and screamed until exhausted 4 nights ago. Temperature was 40°C. Similar episodes without fever have recurred nightly.

Pregnancy was normal, birth weight 2.3 kg. He was diagnosed with Down syndrome at 4 months. Chromosomes are 46,XY,+21. He had croup at 11, 14, and 23 months. "He gets everything that comes along." Red spots on his skin have appeared and disappeared for 1 year. He has been pale for 5 months. He began to walk at 2 years.

Mother (25 years old) is well. Father (33 years old) has asthma. Maternal grandfather died with ruptured aorta.

Weight is 9.5 kg, height 53 cm, temperature 37.1°C, heart rate 140, respiratory rate 24, and blood pressure 90/50 mm Hg. He has epicanthi and flat nasal bridge. Skin looks yellow. Petechiae are on legs. A bruise is on right calf. Respirations are noisy. A systolic heart murmur is present. Soles are furrowed between first and second toes. The rest of the physical findings are normal.

Hematocrit is 0.14. Hemoglobin is 45 g/liter. Red blood cell count is 1.4×10^{12}/liter. MCV is 94 fl. MCH is 33 pg. MCHC is 340 g/liter. Reticulocyte fraction is 2×10^{-3}. White cell count is 3.2×10^9/liter with 0.08 polymorphonuclear cells,

0.25 bands, 0.64 lymphocytes, and 0.03 monocytes. Platelet count is 32×10^9/liter. ESR is 70 mm/hr. Urine specific gravity is 1.004, pH 8. Urine has few epithelial cells/HPF and 0–1 white cell/HPF. Serum sodium is 138 mmol/liter, potassium 5.1, chloride 101, carbon dioxide 25, urea nitrogen 5.0, calcium 2.17, phosphorus 1.32, cholesterol 4.22, and glucose 6.0. Creatinine is 50 µmol/liter, uric acid 500, total bilirubin 5, and direct bilirubin 2. Total protein is 70 g/liter, albumin 41. LDH is 405 U/liter, SGOT 42, and CK 911 (normal: ~40–170).

Little finger curves inward, its middle phalanx is hypoplastic (Figure 30-1A). A gap is between first and second left toes (Figure 30-1B). Ilia flare and neck-shaft angle of femurs is increased (Figure 30-2). Findings in excretory urogram are normal.

Examination of bone marrow shows fibrosis. Two months later, marrow is hypercellular with many blasts, abnormal mitoses, decreased megakaryocytes, and moderate fibrous tissue.

He dies at 32 months.

Diagnosis: Down syndrome, acute myelogenous leukemia.

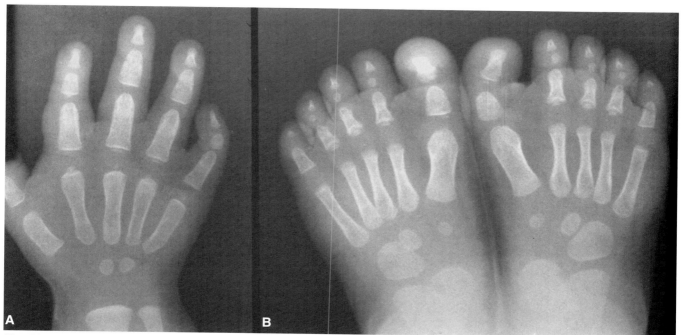

Fig. 30-1

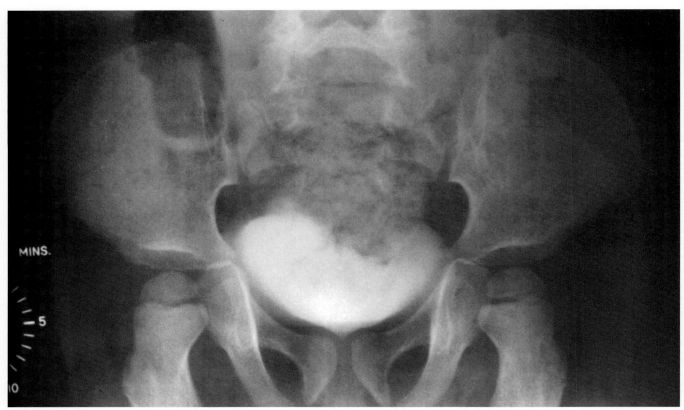

Fig. 30-2

Case 31

A 13½-year-old boy has scoliosis that was found by school nurse.

Term pregnancy was marred by little fetal movement. Birth weight was 1.6 kg. He began to walk at 22 months.

Sister (10 years old) is 138 cm tall.

Height is 136 cm, weight 28 kg. Right side of face and body, right limbs, and right hand and foot are larger than left. Little fingers curve inward. Left little finger lacks distal crease.

Second and third toes are fused. The rest of the physical findings are normal.

Spine is convex left, apex about L1; right hip is higher than left (Figure 31-1). Distal phalanx of left little finger curves inward and bone age in left hand is normal (Figure 31-2).

Diagnosis: Russell-Silver syndrome, scoliosis, Kirner deformity of little finger.

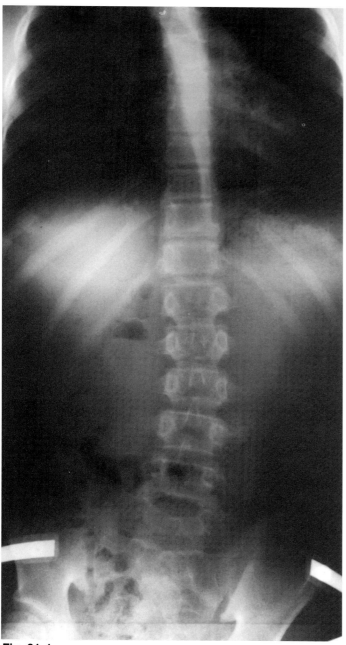

Fig. 31-1

(Continued)

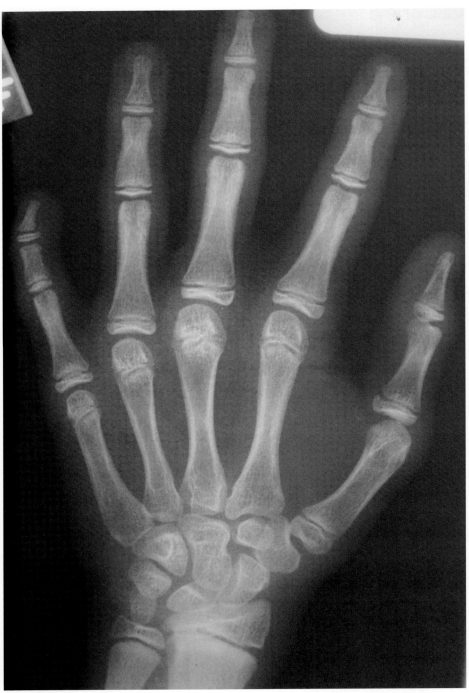

Fig. 31-2

Case 32

A 4-month-old girl is vomiting.

Pregnancy was normal, birth weight 3.5 kg. She began to vomit and had watery stools when switched from breast milk to formula at 2 months. Vomiting has been worse the last 5 days.

Parents and seven siblings are well. Sister (6 years old) is short. A brother died with cough at 3 months.

Weight is 3.9 kg, length 52 cm, head circumference 40 cm, temperature 37.8°C, heart rate 140, respiratory rate 30, and blood pressure 82/50 mm Hg. She has fine hair, depressed anterior fontanel, poor skin turgor, and short limbs. Aphthae are on soft palate. Elbows do not extend fully. A 2-cm scar is on left forearm. Hands deviate medially. The rest of the physical findings are normal.

Hematocrit is 0.33. White cell count is 11.7×10^9/liter with 0.14 polymorphonuclear cells, 0.44 bands, 0.34 lymphocytes, 0.06 monocytes, and 0.02 eosinophils. Platelet estimate is adequate. Urine specific gravity is 1.016, pH 6. Urine has trace ketones, occasional epithelial cells/HPF, 30–35 white cells/HPF, and >100 hyaline casts/LPF. Serum sodium is 134 mmol/liter, potassium 3.2, chloride 91, urea nitrogen 7.5, calcium 2.86, phosphorus 1.61, and glucose 6.5. Alkaline phosphatase is 58 U/liter. IgA is 1.06 g/liter (normal: 0.04–0.80), IgM 0.96 (normal: 0.25–1.00), and complement component 3 0.91 (normal: ~1.112 ± 0.123).

Six-year-old sister has always had sparse, light hair and loose stools. She often has fever and earaches and was hospitalized when she was sick with chickenpox 1 year ago. She sat at 6 months, walked at 14 months, and talked at 18 months.

Sister's height at 6 years is 83 cm, weight 14.4 kg, and head circumference 49 cm. Right eardrum is perforated. The rest of the physical findings are normal.

Sister's hematocrit is 0.33. White cell count is 8.4×10^9/liter with 0.25 polymorphonuclear cells, 0.47 bands, 0.24 lymphocytes, and 0.04 monocytes. Platelet estimate is adequate. Serum calcium is 2.37 mmol/liter, phosphorus 1.55. Alkaline phosphatase is 52 U/liter. Total bilirubin is 5 μmol/liter. T_4 is 99 nmol/liter (normal: ~94–194). T_3 uptake is 0.28 (normal: 0.25–0.35). Albumin is 41 g/liter, α_1-globulin 3 (normal: 1–4), α_2-globulin 10 (normal: 5–12), β-globulin 7 (normal: 5–11), and γ-globulin 24 (normal: 5–17).

Figure 32-1 shows slightly irregular metaphyses of distal ulna, distal tibia, and distal fibula of 4-month-old girl. Ossification centers are already in the proximal femoral epiphyses in Figure 32-1. Figure 32-2 shows irregular metaphyses at knees and ankles and relatively long fibulas of 6-year-old girl.

Diagnosis: Cartilage-hair hypoplasia (metaphyseal chondrodysplasia, McKusick type).

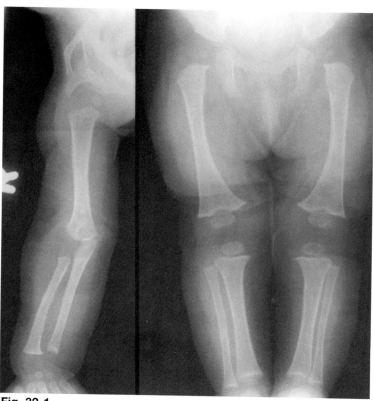

Fig. 32-1

(Continued)

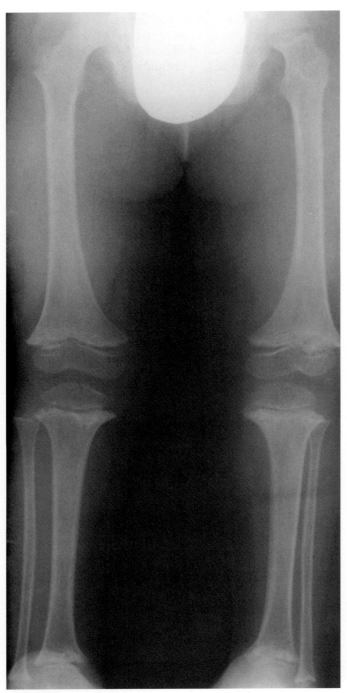

Fig. 32-2

Case 33

A newborn boy has small mandible and cleft soft palate.

Pregnancy of mother (21 years old) was normal. Birth weight is 3.6 kg, length 51 cm, Apgar score 5/8 at 1 and 5 minutes, temperature 32°C, heart rate 110, and respiratory rate 52. He is dusky until given oxygen. He chokes when fed at 2 hours. Small hemorrhages, some with white centers, are in retinas. Liver edge is 2 cm below costal margin. Limbs are short. A 1-cm papule is on left ankle. The rest of the physical findings are normal.

Hematocrit is 0.49. White cell count is 30.1 × 10⁹/liter with 0.71 polymorphonuclear cells, 0.04 bands, 0.15 lymphocytes, 0.08 monocytes, 0.01 eosinophils, and 0.01 basophils. Platelet count is 256 × 10⁹/liter. Serum sodium at 14 hours is 138 mmol/liter, potassium 6.1, chloride 105, carbon dioxide 12, urea nitrogen 3.0, calcium 2.57, phosphorus 2.36, choles-terol 2.40, and glucose 2.0. Creatinine is 80 μmol/liter, uric acid 450, and total bilirubin 54. Total protein is 70 g/liter, albumin 43. Alkaline phosphatase is 273 U/liter, LDH 1,251, and SGOT 132.

Figure 33-1A shows flat vertebrae, mediastinal air separating lobes of thymus from pericardium, and fractured right clavicle. Ends of femurs and tibias are broad at birth (Figure 33-1B) and at 3 years (Figure 33-2). Vertebral height is almost normal at 3 years.

Height is 86 cm at 2½ years, 89 cm at 3 years, when weight is 14.8 kg. He has had ear infections, palatoplasty, and myringotomies. Motor development is normal.

Diagnosis: Weissenbacher-Zweymuller syndrome (questionable infantile Stickler syndrome).

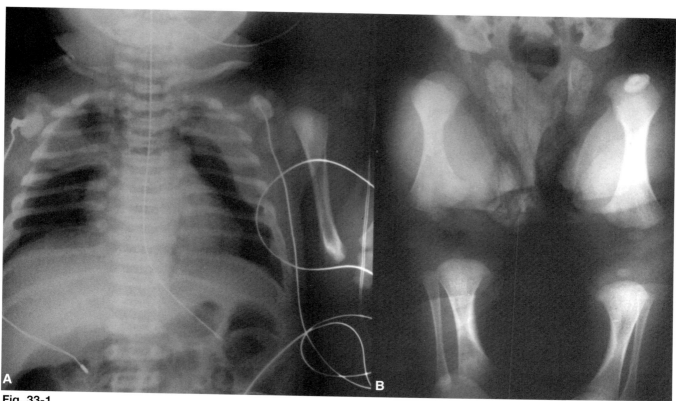

Fig. 33-1

(Continued)

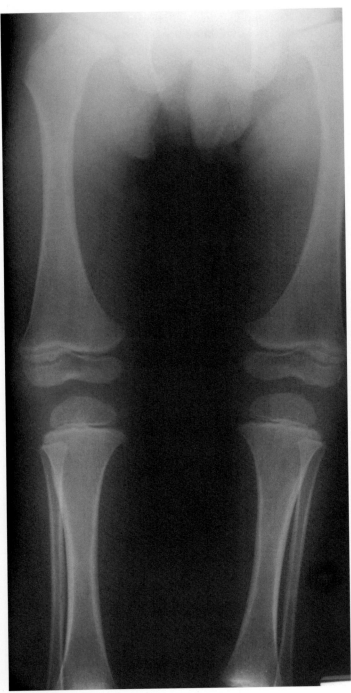

Fig. 33-2

Case 34

A 7-year-old girl, the tallest girl in her class, lacks full rotation at hips and has flat feet.

Mother (35 years old) had pain in hips and knees and took acetaminophen every day during pregnancy and her next pregnancy 2 years later. Birth weight was 4.2 kg, length 53 cm.

Sister (5 years old), who was myopic at 1 month and had epicanthi, depressed nasal bridge, and micrognathia, now has hypotonia, loose joints, and flat feet. Mother has micrognathia, scoliosis, joint pains, and myopia. Maternal aunt has scoliosis, joint pains, and myopia. Maternal grandmother had cleft lip and cleft palate, was blind with retinal detachment at 9 years, and died with hip cancer at 23 years.

The 7-year-old girl has epicanthi, depressed nasal bridge, midface hypoplasia, micrognathia, systolic heart murmur, long fingers, and loose joints, except at hips, where internal rotation is 30 degrees and external rotation 60 degrees. The rest of the physical findings are normal.

Figure 34-1A shows a central defect in head of left femur at 7 years. The defect is still there in examinations 4 months and 1 year later, when she has excellent range of motion at hips and no limp. Defects are gone at 11½ years (Figure 34-1B), when she is 161 cm tall, weighs 58.4 kg, and has full motion at hips.

Diagnosis: Stickler syndrome (hereditary arthro-ophthalmopathy).

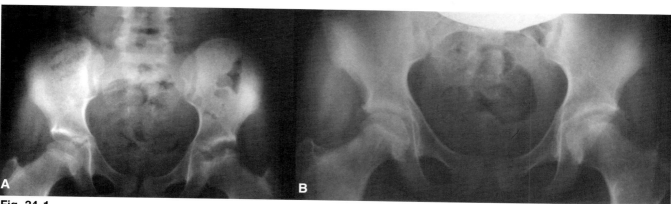

Fig. 34-1

Case 35

Father, daughter, and two sons are short and have limited motion at elbows.

Mother's height is 157 cm, father's 155 cm, daughter's 142 cm at 16 years, one son's 159 cm at 16 years, and other son's 149 cm at 20 years. Father, a carpenter, has pain in elbows. Girl had slight limitation of supination, pronation, and extension at 7 years and short forearms at 10 years. Twenty-year-old boy, whose adult height is 149 cm, was born with large eyes (buphthalmos) and cleft palate. Goniotomies were performed at 4 months for glaucoma. He had otitis media and treatment with myringotomy and tubes. Cleft palate was repaired at 20 months. Vision was only light perception at 10 years. Supination and pronation at elbow were limited, legs bowed. Pain in eyes led to enucleation. He had scoliosis at 15 years.

He has anterior open bite because of short mandibular rami at 20 years. He walks with toes pointed inward.

Roentgenogram of girl's forearms in Figure 35-1 shows bowed radii, acute carpal angles, and dorsal displacement of ulnas at wrists. Roentgenogram in Figure 35-2A shows dorsal displacement of radius at elbow in shorter boy's left forearm. Findings in right forearm are similar. Figure 35-2B shows bowed radii in father's forearms, acute carpal angles, and separate bone between medial epicondyle and trochlea of right humerus.

Diagnosis: Dyschondrosteosis, Madelung deformity, mesomelic dwarfism.

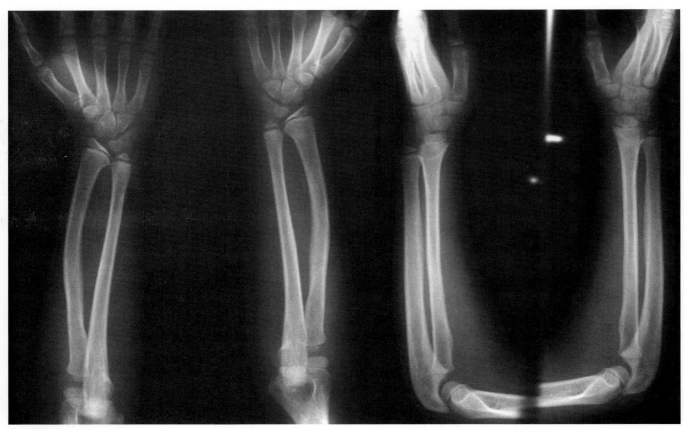

Fig. 35-1

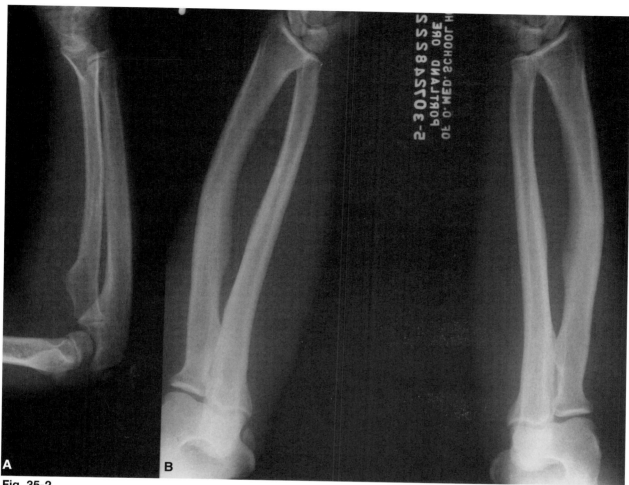

Fig. 35-2

Case 36

An 11-year-old girl tires quickly when she walks but does not become short of breath.

Birth weight was 3.2 kg. She rolled over at 2 months, sat at 6 months, and walked at 12 months. She had ear infections and a staphylococcal infection of neck from 1 to 2½ years. Tonsils and adenoids were removed at 2½ years. She has had 11 tympanostomies with tube placement and 12 dental extractions. She wets bed. She has headaches. Arms, ankles, and feet hurt. She is relieved by heat and bothered by cold.

Mother (36 years old) and sister (6 years old) are well. Father (40 years old) was weak and slow moving, wet bed until he was 13 years old, had hyperesthesia in legs, and felt "awful" until he was in his twenties. His strength is "average" now. He likes to go hunting and to sit in a hot tub.

Weight at 11 years is 24 kg, height 137 cm, and head circumference 54 cm. She lurches to left when she walks. She uses furniture to pull herself up from prone. Grip is weak. She has a hearing aid in left ear. Limbs are thin with little subcutaneous tissue. Skin is velvety; blood vessels are prominent. Motion at shoulders, hips, knees, and ankles is limited. Feet are flat. She can hardly bear to have abdomen and legs touched. Deep tendon reflexes are weak. The attempt to elicit them almost makes her cry. The rest of the physical findings are normal. Blood pressure at 12 years is 110/70 mm Hg. Vision and hearing are normal at 12 years.

Hematocrit is 0.41. White cell count is 7.5×10^9/liter. Platelet count is 368×10^9/liter. Serum sodium is 141 mmol/liter, potassium 4.1, chloride 107, carbon dioxide 21, urea nitrogen 4.3, calcium 2.25, phosphorus 1.19, cholesterol 3.18, and glucose 4.3. Creatinine is 40 µmol/liter, uric acid 170, total bilirubin 7, and direct bilirubin 0. Total protein is 71 g/liter, albumin 42. Alkaline phosphatase is 432 U/liter, LDH 113, and SGOT 13. Free T_4 is 14 pmol/liter (normal: 10–36). TSH is 5 mU/liter (normal: 2–11).

Calvaria and base of skull of daughter (Figure 36-1A) and father (Figure 36-1B) are thick. Her temporal bones are sclerotic (see Figure 36-1A); his are pneumatized (see Figure 36-1B). Her ribs are thick. Figure 36-2A shows thick cortex of bones in girl's arms. Her legs and some metacarpals and metatarsals show similar findings. Figure 36-2B shows thick cortex of father's femur. His radius and ulna are also thick.

Diagnosis: Diaphyseal dysplasia (Engelmann's disease).

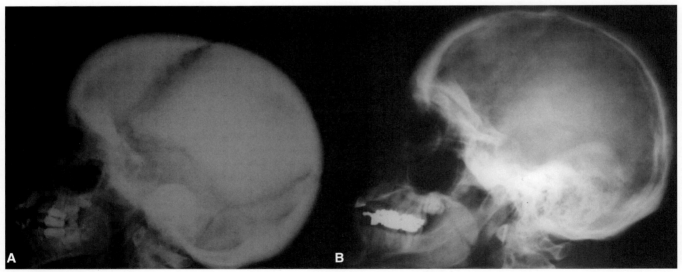

Fig. 36-1

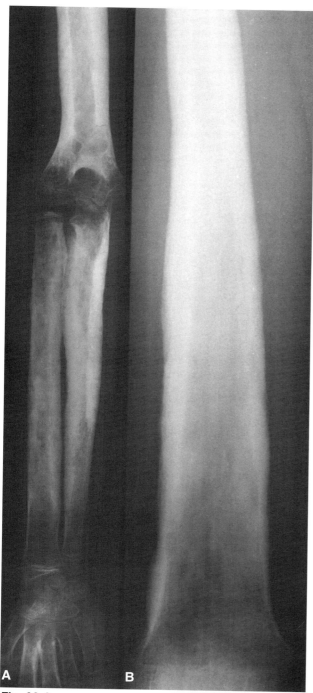

Fig. 36-2

Case 37

A 6-year-old boy has lumps on right scapula, some ribs, and bones of limbs. He has had some of these lumps since he was 22 months old.

Mother is well. Father, father's first cousin, and father's grandfather have bony lumps.

Weight is 20 kg, height 112 cm, temperature 36.9°C, heart rate 80, respiratory rate 20, and systolic blood pressure 80 mm Hg. The rest of the physical findings are normal.

Hematocrit is 0.36. White cell count is 9.3×10^9/liter. Urine specific gravity is 1.030, pH 5.5. Urine has occasional non-squamous epithelial cells/HPF and mucus. Serum sodium is 144 mmol/liter, potassium 4.6, chloride 107, carbon dioxide 25, urea nitrogen 6.4, and glucose 5.1.

Bony lumps deform right scapula and lower left costochondral junctions (Figure 37-1), and bones of limbs (Figure 37-2). Some metacarpals, metatarsals, and phalanges of fingers and toes are also deformed by lumps.

Diagnosis: Multiple cartilaginous exostoses (diaphyseal aclasis).

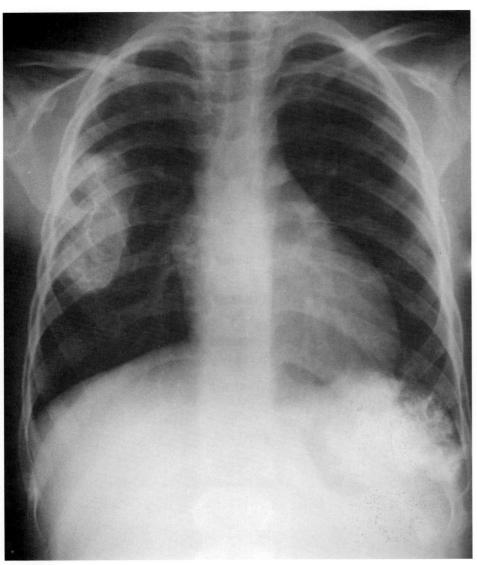

Fig. 37-1

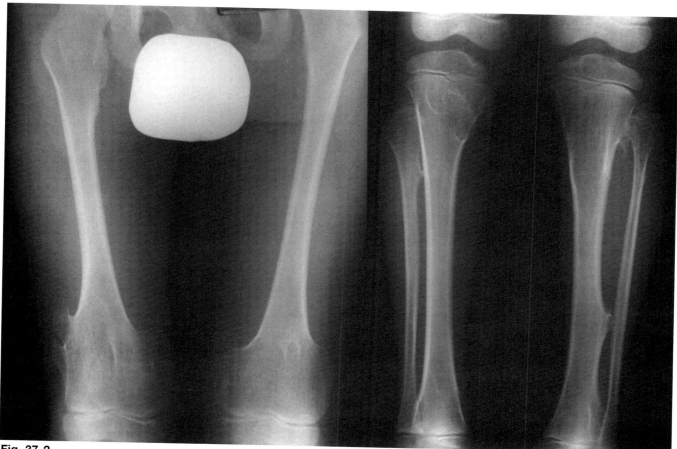

Fig. 37-2

Case 38

A 15-month-old girl has half-closed left eye and lolling head.

Pregnancy was normal, birth weight 3.9 kg. She crawled at 6 months. Ptosis of left upper lid, which first appeared 1 month ago, and neck weakness, which first appeared 3 weeks ago, begin several hours after she wakes up.

Mother and five older siblings are well. Father (57 years old) is 155 cm tall and has had hip trouble since he was 12 years old. Paternal grandfather had hip disease. Paternal uncle and cousin have hip disease.

Temperature is 37.3°C, heart rate 110, respiratory rate 26, weight 9.8 kg, and length 69 cm. Left eye does not adduct past midline. Head lags when she is pulled up to sitting. The rest of the physical findings are normal.

Ptosis disappears briefly after IM edrophonium, longer after subcutaneous neostigmine (Prostigmin). She is treated with oral neostigmine. She has a cold at 3½ years, gets weaker, and after 5 days (1 day after last dose of neostigmine) cannot swallow. Mouth is full of phlegm. She improves quickly after subcutaneous neostigmine (Prostigmin) and waddles away bowlegged.

Hematocrit is 0.34 at 15 months. White cell count is 15.7×10^9/liter with 0.30 polymorphonuclear cells, 0.15 bands, 0.52 lymphocytes, 0.02 monocytes, and 0.01 eosinophils. Platelet estimate is adequate. Urine specific gravity is 1.034, pH 5. Urine has trace ketones, mucus, bacteria, 3–4 epithelial cells/HPF, and 2–3 red cells/HPF. Serum urea nitrogen is 5.0 mmol/liter, calcium 2.52, and phosphorus 1.49. Creatinine is 40 µmol/liter. Alkaline phosphatase is 89 U/liter.

Figure 38-1 shows abnormal epiphyseal ossification centers in carpal bones, hands, and hips at 8 years. Ossification centers are also abnormal in arms, legs, feet, and tarsal bones at 8 years. Knees show erosion and prominent longitudinal striations at 13 years (Figure 38-2). Hips also show erosion. Two brothers and one sister have similar skeletal abnormality. Father's hips show marked degeneration (Figure 38-3).

She no longer needs anticholinesterase at 16 years. She has hip pain at 16 years, lower back pain at 23 years. Height at 23 years is 133 cm.

Diagnosis: Myasthenia gravis, multiple epiphyseal dysplasia.

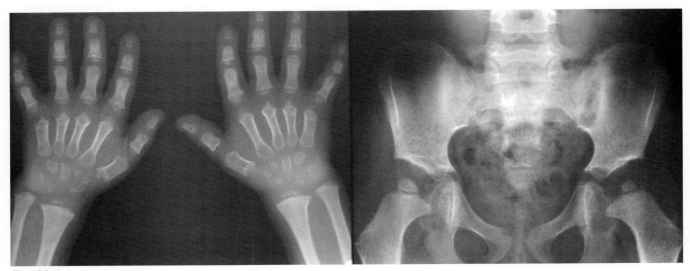

Fig. 38-1

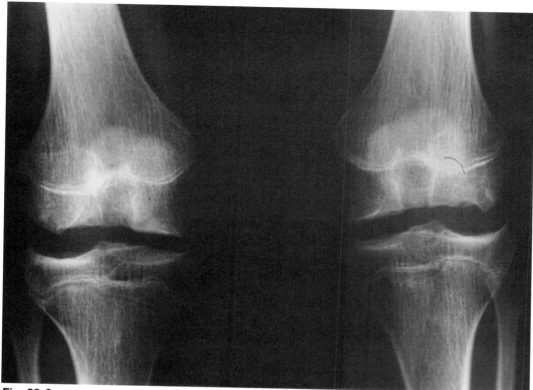

Fig. 38-2

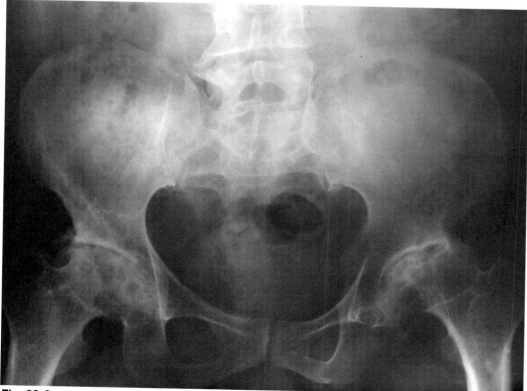

Fig. 38-3

Case 39

A 5-year-old girl is short.

Pregnancy was normal, birth weight 3.6 kg. She had short limbs, cataract in right eye, and Pierre Robin abnormality treated by glossopexy and gastrostomy. At 1½ years she had closure of soft palate and placement of myringotomy tubes. Bone obtained from iliac crest during that operation showed abnormal growth plate with large cartilage cells of variable size, cytoplasmic inclusions in resting chondrocytes, and normal matrix. She has had a lot of ear infections and has sensorineural hearing loss. She wears glasses.

Mother (31 years old) and father (36 years old) are well. The girl is their only child.

Height at 5 years is 84 cm, arm span 89 cm, weight 14 kg, temperature 37.7°C, heart rate 120, respiratory rate 34, and blood pressure 74/58 mm Hg. She breathes through mouth. Neck flexion makes it hard to breathe. Eardrums are dull and immobile. Small lymph nodes are in neck. Upper chest is narrow. Lower ribs flare. A scar is in left side of abdomen.

Femurs abduct 45 degrees. Left femur can be pushed backward out of acetabulum and then abducted into acetabulum. The rest of the physical findings are normal. Pulmonary function test shows normal lung volumes and spirometric values.

Hematocrit is 0.41. White cell count is 8.5×10^9/liter with 0.35 polymorphonuclear cells, 0.57 lymphocytes, 0.07 monocytes, and 0.01 eosinophils.

Roentgenogram at birth shows short limbs, flat vertebrae, and no pubic ossification (Figure 39-1). Metaphyses and some epiphyses, especially at hip, are abnormal at 5 years (Figure 39-2). Vertebrae are flat at 5 years.

C1–C2 fusion is performed at 8 years. Menarche is at 12 years. She has hip and knee pain. She is in seventh grade at 13 years. Height is 99 cm, weight 33 kg, and head circumference 55 cm. She has limited flexion and extension in neck and at hips, pectus carinatum, and thoracolumbar kyphos.

Diagnosis: Spondyloepimetaphyseal dysplasia.

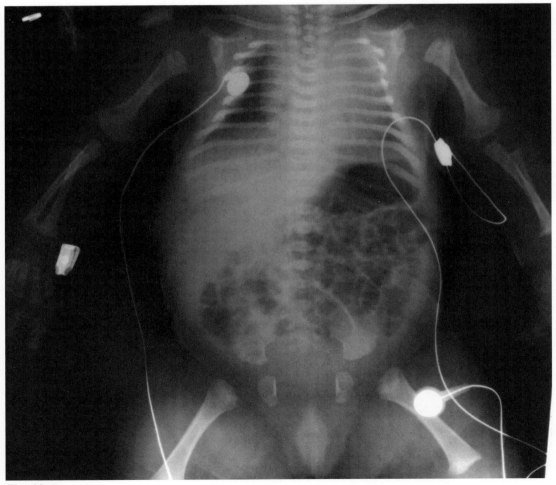

Fig. 39-1

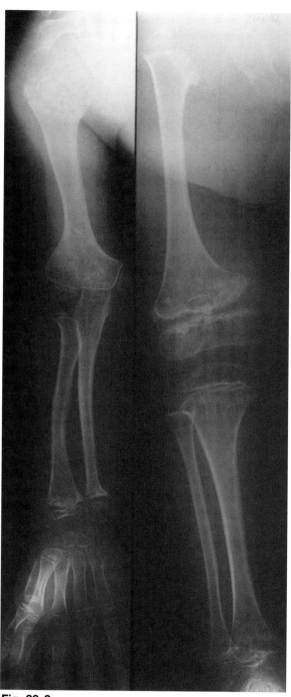

Fig. 39-2

Case 40

A 6-day-old girl has pincer-tight hands, dislocated joints, and clubfeet.

Mother (19 years old) took iron for anemia during pregnancy. Mother had mild clubfoot during infancy; maternal aunt had clubfeet and now has left facial palsy. Child of another maternal aunt has clubfeet. Father (22 years old) has worn glasses for myopia since he was 12 years old.

Birth weight was 2.9 kg. Weight at 6 days is 2.8 kg, temperature 37.2°C, heart rate 140, respiratory rate 32, and head circumference 33 cm. Hard and soft palate is cleft. Liver edge is 1 cm below costal margin. Fingers are long and untapered, thumbnails broad. Left femur is dislocated at hip; right hip is tight. Legs are flexed at knees. Feet are clubbed. The rest of the physical findings are normal.

Hematocrit is 0.48. White cell count is 19.1 × 10⁹/liter with 0.39 polymorphonuclear cells, 0.05 bands, 0.47 lymphocytes, 0.05 monocytes, 0.03 eosinophils, and 0.01 myelocytes. Platelet estimate is adequate. Urine specific gravity is 1.008, pH 6.

Urine has 0–10 epithelial cells/HPF and 70–80 white cells/HPF. Serum urea nitrogen is 8.6 mmol/liter.

Roentgenogram at 7 days shows radius dislocated at elbows (on both sides), clenched fingers, and distal radial epiphyseal ossification center (Figure 40-1A). Figure 40-1B shows flexed knees, clubbed feet, left femur out of acetabulum, fibulas high at knees, and ossification center in proximal epiphysis of right femur and distal epiphyses of tibias.

Weight at 1½ years is 6.6 kg, length 69 cm. She is weak and cranky. Nose is small and flat, midface flat. Simian creases are in palms. Fingers are long, their distal phalanges broader than normal. Distal phalanges of girl's thumbs and mother's thumbs are short and broad.

She has many colds. Palate is repaired at 3¾ years, when she is deemed robust enough for operation.

Diagnosis: Larsen syndrome.

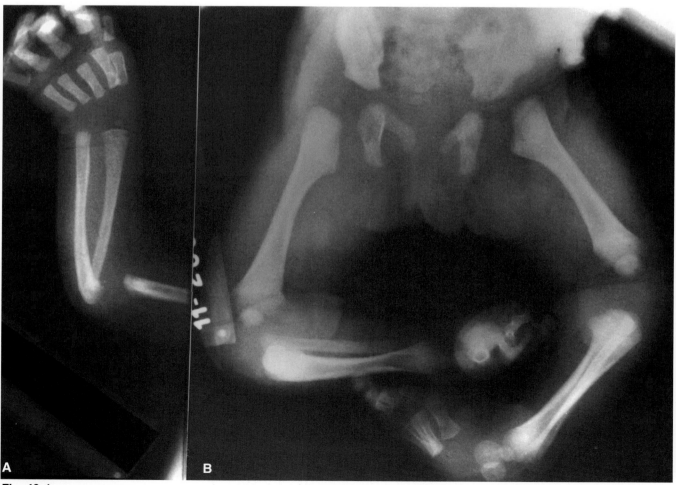

Fig. 40-1

Case 41

A newborn boy is floppy and unresponsive until intubated and given oxygen.

Pregnancy was marred by poor fetal movement, polyhydramnios, and, in last 3 weeks, by proteinuria. Labor was marred by slowing of fetal heart rate to 40.

Mother (37 years old) and father (39 years old) are well. Their only other children, twin boys, who were floppy and unresponsive with chromosomes 46,XY and identical blood group genotypes, died in infancy 9 years ago.

Birth weight is 2.7 kg, head circumference 35 cm, Apgar score 1/1 at 1 and 10 minutes. Temperature at 3 hours is 36.5°C, heart rate 130. Mandible is small. Fingers are flexed, feet clubbed. Right thigh is swollen. Left testis is in inguinal canal, right not palpable. Left second and third toes are partly fused. He moves arms slightly with needle injections, legs not at all. Deep tendon reflexes are absent. The rest of the physical findings are normal.

Hematocrit is 0.55. White cell count is 11.1×10^9/liter with 0.55 polymorphonuclear cells, 0.09 bands, 0.26 lymphocytes, 0.08 monocytes, and 0.02 eosinophils. Platelet count is 271×10^9/liter. Serum sodium at 2 days is 131 mmol/liter, potassium 4.4, chloride 90, carbon dioxide 25, urea nitrogen 11.1, calcium 1.50, phosphorus 2.84, cholesterol 1.89, and glucose 6.0. Creatinine is 80 µmol/liter, uric acid 800, total bilirubin 147, and direct bilirubin 12. Total protein is 47 g/liter, albumin 33. Alkaline phosphatase is 140 U/liter, LDH 428, SGOT 69, and CK 1,260 (normal: ~100–600).

Figure 41-1 shows limbs with little muscle and thin bones, thin ribs, and fractured right femur.

He dies at 16 days. Necropsy shows thin, pale brown skeletal muscle. In microscopic examination, skeletal muscle fibers are in groups of variable size, from small fibers with central nuclei to large fibers with peripheral nuclei and increased fibrous stroma. Number of anterior horn cells in spinal cord is reduced. Many of those present are swollen and chromatolytic. Subarachnoid blood and cerebral periventricular leukomalacia are present. Several swollen neurons with chromatolysis and nuclei off to one side are in hypoglossal nucleus and nucleus ambiguus. Necropsy of one twin, who died at 3 months, showed pale quadriceps muscle and appropriate complement of anterior horn cells in cervical and lumbar enlargements of spinal cord. Necropsy of other twin, who died at 6 months, showed diminished anterior horn cells in spinal cord; mixed segmental atrophy, fatty replacement, and normal striated quadriceps muscle; and pancreatic nodule in wall of duodenum.

Diagnosis: Amyoplasia (arthrogryposis multiplex congenita).

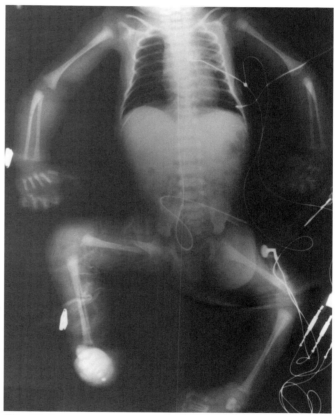

Fig. 41-1

Case 42

A 4-month-old girl has thick tissues behind partly flexed knees.

Pregnancy was marred by hypertension and proteinuria in third trimester. Birth weight was 4.0 kg. Tissues were thick behind knees. A cleft was in hard and soft palate. Thin strands of tissue were between eyelids and in mouth. Feet were clubbed and had four toes: first toe and three webbed toes.

Father and paternal uncle had cleft palate. Father had operations to lengthen calcaneal tendons; paternal uncle had leg amputated for abnormality similar to girl's.

Weight is 7.3 kg, length 63 cm, head circumference 44 cm, temperature 37.2°C, heart rate 144, respiratory rate 32, and systolic blood pressure 100 mm Hg. Eardrums are dull. Small hemangiomas are on body. Strands in mouth prevent full opening. Limb abnormality is like that at birth. The rest of the physical findings are normal.

Hematocrit is 0.29. White cell count is 10.7×10^9/liter. Platelet count is 622×10^9/liter. Urine specific gravity is 1.011, pH 5. Urine has 0.03 g/liter protein and occasional squamous epithelial cells/HPF.

Figure 42-1 shows thick, soft tissues behind knees.

At operation on back of left leg, a fibrous band under subcutaneous tissue overlies anomalous muscle from ischium to calcaneal tendon. Sciatic nerve is under a nerve from high thigh to lateral malleolus. Fibula is farther back than normal. Flexor digitorum longus muscle is pale and atrophic. A large muscle in position of flexor hallucis longus goes lateral to ankle. At operation on back of right leg 1 month later, strands in mouth must first be cut before mouth opens wide enough for endotracheal intubation. Two muscle bellies deep to subcutaneous tissue become tendinous in midcalf with medial insertion in fascia, lateral insertion to calcaneus. Transverse fibrous bands extend from anomalous muscle. Sciatic nerve with high origin of tibial nerve is just below anomalous muscle. Calcaneal tendon inserts in front of normal position.

Microscopic examination of excised tissue shows connective tissue, nerves, normal infant muscle, and focal fibrosis.

At operation at 10 months, anomalous striated muscle is in medial part of feet.

Diagnosis: Popliteal pterygium syndrome.

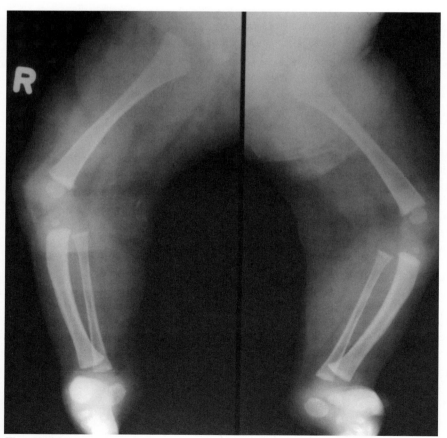

Fig. 42-1

Case 43

An 11-year-old girl has left thigh ache, which becomes worse with movement, better with heat.

Pregnancy was normal. First toes were curved under feet at birth and operated on at 1 year. She walked at 14 months. She had febrile convulsion at 5 years. A tender swelling on left side of neck spread up neck and over front of chest and then became smaller, hard, and nontender. More hard lumps were in neck, shoulders, and lower back at 7 years. She tired easily and napped a lot. Biopsy of neck muscle at 8 years showed small bundles, granulocytes, and loose areolar tissue.

Mother (47 years old) and father (50 years old) are well. The girl is their only child.

Heart rate at 11 years is 112, respiratory rate 20, and blood pressure 122/76 mm Hg. Hard lumps are in back of neck, in left sternocleidomastoid muscle, behind shoulders, and in back. Movement is limited in neck, shoulders, right thumb, first toes, and spine, which is convex right. Left thigh is tender. Thumbs, fifth fingers, and first toes are short. The rest of the physical findings are normal.

At 13 years, back of legs tire. Weight is 49 kg, height 168 cm. Neck flexes only 10–15 degrees. Right arm abducts 30 degrees and does not rotate externally. Left arm abducts 75–80 degrees. She bends forward only at hips. At 30 years, vital lung capacity is 0.68 of predicted normal. Serum bicarbonate is 16 mmol/liter. At 35 years, jaws are fixed almost closed. Spine is immobile. Movement is limited at shoulders, elbows, hips, knees, and ankles.

Bony bars are in subcutaneous tissues of neck and thorax at 11 years (Figure 43-1A) and behind neck at 13 years (Figure 43-1B).

Diagnosis: Fibrodysplasia ossificans progressiva.

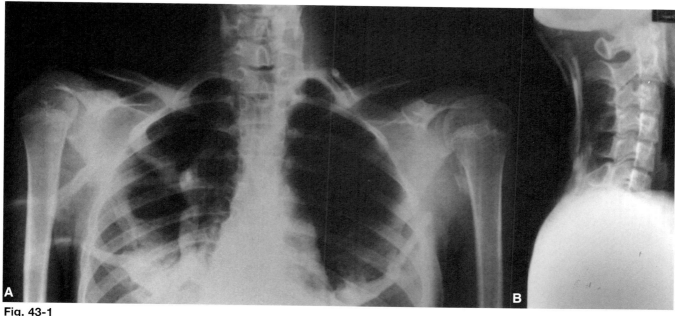

Fig. 43-1

Case 44

A 20-year-old woman, who was just in a car crash, has bruises on face and right leg.

Pregnancy was normal, birth weight 3.2 kg, length 53 cm. At 5 months, head was large. She could lift her head only briefly. At 3 years, umbilical hernia was repaired. At 5 years, she was nearsighted and had ptosis of upper right eyelid. Nasal bridge was depressed, palate high and arched, chin small, and neck short and broad. Voice was throaty. A systolic heart murmur was present. Elbows and knees were lax. Second and third toes were partly fused by soft tissue. The rest of the physical findings were normal. Chromosomes were 46,XX. Toluidine blue screen for mucopolysacchariduria was negative. Tonsils and adenoids were removed. At 10 years, IQ was 94. Menarche was at 11 years. Head circumference was 58 cm. Jaws were small, teeth crowded. At 18 years, partial maxillary osteoplasty was performed.

Mother (now 48 years old) and father were both taking thyroid pills when the girl was born. Father, now dead, had diabetes mellitus. A younger sister is well. Maternal grandmother was hypothyroid.

She is a college sophomore at 20 years. She wears glasses, for myopia, and hearing aids. Height is 140 cm, weight 37 kg, temperature 37.5°C, heart rate 120, respiratory rate 24, and blood pressure 102/74 mm Hg. Nose and right leg are bruised. Upper lip is cut. External acoustic meatuses are small. Nose is broad, nostrils are wide. Blood clot is in left side of nose. She has right nystagmus, slight clumsiness of right arm, atrophy of hand muscles, hypoesthesia across shoulders and upper arms, slight spasticity of left leg, left ankle clonus, and Babinski's sign in feet. Visual-evoked-response test shows impaired conduction in retinas or optic nerves; brain-auditory-response test indicates impaired conduction in auditory nerves or brain stem.

Hematocrit is 0.36. White cell count is 7.6×10^9/liter with 0.77 polymorphonuclear cells, 0.12 bands, 0.07 lymphocytes, and 0.04 monocytes. Platelet count is 233×10^9/liter. Urine specific gravity is 1.018, pH 6. Urine has 0–1 white cell/HPF. Serum sodium is 142 mmol/liter, potassium 4.8, chloride 110, carbon dioxide 25, urea nitrogen 8.6, calcium 2.20, phosphorus 1.16, cholesterol 3.98, and glucose 6.4. Creatinine is 100 μmol/liter, uric acid 160, total bilirubin 7, and direct bilirubin 0. Total protein is 58 g/liter, albumin 37. Alkaline phosphatase is 105 U/liter, LDH 200, and SGOT 30.

Figure 44-1A shows the following findings at 20 years: (1) Sutures and wormian bones are prominent; (2) skull is long, occiput bulges, base is flattened, and pituitary fossa is expanded; (3) frontal sinuses are not developed; and (4) mandibular angles are prominent, condyles small. Figure 44-1B shows C2–C3 zygapophyseal (lateral) joint fused by bone. Figure 44-2 shows acro-osteolysis in distal phalanx of right second digit. Fibula is high at knee. CT scan shows dilated lateral and third ventricles. MRI performed at 27 years because of weakness shows cervicothoracic syrinx.

Diagnosis: Hajdu-Cheney syndrome.

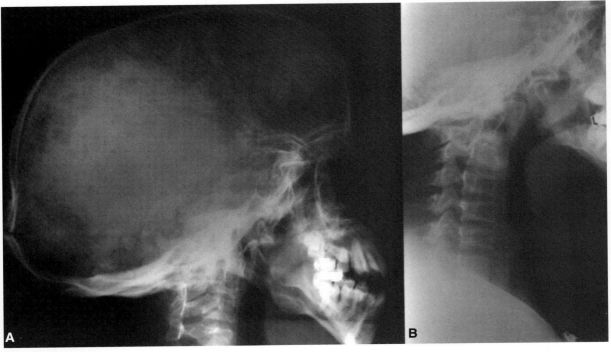

Fig. 44-1

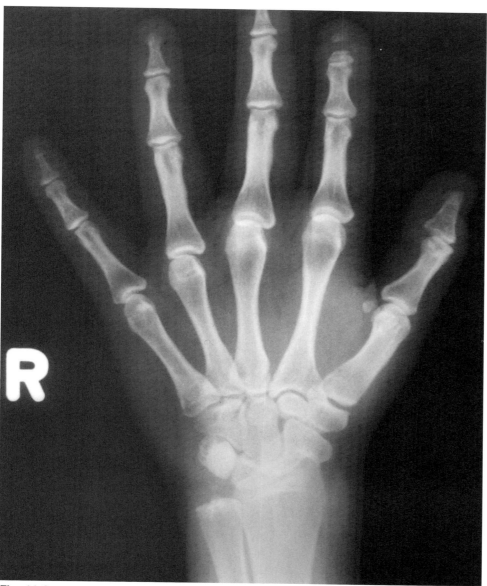

Fig. 44-2

Case 45

A 21-year-old woman has pain when she tries to lift left arm and has never been able to raise it high enough to fix her hair. She has had right exotropia since infancy and has decayed teeth and bleeding gums. Menarche was at 15 years.

Mother (42 years old) has exotropia and skin cancer.

Temperature is 36.9°C, heart rate 72, respiratory rate 18, blood pressure 125/75 mm Hg, weight 71 kg, and height 166 cm. Left shoulder is higher than right. Left arm can be abducted only 90 degrees. A systolic murmur is present. Fourth metacarpal bones are short. The rest of the physical findings are normal.

Hematocrit is 0.35. White cell count is 4.6×10^9/liter with 0.48 polymorphonuclear cells, 0.17 bands, 0.31 lymphocytes, 0.03 monocytes, and 0.01 eosinophils. Urine specific gravity is 1.015, pH 6. Urine has occasional squamous epithelial cells/HPF, 0–2 red cells/HPF, 4–6 white cells/HPF, and bacteria. Serum sodium at 24 years is 144 mmol/liter, potassium 4.4, chloride 108, carbon dioxide 27, urea nitrogen 4.3, calcium 2.69, phosphorus 1.13, cholesterol 4.22, and glucose 5.8. Creatinine is 60 µmol/liter, uric acid 230, total bilirubin 5, and direct bilirubin 0. Total protein is 75 g/liter, albumin 51. Alkaline phosphatase is 105 U/liter, LDH 225, and SGOT 26.

A papule with pearly border and small vessels is on left cheek, near eye, at 22 years, and another 6-mm papule, translucent and telangiectatic, on left breast 3 months later. Small pits are in palms and soles.

Falx cerebri and tentorium cerebelli are calcified at 22 years (Figure 45-1A). Figure 45-1B shows winged and elevated left scapula and asymmetric second ribs. Figure 45-2 shows a cyst and an impacted molar in right angle of mandible. Fourth metacarpals are short. Small defects are in bones of forearms, some metacarpals, and proximal phalanx of left third digit. Left fifth metacarpal is thickened. Defects are in femurs.

Nine tumors are removed from face and upper trunk during the next 2 years. Microscopic examination shows (1) hyperkeratosis of epidermis; (2) focal atrophy of stratum Malpighi; (3) small irregular bands of hyperchromatic basaloid cells without intercellular bridges in papillary dermis; (4) retraction of edematous, fibroblastic stroma from neoplastic cells; and (5) focal lymphocytic infiltrates.

Diagnosis: Nevoid basal cell carcinoma syndrome with Sprengel's deformity at left shoulder.

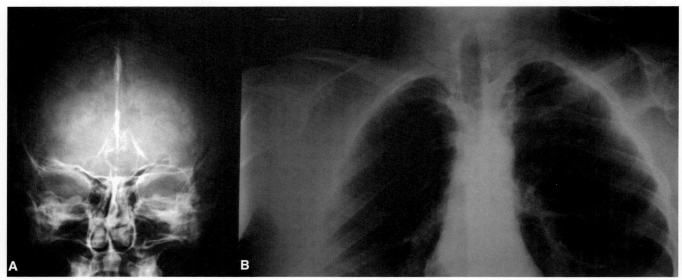

Fig. 45-1

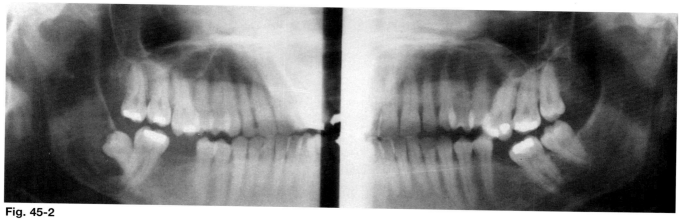

Fig. 45-2

Case 46

An 8-year-old boy has low backache that started 2 days ago when he was taking a bath. Ache is worse with flexion, better when resting on side.

Right ulna was fractured at 4 years when he twisted to get away from sister, who was holding his hand. Roentgenogram showed fracture through a cyst. Microscopic examination of cyst fragments removed with curet was thought to show unicameral bone cyst.

Temperature is 36.7°C. Right paraspinal muscles are in spasm. He can jump on either foot and walk on heels and toes. Motion at right hip hurts.

Right pedicle of lowest lumbar vertebra is sclerotic and enlarged, left pedicle is absent, and vertebra below pedicle is unilateral transitional vertebra (Figure 46-1).

Diagnosis: Absence of pedicle and transitional lumbosacral vertebra.

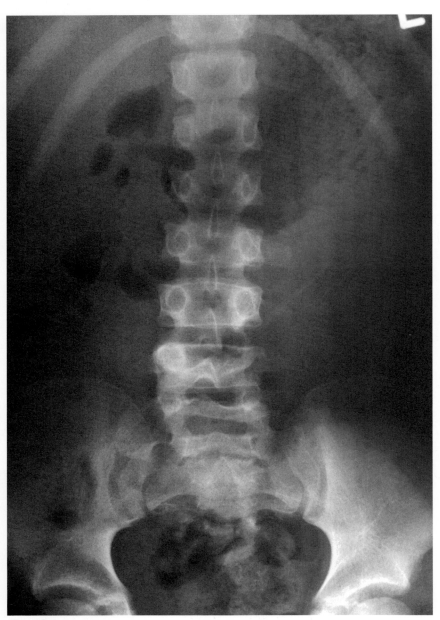

Fig. 46-1

Case 47

A 3½-week-old girl has soft swelling of back at L5–S1 and a strawberry hemangioma just to the left of swelling.

Pregnancy was normal, birth weight 4 kg.

Temperature is 37°C, heart rate 156, respiratory rate 38, blood pressure 98/72 mm Hg, weight 4.6 kg, and head circumference 39 cm. A soft swelling (3- to 4-cm diameter) is at L5–S1. A small, movable, hard lump is in the swelling, and a hemangioma is to the left. Perineal sensation is slightly diminished on left side. Anal wink reflex is absent. The rest of the physical findings are normal. Hematocrit is 0.38.

Examination of chest and abdomen in Figure 47-1A shows abnormal pedicles and increased interpediculate distance in upper sacrum. MRI (Figure 47-1B) shows conus medullaris of spinal cord at L3–L4, high signal in spinal canal behind it, and high signal with inner low signal in dorsal subcutaneous tissues. Ultrasound examination shows normal brain.

At operation, calcified cartilage is in swelling. A fibrovascular stalk goes through lumbodorsal fascia and into spinal canal. Laminae are removed from L3, L4, and L5. A dorsal lipoma continues into spinal canal and into a meningocele. All nerve roots of cauda equina are in front of lipoma and meningocele.

She walks at 1 year. Weight is 10.4 kg, height 71 cm, and head circumference 48 cm. At 2⅓ years, she walks normally and is toilet trained.

Diagnosis: Lipomyelomeningocele (tethered cord).

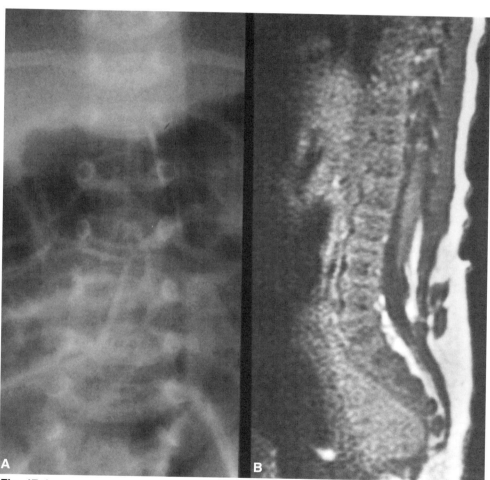

Fig. 47-1

Case 48

A 10-year-old girl, who has always had tight legs and walked on toes, has had increased tightness of right leg for several weeks.

Mother had high blood pressure during pregnancy. Birth weight was 3.2 kg. The girl had lumbosacral meningomyelocele that was closed at 2 days. Head circumference at 6 weeks was 40 cm. Scar and hemangioma were on back. Ventriculoperitoneal shunt was placed at 5 months. She cruised around furniture at 13 months. Legs were tight, feet clubbed. She walked on toes with femurs internally rotated and knees flexed. Sensation to touch and pinprick was diminished in legs. Deep tendon reflexes were exaggerated. Clonus was at ankles, Babinski's sign in feet. She had occipital headaches at 9 years and shunt revision. She is in fourth grade. For the last 3 weeks, legs have tired sooner than they used to, and right leg turns in more.

Mother (33 years old) and father (36 years old) are well. The girl is their only child.

Weight at 10 years is 23.8 kg, height 131 cm, temperature 36.9°C, heart rate 108, respiratory rate 20, and blood pressure 104/60 mm Hg. Shunt is palpable on right side of head. A scar and a patch of hair below it are in lumbosacral midline. Two scars are in right upper quadrant of abdomen. Liver edge is 2 cm below costal margin.

Hematocrit is 0.39. White cell count is 9.0×10^9/liter with 0.42 polymorphonuclear cells, 0.02 bands, 0.52 lymphocytes, and 0.04 monocytes. Platelet count is 390×10^9/liter. Urine specific gravity is 1.024, pH 7. Urine has 0–2 red cells/HPF, 0–2 white cells/HPF, and amorphous phosphates. Serum sodium is 135 mmol/liter, potassium 4.1, chloride 108, carbon dioxide 20, urea nitrogen 2.9, calcium 2.22, phosphorus 1.36, cholesterol 4.22, and glucose 8.1. Creatinine is 50 µmol/liter, uric acid 200, total bilirubin 10, and direct bilirubin 0. Total protein is 54 g/liter, albumin 39. Alkaline phosphatase is 181 U/liter, LDH 177, and SGOT 18.

Plain films at 20 months show abnormal L3 and L4; a small, roughly oval shadow of bone density at abnormal disc between them; and increased sacral and lower lumbar interpediculate distance (Figure 48-1). CT scan at 10 years shows a defect in left side of neural arch at L3–L4 and a spur of bone in spinal canal from vertebral body (Figure 48-2A). MRI at same level shows two collections of CSF in spinal canal (Figure 48-2B).

At operation, bone transects spinal canal at L3 just to left of scar of repaired meningomyelocele. Conus medullaris rises after dura around center of bone spike is divided, spike removed, and filum terminale divided from sacral nerve roots.

Microscopic examination of bone spike shows bone, marrow, cartilage, dense fibrous tissue, and hemorrhage. Microscopic examination of scar shows (1) dense connective tissue, (2) nerve fibers, (3) tangle of degenerated nerves, (4) meningeal fragments that have irregular deposits of calcium and psammoma bodies, and (5) blood vessels.

She is unaware of bladder fullness at 12 years. Sensation below knees is diminished. She walks at 18 years with femurs flexed, adducted, and internally rotated and knees flexed. Height is 159 cm, weight 53 kg.

Diagnosis: Meningomyelocele and diastematomyelia.

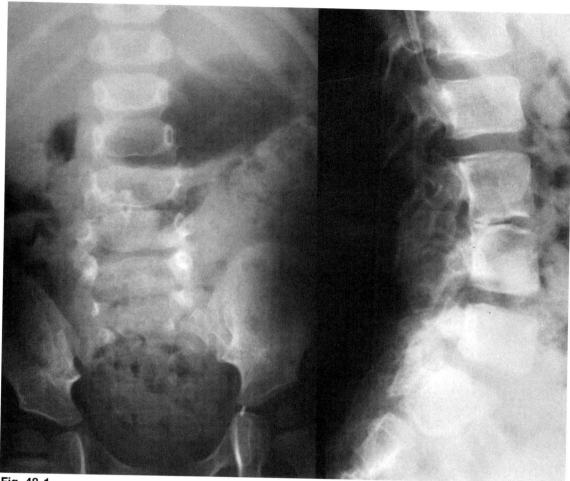

Fig. 48-1

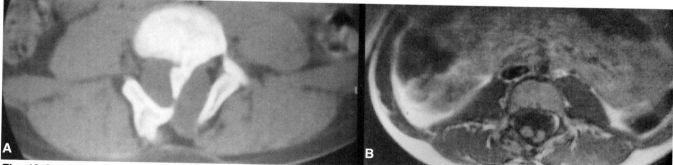

Fig. 48-2

Case 49

A 2-year-old girl turns left foot inward and trips over it when she walks.

Mother took birth control pills until she realized that she was pregnant at approximately 4 weeks gestation. Birth weight was 3.9 kg. A hemangioma covered smaller left buttock and extended to left labium majus. Clear liquid sometimes drains from the hemangioma. She walked at 11 months. She is aware of need to urinate and defecate. She speaks in short sentences.

Mother (23 years old) and father (29 years old) are well. The girl is their only child.

Weight at 2 years is 14 kg, height 91 cm, head circumference 49 cm, temperature 37.9°C, heart rate 140, respiratory rate 22, and systolic blood pressure 90 mm Hg. Left leg and foot are smaller than right. Left foot is cavus. Hemangioma remains on buttock, and another is on lateral side of left ankle. Deep tendon reflexes are diminished in left leg. The rest of the physical findings are normal.

Hematocrit is 0.37. White cell count is 10.6×10^9/liter with 0.18 polymorphonuclear cells, 0.04 bands, 0.68 lymphocytes, 0.06 monocytes, and 0.04 eosinophils. Platelet estimate is adequate. Urine specific gravity is 1.025, pH 5. Urine has few squamous epithelial cells/HPF, 4–6 white cells/HPF, and amorphous urates. Serum sodium is 143 mmol/liter, potassium 5.0, chloride 109, carbon dioxide 24, urea nitrogen 7.1, calcium 2.72, phosphorus 1.87, cholesterol 4.60, and glucose 4.4. Creatinine is 40 μmol/liter, uric acid 210, and total bilirubin 4. Total protein is 67 g/liter, albumin 48. Alkaline phosphatase is 181 U/liter, LDH 247, and SGOT 34.

Roentgenograms at 2 months (Figure 49-1A) and 7 years (Figure 49-1B) show sacral dysplasia and a piece of bone in left side of pelvis. Myelogram at 2 years shows sacral meningocele (Figure 49-2). Angiogram at 2 years shows dilated, tortuous pelvic arteries and veins, and a vascular mass (8.5 × 5.5 cm) in front of left side of sacrum.

She receives no treatment. She has normal bowel and bladder control at 14 years. Height is 166 cm, weight 52 kg. No mass is palpable. A large tuft of hair is just lateral to left side of anus. Left leg and foot are smaller than right. She is pregnant at 18 years.

Diagnosis: Buttock hemangioma, anterior sacral meningocele, teratoma.

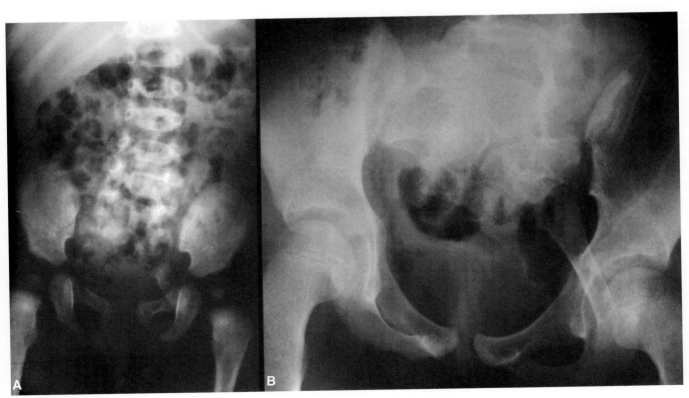

Fig. 49-1

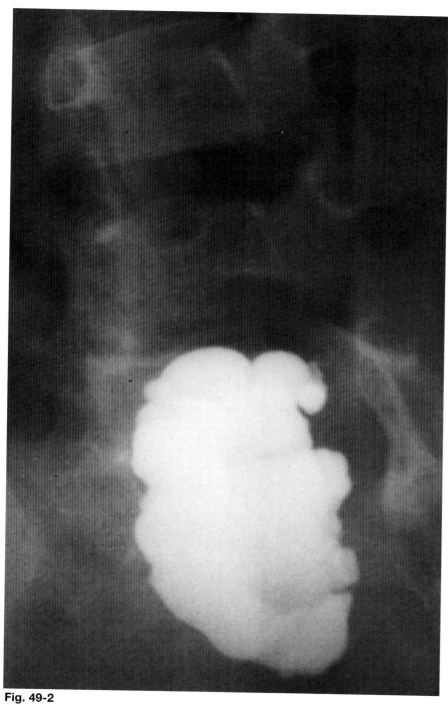

Fig. 49-2

Case 50

A 6½-year-old girl waddles and has storklike shanks.

Birth weight was 3.2 kg, length 46 cm. Examination at 4 days showed midlumbar spinal ridge, buttocks dimpled at greater trochanters, narrow pelvis, legs and feet curled and turned inward, ability only to flex and adduct hips and flex and extend knees, and mild clubfeet. Clubfeet were treated with casts in infancy and with right Turco clubfoot release at 4½ years. She began to walk at 2 years. Schoolmates tease her about her gait. She often wets bed and pants.

Mother (30 years old), father (35 years old), brother (5 years old), and sister (3 years old) are well. Paternal grandmother died with pancreatic cancer; maternal grandfather died with lung cancer.

Weight is 17.7 kg, height 107 cm, and head circumference 52 cm. Gluteal muscles are atrophic. Muscle function is absent below knees. Right foot is clubbed, left flat. Little subtalar motion is in feet. The rest of the physical findings are normal.

Roentgenogram in Figure 50-1 shows fewer than normal lumbar vertebrae, shortened interpediculate distance of lower lumbar spinal canal, no sacrum, butterfly vertebrae in thorax, and slight lateral displacement of femurs.

Menarche is at 13 years. Patellas subluxate. Triple arthrodesis is performed on left foot. At 16 years, she falls two to three times per month because of subluxation of right patella and is treated by medial transfer of patellar tendon in tibia.

Weight at 16 years is 48.5 kg, height 147 cm, and blood pressure 110/88 mm Hg. Hematocrit is 0.32. White cell count is 5.3×10^9/liter. Platelet count is 249×10^9/liter. Urine specific gravity is 1.023, pH 6. Urine has 0.15 g/liter ketones, 3+ hemoglobin/myoglobin, 3–5 white cells/HPF, and 80–100 red cells/HPF. She is well at 22 years and studying for a Ph.D. in theater arts. Knees hurt occasionally.

Diagnosis: Agenesis of sacrum.

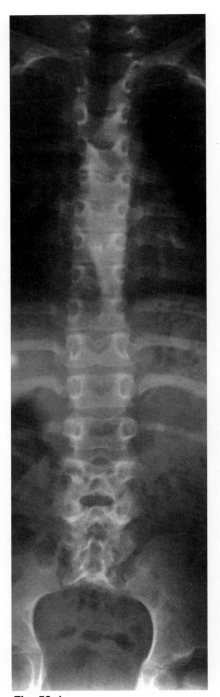

Fig. 50-1

Case 51

A 12-year-old girl cannot straighten her elbows.

Pregnancy was normal, birth weight 2.5 kg. Corneas were cloudy. A systolic heart murmur was heard at 7 days. Iridectomies were performed at 6 weeks. She walked at 20 months. At 2½ years, she was deaf and had nystagmus, cloudy corneas, large pupils, systolic heart murmur, diastolic heart murmur, and limited pronation, supination, and extension at elbows. Ductus arteriosus was ligated and divided. Intraocular pressure at 9 years was 38 mm Hg OD, 42 OS. Gait was wide waddle with knees stiff and feet turned out. A bony lump was on back of each ilium. Patellas were small and moved laterally when knees were flexed.

Knees of mother (40 years old) catch and give way when she descends stairs. Three brothers (11, 14, and 19 years old), sister (17 years old), and maternal grandmother have similar limitation at knees and elbows. Fourteen-year-old brother also has proteinuria, serum urea nitrogen 5.7 mmol/liter, serum creatinine 100 µmol/liter, and, in renal biopsy, proteinaceous eosinophilic matter in Bowman's spaces and hydropic degeneration of epithelial cells of proximal convoluted tubules.

Girl's weight at 12 years is 27 kg, height 134 cm, temperature 36.1°C, heart rate 78, respiratory rate 20, and blood pressure 80/60 mm Hg. Teeth are crowded. A scar is on left side of chest. A systolic heart murmur is present. Fingernails are small.

At 23 years, she has pain in hips, knees, and ankles after walking for long periods. Legs go to sleep after sitting for long periods.

A sclerotic wedge is in midilia at 2½ years. Figure 51-1 shows the sclerotic wedge at 12 years. L5 spondylolysis at 2½ years has changed to third-degree L5–S1 spondylolisthesis at 12 years (Figure 51-2). Sacroiliac joints are unusually oblique and prominent in Figure 51-1. Roentgenogram of 14-year-old brother shows similar sclerotic wedge in ilia and L5–S1 spondylolysis with second degree spondylolisthesis.

Diagnosis: Nail-patella syndrome (Fong disease), spondylolysis and spondylolisthesis, probable congenital rubella.

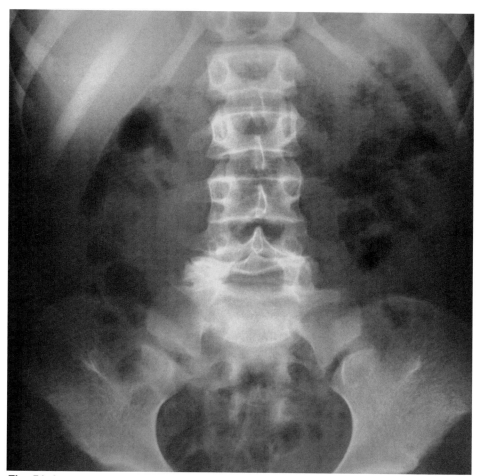

Fig. 51-1

(Continued)

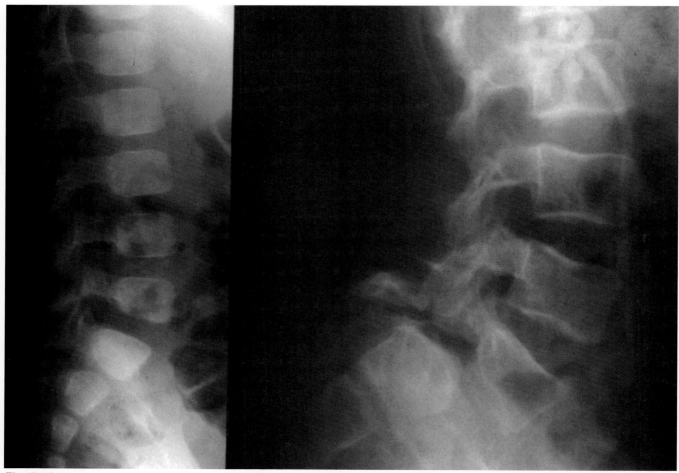

Fig. 51-2

Case 52

A 23-year-old man comes with fiancée for genetic counseling. His brother died at 15 years, father at 32 years, and paternal grandfather at approximately 60 years with kidney disease.

Weight is 61 kg, height 168 cm, and blood pressure 130/90 mm Hg. A soft-tissue web is in front of elbows. Elbows cannot be fully extended. Fingernail lunulae are triangular. Fingernails are dysplastic, especially little fingers, toenails less dysplastic. A bony lump is behind each ilium. Patellas are questionably palpable as small, high, and lateral. Dorsiflexion at ankles is limited. Feet are flat. The rest of the physical findings are normal.

Hematocrit is 0.49. White cell count is 9.1×10^9/liter. Platelet count is 289×10^9/liter. Urine has 3–5 g/liter protein. Serum sodium is 141 mmol/liter, potassium 4.3, chloride 110, carbon dioxide 22, urea nitrogen 6.8, calcium 2.27, phosphorus 1.16, cholesterol 6.41, and glucose 4.8. Creatinine is 90 μmol/liter, uric acid 360, total bilirubin 5, and direct bilirubin 0. Total protein is 58 g/liter, albumin 37. Alkaline phosphatase is 115 U/liter, LDH 230, and SGOT 19.

Roentgenograms at 11 years show back displacement of radii at elbows, hypoplasia of middle phalanges, and clinodactyly of little fingers in Figure 52-1A, and no ossified patellas in Figure 52-1B. Examination also shows normal renal collecting systems and triangles of bone in midilia.

He has palpitations and light-headed spells at 27 years. Blood pressure is 174/120 mm Hg. ECG findings are normal. Urine specific gravity is 1.016, pH 6. Urine has >3.0 g/liter protein, 5.6 mmol/liter glucose, 0–1 hyaline cast/LPF, 0–2 granular casts/LPF, 0–1 cellular cast/LPF, occasional squamous epithelial cells/HPF, and 0–3 white cells/HPF. Serum urea nitrogen is 10.0 mmol/liter. Creatinine is 260 μmol/liter. Antihypertensive treatment is begun. Serum urea nitrogen at 28 years is 18.9 mmol/liter, creatinine 430 μmol/liter. Creatinine clearance is 17 ml/min, 24-hour urinary protein 76 g. He has ankle edema at 28⅓ years. Serum urea nitrogen at 28½ years is 21.4 mmol/liter, calcium 1.95, and phosphorus 1.81. Creatinine is 690 μmol/liter. Peritoneal dialysis is begun at 28¾ years. Cadaveric kidney is transplanted at 31 years. He has a wife, children, and a job at 32 years. He cannot pay Medicare premiums.

Diagnosis: Nail-patella syndrome.

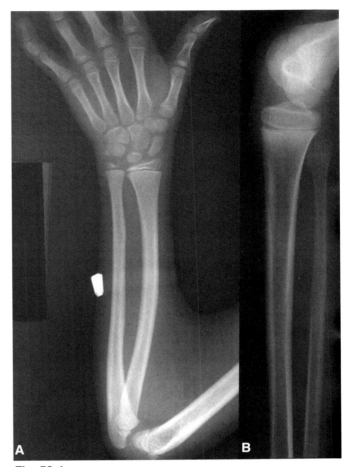

Fig. 52-1

Case 53

A 13-year-old boy, who has been in foster homes much of his life and is in fourth grade, has frontal headache.

He has been treated for clubfeet with casts and braces and has had bilateral inguinal herniorrhaphy. He has worn glasses since age 10 years.

Weight is 39.6 kg, height 150 cm, temperature 37°C, heart rate 60, respiratory rate 15, and blood pressure 100/60 mm Hg. Brow is prominent, with a widow's peak. Eyebrows meet. Auricles are low and cupped and lack antihelices. Eardrums are immobile. Nose is turned up, upper lip long, and mandible small with crowded teeth. Elbows lack full supina-tion. He cannot pat his back. Some fingers are short. Scrotum hoods penis. Ends of fibulas are high at knees. The rest of the physical findings are normal.

Radial heads stick out laterally in Figure 53-1A. In Figure 53-1B, fourth metacarpal bones are short; bone age is normal. Roentgenogram of shanks at 21 years because of painful knees and ankles shows bowlegs, high fibulas, and symmetric tibial exostoses (Figure 53-2).

Height at 21 years is 167 cm, weight 61 kg.

Diagnosis: Aarskog syndrome.

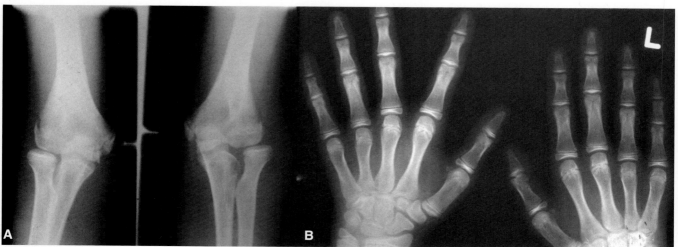

Fig. 53-1

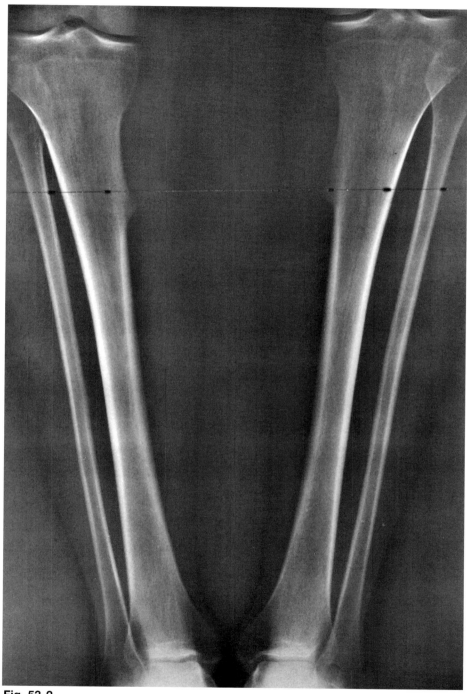

Fig. 53-2

Case 54

A 5-year-old boy has limited motion at elbows.

Mother (20 years old) took phenytoin daily during pregnancy.

Birth weight was 2.6 kg, length 47 cm, head circumference 33 cm, Apgar score 9/9 at 1 and 5 minutes, temperature 36.4°C, heart rate 156, and respiratory rate 56. He was irritable at 4 months and uninterested in surroundings. Muscle tone was increased. Arms were held in bus straphanger's position. Inguinal hernias were repaired at 4 months. He sat at 11 months. He was affectionate at 1 year. Instead of crawling he got up on hands and knees and pulled self to flop. Elbows lacked 30-degree full extension and could not supinate beyond neutral. Fifth fingers and first toes were short. Right little finger was curved inward. Transverse creases were in palms and soles. Scars were in groins. The rest of the physical findings were normal.

He walks and runs normally at 5 years. Elbows lack full extension and do not supinate.

Examination at 5 years shows radii and ulnae fused at elbows (Figure 54-1A) and fused right talar and navicular bones (Figure 54-1B).

Weight at 9 years is 29 kg, height 134 cm.

Diagnosis: Radioulnar synostosis at elbows, right talonavicular coalition.

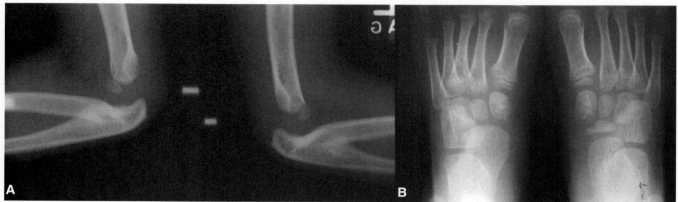

Fig. 54-1

Case 55

A 14-year-old boy's feet turn in. He also has stiff fingers like his father.

Fingers and toes have two phalanges (Figure 55-1). Second, third, and fourth fingers are fused at proximal interphalangeal joints, little fingers at distal interphalangeal joints (Figure 55-1A). Phalanges of left second and third toes are fused (Figure 55-1B). Carpal capitate, hamate, and trapezoid; right scaphoid, trapezium, and first metacarpal; and left scaphoid and trapezium bones are fused (see Figure 55-1A). A bone island is in left fourth finger (see Figure 55-1A).

Diagnosis: Symphalangism and carpal fusion.

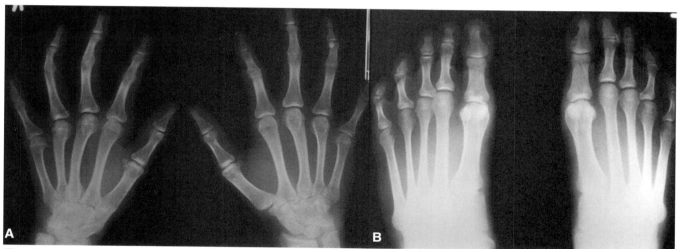

Fig. 55-1

Case 56

A 16-year-old girl has not begun menstruating.

Pregnancy of mother (then 33 years old) was normal, birth weight 2.3 kg, length 46 cm. She walked at 13 months. Cleft palate was repaired at 18 months. She had ear infections until 14 years. Left eye turns in. "She has a little girl voice." Fingers "just stopped growing."

Weight at 16 years is 42 kg, height 135 cm, heart rate 72, and blood pressure 120/80 mm Hg. Neck and trunk are squat, breasts are small, backs of hands and feet are puffy, and fingers and toes are short. She has no pubic hair. The rest of the physical findings are normal.

Left fourth and fifth metacarpal bones, third metacarpal bones to less degree (Figure 56-1A), and fourth metatarsal bones are short (Figure 56-1B). Trabecular pattern of bones in hands is coarse. Bone age in left hand is approximately 13 years, several standard deviations below the mean (see Figure 56-1A).

Chromosomes are 45,XO.

She is treated with estrogen. Height is 140 cm at 18 years.

Diagnosis: Turner's syndrome.

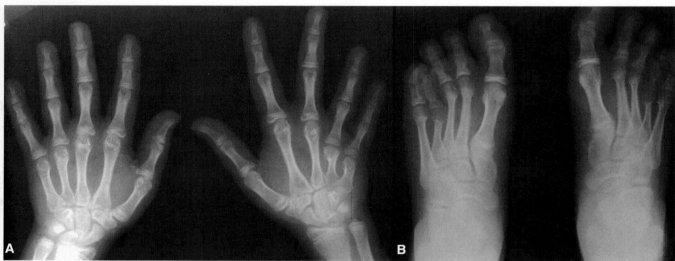

Fig. 56-1

Case 57

A 10-year-old girl has a bruised, swollen right thumb.

A car door was slammed on thumb 2 weeks ago. Thumbnail was removed because of subungual hematoma.

She had a heart murmur at 1 day, heart failure at 8 weeks. Cardiac catheterization at 7 months showed left-to-right ventricular shunt and infundibular pulmonic stenosis. A modified Fontan's operation was performed at 3½ years for functional single ventricle.

A radiolucent band is in distal phalanx of right thumb; distal phalanges of thumbs and middle phalanges of little fingers are short (Figure 57-1).

Diagnosis: Brachydactyly, type A3 (middle phalanx of fifth digit), type D ("stub thumbs"); traumatic acro-osteolysis of right thumb.

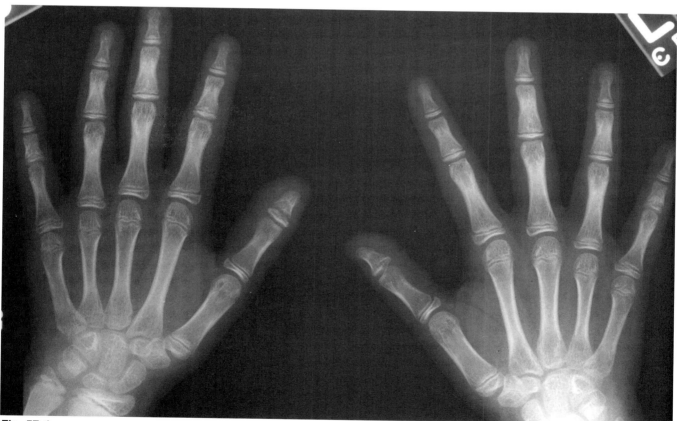

Fig. 57-1

Case 58

An 11-month-old girl has diarrhea.

Parents use illegal drugs. Birth weight was 1.9 kg, length 45 cm, head circumference 31 cm, and Apgar score 3/7 at 1 and 5 minutes. Skin was loose. Hair was whorled on both sides of head and came down almost to glabella. Fontanels were large, sutures wide. Eyebrows were thick. Skin was ridged from cheeks across broad nasal bridge. Auricles were small, low, and lumpy. Lips were thick. An omphalocele was present. Clitoris was swollen. Muscles were hypotonic. Nails and distal phalanges were absent from fourth and fifth fingers and toes. Second and third toes were partly fused. Urine tested positive for methamphetamines. Omphalocele was closed at 1 week. Weight at 2½ months was 2.5 kg, head circumference 34 cm. She was hospitalized for tube feeding at 3 months and for gastrostomy for feeding at 5 months. She crawls at 11 months.

Temperature at 11 months is 37.5°C, heart rate 156, respiratory rate 72, blood pressure 88/55 mm Hg, and weight 4.5 kg. Hair is receding from forehead; head is almost bald. A hemangioma is on head. Anterior fontanel is large. Lips are thick. Skin is loose. Surgical scar and gastrostomy button are on abdomen. Clitoris is large. Muscles are hypotonic, second and third toes are partly fused, fourth and fifth fingers and toes are without nails or distal phalanges.

Hematocrit is 0.37. White cell count is 18.5×10^9/liter with 0.61 polymorphonuclear cells, 0.05 bands, 0.29 lymphocytes, 0.04 monocytes, and 0.01 eosinophils. Platelet count is 603×10^9/liter. Urine specific gravity is 1.030, pH 5. Urine has trace ketones, urobilinogen, 5–10 white cells/HPF, 20–25 red cells/HPF, and few squamous epithelial cells/HPF. Serum sodium is 139 mmol/liter, potassium 5.1. Blood is HIV negative. Chromosomes are 46,XX.

Distal phalanges of fourth and fifth fingers in left (Figure 58-1) and right hands are absent at 11 months; other distal phalanges are small. Bone age is about newborn (see Figure 58-1).

Diagnosis: Coffin-Siris syndrome.

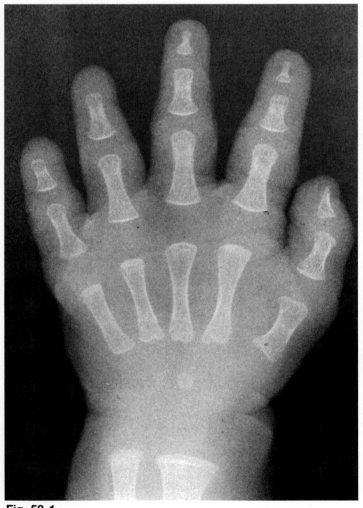

Fig. 58-1

Case 59

A newborn baby has fused legs and a 1-cm external genital stump.

Mother (28 years old) gained 7 kg during pregnancy. Uterine growth stopped at 6 months. No amniotic fluid appeared when membranes were artificially ruptured.

Birth weight is 2.2 kg, length 42 cm, head circumference 34 cm, and Apgar score 1/7 at 1 and 10 minutes. Infant is crying and pale. Breathing is noisy. Thick, yellow, blood-tinged mucus is in nose and mouth. A fleshy lump is in place of right ear. A systolic heart murmur is present. Two vessels are in umbilical cord. Urethra and anus are absent.

Venous blood pH at 1 hour is 7.05 when F_{IO_2} = 0.36. P_{CO_2} is 81 mm Hg, P_{O_2} 43. Serum sodium is 139 mmol/liter, potassium 4.3, chloride 107, urea nitrogen 1.8, and glucose 5.8. Creatinine is 70 μmol/liter. Chromosomes are 46,XX.

Roentgenogram at 5 hours (Figure 59-1) shows that (1) legs and feet are fused, (2) gut is distended with gas, (3) upper thoracic and thoracolumbar vertebrae are dysplastic, (4) 11 ribs are ossified on each side, (5) sacrum is dysplastic, and (6) ischia almost touch.

At necropsy soon after roentgenogram, one vein, one artery, and gut end at umbilicus. Distal aorta is hypoplastic. Kidneys, ureters, bladder, colon, and rectum are absent. Uterus, ovaries, and uterine tubes are present. Vagina is absent. Esophageal atresia and tracheoesophageal fistula are present. Heart is normal. Lungs are half normal weight. Microscopic examination shows (1) hemorrhage, primary atelectasis, and inflammation in lungs; (2) pancreatic islet cell hyperplasia; (3) congestion of cerebral vessels; and (4) normal adrenal glands.

Diagnosis: Sirenomelia.

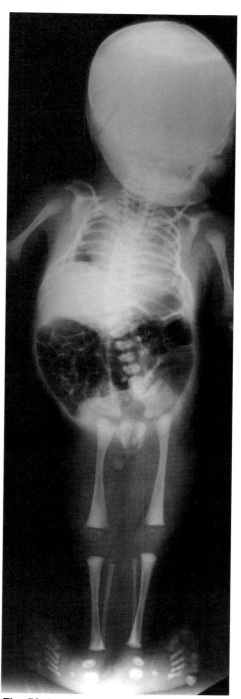

Fig. 59-1

Case 60

An 8-year-old girl has been limping for 1 year. Right thigh was thicker than left and right foot smaller than left when she began to walk at 11 months. Right second and third toes were crowded together, and second toe overlapped third.

Right iliac crest is 3 cm lower than left when she stands. A thickened band of soft tissue is down lateral side of right thigh. Motion at right hip, extension at right knee, and plantar flexion at right ankle are slightly limited. Right foot is narrower and shorter than left. Right second and third toes are crowded together and thickened around metatarsophalangeal joints. The rest of the physical findings are normal.

Hematocrit is 0.39. White cell count is 6.7×10^9/liter with 0.62 polymorphonuclear cells, 0.32 lymphocytes, 0.04 mono-

cytes, and 0.02 eosinophils. Urine specific gravity is 1.016, pH 5. Urine is normal.

Bone at right hip (Figure 60-1), along lateral side of right femur and fibula, including its distal epiphyseal ossification center (Figure 60-2), and in right second and third metatarsals and phalanges (Figure 60-3) is irregularly sclerotic. Bones of right foot are smaller than those of left in Figure 60-3. In examination at 13 years, length of right femur is 40.2 cm, left femur 41.7, right tibia 30.4, and left tibia 32.0.

Diagnosis: Melorheostosis.

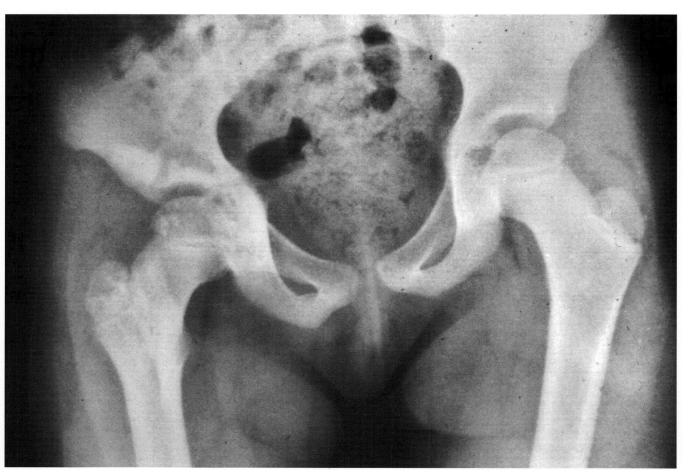

Fig. 60-1

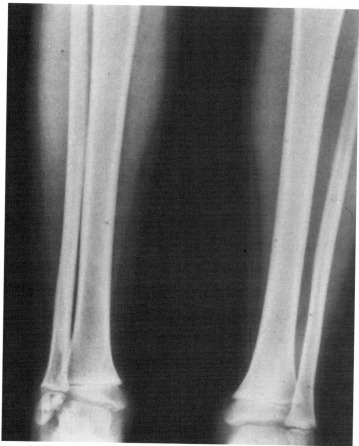

Fig. 60-2

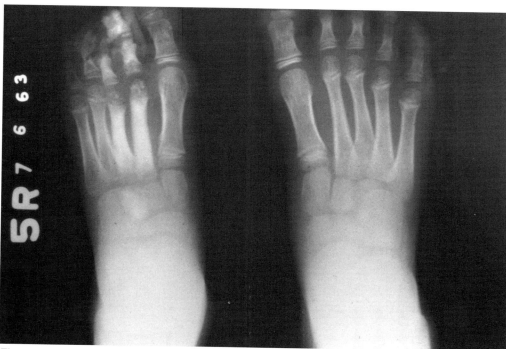

Fig. 60-3

Case 61

An 18-year-old boy, who has just graduated from high school, is short and walks with wide-based waddle on right toes.

Mother (47 years old) has diabetes mellitus, discovered during pregnancy. Birth weight was 4.5 kg. He had cleft palate, hypoplastic mandible, legs of unequal length, and fusion of second and third toes on both feet. Excretory urogram did not show left kidney. Cystoscopy showed no left ureteral opening. Bilateral inguinal herniorrhaphy was performed at 5 months. He sat at 1 year, began to walk at 15 months. He had umbilical hernia at 15 months, groin scars, dimple at each hip, shorter right leg than left, and perhaps no right knee joint. Cleft palate was repaired at 20 months and twice later with pharyngeal flaps.

Father (48 years old) and four siblings are well. Maternal grandmother has diabetes mellitus.

Blood pressure at 16 years was 120/54 mm Hg. Weight at 18 years is 59 kg, height 142 cm. Hips flex to 80 degrees, abduct little. Motion is limited at shoulders, elbows, and partly flexed knees.

Roentgenograms at 1 week (Figure 61-1A) and 2 years (Figure 61-1B) show dysplastic pelvis and femurs and hypoplastic fibulas.

Diagnosis: Proximal femoral focal deficiency.

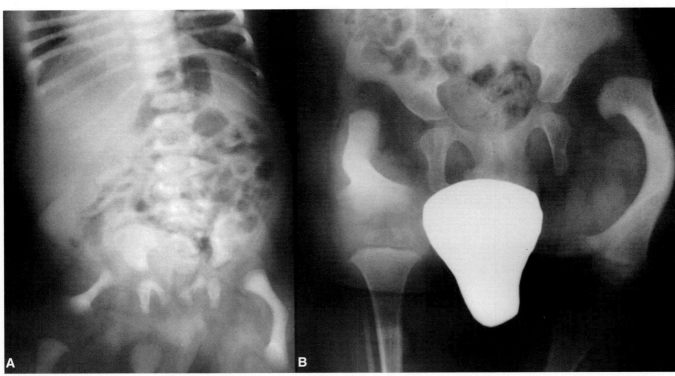

Fig. 61-1

Case 62

A 15-year-old girl is upset because she is short and sexually immature.

She was born with rectovaginal fistula that was repaired in operations at 20 months and 3 years. She had ear infections and urinary tract infections in childhood. Knees swelled intermittently until arthritis "burned out" 5 years ago. She limps sometimes when tired.

Height at 15 years is 136 cm, weight 31.5 kg, head circumference 54 cm, and blood pressure 80/50 mm Hg. Several pigmented nevi are on body. Breasts are 1–2 cm. She has no axillary hair and little pubic hair. Carrying angle at elbows is increased. Scars are around anus. Patellas subluxate. Right knee is loose with lateral pressure. Ends of toenails turn up. The rest of the physical findings are normal.

Chromosomes are 46,X,i,(Xq) (isochromosome of long arm of X chromosome).

In Figure 62-1, medial condyles of femurs are large, medial condyles of tibias are small, and a bony spur is on medial metaphysis of right tibia. Suprapatellar synovial bursas are distended in Figure 62-2.

Diagnosis: Turner's syndrome.

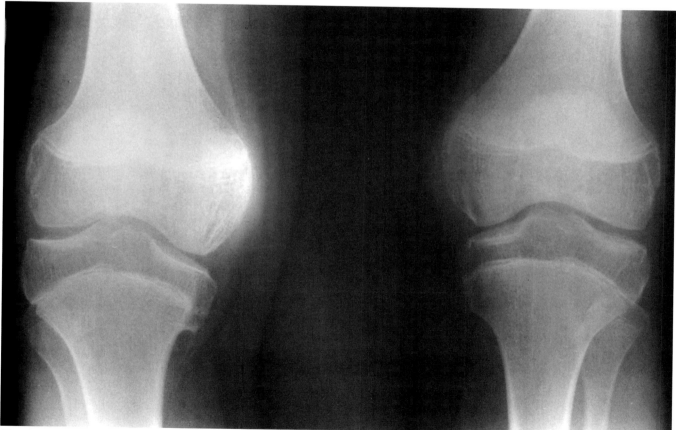

Fig. 62-1

(Continued)

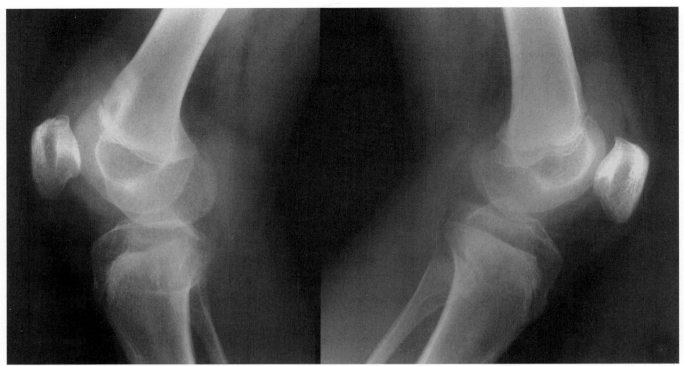

Fig. 62-2

Case 63

A 5-year-old fat boy dribbles urine and often does not get to the toilet in time.

Pregnancy of mother (then 28 years old) was marred by no fetal movement during last 5 days before induced labor. Amniotic fluid was meconium stained, birth weight 2.0 kg, length 44 cm, head circumference 32 cm, and Apgar score 8/8 at 1 and 5 minutes. Temperature at 5 hours was 37°C, heart rate 139, respiratory rate 60, and blood pressure 80/52 mm Hg. He had gastroschisis and an extra left toe. Gastroschisis repair was performed at 10 hours, bilateral inguinal hernia repair and excision of extra toe at 4½ months. He sat at 8 months, walked at 2 years, and said first words at 3 years. He was weak and stumbled a lot. He wheezed often from 6 months to 2 years. He had poor vision at 2 years, tooth cavities, and pulpitis at 3 years.

Brother (13 years old) had an extra finger on each hand and an extra toe on each foot. He was night blind at 3 years and is now fat and retarded.

Weight at 5 years is 36 kg. Eyes are deep set. Nose is upturned. A puckered scar is at umbilicus, in each groin, and on left foot. Genitalia are small. Limbs are thick, hands and feet short. Fine, silvery scales are on flanks and buttocks. The rest of the physical findings are normal. Ophthalmologic examination shows myopia in both eyes, diminished color vision, a broad zone around discs of decreased pigment, mildly granular maculae, and best corrected vision of 20/70. IQ is 82.

Urine specific gravity is 1.024, pH 7. Urine has 0–1 white cell/HPF.

Roentgenogram at 4 months, in Figure 63-1, shows left extra toe. Left fifth metatarsal bone is shorter and broader than right fifth metatarsal bone in Figure 63-1. Excretory urogram at 5 years, in Figure 63-2, shows blunt calyces and excess intra-abdominal fat, which surrounds spleen and displaces ureters medially in pelvis.

Diagnosis: Bardet-Biedl syndrome.

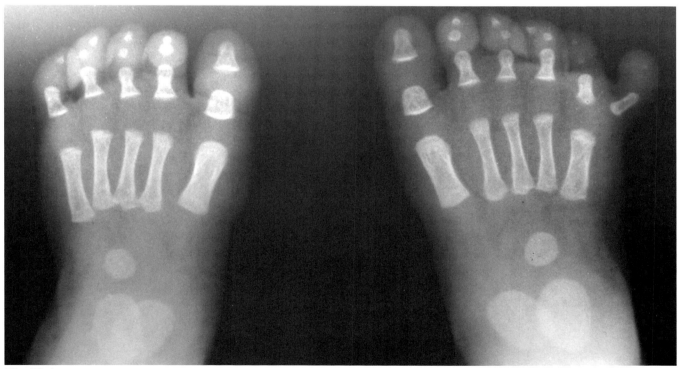

Fig. 63-1

(Continued)

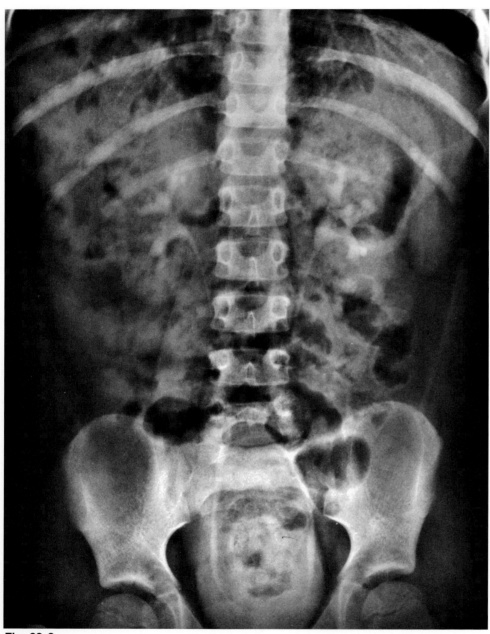

Fig. 63-2

Skeletal Dystrophy

Case 1

A 1½-year-old boy snores and always has a runny nose.

Pregnancy was normal, presentation footling breech, and birth weight 3.9 kg. He has had bilateral inguinal hernia repair. He does not talk. He began to walk at 17 months, unlike his brother (4 years old), who walked at 12 months.

Mother (25 years old), father (25 years old), and brother are well.

Temperature is 37.9°C, heart rate 112, respiratory rate 24, weight 12 kg, height 84 cm, and head circumference 51 cm. Forehead bulges. Face is flat. Corneas are hazy. Nose is small. A small umbilical hernia and inguinal scars are present. Liver edge is 3 cm below costal margin. Back is hairy. Testes are in inguinal canals. The rest of the physical findings are normal.

Hematocrit is 0.38. White cell count is 4.2×10^9/liter with 0.60 polymorphonuclear cells, 0.03 bands, 0.32 lymphocytes, and 0.05 monocytes. Platelet estimate is adequate. Urine specific gravity is 1.007, pH 6. Urine has 0–1 white cell/HPF,

rare epithelial cells/HPF, and bacteria. Urine gives a positive reaction with cetyltrimethylammonium bromide and toluidine blue. Serum sodium is 137 mmol/liter, potassium 4.1, chloride 98, carbon dioxide 23, urea nitrogen 6.1, calcium 1.97, phosphorus 1.61, and glucose 6.1.

Figure 1-1A shows brow bulging beyond face, J-shaped sella turcica, and hypoplastic odontoid. In Figure 1-1B, broad metacarpals are narrow at proximal ends. Ribs are thick, and upper lumbar vertebrae are beaked in Figure 1-2. Bones of arms are thick in Figure 1-3A. In Figure 1-3B, iliac bases are narrow; neck-shaft angle of femurs is greater than normal.

Adenoidectomy is performed at 2 and 3½ years. Liver edge at 3½ years is 6 cm below costal margin, spleen edge 4 cm below costal margin. He dies at 6 years.

Diagnosis: Hurler syndrome (mucopolysaccharidosis I-H).

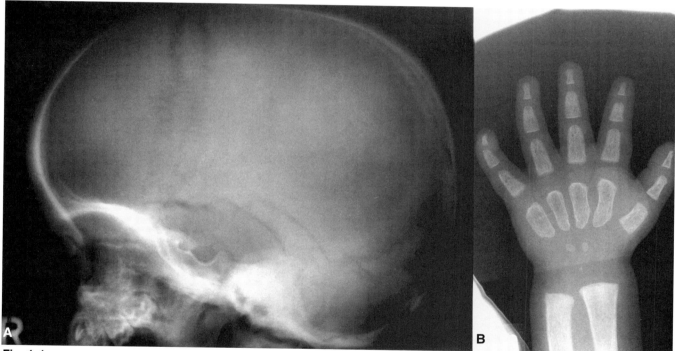

Fig. 1-1

(Continued)

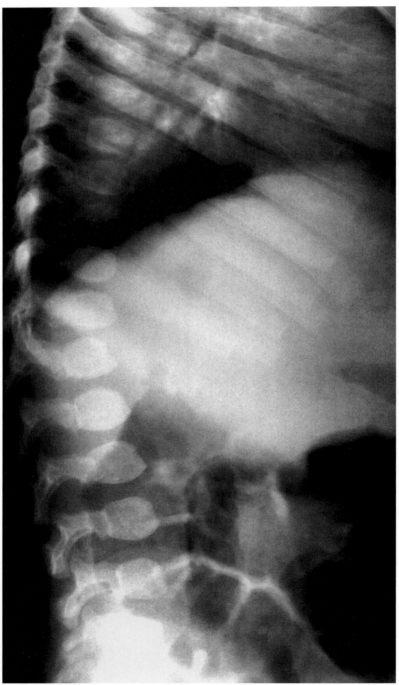

Fig. 1-2

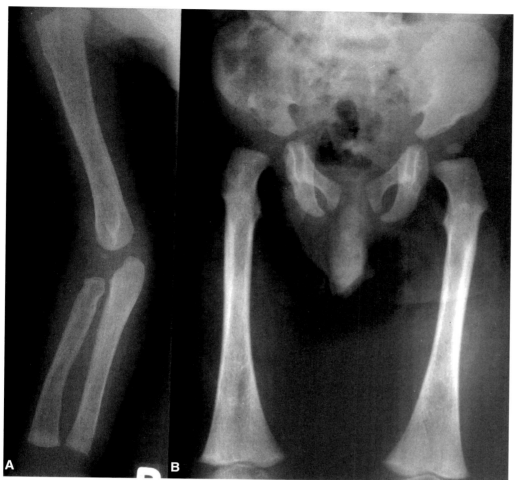

Fig. 1-3

Case 2

A 19-year-old man, who is in twelfth grade, has had headaches for 3 months.

He has had tonsillectomy, herniorrhaphy, and two operations for glaucoma.

Weight is 54 kg, height 152 cm, head circumference 56 cm, temperature 37.2°C, heart rate 124, respiratory rate 18, and blood pressure 120/80 mm Hg. Face is coarse. Right eye turns out. Corneas are cloudy. Lips and tongue are large. Neck is short. He has a systolic heart murmur and umbilical hernia. Thenar muscles are atrophic. Fingers and toes are flexed. The rest of the physical findings are normal.

Hematocrit is 0.44. White cell count is 5.0×10^9/liter with 0.52 polymorphonuclear cells, 0.03 bands, 0.39 lymphocytes, 0.05 monocytes, and 0.01 basophils. Platelet estimate is normal. Serum sodium is 144 mmol/liter, potassium 4.3, chloride 106, carbon dioxide 22, urea nitrogen 5.7, calcium 2.52, phosphorus 1.23, cholesterol 3.93, triglycerides 0.84, and glucose 6.8. Creatinine is 80 μmol/liter, uric acid 290, total bilirubin 13, and direct bilirubin 3. Total protein is 74 g/liter, albumin 48. Alkaline phosphatase is 121 U/liter, LDH 193, SGOT 26, and CK 26.

His sister (17 years old), an A student, is thought to have increased intracranial pressure in ophthalmologic examination.

She had umbilical herniorrhaphy at 6 years, tonsillectomy at 8 years, and operation on right eye for glaucoma at 16 years.

Her weight is 55 kg, height 141 cm, heart rate 84, respiratory rate 12, and blood pressure 120/75 mm Hg. Face is coarse. Corneas are cloudy. Neck is short. A systolic heart murmur is present. Extension is limited in shoulders, knees, hands, and feet. Fingers and toes are flexed. The rest of the physical findings are normal.

Urine specific gravity is 1.012, pH 6. Urine has few squamous and nonsquamous epithelial cells/HPF and bacteria. Her urine tests are positive with cetyltrimethylammonium bromide and toluidine blue.

Her ECG findings are normal.

Mother (53 years old) and sister (27 years old) are well. Father (53 years old) has had arthritis since he was 4 years old, can take only small steps because of hip pain, and has recently begun to use crutches.

Leukocyte α-L-iduronidase levels are the following: 19-year-old man 1.6 nmol/liter/18 hours, 17-year-old sister 0, father 40.3, mother 33.4, and two adult controls 125 and 226.

In Figure 2-1A, the 19-year-old man's pituitary fossa is large, dorsum sellae well defined, condylar processes of mandible eroded, and mandibular notches deep. His ribs are thick, bases of ilia thin, and fingers and toes flexed. Lumbar vertebral bodies are concave toward spinal canal. L5–S1 second-degree spondylolisthesis is present. Figure 2-1B shows 17-year-old sister's large pituitary fossa and well-defined dorsum sellae. Roentgenographic findings in chest, abdomen, pelvis, and limbs are similar to her brother's. She does not have spondylolisthesis.

Ventriculoperitoneal shunts are placed in brother and sister.

He is unable to walk after shunt, is incontinent of urine, and dies with shortness of breath and edema of feet at 19½ years. She is catatonic after shunt and dies at 19⅓ years, 2 years after its placement.

His necropsy shows (1) dermis thickened by dense collagen; (2) shortening and nodular thickening of mitral and pulmonary valve cusps and of chordae tendineae at junction with cusps; (3) endocardial fibrosis in atria and right ventricle; (4) infarction of septal cusp of tricuspid valve; (5) mononuclear infiltrate in myocardium; (6) soft bones; (7) thickened dura; (8) enlarged, spherical cerebral neurons with cytoplasmic deposits that displace Nissl substance to side; (9) Luxol fast blue–positive material in many cerebral neurons but not in Purkinje cells; (10) large perivascular spaces in brain with loose fibrous tissue and large histiocytes that contain granular material; (11) hepatocytes swollen with feathery eosinophilic material that displaces nucleus to side; and (12) cuboidal epithelial cells lining Bowman's space. Her necropsy shows (1) gray-white thickening of right atrial myocardium; (2) thickening of mitral and aortic cusps by myxomatous gray-white nodules; (3) hepatocytes swollen with PAS-positive magenta-staining material, some of it digested by diastase; (4) PAS-positive material, much of it not digested by diastase, in mononuclear phagocytes in lymph nodes and spleen; and (5) round PAS-positive inclusions in many neurons.

Diagnosis: Scheie syndrome (mucopolysaccharidosis I-S).

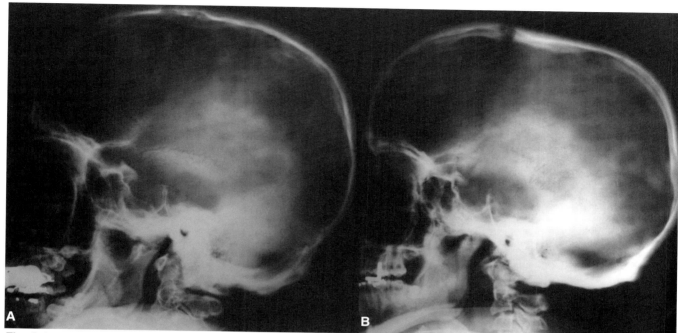

Fig. 2-1

Case 3

An 8-year-old boy has sat gingerly and limped for a year. His few skills have deteriorated for the last 6 months and he is now incontinent of stool and urine.

Mother (then 21 years old) had toxemia of pregnancy. Birth weight was 3.4 kg. Nose has always been stuffy. Bilateral inguinal hernia repair was performed at 3 months. Features coarsened during first year. He sat at 8 months, walked at 17 months. At 9 months, spleen edge was 3 cm below costal margin. He has had ear infections throughout childhood. Eyes were normal at 2½ years. Neck was short. He had a systolic heart murmur, umbilical hernia, large liver and spleen, and spadelike hands. Roentgenograms showed large head, thickened frontal bone, hypoplastic odontoid, broad bones in arms, expanded metacarpals, expanded phalanges in fingers, pinched iliac bases, and small proximal femoral epiphyseal ossification centers. Hair was sparse and coarse at 3½ years. At 4½ years, he could dress and undress, feed himself, and say that he had to go to the toilet. Myringotomies and tube placement were performed at 5 years. Arms and hands were stiff at 6 years. At 7 years, he was hard of hearing. Intelligence and motor skills were at 3-year-old level.

He sits part of the way off chairs with right leg out. After sitting awhile, he gets down on hands and knees before trying to stand. Right hip is immobile.

Figure 3-1A shows expanded metacarpals and phalanges, pinched bases of metacarpals two through five, and small carpal and epiphyseal ossification centers. Figure 3-1B shows eroded epiphysis and metaphysis of right femur and cystic defects in bones of acetabula.

Toluidine blue produces metachromasia of his urine, cetyltrimethylammonium bromide a precipitate. Cultured skin fibroblasts accumulate ^{35}S-mucopolysaccharide, a defect that is corrected by Hunter corrective factor.

Diagnosis: Hunter syndrome (mucopolysaccharidosis II).

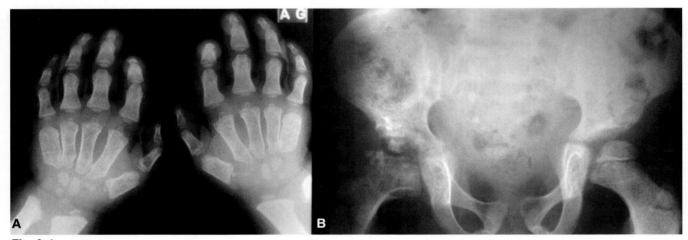

Fig. 3-1

Case 4

A 6-year-old girl walks on her toes, trips over her feet, falls often, and has begun to crawl.

Pregnancy was normal. She sat at 8 or 9 months, walked at 15 months. She had many colds. Face was mildly coarse at 3 years. Nose was stuffy. Elbows extended to 145 degrees. Fingers were short. Language was at level of approximately 20 months, motor function 20–24 months. Urine had excess heparan sulfate. To keep her from hurting herself at 5 years, parents locked her in her room or, on medical advice, tied her to a chair, at which time she screamed so loudly that they were accused of child abuse. She was not toilet trained, could not feed herself, uttered noises but no words, did not understand words, walked on her toes, and had coarse, brittle hair.

Mother (25 years old), father (28 years old), and brother (7 years old) are well.

Weight at 6 years is 21 kg, height 113 cm, and head circumference 55 cm. She is alert, uncooperative, and less disruptive than she used to be. She does not react to loud hand clapping. Hair is wild, brittle, and coarse on head, fine and wavy on arms and back. Forehead is prominent, nasal bridge broad. Lips are large. She drools, with mouth open. Chin rests on sternum. A systolic heart murmur is present. Hands and feet are cool, fingers and toes short. Deep tendon reflexes are hyperactive.

Activity of N-acetyl-α-D-glucosaminidase in serum is 33.6 nmol/ml/hr (control: 8–12).

Figure 4-1A shows thick calvaria and J-shaped sella turcica. In Figure 4-1B, metacarpal bones, especially fifth metacarpals, lack normal waistlike constriction. Figure 4-1B shows short, thick phalanges and undertubulated radii and ulnae.

She cannot walk unaided at 7 years. She chokes on solid food and does not feed herself. She screams for hours at a time. Ophthalmologic examination shows clear corneas and attenuated peripheral vessels and patchy atrophy in retinas. She lies in a heap at 8 years, scissors her legs when held up, makes occasional purposeless movement of arms, and grinds teeth. Gums are thick. Flexion contractures are at elbows and ankles.

Diagnosis: Sanfilippo syndrome (mucopolysaccharidosis III, heparan N-sulfatase deficiency found in biochemical test).

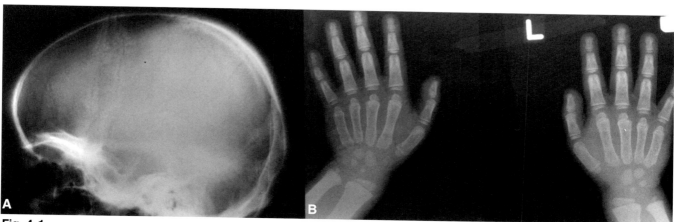

Fig. 4-1

Case 5

A 4-year-old boy, who was limp last night after falling from his scooter, now drags left leg when he walks and barely moves left arm.

Pregnancy was normal, birth weight 2.7 kg. He walked at 1 year. He was "too short" at 1½ years. He has walked stiffly with head back for 1 year and often stumbles. He lies prone when he plays in sandbox. He has quivered for several months.

Mother (29 years old) and father (32 years old) are well. The boy is their only child. Members of father's family have diabetes mellitus.

Weight at 4 years is 12.3 kg, height 86 cm, head circumference 51 cm, temperature 36.7°C, heart rate 120, respiratory rate 20, and blood pressure 115/68 mm Hg. He is talkative. He moves left arm only at shoulder. Neck is extended. Muscle tone is increased in right limbs, decreased in left. Deep tendon reflexes are brisk. Clonus is at ankles, Babinski's sign in feet. The rest of the physical findings are normal. Slit-lamp examination shows small, yellow opacities concentrated in central deep layer of corneas.

Roentgenogram of neck at 2 years shows hypoplasia of odontoid and shallow spinal canal (Figure 5-1A). Roentgenogram of hand at 3 years shows short, expanded metacarpals with pinched bases (Figure 5-1B). Roentgenogram of foot at 3 years shows similar but less marked changes in metatarsal bones. At 3 years, the pelvis has narrow iliac bases and laterally displaced femurs with small, fragmented epiphyseal ossification centers (Figure 5-2A). Myelogram at 4 years shows flat vertebrae, bulging into spinal canal at level of discs (Figure 5-2B), and a block at C2–C3.

Urine contains keratan sulfate. *N*-acetylgalactosamine-6-sulfatase is decreased in cultured fibroblasts.

At operation for suboccipital and cervical decompression, bony overgrowth and atlantoaxial subluxation are found. Spinal cord is compressed at junction with medulla. Ligamentum flavum is normal.

Diagnosis: Morquio syndrome (mucopolysaccharidosis IV).

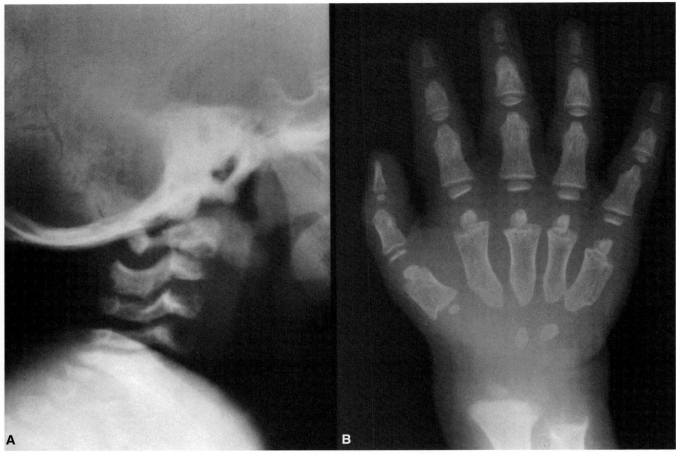

A   B

Fig. 5-1

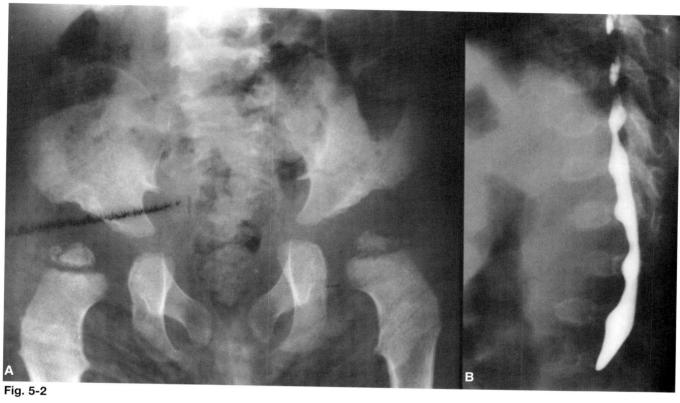

Fig. 5-2

Case 6

A 9-month-old boy has a runny nose and humpback. He sleeps a lot and cannot roll over.

Pregnancy was normal. Inguinal hernias were repaired at 1½ and 2 months. He was hospitalized at 2½ months for noisy breathing.

Mother (27 years old), father (30 years old), and three sisters (2, 4, and 6 years old) are well. Parents belong to an endogamous religious sect. Great-great-grandparents came from same part of Finland. Members of mother's family have allergies.

Weight at 9 months is 7.7 kg, length 64 cm, head circumference 46 cm, heart rate 120, respiratory rate 30, and blood pressure 120/50 mm Hg. Skin is red and flaky. Head is large. Crusts are around ears and nose. Cheeks sag. Gums are thick and without teeth. Breathing is noisy. Liver edge is 2–3 cm below costal margin. Wrists and hands are broad. Head lags when he is pulled toward sitting. The rest of the physical findings are normal.

Hematocrit is 0.38. White cell count is 12.3×10^9/liter with 0.30 polymorphonuclear cells, 0.07 bands, 0.55 lympho-

cytes (one-third with vacuoles or inclusions), 0.04 monocytes, 0.03 eosinophils, and 0.01 basophils. Platelet count is 265×10^9/liter. No Reilly bodies are in peripheral leukocytes. Urine specific gravity is 1.006, pH 7. Urine has 1–2 red cells/HPF, rare white cells/HPF, bacteria, amorphous urates, and no mucopolysaccharide in screening test. Serum hexosaminidase is 124.58 U/liter (normal: 12.89 ± 3.06), hexosaminidase A 33.07 (normal: 8.75 ± 1.13), and hexosaminidase B 91.52 (normal: 0.37 ± 0.17). White cell lysosomal hydrolases are normal. Fibroblast lysosomal enzymes are decreased.

Humeri are expanded at 6½ months, a discovery made in roentgenographic examination of chest for noisy breathing (Figure 6-1A). Bases of ilia are narrow at 7 months. Metacarpals are broad, their proximal ends narrow at 9 months (Figure 6-1B). Bones of feet are normal. Back is humped, L1 beaked at 9 months (Figure 6-2).

Diagnosis: Mucolipidosis II (I-cell disease).

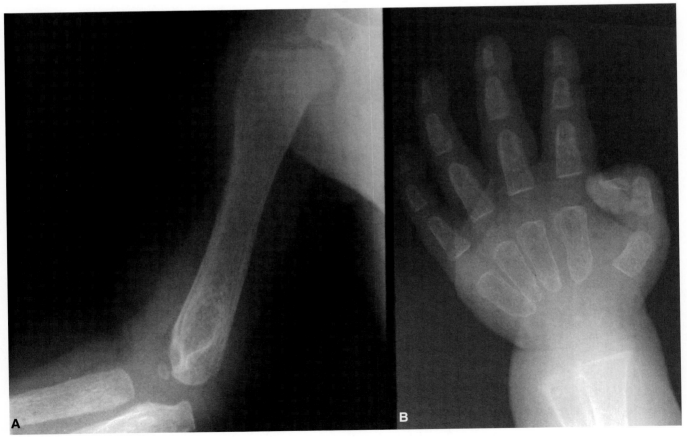

Fig. 6-1

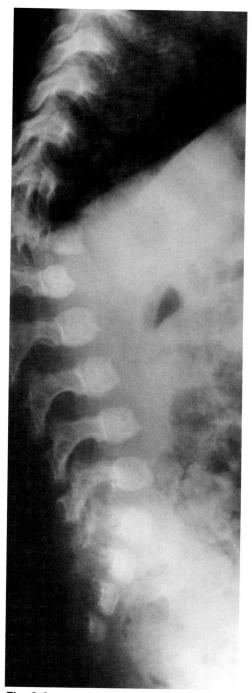

Fig. 6-2

Case 7

A 6-year-old girl walks on her toes, stumbles, has backache, and cannot put her hands flat on a table with palms down. Her grandmother recently pried a gumball from the girl's tight mouth.

Pregnancy was normal, birth weight 2.8 kg, length 48 cm, and head circumference 33 cm. She rolled over at 4 months, sat at 7 months, walked at 13 months, and talked at 2 years. She began to walk on her toes at 3½ years. Hands were tight at 5 years. Back hurt. She has had many sore throats, nose bleeds, and ear infections.

Weight at 6 years is 21 kg, height 108 cm, and systolic blood pressure 88 mm Hg. She is bright and friendly. Abduction at shoulders and extension at elbows, wrists, knees, and interphalangeal joints of third, fourth, and fifth fingers are limited. Hips are stiff. Ankles can be passively dorsiflexed to neutral. The rest of the physical findings are normal.

Hematocrit is 0.39. White cell count is 5.6×10^9/liter. Platelet count is 339×10^9/liter. Urine specific gravity is 1.030, pH 6. Urine is normal. Serum sodium is 139 mmol/liter, potassium 4.2, chloride 104, carbon dioxide 24, urea nitrogen 4.6, calcium 2.42, phosphorus 1.78, cholesterol 3.26, and glucose 5.2. Creatinine is 60 µmol/liter, uric acid 280, total bilirubin 5, and direct bilirubin 0. Total protein is 66 g/liter, albumin 44. Alkaline phosphatase is 247, LDH 320, and SGOT 27. Serum hexosaminidase A is 8.77 U/liter (normal: 0.17 of total), control 4.48 (normal: 0.66 of total), hexosaminidase B 41.80 (normal: 0.83 of total), control 2.27 (normal: 0.34 of total). Her total A and B is 50.57 U/liter, control total A and B 6.75. Mother's serum hexosaminidase B is twice normal. Father is considered an obligate carrier.

At 7 years, she has ear infection, systolic heart murmur, and hazy corneas in slit-lamp examination. Tubes are placed in ears. Heel cords are lengthened. She has spinal kyphosis. She can abduct left femur 45 degrees. Adenoids are removed at 8 years. Left calf is thinner than right at 10 years. She has claw hands, all fingers flexed, at 13 years. Left hip and left knee hurt. Left hip grates and clicks with movement. Spinal fusion is performed at 14 years. Face is coarse at 15 years. Height at 16 years is 135 cm, weight 52 kg. She has shooting pain in legs. Eye examination at 17 years shows stromal haze in corneas and horizontal wrinkles in retinas between disc and fovea centralis.

Roentgenograms of pelvis at 6 years (Figure 7-1A) and 13 years (Figure 7-1B) show erosion at left hip and, to a lesser degree, at right hip. Ilia flare in Figure 7-1. L1 and later T12 erode between 6 years (Figure 7-2A) and 13 years (Figure 7-2B).

Diagnosis: Mucolipidosis III.

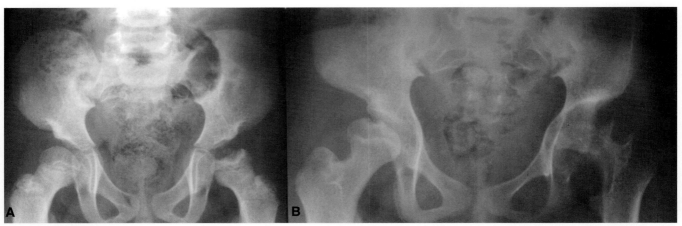

Fig. 7-1

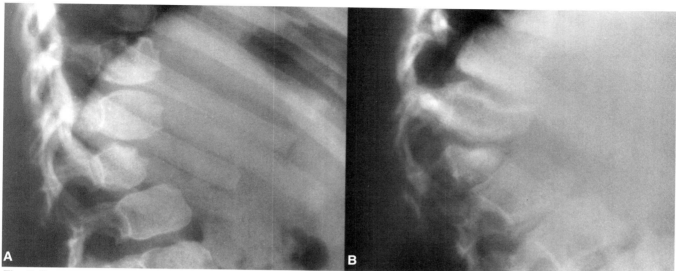

Fig. 7-2

Case 8

A 14-month-old girl has been regressing since she was 6 months old.

Birth weight was 3.5 kg, length 53 cm. She smiled, imitated noises, and sat at 6 months but does not now. Weight was 7.3 kg at 7 months, 8.2 kg at 11 months. She became cranky. Breathing was noisy. She had ear infections before 11 months and myringotomy, tubes, and adenoidectomy at 11 months. Features coarsened, hands thickened, muscles have stiffened for the past 8 months. Results of two screening tests for mucopolysacchariduria were normal. Lymphocytes are vacuolated.

Mother and father are well.

Hair is red. Anterior fontanel is large. Nasal bridge is flat and wide. Upper eyelids are thickened. Epicanthi are present. Small telangiectases are in bulbar conjunctivae and lid margins. Corneas are hazy. Tongue is large. Gums are thick.

Abdomen is distended. Liver edge is 6 cm below costal margin. Joint motion is normal after initial stiffness is overcome. Head lags. Deep tendon reflexes are weak. The rest of the physical findings are normal.

Serum calcium is 2.32 mmol/liter, phosphorus 1.61. Alkaline phosphatase is 140 U/liter.

Figure 8-1A shows hypoplastic dens. Figure 8-1B shows beaked lumbar vertebrae. Metacarpals and phalanges of fingers look like those of Hurler syndrome.

Activity of β-galactosidase in cultured skin fibroblast is 0.13 U/liter (normal: 5.08–15.85). Activity is normal for β-glucosaminidase and β-glucuronidase, slightly above normal for α-galactosidase, β-glucosidase, and α-mannosidase.

Diagnosis: Generalized gangliosidosis.

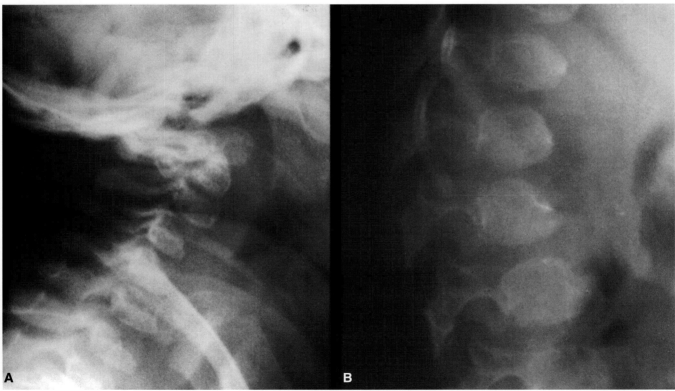

A   B

Fig. 8-1

Case 9

A 15-year-old boy is cheerful, deaf, and mentally retarded.

Father (44 years old) and an older brother are well. Other brothers (11 and 13 years old) are deaf and mentally retarded. Mother became alcoholic after last pregnancy and is said to be schizophrenic.

Weight is 54 kg, height 159 cm, head circumference 57 cm, heart rate 76, and blood pressure 140/70 mm Hg. He walks with toes outward and runs on toes like a robot. Skin is mottled, hair coarse and dry, scalp scaly, and nasal bridge flat. Eyes are wide set and have epicanthi. Mouth is open, lower jaw prominent. Gaps are between teeth, gums thick. Spleen edge is 4 cm below costal margin. Joints are stiff. The rest of the physical findings are normal.

Hematocrit is 0.42. White cell count is 7.3×10^9/liter with 0.69 polymorphonuclear cells, 0.22 lymphocytes, 0.08 monocytes, and 0.01 eosinophils. Urine specific gravity is 1.031, pH 6. Urine has 0–1 epithelial cell/HPF, 0–1 white cell/HPF, and amorphous urates. Serum sodium is 138 mmol/liter, potassium 3.6, chloride 99, carbon dioxide 22, urea nitrogen 6.0, calcium 2.54, phosphorus 1.07, and cholesterol 4.09 (at 13 years). Total bilirubin is 17 μmol/liter, direct bilirubin 3. Total protein is 77 g/liter, albumin 54. Alkaline phosphatase is 61 U/liter, LDH 112, and SGOT 25. Chromosomes are 46,XY.

Audiogram shows 60- to 70-dB sensorineural loss in both ears. IQ is 32.

Most of the physical findings in 11- and 13-year-old brothers are similar to those in 15-year-old boy. Liver edge is 3 cm below costal margin in 13-year-old boy, spleen edge 2 cm. Liver and spleen are not palpable in 11-year-old boy, who has umbilical hernia.

Examination of 15-year-old boy's skull in Figure 9-1 shows thickened diploë, absence of frontal and sphenoidal sinuses, opaque ethmoidal sinuses, and hypoplastic maxillary sinuses. Two younger brothers have thickened diploë to a lesser degree. Examination of youngest brother shows destruction of head of left femur at 7 years (Figure 9-2A) and partial reconstitution at 11 years (Figure 9-2B). Schmorl's nodes are marked in youngest brother's spine at 11 years (Figure 9-3).

Fifteen-year-old brother makes cardboard boxes for a charitable organization when he is 27 years old. He has painful knees. Height is 163 cm, weight 63 kg. At operation on left knee, turbid fluid and thickened synovium are found. Microscopic examination of thickened synovium shows chronic inflammation. Thirteen-year-old brother likes television when he is 25 years old, helps his older brother make boxes, and is hypertensive. Youngest brother dies at 22 years with herpes pneumonia.

Serum α-D-mannosidase activity of 15-year-old boy is 12.6 nmol substrate hydrolyzed/ml serum, 13-year-old boy 13.6, 11-year-old boy 17.7 (normal: 20–28). Leukocyte α-D-mannosidase activity of 15-year-old boy is 0.79 nmol substrate hydrolyzed/mg protein/hr, 13-year-old boy 0.82, 11-year-old boy 0.98, and father 67.8 (normal: 100–203).

Diagnosis: Mannosidosis.

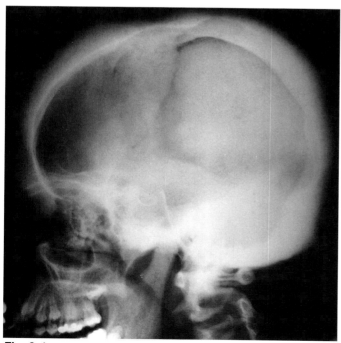

Fig. 9-1

(Continued)

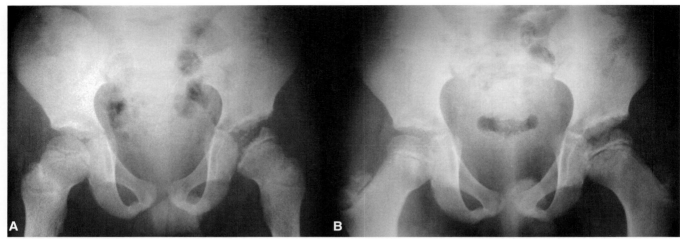

Fig. 9-2

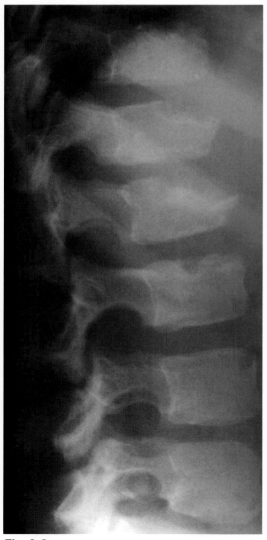

Fig. 9-3

Case 10

A 15-year-old boy has brittle bones.

He has had many fractures since he was 7 years old, four in the last 7 months, some from activity as slight as stepping off a curb. Nose bleeds if he takes aspirin. He was awakened in the middle of the night 2 weeks ago by pain in right thigh caused by 0.5-liter femoral subperiosteal hematoma. He was anemic at 6 years when spleen (weight: 2 kg) was removed. He has had measles, mumps, and right shoulder dislocations.

Mother (41 years old) has high blood pressure. Sister (16 years old) is well. Father died at 38 years with pancreatitis. Maternal grandmother has diabetes mellitus.

Weight at 15 years is 43 kg, height 165 cm, temperature 38°C, heart rate 96, respiratory rate 18, and blood pressure 118/78 mm Hg. He is weak and pale. Crusted blood is in nose. Lower chest and upper abdomen bulge. A scar goes from xiphoid to umbilicus. Liver edge is firm at umbilicus. Right leg is bandaged and tender. The rest of the physical findings are normal.

Hematocrit is 0.25. Hemoglobin is 75 g/liter. Red blood cell count is 2.8×10^{12}/liter. Reticulocyte fraction is 13×10^{-3}. White cell count is 10.1×10^9/liter with 0.55 polymorphonu-clear cells, 0.01 bands, 0.28 lymphocytes, 0.14 monocytes, and 0.02 atypical lymphocytes. Platelet count is 780×10^9/liter. PT is 11.7 seconds (control: 9.8), PTT 35.2 (normal: <40). Blood smear shows Howell-Jolly bodies, burr cells, and ovalocytes. Urine specific gravity is 1.022, pH 7. Urine has rare squamous epithelial cells/HPF and mucous threads. Serum sodium is 132 mmol/liter, potassium 4.8, chloride 106, carbon dioxide 19, urea nitrogen 2.9, calcium 2.20, phosphorus 1.52, cholesterol 3.36, and glucose 4.3. Creatinine is 30 µmol/liter, uric acid 160, total bilirubin 7, and direct bilirubin 2. Total protein is 77 g/liter, albumin 26. Alkaline phosphatase is 1,314 U/liter, LDH 400, and SGOT 120. Leukocyte β-glucosidase is 0.380 nmol substrate hydrolyzed/mg protein/hr (control range: 1.62 ± 0.41). Serum acid phosphatase is 710 nmol substrate hydrolyzed/ml serum/hr (control range: 398 ± 110).

Head and neck of right femur (Figure 10-1A) and proximal part of right tibia are deformed and irregularly mineralized. Proximal part of humeri has similar appearance. Distal parts of femurs have Erlenmeyer flask deformity in Figure 10-1B. Distal tibias show similar deformity.

Diagnosis: Gaucher's disease.

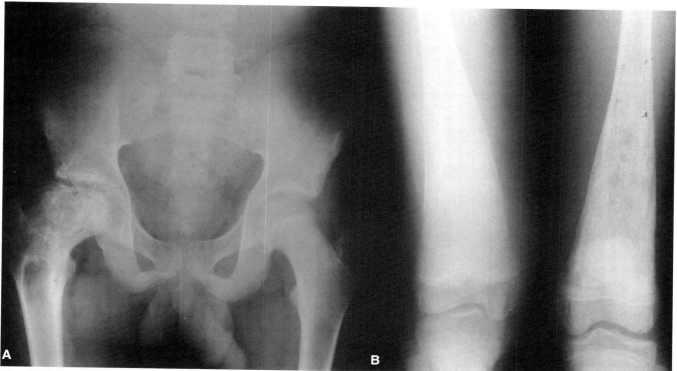

Fig. 10-1

Case 11

A 10-month-old girl is sluggish and underweight. She was a "very even-tempered" child who used to "jabber a lot" until 1 month ago. She has been irritable for 2 weeks.

Delivery was by cesarean section for fetal distress. Birth weight was 2.2 kg. She had trouble swallowing; breast milk, and later formula, often came out of her nose. She has not been given vitamins. She smiled at 2 months, rolled over at 4 months, was "happy and easy going" at 7 months, reached for objects at 8 months, but does not put objects in her mouth or sit at 10 months. Her voice was "deep" at 3 months.

Mother (39 years old), father (38 years old), twin sisters (13 years old), brother (9 years old), and sister (2 years old) are well. Seven years ago, a brother died at 1 day. Paternal great-grandparents have diabetes mellitus.

Temperature is 36.3°C, heart rate 120, respiratory rate 32, systolic blood pressure 100 mm Hg, weight 5.4 kg, length 67 cm, and head circumference 41 cm. She lies still without interest in her surroundings. She has epicanthi, blue irides with stellate pattern, broad nasal bridge, upturned nose, prominent round mouth, cleft uvula and soft palate, and a systolic heart murmur. The rest of the physical findings are normal.

Hematocrit is 0.32. White cell count is 16.8×10^9/liter with 0.29 polymorphonuclear cells, 0.63 lymphocytes, 0.06 monocytes, and 0.02 eosinophils. Platelet count is 492×10^9/liter. Urine specific gravity is 1.005, pH 6.0. Urine is normal. Serum sodium is 136 mmol/liter, magnesium 1.02, potassium 5.0, chloride 107, carbon dioxide 22, calcium 3.77, phosphorus 1.68, cholesterol 3.62, urea nitrogen 9.6, and glucose 4.8. Creatinine is 100 μmol/liter, uric acid 260, and total bilirubin 2. Total protein is 64 g/liter, albumin 42. Alkaline phosphatase is 127 U/liter, LDH 200, and SGOT 40. Ionized calcium is 1.67 mmol/liter (normal: 1.0–1.18); C-terminal parathormone is 79 μlEq/liter (normal: <50) when serum calcium is 3.60 mmol/liter and 88 when calcium is 3.84. T_4 is 158 nmol/liter (normal: 51–142). 25(OH) vitamin D is 2.5 nmol/liter (normal: 78.9 ± 23.2). Six months later, 1,25(OH)$_2$ vitamin D is 139 pmol/liter (normal: 100 ± 28). Serum calcium is 2.47 mmol/liter at 14 months, 2.30 at 15 months.

Figure 11-1 shows dense bones, especially at metaphyses.

Echocardiogram shows normal heart, aorta, and main pulmonary artery.

Diagnosis: Williams syndrome.

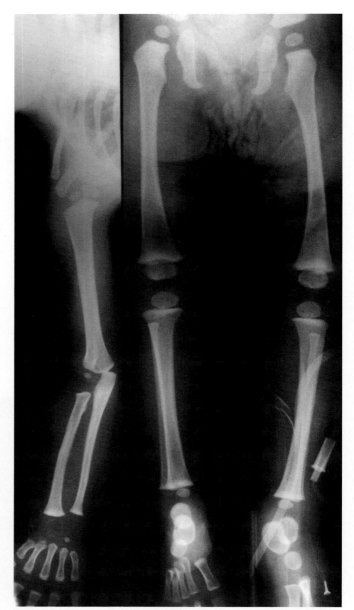

Fig. 11-1

Case 12

A newborn girl is sleepy and will not feed at 6 hours. Nostrils flare, and she grunts occasionally.

Mother (20 years old) is well. Father (28 years old) had an operation on neck for Hodgkin's disease at 7 years. The girl is their only child.

Pregnancy was normal. Birth weight is 3.0 kg, length 48 cm, head circumference 33 cm, and Apgar score 5/8 at 1 and 5 minutes. Temperature at 6 hours is 36.4°C, heart rate 142, and respiratory rate 40. Anterior fontanel is 2.5 × 2.5 cm. Tongue protrudes. The rest of the physical findings are normal.

Hematocrit is 0.57. White cell count is 14.0×10^9/liter with 0.32 polymorphonuclear cells, 0.10 bands, 0.55 lymphocytes, and 0.03 monocytes. Platelet count is 216×10^9/liter. Serum sodium is 151 mmol/liter, potassium 6.9, chloride 115, carbon dioxide 22, urea nitrogen 3.6, calcium 3.32, phosphorus 1.78, cholesterol 1.97, and glucose 3.3. Creatinine is 80 μmol/liter, uric acid 470, total bilirubin 50, and direct bilirubin 2. Total protein is 57 g/liter, albumin 40. Alkaline phosphatase is 154 U/liter, LDH 475, and SGOT 47.

Figure 12-1 shows rarefied bones of thorax. Right and left fourth and fifth ribs and left eighth rib are short, perhaps because of fracture (see Figure 12-1). Limbs are also rarefied.

Serum is nonreactive for syphilis, does not contain IgM antibodies for toxoplasmosis or rubella, and is negative by enzyme immunoassay for cytomegalovirus and by complement fixation for herpes simplex virus. Serum TSH is 14 mU/liter (normal: 2–11). Free T_4 is 42 pmol/liter (normal: 10–36). Serum calcium is between 2.94 and 3.09 mmol/liter in daily determinations during first week, phosphorus 1.26 and 1.32 in two determinations, and ionized calcium 1.75 and 1.80 (normal: 1.00–1.18). Parathyroid hormone is 70.7 pmol/liter (normal: 1.0–6.0) when calcium is 3.00 mmol/liter. A specimen of urine has <2 mg calcium (normal: 100–250 mg). Mother's serum calcium is 2.54 mmol/liter, phosphorus 1.49; father's calcium is 3.19, phosphorus 0.52.

Diagnosis: Neonatal hyperparathyroidism, familial hypocalciuric hypercalcemia.

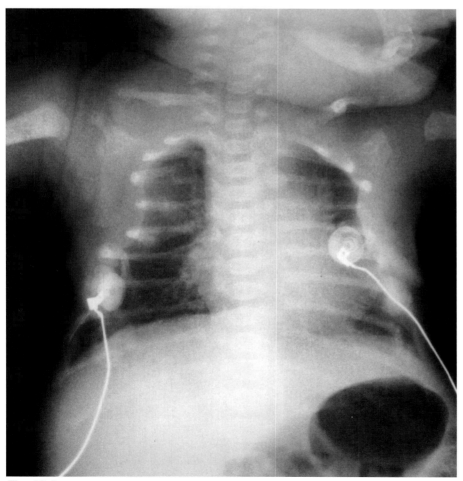

Fig. 12-1

Case 13

A 26-year-old woman has had seizures since she was 17 years old. She stiffens, twitches, breathes noisily, drools for 10–15 minutes, and then is confused. Other times she falls unconscious and lies still. Hands are stiff for days at a time. She has had occipital headaches during the last 3 months.

Birth weight was 2.1 kg. She walked at 1 year, talked at 4 years. She had pains in chest, hands, and feet at 13 years. Legs were weak. Chvostek's and Trousseau's signs were present. Serum calcium was 1.82 and 2.07 mmol/liter. Parathyroid hormone was 7.3 pmol/liter (normal: 1.0–6.0).

Mother (145 cm tall) and maternal grandmother (150 cm tall) have short fingers. Brother and sister have short fingers, cataracts, and seizures. Father has diabetes mellitus.

Height at 26 years is 142 cm, temperature 37°C, heart rate 75, respiratory rate 24, and blood pressure 128/88 mm Hg. She walks unsteadily and has nystagmus, carious teeth, and several short fingers. The rest of the physical findings are normal.

Hematocrit is 0.41. White cell count is 5.3 × 10⁹/liter with 0.47 polymorphonuclear cells, 0.01 bands, 0.41 lymphocytes, 0.07 monocytes, 0.01 eosinophils, 0.01 basophils, and 0.02 atypical lymphocytes. Platelet count is 173 × 10⁹/liter. Serum sodium is 141 mmol/liter, potassium 3.7, chloride 106, carbon dioxide 27, urea nitrogen 2.9, calcium 2.35 (6 days ago: 1.95), phosphorus 2.10, magnesium 0.62, cholesterol 4.71, and glucose 5.3. Creatinine is 100 μmol/liter, uric acid 190, total bilirubin 9, and direct bilirubin 0. Total protein is 57 g/liter, albumin 37. Alkaline phosphatase is 143 U/liter, LDH 143, and SGOT 20.

EEG findings are normal.

Roentgenogram of hands at 7 years (Figure 13-1) shows several short metacarpals and phalanges (serum calcium at time of examination is 1.85 mmol/liter, phosphorus 2.26). CT scan at 26 years shows deposits of calcium density in choroid plexuses and genu and posterior limb of internal capsules (Figure 13-2). Roentgenogram of spine shows calcification of discs between T4–T5 and T5–T6. Distal phalanx of mother's thumbs are short in Figure 13-3A (serum calcium at time of examination is 2.27 mmol/liter, phosphorus 1.23). Third and fourth metatarsal bones of sister (16 years old) are short in Figure 13-3B (serum calcium at the time of examination 2.02 mmol/liter, phosphorus 1.65).

Diagnosis: Albright's hereditary osteodystrophy.

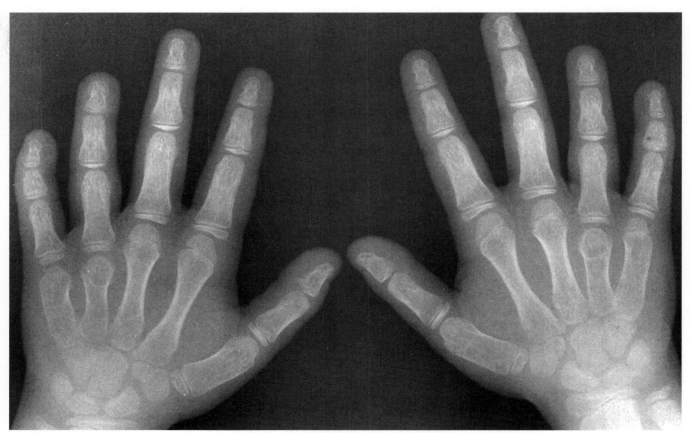

Fig. 13-1

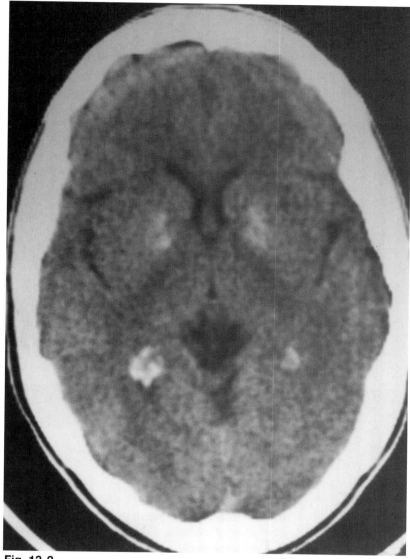

Fig. 13-2

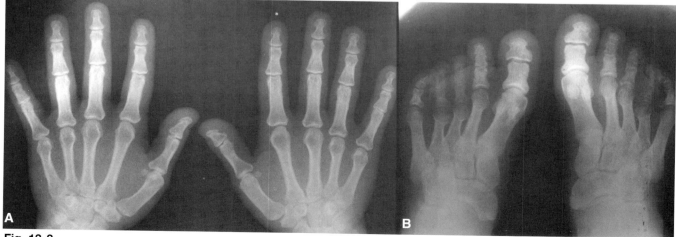

Fig. 13-3

Case 14

A 6-year-old girl "doesn't grow, never gained right, and plays by herself a lot."

Pregnancy was normal, birth weight 4 kg, length 55 cm, and head circumference 37 cm. She had pneumonia twice during first year, has had hematuria, chickenpox, rubella, and, at 2 years, fractured clavicle. She sat at 11 months, walked at 16 months, and began to talk at 3 years. Growth was slow at 3 years. Hands and feet were small, fingers stubby. She and sister (2 years old) are almost the same height.

Mother (28 years old) had a goiter at 13 years and has mitral valve abnormality. Father (31 years old) and two sisters (2 and 7 years old) are well. Maternal grandmother has diabetes mellitus.

Height at 6 years is 95 cm, weight 16 kg, temperature 37.2°C, heart rate 84, respiratory rate 16, and blood pressure 98/68 mm Hg. Speech is hypernasal and hard to understand. Hair is coarse, face puffy, and skin dry and pale. Teeth are decayed. A small umbilical hernia is present. The rest of the physical findings are normal. IQ is 93.

Hematocrit is 0.31. White cell count is 6.4×10^9/liter with 0.53 polymorphonuclear cells, 0.03 bands, 0.37 lympho-cytes, 0.01 monocytes, 0.05 eosinophils, and 0.01 basophils. Urine specific gravity is 1.028, pH 5.5. Urine has mucus, urates, 5–10 white cells/HPF, and few epithelial cells/HPF. Serum urea nitrogen is 7.5 mmol/liter, calcium 2.52, and phosphorus 1.55.

Cranial sutures are prominent; size of pituitary fossa is normal. Nutrient canals in lower thoracic vertebrae are prominent. Ossification of capital femoral epiphyses has barely begun at 6 years (Figure 14-1A) and is fragmentary at 7 years (Figure 14-1B), 1 year after treatment is started.

Protein-bound iodine is 2.2 μg/dl before treatment with thyroid extract, 7.3 μg/dl 1 year later. Four years after treatment is begun, technetium 99m scan and iodine 131 point counts show thyroid gland at base of tongue and no increase in iodine 131 uptake 24 hours after intramuscular injection of 10 U TSH.

Menarche is at 14 years. Height at 17 years is 158 cm, weight 52 kg. School grades are Bs and Cs.

Diagnosis: Primary hypothyroidism, lingual thyroid.

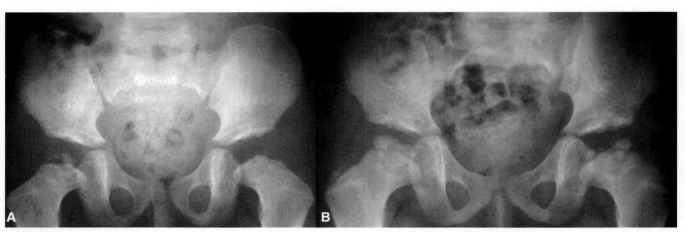

Fig. 14-1

Case 15

Twin sisters (13 years old) have scoliosis.

Pregnancy of mother was normal, amniotic sac single, birth weights 2.2 and 2.4 kg.

Height of one twin is 168 cm, blood pressure 110/50 mm Hg. She has scoliosis, pectus excavatum, and bowlegs. Height of other twin is 165 cm, blood pressure 120/60 mm Hg. She has scoliosis, pectus excavatum, bowlegs, and limitation of abduction of arms.

They have thoracolumbar right convexity in Figure 15-1. Roentgenograms of hands and knees show normal findings.

Taller girl begins to take birth control pills at 16 years. She is confused and has headaches 6 months later, 4 days after taking diazepam, amphetamines, and perhaps phenytoin. Globular lenses are subluxated down and have dot opacities. Diameter of right pupil is 6 mm, left 8 mm. Right side of face and right arm twitch. Right limbs are hypertonic. Doll's eye reflex and right Babinski's sign are present. Blood clot is in left parietal lobe. Use of right limbs returns. She used to write right-handed, now left-handed. At 20 years, she is short of breath. Weight is 64 kg, height 172 cm, heart rate 80, respiratory rate 12, and blood pressure 120/70 mm Hg. A depression is in left parietal bone. Tops of lenses are visible through pupils. Systolic heart murmur and click and diastolic heart murmur are present. Sensation is impaired in right side. Deep tendon reflexes are increased on right side. Clonus is at right ankle. The rest of the physical findings are normal.

Hematocrit at 20 years is 0.36. White cell count is 7.0×10^9/liter with 0.48 polymorphonuclear cells, 0.06 bands, 0.31 lymphocytes, 0.11 monocytes, and 0.04 eosinophils. Platelet count is 312×10^9/liter. Urine specific gravity is 1.020, pH 7. Urine has few squamous epithelial cells/HPF, few nonsquamous epithelial cells/HPF, and 5–7 white cells/HPF. Urine qualitative nitroprusside test is positive. Urine has 588 and 594 µmol homocystine/day (normal: none). Spontaneous and epinephrine-induced platelet aggregation, circulating platelet aggregates, and AT III activity and antigen are normal. Plasma β-thromboglobulin is 51 µg/liter (normal: 12–80).

At 20 years, urine of twin sister has 740 µmol homocystine/day. She is treated with pyridoxine. At 27 years, urinary homocystine is 3 µmol/liter. At 30 years, plasma methionine is 22.0 µmol/liter (normal: 5–40).

Diagnosis: Homocystinuria, pyridoxine responsive.

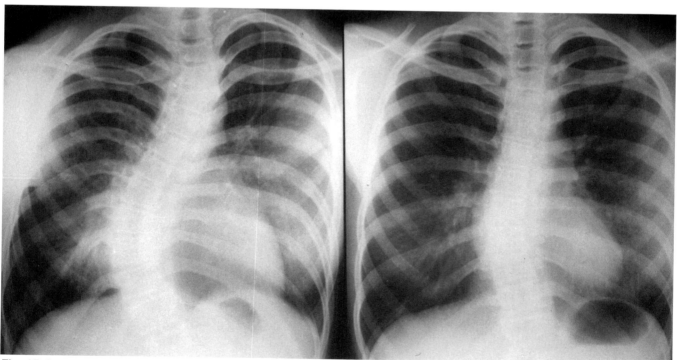

Fig. 15-1

Case 16

A newborn girl, whose twin is normal, has short angled bones that were found in prenatal ultrasound examination. Delivery is by cesarean section.

Birth weight is 1.9 kg, Apgar score 4/8 at 1 and 5 minutes, length 37 cm, head circumference 31 cm, temperature 36.8°C, heart rate 170, respiratory rate 80, blood pressure 58/26 mm Hg, and blood glucose 1.9 mmol/liter. She breathes weakly and has acrocyanosis. Anterior and posterior fontanels are large. Sagittal suture is wide. Orbits are shallow. Neck is short and has loose skin. Sternum is short. Bones of limbs are short and angled. Skin of limbs is loose; it is dimpled over fibular lateral convexities. The rest of the physical findings are normal.

Figure 16-1 shows that (1) skeleton, including skull, is poorly mineralized; (2) vertebrae are slightly flat; (3) bones of limbs are symmetrically angled; (4) 11 ossified ribs are on each side; and (5) lateral part of right seventh rib is thickened as if by an old fracture. Ultrasound examination of head in Figure 16-2 shows cavum veli interpositi between body of fornix above and third ventricle below.

Hematocrit is 0.65. Serum sodium at 2 days is 134 mmol/liter, potassium 4.0, chloride 104, carbon dioxide 18, urea nitrogen 2.5, calcium 2.50, phosphorus 1.74, magnesium 0.80, cholesterol 1.14, and glucose 5.3. Creatinine is 80 µmol/liter, uric acid 300, total bilirubin 66, and direct bilirubin 3. Total protein is 53 g/liter, albumin 36. Alkaline phosphatase is 2 U/liter, LDH 523, SGOT (AST) 45, and SGPT (ALT) 9. Capillary blood pH is 7.34 with oxygen at 100 cc by nasal cannula. P_{CO_2} is 45 mm Hg, P_{O_2} 37. Oxygen saturation is 0.67. At 7 days, urine phosphorylethanolamine is 598 µmol/liter, 4,900 $µmol/g_{creatinine}$ (normal: 140–540). At 14 days, serum calcium is 2.87 mmol/liter, phosphorus 2.49 mmol/liter, and alkaline phosphatase 9 U/liter. At 21 days, serum calcium is 2.64 mmol/liter, phosphorus 2.23 mmol/liter, and alkaline phosphatase 14 U/liter.

Diagnosis: Hypophosphatasia (hypophosphatasemia).

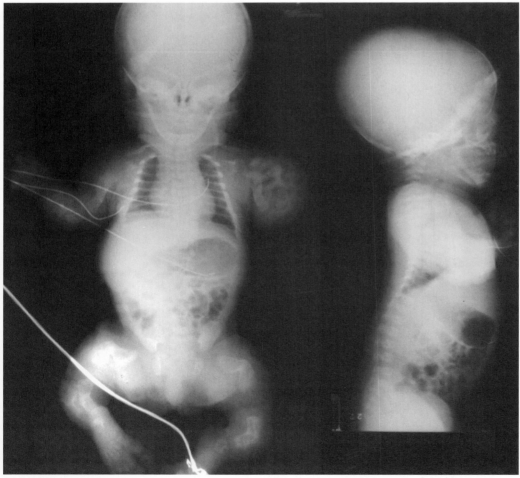

Fig. 16-1

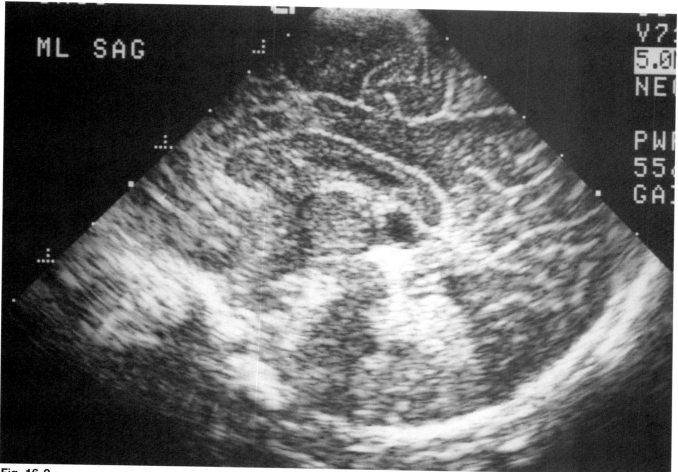

Fig. 16-2

Case 17

A 4-month-old boy, restless and often screaming, is convulsing.

Pregnancy was normal, birth weight 3 kg. He fed poorly, vomited, and was constipated.

Parents and sister are well.

Weight is 4.7 kg, length 57 cm, and head circumference 38 cm. He is quiet and limp at times, crying and thrashing at other times. Calvaria is soft, anterior fontanel large. Cranial sutures are wide. Costochondral junctions, ankles, and knees are thick. Liver edge is 3 cm below costal margin. The rest of the physical findings are normal.

Roentgenographic examination for vomiting at 2 months shows normal GI tract, expanded costochondral junctions, deep triradiate cartilage in innominate bones, and rarefied femoral metaphyses (Figure 17-1A). Roentgenogram of arm at 4 months shows similar metaphyses (Figure 17-1B). Synchondroses and sphenozygomatic and sphenofrontal sutures in base of skull are wide at 4 months (Figure 17-2).

At 2 months, serum calcium is 2.99 mmol/liter, and alkaline phosphatase is 1 U/liter. At 4 months, serum calcium is 2.62–3.19 mmol/liter, phosphorus 1.45–2.03 mmol/liter, and alkaline phosphatase 4 U/liter. Urine has excess phosphoethanolamine. Mother's serum alkaline phosphatase is 24 U/liter; father's and sister's are low normal.

Convulsions recur despite phenobarbital, diazoxide, and valproic acid (Depakene). Blood pressure is 154/90 mm Hg. He dies in status epilepticus.

At necropsy, costochondral junctions and long bone metaphyses are irregular in cross section. Microscopic examination shows distorted enchondral ossification with irregular cords of chondrocytes, irregular areas of fibrosis and osteocyte proliferation, absence of blood vessels, and little calcium in bone. Foci of calcification, neutrophils, and necrosis are in myocardium and renal interstitium, and also with edema in spleen. Centrilobular necrosis is in liver. Bands of fibrous connective tissue and few lymphocytes are in thymus.

Diagnosis: Hypophosphatasia (hypophosphatasemia).

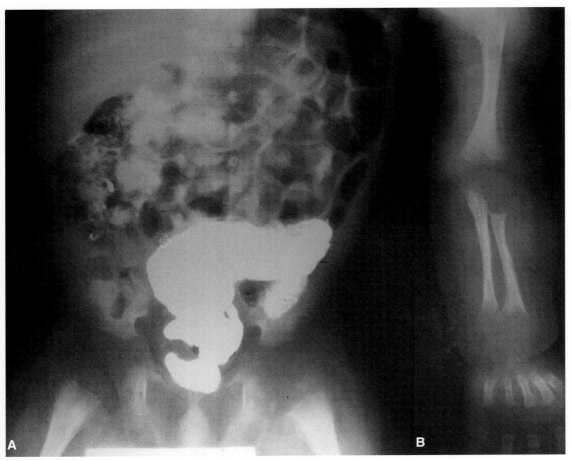

Fig. 17-1

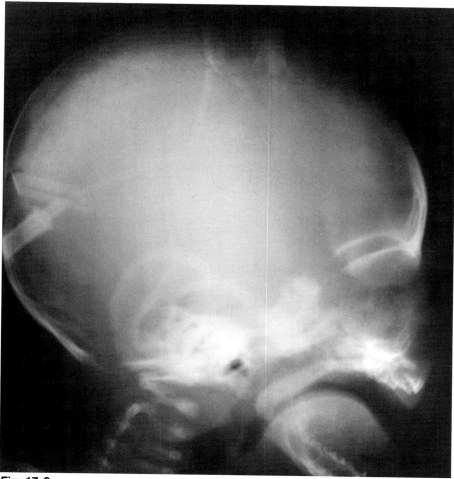

Fig. 17-2

Case 18

A 13-year-old boy, who was adopted 9 weeks ago, has staring spells and sudden lapses of attention. He "falls asleep" while eating, fork halfway to mouth; stares vacuously; and recovers a moment later. He likes frequent small meals and eats fruits and vegetables but not meat.

Pregnancy was normal, birth weight 3.2 kg. He had diarrhea. He had an episode of sweating, agitation, and mydriasis at 5 years. Weight was 11 kg, height 79 cm. At 9 years, intelligence was at the 3–4 year level. He has broken his left arm twice.

Weight at 13 years is 24 kg, height 119 cm, head circumference 54 cm, heart rate 80, and blood pressure 90/60 mm Hg. He looks younger than 13 years. Hair is orange and brittle. Skin is dry. Chest is deep front to back, trunk short. Limbs are thin and freckled. Left arm is crooked. Liver edge is 2 cm below costal margin. Cervical, supraclavicular, and inguinal nodes are prominent. The rest of the physical findings are normal.

Hematocrit is 0.32. Hemoglobin is 113 g/liter. MCV is 87 fl. MCH is 31 pg. MCHC is 350 g/liter. White cell count is 3.8 × 10⁹/liter with 0.22 polymorphonuclear cells, 0.08 bands, 0.58 lymphocytes, and 0.12 monocytes. Reticulocyte fraction is 7 × 10⁻³. Platelet count is 220 × 10⁹/liter. Urine specific gravity is 1.022, pH 5. Urine has 0–1 white cell/HPF, 0–3 red cells/HPF, and mucus. Serum sodium is 140 mmol/liter, potassium 3.4, chloride 107, carbon dioxide 20, urea nitrogen 5.0, calcium 2.30, phosphorus 1.61, cholesterol 4.42, and glucose 4.7. Creatinine is 40 µmol/liter, uric acid 160, total bilirubin 9, direct bilirubin 0, and ammonia 70 and 195 (normal: 5–50). Total protein is 87 g/liter, albumin 49. Alkaline phosphatase is 226 U/liter, LDH 756, SGOT 63, SGPT 53, and GGT 14. Quantitative analysis of amino acids in plasma shows citrulline 59 µmol/liter (normal: 19–52), ornithine 18 (normal: 19–81), lysine 103 (normal: 108–233), and arginine 15 (normal: 44–130). Levels of other amino acids are normal. Quantitative analysis of amino acids in urine shows lysine 458.7 mmol/mol creatinine (normal for child: 31.5–114.9), orotic acid 16.1 µmol/mmol creatinine (normal: 0–5.8).

Vertebral bodies are collapsed in varying degrees, and body of L1 is biconcave in Figure 18-1A. Bone age in a roentgenogram of hand is about 9 years, 4–5 SDs below mean. Roentgenogram of chest at 14 years shows ill-defined nodules of water density in lungs (Figure 18-1B). Subcutaneous tissues of jugular (suprasternal) notch are sunken in Figure 18-1B.

At thoracotomy at 14 years, left lung looks emphysematous. Pink-tan piece of lingula is yellow-brown and consolidated in cross section. Microscopic examination shows alveolar proteinosis.

Diagnosis: Lysinuric protein intolerance with osteoporosis and alveolar proteinosis.

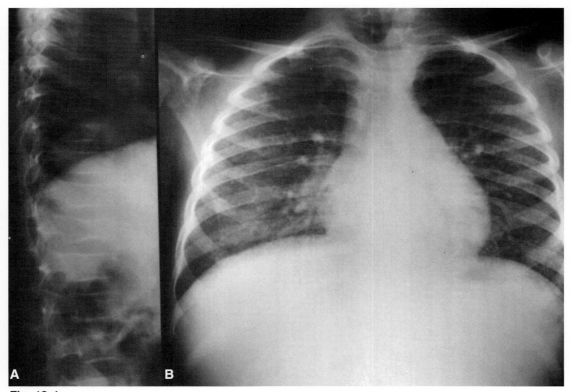

Fig. 18-1

Case 19

A 2½-year-old girl is "sore all over, very nervous, and doesn't eat well."

She stopped walking 2 months ago, cried when moved, became irritable, and would not eat. Feet were swollen. She began to vomit 1 month ago. Hair has been falling out for several weeks.

Pregnancy was normal. She sat at 6 months, walked at 1 year. She has had several colds.

Mother (25 years old) and father (27 years old) are well. The girl is their only child.

Temperature is 37.6°C, weight 10 kg. She is pale and skinny. She lies on her back and moves little. Bones are tender. A systolic heart murmur is present. The rest of the physical findings are normal.

Hemoglobin is 110 g/liter. White cell count is 15.7 × 10^9/liter with 0.37 polymorphonuclear cells, 0.56 lymphocytes, 0.03 monocytes, 0.03 eosinophils, and 0.01 basophils. Reticulocyte fraction is $12 × 10^{-3}$. ESR is 80 mm/45 minutes. Urine specific gravity is 1.002, pH alkaline. Urine has 2+ white cells/HPF, occasional red cells/HPF, 1+ epithelial cells/HPF, bacteria, and amorphous phosphates. Serum urea nitrogen is 4.3 mmol/liter, calcium 2.79, and phosphorus 1.81. Total protein is 68 g/liter, albumin 42. Alkaline phosphatase is 30 U/liter. Serum vitamin A level is 3 µmol/liter after 8 days, 2.2 µmol/liter after 14 days (normal: 0.5–2.1). Serum carotenoids are 2.1 µmol after 8 days, 2.4 µmol/liter after 14 days (normal: 1.5–7.4).

Figure 19-1 shows subperiosteal new bone in right arm. New bone is almost symmetric along ulnas. New bone is also around clavicles and bones of the legs.

Appetite improves and vomiting subsides during the next week. She "is talking all the time" after 6 days. She can pull herself up to sit after 10 days. She runs and plays with other children after 2 weeks and skates and rides her bike after 2 months.

Diagnosis: Hypervitaminosis A. (She was given two solutions containing vitamin A per day since she was 3 months old, an approximate daily total of 99,000 µmol.)

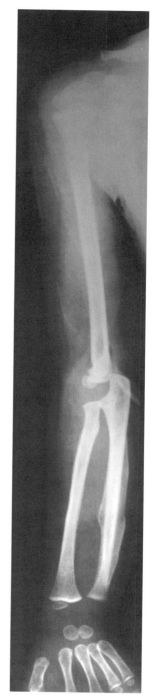

Fig. 19-1

Case 20

A 3-year-old boy has been crying all night the last 3 nights.

He stopped moving legs 3 months ago. Body has been spotted for weeks. He takes water and milk but has had no fruit juice, vegetables, or vitamins for 1 year. Birth weight was 3.2 kg. He was anoxic at birth. He has never sat or tried to walk. He had a bad respiratory infection 1 year ago.

Parents and two siblings are well.

Temperature at 3 years is 38.9°C, heart rate 140, blood pressure 120/80 mm Hg, weight 8 kg, and head circumference 40 cm. He is malnourished and dehydrated. Skin is scaly. Pinpoint brown-red spots are on limbs and abdomen. Arms and legs are flexed, fists clenched. Gums are bloody around teeth. Pharynx is slightly injected. Costochondral junctions are palpable. Abdomen is sunken. The rest of the physical findings are normal.

Hemoglobin is 70 g/liter. White cell count is 14.6×10^9/liter with 0.75 polymorphonuclear cells, 0.02 bands, 0.22 lymphocytes, and 0.01 monocytes. ESR is 25 mm/45 minutes. Urine specific gravity is 1.042, pH acid. Urine has trace albumin, 4+ glucose, amorphous urates, occasional red cells/HPF, occasional white cells/HPF, and epithelial cells/HPF. Serum calcium is 2.40 mmol/liter, phosphorus (3 days later) 1.52. Total protein is 72 g/liter, albumin 50. Alkaline phosphatase is 76.3 King-Armstrong U/liter (normal: 30–120).

In Figure 20-1A, a white band is at end of bones and fragmented at distal femurs, where irregular radiolucencies are in metaphyses (Trümmerfeldzone*). Proximal metaphyses of humeri are fragmented. Subperiosteal new bone is present 13 days after treatment is begun (Figure 20-1B). Diaphysis of left humerus is lateral to lateral epiphyseal ossification center, which is in glenoid fossa (see Figure 20-1B).

Gums stop bleeding 1 day after treatment is begun. Two weeks later, he cries whenever any part of his body except his head is touched.

Diagnosis: Scurvy, ossification of subperiosteal hematoma.

---

*Trümmerfeld: field covered with debris or ruins.

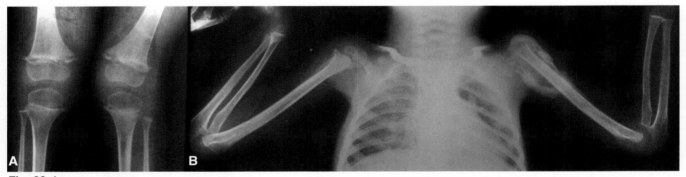

Fig. 20-1

Case 21

A 13-year-old girl has a positive tuberculin test. She came from a Thai refugee camp several weeks ago and speaks English through a bad interpreter. She did not have milk or other dairy products and rarely had fruit. She had a discharge from abdominal wall 1 year ago and has had draining sores on neck for 1 year.

Temperature is 36.9°C, heart rate 80, respiratory rate 20, blood pressure 100/50 mm Hg, weight 25 kg, and height 123 cm. She is short and skinny. Cervical, axillary, and inguinal lymph nodes are large. Scars are in neck, below umbilicus, and in right groin. Breath sounds are diminished at base of left lung. Depigmented, flat, oval spots (3-mm diameter) are on abdomen. An easily reducible umbilical hernia is present. A swelling is on left forearm at site of tuberculin injection. The rest of the physical findings are normal.

Hematocrit is 0.37. White cell count is 5.7×10^9/liter with 0.64 polymorphonuclear cells, 0.06 bands, 0.22 lymphocytes, 0.03 monocytes, 0.03 eosinophils, and 0.02 basophils. Platelet count is 395×10^9/liter. ESR is 52 mm/hr. Urine specific gravity is 1.019, pH 8. Urine has 4–6 white cells/HPF,

mucus, rare hyaline casts/LPF, occasional white cell casts/LPF, and triple phosphates. Serum sodium is 150 mmol/liter, potassium 3.1, chloride 107, carbon dioxide 26, urea nitrogen 2.9, calcium 2.37, phosphorus 1.37, cholesterol 4.00, and glucose 5.4. Creatinine is 50 µmol/liter, uric acid 170, total bilirubin 7, and direct bilirubin 3. Total protein is 70 g/liter, albumin 38. Alkaline phosphatase is 489 U/liter, LDH 256, and SGOT 22. Ova and parasites are not in stool. Sputum and urine cultures have not grown mycobacteria at 8 weeks.

She is treated for tuberculosis. She gets approximately 48% of total calories from school lunch and 49 mg/day vitamin C during the next 8 months.

First examination, in Figure 21-1A, shows compressed vertebrae. Examination also shows left thickened pleura or pleural liquid. Vertebrae are taller 8 months later (Figure 21-1B). In examination 2 months after chest examination, left patella has appearance of bone within a bone (Figure 21-2).

Diagnosis: Scurvy, osteoporosis, healing scurvy.

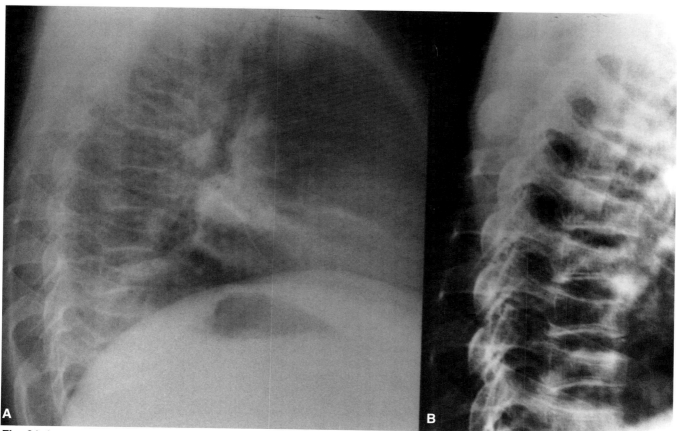

Fig. 21-1

(Continued)

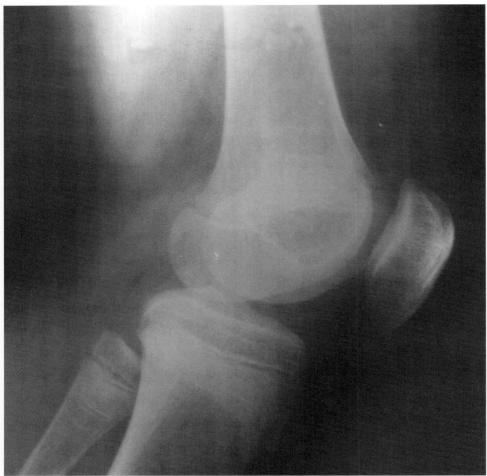

Fig. 21-2

Case 22

A 27-month-old girl, who has been on a high-carbohydrate diet since coma and convulsions at 1 year, has decayed teeth.

Pregnancy was marred by vaginal bleeding several months before birth. Birth weight was 1.9 kg, Apgar score 8/9 at 1 and 5 minutes. She was walking and saying a few words at 1 year. She vomited at 1 year, had temperature of 37.2°C, and then became comatose with blood glucose 0.7 mmol/liter, plasma ammonia 320 µmol/liter (normal: 5–50), and total bilirubin 15 µmol/liter. She then had seizures for 5–10 seconds during which she flexed at waist, grunted, and took deep breaths. She walked stiffly. Deep tendon reflexes in legs were increased. Treatment consisted of frequent high-carbohydrate feedings and phenobarbital, 60 mg/day. Mother substituted cottage cheese for milk. Dental caries appeared at 24 months. Diet was estimated to contain 467 mg/day calcium, 0.58 recommended daily allowance.

Mother (31 years old), father (35 years old), and sister (8 years old) are well.

Weight at 27 months is 13.5 kg, height 86 cm, head circumference 49 cm, temperature 37.2°C, heart rate 120, respiratory rate 32, and blood pressure 82/60 mm Hg. Eight teeth are carious. A systolic heart murmur is present. Liver edge is 2 cm below costal margin. Heel cords are tight. Babinski's sign is in feet. The rest of the physical findings are normal.

Hematocrit is 0.40. White cell count is 10.4×10^9/liter. Urine specific gravity is 1.007, pH 8. Urine has 1–2 red cells/HPF and 1–2 white cells/HPF. Serum sodium is 147 mmol/liter, potassium 4.8, chloride 112, carbon dioxide 19, urea nitrogen 1.4, calcium 1.80, phosphorus 0.87, cholesterol 4.42, triglycerides 1.12, and glucose 5.4. Creatinine is 40 µmol/liter, uric acid 170, total bilirubin 3, and direct bilirubin 0. Alkaline phosphatase is >3,000 U/liter, LDH 435, SGOT 62, and CK 139.

Figure 22-1A shows changes of rickets at knees. Twenty-six days after treatment with vitamin D is begun, changes of healing rickets are prominent at metaphyseal zone of provisional calcification, the müllerian line (Figure 22-1B), about which E.A. Park said, "Müller first called attention to the fact that when rickets healed, calcification took place in a stratum of the proliferative cartilage . . . at the end of the shaft. The lime salts skipped the cartilage adjacent to the end of the shaft and chose cartilage at some distance beyond."*

Seizures continue despite anticonvulsants. Analysis of muscle obtained at 7 years is thought to show carnitine deficiency. She deteriorates despite daily carnitine. Urine smells like sweaty feet. She is blind with optic atrophy at 13 years. She uses a few signs to indicate some of her needs.

Medium-chain acyl coenzyme A dehydrogenase activity, determined in sonic supernatant of a specimen of her muscle by anaerobic electron transfer flavoprotein reduction assay, shows 0.08 nmol/min/mg protein with octanoyl coenzyme A as substrate, 0.05 of mean value in 12 normal controls. Enzymatic activity with butyryl coenzyme A and palmitoyl coenzyme A is normal.

Diagnosis: Vitamin D–deficient rickets; medium-chain acyl coenzyme A dehydrogenase deficiency.

*EA Park. The pathology of rickets. Harvey Lectures 34:157, 1938–9.

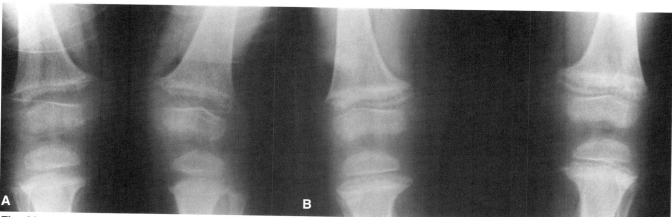

Fig. 22-1

Case 23

A 1-year-old boy is unresponsive. He was crawling and pulling things off a table 3 days ago. Vomiting began that night and persists.

Pregnancy was normal, birth weight 3.1 kg. He has vomited off and on since he was 3 months old. He drinks and urinates a lot. He had measles at 6 months. Two weeks ago, he had a cough, fever, and vomiting for several days.

Parents and sister (3 years old) are well. A first cousin died at 6 years with encephalitis, another at 10 months with pneumonia. Four paternal uncles died before they were 50 years old, two with heart disease.

Temperature at 1 year is 38.9°C, heart rate 156, respiratory rate 60, blood pressure 70/56 mm Hg, and weight 7.4 kg. Respirations are shallow. He is pale. Lips are blue, limbs cool. Hands, feet, and lower legs are swollen. Costochondral junctions bulge. Liver edge is 6 cm below costal margin, spleen edge 1 cm. Deep tendon reflexes are weak. He withdraws from pain. The rest of the physical findings are normal. Slit-lamp examination shows small glittering deposits in corneas.

Hematocrit is 0.25. White cell count is 16.2×10^9/liter with 0.45 polymorphonuclear cells, 0.20 bands, 0.33 lymphocytes, and 0.02 monocytes. Platelet count is 497×10^9/liter. Reticulocyte fraction is 23×10^{-3}. Urine specific gravity is 1.012, pH 6. Urine has glucose, ketones, hemoglobin/myoglobin, 0–1 red cell/HPF, 2–3 white cells/HPF, and 4–5 granular casts/LPF. Urine sodium is 54 mmol/liter, potassium 29, and chloride 64. Serum sodium is 122 mmol/liter, potassium 4.7, chloride 92, urea nitrogen 1.3, calcium 1.15, and glucose 10.2. Alkaline phosphatase is 72 U/liter.

Laminas dura in crypts of unerupted teeth lack mineral in Figure 23-1A. Proximal metaphysis of humerus and distal metaphyses of radius and ulna are frayed and wide in Figure 23-1B.

Leukocyte cystine is 1.3–2.5 µmol/g protein in four determinations (normal: <0.2).

Diagnosis: Cystinosis, rickets.

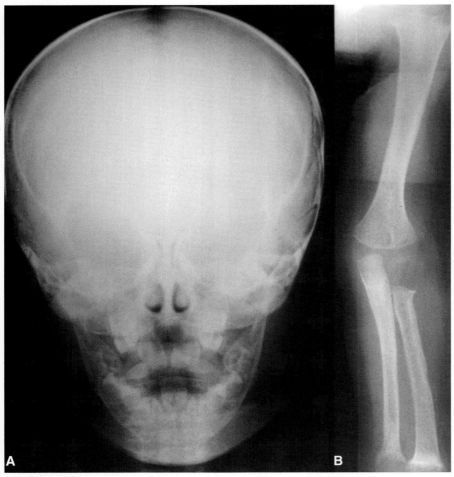

Fig. 23-1

Case 24

A 5-year-old boy, recently adopted, is mentally retarded and the size of a 3-year-old child.

Mother was 24 years old when he was born. Apgar score was 7/9 at 1 and 10 minutes. He had cataracts and proteinuria. At 6 months, superior sector iridectomies were performed. At 15 months, audiometric findings were normal. At 20 months, he tried to crawl and stand, tired after several minutes, and then collapsed for half an hour. Back was hairy. Muscles were thin, joints lax. He had generalized aminoaciduria. At 3 years, weight was 10 kg, height 84 cm, temperature 37.4°C, heart rate 144, respiratory rate 25, and systolic blood pressure 50 mm Hg. A cataract with dense central nucleus attached by thick plaque to back of lens capsule was aspirated from left lens, and 5 months later, similar cataract was extracted from right lens.

He grunts but does not talk at 5 years. He eats a lot: For breakfast he will often eat cereal, milk, two pieces of toast, and three eggs.

Weight at 5 years is 12.7 kg, height 93 cm, and head circumference 49 cm. He is skinny and has nystagmus and operative changes in eyes. The rest of the physical findings are normal.

Serum sodium is 134 mmol/liter, potassium 4.4, chloride 107, carbon dioxide 13, urea nitrogen 1.8, calcium 2.40, phosphorus 0.81, cholesterol 3.83, and glucose 4.0. Creatinine is 40 μmol/liter, uric acid 160, total bilirubin 3, and direct bilirubin 0. Total protein is 70 g/liter, albumin 41. Alkaline phosphatase is 399 U/liter, LDH 408, and SGOT 93. Stool fat is not excessive. Thyroid uptake of radioactive iodine is 0.22 over 24 hours (normal: 0.08–0.30). Total serum T_4 is 194 mmol/liter (normal: 94–194). Urine specific gravity at 7 years is 1.013, pH 7. Urine has 1+ hemoglobin/myoglobin, 1 g/liter protein, amorphous phosphates, 0–1 red cell/HPF, and 2–4 white cells/HPF.

Femurs are rachitic at 5 years (Figure 24-1). Radii at wrists are also rachitic at 5 years, when bone age is 2 years and treatment is begun. Femurs are not rachitic at 7 years, when bone age is approximately 4 years.

He has grand mal convulsions at 9 years, gum hypertrophy and rough skin at 12 years, and biconcave thoracic vertebrae of osteoporosis in roentgenogram of spine at 15 years. At 15 years, he is sociable and able to follow instructions. At 17 years, hematocrit is 0.39. White cell count is 5.9×10^9/liter. Platelet count is 211×10^9/liter. Urine calcium/creatinine is 0.36 (normal: <0.40). Serum urea nitrogen is 4.6 mmol/liter, calcium 2.47, and phosphorus 1.00. Creatinine is 70 μmol/liter.

Diagnosis: Oculocerebrorenal syndrome (Lowe syndrome).

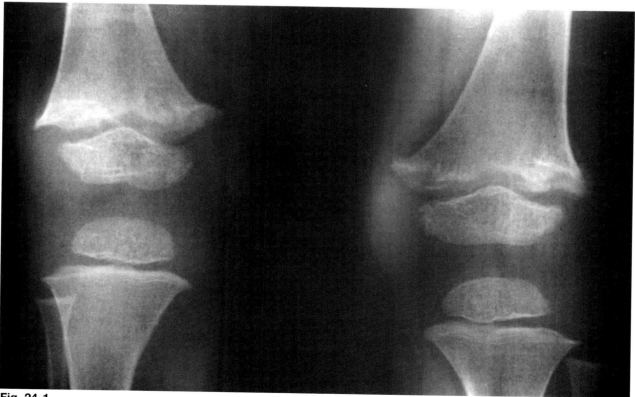

Fig. 24-1

Case 25

A 3½-year-old girl is too short.

Pregnancy was normal, birth weight 4 kg, length 52 cm, and head circumference 35 cm. She had an umbilical hernia. The rest of the physical findings were normal. Height was 79 cm at 2 years (<3rd percentile), weight 12 kg. She wheezed with respiratory infection at 2⅓ years. Knees and shins ached when she played at 2½ years.

Father, three paternal uncles, paternal aunt, paternal grandmother, paternal great-grandmother, and paternal great-uncle are shorter than normal; two paternal uncles are not short.

Height at 3½ years is 89 cm, weight 14 kg. Teeth are discolored. The rest of the physical findings are normal.

Serum sodium is 144 mmol/liter, potassium 4.6, chloride 105, carbon dioxide 24, urea nitrogen 4.3, calcium 2.40 and 2.52, phosphorus 0.81 and 1.03, cholesterol 3.28, and glucose 4.7. Creatinine is 40 μmol/liter, uric acid 270, total bilirubin 7, and direct bilirubin 0. Total protein is 69 g/liter, albumin 32. Alkaline phosphatase is 546 U/liter, LDH 303, and SGOT 34. Plasma C-terminal parathyroid hormone is 88 μlEq/liter (normal <50).

Figure 25-1A shows rachitic femoral and distal tibial metaphyses.

Paternal uncle (22 years old) has pain in lateral part of right thigh and tenderness below right greater trochanter for several days after heavy lifting. He is shorter than normal.

Figure 25-1B shows that (1) paternal uncle's femoral neck-shaft angle is less than normal, (2) a pseudofracture is in medial part of femoral shaft, and (3) shaft of femur is laterally convex.

Girl's height is 149 cm at 16 years.

Diagnosis: Familial X-linked vitamin D–insensitive rickets in child, osteomalacia in adult.

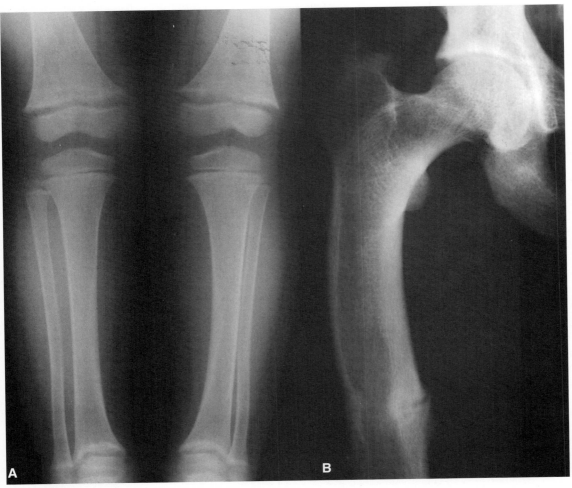

Fig. 25-1

Case 26

A 4½-year-old boy is short and bowlegged. Mother, brother, and maternal grandmother are also short and bowlegged.

Delivery was by cesarean section, birth weight 2.8 kg.

Height of mother (31 years old) and maternal grandmother is 137 cm; father (34 years old) is 173 cm tall and maternal grandfather is 157 cm tall. Parents and brother (7 years old) are well.

Height is 89 cm, weight 13.6 kg. Head is large. Costochondral junctions are prominent. Legs are bowed. The rest of the physical findings are normal.

Serum calcium is 2.50 mmol/liter, phosphorus 1.07 mmol/liter, and alkaline phosphatase 149 U/liter. Mother's serum calcium is 2.40 mmol/liter, phosphorus 0.81 mmol/liter, and alkaline phosphatase 80 U/liter. Brother's calcium is 2.35 mmol/liter, phosphorus 0.84 mmol/liter, and alkaline phosphatase 261 U/liter.

Roentgenograms of skull at 6 months (Figure 26-1A) and 4½ years (Figure 26-1B) show development of scaphocephaly and change from prognathism to retrognathism.

Diagnosis: Vitamin D–resistant rickets, scaphocephaly.

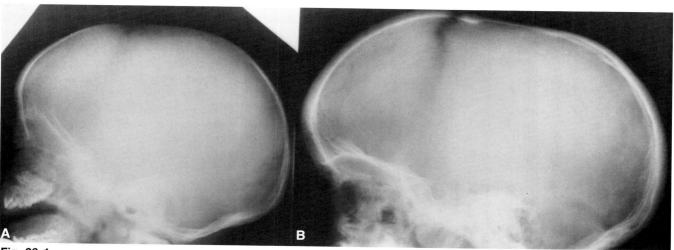

Fig. 26-1

Case 27

A 12-year-old boy convulses for the first time after he vomits, begins to sweat, and says he has a headache. Right hand and arm jerk for a few minutes, body jerks for 5–10 minutes, and then convulsion stops.

He was tired at 7 years. He skipped meals. He gained 5.4 kg in 1 month. Eyelids, face, abdomen, and legs were puffy. He looked waxy and smelled uremic. Blood pressure was 92/50 mm Hg. Gallop rhythm was present. Urine specific gravity was 1.028. Urine had red blood cells and granular casts. Serum potassium was 6.3 mmol/liter, urea nitrogen 27.1. Creatinine was 670 μmol/liter. Albumin was 18 g/liter. Peritoneal dialysis was performed. Serum sodium 3 days later was 138 mmol/liter, potassium 6.1, chloride 107, carbon dioxide 24, urea nitrogen 26.4, calcium 2.10, phosphorus 1.17, triglycerides >5.66, cholesterol 12.28, and glucose 4.2. Creatinine was 140 μmol/liter, uric acid 420, total bilirubin 2, and direct bilirubin 0. Total protein was 46 g/liter, albumin 18. Alkaline phosphatase was 307 U/liter, LDH 355, SGOT 41, CK 833, and GGT 7. Kidney biopsy showed tubulointerstitial inflammation and edema in light microscopy and endothelial cell injury and necrosis of mesangial cells in electron microscopy. Immunoglobulin deposits were absent.

Parents and older sibling are well.

Blood pressure at 12 years is 204/130 mm Hg. He is given IV sodium nitroprusside and furosemide. Blood pressure is then 120/80 mm Hg, heart rate 110, respiratory rate 36, temperature 37.2°C, weight 31.8 kg, and height 142 cm. Liver edge is 2 cm below costal margin. The rest of the physical findings are normal.

Urine specific gravity is 1.009, pH 7. Urine has 1.0 g/liter protein and occasional squamous epithelial cells/HPF. Serum urea nitrogen is 35.2 mmol/liter, calcium 2.27, phosphorus 2.52, and cholesterol 5.07. Creatinine is 410 μmol/liter. Albumin is 39 g/liter. Alkaline phosphatase is 1,662 U/liter.

He is given kidney transplant at 14 years and begins 6 years of treatment for chronic rejection.

Shape of heart in Figure 27-1 suggests dilation of left ventricle when he convulses at 12 years. A fleck of calcium at level of ligamentum arteriosum suggests that ductus arteriosus is closed (see Figure 27-1). Lateral bony ends of clavicles do not meet acromions in Figure 27-1. Edges of middle phalanges of fingers are fuzzy at 13 years, some distal phalangeal heads and tuberosities partly resorbed (Figure 27-2A). Bones are partly remineralized at 15 years (Figure 27-2B). Calcium is in walls of some digital arteries (see Figure 27-2B) when serum calcium is 2.47 mmol/liter, phosphorus 1.32. *N*-terminal parathyroid hormone is 300 ng/liter (normal: 8–24).

Diagnosis: Kidney failure, hypertensive encephalopathy, secondary hyperparathyroidism.

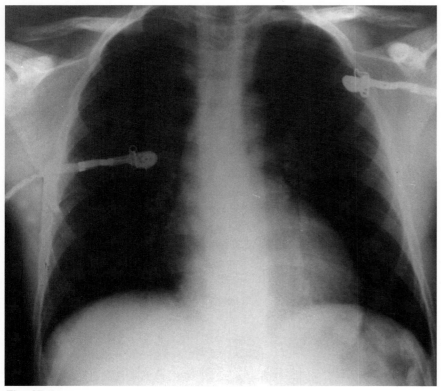

Fig. 27-1

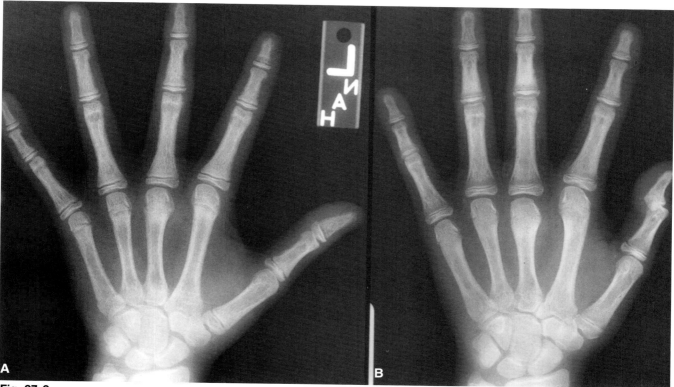

Fig. 27-2

Case 28

A 9-year-old boy "can't run, walks with a waddle," lags behind when walking from school bus, and tires by noon. He has had headache, bellyache, and aches in legs and feet for 3 months.

He walked at 14 months. He has had rubella and two ear infections. He bruises easily. He has always been clumsy. He was 3 years old before he stopped wetting himself during the day. He wets his bed. He drinks more water than his 11-year-old brother and 7-year-old brother, who is as tall as he is.

Mother takes thyroid pills. Maternal great-grandparents and paternal grandmother had diabetes mellitus.

Temperature at 9 years is 37.2°C, heart rate 92, respiratory rate 20, blood pressure 126/78 mm Hg, weight 26 kg, and height 121 cm. A systolic murmur is present. Liver edge is 1 cm below costal margin. The rest of the physical findings are normal.

Hematocrit is 0.29. White cell count is 4.7×10^9/liter with 0.42 polymorphonuclear cells, 0.02 bands, 0.47 lymphocytes, 0.03 monocytes, and 0.06 eosinophils. Platelet estimate is adequate. ESR is 51 mm/45 minutes. Urine specific gravity is 1.008, pH 6. Urine has a few urate crystals. Serum sodium is 137 mmol/liter, potassium 4.3, chloride 101, carbon dioxide <10, urea nitrogen 44.6, calcium 2.50, phosphorus 3.07 (calcium × phosphorus = 7.68), and glucose 5.6. Creatinine is 530 μmol/liter.

Retrograde pyelogram shows contrast material in saclike left pelvis and in dilated right pelvis. Roentgenogram in Figure 28-1 shows rarefaction of vertebral bodies and subchondral sclerosis ("rugger jersey"), probably the result of chronic acidosis. Figure 28-1 also shows resorption of lateral end of clavicles.

Aortography shows hypoplastic renal arteries.

Diagnosis: Renal dysplasia, renal rickets, secondary hyperparathyroidism, "rugger jersey" vertebrae.

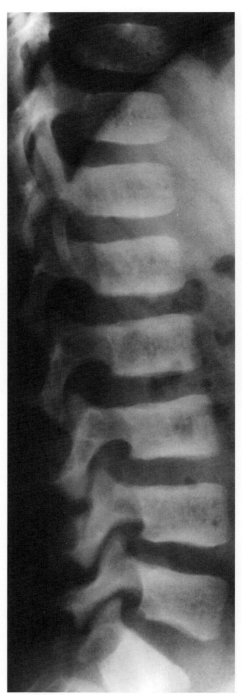

Fig. 28-1

Skeletal Trauma

Case 1

A 5-month-old girl will not move her right arm. She screamed suddenly while her pajamas were being taken off and then refused to move right arm.

Birth weight was 3.2 kg, length 50 cm, head circumference 35 cm, and Apgar score 8/9 at 1 and 5 minutes. Physical findings were normal. Scales and red papules on scalp at 1 month were diagnosed as seborrheic dermatitis. Weight at 4 months was 6.2 kg, length 64 cm. She smiled and had a good grasp. She had bilateral hip click. The rest of the physical and roentgenographic findings at hips were normal.

Roentgenographic findings at 5 months are normal. In lateral examination, right forearm is supinated (Figure 1-1A), left forearm pronated (Figure 1-1B).

She moves right arm soon after roentgenogram, cure having been effected by supination of hand and flexion at elbow for examination.

Diagnosis: Nursemaid's elbow, right.

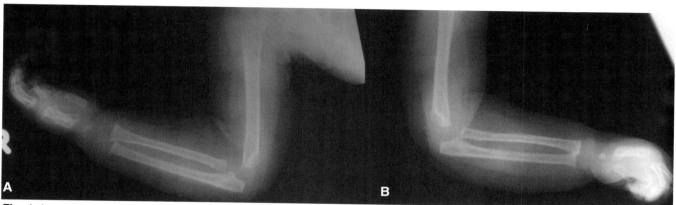

Fig. 1-1

Case 2

A 6-year-old girl has a sore right arm. She fell from a scooter today and hurt right forearm. The arm is not swollen or bruised. Distal part of radius is tender.

Figure 2-1 shows a torus fracture in distal part of radius.

She falls 13 days later while playing soccer. Left arm does not hurt much, but distal part of left forearm is swollen and tender.

In Figure 2-2A, endosteal sclerosis and slight cortical thickening are at healing fracture of right radius. A new torus fracture is in distal part of left radius and distal part of left ulna in frontal and lateral views (Figure 2-2B).

Diagnosis: New and healing torus fractures of forearms.

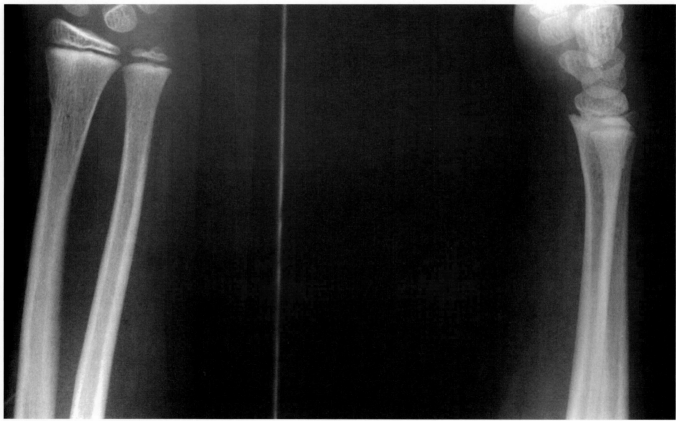

Fig. 2-1

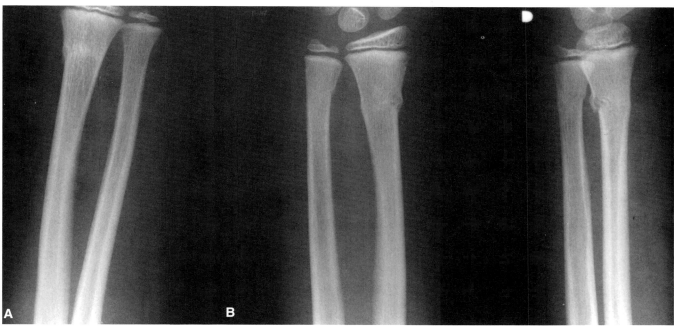

Fig. 2-2

Case 3

A 10-year-old boy, who fell off his bicycle 90 minutes ago, has a swollen left elbow. Front of distal part of left humerus is tender. Left forearm is cooler than right. The rest of the physical findings are normal.

Figure 3-1A shows a transverse fracture between coronoid fossa and lateral epicondyle of left humerus in frontal examination. Figure 3-1B shows swollen soft tissues behind left elbow, subcapsular dorsal fat pad displaced out of left olecra-non fossa, and backward displacement of left capitulum. A line drawn down front of left humerus in lateral examination goes through front third of left capitulum, back third of right (Figure 3-1C).

Diagnosis: Fracture of distal left humerus (epicondylar fracture).

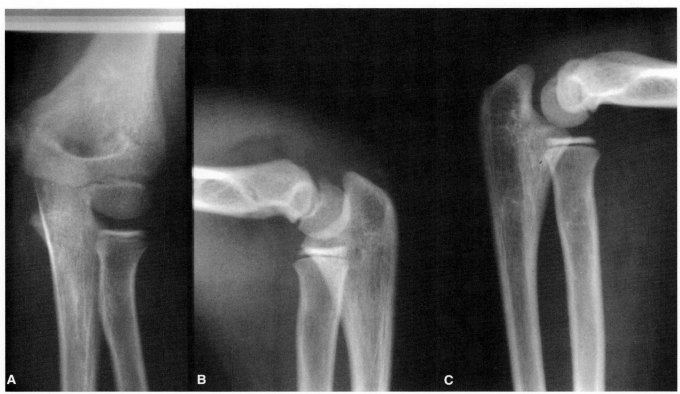

Fig. 3-1

Case 4

An 11-year-old boy has a deformed left arm. He broke his arm when he fell from a tree at 9 years. The fracture was treated with pins, traction, and a cast. He has been hoarse for 4 months.

Temperature is 36.8°C, heart rate 76, respiratory rate 18, blood pressure 86/60 mm Hg, weight 32 kg, and height 122 cm. A nodule is on right true vocal cord. Left arm is laterally convex at elbow and lacks 10-degree flexion. The rest of the physical findings are normal.

Figure 4-1 shows left arm laterally convex at elbow. Left capitulum is displaced backward in lateral roentgenogram. Distal part of left humerus is thickened. Subperiosteal new bone is in dorsal concavity of left humerus.

Diagnosis: Old supracondylar fracture of left humerus with residual gunstock deformity.

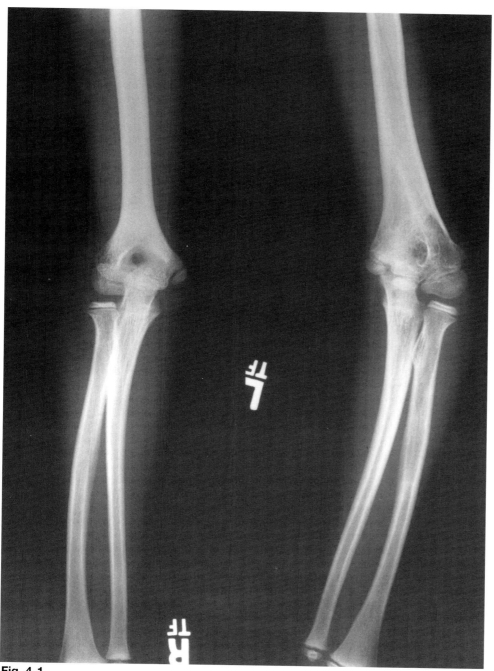

Fig. 4-1

Case 5

A 10½-year-old boy tripped and fell. Now his left arm hurts. Tubes were placed in ears at 8½ years.

Weight is 44 kg, height 143 cm. Small nodes are in neck. A tube is in right ear. Distal part of left forearm is tender and swollen. The rest of the physical findings are normal.

Figure 5-1 shows distal epiphyseal ossification center of left radius displaced laterally and backward.

Diagnosis: Salter 1 fracture of distal growth plate of left radius.

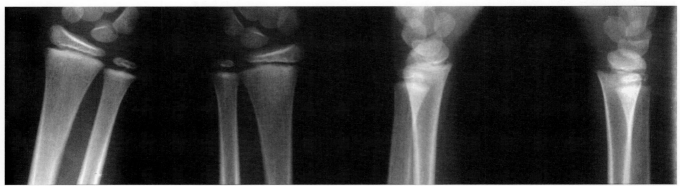

Fig. 5-1

Case 6

A 12-year-old girl has a swollen right little finger that she hurt when she tried to catch a volleyball yesterday. She had pain in right forearm when she fell while roller skating 8 days ago.

Weight is 36 kg, height 143 cm. Right fifth finger is swollen, its mobility decreased. The rest of the physical findings in the hands are normal.

A growth-plate fracture (Figure 6-1) that extends into metaphysis (Figure 6-2) is in proximal phalanx of right fifth digit. A growth-plate fracture that does not involve metaphysis or epiphyseal ossification center is in right radius (see Figure 6-1).

She has no pain or limitation of motion when cast is taken off right hand 20 days later.

Diagnosis: Salter 2 fracture of proximal phalanx of right fifth digit, Salter 1 fracture of right radius.

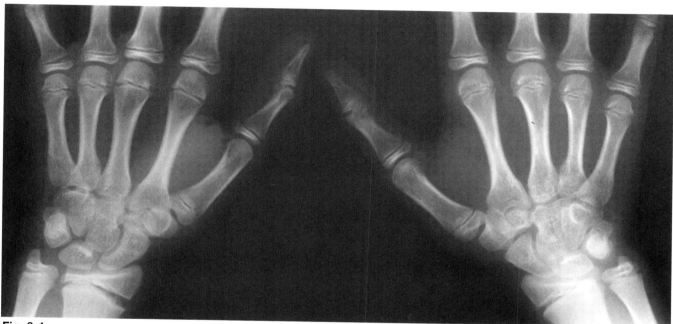

Fig. 6-1

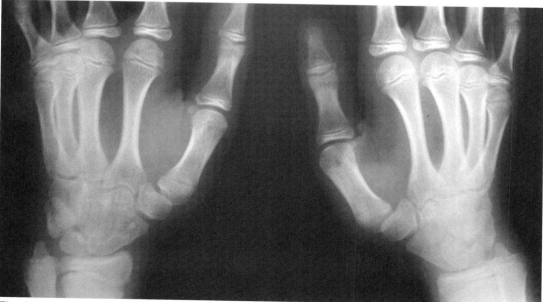

Fig. 6-2

Case 7

A 15-year-old boy has a blue, swollen right little finger. He jammed his finger between a mailbox and handlebar of bicycle he was riding this afternoon. Movement of little finger is decreased; right fifth metacarpophalangeal joint is swollen.

In Figure 7-1, a growth-plate fracture that extends into epiphyseal ossification center is in proximal phalanx of right fifth digit.

Physical findings in hands are normal 1 month later.

Diagnosis: Salter 3 fracture of proximal phalanx of right fifth digit.

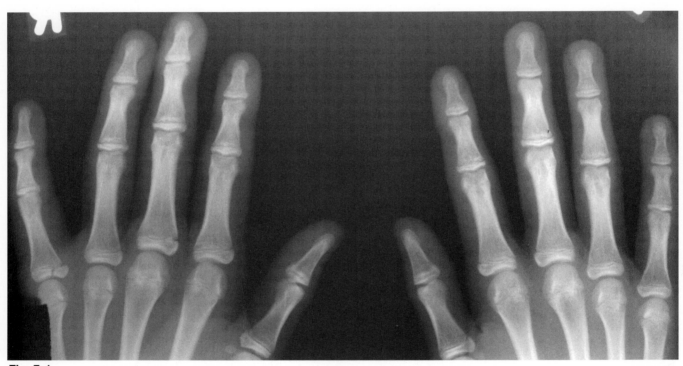

Fig. 7-1

Case 8

A 12-year-old girl has a swollen, painful right ankle after falling over a bush in the park.

Right ankle is tender in front and swollen, especially in front of lateral malleolus. She cannot move right foot because of pain.

Figure 8-1 shows a fracture in lateral part of growth plate of right tibia extending into diaphysis and medial malleolus, and swollen soft tissues around ankle.

She is asymptomatic after cast is removed 2½ months later.

Diagnosis: Salter 4 fracture of right tibia.

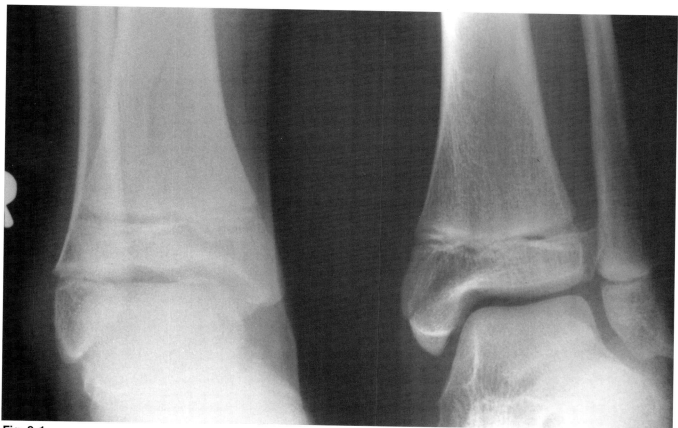

Fig. 8-1

Case 9

An 8-year-old girl has a deformed right wrist.

She was the first born of twins. Mother bruised her head and side in a car crash during second trimester of pregnancy. Birth weight of the girl was 2.9 kg, twin sister 2.7 kg. The girl dragged left leg when she began to crawl at 6 or 7 months. She held objects in her mouth instead of left hand. She uses her right arm for everything, even for breaking a fall when she trips. She holds left arm at her side when she runs and pushes off with toes of left foot. She limps. She has hay fever. Her school work is average.

Mother (39 years old), father (38 years old), sister (11 years old), and twin are well.

Movement of eyes is occasionally disconjugate. Movement at all joints is normal. Right wrist bulges. Sensation to pinprick is diminished in left hand.

In Figure 9-1, carpal ossification of right hand is greater than that of left; right radius is short at wrist; ulna protrudes medially; growth plates of right radius and right first, second, and fifth metacarpal bones are shallow; and metaphyses flare. Similar findings are at right elbow.

Diagnosis: Left hemiparesis with Salter 5 fractures of right arm and hand.

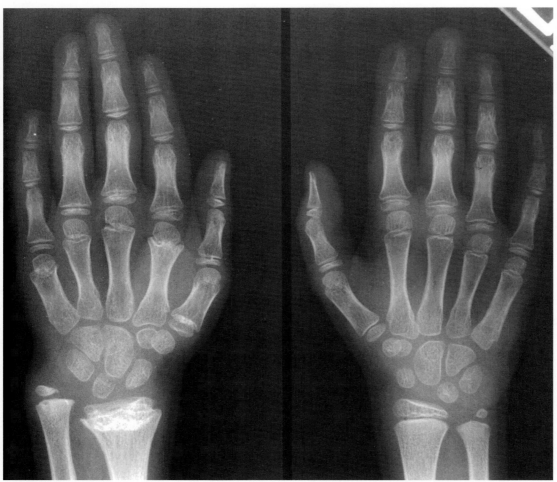

Fig. 9-1

Case 10

A 5-year-old girl hurt left arm when she fell off a cow this evening.

Physical examination shows bent radius.

Figure 10-1A shows a fracture in concave distal part of shaft of left radius. Figure 10-1B shows swollen medial soft tissues along ulnar metaphysis.

Arm is put in a cast for 4 weeks. She hits left elbow on a pipe while wrestling at 12 years. Left elbow hurts 6 days later.

Figure 10-1C shows short ulna with radius bent toward it.

Diagnosis: Greenstick (or, strictly, reverse greenstick) fracture of left radius and Salter 5 fracture of left ulna, at 5 years.

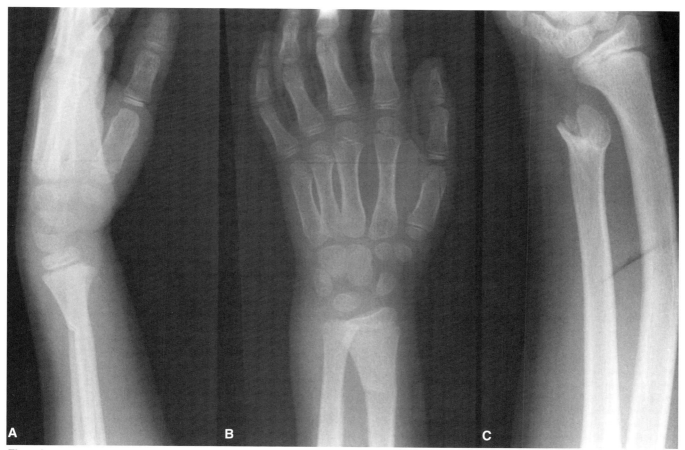

Fig. 10-1

Case 11

A 10-year-old girl has pain in left ankle when she walks.

She fell and hurt left ankle 4 weeks ago. A cast was put on then and taken off yesterday. She turned left foot inward when she tripped today. She fractured left fibula 2¼ years ago.

Pain is just above left lateral malleolus and worsens when she turns foot from side to side. The rest of the physical findings at ankles are normal.

Roentgenographic findings at ankles are normal. In Figure 11-1A, a sclerotic band is in left tibia. Lateral roentgenogram of left ankle 2¼ years ago shows small fracture of metaphysis of left fibula (Figure 11-1B).

Diagnosis: Postarrest growth line in left tibia 2¼ years after fracture of left fibula.

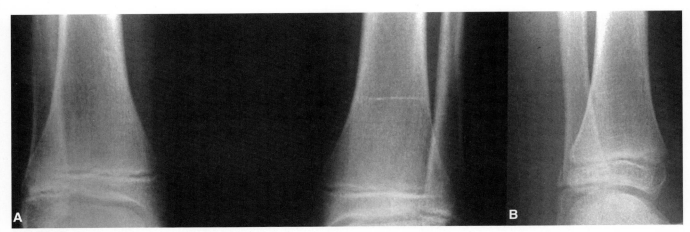

Fig. 11-1

Case 12

A 10-year-old boy's left little finger is shorter than the right. He thinks that its growth slowed when he was kicked by his brother 1 year ago.

Weight is 28 kg, height 132 cm. The rest of the physical findings in hands are normal.

In Figure 12-1, growth plates of all distal phalanges of left hand and middle phalanx of fifth digit are closed; growth plate of middle phalanx of left second digit is partly closed. The rest of the physical findings in hands, including bone age, are normal.

Impression: Injury to growth plates of left hand, probable frostbite.

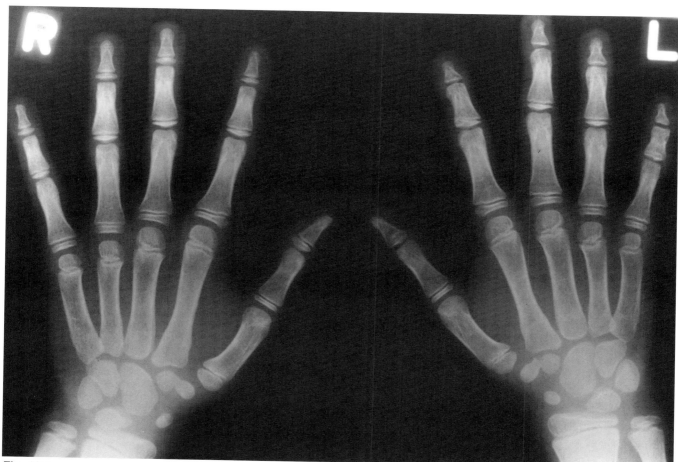

Fig. 12-1

Case 13

A 28-month-old girl cried all night and will not move left arm this morning.

She fell on left shoulder yesterday.

Birth weight was 1.4 kg. She was hospitalized for the first 3 months. She walked at 15 months. She burned left leg on radiator 1 year ago. Chorioretinal scars were found 2 months ago. She took aspirin 1 month ago and was given ipecac.

Temperature is 35.4°C, heart rate 140, respiratory rate 28, blood pressure 106/58 mm Hg, and weight 12.5 kg. Left shoulder is swollen, left humerus high, and left arm held against body. A scar is on left calf. The rest of the physical findings are normal.

Hematocrit is 0.34. White cell count is 16.8×10^9/liter with 0.63 polymorphonuclear cells, 0.01 bands, 0.29 lymphocytes, and 0.07 monocytes. Platelet count is 469×10^9/liter. Urine specific gravity is 1.024, pH 6. Urine has 1+ ketones. Serologic toxoplasmosis IFA titer is 1:8,192.

Figure 13-1 shows fractured left humerus, epiphyseal ossification centers in glenoid fossa, and diaphysis displaced laterally and upward.

Diagnosis: Salter 1 fracture of left humerus (anatomic neck), questionable child abuse; posterior uveitis, congenital toxoplasmosis.

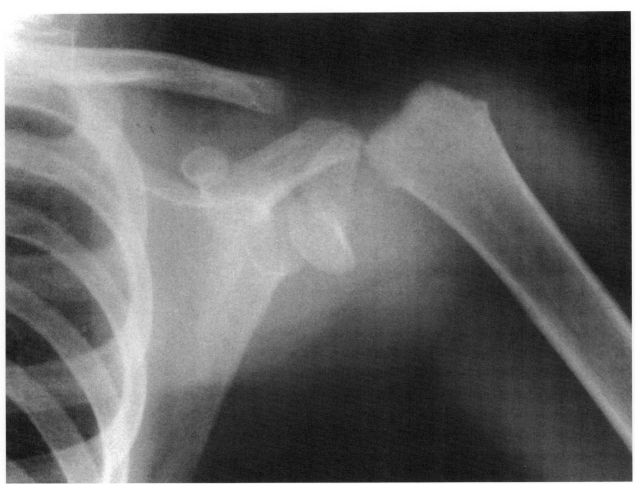

Fig. 13-1

Case 14

A 9-year-old girl, who tripped and fell on left shoulder last night, has pain in left arm.

Left arm is swollen and tender near shoulder. The rest of the physical findings in left arm are normal.

In Figure 14-1, cortex of left humerus is angulated along medial side approximately 1.5 cm below growth plate, a faint linear radiolucency extends obliquely down to lateral side of cortex, and a thin, radiolucent longitudinal strip is slightly lower in shaft.

Diagnosis: Fracture at surgical neck of left humerus, nutrient canal in shaft.

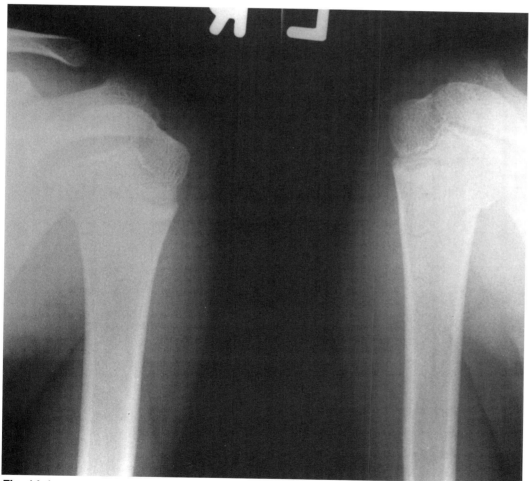

Fig. 14-1

Case 15

A 13-year-old boy cannot completely extend right elbow. Three weeks ago, he hyperextended and twisted right arm while heaving a shot put. He can flex right elbow to 135 degrees but cannot extend it beyond 60-degree flexion. Pronation is painful. Medial epicondyle of right humerus is tender.

In Figure 15-1, cortical new bone is along medial supracondylar crest of right humerus, a gap is between right humerus and medial epicondyle, and right elbow is not as extended as left.

Diagnosis: Avulsion of medial epicondyle of right humerus.

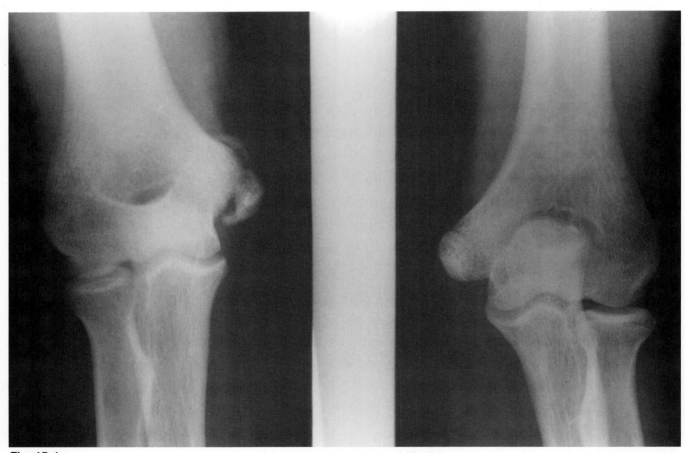

Fig. 15-1

Case 16

A 5-year-old girl has lacked full motion at right elbow since breaking right arm 3 months ago. Standing on a table, she was batting a balloon with a baby-sitter when she fell, right arm flexed behind her back, and hit arm on edge of table. Right arm was put in a cast.

Weight is 21.5 kg, temperature 37.4°C, heart rate 100, respiratory rate 24, and blood pressure 90/60 mm Hg. Right elbow lacks 30–40 degrees of full extension. Right forearm does not supinate beyond neutral. Head of right radius is tender. The rest of the physical findings are normal.

Hematocrit is 0.36. White cell count is 6.9×10^9/liter with 0.39 polymorphonuclear cells, 0.03 bands, 0.42 lymphocytes, 0.08 monocytes, and 0.08 eosinophils. Platelet count is $370 \times$

10^9/liter. Urine specific gravity is 1.015, pH 5. Urine has 0–2 white cells/HPF and mucus.

Figure 16-1 shows a healing fracture in right ulna, ulna convex backward at fracture, and head of right radius displaced forward.

At operation, radial head cannot be placed in elbow joint until torn annular ligament and scar tissue in joint are removed and ulnar osteotomy at level of fracture is performed. Annular ligament is reconstructed with partial tendon graft.

Diagnosis: Fracture of ulna, dislocation of radial head (Monteggia fracture).

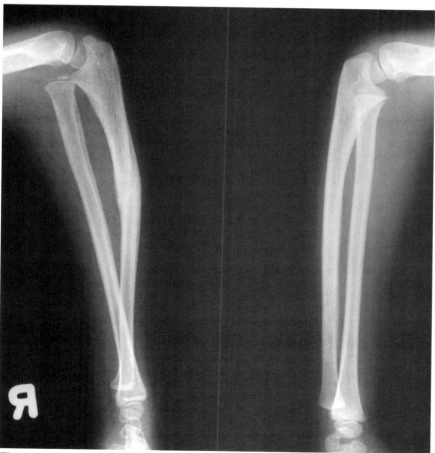

Fig. 16-1

Case 17

A 15-year-old boy has swollen left hand.

Left hand and head hit pavement when he fell from bicycle last night; then he rolled and scraped right arm and hand. Left hand was swollen within 1 hour.

Weight is 83 kg. Swelling of left hand is around thumb and halfway across palm and dorsum. Abduction of left thumb is limited to 5–10 degrees, apposition to 60 degrees. Adduction is full and painless. Left first metacarpal bone is tender. Pushing and pulling left thumb does not hurt. Forehead, hands, and right arm are scraped.

Figure 17-1 shows a longitudinal fracture in proximal part of left first metacarpal bone and lateral displacement of metacarpal bone at joint between metacarpal bone and trapezium.

Diagnosis: Bennett's fracture-subluxation.

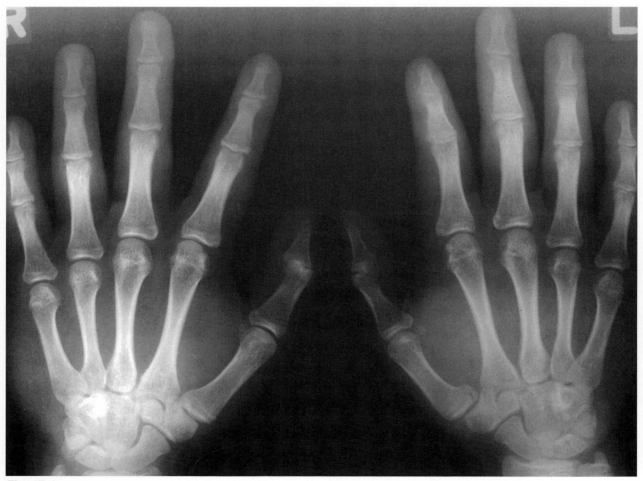

Fig. 17-1

Case 18

An 11-year-old boy, who was pushed by his friend against a desk and then hit his friend in the head, has swollen, painful right hand.

Figure 18-1 shows fractured right fifth metacarpal bone.

Diagnosis: "Slasher's" fracture of right fifth metacarpal bone.

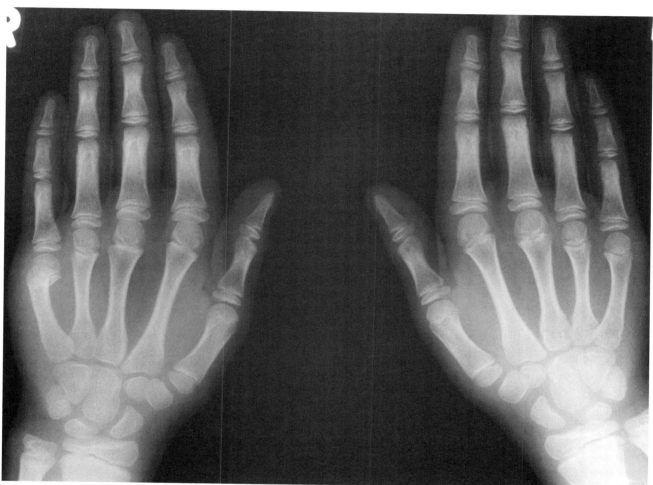

Fig. 18-1

Case 19

A 2½-year-old girl has had a red, tender bump, which sometimes drains, in palm of right hand, since injuring palm 1 month ago.

Weight is 18 kg, height 95 cm. The rest of the physical findings are normal.

Figure 19-1 shows an angular radio-opaque object between capitate and base of second metacarpal bone. Bone age, which is based on standards for left hand, is approximately 4 years in Figure 19-1.

Diagnosis: Glass fragment in palm.

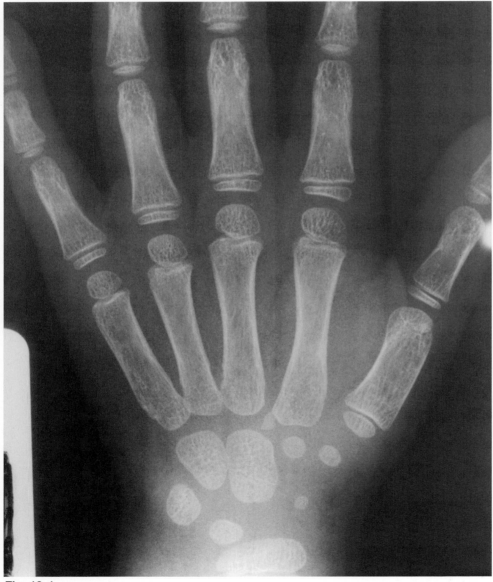

Fig. 19-1

Case 20

A 16-year-old boy has had a swollen, tender left index finger for 2 months.

He scraped the finger 2 months ago when he fell off a motorcycle. He pulled a piece of wood from it 1 week later.

Mother (42 years old) and stepfather are being treated for tuberculosis.

Weight is 52 kg, height 165 cm, temperature 35.8°C, heart rate 60, respiratory rate 24, and blood pressure 100/50 mm Hg. Distal part of left second digit is tender, slightly red, and swollen hard. A nick is on ulnar side of dorsum at base of distal phalanx. Flexion at distal interphalangeal joint is limited to 60 degrees. The rest of the physical findings are normal.

Hematocrit is 0.43. White cell count is 8.9×10^9/liter with 0.48 polymorphonuclear cells, 0.11 bands, 0.35 lymphocytes, 0.03 monocytes, 0.01 eosinophils, and 0.02 basophils. Platelet estimate is adequate. ESR is 4 mm/hr. Urine specific gravity is 1.029, pH 7. Urine has rare squamous epithelial cells/HPF.

Figure 20-1 shows thickened soft tissues of distal half of left second digit, a defect in base of distal phalanx, and thickened cortex of middle phalanx.

At operation, a cavity (0.5- to 0.7-cm diameter) in base of distal phalanx contains pink, granular tissue and a tapered, brown foreign body.

After fixation in formalin, the resected tissue is white, fibrillar, and friable and has a black object (1.5×0.1 mm) on its irregular surface. Microscopic examination shows no yeast or fungal elements. Culture does not grow bacteria or mycobacteria.

Diagnosis: Foreign body with foreign body reaction, chronic inflammation, and fibrosis.

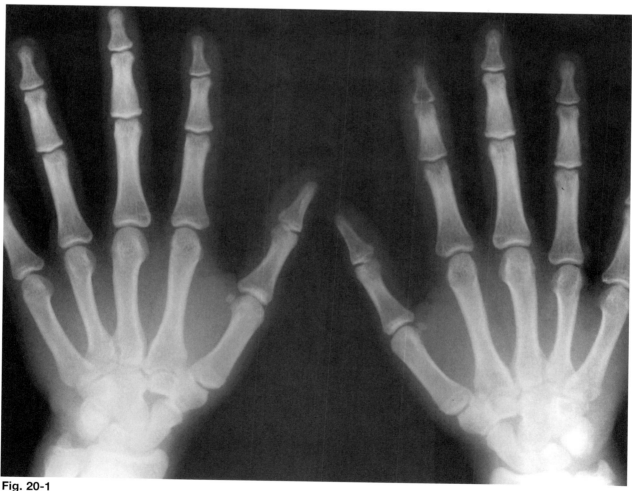

Fig. 20-1

Case 21

A 12-year-old boy has an ache along lateral right thigh. He kicked a ball today, felt a pop in his right hip, and now has a dull ache that is worse with walking.

Temperature is 37.4°C, heart rate 96, respiratory rate 28, and blood pressure 138/76 mm Hg. Right groin is tender, flexion beyond 90 degrees at right hip painful. The rest of the findings at the right hip are normal.

Figure 21-1 shows a fragment of bone lateral to head of right femur and a secondary ossification center in superior margin of both acetabula just below anterior inferior iliac spines.

He has no pain and goes swimming 3 weeks later.

Diagnosis: Avulsion of bone at origin of reflected (posterior) tendon of rectus femoris in groove above brim of acetabulum behind anterior inferior iliac spine; normal ossification of acetabulum.

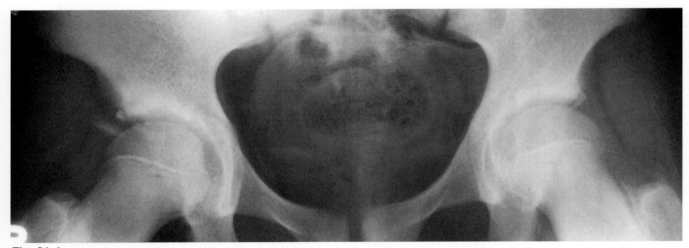

Fig. 21-1

Case 22

A 15-year-old boy, who was just thrown from the back of a pickup truck that rolled over, has pain in abdomen and left hip.

Heart rate is 74, respiratory rate 24, and blood pressure 150/80 mm Hg. Nose is scraped. Blood is in mouth. Left side of abdomen is tender. Pelvis is tender and unstable. Legs resist movement. Left thigh is punctured, left ankle scraped. The rest of the physical findings are normal.

Hematocrit is 0.34. White cell count is 16.6×10^9/liter. Platelet count is 738×10^9/liter. Catheterized specimen of urine is bloody. Eight hours after injury, serum sodium is 142 mmol/liter, potassium 4.9, chloride 104, carbon dioxide 25, urea nitrogen 3.9, calcium 2.62, phosphorus 1.80, cholesterol 2.28, and glucose 8.3. Creatinine is 80 μmol/liter, uric acid 410, total bilirubin 19, and direct bilirubin 3. Total protein is 54 g/liter, albumin 30. Alkaline phosphatase is 156 U/liter, LDH 378, and SGOT 45. Urine specific gravity 18 hours after injury is 1.029, pH 6. Urine has 0.30 g/liter protein, 1–3 white cells/HPF, 0–1 squamous epithelial cell/HPF, and 50–75 red cells/HPF.

Figure 22-1 shows fractured rami of pubic bones and ischia. Sacroiliac joints are widened in plain film (see Figure 22-1) and in CT scan (Figure 22-2), which shows bone fragments at left sacroiliac joint. Iliopsoas muscles are thickened and of varying density in Figure 22-2.

At operation, left posterior sacroiliac ligaments are torn. Pelvis is fixed with two Harrington rods.

Diagnosis: Fractures and dislocations of pelvic ring.

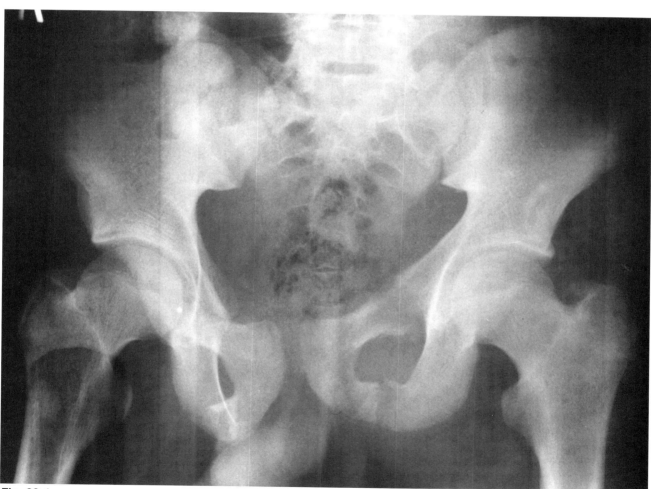

Fig. 22-1

(Continued)

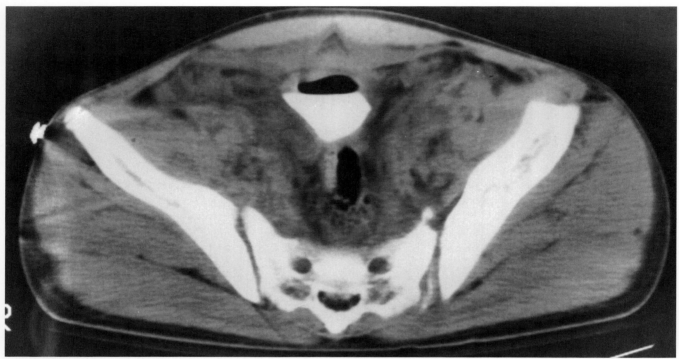

Fig. 22-2

Case 23

A 10-year-old boy riding his bicycle today was hit by a car and thrown 20 ft. Head, chest, and right leg hurt.

Heart rate is 128, respiratory rate 38, and systolic blood pressure 100 mm Hg. Lacerations are on head, inside mouth, on left forearm, and on bent right shank. Bruises and lacerations are on left side of chest. Sternum, left ribs, upper abdomen, and left thigh near hip are tender. Diminished breath sounds and rales are in left side of chest. The rest of the physical findings are normal.

Hematocrit is 0.34. White cell count is 19.4×10^9/liter. Platelet count is 620×10^9/liter. Urine specific gravity is 1.020, pH 5. Urine has 3+ hemoglobin/myoglobin, 5.6 mmol/liter glucose, few nonsquamous epithelial cells/HPF, 100+ red cells/HPF, and 20–30 white cells/HPF. Serum sodium is 140 mmol/liter, potassium 2.7, chloride 110, urea nitrogen 6.1, and glucose 11.0. Creatinine is 80 µmol/liter. CK is 704 U/liter.

Open fracture of right tibia is reduced at operation. Pelvis and right leg are put in plaster cast.

He limps and has pain in left hip and leg after cast is taken off. He lies with left leg externally rotated. Movement of left femur hurts. He can abduct left femur 30 degrees and flex it 110 degrees.

Figure 23-1 shows a transverse fracture in neck of left femur immediately after injury. Figure 23-2 shows subluxated left femur 1 year after injury. Head of left femur is flattened and sclerotic, medial edge is not well defined, and a fragment of bone is along lateral edge in Figure 23-2.

Diagnosis: Fracture of neck of left femur, traumatic avascular necrosis of head of left femur.

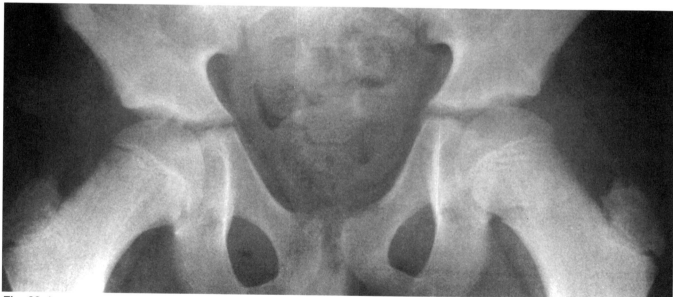

Fig. 23-1

(Continued)

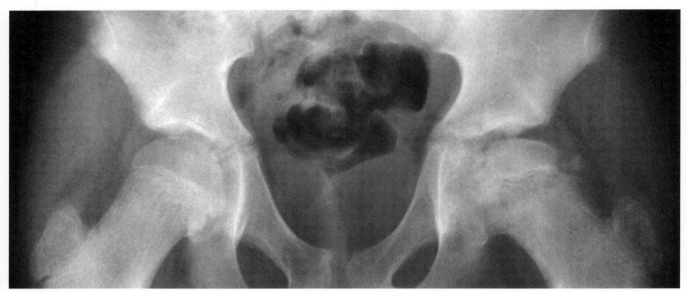

Fig. 23-2

Case 24

A 2½-year-old girl is knock-kneed. She jumped from her crib at 2 years and broke her left tibia.

Temperature is 37.3°C, heart rate 120, respiratory rate 36, blood pressure 84/50 mm Hg, weight 13.7 kg, and height 85 cm. Small bruises are on arms and legs. The rest of the physical findings are normal.

Roentgenogram at 2 years shows an oblique fracture in proximal part of right tibia (Figure 24-1). Roentgenogram at 2½ years shows knock-knees, left more so than right (Figure 24-2). Proximal part of left tibia is thickened along medial aspect in Figure 24-2. Postarrest growth lines are in distal part of left tibia (see Figure 24-2) and fibula.

Diagnosis: Knock-knees, left more than right because of fracture 6 months ago.

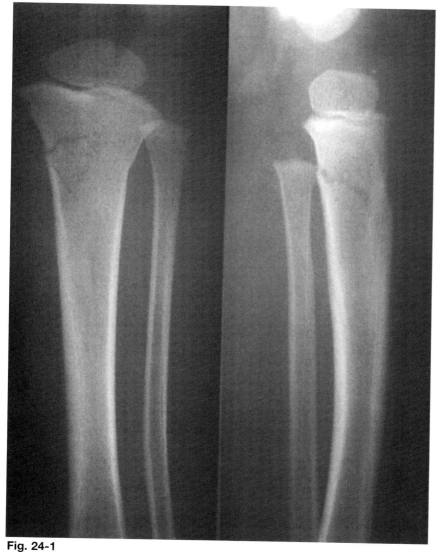

Fig. 24-1

(Continued)

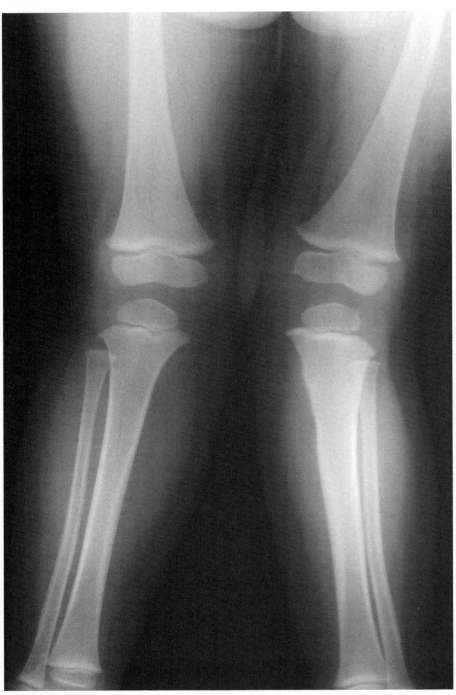

Fig. 24-2

Case 25

A 3¼-year-old girl has right knock-knee.

She broke right leg 10 months ago when she jumped on her bed and bounced to the floor.

Right leg is 0.6 cm longer than left. Medial condyle of right femur is prominent when right knee is fully flexed. Movement is normal. Right knock-knee is 13–15 degrees. Medial malleoli are 8 cm apart when she stands with knees together.

Three years later, father says that he would not know "anything was wrong unless . . . particularly looking at her." An orthopedist sees no asymmetry 5 years after fracture.

Roentgenogram of knees and shanks 10 months after fracture of proximal part of right tibia (Figure 25-1A) shows knock-knee. Roentgenogram 5 years after fracture shows no knock-knee (Figure 25-1B).

Diagnosis: Unilateral knock-knee after proximal tibial fracture and self-correction.

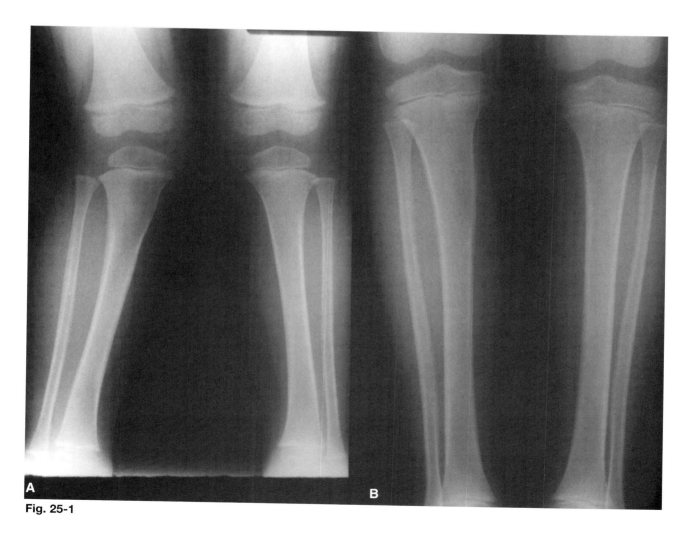

Fig. 25-1

Case 26

An 18-month-old girl stopped walking 4 days ago, began to walk again today, fell, and now will not walk.

Birth weight was 3.5 kg. She began to walk at 15 months. Her right foot was caught under a piece of furniture when she fell backward 4 days ago, and then she would not walk until today, when she fell again.

She cried when her right ankle was handled after she fell 4 days ago. The rest of the physical findings at ankles 4 days ago were normal. All physical findings in legs are now normal.

Roentgenographic examination of legs in lateral view shows slight fuzziness of subcutaneous fat–deep soft-tissue plane in front of lower part of right tibia (Figure 26-1). Examination in frontal view shows a faint oblique fracture going up laterally from medial part of metaphysis (Figure 26-2A). Examination in frontal view 15 days later shows fracture more clearly and thickening of tibial cortex (Figure 26-2B).

Diagnosis: Toddler's fracture.

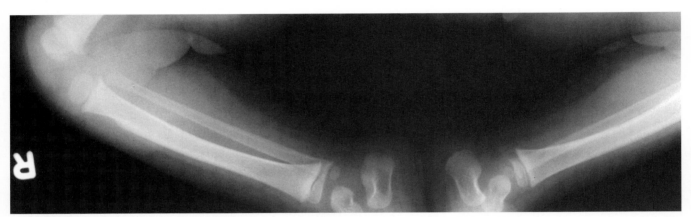

Fig. 26-1

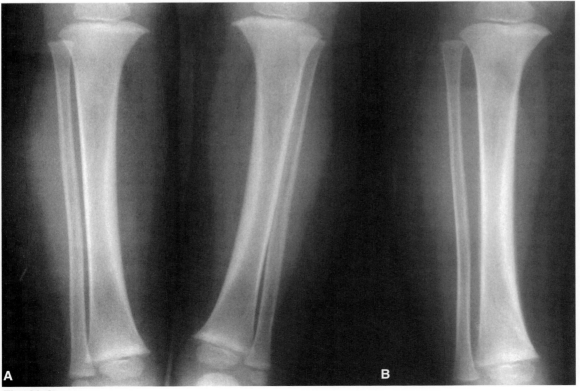

Fig. 26-2

Case 27

A 3-year-old boy limps and holds right arm flexed.

He has been in a foster home for the last 2 years with other children, including teenagers. His foster mother brought him for examination 10 months ago "to see why he doesn't grow" despite eating everything and drinking constantly. He was diagnosed as having panhypopituitarism after insulin-arginine growth hormone–stimulation test. Treatment with levothyroxine, hydrocortisone, and growth hormone was begun. He fell, hit his head, and was knocked out 1 month ago. Abrasions were noticed this week. He has been limping for 4 days.

Weight at 3 years is 11.7 kg, height 87 cm, head circumference 51 cm, temperature 37.2°C, heart rate 104, respiratory rate 18, and blood pressure 104/54 mm Hg. He smells bad. Dirt is caked under fingernails. Right shoulder is red, right upper arm blistered. A red welt crosses front of chest, goes under arms, and up along scapulas. Right heel is tender. The rest of the physical findings are normal.

Hematocrit is 0.30. White cell count is 6.7×10^9/liter with 0.45 polymorphonuclear cells, 0.43 lymphocytes, 0.07 monocytes, 0.03 eosinophils, 0.01 basophils, and 0.01 atypical lymphocytes. Platelet count is 468×10^9/liter. Urine specific gravity is 1.025, pH 8. Urine has trace protein, occasional squamous epithelial cells/HPF, 3–5 white cells/HPF, amorphous and triple phosphates, bacteria, and yeast buds. Serum sodium is 140 mmol/liter, potassium 4.4, chloride 106, carbon dioxide 24, urea nitrogen 4.3, calcium 2.32, phosphorus 1.42, cholesterol 3.18, and glucose 3.7. Creatinine is 40 µmol/liter, uric acid 290, total bilirubin 3, and direct bilirubin 2. Total protein is 59 g/liter, albumin 37. Alkaline phosphatase is 163 U/liter, LDH 192, and SGOT 39.

Figure 27-1 shows a defect in right calcaneus, bent right fibula, and postarrest growth lines in distal femoral and proximal tibial metaphyses. Roentgenographic findings in rest of skeleton are normal.

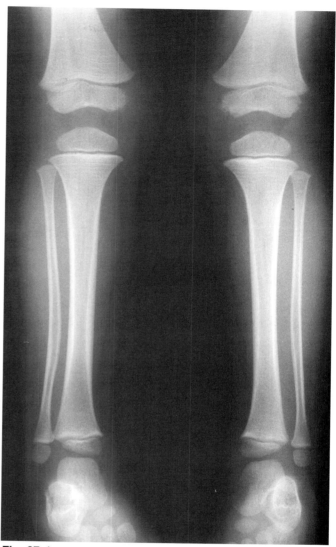

Fig. 27-1

The first day in hospital he "takes food as though he is never fed . . . very fast . . . gulps fluid," according to nurses; vomits; keeps asking for food; and gains 0.8 kg.

Diagnosis: Fracture of right calcaneus; plastic fracture of right fibula; abused, starved child.

Case 28

An 11-year-old boy has had pain in right foot since turning it in yesterday when he tripped while going down stairs in school. Foot swelled and hurt more last night.

Right foot is swollen, bruised, and tender along fifth metatarsal bone, especially proximal part. Any movement there is painful.

Figure 28-1 shows a transverse fracture near proximal end of right fifth metatarsal bone and a scale apophysis below and lateral to proximal part of both fifth metatarsal bones.

Diagnosis: Fracture of right fifth metatarsal bone.

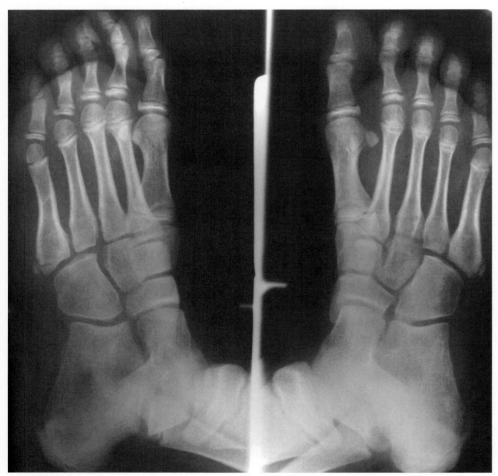

Fig. 28-1

Case 29

A 15-year-old girl has pain in right foot.

She jogs every day and likes to play tennis. Right foot began to hurt 2 weeks ago when she got up from the dinner table.

Right foot is tender and swollen over second and third metatarsal bones. The rest of the findings in feet are normal.

Cortex of right second metatarsal bone is slightly thickened along medial aspect in first examination 2 weeks after foot began to hurt (Figure 29-1A). Cortex is thicker 19 days later (Figure 29-1B), approximately 1 month after it began to hurt.

Diagnosis: Stress fracture of right second metatarsal bone.

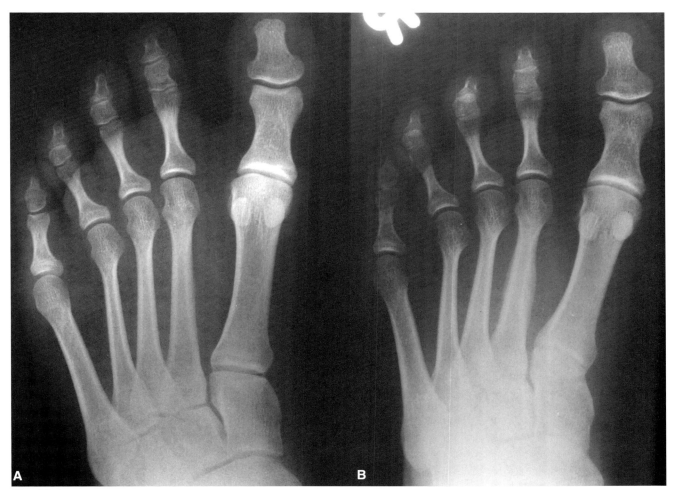

Fig. 29-1

Case 30

A 13-year-old girl has had pain in right foot since running 1.5 miles 1 month ago. Dorsum of foot was slightly swollen for a while.

Distal one-third of right third metatarsal bone is tender. Motion at toes and ankle is normal.

Head of right third metatarsal bone is slightly sclerotic and flattened in Figure 30-1.

Diagnosis: Freiberg infraction of right third metatarsal bone.

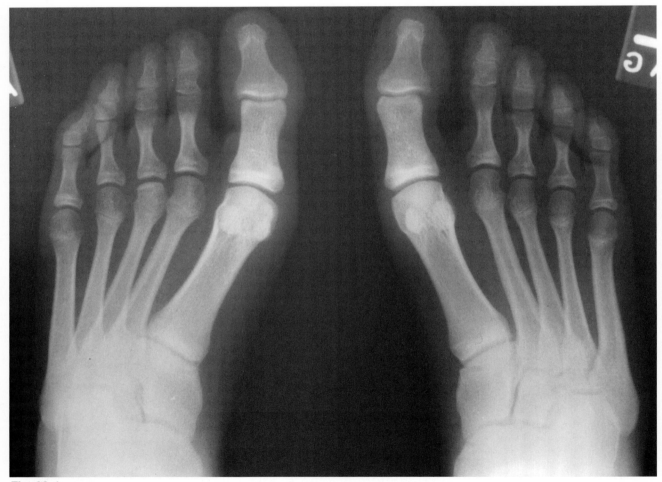

Fig. 30-1

Case 31

A 14-year-old boy has pain in right arm that began suddenly when he threw a basketball this morning.

He wrestles for his high school team and plays basketball and football. He had bronchitis last month and sprained his left ankle a few days ago.

Weight is 70.5 kg, height 177 cm, temperature 36.5°C, heart rate 88, respiratory rate 18, and blood pressure 110/70 mm Hg. Right upper arm is tender and hurts when abducted. Medial left ankle is tender. The rest of the physical findings are normal.

Hematocrit is 0.43. White cell count is 10.4×10^9/liter with 0.62 polymorphonuclear cells, 0.05 bands, 0.21 lymphocytes, 0.08 monocytes, and 0.04 eosinophils. ESR is 2 mm/hr. Serum sodium is 137 mmol/liter, potassium 4.2, chloride 101, carbon dioxide 24, urea nitrogen 6.8, calcium 2.45, phosphorus 1.61, cholesterol 3.41, and glucose 5.5. Creatinine is 70 μmol/liter, uric acid 230, total bilirubin 7, and direct bilirubin 0. Total protein is 69 g/liter, albumin 45. Alkaline phosphatase is 166 U/liter, LDH 202, and SGOT 12.

Figure 31-1 shows an oblique hairline fracture and small defects in right humerus.

At operation, necrotic tissue under periosteum of right humerus is removed with a curet.

Microscopic examination of reddish-tan, granular tissue shows (1) cells with indistinct boundaries, light basophilic cytoplasm, and hyperchromatic pleomorphic nuclei; (2) bizarre mitoses; (3) poorly formed osteoid; (4) giant cells; and (5) osteoclasts.

He is treated with drugs, irradiation, resection of proximal 17.3 cm of right humerus, and replacement with prosthesis. He dies at 18 years.

Diagnosis: Osteosarcoma, pathologic fracture.

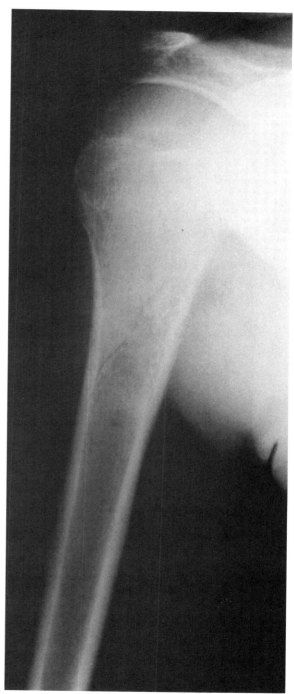

Fig. 31-1

Case 32

A 9-month-old boy has "screaming nightmares," does not want to be touched or held, and seems to be in pain when diapers are changed. Mother says that "he reacted to all foods the first 2 weeks" and that he has trouble swallowing, has breath-holding spells, and is always irritable. He stopped trying to stand at 3 months and stopped trying to crawl at 7 months. His left leg and ankle swell periodically.

Mother (26 years old) is well; father (29 years old) is in "fair health." The boy is their only child. Mother says father is unreasonable. A psychologist says mother is manic, paranoid, and hysterical, and father a born loser.

Weight at 9 months is 8.1 kg, length 72 cm, and head circumference 46 cm. He sits with right leg extended and cries when left leg is moved. Flexion at knees is resisted, movement at other joints full. He is reluctant to put weight on either leg when held up. Bruises are on back. The rest of the physical findings are normal.

Hematocrit is 0.33. White cell count is 8.4×10^9/liter with 0.20 polymorphonuclear cells, 0.08 bands, 0.65 lymphocytes, 0.06 monocytes, and 0.01 eosinophils. Platelet count is 390×10^9/liter. Serum sodium is 141 mmol/liter, potassium 4.9, chloride 105, carbon dioxide 25, urea nitrogen 7.9, calcium 2.45, phosphorus 1.81, and glucose 4.7. Creatinine is 30 μmol/liter, uric acid 190, total bilirubin 3, and direct bilirubin 3. Total protein is 61 g/liter, albumin 40.

Figure 32-1 shows "bucket handles" in frontal view. Figure 32-2, in lateral view, shows "chips" at distal metaphyses of tibias. Figures 32-1 and 32-2 show subperiosteal new bone around left tibia. Distal part of left femur is thickened by old fracture, and deep soft tissues in front of distal left femur are swollen in Figure 32-2.

Diagnosis: Older and newer fractures of tibias, recurrent trauma in battered child.

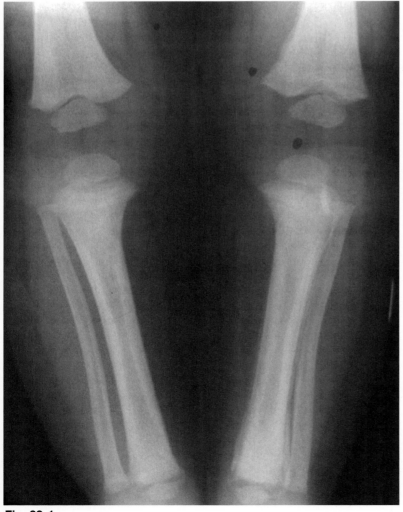

Fig. 32-1

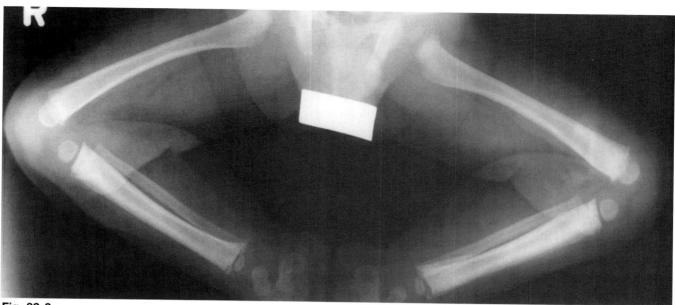

Fig. 32-2

Case 33

A 12-year-old boy has pain in left knee. He hurt left knee while wrestling 1 year ago. He felt a "crack" in left knee while climbing out of a swimming pool 3 months ago, had sudden sharp pain, and then limped for a few days. Left knee hurts sometimes when he runs.

Weight is 57 kg, height 164 cm, temperature 37°C, heart rate 72, respiratory rate 16, and blood pressure 98/54 mm Hg. Crepitus is along lateral aspect of left knee, which hurts when knee is twisted while flexed. Circumference of left thigh, 10 cm above patella, is 1 cm less than that of right thigh. The rest of the physical findings are normal.

Hematocrit is 0.42. White cell count is 4.7×10^9/liter. Platelet count is 260×10^9/liter.

Figure 33-1 shows a small piece of bone in left knee. A postarrest growth line is 12–13 mm below left tibial growth plate in frontal view (Figure 33-1A) and 15 mm below fibular growth plate in lateral view (Figure 33-1B).

At arthroscopy, back part of medial meniscus is stable but slightly irregular. A firm nodule is in contiguous synovium. No free foreign body or other abnormality is present.

He is skateboarding 2 weeks later.

Diagnosis: Osteocartilaginous foreign body *(joint mouse)* in knee.

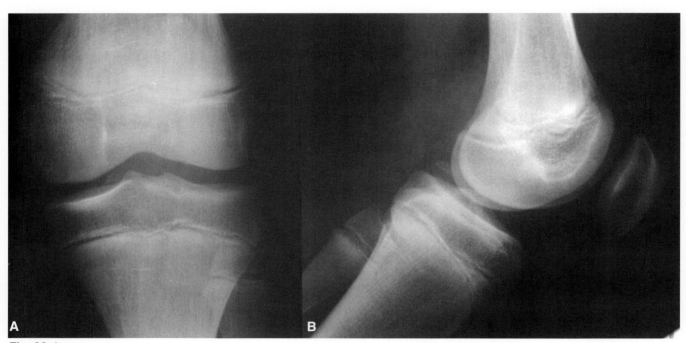

Fig. 33-1

Case 34

A 9-year-old boy has sore ankles in the afternoon, after he has been walking for a while.

Puffy eyelids and tight clothes 2 years ago led to diagnosis of nephrotic syndrome. He hits siblings and breaks things when taking high doses of prednisone, becomes edematous when not. Pain in right ankle and slight limp appeared 4 months ago. Both ankles hurt a little now. Biopsy of tissue from right kidney, obtained 2 months ago with percutaneous needle, shows normal findings in light microscopy, and variable thickness of glomerular basement membrane and slight focal collapse of epithelial cell foot processes in electron microscopy.

Mother (35 years old), father (40 years old), sister (14 years old), and brother (8 years old) are well. Two maternal great-aunts have diabetes mellitus.

Weight at 9 years is 55 kg, height 137 cm, heart rate 80, and blood pressure 96/58 mm Hg. He is fat and has buffalo hump. The rest of the physical findings are normal.

Hematocrit is 0.38. White cell count is 8.1×10^9/liter with 0.83 polymorphonuclear cells, 0.13 lymphocytes, 0.03 mono-cytes, and 0.01 basophils. Platelet count is 370×10^9/liter. Serum sodium is 142 mmol/liter, potassium 4.8, chloride 108, carbon dioxide 24, urea nitrogen 5.4, calcium 2.42, phosphorus 1.42, cholesterol 5.20, and glucose 6.3. Creatinine is 50 μmol/liter, uric acid 270, total bilirubin 9, and direct bilirubin 2. Total protein is 64 g/liter, albumin 44. Alkaline phosphatase is 175 U/liter, LDH 297, and SGOT 21.

Figure 34-1 shows sclerotic and fragmented navicular bones. Roentgenographic findings are similar 1½ years later, when he still has slight ankle soreness.

Biopsy of kidney at 16 years shows normal findings in light microscopy and extensive collapse of foot processes in electron microscopy.

Diagnosis: Minimal-change nephrotic syndrome, steroid-induced necrosis of navicular bones.

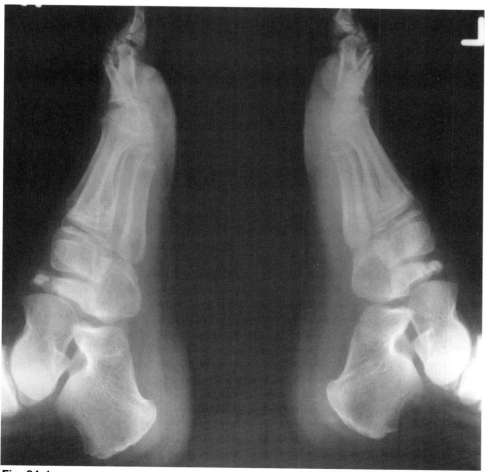

Fig. 34-1

Case 35

A 14-year-old girl cannot move right leg.

She fell 5 months ago and could not move right leg the next morning. Paralysis lasted 2 months, abated for 1 month after she was treated with acupuncture, returned 2 months ago, and persists. She has a feeling like "air and water" in right leg and like a "razor blade cutting my muscles." She uses crutches and rides horseback. She smokes 1 pack of cigarettes per day.

At 7 years, she was hospitalized 1 week for pelvic injury. Menarche was at 10 or 11 years. She ran away from home at 12 years and slept in the woods for 9 days after her mother beat her with a stick for smoking. She had abdominal pain for several months at 13 years. She quit school 1 year ago.

She lives on a farm with her mother and two older brothers and fights with all of them. They keep two horses. She has not seen her father since he left the family 10 years ago.

Temperature at 14 years is 36.6°C, heart rate 100, respiratory rate 20, blood pressure 100/65 mm Hg, weight 58 kg, and height 163 cm. She is "seductive, angry, depressed," according to psychologist, and seems unconcerned about the paralysis. Back of right thigh is discolored brown. Scratches "from shaving" are on right leg. A puncture mark is on right thigh, another on calf. Crepitus extends from right thigh to ankle. She does not feel pinprick in right leg or vibration at medial malleolus. Muscles in right leg contract when she moves left leg. Deep tendon reflexes in right leg are diminished to absent. The rest of the physical findings are normal.

Hematocrit is 0.36. White cell count is 10.0×10^9/liter with 0.37 polymorphonuclear cells, 0.12 bands, 0.24 lymphocytes, 0.04 monocytes, 0.22 eosinophils, and 0.01 basophils. Platelet estimate is adequate. ESR is 7 mm/hr. Urine specific gravity is 1.022, pH 6. Urine has few epithelial cells/HPF, 8–10 white cells/HPF, few bacteria, and amorphous matter. Serum sodium is 139 mmol/liter, potassium 4.4, chloride 106, carbon dioxide 23, urea nitrogen 4.6, calcium 2.42, phosphorus 1.49, and glucose 4.8. Creatinine is 60 µmol/liter, uric acid 230, total bilirubin 7, and direct bilirubin 3. Total protein is 62 g/liter, albumin 40.

Figure 35-1 shows gas in subcutaneous tissues of right leg. Gas is gone 6 days later, while she is still in hospital.

She walks in for electromyography 3 months after her mother has signed her out of hospital. Examination shows no evidence or abnormality of nerves but few or no action potentials on volitional contraction in right leg.

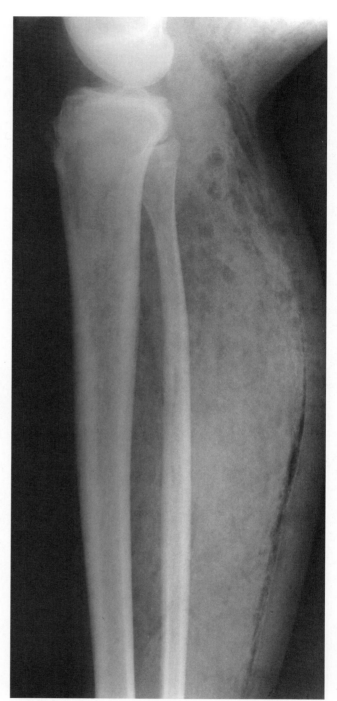

Fig. 35-1

Diagnosis: Personality disorder, conversion reaction, injection of air into right leg.

Case 36

A 6½-year-old girl has pain in left thigh that began while she was swimming 2 weeks ago. She has to be lifted out of bed in the morning because of pain that subsides in several hours.

She can abduct left femur to 25 degrees, right to 60 degrees; she can internally rotate left femur 30 degrees when hip is flexed, right femur 45 degrees; and she can externally rotate left femur 45 degrees, right femur 90 degrees.

Roentgenogram 2 weeks after pain began shows left femur laterally displaced from acetabulum with a subchondral fracture in front half of epiphysis (Figure 36-1).

She swims, rides her bike, and has no pain 5 months later.

In Figure 36-2A, epiphyseal ossification center is flatter and more sclerotic 5 months after first roentgenogram. In Figure 36-2B, 16 months after first roentgenogram, ossification center is partly replaced by nonbony tissue, when sclerotic irregularity is in metaphysis. In Figure 36-3 at 10 years, ossification center is almost completely reossified above a short, broad metaphysis.

Diagnosis: Perthes' disease, left hip.

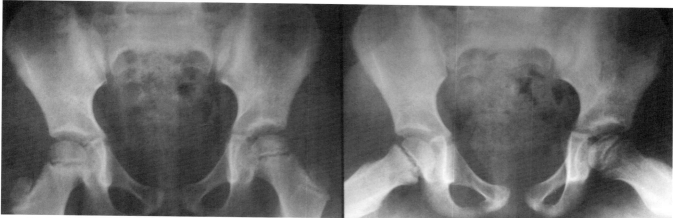

Fig. 36-1

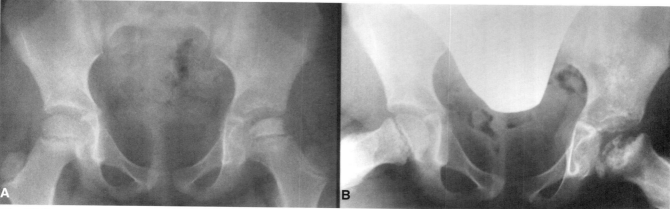

Fig. 36-2

(Continued)

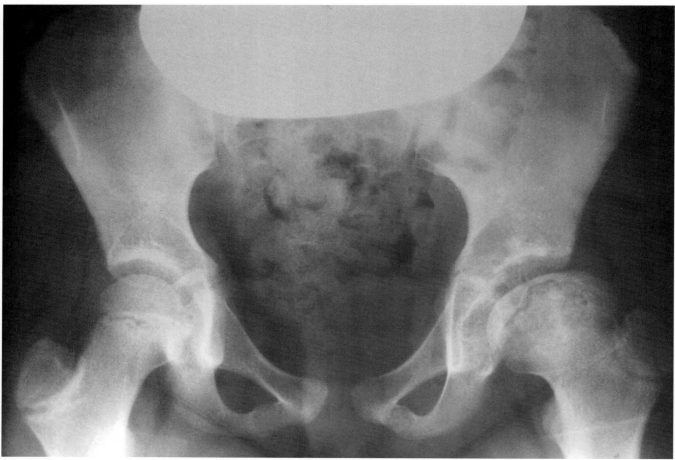

Fig. 36-3

Case 37

A 12-year-old boy has pain near left knee that began when he was playing baseball 5 months ago.

Temperature is 36.7°C, heart rate 80, respiratory rate 20, blood pressure 110/50 mm Hg, height 148 cm, and weight 40 kg. Flexion is limited at left hip, extension at left knee. Muscles behind left femur are weak. The rest of the physical findings are normal.

Hematocrit is 0.35. White cell count is 2.9×10^9/liter. Urine specific gravity is 1.021, pH 8. Urine is normal.

In adduction view, growth plate (physis) of left femur is deeper and more oblique than that of right, and neck of left femur is displaced slightly upward (Figure 37-1A). Abduction view in Figure 37-1B confirms abnormal relation between left femoral epiphysis and metaphysis.

Diagnosis: Slipped left capital femoral epiphysis.

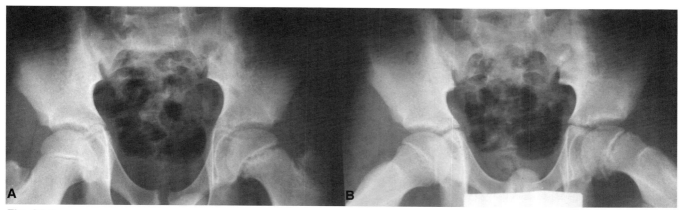

Fig. 37-1

Case 38

A 12½-year-old boy has pain below right patella that began 1 month ago, when he was running at school. The pain is now worse with activity.

Weight is 52 kg, height 159 cm. The findings in physical examination are normal.

Figure 38-1 shows swollen soft tissues and a small shell of bone in front of each tibial tuberosity.

Diagnosis: Early Osgood-Schlatter abnormality, bilateral.

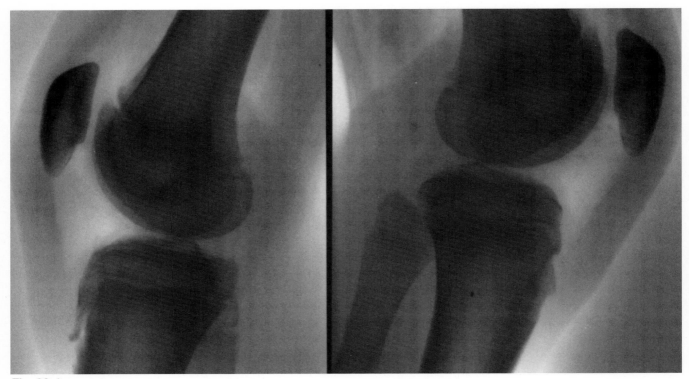

Fig. 38-1

Case 39

A 13-year-old girl has had pain in left knee since twisting it yesterday.

She has had "problems" and pain at left knee that she thinks started 3 years ago when she was riding a bicycle. Six months ago, she fell 12 ft from a loft and bruised her ribs and right knee.

Weight is 75 kg, height 168 cm. Knees are not swollen or bruised. Motion at knees is normal.

Findings at right knee are normal (Figure 39-1A). A bony extension from left tibial tuberosity is in patellar tendon of left knee (Figure 39-1B), and overlying soft tissues are slightly swollen.

Diagnosis: Old Osgood-Schlatter avulsion, left knee.

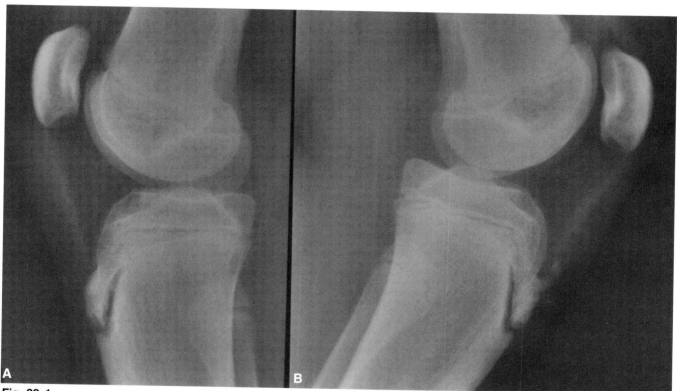

Fig. 39-1

Case 40

A 2-year-old girl will not flex her back. She squats with straight back to pick up toys. She will not sit to eat and is reluctant to sit on the toilet to urinate.

She fell on buttocks 2 weeks ago but got up immediately and seemed all right. Four days later she crawled rather than walked to her room. She was fussy the next night, had a fever of 38.3°C when she woke up, and would not sit.

Birth weight was 3.9 kg. She walked at 9–10 months.

Mother (21 years old), father (22 years old), and sister (6 months old) are well.

Temperature is 36.4°C, heart rate 130, respiratory rate 28, blood pressure 100/72 mm Hg, height 92 cm, and weight 14.1 kg. She will not flex back and resists flexion. The rest of the physical findings are normal.

ESR is 6 mm/hr. Two blood cultures are sterile after 1 week.

She will not flex back or sit with knees extended 3 weeks later and cries whenever anyone tries to move her. She wakes up at night and shakes with pain for approximately 20 minutes. She arches back when she urinates. She has not had fever.

Back is arched. Babinski's sign is in feet. The rest of the physical findings are normal.

Hematocrit is 0.37. White cell count is 6.8×10^9/liter with 0.26 polymorphonuclear cells, 0.02 bands, 0.54 lymphocytes, 0.16 monocytes, and 0.02 eosinophils. Platelet count is 412×10^9/liter. ESR is 7 mm/hr. CSF is clear and colorless with 1×10^6/liter red cell, 1×10^6/liter white cell, 2.8 mmol/liter glucose, and 0.04 g/liter protein. It is sterile after 3 days. Serum sodium is 144 mmol/liter, potassium 4.9, chloride 112, carbon dioxide 24, urea nitrogen 2.9, calcium 2.42, phosphorus 1.68, cholesterol 3.65, and glucose 4.8. Creatinine is 30 µmol/liter, uric acid 280, total bilirubin 5, and direct bilirubin 0. Total protein is 62 g/liter, albumin 35. Alkaline phosphatase is 294 U/liter, LDH 314, and SGOT 73.

Figure 40-1A shows normal findings in lumbar spine 16 days after girl fell on her buttocks and 11 days after she began to arch back. Disc between L3 and L4 is less high and contiguous vertebral end plates less well defined in excretory urogram (Figure 40-1B) 33 days after she began to arch back. Isotope scan at same time shows increased uptake at L3 and L4 (Figure 40-2A). Myelogram in Figure 40-2B shows backward displacement of theca and slight constriction at L3 and L4 in frontal view.

Diagnosis: Discitis.

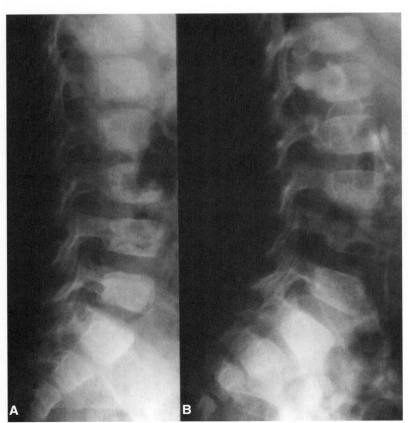

Fig. 40-1

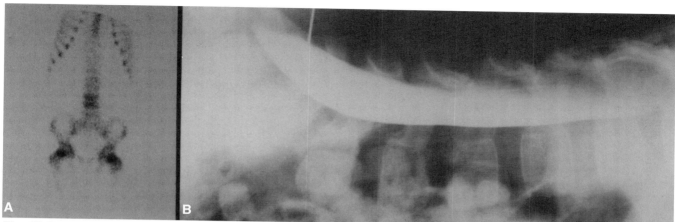

Fig. 40-2

Case 41

A 20-year-old woman has backache.

She thinks she had tuberculosis of the spine when she was an infant. She wriggled across floor to her mother at 21 months. She walked with legs apart and back stiff. She would not bend over to pick up toys. She slept prone with rump up and hands on back. She was better after several days. She stopped horseback riding at 10 years and slept prone because of backache, which was worse at night. She was afebrile. Movement of spine was normal. She had inconstant thoracolumbar spinal tenderness. Right leg was 2 cm longer than left. The rest of the physical findings were normal. Blood cultures were sterile. Skin tests for tuberculosis, histoplasmosis, blastomycosis, and coccidioidomycosis were negative.

Mother had Crohn's disease; father had bone disease in his hand and was treated for tuberculosis. Paternal grandfather died with tuberculosis.

Mobility of spine is normal at 20 years. Lateral bending causes discomfort. Spine is not tender. Movement of legs is normal.

Figure 41-1 shows shallow L2–L3 disc space at 2 years, irregular contiguous vertebral end plates, and, in lower thoracic vertebrae, prominent vascular grooves. L2 and L3 are fused at 10 years (not illustrated) and 20 years (Figure 41-2).

Diagnosis: Discitis.

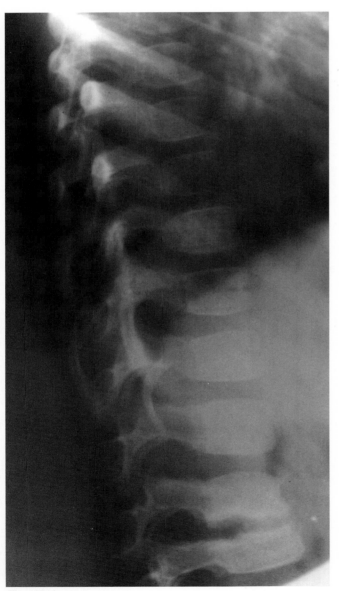

Fig. 41-1

Skeleton and Blood Dyscrasias

Case 1

A 2½-year-old boy has a runny nose and eyes and will not walk. He said, "Feet hurt," and would not wear shoes 2 days ago. Feet were swollen yesterday. Appetite is decreased. He had chickenpox 1 year ago. He has had four or five colds in the last 2 months.

Mother (21 years old), father (22 years old), and two sisters (1 and 4 years old) are well. Maternal great-grandmother and maternal cousin have diabetes mellitus. Members of father's family have heart disease.

Temperature is 37.9°C, heart rate 120, respiratory rate 32, blood pressure 124/60 mm Hg, weight 12.6 kg, and height 59 cm. Dark spots from chickenpox are on body. Nose is runny. Sclerae are slightly yellow. Cervical lymph nodes are prominent. Abdomen is distended and tender. Spleen edge is 2–3 cm below costal margin. Dorsa of feet are red, swollen, tender, and warm. The rest of the physical findings are normal.

Hematocrit is 0.26. White cell count is 18.2×10^9/liter with 0.18 polymorphonuclear cells, 0.07 bands, 0.46 lymphocytes, 0.27 monocytes, 0.01 eosinophils, and 0.01 metamyelocytes.

Platelet count is 700×10^9/liter. Blood smear shows sickle cells. Serum sodium is 136 mmol/liter, potassium 4.9, chloride 104, carbon dioxide 20, urea nitrogen 2.1, calcium 2.50, phosphorus 1.55, cholesterol 4.53, and glucose 8.9. Creatinine is 40 µmol/liter, uric acid 240, total bilirubin 34, and direct bilirubin 3. Total protein is 73 g/liter, albumin 44. Alkaline phosphatase is 206 U/liter, LDH 1,160, SGOT 76, and CK 56. Hemoglobin electrophoresis shows 0.08 HbA_2, 0.72 HbS, and 0.20 HbF.

He will not stand or walk, and feet are swollen but less tender 4 days after first refusal to walk. He walks and rides a tricycle 2 days later. Feet are still puffy.

Figure 1-1A shows normal findings 2 days after refusal to walk. Figure 1-1B shows thickened cortex of first metatarsals 3 weeks later, when physical findings are normal.

Diagnosis: Hand-foot syndrome in boy with sickle cell anemia.

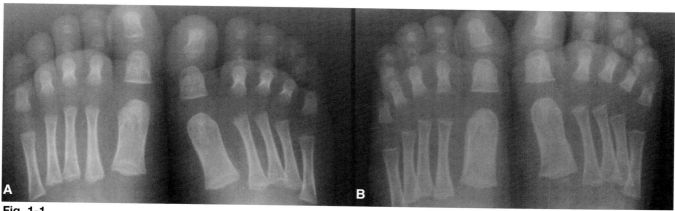

Fig. 1-1

Case 2

A 10-year-old boy has backache. He landed on his back on the hood of a slow-moving car that hit him this evening.

Temperature is 37.5°C, heart rate 120, respiratory rate 20, blood pressure 110/70 mm Hg, weight 25 kg, and height 131 cm. Arms are bruised. Midthoracic spine and right elbow are painful and tender. A systolic heart murmur is present. The rest of the physical findings are normal.

Hematocrit is 0.23. White cell count is 9.3×10^9/liter with 0.53 polymorphonuclear cells, 0.38 bands, 0.08 lymphocytes, and 0.01 monocytes. Blood smear shows sickle cells and 20 nucleated red blood cells per 100 white cells. Urine specific gravity is 1.020, pH 7. Urine is normal. Serum sodium is 140 mmol/liter, potassium 4.3, chloride 110, carbon dioxide 18, urea nitrogen 3.0, calcium 2.25, phosphorus 1.49, cholesterol 3.36, and glucose 4.9. Creatinine is 50 µmol/liter, uric acid 260, total bilirubin 48, and direct bilirubin 9. Total protein is 65 g/liter, albumin 40. Alkaline phosphatase is 217 U/liter, LDH 1,260, and SGOT 59.

Figure 2-1 shows steplike insets in thoracic and lumbar vertebral bodies.

Diagnosis: Vertebral changes (questionable infarction) in boy with sickle cell anemia.

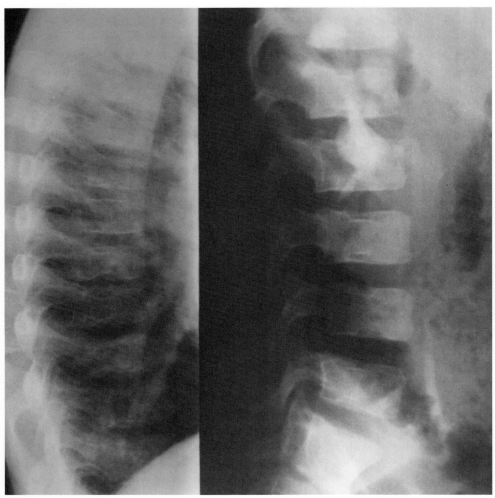

Fig. 2-1

Case 3

A 6-year-old boy limps with left knee flexed.

Birth weight was 3.6 kg. Right forearm was bruised at 5 months; shins were bruised at 9 months. He walked at 12 months. He hit his mouth in a fall at 3 years and bled so much that he was given a blood transfusion. He fell and hit his mouth 10 months ago and bled until he was given herbs by a Chinese apothecary. Thigh was swollen after diphtheria-pertussis-tetanus vaccination 5 months ago. Painful swelling of knees comes and goes every 6 months or so. Occasionally, nose bleeds for 1–2 days.

Parents, two brothers (9 and 10 years old), and two sisters (4 and 12 years old) are well.

Weight at 6 years is 15 kg, height 102 cm, temperature 37.2°C, heart rate 130, respiratory rate 24, and blood pressure 100/54 mm Hg. Left knee is swollen and has limited motion. The rest of the physical findings are normal.

Hematocrit is 0.37. White cell count is 9.8×10^9/liter with 0.40 polymorphonuclear cells, 0.08 bands, 0.45 lymphocytes, 0.05 monocytes, and 0.02 eosinophils. Platelet count is 379×10^9/liter. Urine specific gravity is 1.016, pH 5. Urine is normal. PT is 10 seconds (control: 9.8), PTT 66.4 (normal: <40). Plasma factor VIII is 0.04 (normal: 0.5–2.0).

Joints, especially left knee and elbow, often swell and ache despite treatment. Motion at left elbow is limited at 7, 13, and 23 years. Left leg is 2.5 cm longer than right at 8 and 13 years. Left quadriceps is smaller than right, synovium in left knee is thickened, and left knee cannot be fully extended at 13 years. Left knee has full range of motion at 23 years. He tests positive for HIV at 23 years. CD4 count is 0.5×10^9/liter.

Figure 3-1A shows excavated olecranon and/or coronoid fossa of left humerus at 9 years. Left knee lacks joint cartilage and patellar surface of left femur is excavated at 13 years (Figure 3-1B).

Diagnosis: Hemophilia A.

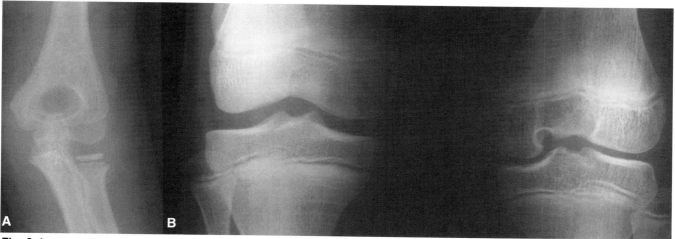

Fig. 3-1

Case 4

A 24-year-old man has pain and morning stiffness in left elbow and ankle and also pain in ankles when he stands or walks for a while.

He was not circumcised because a half brother of his mother died at 10 years with intracranial bleeding and a maternal male cousin has hemophilia. He bled from tongue when he was an infant. He bled into left hip at 4 years, into ankles repeatedly at 6 years, and later into elbows, sometimes when he threw a ball or just straightened his arm quickly. At 16 years, he had dark streaks in skin on back of hands over veins used for infusion of cryoprecipitate. Biopsy showed coarse black granules in dermis that did not polarize light or stain for iron or melanin. Streaks disappeared. At 17 years, small cysts were along medial sides of elbows.

Weight at 21 years was 71.3 kg, height 175 cm, and blood pressure 132/80 mm Hg.

At 24 years, he swims and lifts weights. He infuses cryoprecipitate every 1–2 weeks. Small lymph nodes are in neck and groin. Elbows are flexed, right more than left. Internal rotation is limited at left hip. Skin along outside at ankles is thick. Left leg is 2 cm shorter than right. The rest of the physical findings are normal.

Hematocrit is 0.42. White cell count is 5.3×10^9/liter with 0.47 polymorphonuclear cells, 0.03 bands, 0.45 lymphocytes, and 0.05 monocytes. Platelet count is 242×10^9/liter. Urine specific gravity is 1.019, pH 6. Urine has occasional squamous epithelial cells/HPF and 0–2 white cells/HPF. Serum sodium is 142 mmol/liter, potassium 4.8, chloride 104, carbon dioxide 26, urea nitrogen 5.0, calcium 2.32, phosphorus 1.03, cholesterol 3.05, and glucose 3.0. Creatinine is 70 μmol/liter, uric acid 200, total bilirubin 9, and direct bilirubin 0. Total protein is 66 g/liter, albumin 40. Alkaline phosphatase is 60 U/liter, LDH 197, and SGOT 15. Factor VIII <0.01 (normal: 0.5–2.0). Serum has HBsAb. Nine months later, blood has 0.3×10^9/liter CD4 + lymphocytes and 0.5×10^9/liter CD8+ lymphocytes. Serum has HIV antibody.

Left femur is displaced outward and upward at 14 years (Figure 4-1A). Left epiphyseal ossification center is focally sclerotic and smaller than right (see Figure 4-1A). Figure 4-1B shows uneven and expanded left femoral epiphysis and shortened left femoral neck at 24 years.

Diagnosis: Hemophiliac arthropathy at left hip.

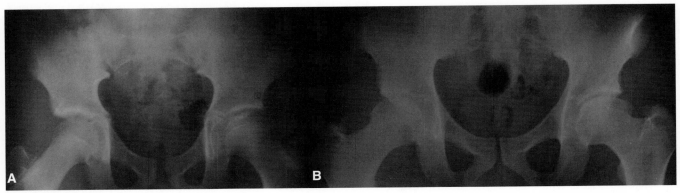

Fig. 4-1

Case 5

A 6½-year-old boy with hemophilia has a hard swelling of left hand 1 month after hand was kicked by a horse. One thousand units of factor VIII have been infused IV every day for the last 2 weeks.

Mother, father, and sister (8 years old) are well. A maternal half uncle has hemophilia.

Swelling is not tender. Sensitivity in left hand is normal, movement slightly diminished.

Hematocrit is 0.36. White cell count is 5.9×10^9/liter with 0.35 polymorphonuclear cells, 0.01 bands, 0.47 lymphocytes, 0.14 monocytes, 0.01 eosinophils, and 0.02 atypical lymphocytes. Urine specific gravity is 1.022, pH 6. Urine has occasional white cells/HPF. Serum sodium is 139 mmol/liter, potassium 3.8, chloride 104, carbon dioxide 24, urea nitrogen 4.3, calcium 2.52, phosphorus 1.39, cholesterol 3.28, and glucose 6.1. Creatinine is 40 μmol/liter, uric acid 170, total bilirubin 7, and direct bilirubin 0. Total protein is 69 g/liter, albumin 42. Alkaline phosphatase is 242 U/liter, LDH 269, and SGOT 37.

Roentgenogram after horse kick 1 month ago shows fractured left third metacarpal bone (Figure 5-1A). The bone is divided, distorted, and swollen now (Figure 5-1B).

Daily infusions of factor VIII are continued for 2 more weeks and then tapered. A small lump is on back of left hand 1 year later. The rest of the physical findings are normal.

Diagnosis: Pseudotumor in boy with hemophilia.

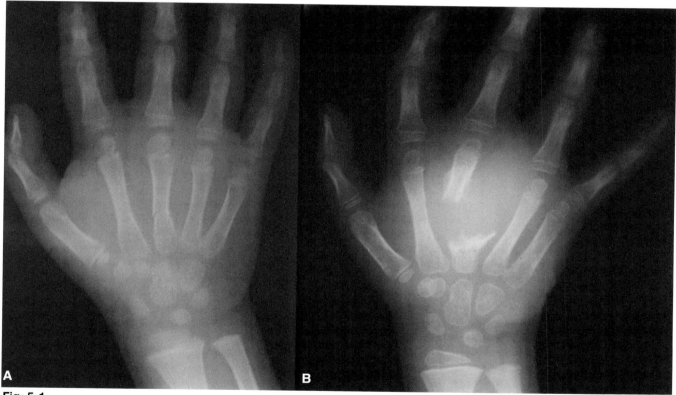

Fig. 5-1

Joints

Case 1

A newborn girl has a hip click.

Mother (22 years old), father (30 years old), and sister (2 years old) are well.

Pregnancy was normal. Birth weight is 3.0 kg, length 46 cm, and head circumference 32 cm. Elbows are flexed and can be extended to 140 degrees. Fingers are flexed with thumbs inside. Femurs abduct to 60 degrees, adduct to 20 degrees, and click at hips when pulled down and abducted more. Head of talus is medially palpable in both feet and can be pushed into place. The rest of the physical findings are normal.

Figure 1-1 shows contrast medium in right hip and soft tissue outside hip. In fluoroscopic image on reader's right, head of femur, surrounded by contrast medium, is lateral to acetabular labrum until it "clicks" into acetabulum when femur is externally rotated and more abducted in image on left (see Figure 1-1). Roentgenogram in Figure 1-2 is of a 5-month-old girl who has bilateral hip click because of gas entering joint when femurs are abducted.

Diagnosis: Ortolani click, questionable dislocatable hip; rocker-bottom feet. Antivacuum phenomenon in 5-month-old girl.

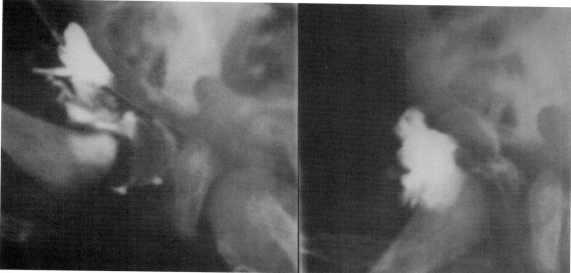

Fig. 1-1

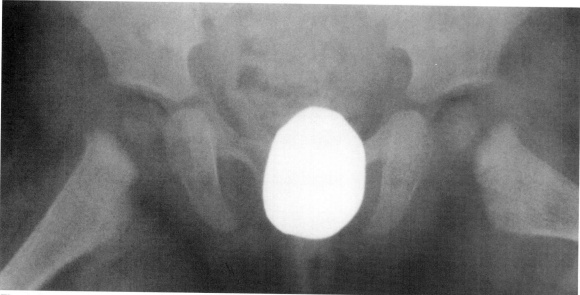

Fig. 1-2

Case 2

A 1½-year-old boy, who began to walk 4 months ago, limps.

Mother noticed when he was born that left leg was shorter than right; at 6 months, it was also thinner. He had right inguinal hernia repair at 4 months and was hospitalized with gastroenteritis at 9 months. He is her only child.

Temperature is 36°C, heart rate 128, respiratory rate 28, systolic blood pressure 96 mm Hg, weight 10.9 kg, and height 80 cm. Abduction at left hip is limited. Spine is concave left when he stands (Galeazzi's sign). The rest of the physical findings are normal.

Hematocrit is 0.38. White cell count is 13.5×10^9/liter. Platelet count is 379×10^9/liter. Serum sodium is 142 mmol/liter, potassium 5.0, and chloride 114.

Plain film in Figure 2-1 shows lateral and upward displacement of left femur, delayed ossification of left femoral epiphysis, and higher slope of left bony acetabulum than that of right (Putti triad). Left arthrogram shows fibrocartilaginous labrum of left acetabulum between bony acetabulum and contrast medium around cartilaginous epiphysis of left femur when femur is abducted and internally rotated (Figure 2-2A) and when it is abducted and externally rotated (Figure 2-2B).

At operation, "redundant limbus," according to orthopedic surgeon, keeps left femur out of acetabulum.

Examination of resected labrum shows adipose tissue, fibrocartilage, and focal myxoid degeneration. Examination of resected ligamentum teres shows dense fibrous tissue and myxoid degeneration.

Diagnosis: Dislocation at left hip.

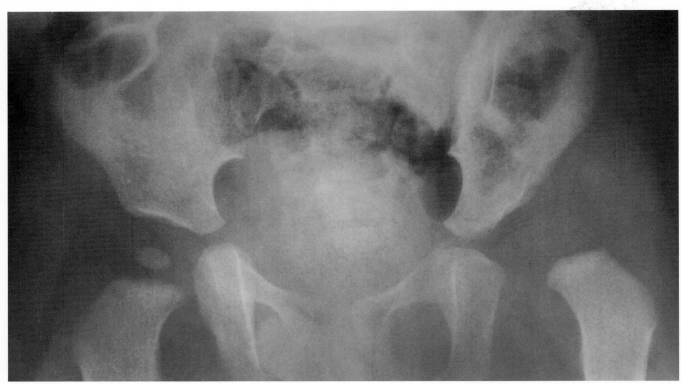

Fig. 2-1

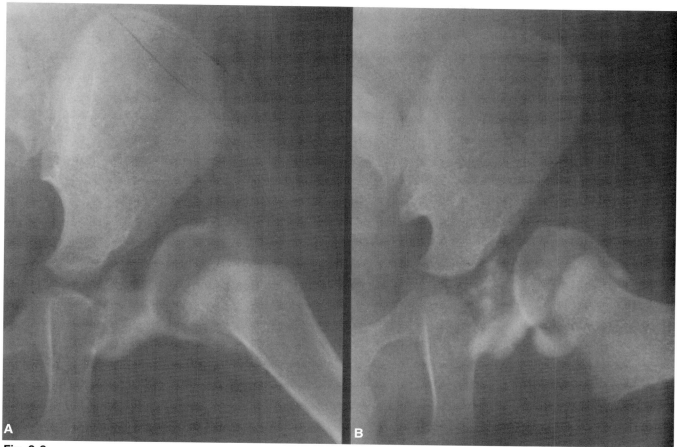

Fig. 2-2

Case 3

A 4-year-old girl has cerebral palsy.

Pregnancy was marred by cervical cerclage, cesarean section 12 days after spontaneous rupture of membranes, and hysterectomy for placenta accreta.

Mother (33 years old) and father (29 years old) are well. The girl is their only child.

Birth weight was 1.5 kg, length 42 cm, head circumference 28 cm, and Apgar score 7/8 at 1 and 5 minutes. She had respiratory distress and was intubated at 30 minutes, extubated at 3 days. She had episodic apnea and bradycardia until 4½ weeks. At 5 weeks, a ridge and arborized vessels were in temporal part of both retinas with adjacent small hemorrhage in right eye. At 5 months, she had strabismus and muscle hypertonia. At 1 year, she could transfer objects awkwardly from hand to hand but still had asymmetric tonic neck and Moro's reflexes. Legs extended and toes pointed down when she was picked up. At 15 months, she was operated on for strabismus. At 16 months, auditory responses were normal. At 3 years, adductor transfer from pubis to ischium for tight hips was performed.

Weight at 4 years is 17 kg, length 104 cm, head circumference 51 cm, temperature 36.4°C, heart rate 112, respiratory rate 24, and blood pressure 110/70 mm Hg. She is alert and speaks in sentences. She has alternating exotropia. Trunk is weak. She sits with back arched. She can "commando crawl." Legs are spastic. A scar is on inside of each thigh. The rest of the physical findings are normal.

CT scan shows blood in lateral ventricles at 4 days. Figure 3-1, at 4 years, shows subluxated left femur and greater-than-normal neck-shaft angle of femurs.

Diagnosis: Spastic diplegia.

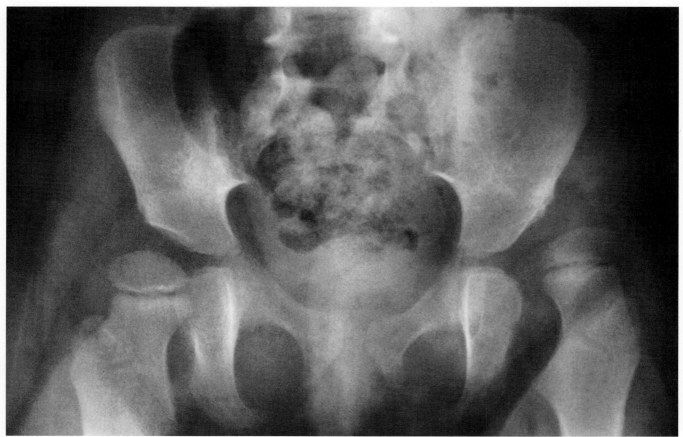

Fig. 3-1

Case 4

A newborn girl's right shank is turned out.

Mother (20 years old) and father (24 years old) are well. The girl is their only child.

Birth weight is 2.3 kg, Apgar score 7/10 at 1 and 5 minutes. Right shank is turned out at knee. Right patella is palpable outside lateral condyle of femur. Right foot is flat. Hip adductors are tight. The rest of the physical findings are normal.

Figure 4-1 shows (1) pelvis, femurs, and left shank in frontal projection, while right shank is in lateral projection; (2) flat right foot; and (3) plantar flexed right talus.

She has pyloromyotomy for pyloric stenosis at 5 weeks. At operation at 3 months, right patella is lateral to lateral condyle of right femur. Right iliotibial tract is connected to lateral part of patella. Patella cannot be placed in groove between femoral condyles until adhesions between quadriceps tendon, lateral patellar retinaculum, and contiguous soft tissues are broken. She has adductor tenotomy for dislocation at left hip at 10 months.

Diagnosis: Congenital dislocation of right patella.

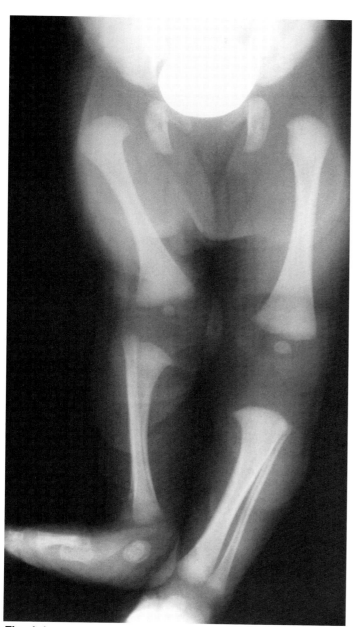

Fig. 4-1

Case 5

An 8½-year-old girl has right bowleg.

Mother had high blood pressure during pregnancy. Birth weight was 4 kg, length 49 cm. Tonsils and adenoids were removed at 2 years.

Mother and father (both 37 years old), brother (14 years old), and sister (10 years old) are well.

Right leg is bowed 5–10 degrees at knee. The rest of the physical findings are normal.

Figure 5-1A shows bowed legs at 3 years. Right tibial epiphysis and metaphysis slope medially downward at 8½ years (Figure 5-1B).

Diagnosis: Blount's disease in right leg, normal left bowleg at 3 years.

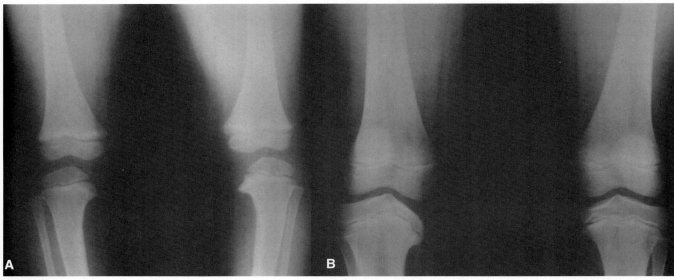

Fig. 5-1

Case 6

A 5-year-old girl walks pigeon-toed.

Pregnancy was normal, birth weight 3.4 kg. Feet were clubbed at birth. Lengthening of calcaneal tendons was performed at 15 months. She then wore shoes that flared outward and slept in Denis Browne splint.

Mother (29 years old), father (33 years old), and sister (3 years old) are well.

Weight at 5 years is 18.8 kg, height 102 cm. Forefeet are adducted. Right forefoot can be passively abducted to neutral, left forefoot almost to neutral. Hindfeet are inverted. Heels are equinus. The rest of the physical findings are normal.

Head of talus in Figure 6-1A points to second or third metatarsal bone and not, as is normal, to first. Small navicular bone is high on head of talus in Figure 6-1B. Calcaneus is almost horizontal in Figure 6-1B.

Diagnosis: Clubfeet.

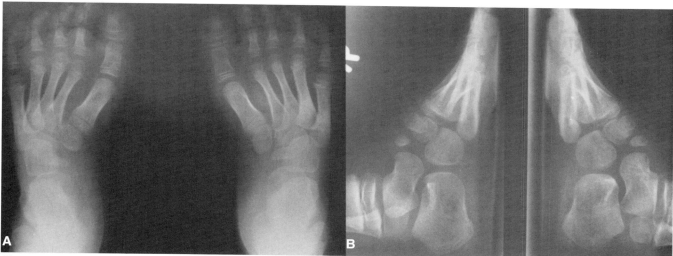

Fig. 6-1

Case 7

A newborn boy has a bump on medial side of right foot.

Pregnancy of mother (16 years old) was normal. Birth weight is 3.3 kg, length 50 cm, head circumference 33 cm, Apgar score 8/9 at 1 and 5 minutes, temperature 35.7°C, heart rate 150, respiratory rate 56, and hematocrit 0.56. Right foot is dorsiflexed and flexible. Head of talus makes a bump on medial side of arch of right foot. The rest of the physical findings are normal.

The foot is manipulated and casts are changed periodically. Right foot can be plantar flexed to 45 degrees at 6 months.

Figure 7-1 shows head of right talus pointing medially and downward and normal left foot at 6 months.

At operation at 8 months, talus is plantar flexed and immobile until soft-tissue release, when it can be moved 15 degrees, and navicular can be moved into place at head of talus.

Diagnosis: Plantar-flexed right talus (rocker-bottom foot).

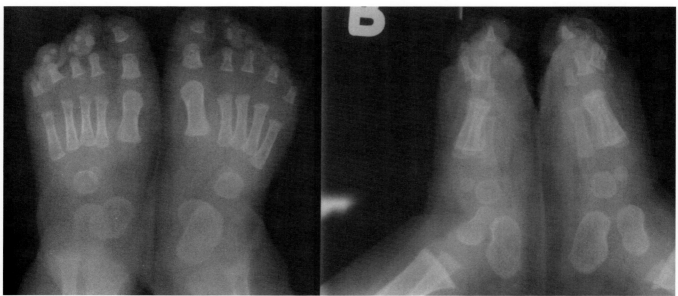

Fig. 7-1

Case 8

A 12-year-old boy cannot supinate forearms.

Birth weight was 3.1 kg. Right forefoot was adducted. Fingers and toes were long at 2 years. Chest and limbs ached during play at 4 years. He wore glasses. Teeth were carious. He was pigeon-breasted. He could not supinate forearms and had a lump behind elbows at 5 years.

Mother was 183 cm tall and weighed 97 kg. She had subluxated lenses, decayed teeth, scoliosis, pectus carinatum, systolic heart murmur, diastolic heart murmur, and long fingers and toes. She fell over dead at 32 years while talking with husband in kitchen. Maternal great-grandmother; maternal grandfather; and two maternal aunts died suddenly, one during her second pregnancy.

Height at 12 years is 170 cm, weight 55 kg, heart rate 70, and blood pressure 118/70 mm Hg. Lenses are subluxated upward. Teeth are capped. A systolic heart murmur is present. Bony spurs are behind elbows. Striae are on thighs. The rest of the physical findings are normal.

Figure 8-1A shows normal bone age in left hand. Metacarpal index (the average of length in millimeters of metacarpals two through five divided by width at midpoint, which should be determined in right hand) is more than upper normal limit of 8 (see Figure 8-1A). Figure 8-1B shows left radial head displaced backward. Right radial head shows similar displacement.

At 14 years, radial heads are excised because lumps bother him. At 24 years, he tires after ascending one flight of stairs. Height is 199 cm, weight 117 kg, heart rate 96, and blood pressure 150/84 mm Hg. Vision is blurred in left eye, 20/40 with glasses in right eye. He has pectus carinatum, slight scoliosis, loose joints, midsystolic click, and striae on back and abdomen. Ultrasound examination shows diameter of aorta 3–4 cm above root to be 4 cm.

Diagnosis: Marfan syndrome.

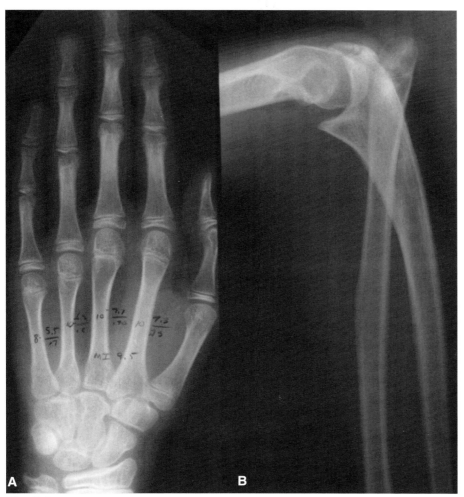

Fig. 8-1

Case 9

A 13-year-old girl has a stiff neck.

Neck started to ache 3 years ago. Hips and legs have ached for 2 years. Head was tilted left at age 11, rotation to right limited. She splinted neck with hands. Arms had "give-way" weakness. Extended fingers twitched. She walked slowly with toes in and could not hop. Deep tendon reflexes were absent.

Mother (40 years old), father (42 years old), and five siblings are well.

Weight at 13 years is 47 kg, height 155 cm. Grip waxes and wanes. Lumbar spine is straightened. Flexion and abduction at right hip are limited. She steps heavily when walking.

Hematocrit is 0.36. White cell count is 7.5×10^9/liter with 0.58 polymorphonuclear cells, 0.02 bands, 0.33 lymphocytes, 0.02 monocytes, and 0.05 eosinophils. Serum sodium is 144 mmol/liter, potassium 4.5, chloride 104, carbon dioxide 28, urea nitrogen 4.3, calcium 2.59, phosphorus 1.52, cholesterol 4.50, triglycerides 1.57, and glucose 4.3. Creatinine is 80 µmol/liter, uric acid 300, total bilirubin 5, and direct bilirubin 0. Total protein is 73 g/liter, albumin 45. Alkaline phosphatase is 148 U/liter, LDH 167, SGOT 19, and CK 60. Serum is neg-ative for antinuclear antibodies at 11 years and for rheumatoid factor at 11 and 13 years. At 13 years, serum complement com-ponent 3 is 0.9 g/liter (normal: 0.7–1.6) at 13 years. Blood tests positive for human leukocyte antigen–B27.

She becomes more active. She has occasional lower back-ache. Weight at 14 years is 51 kg, height 157 cm. Rotation of neck and abduction and external rotation at hips are limited. Chest expansion is 4 cm. Lower thoracic spine is tender. She is "not handicapped in any way," according to examining physician. She has iritis at 17, 20, and 23 years. Pulmonary function test at 17 years shows mild restriction. Right tem-poromandibular joint is operated on at 23 years.

Neck is normal at 13 years (Figure 9-1A). C2–C3 and C3–C4 zygapophyseal joints are fused at 18 years (Figure 9-1B). Sacroiliac joints are not well defined at 14 years (Figure 9-2). Figure 9-3 shows fused sacroiliac joints at 21 years, irregular symphysis pubis, sclerotic contiguous bone, and pointed lateral aspects of femoral epiphyses. A defect is in left greater trochanter.

Diagnosis: Ankylosing spondylitis.

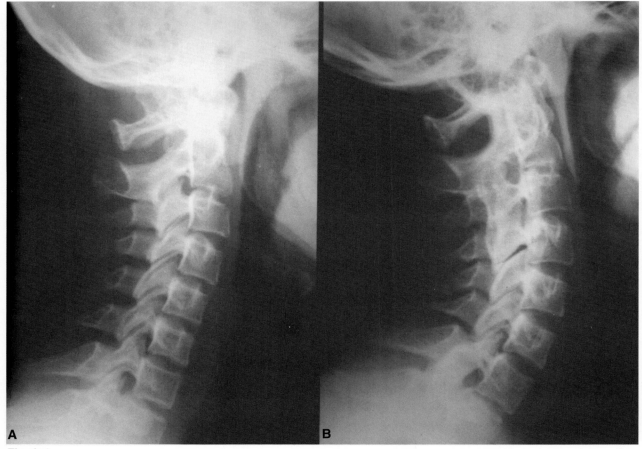

A   **B**

Fig. 9-1

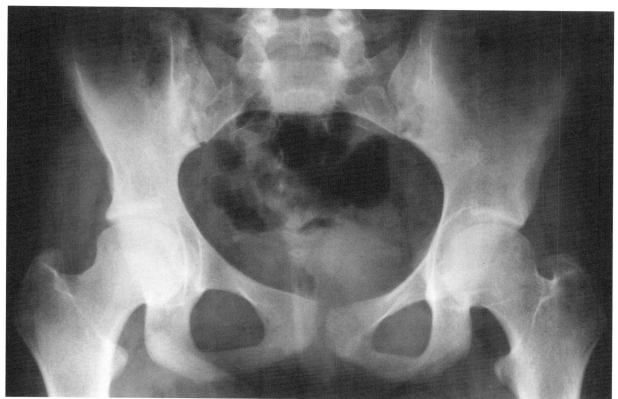

Fig. 9-2

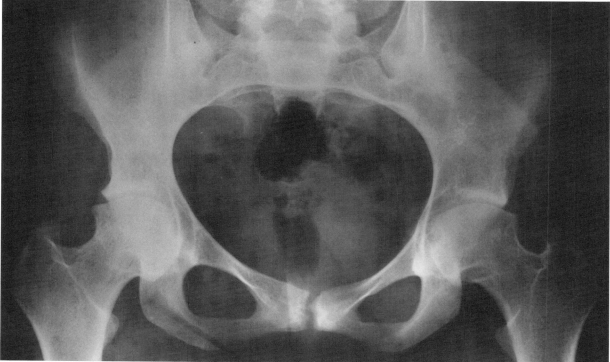

Fig. 9-3

Case 10

A 14-year-old girl has had pain and tingling "like falling asleep" in left arm and left hand for 4 days, swelling for 2 days, and now cannot move left hand.

Mother had rubella during first trimester. Birth weight was 3.9 kg. Infant was upset when arms were moved to dress her. At 2 years, right elbow was swollen and lacked motion. Pupils were unequal. Knees hurt and were swollen after she walked. At 6 years, she could not open mouth wide. Mandible was small. Limb muscles were weak. Elbows, left wrist, fingers, knees, and ankles were swollen. Flexion contractures were at knees. At 10 years, she was too stiff in the morning to go to school. At 11 years, cataract was extracted from right eye. She could not touch palms with tip of flexed index finger. She had knock-knees and flat feet.

Mother (39 years old), father (42 years old), and brother (17 years old) are well. Paternal grandfather has rheumatoid arthritis.

Temperature at 14 years is 37°C, heart rate 90, respiratory rate 20, blood pressure 98/60 mm Hg, weight 31.1 kg, and height 145 cm. Pigmented nevi are on back and legs. Pupils are small and irregular. Right pupil is nonreactive. Pharynx and left eardrum are slightly red. Braces are on teeth. Neck is tender. Left wrist and fingers are swollen, warm, and almost immobile. Deep tendon reflexes are absent in left arm. Perineum is red. The rest of the physical findings are normal.

Hematocrit is 0.33. White cell count is 10.0×10^9/liter with 0.85 polymorphonuclear cells, 0.01 bands, 0.08 lymphocytes, 0.04 monocytes, and 0.02 eosinophils. Platelet count is 729×10^9/liter. ESR is 72 mm/hr. Serum sodium is 139 mmol/liter, potassium 4.3, chloride 108, carbon dioxide 24, urea nitrogen 7.5, calcium 2.40, phosphorus 1.68, cholesterol 3.57, and glucose 5.2. Creatinine is 40 μmol/liter, uric acid 210, total bilirubin 5, and direct bilirubin 2. Total protein is 77 g/liter, albumin 36. Alkaline phosphatase is 108 U/liter, LDH 128, and SGOT 11.

Figure 10-1 shows rarefied bones, swollen left wrist, fusiform swelling around some proximal and distal interphalangeal joints of both hands, and small carpal bones. Little joint cartilage and subchondral erosions are in hands (see Figure 10-1), knees (Figure 10-2), and ankles.

She is treated with prednisone. Left arm and leg are back to usual state in 2 days.

Serum titers for rheumatoid factor and antinuclear antibody are negative.

Weight at 19 years is 37.9 kg, height 147 cm. She plans to become a certified public accountant. Knees are replaced by prostheses.

Diagnosis: Juvenile rheumatoid arthritis, chronic iridocyclitis, vaginal candidiasis.

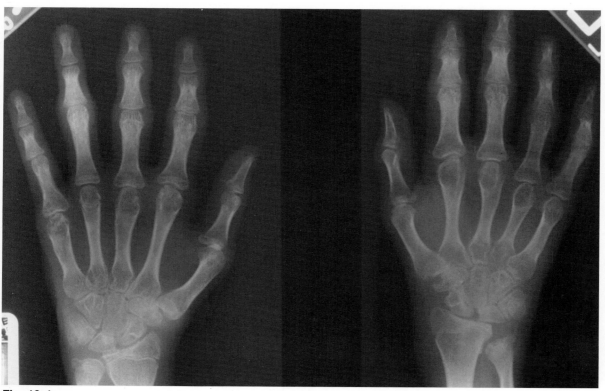

Fig. 10-1

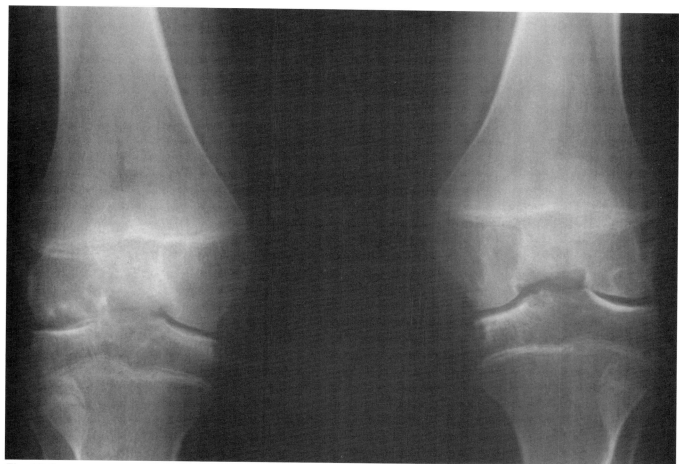

Fig. 10-2

Case 11

A 9-year-old boy has fever and a painful, swollen left knee.

He fell and scraped left knee 1 month ago. He had a cough 2 weeks ago. Physical findings were normal except for healing scrapes, systolic heart murmur, and impalpable left testis. He was hit on left knee by a soccer ball 9 days ago. It hurt his knee to pedal his bicycle home that afternoon. Left knee was swollen that evening. Temperature was 39.4°C 8 days ago. He took an antibiotic from 7 days to 3 days ago. Aspirate of left knee 6 days ago was clear yellow and contained a few white cells and no bacteria in Gram's stain.

Parents, two brothers, and one sister are well.

Temperature is 39°C, heart rate 108, respiratory rate 24, blood pressure 138/60 mm Hg, weight 27.2 kg, and height 127 cm. Lips are chapped, tonsils hyperemic. A systolic heart murmur is present. Groins are tender. Left testis is not in scrotum. He will not move left knee. The rest of the physical findings are normal.

Hematocrit is 0.35. White cell count is 15.1×10^9/liter with 0.65 polymorphonuclear cells, 0.12 bands, 0.15 lymphocytes, and 0.06 monocytes. Platelet estimate is adequate. ESR is 125 mm/hr. C-reactive protein is 4+. ASO titer is 166 Todd units. Urine specific gravity is 1.022, pH 5. Urine has 1+ ketones, amorphous matter, and rare white cells/HPF. Serum sodium is 137 mmol/liter, potassium 4.9, chloride 96, urea nitrogen 3.2, calcium 2.87, and phosphorus 1.26. Creatinine is 50 µmol/liter, uric acid 200, total bilirubin 9, and direct bilirubin 0. Total protein is 73 g/liter, albumin 40. Alkaline phosphatase, LDH, and SGOT are not determined.

Figure 11-1 shows (1) left knee joint and suprapatellar synovial bursa distended by liquid or thickened synovium, (2) overlying left suprapatellar fat body not visible, and (3) patellas ossifying normally.

Aspirate of left knee is bloody and viscous. It contains 1.0 mmol/liter glucose, 43 g/liter protein, 105×10^9/liter white cells, 0.92 polymorphonuclear cells, 0.03 lymphocytes, and 0.05 monocytes. Culture grows β-hemolytic group C streptococci.

He is given an antibiotic. At operation 1 week later, a blood clot and swollen, hemorrhagic synovium are in left knee and suprapatellar synovial bursa.

Microscopic examination of yellow to red-brown synovium shows thrombi, granulation tissue, and chronic inflammation.

Three months later, left knee is normal except for operative scar. Left testis cannot be found at operation.

Diagnosis: Septic arthritis, left knee.

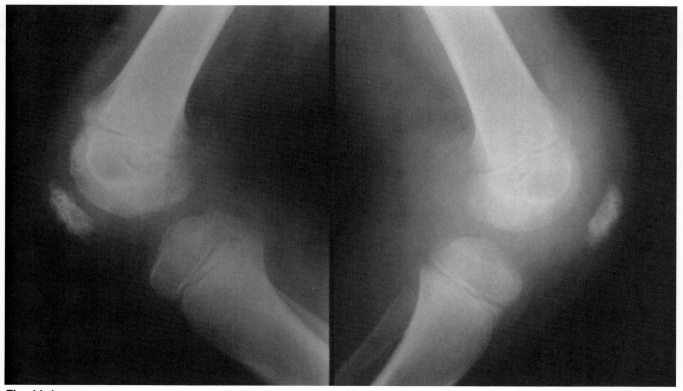

Fig. 11-1

Overgrowth and Soft Tissues

Case 2

A 3-month-old boy has nevi and difference in size of legs and feet.

Pregnancy was normal, birth weight 4 kg. Skin of right shoulder and right arm was rough. A port-wine nevus was on left thigh.

Mother (31 years old), father (29 years old), and two half sisters from mother's previous marriage are well. Members of father's family have webbed toes.

Weight at 3 months is 5.3 kg, length 60 cm, and head circumference 40 cm. Skin of right shoulder and arm down to back of fingers is scaly, yellow, and sharply demarcated. A hemangioma (1.5 cm) is in crease above anus. A small hemangioma is on back of left hand. A left scrotal hydrocele is present. A large, rust-colored patch with central, tortuous distended vein is on left thigh. A hemangioma is on left fifth toe, a smaller one on left fourth toe. Left second, third, and fourth toes and right second and third toes are enlarged and partly fused by soft tissue. Left leg is larger than right. The rest of the physical findings are normal.

At 3 months, deep soft tissues in lateral left thigh and shank, where they are of mixed muscle and fat density, are abnormal (Figure 2-1). Some toes are enlarged and left third metatarsal is slightly angled (Figure 2-2).

Right hand is larger than left at 4 years. Duplex scan of veins of legs at 5 years shows normal veins in right leg, and, in left leg, small superficial veins, large femoral vein, incompetent valves, and superficial varicosities (some thrombosed) in lateral calf.

Diagnosis: Proteus syndrome; syndactyly of toes.

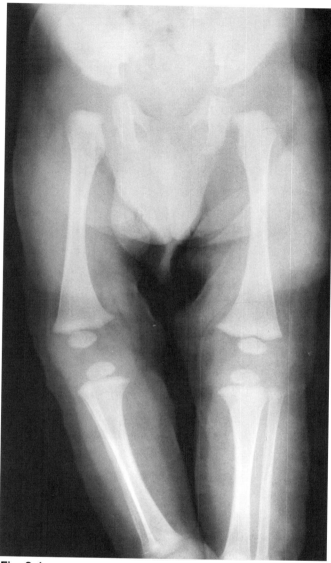

Fig. 2-1

(Continued)

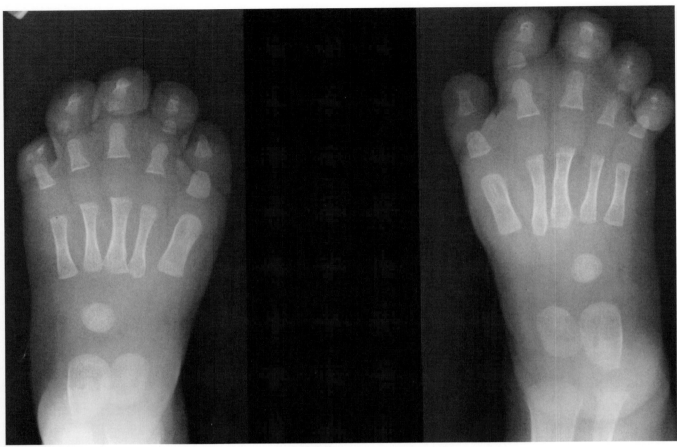

Fig. 2-2

Case 3

An 8-year-old boy has purple lumps on left leg and pain in left leg after vigorous play.

Purple lumps appeared when he was 3–4 months old and have enlarged. He had a tonsillar abscess at 2 years and left inguinal herniorrhaphy at 3 years. At 6 years, large veins were in groins, in left side of scrotum, and down medial side of left thigh to a purple bulge on medial side of left knee.

Temperature at 8 years is 37.4°C, heart rate 88, respiratory rate 20, and blood pressure 108/60 mm Hg. Purple lumps are in groins, on left side of scrotum, and along medial side of left leg almost to ankle. The rest of the physical findings are normal.

Left common and superficial femoral, popliteal, posterior tibial, and saphenous veins are normal in Doppler examination.

Angiography shows dilated superficial veins and small peripheral arterial feeders.

Leg length examination in Figure 3-1 shows bulging soft tissues at medial side of left knee and longer bones in left leg than in right.

He is treated with sclerosing injections in veins. Left leg hurts at 13 years. He is embarrassed by its appearance. Bumps cause bleeding. Swelling diminishes with elevation of leg. Purple swelling has spread to both sides of scrotum, base of penis, and left ankle.

Diagnosis: Klippel-Trénaunay syndrome.

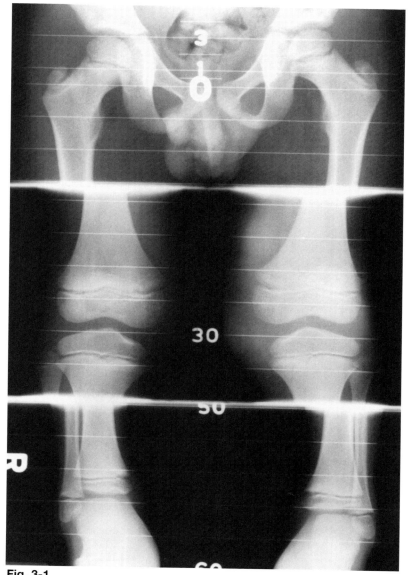

Fig. 3-1

Case 4

A 6-year-old girl has a painful, swollen left calf and will not walk.

She has had left calf pain three or four mornings in a row several times in the last 2 years. The pain goes away a few minutes after she wakes up and moves around.

Mother bled from vagina during first trimester of pregnancy. Birth weight was 3.3 kg. A strawberry hemangioma was on back of left leg just above knee at 2 weeks.

Parents and two siblings (3 and 7 years old) are well.

Temperature at 6 years is 37.4°C, heart rate 96, respiratory rate 24, blood pressure 114/80 mm Hg, weight 20.5 kg, and height 110 cm. She holds left leg flexed at knee and resists extension at knee and dorsiflexion at ankle. Upper left calf is tender and 1 cm larger than right. The rest of the physical findings are normal.

Hematocrit is 0.35. White cell count is 7.3×10^9/liter with 0.41 polymorphonuclear cells, 0.03 bands, 0.50 lymphocytes, 0.02 monocytes, and 0.04 eosinophils. Platelet count is 259×10^9/liter. PT is 13 seconds (normal: 11–13), PTT 30.6 (normal: 27–37), and thrombin time 40.7 (control: 26.3). Fibrinogen is 1.5 g/liter (normal: 1.5–3.5). Urine specific gravity is 1.007, pH 6. Urine is normal. Serum sodium is 143 mmol/liter, potassium 4.4, chloride 108, carbon dioxide 22, urea nitrogen 3.6, calcium 2.50, phosphorus 1.68, cholesterol 3.93, and glucose 6.4. Creatinine is 40 μmol/liter, uric acid 110, total bilirubin 2, and direct bilirubin 0. Total protein is 67 g/liter, albumin 41. Alkaline phosphatase is 232 U/liter, LDH 253, and SGOT 31.

Small round shadows of calcium density are in soft tissues below left knee (Figure 4-1A). Venogram shows deep venous aneurysms, some with clots, in upper two-thirds of left shank (Figure 4-1B).

She has a slight limp and no pain when she is allowed to walk 9 days later. Venogram 5 months later shows aneurysms and capillary blush in back of left thigh where strawberry hemangioma used to be. Angiogram shows normal arteries. She later has recurrent calf pain, clinical thrombosis with swelling, and Homans' sign despite anticoagulants and elastic stocking, including an episode at 15 years when PT is 25.7 seconds after a 7-hour car ride.

Diagnosis: Deep venous malformation of left shank.

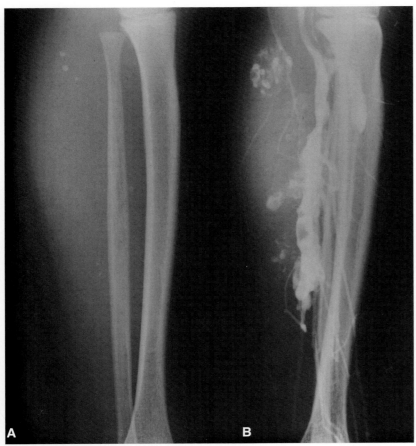

Fig. 4-1

Case 5

A 12-year-old boy has a swollen left leg. Left ankle swelled 2 weeks ago; the next day, entire left leg was swollen.

He has occasional headache. He has had rubella, mumps, and chickenpox.

Mother (30 years old), father (33 years old), and sister (11 years old) are well. Maternal grandmother had diabetes mellitus.

Weight is 53.6 kg, height 165 cm, temperature 37.2°C, heart rate 68, respiratory rate 16, and blood pressure 118/86 mm Hg. Left leg is slightly dusky. Circumference of left thigh is 50 cm, right thigh 46.5, left calf 33, right calf 29.5. Left groin is boggy. Pitting edema is at left ankle. Femoral pulses are normal. The rest of the physical findings are normal.

Hematocrit is 0.40. White cell count is 6.1×10^9/liter with 0.68 polymorphonuclear cells, 0.25 lymphocytes, 0.04 monocytes, 0.02 eosinophils, and 0.01 basophils. Platelet count is 324×10^9/liter. ESR is 3 mm/hr. Total serum protein is 61 g/liter, albumin 41. Urine specific gravity is 1.032, pH 5. Urine is normal.

Lymphangiogram in Figure 5-1 shows sparse lymphatics and small lymph nodes on left side.

Diagnosis: Late-onset lymphedema (Meige's disease).

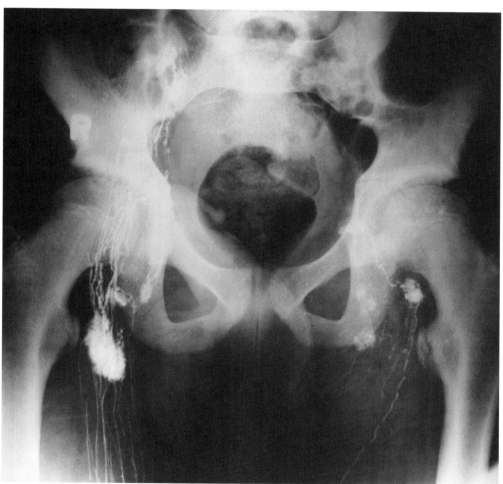

Fig. 5-1

Case 6

A 15-year-old girl limps and has a painful, swollen finger.

A red papule was on right hand 1 week ago. Right knee hurt when she woke up 6 days ago. She had a fever a few nights ago and early morning chills. Left third finger was swollen 2 days ago. Joint aches have kept her awake. She is nauseated.

She had kidney operation at 7 years. She has had chickenpox. She fainted several months ago. She fell and hit back of head a few days ago. Menarche was at 12 years.

Mother has kidney problem. Father died of drug overdose at 28 years. A brother (14 years old) is well. Paternal grandmother has diabetes mellitus.

Temperature at 15 years is 36.4°C, heart rate 74, respiratory rate 20, blood pressure 120/90 mm Hg, weight 73 kg, and height 165 cm. Pustules, some crusted, are on right elbow, right hand, and on immobile, swollen, red, and tender left third fin-ger. Flexion of other left fingers is painful. Right second finger and right knee are swollen and tender. Left calcaneal tendon is tender. The rest of the physical findings are normal.

Hematocrit is 0.43. White cell count is 11.3×10^9/liter with 0.63 polymorphonuclear cells, 0.09 bands, 0.20 lymphocytes, 0.05 monocytes, and 0.03 eosinophils. ESR is 48 mm/hr. Urine specific gravity is 1.020, pH 5. Urine has moderate squamous epithelial cells/HPF, 4–6 white cells/HPF, and bacteria.

Left third digit is swollen, phalanges normal (Figure 6-1).

Left ankle and left third toe hurt the next day.

Culture of a pustule grows coagulase-negative staphylococci. Cultures of two rectal swabs grow *Neisseria gonorrhoeae*.

Diagnosis: Gonococcemia.

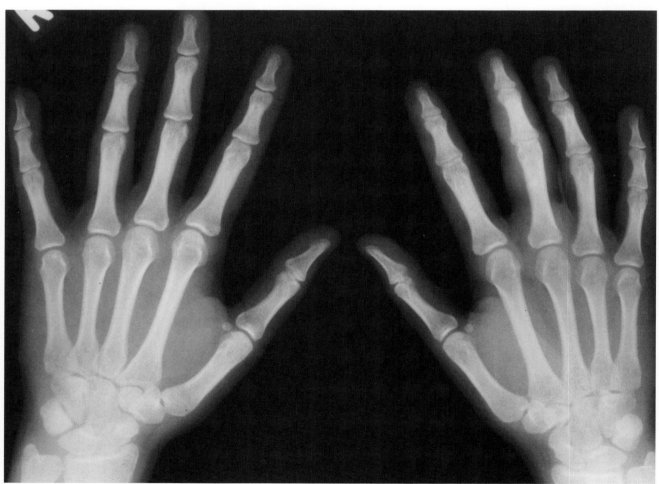

Fig. 6-1

Case 7

A 3-year-old girl has hard, nontender lumps on her legs.

Pale mottling of arms, shanks, and chin and red welts on legs were noticed about 1 year ago. Hard lumps then replaced welts. Two months ago, she limped and had hives on legs for 1 day. She runs, rides her bicycle, and plays normally. Pregnancy of mother was normal, birth weight 3.37 kg.

Mother (24 years old) and father (26 years old) are well. Paternal great-grandmother, paternal grandfather, and maternal great-uncle have arthritis. Paternal grandmother has diabetes mellitus.

Weight at 3 years is 14.2 kg, height 97 cm, and blood pressure 80/50 mm Hg. Many lumps are palpable in legs. The rest of the physical findings are normal.

Hematocrit is 0.38. White cell count is 8.5×10^9/liter with 0.26 polymorphonuclear cells, 0.02 bands, 0.61 lymphocytes, 0.09 monocytes, 0.01 basophils, and 0.01 atypical lymphocytes. Platelet count is 359×10^9/liter. ESR is 2 mm/hr. Serum sodium is 139 mmol/liter, potassium 4.3, chloride 108, carbon dioxide 18, urea nitrogen 6.8, calcium 2.42, phosphorus 1.71, cholesterol 4.76, and glucose 4.1. Creatinine is 40 µmol/liter, uric acid 210, total bilirubin 2, and direct bilirubin 0. Total protein is 72 g/liter, albumin 48. Alkaline phosphatase is 176 U/liter, LDH 309, SGOT 36, and CK 54. Antinuclear antibody test is negative. Urine creatinine is 125 µmol/kg/day (normal: 71–194), creatine 0.04 mol/kg/day (average: 0.03), and phosphoethanolamine 140 $\mu mol/g_{creatinine}$ (normal: 80–220). Urine does not contain oxalic or glycolic acid. Midmolecule parathormone is 105 pmol/liter (normal: 30–80) when serum calcium is 2.45 mmol/liter. $1,25(OH)_2$ vitamin D is 86 pmol/liter (adult normal: 100 ± 28), 25(OH) vitamin D 81.9 nmol/liter (normal: 78.9 ± 23.2).

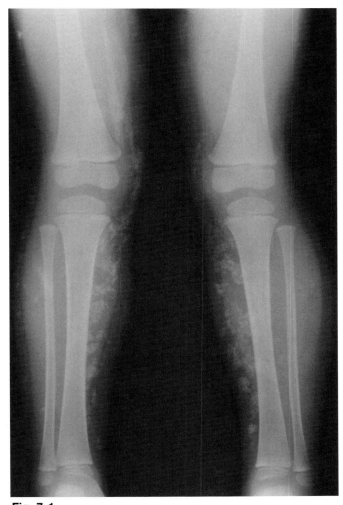

Fig. 7-1

Deposits of calcium are in subcutaneous fat and perhaps muscle in legs (Figure 7-1). Findings in arms are similar to a lesser extent.

Punch biopsy shows calcium in subcutaneous fat lobules.

Diagnosis: Calcinosis cutis, questionable dermatomyositis.

Case 8

A 7½-month-old girl has had swelling in left groin and thigh for several days.

Pregnancy was normal, birth weight 4.2 kg. Intermittent duskiness of left leg at 3 months was followed 1 week later by swelling (4-cm diameter) in left thigh that, at excision, extended from left obturator foramen to lesser trochanter of left femur and stretched and pushed femoral vessels, except saphenous vein, laterally.

Weight at 7½ months is 9.3 kg, length 69 cm, head circumference 44 cm, temperature 36.9°C, heart rate 136, respiratory rate 30, and systolic blood pressure 114 mm Hg. A healed scar is in left inguinal crease. A firm, nonmobile mass (4- to 6-cm diameter) is in left groin and upper thigh. The rest of the physical findings are normal.

Hematocrit is 0.36. White cell count is 16.9×10^9/liter. Platelet count is 514×10^9/liter. Serum sodium is 141 mmol/liter, potassium 5.0, chloride 110, carbon dioxide 14, urea nitrogen 4.3, calcium 2.52, phosphorus 2.26, cholesterol 4.47, and glucose 5.6. Creatinine is 40 μmol/liter, uric acid 270, total bilirubin 3, and direct bilirubin 0. Total protein is 62 g/liter, albumin 47. Alkaline phosphatase is 242 U/liter, LDH 311, and SGOT 44.

CT scan shows septate tumor of fat density in left thigh and groin (Figure 8-1).

At operation, a white, lobed tumor ($7 \times 5 \times 4$ cm) is over adductors from obturator foramen to femoral canal.

Microscopic examination of both excised tumors shows (1) fibrous capsule; (2) fibrous septa of varying thickness with vessels in them; (3) lobules that contain fat cells of various size and a mixture of mature adipocytes and lipoblasts (some lipoblasts almost like signet rings with fat droplet displacing nucleus); and (4) rare mesenchymal cells.

Weight at 8 years is 42 kg, height 131 cm. Left thigh is slightly fuller than left. Gait is normal.

Diagnosis: Lipoblastoma.

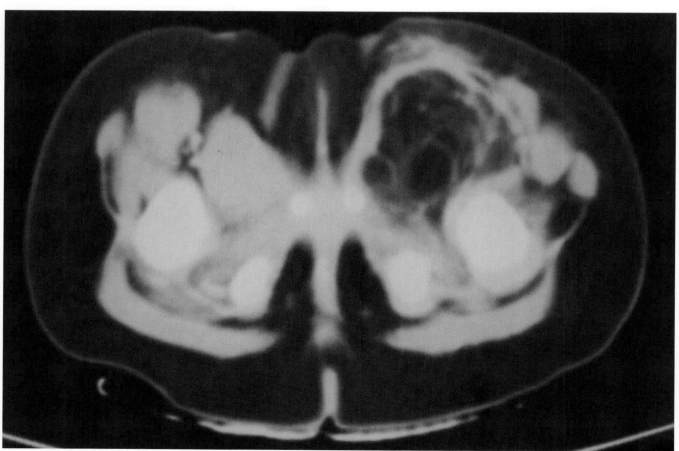

Fig. 8-1

Infection

Case 1

A boy is delivered by cesarean section because of fetal bradycardia.

Mother (19 years old) had fever and aches during first trimester. Onset of labor was spontaneous. Heart rate slowed from 132 to 43 and remained below 80 after amniotomy.

Birth weight is 2.2 kg, length 44 cm, head circumference 33 cm, and Apgar score 3/7 at 1 and 5 minutes and 8 at 10 minutes. Temperature is 36.6°C, heart rate 152, and respiratory rate 48. Infant is pale. Nonblanching red spots (2- to 4-mm diameter) are on face, body, and limbs. Liver edge and spleen edge are 2 cm below costal margin. The rest of the physical findings are normal. Left arm and leg extend at 3½ hours; head turns left.

Hematocrit is 0.43. White cell count is 9.0×10^9/liter. Platelet estimate is slightly decreased. Serum sodium is 135 mmol/liter, potassium 4.7, calcium 2.05, and glucose 5.1. Total bilirubin is 55 μmol/liter. CSF glucose is 4.1 mmol/liter with no white cells and 2.6×10^9/liter red cells.

Longitudinal striations are prominent in bones of arms and legs, especially in distal part of femurs (Figure 1-1).

He is given phenobarbital for thrashing seizures, which stop at 7 days. At 15 days, a systolic heart murmur is present, and liver edge is 5 cm below costal margin, spleen edge 3 cm below costal margin. He dies at 6 weeks.

Necropsy shows (1) absence of most of septum pellucidum; (2) atrophy of thymus; (3) large ductus arteriosus; (4) inflammation, congestion, and hyaline membranes in lungs; and (5) chronic passive congestion in liver.

Six specimens of urine do not contain cytomegalovirus. Rubella virus is in blood obtained during first week.

Diagnosis: Congenital rubella syndrome.

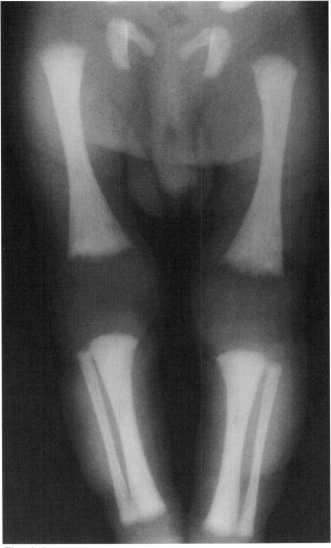

Fig. 1-1

Case 2

A newborn girl has 1.0- to 1.5-cm silvery blue spots on body that peel when rubbed, peeling palms and soles, red bumps on knuckles of right hand, bumps at angles of mouth, and large liver and spleen.

Mother (17 years old) had genital sore 20 months ago, blisters on palms 18 months ago. She was given two injections of penicillin. Serum was reactive in fluorescent treponemal antibody absorption test 18 days ago, its VDRL titer 1:16. Serum VDRL titer is now 1:64.

Amniotic fluid is meconium stained, birth weight 2.5 kg, Apgar score 4/8 at 1 and 5 minutes, length 47 cm, head circumference 33 cm, temperature 35.8°C, heart rate 150, and respiratory rate 45. The rest of the physical findings are normal. Ophthalmologic findings are normal.

Alternating bands of increased and decreased density are in bones of arms and legs (Figures 2-1 and 2-2).

Hematocrit is 0.36. White cell count is 13.2×10^9/liter with 0.55 polymorphonuclear cells, 0.01 bands, 0.39 lymphocytes, 0.04 monocytes, and 0.01 eosinophils. Platelet count is 65 × 10^9/liter. Urine specific gravity is 1.008 at 4 days. Urine has few squamous epithelial cells/HPF and occasional white cells/HPF. Serum sodium at 3 days is 145 mmol/liter, potassium 5.0, chloride 113, carbon dioxide 18, urea nitrogen 7.1, calcium 2.17, phosphorus 1.19, cholesterol 6.27, and glucose 4.2. Creatinine is 120 μmol/liter, uric acid 370, total bilirubin 32, and direct bilirubin 24. Total protein is 62 g/liter, albumin 24, and IgM 17.60 (normal: <0.25). Alkaline phosphatase is 200 U/liter, LDH 588, and SGOT 88. CSF has 6×10^6/liter red cells, 10×10^6/liter white cells, 0.25 polymorphonuclear cells, 0.38 lymphocytes, 0.35 pia-arachnoid cells, 1.04 g/liter protein, and VDRL titer 1:8. Serum is reactive in fluorescent treponemal antibody absorption test, its VDRL titer 1:512.

Weight is 35 kg at 8 years, when she comes in for examination for earaches. An otorhinolaryngologist finds slight retraction and diminished motility of left eardrum and normal hearing in audiography.

Diagnosis: Congenital syphilis.

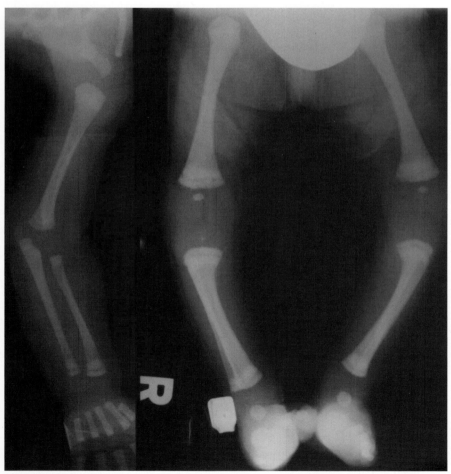

Fig. 2-1

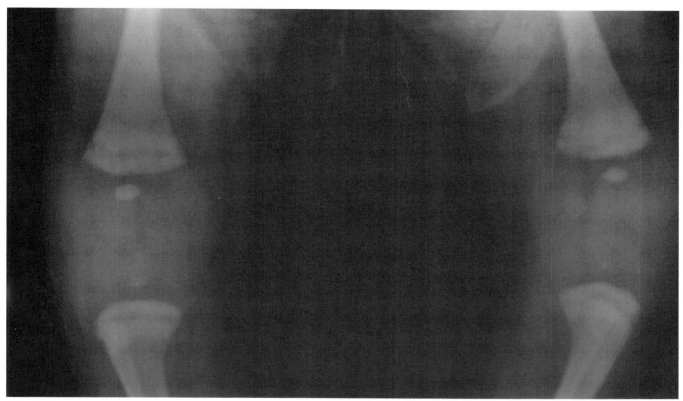

Fig. 2-2

Case 3

A 12-year-old boy uses crutches because of pain in right foot. One month ago, he stepped on a nail with his right heel, while wearing tennis shoes. The right heel around nail puncture was swollen, red, and tender 2 weeks later.

Temperature is 37.6°C, heart rate 124, respiratory rate 20, blood pressure 100/62 mm Hg, and weight 36 kg. Right heel is red, swollen, tender, and not fluctuant. The rest of the physical findings are normal.

Hematocrit is 0.38. White cell count is 8.8×10^9/liter. Platelet count is 532×10^9/liter. ESR is 87 mm/hr. Serum sodium is 142 mmol/liter, potassium 4.2, chloride 102, carbon dioxide 24, urea nitrogen 4.6, calcium 2.45, phosphorus 1.36, cholesterol 2.92, and glucose 6.3. Creatinine is 60 μmol/liter, uric acid 340, total bilirubin 5, and direct bilirubin 0. Total protein is 86 g/liter, albumin 44. Alkaline phosphatase is 178 U/liter, LDH 343, and SGOT 25.

Bones of right foot are rarefied and right calcaneal apophysis is partly resorbed in Figure 3-1.

At operation, an abscess in subcutaneous fat goes up approximately 1 cm into tuberosity of calcaneum. Necrotic bone is debrided.

Culture obtained at operation grows *Pseudomonas aeruginosa* from plantar soft tissue and calcaneum and also coagulase-negative staphylococci from calcaneum.

Diagnosis: Tennis shoe nail puncture, *Pseudomonas* osteomyelitis.

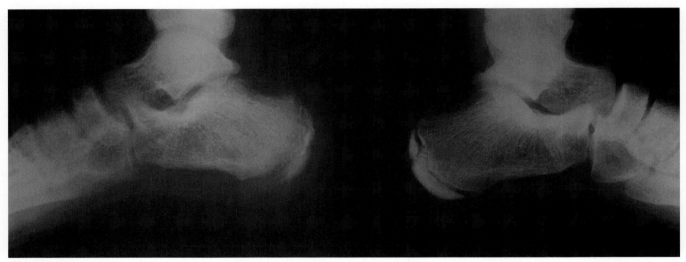

Fig. 3-1

Case 4

A 6-year-old boy walks with flexed knees.

Pregnancy of mother was normal. He had meningococcal meningitis at 3 months and has had "staring" seizures since then. He sat at 18 months and walked at 20 months. He uses left arm and leg more than right.

Mother (25 years old), father (26 years old), and two sisters are well.

Height at 6 years is 100 cm, temperature 37.4°C, heart rate 100, respiratory rate 20, and blood pressure 78/42 mm Hg. Fingers are short, their ends bulbous. Knees extend only 45 degrees. He has right knock knee, bulge of right fibula at

knee, and lateral convexity at right ankle. Ankles flex 20 degrees; right ankle extends to neutral, left 5 degrees beyond neutral. Right third, fourth, and fifth toes are short and lack nails. The rest of the physical findings are normal.

Some growth plates in legs are gone at 3 years and epiphyses and metaphyses are distorted (Figure 4-1). Distal phalanges are gone from fingers but not thumbs at 6 years. Some middle phalanges are only small spikes.

Diagnosis: Meningococcemia at 3 months with necrosis of bone and cartilage.

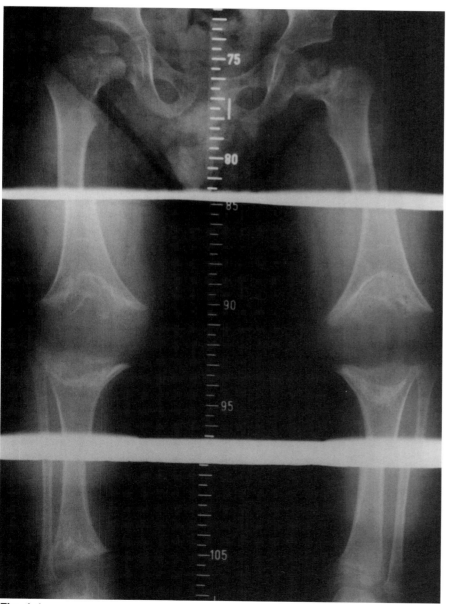

Fig. 4-1

Case 5

A 10-year-old girl has had pains in left arm that last a few days for the last 3 months. The pains are relieved by rubbing and do not limit her activity.

Parents and two brothers are well.

Temperature is 36°C, heart rate 88, respiratory rate 20, blood pressure 98/60 mm Hg, weight 31.2 kg, and height 143 cm. A hard, slightly tender mass is fixed to left humerus. The rest of the physical findings are normal.

Hematocrit is 0.46. White cell count is 7.1×10^9/liter with 0.57 polymorphonuclear cells, 0.01 bands, 0.37 lymphocytes, and 0.05 monocytes. Platelet count is 278×10^9/liter. ESR is 62 mm/hr. Urine specific gravity is 1.020, pH 6. Urine has 0–1 white cell/HPF and many amorphous urates. Serum sodium is 136 mmol/liter, potassium 4.3, chloride 102, carbon dioxide 21, urea nitrogen 4.3, calcium 2.37, phosphorus 1.52, cholesterol 3.36, and glucose 6.4. Creatinine is 60 µmol/liter, uric acid 290, total bilirubin 5, and direct bilirubin 0. Total protein is 85 g/liter, albumin 43. Alkaline phosphatase is 250 U/liter, LDH 309, and SGOT 42.

Cortex is thickened and cystlike defects are in upper humerus (Figure 5-1).

At operation, sclerotic bone is around humerus and defects in medulla. Microscopic examination shows (1) cancellous bone, (2) neutrophils, (3) lymphocytes, (4) occasional plasma cells, (5) myxoid degeneration, and (6) hemorrhage. Cultures are sterile. Another biopsy 1 month later shows fibrous connective tissue with an inflammatory infiltrate of plasma cells in places and a mixture of neutrophils and single multinucleated histiocytes in other places without granulomas or microorganisms. Cultures are sterile.

Diagnosis: Chronic sclerosing osteomyelitis (Garré's disease) with negative cultures.

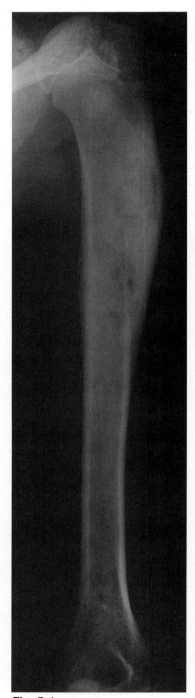

Fig. 5-1

Case 6

A 13-year-old boy cannot stand on right leg. He began to have pain in right groin and down front of right thigh 10 days ago, while playing basketball. Pain is worse and has shifted to right buttock and back of right thigh.

Temperature is 37.8°C, heart rate 75, respiratory rate 20, blood pressure 130/75 mm Hg, and weight 59.7 kg. Adduction and extension are limited at right hip. Right buttock and right ischiorectal fossa are tender. Rectal palpation finds tenderness behind and to right. The rest of the physical findings are normal.

Hematocrit is 0.37. White cell count is 21.4 × 10⁹/liter with 0.58 polymorphonuclear cells, 0.28 bands, 0.10 lymphocytes, 0.03 monocytes, and 0.01 basophils. Platelet count is 548 × 10⁹/liter. ESR is 109 mm/hr. Urine specific gravity is 1.015, pH 5. Urine has trace protein. Serum sodium is 140 mmol/liter, potassium 5.0, chloride 98, carbon dioxide 23, urea nitrogen 3.9, calcium 2.68, phosphorus 1.38, cholesterol 3.88, and glucose 5.5. Creatinine is 60 μmol/liter, uric acid 230, total bilirubin 7, and direct bilirubin 3. Total protein is 67 g/liter, albumin 34. Alkaline phosphatase is 360 U/liter, LDH 258, and SGOT 48. Blood culture shows no growth.

Roentgenogram of pelvis shows moth-eaten tuberosity and lower part of right ischium and cortical thickening along upper part at right obturator foramen (Figure 6-1). CT scan shows irregularity of back part of right ischium and swelling of adjacent muscles (Figure 6-2A). T1-weighted MRI shows increased signal and swelling in posteromedial aspect of right thigh (Figure 6-2B).

Approximately 75 ml pus with bits of bone is found at operation. Gram's stain of pus shows gram-positive cocci and white cells. Microscopic examination shows acute and chronic inflammation.

Culture of pus grows *Staphylococcus aureus*.

Diagnosis: Osteomyelitis.

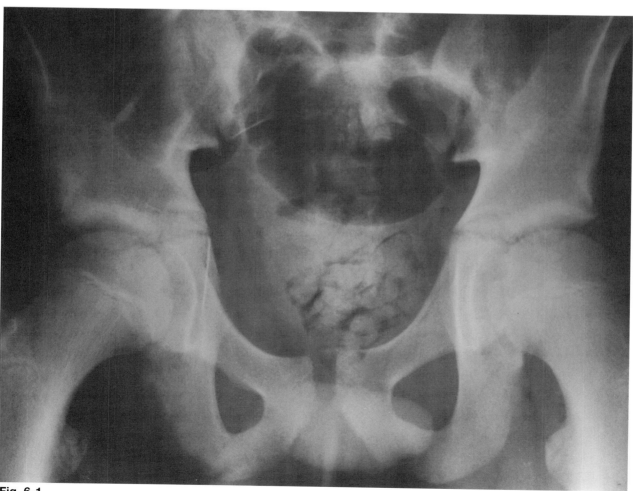

Fig. 6-1

(Continued)

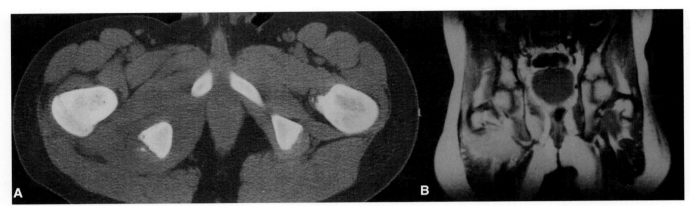

Fig. 6-2

Case 7

An 11-month-old girl is breathing fast and deep.

For 1 week, she has had a cough and fever, for which her mother has given aspirin. She sat at 6 months.

Parents and three siblings are well.

Temperature is 38.5°C, heart rate 148, respiratory rate 70 without retraction, blood pressure 130/70 mm Hg, weight 8.2 kg, and length 72 cm. She will not sit up and arches back. A systolic heart murmur is present. Liver edge is 2 cm below costal margin. The rest of the physical findings are normal.

Hematocrit is 0.35. White cell count is 26.5 × 10⁹/liter with 0.26 polymorphonuclear cells, 0.45 bands, 0.10 lymphocytes, and 0.19 monocytes. Urine specific gravity is 1.010, pH 5. Urine has protein, glucose, rare epithelial cells/HPF, and 0–2 white cells/HPF. Serum sodium is 134 mmol/liter, potassium 3.7, chloride 111, urea nitrogen 4.6, salicylate 2.17 (normal therapeutic level: <1.45), and glucose 6.6. CSF has 2 × 10⁶/liter small lymphocytes, 5.2 mmol/liter glucose, and 0.04 g/liter protein. CSF and blood cultures show no growth.

She is given ampicillin for 2 days. Fever persists. Eardrums are opaque and retracted the fourth day. Temperature the tenth day is 39.4°C, hematocrit 0.28, platelet count 1.0 × 10¹²/liter, reticulocyte fraction 50 × 10⁻³, and ESR 111 mm/hr. A nurse notices that when baby is in a walker, she pushes herself with left leg and foot, holds right leg off floor, and will not use right foot at all. Treatment with erythromycin is begun for otitis media. Mother brings her back the sixteenth day because she still has fever and will not bear weight on right leg. She holds right leg flexed and externally rotated and resists movement at right hip. Right groin is tender. ESR is 95 mm/hr. Bloody aspirate, 0.5 ml, from right hip is sterile.

Figure 7-1A shows laterally displaced right femur and swollen deep soft tissues along right greater trochanter 16 days after first admission. Figure 7-1B, at 11 years, shows most of neck of right femur gone, ectopic bone below it, and fused right greater trochanter higher than acetabulum, when right femur is 3 cm shorter than left and movement at right hip is limited to 0 degrees of abduction, 15 degrees of adduction, and 90 degrees of flexion.

Diagnosis: Salicylism, osteomyelitis of right femur, secondary infectious arthritis of right hip.

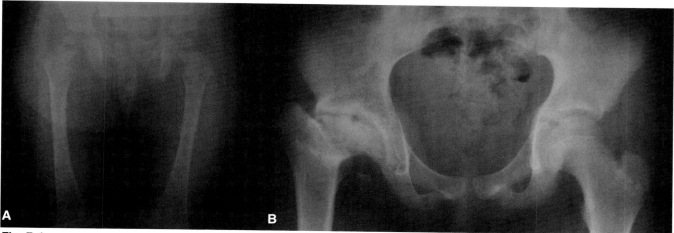

Fig. 7-1

Case 8

A 7-year-old girl will not walk. She had a fever and headache 2 days ago, and right ankle ache yesterday. She limped to bathroom on right toes. She did not sleep well last night and will not walk today.

Mother, two half sisters (17 and 18 years old), and brother (10 years old) have spherocytosis; a half brother (11 years old) does not.

Pregnancy was normal, birth weight 3.6 kg. Blood smear at 3 days showed spherocytes. A systolic heart murmur was present at 13 days, liver edge 2 cm below costal margin, spleen edge 2 cm below costal margin, hematocrit 0.16, and reticulocyte fraction 4×10^{-3}. White cell count was 12.7×10^9/liter, total bilirubin 100 μmol/liter. Blood was Rh negative, Coombs' negative, and ABO compatible. At 3 years, weight was 14 kg, height 96 cm, and blood pressure 96/72 mm Hg. Liver edge was 2 cm below costal margin, spleen edge 3 cm below costal margin. Hematocrit was 0.30, reticulocyte fraction 13×10^{-3}. Spleen, twice normal size, and two accessory hilar spleens were removed. She has had only respiratory infections, some with otitis media, since then.

Temperature at 7 years is 37.7°C, heart rate 88, respiratory rate 18, weight 23 kg, and height 133 cm. A systolic heart murmur is present. A transverse scar is in left upper quadrant of abdomen. A warm, very tender swelling is contiguous to right fibula just above minimally tender malleolus. Movement at right ankle is limited. The rest of the physical findings are normal.

Hematocrit is 0.39. Hemoglobin is 146 g/liter. Red blood cell count is 4.4×10^{12}/liter. MCV is 85 fl. MCH is 32 pg. MCHC is 380 g/liter. White cell count is 10.9×10^9/liter with 0.46 polymorphonuclear cells, 0.22 bands, 0.25 lymphocytes, and 0.07 monocytes. ESR is 63 mm/hr. Two blood cultures are sterile. Urine specific gravity is 1.002, pH 6.5. Urine has 0–1 squamous epithelial cell/HPF, rare nonsquamous epithelial cells/HPF, and 0–1 white cell/HPF. Serum sodium is 136 mmol/liter, potassium 3.8, chloride 93, carbon dioxide 28, urea nitrogen 3.9, and glucose 7.0.

Deep soft tissues along distal metaphysis of right fibula are swollen (Figure 8-1A). Examination 1½ years later, when she has right ankle pain for 1 day that is gone the next and ESR is 17 mm/hr, shows postarrest growth lines because of illness, the one in the right tibia slightly deeper because of ipsilateral hyperemia (Figure 8-1B).

Diagnosis: Osteomyelitis, right fibula, at 7 years; hereditary spherocytosis.

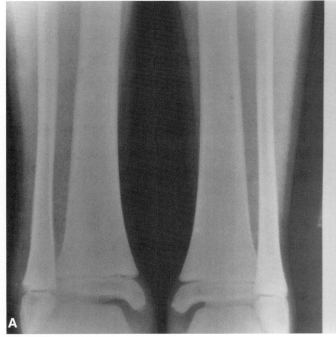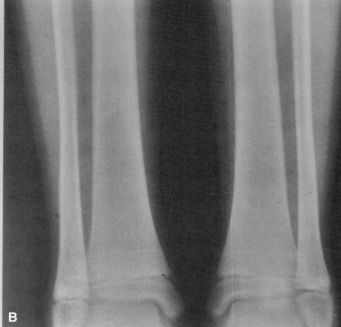

Fig. 8-1

Case 9

A 7-year-old girl has had pain at left knee for 2 years. Pain is worse at night and sometimes wakes her. She runs and plays without pain. Knee is stiff in evening and early morning.

Birth weight was 1.2 kg. She was in hospital nursery for 2 months. While there, cultures of a sore on left leg and left side of chest grew *Staphylococcus aureus*. Bile vomit and abdominal distention at 3 weeks were found to be caused by necrotizing enterocolitis at operation. Perforated cecum and necrotic 5 cm of distal ileum were removed, gastrostomy and central venous catheter placed. Cultures of catheter and blood grew *S. epidermidis*. Cultures of stoma grew *Escherichia coli*, *S. aureus*, and *Micrococcus*. At 2 months, gastrostomy was removed, and she went home. At 3 years, she had a stitch abscess. At 4 years, she was well. Weight was 14.7 kg, height 99 cm. At 7 years, she is in second grade.

Temperature at 7 years is 36.8°C, heart rate 100, respiratory rate 24, blood pressure 80/60 mm Hg, weight 20.5 kg, and height 118 cm. Scars are in upper quadrants of abdomen. A small, tender swelling is under left patella. The rest of the physical findings are normal.

Hematocrit is 0.41. White cell count is 8.8×10^9/liter. Platelet count is 325×10^9/liter. Urine specific gravity is 1.022, pH 8. Urine is normal.

A defect is in proximal metaphysis of left tibia (Figure 9-1).

At operation, brown-gray, mucinous, gelatinous matter is in a cavity beneath cortex of tibia. Growth plate at top of cavity looks normal.

Microscopic examination of lining of cavity shows chronic inflammation. Culture of matter removed from cavity grows 4+ coagulase-positive and 1+ coagulase-negative staphylococci.

Diagnosis: Chronic osteomyelitis (Brodie's abscess).

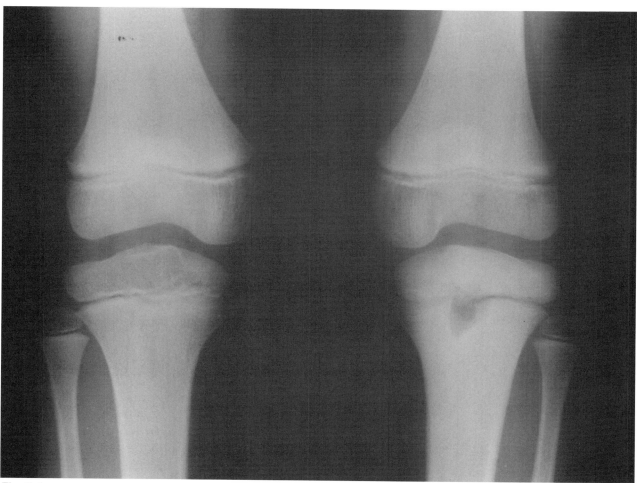

Fig. 9-1

Skeletal Tumors

Case 1

A 4½-month-old boy is fussy and has not been eating well for 4 days. He would not put weight on left leg 1 month ago. Left shank was swollen and tender 1 week ago.

Birth weight was 3.1 kg. He had a diphtheria-pertussis-tetanus vaccination in left thigh 2 months ago.

Temperature is 37.4°C, heart rate 125, respiratory rate 30, systolic blood pressure 90 mm Hg, weight 5.8 kg, length 62 cm, and head circumference 40 cm. Jaw is large and square. A mongolian spot is on lower back. Left shank is swollen and tender from just below knee to ankle. The rest of the physical findings are normal.

Hematocrit is 0.26. White cell count is 17.6 × 10⁹/liter with 0.34 polymorphonuclear cells, 0.04 bands, 0.56 lymphocytes, and 0.06 monocytes. ESR is 79 mm/hr. Red cells are microcytic. Urine specific gravity is 1.025, pH 5. Urine has trace protein and 0–1 white cell/HPF. Two blood cultures are sterile. VDRL test is nonreactive.

He is smiling 2 months later. ESR is 22 mm/hr.

At 4½ months, mandible, cortex of left tibia, and lower left medial calf muscles are thickened, and sphenofrontal suture and spheno-occipital synchondrosis are prominent (Figure 1-1). Findings are similar at 7 months. Roentgenographic findings in rest of skeleton are normal at 7 months.

Diagnosis: Caffey's disease (infantile cortical hyperostosis).

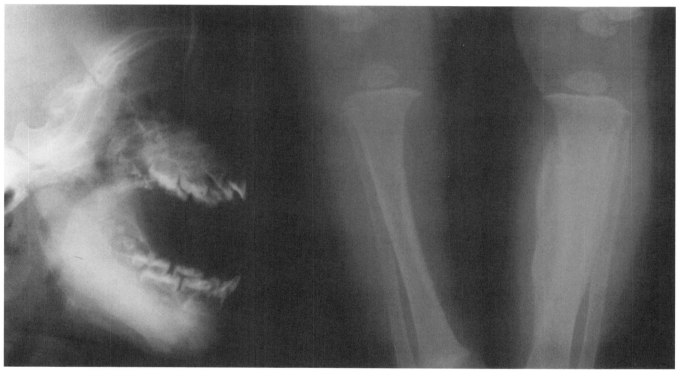

Fig. 1-1

Case 2

A newborn girl has heart disease that was found in prenatal ultrasound examination.

Mother (20 years old) has been operated on for Fallot's tetrad.

Birth weight is 1.7 kg, Apgar score 8/9 at 1 and 5 minutes, heart rate 170, respiratory rate 50, and blood pressure 63/47 mm Hg. Right side of face is smaller than left. Skin tags are in front of ears. Left auricle is cupped. A systolic heart murmur is present. Left thumb is hypoplastic; right thumb is a small piece of soft tissue. The rest of the physical findings are normal.

Hematocrit is 0.39. White cell count is 14.3×10^9/liter with 0.71 polymorphonuclear cells, 0.02 bands, 0.13 lymphocytes, 0.12 monocytes, and 0.02 eosinophils. Platelet count is 279×10^9/liter. Serum sodium is 136 mmol/liter, potassium 3.5, chloride 100, carbon dioxide 17, urea nitrogen 3.2, calcium 2.42, phosphorus 1.87, cholesterol 1.53, and glucose 13.4 (IV fluids). Creatinine is 50 μmol/liter, uric acid 310, total bilirubin 80, and direct bilirubin 5. Total protein is 43 g/liter, albumin 29. Alkaline phosphatase is 87 U/liter, LDH 406, and SGOT 27. Chromosomes are 46,XX.

Echocardiogram and cine angiocardiogram show (1) single ventricle, (2) small subaortic chamber, (3) common atrioventricular valve, (4) aorta in front and to left of atretic pulmonary valve, and (5) right aortic arch.

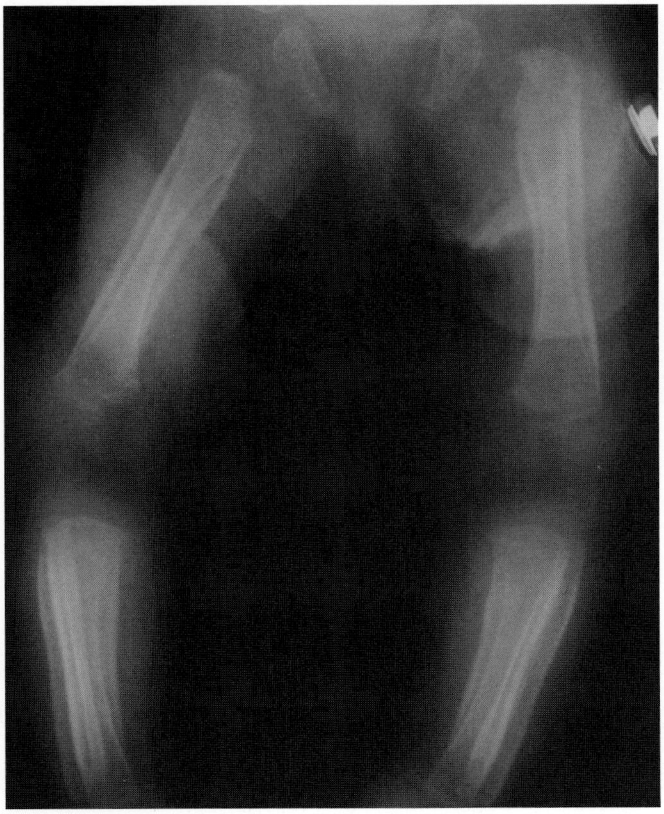

She is blue and has apneic spells. IV prostaglandin E_1 is begun at 23 hours. Edema of feet is present at 9 days, nonpitting swelling of legs at 20 days. Legs will not extend fully at 28 days. She cries when diapered. Oxygen saturation is below 0.70 at 37 days despite continuance of prostaglandin and extra oxygen. Red spots and bumps are on arms and thighs. Blalock-Taussig shunt operation is performed at 56 days, and administration of prostaglandin is stopped.

Serum alkaline phosphatase is 86 U/liter at 3 days; 123 at 7 days; 273 at 19 days, when calcium is 2.32 mmol/liter, phosphorus 1.74 mmol/liter, and total bilirubin 9 μmol/liter; 1,098 at 45 days, when calcium is 2.27 mmol/liter, phosphorus 1.49 mmol/liter, and total bilirubin 9 μmol/liter; 957 at 52 days; and 632 at 58 days.

Cortex of bones of legs is thickened at 42 days (Figure 2-1). Findings are similar in arms. Roentgenograms of chest show thickening of cortex of clavicles but not mandible at 25 days, thickening of cortex of ribs and humeri at 39 days.

Diagnosis: Prostaglandin E_1–induced cortical hyperostosis.

Fig. 2-1

Case 3

A 2⅔-year-old girl limps, cannot stand on tiptoes, and pushes herself up with arms when supine.

Birth weight was 4 kg. Light brown spots were on chest at 3 months. She sat at 6 months and began to walk at 10 months. Right heel was softer than left at 1½ years. She began to limp at 2⅓ years. Mother noticed that right leg was longer than left.

Mother (26 years old) and sister (6 years old) are well. Father (31 years old) has skin tags in right axilla, a tan spot (4 × 2 cm) below left scapula, a dark spot (2 × 1 cm) on right thigh, a hard subcutaneous lump on left thigh, and another lump on abdominal wall. A paternal aunt has five red-brown lumps on her arms and a small tan spot.

Weight at 2⅔ years is 14.5 kg, height 95 cm, head circumference 52 cm, temperature 37.6°C, heart rate 98, and respiratory rate 26. She has café au lait spots (up to 5 × 3 cm) on chest, freckles in both axilla, tan macules on thighs, and port-wine nevus on back of right ankle. Abdominal and leg muscles are weak. Right leg is 2 cm longer than left, right calf thinner than left. The rest of the physical findings are normal.

Hematocrit is 0.38. White cell count is 12.1×10^9/liter with 0.43 polymorphonuclear cells, 0.06 bands, 0.36 lymphocytes, 0.13 monocytes, and 0.02 basophils. Platelet estimate is adequate. Urine specific gravity is 1.026, pH 6. Urine has 1–2 red cells/HPF, 5–6 white cells/HPF, and occasional epithelial cells/HPF.

She reads at third-grade level at 11 years. Heart rate is 72, respiratory rate 16, and blood pressure 100/68 mm Hg. Eyes are normal. Coarse, thick hair is on left side of head. Right heel is soft and elephantine. Joints are hyperextensible. She has a lump on left side of head at 24 years. She can stand at work for 2 hours if she wears an elastic stocking on right leg.

Figure 3-1 shows right tibia and fibula longer than left, medially convex right tibia, and thickened soft tissues at right ankle at 7 years.

Diagnosis: Neurofibromatosis.

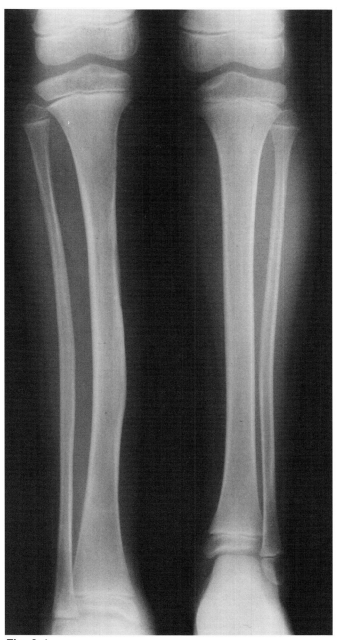

Fig. 3-1

Case 4

A 1-year-old boy cannot be aroused in postoperative recovery room.

Mother bled from vagina during pregnancy. He was born with bowed left shank and turned-in, deformed left foot. Operation was performed to provide a stump for prosthesis.

Mother (26 years old), father (29 years old), and sister (4 years old) are well.

Temperature is 37.4°C, heart rate 160, respiratory rate 35, weight 9.8 kg, and length 78 cm. Systolic blood pressure in arm is 200 mm Hg, in leg 108. Eyes wander. Systolic heart murmur and gallop rhythm are present. Hyperpigmented skin with a few dark papules is in diaper area. A bandage is on stump of left leg. The rest of the physical findings are normal.

Hematocrit is 0.35. White cell count is 9.9×10^9/liter with 0.74 polymorphonuclear cells, 0.09 bands, 0.13 lymphocytes, and 0.04 monocytes. Platelet estimate is normal. Urine sodium is 4 mmol/liter, potassium 48, chloride 5, and osmolality 608. Serum sodium is 139 mmol/liter, potassium 4.1, chloride 107, carbon dioxide 19, urea nitrogen 10.7, calcium 2.52, phosphorus 1.32, cholesterol 2.30, and glucose 11.3. Creatinine is 70 µmol/liter, uric acid 540, total bilirubin 7, and direct bilirubin 0. Total protein is 58 g/liter, albumin 43. Alkaline phosphatase is 499 U/liter, LDH 478, and SGOT 45.

ECG shows left ventricular hypertrophy; echocardiogram shows left ventricular hypertrophy and left atrial enlargement.

Roentgenogram at 7 weeks shows deformity of left shank and foot (Figure 4-1). Figure 4-2 shows large heart at 1 year, when aortogram in Figure 4-3 shows stenosis of abdominal aorta, celiac, superior mesenteric, and renal arteries, and no flow in inferior mesenteric artery. Left kidney is small.

Examination of arteriole in left foot shows proliferation of smooth muscle in intima. Biopsy of hyperpigmented skin shows epidermal hyperpigmentation.

Blood pressure remains high despite medicine. Oliguria results from too much medicine. Blood pressure is 180/120 mm Hg at 6 years. He has pain and tenderness above right lateral malleolus that begins at 7⅔ years and is still present 9 months later.

A defect in shaft of right fibula at 7 years, 11 months (Figure 4-4A) is larger at 8 years, 4 months (Figure 4-4B).

A large capillary hemangioma is on chest at 10 years. His sister (13 years old) has a hyperpigmented spot on right foot. His buttocks get numb when he walks at 12 years. Numbness sometimes goes down leg, is sometimes associated with urinary incontinence, and subsides with rest. Weight at 13 years is 44 kg, temperature is 37.2°C, heart rate 103, respiratory rate 24, and blood pressure 190/116 mm Hg. He has midline abdominal bruit, no femoral pulses, and scars on legs. Aorta-aorta, aorta-right renal artery, and aorta-superior mesenteric artery bypasses are performed. Left kidney is removed because left renal artery is occluded.

Diagnosis: Neurofibromatosis; arterial stenoses; congenital pseudoarthroses, left tibia and left fibula; pseudoarthrosis, right fibula.

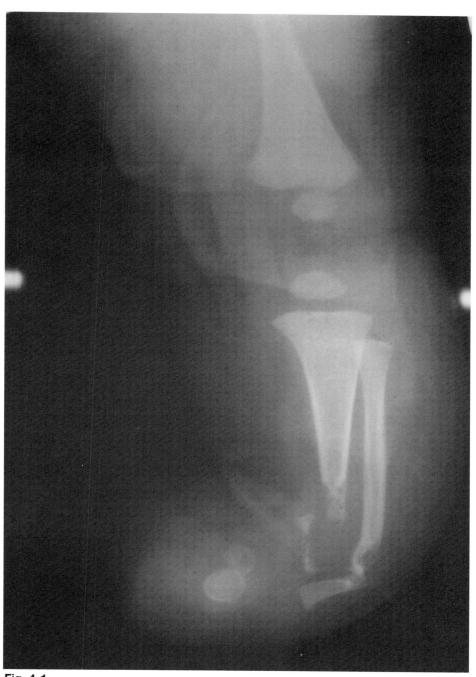

Fig. 4-1

(Continued)

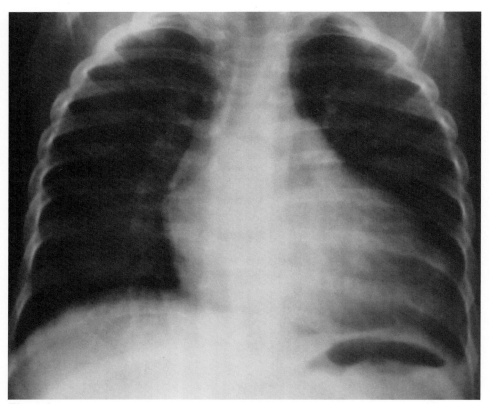

Fig. 4-2

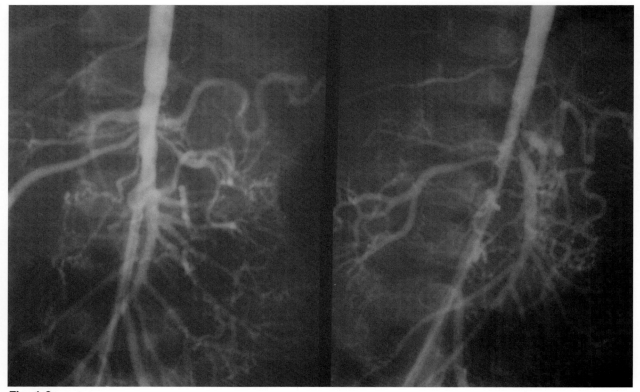

Fig. 4-3

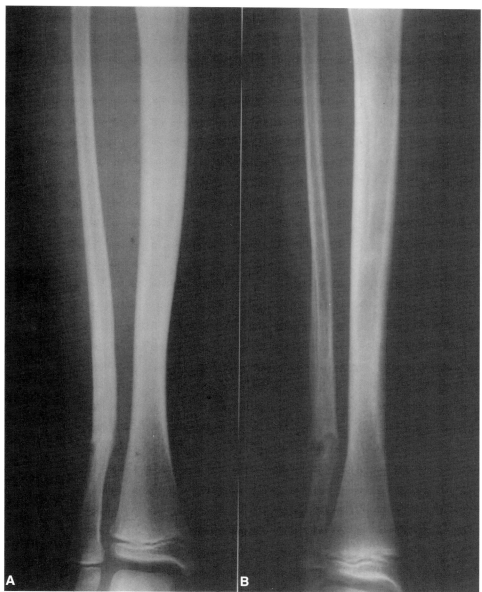

Fig. 4-4

Case 5

A 5½-year-old boy, who has limped since he started to walk, has had pain around right knee for the last 6 months when he walks a lot.

Pregnancy was normal, birth weight 2.9 kg. Brown spots with rough margins were on scalp and back at 1 month. He swung right leg out when he ran at 3 years.

Mother (35 years old), father, and sister (13 years old) are well. Brother (9 years old) has seizures. Two maternal aunts and two maternal cousins have brown spots.

Weight at 5½ years is 20.4 kg, height 113 cm, temperature 37.1°C, heart rate 104, respiratory rate 20, and blood pressure 106/58 mm Hg. Small dark spots are on scalp; larger spots, one as large as 10 × 9 cm, are on back. The rest of the physical findings are normal.

Hematocrit is 0.39. White cell count is 8.9×10^9/liter with 0.43 polymorphonuclear cells, 0.08 bands, 0.37 lymphocytes,

0.08 monocytes, 0.02 eosinophils, and 0.02 basophils. Platelet count is 395×10^9/liter.

Cystic defects are in neck of right femur at 3½ years (Figure 5-1A) and 5½ years (Figure 5-1B). He has an intertrochanteric fracture at 5½ years (see Figure 5-1B). Base of skull, including petrous part of right temporal bone, is sclerotic at 3½ years (Figure 5-2).

Biopsy of expanded right fibula at 4 years shows irregular bone trabeculae in odd patterns, with fibrous connective tissue between them and inside some of them, no rim of osteoblasts, and no lamination.

Diagnosis: Fibrous dysplasia, pathologic fracture.

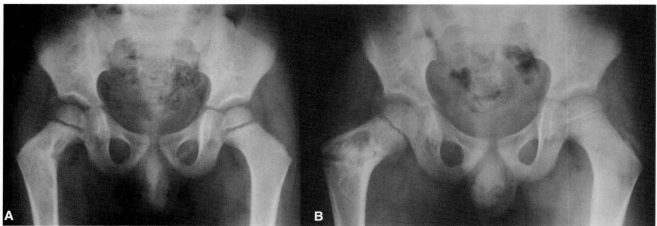

Fig. 5-1

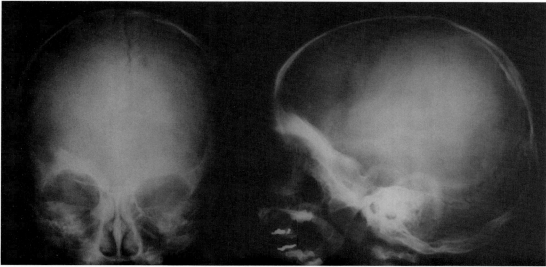

Fig. 5-2

Case 6

A 3-month-old boy has been fussy and has refused to eat for several days.

Mother bled from vagina during second trimester. Birth weight was 4 kg, length 53 cm, head circumference 36 cm, and Apgar score 8/9 at 1 and 5 minutes. He was "breast-feeding all the time." Weight was 4.5 kg at 6½ weeks. Face was chubby.

Mother, father, brother (6 years old), and sister (3 years old) are well. Mother has occasional swelling of airway, hands, and feet with stress.

Weight at 3 months is 4.6 kg, length 54 cm. Cheeks, neck, and insteps are fat. Liver edge is 1 cm below costal margin. Limbs are short, muscles weak. The rest of the physical findings are normal. Weight at 4 months is 4.6 kg, length 57 cm, temperature 37°C, heart rate 180, and blood pressure 68/54 mm Hg.

Serum sodium at 4 months is 134 mmol/liter, potassium 4.8, chloride 105, carbon dioxide 16, urea nitrogen 2.1, calcium 2.54, phosphorus 1.36, cholesterol 10.34, and glucose 5.1. Creatinine is 40 μmol/liter, uric acid 280, total bilirubin 14, and direct bilirubin 0. Total protein is 61 g/liter, albumin 34. Alkaline phosphatase is 759 U/liter, LDH 601, SGOT 388, SGPT 702, GGT 2,184, and CK 31. Serum is negative for hepatitis A, HBsAg, HBsAb, HBcAb, and hepatitis C antibody. No virus is isolated from urine. Serum adrenocorticotropic hormone is 0.7 and 0.4 pmol/liter (normal: 4–22). Cortisol is 520, 470, and 590 nmol/liter (normal: 30–660), 720 and 700 with low-dose dexamethasone suppression (80 μg q6h for 2 days), and 730 and 790 with high-dose suppression (320 μg q6h for 2 days). Urine cortisol is 180 and 160 nmol/day (normal: 6–74), 230 and 220 with low suppression, and 190 and 380 with high suppression.

CT scan at 4 months shows fat around adrenal glands (Figure 6-1).

At bilateral adrenalectomy at 7 months, size of adrenal glands is normal.

Right adrenal gland weighs 1.5 g, left 2.0. Cortical and medullary tissue is distinct and looks normal. Microscopic examination shows diffuse nodular prominence of zona fasciculata and zona reticularis with slight focal pigmentation and cellular atypia. Liver shows fatty infiltration.

He is treated with hydrocortisone and fludrocortisone.

Serum enzymes at 2 years are alkaline phosphatase 552 U/liter, LDH 473, SGOT 156, and GGT 1,100.

Weight at 3 years is 15.7 kg, height 91 cm. An operative scar is in upper abdomen. The rest of the physical findings are normal. Serum calcium is 2.82 mmol/liter, phosphorus 1.29, cholesterol 4.06. Total bilirubin is 10 μmol/liter, direct bilirubin 0. Alkaline phosphatase is 611 U/liter, LDH 430, and SGOT 277.

Proximal part of shaft of left humerus is rarefied and expanded at 3 years (Figure 6-2). Mineralization of neck of left femur is slightly irregular, and endosteal cortical thickening and slight lateral convexity are in distal part of shaft of left femur (Figure 6-3).

Diagnosis: Cushing's syndrome, diffuse nodular dysplasia of adrenal glands, chronic elevation of serum hepatocellular enzyme levels, McCune-Albright polyostotic fibrous dysplasia.

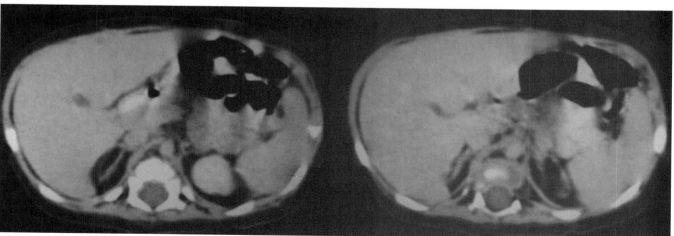

Fig. 6-1

(Continued)

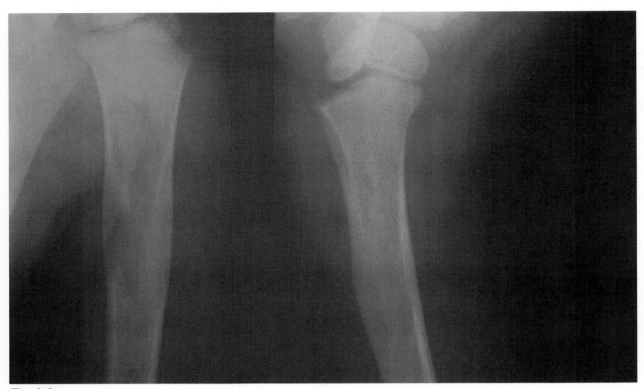

Fig. 6-2

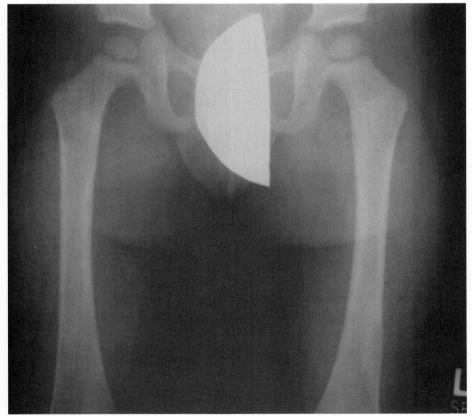

Fig. 6-3

Case 7

A 10-month-old boy has a bowed right shank.

Pregnancy was normal, birth weight 3.7 kg. Physical findings were normal. He hurt his right leg when he fell from a couch 3 weeks ago.

Mother and half sister (2 years old) are well. A sibling died at 7 months.

Right shank is convex forward. The rest of the physical findings are normal.

Hemoglobin is 93 g/liter. White cell count is 11.3×10^9/liter with 0.16 polymorphonuclear cells, 0.81 lymphocytes, 0.02 monocytes, and 0.01 basophils. ESR is 10 mm/hr.

Fracture and cystic defects are in bowed diaphysis of right tibia; a radiolucent growth arrest line is in its distal metaphysis (Figure 7-1).

Biopsy of right tibia above fracture shows long and broad trabeculae of woven bone covered by osteoblasts and separated by fibrous connective tissue.

Weight at 2 years is 13 kg, temperature 36.9°C, heart rate 96, respiratory rate 30, and systolic blood pressure 90 mm Hg. Right tibia is convex forward. The rest of the physical findings are normal.

Hematocrit at 2 years is 0.35. White cell count is 11.6×10^9/liter. Platelet count is 364×10^9/liter. Serum sodium is 136 mmol/liter, potassium 4.2, and chloride 107. Tibial osteotomy and external fixation are performed.

Diagnosis: Osteofibrous dysplasia, pathologic fracture, growth arrest line.

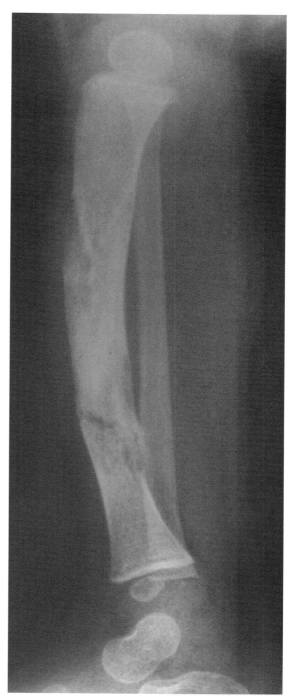

Fig. 7-1

Case 8

An 11-year-old boy has seizures during which he stiffens with arms flexed and fists clenched, stares, stops breathing for 30–40 seconds, and then is briefly confused.

Birth weight was 3.6 kg. He had seizures at 13 and 25 months. He did not talk until he was 4 years old. He could not button his clothes or tie his shoes at 8 years. He had 1- to 2-minute seizures during which he froze and stared, or turned his head from side to side and smacked his lips.

Mother (50 years old) has headaches. Father had narcolepsy and ichthyosis and died at 55 years with heart disease. Two sisters (24 and 27 years old) have ichthyosis. Paternal grandmother had ichthyosis and seizures.

Weight is 35.6 kg, height 140 cm, and blood pressure 110/60 mm Hg. Pimples are on cheeks and nose. Teeth are carious.

Limbs are dry and scaly. Back and arms are hairy. A depigmented patch (5 × 3 cm) is on right flank. Fingernail and end of fourth digit of right hand are broad. Deep tendon reflexes are hyperactive. Babinski's sign is in feet. The rest of the physical findings are normal.

Hematocrit is 0.37. White cell count is 6.9×10^9/liter with 0.43 polymorphonuclear cells, 0.16 bands, 0.36 lymphocytes, 0.02 monocytes, 0.02 eosinophils, and 0.01 basophils.

Figure 8-1 shows broad and long distal phalanx of right fourth digit, hooked tuberosity, enlarged end of finger, and slightly thickened cortex of fifth metacarpal bone.

Diagnosis: Tuberous sclerosis, subungual fibroma.

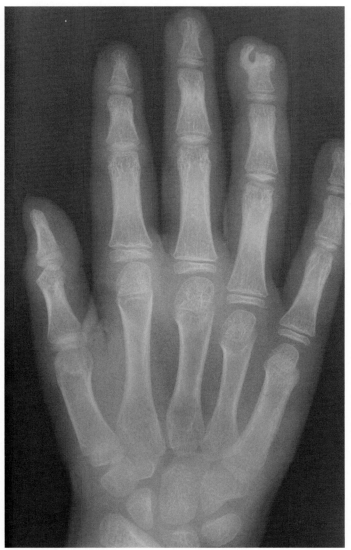

Fig. 8-1

Case 9

A 6-week-old girl has held right leg flexed at knee for 5 days. She cries whenever leg is moved or diapers are changed.

Parents and brother (2 years old) are well.

Pregnancy was normal, birth weight 3.0 kg. Pimply red spots were on face, head, back, and perineum; some were enlarged and filled with clear liquid, some ulcerated and formed scabs. Other spots cleared while new ones appeared. She began to cough and breathe noisily at 4 weeks. Abdomen got larger. Stools were streaked with blood.

Weight at 4 weeks was 4.3 kg, length 52 cm, temperature 36.2°C, heart rate 140, respiratory rate 72–90, systolic blood pressure 90 mm Hg, and head circumference 37 cm. Sores were on gums, mucous membranes, body, and limbs. The largest (1 cm) was on right labium majus. Some sores were crusted; some contained pus or blood. Many small sores (3–4 mm) were umbilicated. Palms and soles were free of sores. Liver edge and spleen edge were 4 cm below costal margin. Blood was in rectum. The rest of the physical findings were normal.

Hematocrit at 4 weeks was 0.27. White cell count was 11.2 × 10⁹/liter with 0.30 polymorphonuclear cells, 0.08 bands, 0.56 lymphocytes, 0.05 monocytes, and 0.01 eosinophils. Platelet count was 397 × 10⁹/liter. Urine specific gravity was 1.003, pH 5. Urine was normal. Serum sodium was 138 mmol/liter, potassium 4.6, chloride 108, carbon dioxide 22, urea nitrogen 4.3, calcium 2.57, phosphorus 1.81, cholesterol 2.35, and glucose 5.4. Creatinine was 20 μmol/liter, uric acid 240, total

bilirubin 9, and direct bilirubin 2. Total protein was 53 g/liter, albumin 36. Alkaline phosphatase was 285 U/liter, LDH 301, and SGOT 33.

An ulcer was Tzanck positive for multinucleated giant cells. Labial ulcer was dark-field negative for spirochetes. VDRL and rapid plasma reagent tests for syphilis were negative. Toxoplasma IFA-IgM test and rubella IgM (enzyme immunoassay) tests were negative. Cytomegalovirus complement fixation titer and herpes simplex virus complement fixation titer were <1:8. Stool tested positive for rotavirus by enzyme immunoassay.

Proctosigmoidoscopic examination showed small ulcers. Biopsy of an ulcer showed (1) infiltrates of large histiocytes with irregular, indented nuclei and prominent nucleoli; (2) plasma cells; (3) eosinophils; and (4) small lymphocytes.

Distal part of right femur is expanded posteromedially (Figure 9-1A). T5 vertebral body is flat (Figure 9-1B).

Punch biopsy of a sore shows large round histiocytes with eosinophilic cytoplasm and eccentric, kidney-shaped nuclei. Electron microscopy shows macrophage-like cells that have Langerhans' cell granules. Biopsy of right femur shows clot, histiocytes, and eosinophils.

Diagnosis: Infection with herpes simplex virus type I, Langerhans' cell histiocytosis, Calvé's vertebra plana.

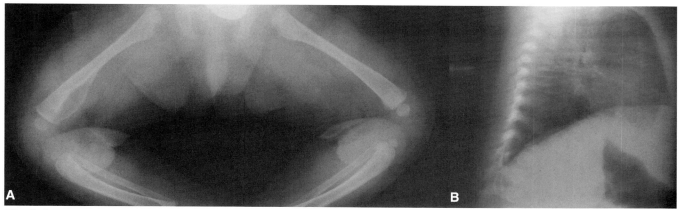

Fig. 9-1

Case 10

A 4-year-old boy wakes up at night with pain in right thigh and has a limp that was barely perceptible 6 weeks ago, obvious 2 weeks ago.

Parents and sister (7 months old) are well.

Temperature is 37°C, heart rate 120, respiratory rate 20, blood pressure 90/58 mm Hg, weight 16.1 kg, and height 103 cm. Physical findings are normal.

Hematocrit is 0.40. White cell count is 8.5 × 10⁹/liter. Platelet count is 472 × 10⁹/liter. Serum sodium is 140 mmol/liter, potassium 4.3, chloride 107, carbon dioxide 21, urea nitrogen 3.6, calcium 2.47, phosphorus 1.55, cholesterol 5.30, and glucose 6.8. Creatinine is 40 μmol/liter, uric acid 110, total bilirubin 3, and direct bilirubin 0. Total protein is 64 g/liter, albumin 45. Alkaline phosphatase is 292 U/liter, LDH 223, and SGOT 33.

Laminated new bone is around a defect in shaft of right femur, and entry point for nutrient artery is in center of defect (Figure 10-1).

At operation, dark gray matter is in medulla of right femur.

Microscopic examination shows (1) many histiocytes, some with notched and grooved nuclei; (2) polymorphonuclear cells; (3) eosinophils; (4) lymphocytes; (5) hemorrhage; (6) scattered multinucleated giant cells; and (7) new and old bone. Electron microscopy shows (1) many cytoplasmic liposomes, mitochondria, and projections; (2) inconspicuous cell junctions; and (3) no Birbeck granules.

Diagnosis: Langerhans' cell histiocytosis.

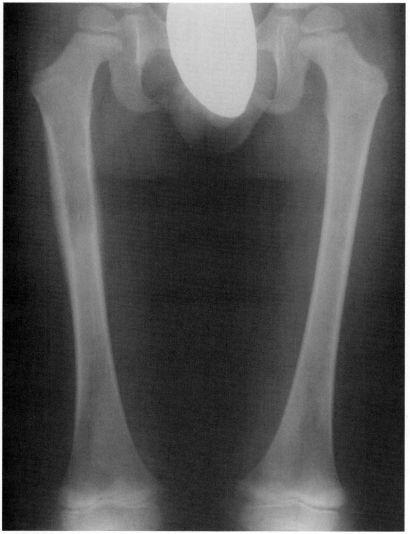

Fig. 10-1

Case 11

An 11-year-old boy has painless lumps on some fingers that have not changed since he noticed them 15 months ago. He fractured proximal phalanx of left fourth finger several years ago.

Left fingers diverge when he grips tightly. Movement at wrists is normal. The rest of the physical findings in arms and hands are normal.

"Scooped-out" defects are in phalanges of left third finger and proximal and middle phalanges of left fourth finger (Figure 11-1). Left third metacarpal bone is shorter and broader than right (see Figure 11-1). A defect is in the shortened, broadened left ulna (Figure 11-2).

Diagnosis: Enchondromas of phalanges, metacarpal, and ulna.

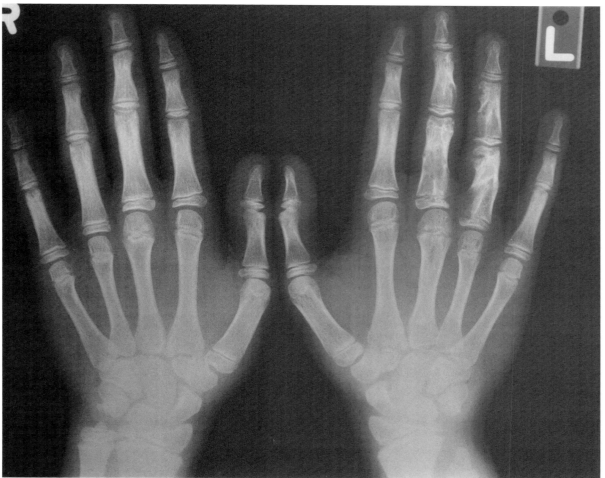

Fig. 11-1

(Continued)

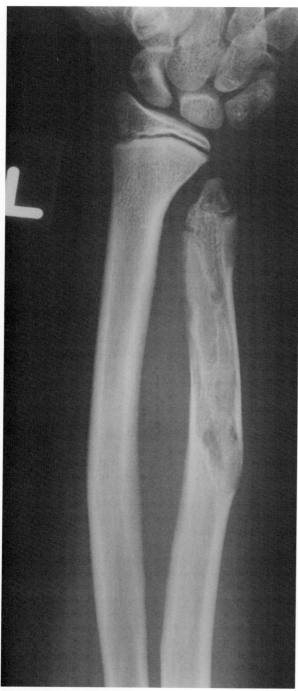

Fig. 11-2

Case 12

An 11-year-old girl, who has limped since age 3 years, has had pain in left leg for 3 months.

Weight is 25.5 kg, height 137 cm, temperature 37.1°C, heart rate 68, respiratory rate 20, and blood pressure 110/68 mm Hg. Dark, deep induration is along medial side of left leg from groin to instep. Left ankle is tender. Left ankle and foot are stiff and swollen. Distance from anterior superior iliac spine to medial malleolus is 79 cm on right, 73 on left. Maximal circumference of right calf is 29.5 cm, left calf 20. The rest of the physical findings are normal.

Hematocrit is 0.38. White cell count is 7.9×10^9/liter with 0.72 polymorphonuclear cells, 0.01 bands, 0.19 lymphocytes, and 0.08 monocytes. Urine specific gravity is 1.007, reaction acid. Urine has trace albumin, 5–7 white cells/HPF, and 5–7 epithelial cells/HPF. Serum calcium is 2.52 mmol/liter, phosphorus 1.29, urea nitrogen 5.0, cholesterol 4.14, and glucose 3.9. Uric acid is 210 µmol/liter, total

bilirubin 5, and direct bilirubin 0. Total protein is 73 g/liter, albumin 46. Alkaline phosphatase is 230 U/liter, LDH 190, and SGOT 20.

Roentgenogram shows defects in left os calcis at 3 years (Figure 12-1A) and disappearing bones in left leg and foot and bend at fracture of tibia at 11 years (Figure 12-1B).

Biopsy of left os calcis at 3 years shows (1) bone; (2) fatty marrow; (3) fibrous connective tissue; and (4) many varyingly dilated vascular channels with single layer of normal, flat epithelium, some with red blood cells, other with thick muscular walls.

Below-knee amputation is performed, and she is given prosthesis.

Diagnosis: Hemangiomas, Gorham-Stout disappearing bone disease, pathologic fracture.

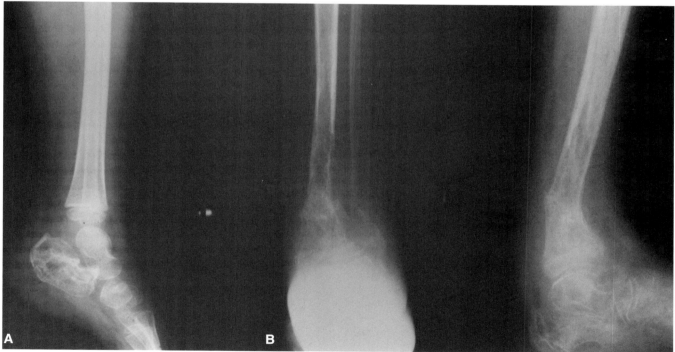

Fig. 12-1

Case 13

A 12-year-old girl has had a backache for several months. Scoliosis was found when she went to school nurse because of ache.

Weight is 41 kg, height 163 cm, heart rate 100, respiratory rate 20, and blood pressure 100/70 mm Hg. A firm, non-tender mass is in left side of abdomen. Lumbar spine is convex right. The rest of the physical findings are normal.

Hematocrit is 0.38.

Body of L3 is flattened, elongated, and cystic (Figure 13-1). Ultrasound examination shows a cyst without internal echoes and a track to spine. CT scan shows an avascular cyst separate from kidney and spleen and contiguous to a defect in body of L3 (Figure 13-2).

At operation, a cyst with serous, straw-colored liquid in left retroperitoneum between spleen and pelvic brim pushes transverse colon downward and left ureter laterally. Cyst extends into body of L3, where contiguous discs can be felt. Cyst is removed, L3 packed with bone chips from left ilium.

Cyst wall is pink to tan to brown fibromembranous tissue (0.1–0.6 cm thick) and contains firm nodules. Microscopic examination shows (1) bland, mature connective tissue; (2) lymphoid follicles with germinal centers; and (3) small spaces that are lined by thin endothelium and contain amorphous eosinophilic material, aggregates of mature lymphocytes, hemorrhagic foci, and no giant cells.

Diagnosis: Lymphangioma.

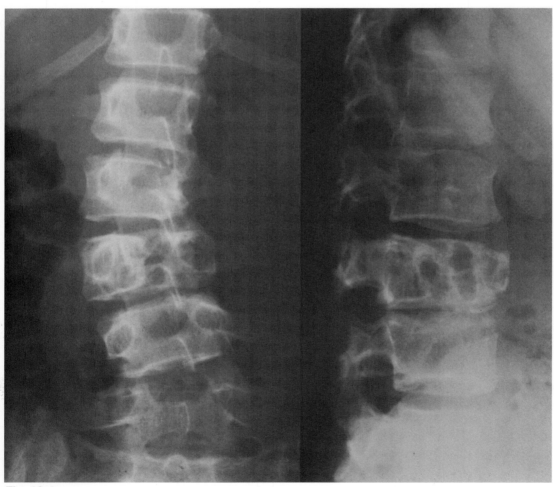

Fig. 13-1

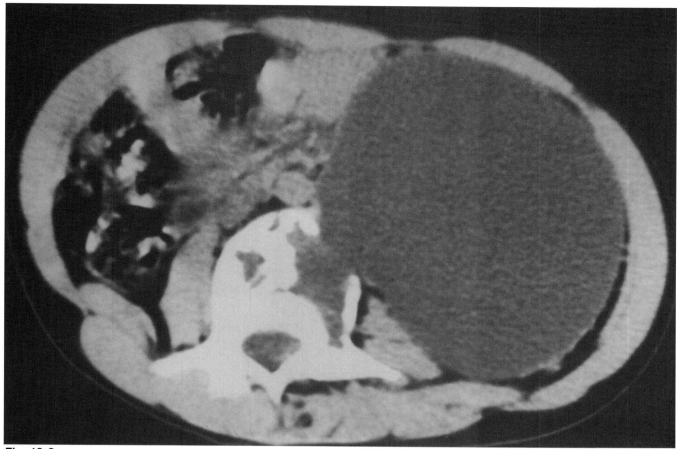

Fig. 13-2

Case 14

A 12-day-old boy has lumps on cheek, back, and hip.

Mother bled from vagina during fourth month of pregnancy. Birth weight was 2.2 kg. The lumps, present at birth, are now larger.

Mother (21 years old) and father (20 years old) are well. The boy is their only child.

Weight is 2.3 kg. A firm, mobile lump (1-cm diameter) is on left cheek, a cystic lump (2.5 × 1.5 cm) on back, and a firm lump (1-cm diameter) over left greater trochanter.

Weight at 4 weeks is 2.9 kg, length 54 cm, head circumference 36 cm, temperature 37.2°C, heart rate 168, respiratory rate 56, and systolic blood pressure 74 mm Hg. A hard lump (2-cm diameter) is on left cheek, a lump is on chest, four lumps are on back, a lump is over left greater trochanter, and a lump is in each thigh. The lumps are firm, fixed, and nontender. He has systolic heart murmur and diastolic heart murmur. The rest of the physical findings are normal. ECG findings are normal.

Hematocrit at 4 weeks is 0.43. White cell count is 15.3 × 10^9/liter with 0.25 polymorphonuclear cells, 0.10 bands, 0.40 lymphocytes, 0.19 monocytes, 0.04 eosinophils, 0.01 basophils, and 0.01 myelocytes. Urine specific gravity is 1.003, pH 6. Urine has occasional white cells/HPF and bacteria. Serum sodium is 141 mmol/liter, potassium 6.6, chloride 111, carbon dioxide 21, urea nitrogen 1.0, calcium 2.50, phosphorus 2.00, cholesterol 1.81, and glucose 4.5. Creatinine is 50 μmol/liter, uric acid 190, total bilirubin 20, and direct bilirubin 5. Total protein is 48 g/liter, albumin 35. Alkaline phosphatase is 309 U/liter, LDH 444, and SGOT 39.

Defects in proximal humeral and both ulnar metaphyses of right arm at 12 days are about the same size at 1 month (Figure 14-1A) and larger at 5 months (Figure 14-1B). Right acromion and part of right fourth rib are expanded at 5 months. Defects are at proximal metaphyses of left humerus and left ulna at 5 months. Similar defects that were small at 12 days in femurs and tibias are larger at 5 months (Figure 14-2). Defects are in innominate bones (see Figure 14-2) and calvaria (Figure 14-3) at 5 months, and body of L4 is collapsed (Figure 14-4).

Microscopic examination of pale gray, firm, fixed lump (1.0 × 0.8 × 0.3 cm), removed from subcutaneous tissue and muscle

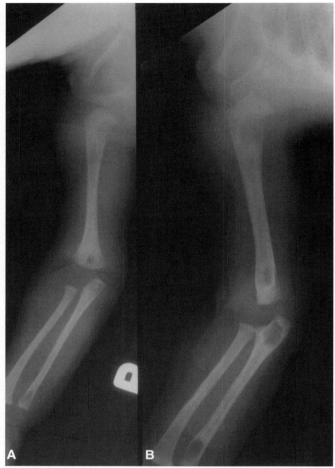

Fig. 14-1

of right side of chest at 1 month, shows (1) aggregates of oval to spindle cells with little cytoplasm, oval to spindle vesicular nuclei, and nucleoli; (2) bands of spindle cells; (3) thick walled vascular channels; (4) necrosis; (5) focal hyalinization; and (6) up to 3 mitoses/HPF.

Three more lumps and no heart murmur are present at 2 months. He is well and without lumps at 1 year.

Diagnosis: Multicentric infantile myofibromatosis.

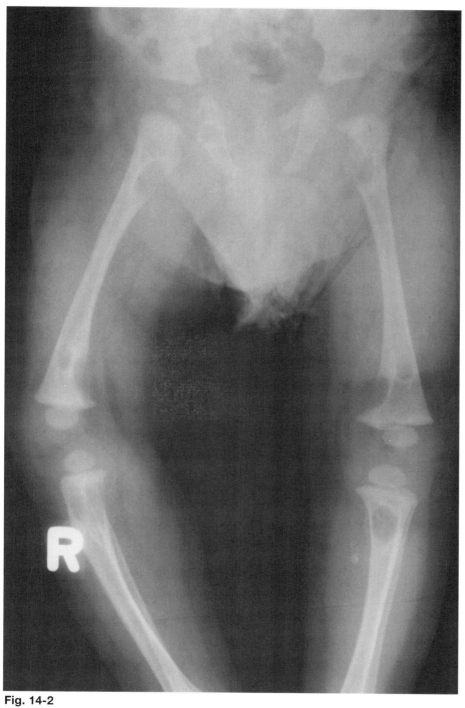

Fig. 14-2

(Continued)

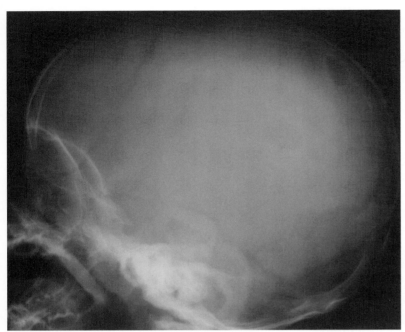

Fig. 14-3

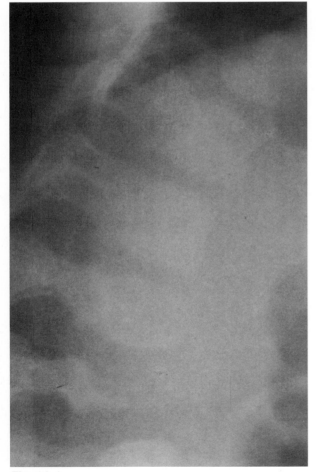

Fig. 14-4

Case 15

A 6-year-old boy has occasionally limped on left leg for several months.

Omphalocele was repaired soon after birth, right inguinal hernia at 1 month. Operation for intestinal obstruction was performed at 3 years.

Temperature at 6 years is 36.2°C, heart rate 76, respiratory rate 24, blood pressure 97/58 mm Hg, weight 18.9 kg, and height 111 cm. Scars are on abdomen. The rest of the physical findings are normal.

Hematocrit is 0.36.

A septate defect is in neck of left femur and proximal part of shaft of left femur (Figure 15-1). Cyst is farther from growth plate in roentgenogram 4 years later.

After 10 ml serosanguineous liquid is aspirated from cyst, contrast medium flows throughout cyst. Methylprednisolone is injected into cyst at 6 years.

He limps occasionally 4 years later. Physical findings at left hip are normal.

Diagnosis: Unicameral (simple) bone cyst.

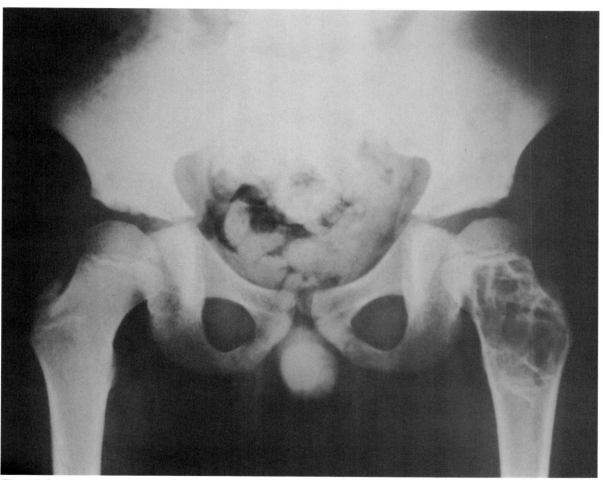

Fig. 15-1

Case 16

A 10-year-old boy has a tumor in right radius that was found 5 months ago, when he fell and broke his arm.

Temperature is 36.1°C, heart rate 76, respiratory rate 24, blood pressure 98/60 mm Hg, weight 33 kg, and height 139 cm. Distal part of right forearm is enlarged, firm, and non-tender. Flexion and extension at right wrist are limited. The rest of the physical findings are normal.

Hematocrit is 0.39. White cell count is 6.8×10^9/liter. Platelet count is 374×10^9/liter. Urine specific gravity is 1.027, pH 6. Urine is normal.

An expanded defect that thins cortex and abuts growth plate is in metaphysis and shaft of right radius (Figure 16-1A).

Right carpal bones are rarefied in Figure 16-1A. Angiogram shows twigs of common interosseous artery around defect and no neovascularity or early draining veins (Figure 16-1B).

Biopsy shows (1) cysts filled with blood and stained with hemosiderin, (2) osteoid trabeculae, (3) normal mitoses, (4) multinucleated giant cells, and (5) inflammatory cells on a fibrous background.

Treatment is with curettage and iliac bone autograft.

Diagnosis: Aneurysmal bone cyst.

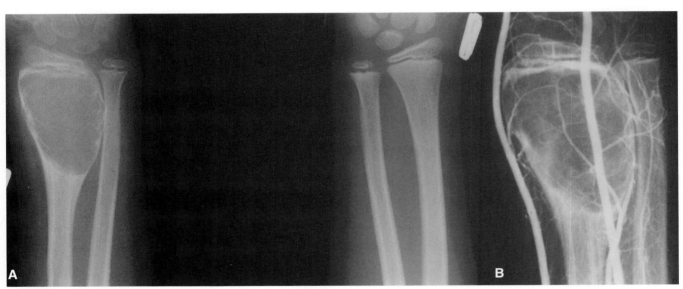

Fig. 16-1

Case 17

A 14-year-old boy has pain in left shin that began several months ago, is worse after exercise, wakes him up crying at night, and forced him from karate class 2 weeks ago.

He wheezed from ages 5 to 10 years. Adenoids were removed at 4 years. A nevus in right groin was excised and left inguinal hernia repaired at 9 years.

Lower right tibia has a tender 5-cm swelling. The rest of the physical findings in right shank are normal.

Hematocrit is 0.39. White cell count is 6.3×10^9/liter. Platelet count is 238×10^9/liter. ESR is 3 mm/hr.

Figure 17-1 shows sclerotic thickening in front part of distal left tibia.

Pain is relieved by nonsteroidal anti-inflammatory drugs, such as aspirin, and even more by ibuprofen during next 7 months. His school work deteriorates.

Weight at 15 years is 54 kg, height 167 cm, temperature 36.4°C, heart rate 62, respiratory rate 20, and blood pressure 100/74 mm Hg. Left tibia is thickened by a firm, nontender swelling (2 cm) centered 13 cm above ankle. The rest of the physical findings are normal.

At operation, removal of swollen bone by means of drill holes and bone cutter exposes a vascular nidus surrounded by sclerotic bone. Bone fragments from left ilium are packed in defect in left tibia.

Diagnosis: Osteoid osteoma.

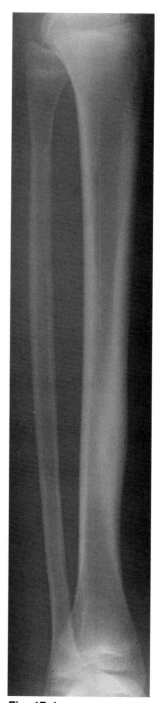

Fig. 17-1

Case 18

A 6-year-old girl has had pain in left arm for 4 months.

Temperature is 35.9°C, heart rate 96, respiratory rate 24, blood pressure 80/58 mm Hg, and weight 27.5 kg. A hard, tender swelling is along anterolateral aspect of left humerus. The rest of the physical findings are normal.

Hematocrit is 0.40. White cell count is 5.3×10^9/liter. Platelet count is 361×10^9/liter.

A fusiform expansion with thinned cortex, slight radiolucency, and trabecular irregularity is in midpart of left humerus (Figure 18-1).

Specimen obtained by needle aspiration shows (1) degenerated chondroid tumor of blue myxoid debris, (2) pyknotic nuclei, (3) abnormal cartilage surrounded by myxoid tissue, and (4) sheets of uniform round cells with small dark nuclei and abundant cytoplasm. Contents of medullary canal bulge when cortex is cut through at operation. Vascular, gelatinous tumor has (1) trabeculae of new bone; (2) cellular fibrous tissue; (3) myxoid lobules of uniform cells with dark, small, round nuclei and stellate tapering of eosinophilic cytoplasm; and (4) foci that suggest formation of cartilage.

Diagnosis: Chondromyxoid fibroma.

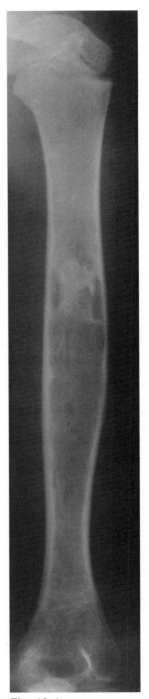

Fig. 18-1

Case 19

A 17-year-old boy has a right knee ache. It was sporadic when it started 2 months ago; it has been constant for 3 weeks. Ache is mostly at medial condyle of femur, but sometimes extends up the leg.

Temperature is 36.6°C, heart rate 88, respiratory rate 16, blood pressure 130/80 mm Hg, weight 64 kg, and height 183 cm. Right knee joint is full, its circumference 0.5 cm more than left. Right medial condyle is tender. Right knee is held slightly flexed. Flexion and extension of right knee are painful. The rest of the physical findings are normal.

Hematocrit is 0.42. White cell count is 7.8×10^9/liter with 0.50 polymorphonuclear cells, 0.14 bands, 0.26 lymphocytes, 0.05 monocytes, 0.04 eosinophils, and 0.01 basophils. ESR is 12 mm/hr. Urine specific gravity is 1.023, pH 7. Urine has few squamous epithelial cells/HPF.

Figure 19-1 shows a small, bubblelike radiolucency spanning medial side of femoral growth plate and a defect higher in diaphysis that is more sclerotic along its upper edge than lower edge.

A yellow-white mass (0.5 × 0.5 cm) erodes epiphyseal surface at operation.

Microscopic examination of the rubbery, translucent white specimen shows a cellular tumor of (1) closely packed polygonal or rounded cells with a distinct border in most areas, slightly basophilic cytoplasm, small clear vacuoles, rounded nuclei with granular chromatin, nucleoli, some nuclear pleomorphism with uniform staining characteristics; (2) few mitoses; (3) wide intercellular bands of eosinophilic cartilage; and (4) many multinucleated giant cells.

Diagnosis: Benign chondroblastoma at physis, benign cortical defect in diaphysis.

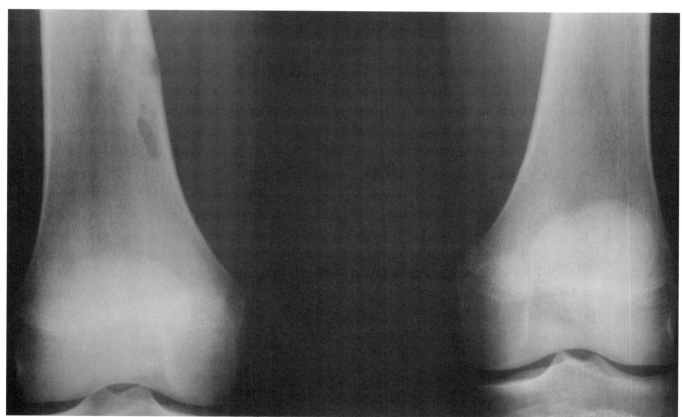

Fig. 19-1

Case 20

A 16-year-old girl has pain and swelling at right knee that began 10 months ago. She likes to dance but is now on crutches.

Tonsils were removed at 12 years.

Father has porphyria.

Temperature is 36.5°C, heart rate 72, respiratory rate 20, blood pressure 96/68 mm Hg, weight 53 kg, and height 168 cm. A swelling (2.0 × 1.5 cm) is along lateral aspect of right tibia just below knee. The rest of the physical findings are normal.

Hematocrit is 0.41. White cell count is 6.8 × 10⁹/liter. Platelet count is 337 × 10⁹/liter. Serum sodium is 139 mmol/liter, potassium 4.4, chloride 103, carbon dioxide 28, urea nitrogen 2.9, calcium 2.42, phosphorus 1.26, cholesterol 3.18, and glucose 4.1. Creatinine is 60 μmol/liter, uric acid 180, total bilirubin 17, and direct bilirubin 3. Total protein is 70 g/liter, albumin 45. Alkaline phosphatase is 122 U/liter, LDH 136, and SGOT 14.

A defect, in which bone trabeculae are effaced in proximal metaphysis and diaphysis of right tibia, occupies all but a narrow, medial strip and is covered by a thin, displaced layer of subperiosteal new bone (Figure 20-1). Delayed bone scan shows increased uptake above and below right knee (Figure 20-2A). CT scan shows expanded defect in tibia (Figure 20-2B).

At operation, soft, dark brown matter deep to periosteum is removed from right tibia and replaced by autologous "matchstick" graft from right ilium. She is dancing 1 year later and well 4 years later.

Microscopic examination shows (1) blood vessels, (2) extravasated blood, (3) foci of osteoid, (4) rare foci of necrosis, (5) stromal cells with round to spindle-shaped nuclei, (6) few mitoses, and (7) scattered giant cells, some quite large with almost countless nuclei.

Diagnosis: Giant cell tumor.

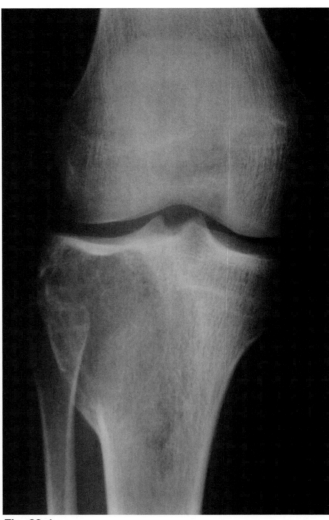

Fig. 20-1

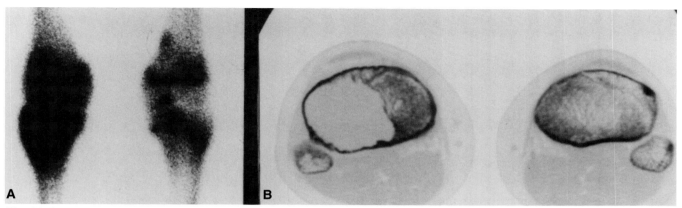

Fig. 20-2

Case 21

A 7-year-old girl has had pain in left knee since she fell on it yesterday. Right knee hurt 1 year ago. Pressure on right patella then caused crepitus.

Weight is 28 kg, height 130 cm. A scar is on forehead. Left knee is tender. The rest of the physical findings are normal.

Front of right femur is scalloped (Figure 21-1A). Roentgenographic findings at left knee are normal (Figure 21-1B).

Diagnosis: Juxtacortical chondroma, distal right femur.

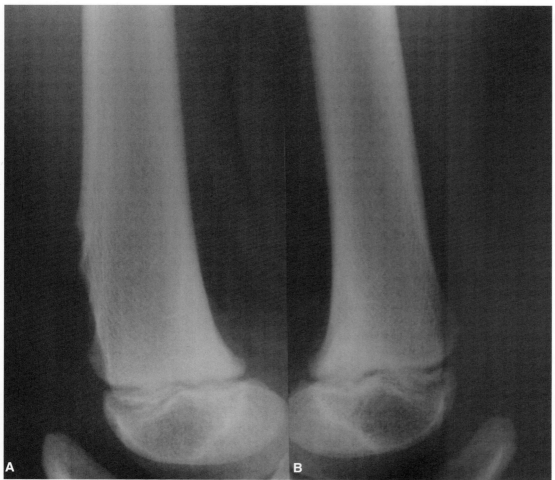

Fig. 21-1

Case 22

An 8-year-old boy has pain at left hip that was brief 1½ years ago, is more frequent now, and lasts for 1 hour or more after activity.

Weight is 25.6 kg, temperature 36°C, heart rate 78, respiratory rate 18, and blood pressure 110/55 mm Hg. Flexion at left hip is slightly limited, internal rotation slightly painful. The rest of the physical findings are normal.

Hematocrit is 0.42. White cell count is 6.0×10^9/liter with 0.41 polymorphonuclear cells, 0.02 bands, 0.40 lymphocytes, 0.12 monocytes, 0.02 eosinophils, and 0.03 basophils. Alkaline phosphatase is 152 U/liter, LDH 203.

Left femur is displaced laterally from acetabulum, and radiolucent defects are in body of left ischium (Figure 22-1). T1-weighted MRI shows low-signal matter with signal voids in it at left hip (Figure 22-2A). T2-weighted MRI shows high-signal matter with signal voids in left hip (Figure 22-2B).

Arthroscopy shows proliferation of diffusely pigmented synovium at left hip.

Biopsy shows acutely and chronically inflamed synovium with deposits of hemosiderin in papillary outgrowths of synovium.

Diagnosis: Pigmented villonodular synovitis, left hip.

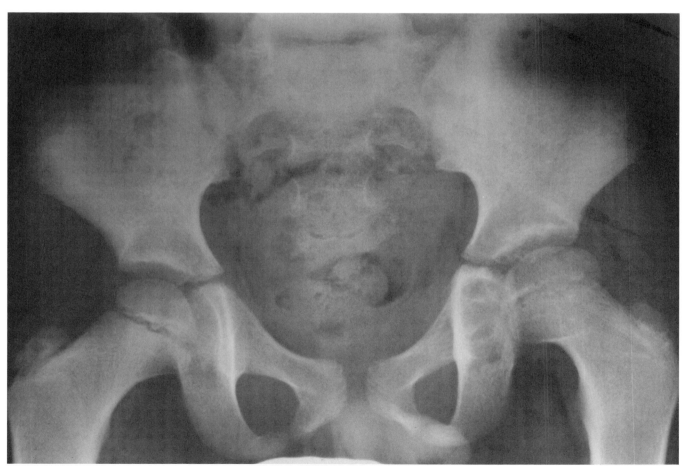

Fig. 22-1

(Continued)

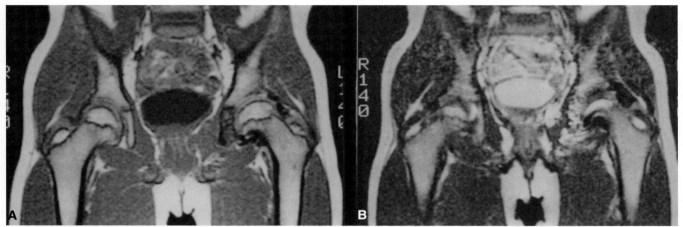

Fig. 22-2

Case 23

A 7-year-old boy has swelling of left buttock that was noticed by his mother 1 week ago while he was getting out of the bathtub.

Left fifth toe has been swollen for several weeks. Left foot hurt for a while after he hit it on a chair at 5½ years. He has had three operations for cross-eyes. Tonsils and adenoids were removed 2 years ago.

Weight at 7 years is 23.8 kg, height 122 cm, temperature 36.2°C, heart rate 96, respiratory rate 24, and blood pressure 100/60 mm Hg. A firm, nontender mass (12 × 10 × 8 cm) is in left buttock. Proximal half of left fifth toe is swollen. The rest of the physical findings are normal.

Hematocrit is 0.39.

CT scan shows a mass in left gluteus maximus muscle (Figure 23-1A).

At operation on left buttock, a firm, gritty tumor in gluteus maximus muscle is excised.

Microscopic examination of encapsulated gray-white to yellow tumor shows whorls and random, interlacing bands of fibrous tissue that contain cells that have ill-defined, eosinophilic cytoplasm; some cells have elongated-to-spindled, pleomorphic nuclei, some have plump, monomorphic nuclei in amphophilic stroma. Bands of fibrous tumor infiltrate surrounding fat. Mitoses are few.

Left fifth toe begins to hurt 3 months after its swelling appears. Gait is normal 6 months after swelling. A firm, tender mass (2 × 1 cm) is on the toe.

A defect is in proximal phalanx of left fifth toe (Figure 23-1B). Soft-tissue swelling is approximately the same size as it was 6 months earlier.

At operation, gritty tumor over proximal phalanx extends slightly beyond joint at either end and surrounds extensor tendon.

Microscopic findings in the mottled tan and yellow tumor of toe are like those of buttock.

Diagnosis: Benign musculoaponeurotic fibromatosis (desmoid tumor) of buttock and toe.

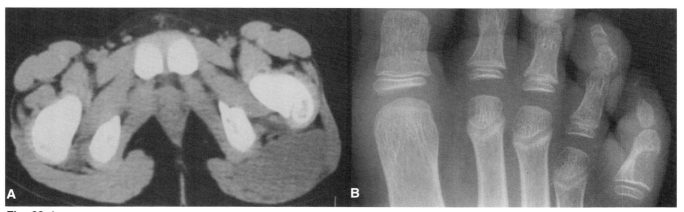

Fig. 23-1

Case 24

A 10½-year-old girl has had pain at right knee since she was kicked there 3 weeks ago. Right leg hurts when she straightens it or stands too long.

She has had roseola and chickenpox. She had pneumonia at 7 years, and a concussion at 9 years.

Mother (30 years old), father (32 years old), brother (13 years old), and two sisters (2 and 12 years old) are well.

Weight is 22 kg, height 130 cm, temperature 36.7°C, heart rate 84, respiratory rate 16, and blood pressure 120/80 mm Hg. Medial side of right leg just above knee is red, swollen, warm, and tender. The rest of the physical findings are normal.

Hematocrit is 0.42. White cell count is 9.6×10^9/liter with 0.50 polymorphonuclear cells, 0.44 lymphocytes, 0.05 monocytes, and 0.01 eosinophils. Platelet count is 500×10^9/liter. ESR is 5 mm/hr. Urine specific gravity is 1.016, pH 5. Urine has occasional squamous epithelial cells/HPF, occasional white cells/HPF, and bacteria. Serum sodium is 147 mmol/liter, potassium 4.0, chloride 101, urea nitrogen 6.4, and glucose 6.3. Alkaline phosphatase is 100 U/liter.

A defect in distal medial part of right femur with irregular margin in diaphysis and epiphyseal ossification center is associated with amorphous bits of bone in defect and in adjacent swollen soft tissues (Figure 24-1A). Lateral view shows these findings as well as cortical new bone.

Biopsy shows (1) friable white mass of densely cellular nests; (2) bizarre mitoses separated by disorganized eosinophilic staining osteoid, fat, and hemorrhage; (3) spicules of dead bone; (4) fibroblastic spindle cells; (5) chondroblast-like cells in poorly organized cartilage matrix; and (5) giant cells with dark eosinophilic cytoplasm and many small round nuclei.

Right leg is disarticulated at hip and removed 5 months after treatment is begun.

Microscopic examination of femur shows (1) whorls, strands, and clumps of spindle- and tadpole-shaped anaplastic cells with indistinct margins, little eosinophilic cytoplasm, pleomorphic hyperchromatic nuclei with prominent membrane and occasional nucleoli; (2) necrosis; (3) fibrosis; (4) granulation tissue; and (5) no mitoses.

Left upper lobe is atelectatic at 11 years, 7 months. She has dull ache in right side of abdomen at 12 years that suddenly worsens several weeks later. She cannot move, eat, or sleep. It hurts to urinate. Temperature is 37.8–38.3°C. She is hairless. Rales are in lungs. A firm mass (10×7 cm) is in right side of abdomen.

Shadows of water density are in lungs. Air is in left pleural space. A mass with calcium in it displaces gut from right side of abdomen (Figure 24-1B).

She convulses and dies at 12 years, 3 months. Necropsy shows (1) blood and blood clot in abdomen; (2) crumbly calcified tumor in mesentery near cecum; (3) tumor attached to small bowel, diaphragm, and aorta; (4) tumor in lungs and on pleura; (5) pericardial effusion; and (6) pleural hemorrhage and adhesions. Microscopic examination of mesenteric tumor shows (1) pleomorphic cells with little cytoplasm, hyperchromatic nuclei, and rare mitoses; (2) osteoid; and (3) calcification.

Diagnosis: Osteosarcoma.

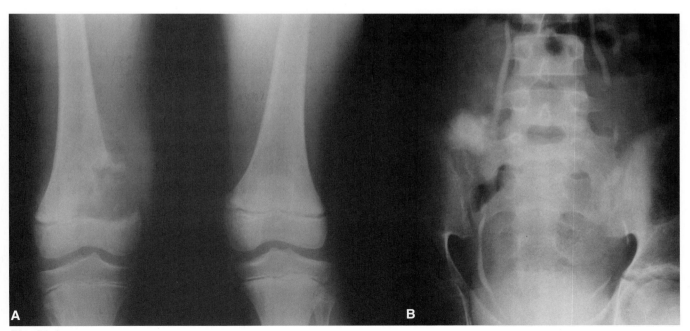

A   B

Fig. 24-1

Case 25

A 15-year-old boy cannot completely flex his right knee and has had pain for 4 or 5 months when he flexes it more than 90 degrees. He plays ball. He does not limp.

Temperature is 36.5°C, heart rate 72, respiratory rate 18, blood pressure 102/68 mm Hg, and weight 76.2 kg. He can jump on either leg. Flexion at right knee hurts behind knee and stops at 95 degrees. A firm, fixed, nontender mass (4-cm diameter) is in right popliteal fossa. The rest of the physical findings are normal.

Hematocrit is 0.42. White cell count is 5.1×10^9/liter. Serum sodium is 142 mmol/liter, potassium 4.3, chloride 106, carbon dioxide 27, urea nitrogen 5.0, calcium 2.32, phosphorus 1.03, cholesterol 3.67, and glucose 5.1. Creatinine is 90 μmol/liter, uric acid 240, total bilirubin 9, and direct bilirubin 2. Total protein is 69 g/liter, albumin 45. Alkaline phosphatase is 292 U/liter, LDH 179, and SGOT 20.

An irregular, fragmented mass of bone with cortical thickening, much of it endosteal, is behind distal part of shaft of right femur (Figure 25-1).

At operation, a soft, multilobed mass in right popliteal fossa has bone at base and glistening capsule. Three large mobile fragments look like benign fibrous tissue. Base is attached by bone to cortex of femur between condyles. Hard gray fragments are removed from soft attachments at base. Soft white translucent pieces of cartilage, with hard, white to gray fragments between them, are near apex.

Microscopic examination shows benign reactive fibrous tissue at apex. Tumor is multinodular with interlacing bands of connective tissue and consists of (1) fibrocartilage of loose matrix and bland nuclei; (2) foci of osteoid with round, pale, basophilic nuclei that show little atypia; (3) mature hyaline cartilage with nuclei that show little atypia in lacunae; (4) mature osteoid with nuclei that show little atypia in scattered lacunae; and (5) parts that are almost all cartilage or osteoid.

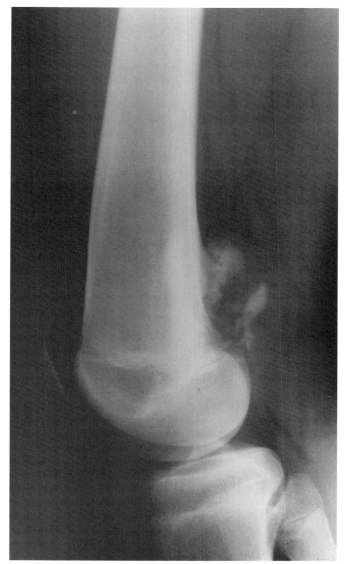

Fig. 25-1

Diagnosis: Parosteal osteosarcoma (juxtacortical osteogenic sarcoma).

Case 26

A 9-year-old girl has had pain in right thigh since she jumped from a platform at school 2 weeks ago. She has limped since then. Pain is worse at rest and sometimes wakes her up.

Parents and brother (2 years old) are well. A grandfather had lung cancer.

Temperature is 35.1°C, heart rate 72, respiratory rate 20, blood pressure 100/60 mm Hg, and weight 26.4 kg. Extremes of motion at right hip hurt her. A hard lump (5- to 6-cm diameter) is in front of femur in midright thigh and a diffuse swelling is behind femur at same level. The rest of the physical findings are normal.

Hematocrit is 0.45. White cell count is 6.3×10^9/liter with 0.42 polymorphonuclear cells, 0.05 bands, 0.45 lymphocytes, and 0.08 monocytes. Platelet count is 398×10^9/liter. Urine specific gravity is 1.025, pH 5. Urine has few squamous epithelial cells/HPF and 0–3 white cells/HPF. Serum sodium is 140 mmol/liter, potassium 4.5, chloride 105, carbon dioxide 25, urea nitrogen 5.4, calcium 2.52, phosphorus 1.26, cholesterol 3.59, and glucose 4.4. Creatinine is 60 µmol/liter, uric acid 260 µmol/liter, total bilirubin 10, and direct bilirubin 2. Total protein is 73 g/liter, albumin 48. Alkaline phosphatase is 480 U/liter, LDH 220, and SGOT 32.

Cortex of right femur is thickened medially and a haze of calcium density is in soft tissues around femur (Figure 26-1).

Biopsy of tumor shows neoplastic cartilage and aggregates of spindle cells. Cartilage is cellular; many chondrocytes have double, hyperchromatic nuclei with clumps of chromatin and occasional prominent nucleoli. Electron microscopy shows (1) loose, collagenous, ground substance and stromal clearing around tumor cells, which have cytoplasmic villous-like projections and scalloped cell membranes; (2) lipid droplets and abundant dilated round endoplasmic reticulum in cytoplasm; and (3) irregular, cleft nuclei with clumped chromatin and prominent nucleoli.

She is given five courses of chemotherapy. Right leg is removed 2 months later.

A fusiform mass in femur is covered by gray-white periosteum and mottled by yellow streaks perpendicular to shaft. Microscopic examination shows (1) atypical osteocytes in an osteoid matrix, pleomorphic and crowded in places; (2) tumor giant cells; (3) acellular osteoid and cartilage; and (4) scattered vascular spaces.

Diagnosis: Periosteal osteogenic sarcoma.

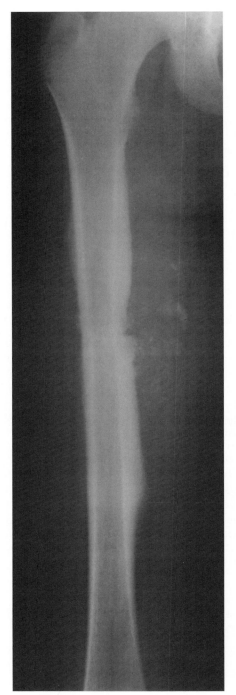

Fig. 26-1

Case 27

A 4-year, 10-month-old boy has swelling near left knee. He has limped and had swelling since he fell off his bicycle 2 weeks ago. He has had some ear infections.

Mother (30 years old), father (33 years old), and two sisters (3 and 9 years old) are well.

Temperature is 36°C, heart rate 96, respiratory rate 20, blood pressure 98/70 mm Hg, weight 18 kg, and height 109 cm. Lower left thigh is swollen. Left knee stops 5 degrees short of full extension. The rest of the physical findings are normal.

Hematocrit is 0.37. White cell count is 6.9×10^9/liter with 0.58 polymorphonuclear cells, 0.26 lymphocytes, 0.07 monocytes, 0.07 eosinophils, and 0.02 basophils. Platelet count is 313×10^9/liter. Urine specific gravity is 1.025, pH 5. Urine has 1–2 white cells/HPF. Serum sodium is 141 mmol/liter, potassium 4.8, calcium 2.15, phosphorus 1.45, cholesterol 3.54, and glucose 4.3. Creatinine is 40 µmol/liter, uric acid 280, total bilirubin 9, and direct bilirubin 2. Total protein is 66 g/liter, albumin 39. Alkaline phosphatase is 4,560 U/liter, LDH 1,116, and SGOT 39.

Isotope scan shows increased uptake in left femur. Roentgenogram at 4 years, 10 months, shows cortical thickening and dense, fluffy calcification both inside and outside distal part of left femur (Figure 27-1). At 5 years, 1 month, proximal epiphysis of right tibia is sclerotic. At 5 years, 6 months, sclerotic bone is in proximal part of both humeri and right scapula. One month later, sclerotic bone is in right ilium, right ischium, and left pubic bone. At 6 years, 1 month, sclerosis is more marked in right ilium, right ischium, left pubic bone, and proximal epiphysis of right tibia, and is also in right pubic bone and metaphysis of right tibia. Sclerotic bone is in several vertebrae and at right shoulder (Figure 27-2).

Serum alkaline phosphatase at 6 years, 2 months, is 8,800 U/liter, LDH 2,280, and SGOT 71.

Biopsy of left femur at 4 years, 10 months, shows large vessels over calcified tumor that consists of large cells with much eosinophilic cytoplasm; large, dark, pleomorphic nuclei; rare mitoses; and islands of osteoid.

He is treated with chemotherapy and left above-knee amputation at 5 years, 2 months. He dies at 6 years, 4 months.

Diagnosis: Multicentric osteosarcoma.

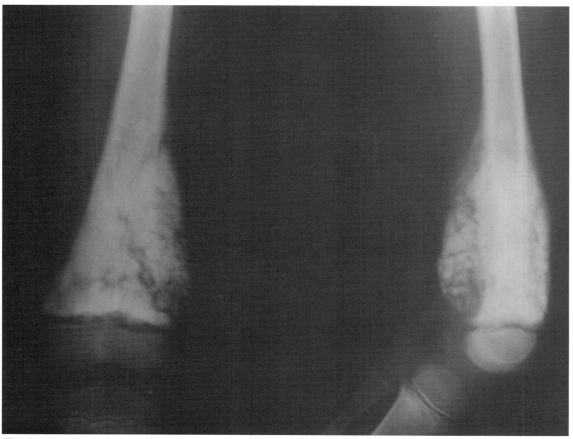

Fig. 27-1

(Continued)

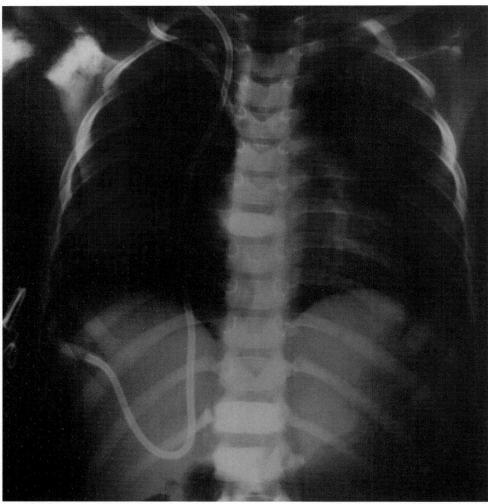

Fig. 27-2

Case 28

A 4-year-old girl limps and has pain in left leg.

She has complained of pain in left leg for 6 months, initially several times per week, usually in the evening, and, during last 2 months, several times per day. She began limping occasionally 2 weeks ago and has limped all day today.

Mother had toxoplasmosis during pregnancy. Father and sister (2 years old) are well. Maternal grandfather had "brown tumor"; paternal grandfather had colon cancer.

Temperature is 38°C, heart rate 124, respiratory rate 22, blood pressure 88/52 mm Hg, weight 11.8 kg, and height 95 cm. Upper lateral part of left calf is swollen, warm, firm, and tender. Circumference of upper left calf is 21 cm, right calf 18. Right knee jerk is 1+, left knee jerk 2+. The rest of the physical findings are normal.

Hematocrit is 0.38. White cell count is 19.3×10^9/liter with 0.60 polymorphonuclear cells, 0.04 bands, 0.28 lymphocytes, 0.07 monocytes, and 0.01 atypical lymphocytes. Platelet count is 602×10^9/liter. ESR is 40 mm/hr. Urine specific gravity is 1.031, pH 6. Urine has 1+ ketones, mucus, and few squamous epithelial cells/HPF. Serum sodium is 138 mmol/liter, potassium 4.3, chloride 106, carbon dioxide 20, urea nitrogen 3.9, calcium 2.40, phosphorus 1.49, cholesterol 2.46, and glucose 5.9. Creatinine is 50 µmol/liter, uric acid 200, total bilirubin 3, and direct bilirubin 0. Total protein is 75 g/liter, albumin 41. Alkaline phosphatase is 258 U/liter, LDH 648, and SGOT 45.

Irregular cortical new bone is around partly destroyed upper half of left fibula (Figure 28-1).

At operation, soupy necrotic tumor oozes from incised fibula.

Microscopic examination shows nests and sheets of uniform small cells with little amphophilic cytoplasm, round-to-oval hyperchromatic nuclei, and many mitoses. Tumor cells are PAS positive. Electron microscopy shows (1) uniform cells, (2) irregular nuclei, (3) prominent nucleoli, (4) many mitochondria, (5) slightly rough-surfaced endoplasmic reticulum, (6) microfibrils, and (7) glycogen aggregates.

Left above-knee amputation is performed. She receives chemotherapy for 19 months. She has a dry cough, looks good, and goes skiing at 13 years, 3 months.

Weight at 13 years, 4 months, is 39 kg, height 142 cm, temperature 37°C, heart rate 106, respiratory rate 20, and blood pressure 115/50 mm Hg. Breath sounds are diminished at left base. Left above-knee amputation is healed.

Roentgenograms show mass in left lower lobe. CT scan shows mass of varying radio-opacity in left lower lobe and in front of aorta (Figure 28-2).

At left lower lobectomy, firm, tan tumor ($11.0 \times 7.0 \times 5.5$ cm) is in left lower lobe and along pulmonary vein into pericardium. Tan nodules (0.1–0.4 cm) are on pleura.

Microscopic examination shows small blue-cell tumor with vascular and pleural spread. PAS-positive tumor cells lose stain when digested by diastase. Nineteen of 20 tumor cells are aneuploid, 18 are t(11;22), and two have an extra chromosome 8.

She is treated with chemotherapy, autologous marrow infusion, and granulocyte colony-stimulating factor. Weight is 36.6 kg when she has a cold at 15 years. Hematocrit is 0.31. White cell count is 4.5×10^9/liter with 0.42 polymorphonuclear cells, 0.37 lymphocytes, 0.18 monocytes, and 0.03 eosinophils. Platelet count is 80×10^9/liter.

Diagnosis: Ewing's sarcoma.

(Continued)

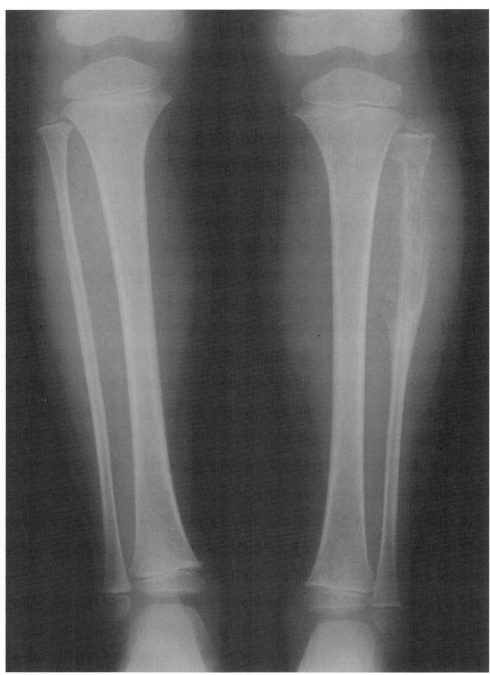

Fig. 28-1

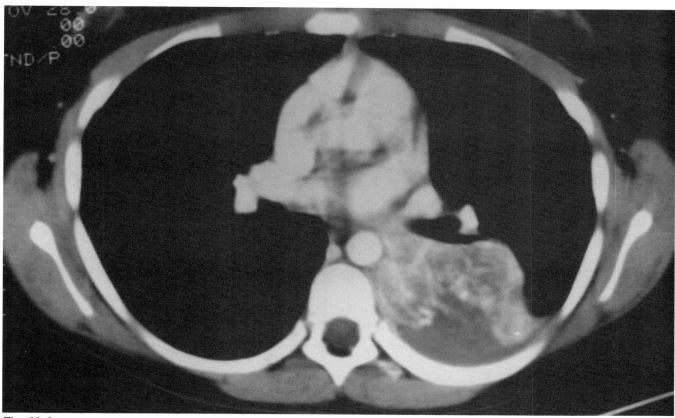

Fig. 28-2

Case 29

A 14-year-old boy has lower thoracic backache that began 4 months ago, woke him during nights 2 months ago no matter what position he slept in, and has been getting worse for 2 weeks. Deep ache is centered at spine and less intense lateral to it. He has lost 1.4 kg in 2 weeks and has felt full the last 2 days. Legs were numb, tingly, and weak during 2-hour ride to hospital, and a band across abdomen at level of umbilicus began to itch.

He had cold and ear infection 4 months ago.

He is in ninth grade and wrestles for school team.

Weight is 53.3 kg, height 157 cm, temperature 37°C, heart rate 120, respiratory rate 20, and blood pressure 118/70 mm Hg. He walks slowly, back straight, is tender at T10, and has slight hypoesthesia at level of umbilicus and several centimeters above and below it. Deep tendon reflexes are increased in legs. Unsustained clonus is at ankles. Babinski's sign is in feet, diminished position sense in first toes. Liver edge is 1–2 cm below costal margin. The rest of the physical findings are normal.

Hematocrit is 0.46. White cell count is 13.7×10^9/liter with 0.64 polymorphonuclear cells, 0.03 bands, 0.19 lymphocytes, 0.11 monocytes, 0.01 eosinophils, 0.01 basophils, and 0.01 atypical lymphocytes. ESR is 12 mm/hr. Serum sodium is 144 mmol/liter, potassium 4.7, chloride 100, carbon dioxide 29, urea nitrogen 4.6, calcium 2.54, phosphorus 1.78, cholesterol 2.33, and glucose 6.2. Creatinine is 80 μmol/liter, uric acid 310, total bilirubin 9, and direct bilirubin 0. Total protein is 73 g/liter, albumin 48. Alkaline phosphatase is 160 U/liter, LDH 255, and SGOT 32. Bone marrow is normal.

Figure 29-1 shows thickened paraspinal soft tissues around T10 and slightly wedged body of T10, its left pedicle indistinct.

At operation, brown-red epidural tumor is along left side of spinal cord at T10 and several centimeters above and below T10.

Microscopic examination shows sheets of cells with indistinct borders and stroma of delicate connective tissue. Cell cytoplasm is lightly basophilic and magenta with PAS stain, less so after digestion with diastase; nuclei are round to oval, mildly pleomorphic, with prominent membrane, coarse chromatin with clearing, many small nucleoli, and 0–3 mitoses/HPF. Many blood vessels, foci of necrosis, and distorted and fragmented reticulin fibers are in the tumor.

He is treated with drugs and local irradiation.

Backache at same level recurs 2½ years later, 7 months after drug treatment is stopped. Bone marrow is normal. Biopsy of new paraspinal mass shows similar tumor. He dies at 17 years.

Diagnosis: Ewing's sarcoma.

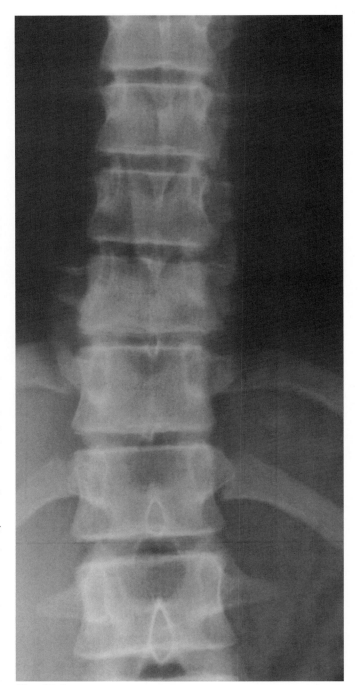

Fig. 29-1

Case 30

A 17-year-old boy has pain at right wrist and pain in left foot when he walks a lot. He is worried about being a "shrimp."

Tonsils and adenoids were removed at 5 years, and cartilaginous exostoses at 8, 9, 13, and 14 years. He was found to have a large, normal left kidney and no right kidney when he had hematuria at 9 years. He fractured right arm at 15 years.

Mother and maternal grandfather have glaucoma.

Height at 17 years is 160 cm, weight 44 kg, temperature 37.2°C, heart rate 64, respiratory rate 18, and blood pressure 126/88 mm Hg. He has bony lumps and scars. Right hand deviates medially. Fingernails are ridged and distorted by phalangeal exostoses. Pronation and supination of forearms and abduction and rotation at hips are limited. Left first metatarsal bone is tender. Left extensor hallucis longus tendon "pops over" an exostosis, according to orthopedist. The rest of the physical findings are normal.

Hematocrit is 0.40. White cell count is 6.1×10^9/liter with 0.27 polymorphonuclear cells, 0.21 bands, 0.40 lymphocytes, 0.11 monocytes, and 0.01 eosinophils. Platelet count is 354×10^9/liter.

At operation, distal part of left first metatarsal bone, sesamoid bone medial to left flexor hallucis longus tendon, and part of an exostosis of proximal part of right fibula are removed.

Microscopic examination of the tan-pink fragments, including sesamoid bone, shows bone, perichondrium, and orderly ossification of cartilage. Nuclei of occasional chondrocytes are hyperchromatic. No mitoses and no binucleated chondrocytes are present.

Right ankle is swollen 3 months later. Swelling enlarges and hurts when he walks.

Fragments of bone density are in swelling at right ankle (Figure 30-1).

At operation, distal right fibula and an attached glistening white mass ($10 \times 8 \times 5$ cm) are removed.

Microscopic examination shows cartilage islands, bone trabeculae, fibrous connective tissue, fat, and marrow. Cartilage lacunae are closely packed and contain one to three and occasionally more chondrocytes with distinct cell membranes and eosinophilic cytoplasm that is more basophilic at periphery. Most chondrocytes have one nucleus, some two or three. Nuclei are round to oval, hyperchromatic, and basophilic. A few are enlarged, and several are mitotic.

Below-knee amputation is performed at 21 years for new growth along lateral aspect of right tibia. Occasional chondrocytes have three to four nuclei of variable size and shape. A few are mitotic. He has "electric shocks" where right foot used to be, and 90 days after amputation he says, "If I had a gun, I'd shoot myself." He still has pain at 28 years that he has

"learned to deal with" and a mass that has been growing for 2 years and "feels funny" above left nipple. Height is 168 cm, weight 57 kg, and blood pressure 130/82 mm Hg. Mass and part of left second rib are resected. Microscopic examination of mass shows chondrocytes oriented like cells in normal epiphysis and thin bony septa. He is a guitar teacher at 36 years.

Diagnosis: Multiple cartilaginous exostoses, chondrosarcoma of right tibia and right fibula.

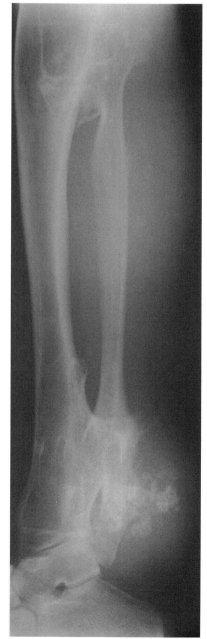

Fig. 30-1

Case 31

A 17-year-old boy has had a tender lump in left thigh for 5 months. He woke up with pain a few nights ago. He limps now. He had similar pain 2 years ago and 10 months ago, both times ascribed to a pulled muscle from wrestling.

Temperature is 37.4°C, heart rate 108, respiratory rate 18, blood pressure 108/80 mm Hg, weight 57.2 kg, and height 166 cm. A mobile, tender mass (8 cm long), its top at groin, is in left thigh under sartorius muscle. The rest of the physical findings are normal.

Hematocrit is 0.47. White cell count is 6.2×10^9/liter with 0.44 polymorphonuclear cells, 0.46 lymphocytes, 0.06 monocytes, and 0.03 eosinophils. Platelet count is 262×10^9/liter. Serum sodium is 144 mmol/liter, potassium 4.3, chloride 108, carbon dioxide 26, urea nitrogen 6.8, calcium 2.37, phosphorus 1.32, cholesterol 3.34, triglycerides 0.78, and glucose 4.2. Creatinine is 80 μmol/liter, uric acid 380, total bilirubin 14, and direct bilirubin 0. Total protein is 75 g/liter, albumin 42. Alkaline phosphatase is 32 U/liter, LDH 635, and SGOT 31.

CT scan shows tumor between femur and anterior muscles of left thigh (Figure 31-1). Roentgenogram shows lung metastases (Figure 31-2).

At operation, incision of pseudocapsule over mass reveals gray, friable tumor. Biopsy shows (1) anaplastic ovoid and spindle cells in trabeculae and nests separated by fibrovascular septa; (2) many mitoses; and (3) in electron microscopy, epithelial differentiation by presence of tight junctions, microvilli, and a cilium.

Tumor (10.5 × 6.0 × 3.5 cm), its outer surface red-brown and rough, cut section surface light beige, lobular, and vascular, is removed 10 days later.

He dies at 20 years.

Diagnosis: Synovial sarcoma.

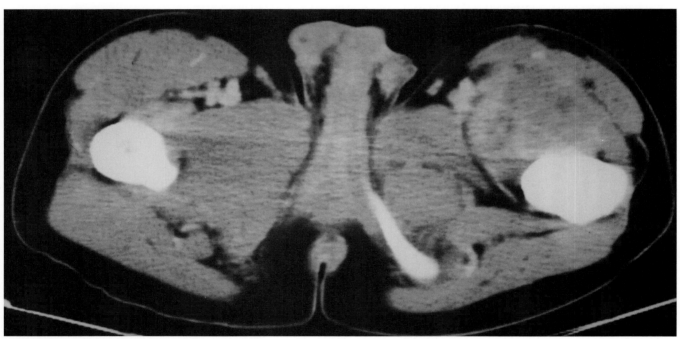

Fig. 31-1

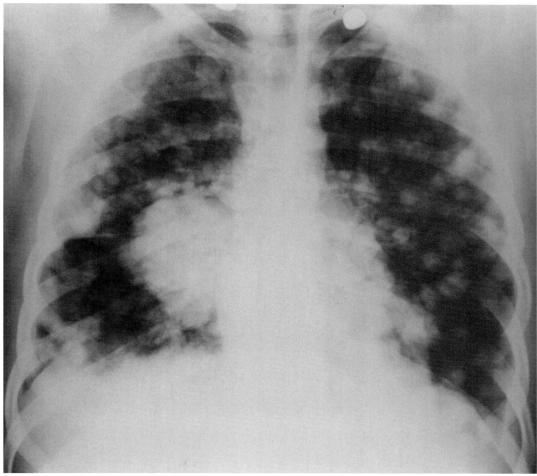

Fig. 31-2

Case 32

A 5-year-old girl will not walk or play, and aches all over. Legs began to hurt 2 months ago. She has night fever to 38.9°C.

Weight is 17 kg, height 107 cm, temperature 37.9°C, heart rate 172, respiratory rate 20, and blood pressure 94/60 mm Hg. She is pale and wants to lie undisturbed. Liver edge is 1 cm below costal margin. The rest of the physical findings are normal.

Hematocrit is 0.23. Hemoglobin is 76 g/liter. Red blood cell count is 3.1×10^{12}/liter. MCV is 74 fl. MCH is 25 pg. MCHC is 330 g/liter. Red-blood-cell distribution width is 18.5% (normal: 11.5–15.0). ESR is 135 mm/hr. White cell count is 8.0×10^9/liter with 0.53 polymorphonuclear cells, 0.11 bands, 0.32 lymphocytes, 0.03 monocytes, and 0.01 eosinophils. Platelet count is 489×10^9/liter. Bone marrow aspirate is normal. Serum does not contain rheumatoid factor.

Figure 32-1 shows rarefied bones of legs, especially metaphyses at knees, and slightly thickened cortex of right fibula and lateral proximal tibias. Bones of feet are also rarefied.

Bone marrow aspirate obtained 16 days later is hypercellular with replacement of normal elements by blasts. Smear shows blasts with little cytoplasm and large nuclei with fine chromatin, blunted outlines, and occasional folded appearance. Blasts stain with TdT, CALLA, and B1 and B4 pan–B cell antibodies in surface marker analysis but do not stain with antibodies to surface immunoglobulins, T-cell antigens, or myelomonocyte antigens.

Diagnosis: Acute lymphoblastic leukemia, leukemic lines ("sick child lines") in distal femoral and proximal tibial metaphyses, a zone in which presumably is a mixture of trabecular poverty, wide spongy marrow spaces that contain lymphoblasts, and lack of endochondral ossification.

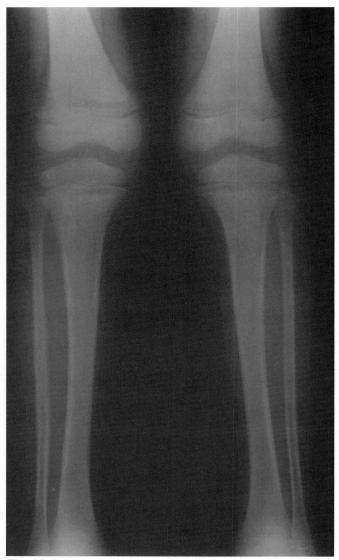

Fig. 32-1

Case 33

A 4-year-old boy has refused to walk for 1 month. He started to limp 5 months ago. He has been pale for several months. Left knee has been swollen for 1 month.

Parents are well. He is their only child.

Temperature is 37.3°C, heart rate 90, respiratory rate 24, blood pressure 105/60 mm Hg, weight 18.6 kg, and height 106 cm. Bruises and petechiae are on body. Small lymph nodes are in neck, axilla, and right groin. Liver edge is 3 cm below costal margin. A firm, nontender mass (6 × 5 cm) is in left lower quadrant of abdomen. The rest of the physical findings are normal.

Hematocrit is 0.21. Hemoglobin is 74 g/liter. White cell count is 5.9×10^9/liter with 0.10 polymorphonuclear cells, 0.01 bands, 0.83 lymphocytes, and 0.06 monocytes. Platelet count is 55×10^9/liter. Reticulocyte fraction is 39×10^{-3}.

Figure 33-1 shows defects and a pathologic fracture in distal part of left femur, a cloud of bone density higher along medi-al side of cortex, and an irregular defect in medial part of metaphysis of right femur. In excretory urogram, a mass compresses left side of bladder. Pelves, calyces, and position of kidneys are normal.

Urine vanillylmandelic acid is 93 μmol/day (normal: <25), homovanillic acid 150 (normal: 8–24).

Microscopic examination of iliac marrow smear shows clumps of degenerating cells and cells that have little cytoplasm, large nuclei with fine chromatin, and as many as four nucleoli. Needle biopsy of tumor in left lower quadrant of abdomen shows (1) small, densely hyperchromatic cells with little cytoplasm, round nuclei, and mitoses; (2) little stroma; (3) tumors around blood vessels and plugging a vessel; (4) pseudorosettes; and (5) rare small tapered cells with argyrophilic fibrils. Wright's stain shows many tapered tumor cells with distinct processes.

Diagnosis: Neuroblastoma.

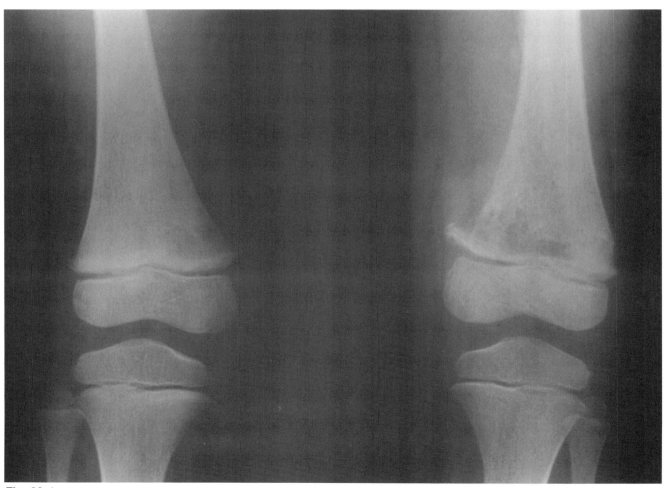

Fig. 33-1

Case 34

A 4-year-old girl has backache.

Two years ago and again 1 year ago, she had fever and knee pain for 2 weeks. Three months ago and again 2 months ago, she had backache and fever for 2 weeks and then ran and played normally until 1 month ago, when back ached for 1 week. Now she cannot take a deep breath because of backache and does not want to be moved. She has lost 3 kg in 3 months.

Mother (28 years old) and father (29 years old) are well. The girl is their only child. One maternal great-aunt had breast cancer; another had cervical cancer.

Weight at 4 years is 13.2 kg, height 102 cm, temperature 37.6°C, heart rate 144, respiratory rate 28, and blood pressure 95/68 mm Hg. She is pale. Head and limbs are tender. The rest of the physical findings are normal.

Hemoglobin is 82 g/liter. Hematocrit is 0.25. MCV is 77 fl. MCH is 26 pg. MCHC is 330 g/liter. Reticulocyte fraction is 26×10^{-3}. White cell count is 3.4×10^9/liter with 0.55 polymorphonuclear cells, 0.13 bands, 0.16 lymphocytes, 0.14 monocytes, 0.01 eosinophils, and 0.01 basophils. Platelet count is 220×10^9/liter. ESR is 71 mm/hr. Urine specific gravity is 1.021, pH 6. Urine has 1+ ketones, 2–3 white cells/HPF, amorphous urates, and moderate uric acid crystals.

Examination of bone marrow aspirated from left iliac crest shows replacement by small cells that have diffusely homoge-neous magenta cytoplasm and eccentric, grooved, large, moderately basophilic nuclei with thin membrane, fine chromatin clumping, and small, often many, nucleoli. Cytoplasm and nuclei are PAS positive.

She has no pain 3 months after treatment is begun. Hematocrit is 0.32. White cell count is 4.0×10^9/liter. Platelet count is 325×10^9/liter. Reticulocyte fraction is 13×10^{-3}. Serum sodium is 143 mmol/liter, potassium 4.2, chloride 108, carbon dioxide 18, urea nitrogen 5.7, calcium 2.64, phosphorus 1.52, cholesterol 4.37, triglycerides 1.10, and glucose 5.0. Creatinine is 50 µmol/liter, uric acid 230, total bilirubin 7, and direct bilirubin 0. Total protein is 72 g/liter, albumin 56. Alkaline phosphatase is 200 U/liter, LDH 354, and SGOT 42. Bone marrow aspirate is normocellular.

Defects with ill-defined margins are in calvaria, and vertebral bodies are collapsed 3 months after treatment is begun (Figure 34-1). Defects are also in bones of pelvis and femurs. Vertebral bodies were normal in roentgenogram when backache first appeared 6 months ago.

She dies at 5 years.

Diagnosis: Undifferentiated small-cell malignant tumor, questionable lymphocytic lymphoma, questionable Ewing's sarcoma.

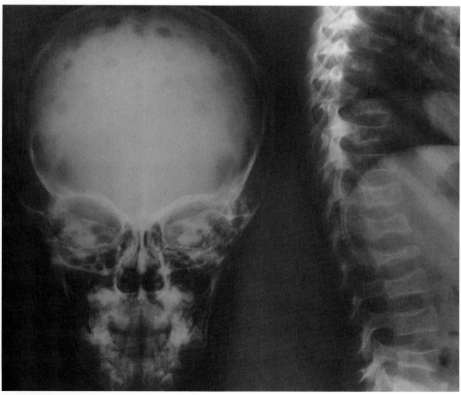

Fig. 34-1

Spine

Case 1

A 14½-year-old girl has scoliosis.

Parents and nine siblings are well.

Pregnancy was normal, birth weight 2.8 kg. Mother thought that the girl had too fast a heartbeat at 4 months. The girl tired quickly with feedings. A systolic heart murmur was present. Liver edge was 3 cm below right costal margin. Ductus arteriosus was divided. Continuous murmur, thrill, and S_3 were present at 6 years. Weight at 10⅓ years was 27 kg, height 137 cm. Systolic heart murmur and diastolic heart murmur were present. Commissurotomy of stenotic bicuspid aortic valve and resection of subaortic band were performed at 10⅚ years. Mother noticed swelling of girl's right shoulder at 11 years. The girl began to menstruate at 12 years. Blood pressure was 154/70 mm Hg at 13½ years. Coarctation of the aorta was resected.

Weight at 14½ years is 51 kg, height 156 cm, temperature 37.6°C, heart rate 92, respiratory rate 16, and blood pressure 116/90 mm Hg. She has precordial thrill, systolic heart murmur, scoliosis, and operative scars. The rest of the physical findings are normal.

Hematocrit is 0.41. White cell count is 6.2×10^9/liter with 0.37 polymorphonuclear cells, 0.07 bands, 0.50 lymphocytes, 0.05 monocytes, and 0.01 eosinophils. Urine specific gravity is 1.022, pH 6. Urine has 0–4 white cells/HPF, 0–3 epithelial cells/HPF, and mucus. Serum sodium is 141 mmol/liter, potassium 4.5, chloride 107, carbon dioxide 25, urea nitrogen 5.0, and glucose 4.9. SGOT is 120 U/liter, CK 70.

Pulmonary function test shows restrictive impairment, vital capacity 0.33 predicted, without obstruction, FEV_1 0.81 vital capacity.

Spine is straight in examination at 9 years. At 10⅓ years, thoracic spine is convex right, apex T8, and thoracolumbar spine convex left, apex L1–L2 (Figure 1-1A). The curves show progressive increase at 11 and at 14½ years (Figure 1-1B).

Diagnosis: Idiopathic scoliosis.

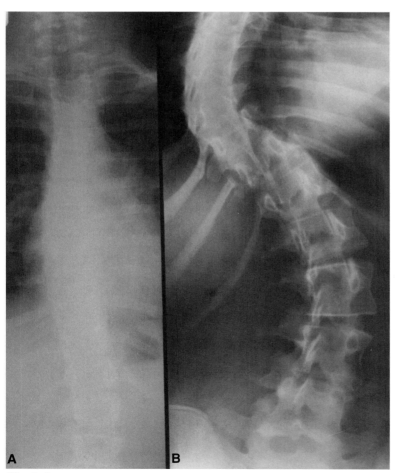

Fig. 1-1

Case 2

A 16-year-old girl has scoliosis.

Pregnancy was normal. Health is good. Menarche was at 13 years.

Weight is 52.9 kg, height 165 cm. She has right rib hump and left flank hump.

Mother noticed scoliosis in girl's 14-year-old sister. Pregnancy was normal. Health is good. Menarche was at 13 years.

Weight of 14-year-old is 56.4 kg, height 154 cm. She has slight right rib hump, moderate left flank hump. Spine is flexible.

A 13-year-old sister has scoliosis. Birth weight was 3.5 kg. Health is good except for hay fever. She has not begun to menstruate.

Weight of 13-year-old is 45 kg, height 151 cm. Physical findings are like those of two older sisters.

Their 18-year-old sister has had spinal fusion for scoliosis. The remaining sibling, a 17-year-old girl, has scoliosis. A paternal aunt has scoliosis. Parents, three paternal aunts, two paternal uncles, four maternal aunts, and four maternal uncles do not have scoliosis.

Spines of 13-year-old (Figure 2-1), 14-year-old (Figure 2-2), and 16-year-old (Figure 2-3) show thoracic right convexity, apex at approximately T8, and thoracolumbar left convexity, apex at L2.

Diagnosis: Familial idiopathic adolescent scoliosis.

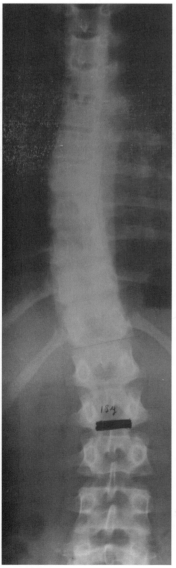

Fig. 2-1

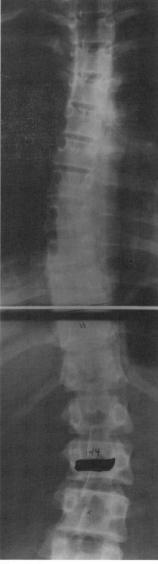

Fig. 2-2

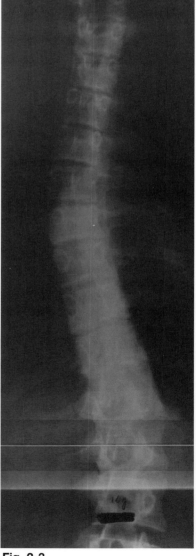

Fig. 2-3

Case 3

A 7-year-old boy has café au lait spots.

Mother and one brother have scoliosis; father and other brother do not.

Pregnancy was normal, birth weight 2.6 kg. He sat at 7 months, walked at 15 months, and used sentences at 2 years. He has had chickenpox.

Weight at 7 years is 21 kg, height 110 cm. Thoracic spine is slightly prominent. Café au lait spots are on body. The rest of the physical findings are normal.

Figure 3-1 shows a short right convexity at T5–T7.

Diagnosis: Scoliosis of neurofibromatosis.

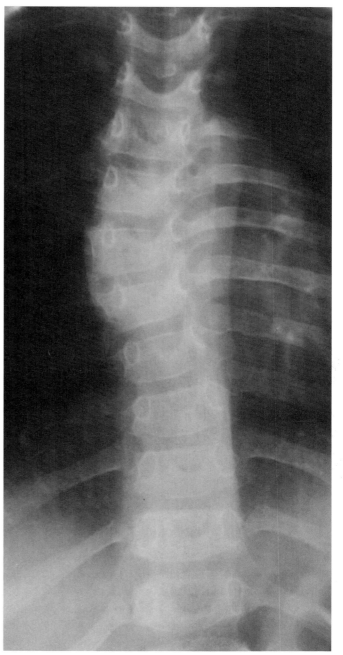

Fig. 3-1

Case 4

A 13-day-old girl stiffens episodically with jaws clenched and arms adducted and flexed, urinates, and has fever.

Mother is para 7007. Pregnancy was normal, delivery at home. The girl breathed and cried quickly. Umbilical cord was tied with a string, cut with scissors, smeared with breast milk, and covered with an adhesive bandage. She had blue spells and jaw jerks for 1–2 minutes at a time last night and then slept. She is breast-fed.

Temperature at 13 days is 38.3°C, heart rate 180, respiratory rate 50, systolic blood pressure 83 mm Hg, weight 3.3 kg, length 48 cm, and head circumference 35 cm. She is pale gray. Hands clench and shake. Neck is supple, abdomen rigid. Rustling of bed clothes causes opisthotonus, stiffening, and jaw clenching. Pupils react sluggishly to light. The rest of the physical findings are normal.

Hematocrit is 0.47. White cell count is 23.6×10^9/liter with 0.44 polymorphonuclear cells, 0.32 bands, 0.16 lymphocytes, and 0.08 monocytes. Platelet estimate is adequate. Urine specific gravity is 1.021, pH 5. Urine has 1 white cell/HPF, rare granular casts/HPF, and 3+ protein. Serum sodium is 158 mmol/liter, potassium 5.3, chloride 120, carbon dioxide 24, urea nitrogen 17.1, calcium 2.37, and glucose 3.2. Venous blood pH is 7.31. P_{CO_2} is 47 mm Hg, P_{O_2} 30. CSF has 4.0 mmol/liter glucose, 1 g/liter protein, 154×10^6/liter red cells, 6×10^6/liter white cells, 0.80 polymorphonuclear cells and 0.20 small lymphocytes, and is sterile.

Spine has focal thoracolumbar left convexity (Figure 4-1).

Culture of umbilicus grows *Pseudomonas aeruginosa*, *Bacteroides incommunis*, anaerobic diphtheroids, and coagulase-negative staphylococci.

She is treated with curare, sedative, endotracheal intubation, and gastrostomy. Muscle tone is normal without curare 2 months later. She lifts and turns her head.

Diagnosis: Tetanus neonatorum.

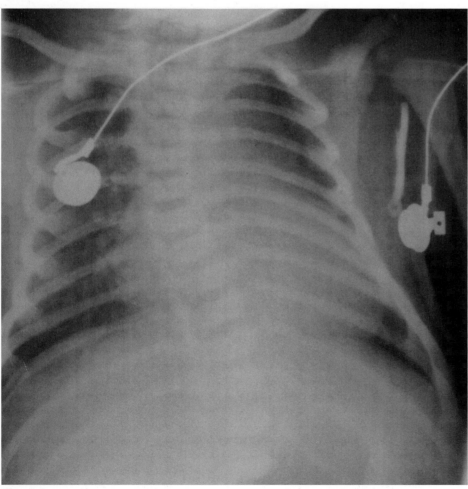

Fig. 4-1

Case 5

A 12¾-year-old boy has scoliosis.

Pregnancy of mother (at 20 years) was normal, birth weight 3.2 kg. He did not crawl. He began to walk at 14 months but fell often, unable to catch himself. It was hard for him to stand up from sitting or supine. He moved his hands up his legs as he rose to stand. He walked with deep lumbar lordosis, ankles turned inward, flat feet, and slight foot drop. He crawled up stairs. He walked fast when asked to run at 4 years. He could not close his eyes tightly. Muscles at shoulders and hips were small. Calf muscles were tight. Deep tendon reflexes were weak. He walked on his toes at 6 years and could climb stairs. ECG showed left ventricular hypertrophy and left ventricular diastolic overload. Serum CK was 1,630 U/liter at 4 years, 1,496 at 7 years; serum CK of parents and sister was normal. Muscle biopsy during bilateral iliotibial band resection at 6 years showed random atrophic and degenerating fibers surrounded by mild chronic inflammation and fiber regeneration with basophilic cytoplasm and central nuclei. He could not climb stairs as well at 9 years and fell more often. Hips, knees, and heel cords were tighter. Limb muscles were small and soft. He had to be helped out of a chair and in and out of the bathtub at 10 years. He could not fasten snaps on his pants. He stopped walking at 11 years. He could raise his hands above his head if he locked them together. He could roll over in bed but sometimes asked his mother to straighten an arm or a leg if he rolled on it. He could feed himself at 12 years but needed help cutting food. He used a urinal at fixed intervals. He had flexible scoliosis that quickly increased. Contractures were worse.

Hematocrit at 12¾ years is 0.44. White cell count is 3.4 × 10^9/liter with 0.17 polymorphonuclear cells, 0.12 bands, 0.61 lymphocytes, 0.07 monocytes, 0.02 eosinophils, and 0.01 metamyelocytes. Urine specific gravity is 1.027, pH 5. Urine has trace ketones, 0–2 white cells/HPF, mucus, and bacteria. Serum sodium is 143 mmol/liter, potassium 4.4, chloride 104, carbon dioxide 27, and urea nitrogen 4.0. Creatinine is 50 µmol/liter. ECG shows flattened T waves in leads 1, V5, and V6. Pulmonary function test shows restrictive lung disease with static lung volume 0.47 predicted and FEV_1 0.54 predicted.

Figure 5-1 at 12½ years shows boy leaning right when he sits and long left convexity in spine.

At placement of Harrington rod, muscles are thin and pale. Iliac bone is soft.

A systolic heart murmur is present at 15 years. ECG shows flattened T waves and right ventricular hypertrophy. He cannot lift a glass of water at 16 years. He is constipated. He coughs up blood, is in shock, and dies at 18⅓ years.

Diagnosis: Duchenne's muscular dystrophy, scoliosis.

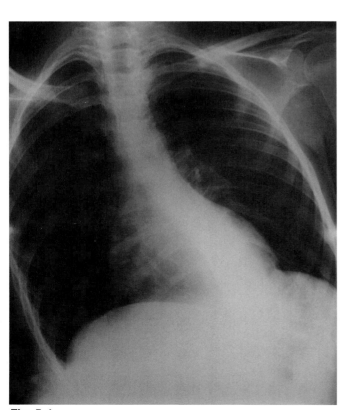

Fig. 5-1

Case 6

A 9-year-old girl has a fever, headache, and sore throat.

She drank from a stream and was bitten by bugs 10 days ago. She has been around dogs, horses, goats, and rabbits recently. She has had sore throat, pain in neck, and large nodes in neck for 5 days.

She has had throat infections, broken arm, broken finger, and, 2 months ago, chickenpox.

Parents and three siblings are well.

Temperature is 37.9°C, heart rate 108, respiratory rate 22, blood pressure 84/40 mm Hg, and weight 23.6 kg. She is jaundiced. Conjunctivae, eardrums, and throat are red. Anterior cervical lymph nodes are large. Neck is supple but hurts on left side. Small, itchy spots are on abdomen. Right upper quadrant is tender. Liver edge is 2 cm below costal margin. The rest of the physical findings are normal.

She has abdominal pain when she breathes 2 days later and vomits twice. Rash is gone. Joints hurt the next day and feet are slightly edematous. Temperature is 39.5°C 10 days after illness begins. Conjunctivae, eardrums, and throat are red. Neck is sore, and she is reluctant to move it. Tender liver edge is 3 cm below costal margin. Left elbow is swollen. A tender cyst (3–4 × 2 cm) is in right popliteal fossa, slightly to medial side. No bruit is heard. Right knee lacks 10 degrees of full extension. Neck is still sore 2 weeks after illness begins.

Hematocrit is 0.40. White cell count is 14.7 × 10⁹/liter with 0.57 polymorphonuclear cells, 0.32 bands, 0.08 lymphocytes, and 0.03 monocytes. ESR is 80 mm/hr. Urine specific gravity is 1.010, pH 6. Urine has 1+ protein, trace acetone, small amount occult blood, moderate bile, 5–10 white cells/HPF, 0–5 red cells/HPF, and 0–5 epithelial cells/HPF. Serum sodium is 133 mmol/liter, potassium 4.2, chloride 94, urea nitrogen 3.9, calcium 2.27, phosphorus 1.58, cholesterol 3.62, and glucose 4.7. Creatinine is 60 μmol/liter, uric acid 200, total bilirubin 116. Total protein is 78 g/liter, albumin 42. Alkaline phosphatase is 389 U/liter, LDH 260, SGOT 135, and amylase 77. Group A β-hemolytic streptococci do not grow in throat culture. Serologic tests for hepatitis A and B, Epstein-Barr virus, parvovirus, echo virus, coxsackie virus, cytomegalovirus, tularemia, Lyme disease, and leptospirosis are negative. Blood cultures are sterile. Urine culture grows 1+ *Staphylococcus aureus*. Dark-field examination of urine does not show leptospira. Slightly bloody, purulent liquid aspirated from right popliteal cyst is sterile.

Ultrasound examination of right popliteal fossa 3 days after discovery of cyst shows a hypoechoic mass behind tibial epiphysis (Figure 6-1). Plain film of knees shows slight bulge behind right knee. Examination of neck at 2 weeks (Figure 6-2) shows head tilt to right and in open mouth view non–straight line relation between tip of odontoid, tip of spinous process of C2, and symphysis of mandible.

Total bilirubin 2½ weeks after illness begins is 15 μmol/liter, and direct bilirubin 9. Herpes simplex virus is cultured from throat swab.

Diagnosis: Fever of unknown (questionable herpetic) origin; rotatory subluxation of C1 on C2; right Baker's cyst.

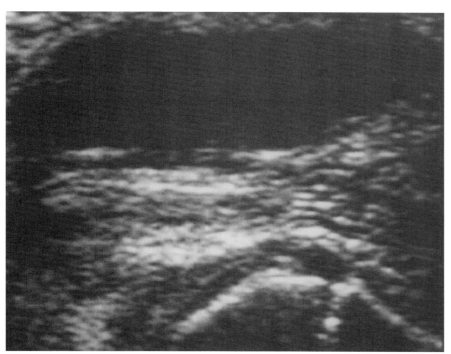

Fig. 6-1

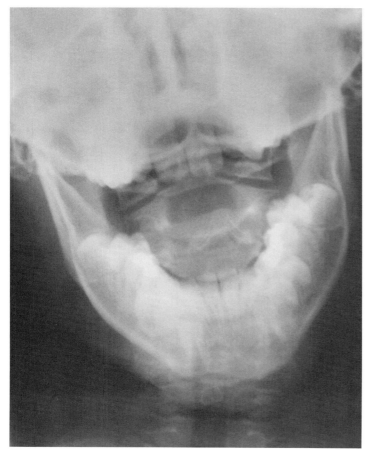

Fig. 6-2

Case 7

A 10-year-old boy is humpbacked.

He was treated for tuberculosis for 2 years in early childhood. He had backache 5 months ago. Body of T11 was removed with a rongeur 5 months ago, and parts of left ninth, tenth, eleventh, and twelfth ribs were separated from periosteum, removed, and used as anterior struts. The surgeon found it "not possible to obtain much of a correction . . . due to probable fusion of posterior fasciculus."

Temperature at 10 years is 37.7°C, heart rate 92, respiratory rate 22, and blood pressure 110/70 mm Hg. He has lower thoracic hump. A longitudinal scar is on left side of back. The rest of the physical findings are normal.

Hematocrit is 0.41. White cell count is 8.0×10^9/liter with 0.48 polymorphonuclear cells, 0.03 bands, 0.39 lympho-

cytes, 0.06 monocytes, and 0.04 eosinophils. ESR is 8 mm/hr. Serum sodium is 141 mmol/liter, potassium 4.0, chloride 105, carbon dioxide 27, urea nitrogen 4.0, calcium 2.45, phosphorus 1.55, cholesterol 4.53, and glucose 4.6. Creatinine is 40 µmol/liter, uric acid 200, total bilirubin 5, and direct bilirubin 0. Total protein is 73 g/liter, albumin 46. Alkaline phosphatase is 233 U/liter, LDH 273, and SGOT 91. Urine specific gravity is 1.031, pH 5. Urine has 0–1 white cell/HPF and mucus.

Spine is kyphotic and convex slightly to left, apex at T11, and contrast medium is in spinal canal and along sacral nerve roots (Figure 7-1).

Diagnosis: Tuberculosis of spine (Pott's disease).

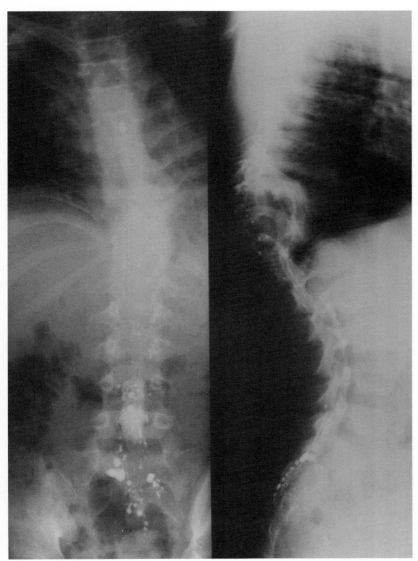

Fig. 7-1

Case 8

A newborn girl has a large hemangioma on left flank; a red, swollen left leg; and a port-wine stain on right side of neck and chest and on right arm.

Mother (22 years old) and father (23 years old) are well. Father has three small flat hemangiomas on chest and head circumference at ninety-eighth percentile.

Pregnancy was normal. Birth weight is 3.5 kg, Apgar score 8/9 at 1 and 5 minutes, length 49 cm, and head circumference 33 cm. Temperature at 1 day is 36.8°C, heart rate 151, respiratory rate 100, and blood pressure 69/32 mm Hg. A soft mass (5 × 4 × 3 cm) is on left flank. Left side of perineum; left labium majus; and left hip, leg, and foot are red. Little fingers curve in. Left foot is 1 cm longer than right foot. A systolic heart murmur is present. The rest of the physical findings are normal.

Hematocrit is 0.49. White cell count is 20.1×10^9/liter with 0.42 polymorphonuclear cells, 0.10 bands, 0.32 lymphocytes, 0.07 monocytes, and 0.09 eosinophils. Platelet count is 234×10^9/liter. Capillary blood pH is 7.39. P_{CO_2} is 47 mm Hg, P_{O_2} 37. Bicarbonate is 28 mmol/liter. Serum sodium is 140 mmol/liter, potassium 5.2, chloride 111, carbon dioxide 25, urea nitrogen 3.2, calcium 2.32, phosphorus 2.39, cholesterol 2.92, and glucose 3.2. Creatinine is 80 μmol/liter, uric acid 340, and total bilirubin 186 (day 5: total bilirubin 350, direct bilirubin 12; day 6: peak total bilirubin 373). Total protein is 53 g/liter, albumin 35. Alkaline phosphatase is 108 U/liter, LDH 754, and SGOT 51.

Ultrasound examination shows vascular mass in left flank that has feeding artery at upper end and that pushes left kidney forward. Echocardiogram shows dilation of left ventricle, small ventricular and atrial septal defects, and regurgitation at mitral and tricuspid valves.

She is treated with digitalis. At 6 months, she has systolic heart murmur, gallop rhythm, and liver edge 3 cm below costal margin. Diameter of left leg is twice that of right. She moves left leg less than right. Deep tendon reflexes are normal. She walks at 18 months. She has systolic heart murmur and liver edge 1 cm below costal margin. Echocardiogram shows small ventricular septal defect and increased blood flow in inferior vena cava and pulmonary arteries and veins.

MRI at 2 years shows large intraspinal vein from T11 to lower lumbar exit (Figure 8-1). Vein ramifies into small left pelvic veins at lumbar exit. Arteriogram shows feeding artery, a large lumbar artery, at L1.

Wire coils are placed in feeding artery. According to pediatric neurosurgeon, she is "developmentally quite normal" at 3 years. Weight is 13 kg, height 87 cm, heart rate 116, and blood pressure 92/49 mm Hg. She does not have heart murmur. Echocardiogram shows all heart chambers slightly enlarged, little regurgitation at mitral and tricuspid valves, and fractional shortening 0.27.

Diagnosis: Parkes Weber syndrome (angio-osteo-hypertrophy).

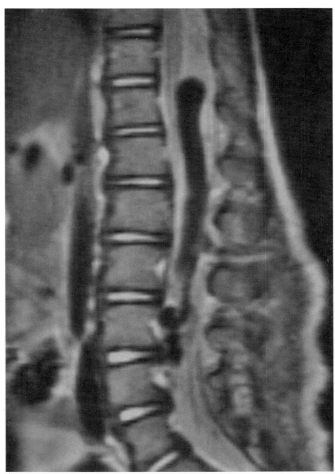

Fig. 8-1

Case 9

A 4-year-old boy, who was in back seat wearing a lap belt in car crash 5 days ago, is paraplegic. Brother (6 years old) was killed, mother injured.

He could move arms and legs after car crash. He complained of lower abdominal pain. Lower abdomen, flanks, and hips were bruised. Paraspinal tenderness was maximal at thoracolumbar junction. Abdomen was distended and rigid the second day, soft and tender the third day. He could not urinate. He was alert, smiling, and unable to move legs the fourth day. He arched his back to move pelvis. CSF was bloody.

Temperature is 37.7°C, heart rate 116, respiratory rate 32, blood pressure 116/54 mm Hg, and weight 18 kg. Legs are flaccid. He is hypersensitive from T11–T12 to knees. Deep tendon reflexes at knees and ankles are absent. The rest of the physical findings are normal.

Hematocrit is 0.34. White cell count is 9.7×10^9/liter with 0.59 polymorphonuclear cells, 0.11 bands, 0.20 lymphocytes, 0.06 monocytes, and 0.04 atypical lymphocytes. Platelet count is 552×10^9/liter. Urine specific gravity is 1.015, pH 6.

Urine has 0.15 g/liter ketones and 0–1 white cell/HPF. Serum sodium is 138 mmol/liter, potassium 5.0, chloride 101, carbon dioxide 20, urea nitrogen 3.9, calcium 2.37, phosphorus 1.58, cholesterol 4.73, and glucose 6.3. Creatinine is 40 µmol/liter, uric acid 300, total bilirubin 15, and direct bilirubin 3. Total protein is 67 g/liter, albumin 42. Alkaline phosphatase is 196 U/liter, LDH 328, and SGOT 35.

Plain film of pelvis shows fracture of ilia at about level of anterior superior spines. CT scan shows high attenuation in left side of spinal canal and at T11 in center of spinal canal (Figure 9-1A). T1-weighted MRI shows high signal in left side of thecal sac at T10–T12 (Figure 9-1B).

At operation, spinous processes and laminas of T10 and T11 are resected; ligamentum flavum and dark blue, tense, pulseless dura are opened to reveal organized clot, hematomyelia, and, predominantly at T11, edematous, necrotic spinal cord.

Diagnosis: Spinal cord necrosis and hemorrhage.

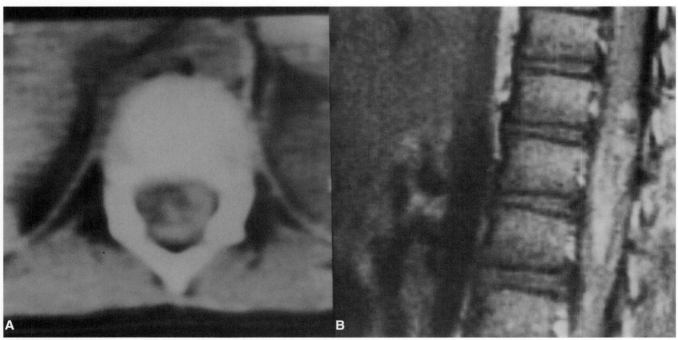

Fig. 9-1

Case 10

A 5-year-old boy has had abdominal pain for 1 month, often causing him to wake screaming at night. Pain was episodic at first, lasting 15 minutes to 1 hour; now it is almost continuous.

"He just lies on the couch all day," prone with pillow under chest. He will not sit or bend forward. He eats lying down and has lost 1.4 kg in past month. He has trouble urinating.

He is an adopted child. Health of parents is not known.

Weight is 15.8 kg, height 103 cm, temperature 36.5°C, heart rate 104, respiratory rate 20, and blood pressure 110/70 mm Hg. He is pale. He holds neck stiff and straight, zealously maintains lumbar lordosis, moves cautiously, and swings stiff left leg when he walks. Superficial abdominal reflexes, right knee jerk, and left ankle jerk are absent. Vibration sense in shanks is diminished. Toes do not move when sole is scratched. He withdraws feet slowly when soles are pinched. The rest of the physical findings are normal.

Hematocrit is 0.37. White cell count is 6.0×10^9/liter with 0.35 polymorphonuclear cells, 0.01 bands, 0.58 lymphocytes, 0.05 monocytes, and 0.01 basophils. Platelet count is 556×10^9/liter. ESR is 120 mm/hr. Urine specific gravity is 1.021, pH 6. Urine has 0–2 white cells/HPF. Serum sodium is 138 mmol/liter, potassium 3.9, chloride 107, and glucose 6.0.

T1-weighted MRI shows cylindrical expansion of conus medullaris (Figure 10-1).

At laminectomy of T10–L1, spinal cord is swollen. Myelotomy releases a gelatinous, vascular tumor with a vascular node in it.

Microscopic examination of dark red and tan tumor shows clot, hemorrhage, and neutrophils. Many small vascular channels lined by plump endothelial cells are along clot edge on a stroma of moderate-sized polyhedral cells that have eosinophilic cytoplasm and oval nuclei. Proliferating vessels are along an edge of neural tissue that contains glial cells with indistinct borders, bubbly eosinophilic cytoplasm, and oval nuclei with clumped chromatin that do not stain with glial fibrillary acidic protein.

Weight is 39 kg at 13 years. He is an "all-star" baseball player who pitches and plays shortstop and third base. Left leg is 2 cm shorter than right. Sensation in first toes is mildly impaired. The rest of the neurologic findings are normal.

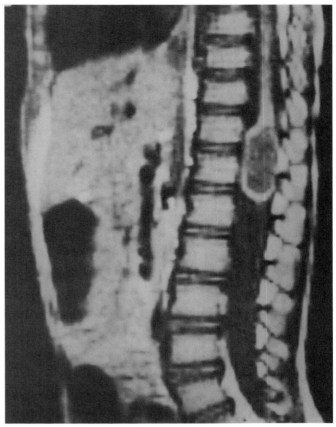

Fig. 10-1

Diagnosis: Hemangioblastoma with hemorrhage and gliosis.

Index